SIXTH EDITION

Outdoor Emergency Care

A Patroller's Guide to Medical Care

NATIONAL SKI PATROL ®

Editor: Edward C. McNamara, BS, NRP
Medical Editor: David H. Johe, MD
Associate Editor: Deborah A. Endly, BA, DH, NREMT

Effective July 1, 2025: The Outdoor Emergency Care (OEC) course is now fully administered through NSP's Center for Learning on the nsp.org website. The Navigate Advantage Access version is no longer in use. All students should enroll directly through the NSP Center for Learning platform. You will access your course materials through the NSP Center for Learning once enrolled. Please consult your instructor or Instructor of Record if you have any questions about accessing the course or selecting the correct textbook format.

JONES & BARTLETT LEARNING

World Headquarters
Jones & Bartlett Learning
25 Mall Road
Burlington, MA 01803
978-443-5000
info@jblearning.com
www.jblearning.com

Jones & Bartlett Learning books and products are available through most bookstores and online booksellers. To contact Jones & Bartlett Learning directly, call 800-832-0034, fax 978-443-8000, or visit our website, www.jblearning.com.

Substantial discounts on bulk quantities of Jones & Bartlett Learning publications are available to corporations, professional associations, and other qualified organizations. For details and specific discount information, contact the special sales department at Jones & Bartlett Learning via the above contact information or send an email to specialsales@jblearning.com.

To order this product, use ISBN: 978-1-284-32958-2

Production Credits

General Manager and Executive Publisher: Kimberly Brophy
VP, Product Management: Christine Emerton
Senior Managing Editor: Donna Gridley
Product Manager: Tiffany Sliter
Senior Editor: Amanda Mitchell
VP, Sales, Public Safety Group: Matthew Maniscalco
Project Specialist: Nora Menzi
Project Specialist, Navigate: Nora Menzi
Senior Digital Project Specialist: Angela Dooley
Director of Marketing Operations: Brian Rooney
VP, Manufacturing and Inventory Control: Therese Connell
Composition: S4Carlisle Publishing Services
Cover Design: Kristin E. Parker
Text Design: Kristin E. Parker
Senior Media Development Editor: Troy Liston
Media Development Editor: Faith Brosnan
Rights Specialist: Rebecca Damon
Cover Image (Title Page): Edward McNamara
Back Cover Images: © iStock/Getty Images Plus/Getty, © iStock / Getty Images Plus/Getty, © National Ski Patrol
Historical Timeline Images: National Ski Patrol
Design Features: © thianchai sitthikongsak/Getty Images.; © Erlon Silva - TRI Digital/Getty Images
Printing and Binding: Lakeside Book Company

Library of Congress Cataloging-in-Publication Data
LCCN: 2020011601

6048

Printed in the United States of America
29 28 27 26 25 10 9 8 7 6 5

BRIEF TABLE OF CONTENTS

EXTENDED TABLE OF CONTENTS

CHAPTER 6

CHAPTER 7

CHAPTER 8

CHAPTER 9

CHAPTER 10

CHAPTER 11

CHAPTER 12

CHAPTER 13

CHAPTER 14

CHAPTER 15

CHAPTER 16

CHAPTER 17

CHAPTER 18

CHAPTER 19

CHAPTER 20

CHAPTER 28

CHAPTER 29

CHAPTER 30

CHAPTER 34

OUTDOOR EMERGENCY CARE SKILLS

CHAPTER 3

CHAPTER 5

CHAPTER 7

CHAPTER 9

CHAPTER 10

CHAPTER 13

CHAPTER 14

CHAPTER 15

CHAPTER 17

CHAPTER 19

CHAPTER 20

CHAPTER 21

CHAPTER 22

CHAPTER 24

CHAPTER 33

LETTER TO STUDENTS

Outdoor Emergency Care, referred to simply as OEC throughout this text, has completed its sixth revision. OEC has evolved to its present form using information from evidence-based prehospital care. No other program provides specific emergency medical responder (EMR) training for skiers, mountain bikers, and other outdoor enthusiasts in a comprehensive manner. The *Sixth Edition* also includes unique information, such as wilderness splinting techniques, that is not present in other EMR programs. The goal of the OEC program is to prepare you to handle any medical situation you may encounter as an OEC technician. This unique program trains you to provide care in the outdoor environment, during all seasons.

Providers working for other agencies may also find useful information in this text, complementing their knowledge of prehospital care. The content has been written and reviewed by highly respected doctors and other medical personnel who are experts in education in the outdoor emergency care community. The majority of these providers are actively practicing, providing the most recent medically accepted care for patients. The editors' goal is to provide you with up-to-date and practical training. Following an introduction to EMS systems and the role of OEC within EMS, this text provides a basic overview of human anatomy and physiology before examining the different types of medical conditions and traumatic injuries OEC technicians may encounter. During this examination, you will learn what causes these emergencies, how patients are affected, and how to care for them.

By understanding what is going on with the patient, you can form a plan of care to move the patient successfully to the next, higher level of care. The better you understand the "why" of a patient's symptoms, the better your care will be.

The content is organized to embrace continuity as you move through the material. Each chapter begins with a list of objectives. It is important to review the objectives first because they describe what you should have learned upon completion of each chapter. Each chapter also includes key terms and their definitions. You must master these terms to communicate among peers and with other medical personnel. In addition, you must master the OEC Skills described throughout the text because you will use these skills in your experience as a patroller. At the end of the course, your evaluation is based on the objectives, key terms, and OEC Skills.

During this sixth revision of the text, many patrollers, OEC instructors, prehospital providers, and physicians involved with both ski patrols and other outdoor medical care organizations were consulted to help determine what information would be most valuable to this program and how best to present it to you. The editors want to make the OEC program both educational and enjoyable. This content will be used throughout your initial training and during refresher training, and the text serves as a valuable reference manual for future use.

After you have completed your OEC training, we truly hope you have the tools to enjoy many years as an OEC technician, providing the outdoor public with excellent care.

Ed McNamara, Editor
David Johe, Medical Editor
Deb Endly, Associate Editor

PREFACE

Medical education for ski patrollers has evolved over the years. Initially, ski patrollers were required to take an American Red Cross first aid course. In 1985, Warren Bowman, MD, wrote a textbook, *Winter Emergency Care*, specifically for the training of ski patrollers. Dr. Bowman later changed the title of the text to *Outdoor Emergency Care*, as patrollers, or "OEC technicians," began to provide care for other entities during all four seasons. He was also the principal author for the next two editions of the text.

Today, many ski resorts have year-round sporting and recreational activities. In addition, prehospital care in both urban and wilderness settings has changed, modifying the care provided, and newer technology has provided EMRs with new tools for providing care. The OEC program has evolved to reflect these important changes.

Revisions to this program took place over a 2-year period. First, in 2018, a survey was completed by the National Ski Patrol (NSP) national office, asking patrollers to provide feedback on the current (fifth) edition of *Outdoor Emergency Care*. Next, the NSP National Board appointed the editors to use the survey results and begin the revision.

This *Sixth Edition* is an extensive revision of the *Fifth Edition*, as editors Ed McNamara and David Johe incorporated many new concepts using evidence-based medicine. The new edition also includes recommendations made by the NSP National Medical Committee. This committee includes physician experts in prehospital care, nearly all of whom are patrollers or advisors to patrols.

Using the information gathered by the NSP survey and the recommendations made by the NSP National Medical Committee, chapters were revised, reorganized, condensed, or rewritten. The objectives and key terms at the start of each chapter were carefully reviewed and modified, so the OEC student will understand what information is most important to learn in becoming an effective OEC technician.

Once the chapters were revised, the manuscript was sent for peer review by the NSP. Bill Devarney, the NSP Review Coordinator, assigned each chapter to a minimum of three reviewers—a physician; an NSP Instructor, Instructor/Trainer (I/T), or patroller; and another member of the health care field (a registered nurse, EMT, or paramedic). The legal chapter was reviewed by the NSP legal advisor. The manuscript was revised a final time based on the peer review comments, and the manuscript was then submitted to the publisher. The publisher reviewed the manuscript and conducted additional editing by members of the healthcare field, including physicians and paramedics. Recommendations were made to the editors, who reviewed the comments and made appropriate changes. The manuscript was then finalized for production.

From here, OEC Skills and Skill Guides were designed; diagrams, tables, and other illustrations were rendered; and photo logs were created. Deb Endly was primarily responsible for recommending and incorporating photos into the chapters. Ed McNamara and others completed numerous photo shoots because it was important to obtain new photos for this edition. Later, other educational elements peripheral to the text were completed under the guidance of Bill Devarney, including an online course, lecture outlines, lectures in PowerPoint format, a test bank, and instructor information.

This text contains material that has not been in previous editions. Some of the key revisions and additions to the *Sixth Edition* include the following:

- The use of a new protocol on spinal motion restriction that limits the use of backboards in treating patients
- Use of pulse oximeters to identify patients in need of oxygen treatment
- Modifications to the patient assessment protocol—specifically, moving the identification of life-threatening hemorrhage to the top of the list
- Introduction of a new technique in the care of pelvic trauma
- New content about the administration of naloxone (Narcan)
- New *Adaptive Athletes* chapter

Features of the *Sixth Edition* intended to enhance learning and ensure students are receiving the most authoritative, current information possible include the following:

- *A straightforward, consistent patient assessment process.* The patient assessment process is presented in the same way patients are assessed in the healthcare system. Flowcharts are provided throughout the *Patient Assessment* chapter to keep the reader focused on each step of the process.
- *Up-to-date content.* As you read through each chapter, you will find new information that is current with present prehospital patient care.
- *Subject matter that meets and, in many cases, exceeds the National Emergency Medical Responder criteria.* Information unique for ski and bicycle patrollers, including extrication, is included. This material is presented in a format that combines the disciplines of urban EMS and wilderness medical rescue.
- *Continuous case studies.* A continuous case study is included in each chapter to encourage critical thinking and application of the information as readers proceed through the chapter.
- *End-of chapter review questions.* The review questions included at the end of each chapter allow students to evaluate the knowledge they have gained while reading the chapter.
- *Learning objectives.* Specific objectives listed at the beginning of each chapter tell students at the outset what they are expected to learn as they move through the chapter.

The NSP is a unique organization that has provided medical training for the outdoor environment to countless individuals. Nearly all the ski areas in the United States, and many in other countries, use OEC to train patrollers. As ski patrollers have joined other first responder organizations, they have found their training is widely accepted by those organizations, and in many states, successful completion of an OEC course allows the individual the opportunity through reciprocity to obtain an EMS first responder card (EMR). Because of the strength of the OEC program, other agencies now look to the NSP for OEC courses to serve as the primary education program for their first responders. We expect this audience to expand following the publication of this edition.

Completion of this program has been a pleasurable task, taking over 2 years. We think many present and future patrollers will find the knowledge in this text beneficial as they help the public in prehospital care situations.

Edward McNamara, BS, NRP
Editor
David H. Johe, MD
Medical Editor

ACKNOWLEDGMENTS

We wish to acknowledge the remarkable talents and efforts of the following people who contributed to and reviewed this edition of *Outdoor Emergency Care*. Individually, they worked with extraordinary commitment to this program. Together, they form a team of highly dedicated professionals who have upheld the highest standards of EMS instruction.

AUTHORS

Two new authors have joined the author team for the *Sixth Edition*. We thank them for their work on *Chapter 32, Adaptive Athletes*.

Ty Damon II, MBA
OEC Instructor, PSIA Adaptive Instructor
Member, Pine Knob Ski Patrol
Clarkston, MI
National Appointment #7880

Stephen Werner, MD
National Medical Committee
OEC Instructor
Member, Pine Knob Ski Patrol
Clarkston, MI
National Appointment #8006

In addition, the editors would like to extend their appreciation for the work done by the previous (fifth) edition author team:

Paul S. Auerbach, MD, MS, FACEP, FAWM
Gregory A. Bala, MS
Michael Bateman, EMT, OEC Technician
Eric P. Bowman, MD, FACEP, FAWM
Warren Bowman, MD
Brigitte Schran Brown, MEd, MA, EMT
Jonathan Busko, MD, MPH, EMT-P
Jennifer Dow, MD, FACEP, FAWM
Jeffrey Druck, MD
Bruce Evans, MD
Jane Lee Fansler, MD
Luanne Freer, FACEP, FAWM
Matthew Fulton, BA, NREMT-P
James Geiling, MD, FACP, FCCM
Jamie A. Goodis, MD
Colin K. Grissom, MD
Seth C. Hawkins, MD, FAWM
Rick King, NSP National Mountain Travel & Rescue Program Director, National Ski Patrol System, Inc.
Joshua Kucker, MD
Ricky C. Kue, MD, MPH
Eric M. Lamberts, MD, FAAFP, ASAM
Howard M. Laney, National Avalanche Program Director, National Ski Patrol System, Inc.
John Latimer, MD
Roxanne Latimer, MD
Matthew J. Levy, DO, MS, NREMT-P
Michael Levy, MD, FACP, FAAEM
David Markenson, MD, FAAP, EMT-P
Marion C. McDevitt, DO
Scott McIntosh, MD, MPH
Denis Meade, MA, EMT-P
Michael G. Millin, MD, MPH, FACEP
Paul Murphy, MS, MA, EMT-P
John S. Nichols, MD, PhD, FACS, FAANS
Jonathan Politis, MPA, NREMT-P
Frank Rossi, Pacific Northwest Division Mountain Travel and Rescue Advisor, National Ski Patrol System, Inc.
Robert Scarlett, Esq
Fred Severyn, MD, FACEP
Nici Singletary, MD, FACEP
Maurus Sorg, MD, MPH
David Walker, MD

REVIEWERS

William Devarney, CSP, NREMT
Review Coordinator
OEC National Program Director
Eastern Division Admin Patrol
West Boylston, MA

Wendy Aarnio, RN
National Board of Directors
National Appointment #8308
Eastern Division, Bromley Mountain, VT

Douglas K. Adams, CPCU, EMT, OEC IT, SR OEC T/E
Regional Director Central NY
National Appointment #11604, Eastern Division
Song Mountain
Tully, NY

Charles Allen, DO, FACOEP
NSP National Medical Advisor
OET-IT, OEC-IT, National Appointment #11444
Huff Hills Ski Patrol or Area
Mandan, ND

George Angelo, MEd, BS, LAT
Sports Medicine Director, Judge Memorial High School
Utah Olympic Park Ski Patrol
Park City, UT

Kimberly Beadle Baker, BS, NR-AEMT
OEC Instructor, Instructor Development IT
Black Mountain
Jackson, NH

Peter Bayer, MSME, PE, OEC IT, OETI
Connecticut Region ROA
Eastern Division, Mohawk Mountain Ski Patrol
Cornwall, CT

James Bender, PhD
OEC Instructor
Alpine Patroller
Central Division, Villa Olivia
Bartlett, IL

Jeff Birks, FP-C, TP-C, NRP
OEC Instructor
Beech Mountain Ski Patrol
Beech Mountain, NC

David Bolstad
OEC Instructor, OET IT
Central Division, Spirit Mountain Patrol
Duluth, MN

Paul D. Brooks, MICP
Alaska Division OEC Supervisor
OEC IT
National Appointment #5471
Alyeska Ski Patrol
Girdwood, AK

Deborah A. Brown, MSN, APRN, ONP-C, OEC TE, MTR TE, OET TE
Avalanche, Level 1 Instructor
National Appointment #12036
Ragged Mountain Ski Area
Danbury, NH

Patricia A. Burns, RN, EMT
Southern NY Region ROA
OEC IT
Eastern Division, Sterling Forest Ski Patrol
Tuxedo Park, NY

David Callaghan, MS PT, OCS, Board Certified Clinical Specialist, Orthopedic Physical Therapy
OEC IT
Instructor Development IT, OET Instructor
National Appointment #12111
Mont Ripley Ski Patrol
Ripley, MI

Timothy Carey, MD
OEC Instructor
National Appointment #264650
PNW Division
Alpental Ski Area
Snoqualmie Pass, WA

Aileen Cassidy, PA-C
OEC Supervisor, Southern Division
National Appointment #11960
Southern Division, Wintergreen Patrol
Nellysford, VA

Keith Cassidy, Esq
Former Assistant National Chair and Legal Advisor
Wintergreen, VA

Carl Chaplin, NREMT, CSM
New Hampshire Region Director
NSP Certified #701, PSPA Certified
OEC IT, OEC TE, OET ATI, ID Instructor
National Appointment #11618
Eastern Division, Mount Sunapee Ski Patrol
Newbury, NY

Stefanie Costello, EMT
Pats Peak Ski Patrol Director
NH Region OEC Administrator, OEC IT/TE, Senior Patroller
Eastern Division, Pats Peak
Henniker, NH

Garreth Debiegun, MD, FACEP, FAWM
Maine Region NSP Medical Advisor
National Appointment #228048
Saddleback Ski Patrol, Maine Region, Eastern Division
Rangeley, ME

Sue Dennison
OEC IT, Far West Division OEC Supervisor
Sugar Bowl Ski Resort
Norden, CA

Bob Elling, EMT-P, MPA
Educator, Author, and Provider
High Quality Endeavors, Ltd.
Whiteface Medical Services
Hudson Valley Community College
North Country Community College
Lake Placid, NY

Jason Erdmann, BS
OEC IT, OEC Refresher Committee
Tyrol Basin Ski Area
Mount Horeb, WI

Deborah Foss, AS, RT, EMT
Eastern Division OEC Supervisor
Wachusett Mountain Ski Area
Princeton, MA

Roberta Fox
OEC IT, OEC Trainer/Evaluator, ID Instructor
National Appointment #5931
Eastern Division, Royal Mountain
Caroga Lake, NY

John T. Fradette, BA
OEC IT, OEC Division Supervisor
Sr. Advisor to the OEC National Program Director
University of Montana/Great Divide Ski Area
Helena, MT

Jeffrey R Gagliano, MD
Physician-Partner Eldora Ski Patrol
Orthopedic Surgeon
Boulder Bone and Joint
Boulder, CO

Kirsten Gannon
National Sports Center for the Disabled
Winter Park, CO

Janet Glaeser, MEd
Ohio Region Senior OEC Coordinator
OEC IT, Instructor Development IT
National Appointment #7409
Central Division, Boston Mills/Brandywine/Alpine Valley Ski Patrol
Brecksville, OH

Kathy Glynn
OEC Refresher Committee, OEC Instructor
Instructor Development IT
Hyland Hills/Three Rivers Ski Area
Bloomington, MN

Cal Goldsmith
EMARI Region Director/Eastern Division Assistant Director
National Appointment #11288
Wachusett Mountain Ski Patrol
Princeton, MA

Michelle Goldsmith, RDH
Eastern Division OEC Assistant Supervisor
OEC IT, CPR Instructor, Toboggan Instructor
National Appointment #11122
Wachusett Mountain Ski Patrol
Princeton, MA

Mark Goldstein, MSN, RN, EMT-P I/C
St. Anthony Hospital, Emergency Department
OEC Instructor
Copper Mountain Ski Patrol
Denver, CO

Colin K. Grissom, MD
National Medical Committee, NSP
Alumni/Admin Intermountain Division
Senior Medical Director Critical Care, Intermountain Healthcare, Utah
Professor of Medicine, University of Utah
Park City, UT

Jim Gunderson, BA, BSc
Assistant Director of Training, Divers Alert Network (DAN)
DAN Examiner #15898
NAUI Course Director Trainer #53243
NSP Certified #171990
OEC Instructor
Riverview, FL

Dayle Hadden, BBA
OEC Instructor
American Heart Association BLS Instructor
Central Division Timber Ridge Ski Patrol, Alumni
National Appointment #10928
Gobles, MI

Karen Anderson Hadden, RN
OEC Instructor
American Heart Association BLS Faculty
Central Division Timber Ridge Ski Patrol, Alumni
Leadership Commendation Appointment #8329
Plainwell, MI

Frauke V. Haertel, PhD, Research Associate
Division OEC Program Supervisor
OEC IT, OET I
International Division, Zürich Ski Patrol
National Appointment #12070
Zürich, Switzerland

Bryant F. Hall, MBA, BS (MT), PMP, NRP
QA/QI/Peer Review Chairperson
National Appointment #10076
OEC IT, Senior EMM TE
Canaan Valley Ski Patrol
Wisp Ski Patrol
Canaan Valley, WV

James J. Hamilton, MD
PNWD Medical Advisor, Wy'East Medical Advisor
OEC Instructor
National Appointment #5005
PNWD Mt. Hood Ski Patrol
Portland, OR

Brett H. Hamlin, PhD
Senior Administrator, North Central Region
Mont Ripley Ski Area, Michigan Tech University
Houghton, MI

Susan C. Hayes, MS, RN
OEC IT, Instructor Development IT
Central Division, Welch Village Ski Patrol
National Appointment #11322
Welch, MN

David Hemendinger, MBA, EMT
National Refresher Committee
Eastern Division Assistant OEC Administrator
OEC IT, ID IT
Yawgoo Valley Ski Patrol
National Appointment #11230
Exeter, RI

Kelly Hurlbut, ACA, EMT
OEC Instructor
Wachusett Mountain Ski Patrol
Princeton, MA

Mami Iwamoto, MD
Clinical Instructor of Ophthalmology, Harvard Medical School
OEC TE, OET TE
Eastern Division
Sunday River Ski Patrol
Newry, ME

Greg Jellinek, MD, OEC Instructor
Retired NSP Patroller/OEC Instructor
49 Degrees North Ski Patrol
Chewelah, WA

William Jordan, DO
Associate Professor of Ophthalmology GCMC
OEC Instructor, Past Certified ED Chair,
NSP Certified #369
National Appointment #9120
Elk Mountain
Union Dale, PA

Bill Kane, BA, NR AEMT, Wilderness EMT, Licensed EMS Instructor Coordinator NH and ME
Founder, Director, The Kane Schools, Wild & Rescue Medicine
Fryeburg, ME

Kristiana Kaufmann, MD, MPH
Senior Alpine Patroller, OEC Instructor, Eastern MI Region Medical Advisor,
Division, Eastern MI Region, Alpine Valley East Patrol
Elkhorn, WI

Kevin Kent, MD, FACEP
Department of Emergency Services
Milford Regional Medical Center
Assistant Professor of Emergency Medicine
University of Massachusetts Medical School
Wachusett Mountain Ski Patrol
Princeton, MA

Paula Knight, Retired Educator
National OEC Program Sr. Advisor
Eastern Division Assistant OEC Supervisor
OEC IT, ID IT
National Appointment #7249
Eastern Division, Connect Region, Mt. Southington Ski Patrol
Plantsville, CT

Eva Kunkel, MS
OEC Instructor
Western Appalachian Region
Seven Springs Resort
Champion, PA

Jenn Laitala, CDA
NSP Certified #765
National Appointment #10738
OEC Inst, Sr EMM TE
Patrol Director
Wachusett Mountain Ski Patrol
Princeton, MA

Michael Levy, MD, FACP, FAAEM
Alaska Division Medical Advisor
Alaska Admin Patrol
Eagle River, AK

Chuck Lollar, Esq
NSP National Legal Advisor
Southern Division
Norfolk, VA

Trudy Malone, MD
Heiliger Hügel Ski Patrol
Hubertus, WI

James Margolis, MD
Clinical Professor in Psychiatry at University of California Davis and California Northstate University Medical Schools
Leadership Commendation Appointment #8387, OEC IT
Medical Advisor for ESR and Homewood Ski Patrol
Far West Division
Homewood, CA

Stu Mavros, EMT
OEC IT
Eastern Division
Patrol Director, High Point Nordic Ski Patrol
Sussex, NJ

Edee McNamara, RN
OEC IT, Sr EMM TE, OET Inst
National Appointment #8068
Wachusett Mountain Ski Patrol
Princeton, MA

Jeannine Mogan, BS, NR-EMT
Risk Manager
Giants Ridge Resort
Biwabik, MN

David L. Mooney, RA, LEED AP
NJ Region OEC Administrator
Eastern Division, Delaware Valley Ski Patrol
National Application #11874
Lambertville, NJ

Michael D. Most, MD, FACS
Medical Director, OEC Instructor
Eastern Division, Magic Mountain Ski Patrol
Londonderry, VT

John S. Nichols, MD, PhD, FACS, FAANS
Neurological Surgeon
Medical Advisor Rocky Mountain Division
Medical Director, Winter Park Ski Patrol
Winter Park, CO

Stephen Oliver, MD
Division Medical Advisor
Senior Advisor, Division Senior Program Administrator, OEC Instructor, OET Instructor
National Appointment #91140
International Division, Zürich Ski Patrol
Zürich, Switzerland

Ryan Overberger, DO, EMT-PHP
Medical Advisor, OEC/OET Instructor
Senior Patroller
Eastern Division
Big Boulder, Harmony, PA; Jack Frost Ski Patrols, White Haven, PA

Kevin Qualseth
CPVSP Director
OEC IT, OET Instructor
National Appointment #11302
Far West Division, Mother Lode Region
China Peak Mountain Resort
Lakeshore, CA

Marc Restuccia, MD, FACEP, FAEMS
Associate Professor of Emergency Medicine (Retired)
University of Massachusetts Medical School
Worcester, MA

James L. Riedemann
OEC IT, Senior OEC Evaluator, CPR Instructor
National Appointment #11056
Central Division, South Central Region
Cascade Mountain Ski Patrol
Portage, WI

Jane San Romani, RDH
Division OEC Supervisor, OEC IT
National Appointment #9894
Pacific Northwest Division
Santiam Pass Ski Patrol
Sisters, OR

Reid Roper, BS, NREMTP, OEC IT
Appalachian Ski Mountain
Blowing Rock, NC

David Shatz, MD
Trauma Surgeon/Surgical Intensivist
University of California, Davis Medical Center
OEC Instructor
Far West Division, Sierra Ski Patrol
Twin Bridges, CA

Jeb Sheidler, DMSc, MPAS, PA-C, ATC, NPR, TP-C
Network Vice President Trauma and Emergency Services Lutheran Health Network
Captain, Bath Township Fire Department
SWAT Medic, Allen County Sheriff's Office
Alpine Patroller, Mad River Mountain
Valley Hi, OH

Eric Silva, MD, FACEP
Eastern Division Medical Advisor
OEC Instructor
Sterling Forest, Tuxedo Park, NY; Belleayre Ski Patrol, Highmount, NY

Paul A. Skudder, MD, FACS, FSVS
Southeastern Vascular Associates/VOHRA Wound Physicians
Eastern NY Regional Medical Advisor
OEC Instructor
Gore Mountain
North Creek, NY

Amy Slichter
NSCD Programs Lead
PSIA Adaptive I, CADS Examiner
National Sports Center for the Disabled
Winter Park, CO

Will Smith, MD, Paramedic, FAEMS
Medical Director, Grand Teton National Park, Teton County Search and Rescue, Jackson Hole Fire/EMS, USFS-BTNF
Clinical Assistant Professor, University of Washington School of Medicine
Emergency Medicine, St. John's Medical Center
Colonel, MC, US Army Reserve, 62A (Emergency Medicine)
Jackson, WY

Ray Smittle, EMT
Rocky Mountain Division OEC Supervisor
OEC IT, ID Instructor, BLS Instructor
Loveland Ski Patrol
Georgetown, CO

Scott Spillane
Region OEC Advisor
Titus Mountain
Eastern NY Region
Malone, NY

Walt Stoy, PhD, EMT-P
Western Appalachian Region Medical Consultant
OEC IT and Senior EMM TE
Eastern Division, Hidden Valley Ski Patrol
Professor, Emergency Medicine, University of Pittsburgh
Director Emeritus, Center for Emergency Medicine, UPMC
Pittsburgh, PA

Susan M. Swapp-Trueblood, PhD
OEC IT
Regional OEC Advisor
Snowy Range Ski Patrol, Rocky Mountain Division
Leadership Commendation Appointment #8297
Centennial, WY

David K. Tan, MD, FAAEM, FAEMS
Associate Professor & Chief, Division of EMS
Department of Emergency Medicine
Washington University School of Medicine
St. Louis, MO

Tim Thayer, BS
OEC Instructor, OEC Refresher Committee
Afton Alps Ski Area
Hastings, MN

Jay S. Van Zeeland, Paramedic, EMS Instructor Coordinator
Pine Mountain Ski Patrol Director, Regional YAP Advisor
OEC-IT
National Appointment #12046
North Central Region, Central Division
Pine Mountain Ski Patrol
Iron Mountain, MI

Bill Welch
OEC IT, STC
Eastern Division, Butternut
Great Barrington, MA

Ron Wenzel, EMT, PHTLS, TCCC
Police Officer (Retired)
US Coast Guard Reserve 2004–2016
Bigfork, MT

Robert West, NREMT Paramedic
EMARI Region ROA
OEC IT, Senior OEC TE, Avalanche Instructor
Eastern Division, Wachusett Mountain
Princeton, MA

Kevin Whitney, DNP, RN, NEA-BC
OEC Instructor and Development Instructor
Pro Division
Loon Mountain Ski Patrol
Lincoln, NH

David Willett, BSN, RN, LTC(R) AN
Alpine Patroller, OEC IT
Central Division, Seven Oaks
Boone, IA

Jason Williams, BS, NRP, DiMM
University of New Mexico, International Mountain Medicine Center
Department of Emergency Medicine
Albuquerque, NM

Debra Wright, AEMT
Idaho EMT Instructor
Intermountain Division OEC Supervisor
OEC IT, ID Instructor
Kelly Canyon Patrol
Ririe, ID

Jake Zadra, MD
Medical Advisor
Alpine Patroller
Central Division, Devil's Head Ski Patrol
Merrimac, WI

Vicki Zierden
OEC Instructor, ID Instructor
OEC MSP T/E
Western Region Section Chief
Central Division: Three Rivers
Leadership Commendation Appointment #8437
Bloomington, MN

NATIONAL MEDICAL COMMITTEE REVIEWERS

Charles Allen, DO, FACOEP
NSP National Medical Advisor
OET-IT, OEC-IT, National Appointment #11444
Huff Hills Ski Patrol or Area
Mandan, ND

Charles Clements II, MD
Chair, Medical Advisory Committee, Southern Division
OEC Instructor
New Winterplace Ski Patrol, Southern Division
Ghent, WV

Stefan Hamelin, MD
Central Division
Saint Charles, MO

Adam Johnson, MD
Intermountain Emergency Department
St. John's Medical Center
Teton Ridge Emergency Medicine
Jackson, WY

Michael Levy, MD, FACP, FAAEM
Alaska Division Medical Advisor
Alaska Admin Patrol
Eagle River, AK

John S. Nichols, MD, PhD, FACS, FAANS
Rocky Mountain
Intermountain Neurosurgery & Neuroscience
Denver, CO

Stephen Oliver, MD
Division Medical Advisor
Senior Advisor, Division Senior Program Administrator, OEC Instructor, OET Instructor
International Division, Zürich Ski Patrol
Zürich, Switzerland

Eric Silva, MD, FACEP
Eastern Division Medical Advisor
OEC Instructor
Sterling Forest, Tuxedo Park, NY; Belleayre Ski Patrol, Highmount, NY

Keith Tatsukawa, MD
Far West Division
Truckee, CA

Stephen Werner, MD
National Medical Committee
OEC Instructor
Member, Pine Knob Ski Patrol
National Appointment #8006
Clarkston, MI

NATIONAL MEDICAL COMMITTEE MEMBERS AT LARGE

Paul S. Auerbach, MD, MS
Member, National Medical Committee
Editor, *Wilderness Medicine*
Sugar Bowl Resort Doctor Patrol
National Appointment #378142
Norden, CA

Colin Grissom, MD
Park City, UT

James A. Katz, MD
The Midwest Center for Sight
Des Plaines, IL

PHOTOGRAPHERS

Deb Endly, BA, DH, NREMT
Hyland Hills/Three Rivers Ski Area

Kathy Glynn
Hyland Hills/Three River Ski Area

David H. Johe, MD
Holiday Valley Ski Area

Edward McNamara, BS, NRP
Wachusett Mountain Ski Area

Chris Pringle
National Board
Bradford Ski Area

Cenanne Sanders, MEd
Canterbury, NH

Vicki Zierden
Hyland Hills/Three River Ski Area

MODELS

Kelsey Andvik
Hyland Hills/Three Rivers Ski Area
Bloomington, MN

Luke Andvik
Hyland Hills/Three Rivers Ski Area
Bloomington, MN

Marc Andvik
Hyland Hills/Three Rivers Ski Area
Bloomington, MN

Meghan Arnold
Senior Alpine Patroller
Wachusett Mountain
Princeton, MA

Chris Bierfeldt
Alpine Patroller
Holiday Valley
Ellicottville, NY

Leo Bierfeldt
Alpine Patroller
Holiday Valley
Ellicottville, NY

Kevin Brody
Senior Alpine Patroller
Wachusett Mountain
Princeton, MA

Beth Glynn Chambers
St. Paul, MN

Michael Ciccone
EMT
Wachusett Mountain
Princeton, MA

Edwin "Red" Clark
Alpine Patroller
Holiday Valley
Ellicottville, NY

John D. Curtin
Hyland Hills/Three Rivers Ski Area
Bloomington, MN

Amy Fantoni
Alpine Patroller
Wachusett Mountain
Princeton, MA

William Foley
Alpine Patroller
Wachusett Mountain
Princeton, MA

Deborah Foss
Senior Alpine Patroller
National Appointment #9824
Wachusett Mountain
Princeton, MA

Jenny Glynn
Seattle, WA

Mark Glynn
Seattle, WA

Calvin Goldsmith
Senior Alpine Patroller
National Appointment #11288
Wachusett Mountain
Princeton, MA

Dana Gray
Senior Alpine Patroller
Wachusett Mountain
Princeton, MA

Victoria Gunning
Alpine Patroller
Wachusett Mountain
Princeton, MA

Mathew Haddad
Senior Alpine Patroller
Wachusett Mountain
Princeton, MA

Ted R. Hanna, Jr.
Senior Alpine Patroller
Hyland Hills/Three Rivers Ski Area
Bloomington, MN

Nathan Harvey
Young Adult Patroller
Wachusett Mountain
Princeton, MA

Derek Hersey
Alpine Patroller
Wachusett Mountain
Princeton, MA

Jeff Holmes
Hyland Hills/Three Rivers Ski Area
Bloomington, MN

Gabrielle Hunt
Millbury, MA

Kelly Hurlbut
Patroller
Wachusett Mountain
Princeton, MA

Tarik Huseinbegovic
Alpine Patroller
Wachusett Mountain
Princeton, MA

Roslyn Johe
Holiday Valley, NY
St Marys, PA

Kevin Kent, MD
Alpine Patroller
Wachusett Mountain
Princeton, MA

Avery Laitala
Young Adult Patroller
Wachusett Mountain
Princeton, MA

Jenn Laitala
Patrol Director
NSP Certified #765
National Appointment #10738
Wachusett Mountain
Princeton, MA

John Laitala
Senior Alpine Patroller
Wachusett Mountain
Princeton, MA

Reilly Laitala
Young Adult Patroller
Wachusett Mountain
Princeton, MA

Craig Larson
Senior Alpine Patroller
National Appointment #11938
Wachusett Mountain
Princeton, MA

Ryan Larson
Buck Hill Ski Area
Burnsville, MN

Joseph Lau
Alpine Patroller
Holiday Valley
Ellicottville, NY

Grace Leppink
Bloomington, MN

Jon Longley
Senior Alpine Patroller
Wachusett Mountain
Princeton, MA

Kevin McDonald
Safety Manager
National Appointment #11990
Wachusett Mountain
Princeton, MA

Jim McGuiness
Alpine Patroller
Wachusett Mountain
Princeton, MA

Edee McNamara
Senior Alpine Patroller
National Appointment #8068
Wachusett Mountain
Princeton, MA

Emily McNamara
Young Adult Patroller
Wachusett Mountain
Princeton, MA

Johannah Medeiros
Senior Alpine Patroller
Wachusett Mountain
Princeton, MA

Jeff Morris
Senior Alpine Patroller
Wachusett Mountain
Princeton, MA

Ashley O'Rourke
Hyland Hills/Three Rivers Ski Area
Bloomington, MN

Alexandria Pariseau
EMT
Wachusett Mountain
Princeton, MA

Cenanne Sanders, MEd
Canterbury, NH

Robert Scarlett, Esq
Former National Legal Advisor
National Board Rep
Ski Liberty
Fairfield, PA

Leslie Snyder
Alpine Patroller
Wachusett Mountain
Princeton, MA

Soroush Sotoudeh
Hyland Hills/Three Rivers Ski Area
Bloomington, MN

Terry Spohn
National Appointment #8334, NSP Certified #473
Hyland Hills/Three Rivers Ski Area
Bloomington, MN

Aidan Tamulen
Young Adult Patroller
Wachusett Mountain
Princeton, MA

Joshua Tamulen
Alpine Patroller
NSP Certified #763
Wachusett Mountain
Princeton, MA

Logan Tamulen
Young Adult Patroller
Wachusett Mountain
Princeton, MA

Michael Testa
Alpine Patroller
Wachusett Mountain
Princeton, MA

Kathy Tobey
Princeton, MA

Christopher Tota
Senior Alpine Patroller
Wachusett Mountain
Princeton, MA

Laura Tota
Ayer, MA

Debbie Truman
Alpine Patroller
Holiday Valley
Ellicottville, NY

Bernard Vallie
Senior Alpine Patroller
Wachusett Mountain
Princeton, MA

Jill Wanous
Hyland Hills/Three Rivers Ski Area
Bloomington, MN

John Woudenberg
Alpine Patroller
Wachusett Mountain
Princeton, MA

John Yager
Hyland Hills/Three Rivers Ski Area
Bloomington, MN

Scott Young
National Appointment #9020
Hyland Hills/Three Rivers Ski Area
Bloomington, MN

Vicki Zierden
Leadership Commendation Appointment #8437
Hyland Hills/Three Rivers Ski Area
Bloomington, MN

Front Cover Models

Reilly Laitala
Young Adult Patroller
Wachusett Mountain Ski Patrol

Craig Larson
Senior Patroller
Wachusett Mountain Ski Patrol

Emily McNamara
Young Adult Patroller
Wachusett Mountain Ski Patrol

Aidan Tamulen
Young Adult Patroller
Wachusett Mountain Ski Patrol

ABOUT THE EDITORS

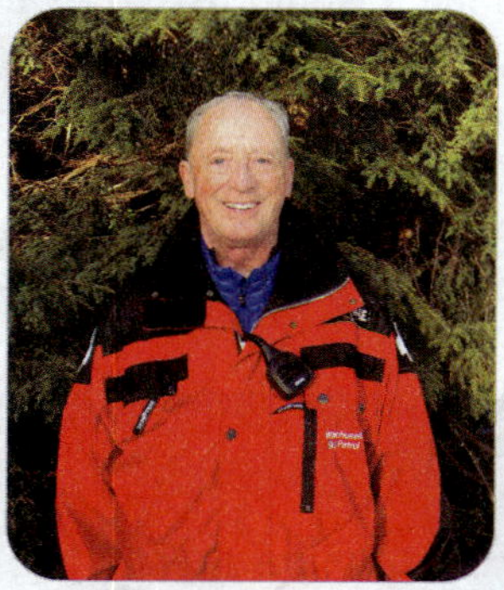

EDWARD C. MCNAMARA, BS, NRP—EDITOR

Edward McNamara is the former Executive Director of the Central Massachusetts EMS Corporation. Now retired, he spends his time with his wife, Edee, enjoying their hobbies of skiing, horse riding, motorcycling, and other outdoor activities. He is a retired Deputy Chief of the Sterling Massachusetts Fire Department and currently the Safety Officer for Massachusetts' 2 DMAT (Disaster Medical Assistance Team). He has also served since 1974 as an EMT and as a paramedic for the past 25 years.

Before beginning his career in health administration, Ed received his BS in education from Norwich University and then spent 3 years in the US Army. In 2001, he retired as a colonel after 30 years of service from the Massachusetts Army National Guard.

Ed is a former Wachusett Mountain Ski Patrol Director, OEC Instructor Trainer and Senior Trainer Evaluator, Eastern Division OEC Chief Supervisor, National OEC Program Director, National Board Member, and Past National Board Chair. He currently is serving his 41st year as an NSP patroller at the Wachusett Mountain Ski Area in Princeton, Massachusetts. He was recently elected as the Eastern Massachusetts and Rhode Island (EMARI) Region Director of the NSP.

Ed's national leadership awards include National Appointment #7858, Meritorious Service Award, Distinguished Service Award, National Outstanding Administrator Award, Service Excellence Award, Minnie Dole Award, and induction into the National Ski Patrol Hall of Fame Class of 2016.

Personal Acknowledgment

As the editor of *Outdoor Emergency Care*, this edition will conclude my editorial work on NSP OEC texts. It has been an honor to have been selected by the NSP Board of Directors to serve as the OEC Textbook Editor of the *Fifth* and *Sixth Editions*. I have enjoyed the opportunity to serve with my good friends and coworkers, David Johe and Deb Endly. Without their knowledge, expertise, and hard work, the fifth and sixth OEC texts could not have been produced.

To all the reviewers, photographers, models, and other collateral support personnel, know that you have provided a remarkable product for the NSP and that your dedicated service is recognized and appreciated.

To my daughters Jenn Laitala and Kelly Hurlbut; son-in-law Johnny Laitala; and granddaughters Emily McNamara, Reilly Laitala, and Avery Laitala, who responded on the spur of the moment to review a chapter, help set up scenarios, appear in photographs as patrollers or patients, and assist in many other ways, I can't thank you enough. We are a family of eight Wachusett Mountain Ski Patrollers who continue to proudly serve the NSP.

To my wife Edee, you have once again been kind enough to allow me to pursue my passion with the NSP and its OEC program. I commandeered the guest bedroom as my second office, which was dedicated to the *OEC Sixth Edition* project, and it is filled with textbooks, computers, equipment, supplies, cameras, and much more. Thanks for your patience and your support in reviewing materials and modeling in photographs on the spur of the moment. Serving together for over 41 years on the NSP has been a fantastic experience. Thank you, Edee, for your support and encouragement these past 2 years.

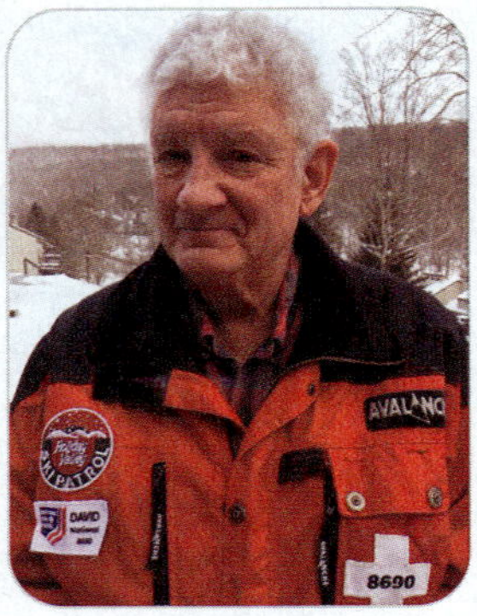

DAVID H. JOHE, MD—MEDICAL EDITOR

David Johe retired from the practice of orthopedic surgery in rural western Pennsylvania in 2013. He was in private practice in Saint Marys, Pennsylvania, for over 30 years. After graduating from West Virginia University Medical School in his birth state, he completed an internship at Hartford Hospital in Connecticut. His residency in orthopedic surgery was at University Hospitals (Case Western Reserve) in Cleveland, Ohio.

David began his ski patrol career in 1990 in western New York at Holiday Valley Ski Resort, where he still patrols today. Following stints as Western New York Region and Eastern Division Medical Advisor, David took over for Warren Bowman as national Medical Advisor in 2001 and retired from that position in 2019. As a Senior Patroller, OEC Instructor, Senior Trainer Evaluator, and Instructor Trainer, he continues to be active at the local level. He teaches both Outdoor First Care (OFC), which he created, and OEC annually; is an instructor of record and proctor for refreshers; and examines for OFC and OEC. He has National Appointment #8690 and was inducted into the National Ski Patrol Hall of Fame Class of 2015. He continues to help his local ski area as the medical advisor.

David's other interests include breeding, training, and hunting Braque d'Auvergne French bird dogs; restoring antique, foreign, and muscle cars; and working with local Boy Scouts to obtain the winter snow sports merit badge. He continues to serve on several boards in his local area.

Personal Acknowledgment

Many people, both patrollers and nonpatrollers, have given me the opportunity to serve the NSP through the years. The list is too long to include here, but these folks know who they are. Without all these people who have helped me in so many ways, I could not have been a part of the NSP. To each one, thank you for believing in me and allowing me to be part of the NSP. Thanks to Ed and Deb for believing in me. I would like to thank my wife, Roslyn, for giving me her support and patience during the process of writing, editing, and completing this text. Her encouragement has been unwavering.

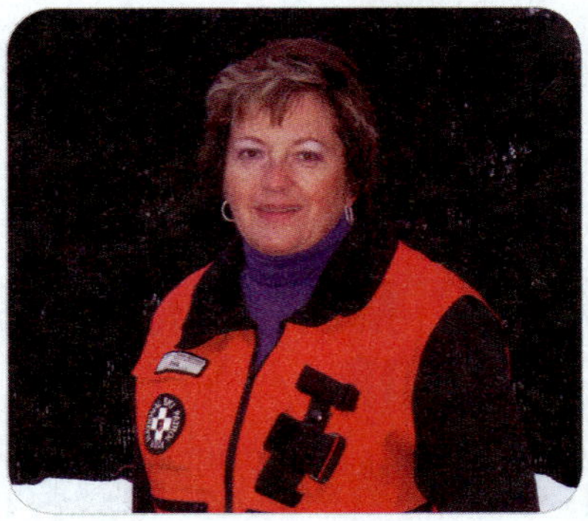

DEBORAH A. ENDLY, BA, DH, NREMT—ASSOCIATE EDITOR

Deborah Endly is currently a Senior Investigator for the State of Minnesota and has been the Compliance Officer for the Minnesota Board of Dentistry since 1995. Deb received her associate of science degree in dental hygiene from Normandale Community College and a bachelor of arts degree focusing on business administration and human resources administration from Metropolitan State University in St. Paul, Minnesota. Prior to working for the State of Minnesota, Deborah practiced clinical dental hygiene and taught university-level dental hygiene courses at Argosy University, Eagan, Minnesota.

Deb is a Minnesota licensed dental hygienist as well as an NREMT and a Basic Life Support Instructor for the American Heart Association. Prior to becoming an EMT, Deb was an EMR and is active in her local Citizen Emergency Response Team as well as Hennepin County Medical Reserve Corp. During her free time, when she is not patrolling, Deborah likes to be outside gardening, boating, or riding her bike.

Deb has been with the NSP since 1993, with the Hyland Hills Ski Patrol at Three Rivers in

Bloomington, Minnesota. She has been a Hill Captain/Shift Leader for 20 years and is the Assistant Patrol Director. Deb has served as the Western Region OEC Administrator and Central Division OEC Supervisor. She has also served on the National OEC Refresher Committee and as the Assistant National OEC Program Director. Deb was an Associate Editor for the *OEC Fifth Edition* text and headed up the Collateral Committee of the book. Deb was the National Program Director for the OEC program from 2013 to 2019. Her National Awards include Leadership Commendation Appointment #8305, the Distinguished Service Award, the Service Excellence Award, and a Gold Merit Star, along with numerous Yellow Merit Stars.

Personal Acknowledgment

I want to thank my sister Vicki, who has supported me with some of the tasks and has given me pep talks along the way as things seemed impossible and tasks were mounting. Thanks also to my Hyland patrol friends who helped pose for photos at the last minute. I want to especially thank my good friends and coeditors Ed McNamara and David Johe. Over the years, as we have worked on these tasks, we have become great friends. We have spent uncountable hours on conference calls, individual phone calls, text messaging, and thousands of emails, developing the best OEC program possible. We are proud of the final product.

CHAPTER 1

INTRODUCTION TO OUTDOOR EMERGENCY CARE

OBJECTIVES

Upon completion of this chapter, the OEC technician will be able to:

1-1 Describe the evolution and purpose of the National Ski Patrol's OEC program.
1-2 Identify the founder of the National Ski Patrol.
1-3 Describe the OEC certification and recertification processes.
1-4 Describe the impact of Good Samaritan laws on volunteer rescuers.
1-5 Contrast the standard of training and standard of care.
1-6 Define the following legal terms:
- Abandonment
- Duty to act
- Negligence
- Breach of duty
- Consent
- Assault
- Battery

1-7 Describe the following concepts relating to consent:
- Informed consent
- Expressed consent
- Implied consent
- Minor consent

KEY TERMS

Abandonment, p. 12
Assault, p. 17
Battery, p. 17
Breach of duty, p. 13
Charles Minot "Minnie" Dole, p. 2
Consent, p. 15
Doctrine of public reliance, p. 11
Duty to act, p. 12
Ethics, p. 10
Expressed content, p. 15
Good Samaritan laws, p. 10
Gross negligence, p 11
Health Insurance Portability and Accountability Act (HIPAA), p 17
Implied consent, p. 15
Informed consent, p. 15
Minor consent, p. 16
National Medical Advisor, p. 4
National Medical Committee, p. 8
National OEC Program Committee, p. 8
National OEC Program Director, p. 8
National OEC Refresher Committee, p. 8
National Ski Patrol System, Inc. (NSP), p. 3
Negligence, p. 12
Outdoor Emergency Care (OEC), p. 2
Prehospital care, p. 2
Refresher, p. 8
Standard of care, p. 14
Standard of training, p. 14
Winter Emergency Care, p. 2

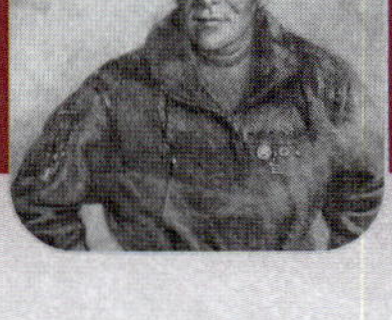

HISTORICAL TIMELINE 1938. Portrait of Minnie Dole, founder of the National Ski Patrol.

CHAPTER OVERVIEW

For over 80 years the National Ski Patrol (NSP) has trained people who have successfully cared for thousands of injured snow sports enthusiasts. Early in its history, an Advanced Red Cross first-aid course was used for training. Since that time, prehospital care has significantly changed. The public has greater expectations of care now, so the NSP has improved the patroller's level of training to that of a National Highway Traffic Safety Administration (NHTSA) emergency medical responder.

Today there are a variety of outdoor activities available at ski areas, bike parks, and other land management areas that occur during all seasons of the year. As a result, the NSP changed the medical training of patrollers to cover not just snow sports, but a variety of other nonwinter activities, including mountain biking, ziplining, downhill bike racing, and riding at bike parks.

In the mid-1980s Dr. Warren Bowman, the National Medical Advisor for the NSP, created a text called ***Winter Emergency Care*** and a corresponding program that provided prehospital medical care training for ski patrollers. Today, the program, aptly named **Outdoor Emergency Care (OEC)**, is the backbone of the NSP's medical training. It is also the standard of training for other organizations using an emergency medical responder curriculum involved with outdoor recreation. Its corresponding textbook of the same title is the primary resource for a student who wants to become a ski or bicycle patroller, or prehospital first responder, called an OEC technician (**Figure 1-1**).

The OEC program also has value for other outdoor enthusiasts. It bridges the gap between urban medical responders with immediate access to an ambulance and advanced equipment, and wilderness search-and-rescue personnel who are several hours from advanced care. No other comprehensive medical textbook covers this niche of **prehospital care**. River rafters, rope-course rescuers, cavers, park rangers, mountain bike race personnel, search-and-rescue personnel, and rescuers at large sporting events and outdoor concerts will find the information in this text invaluable when providing care for patients.

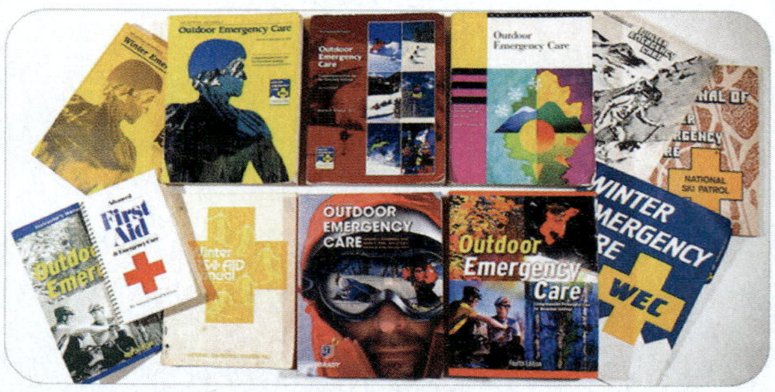

Figure 1-1 These covers show the evolution of the NSP's emergency medical care program from the American Red Cross First Aid Course to the fifth edition of Outdoor Emergency Care.

The prospective OEC technician will learn how to function with minimal equipment in any environment while assessing and caring for the sick and injured. The student will also learn to interact with patients and their families, the public, peers, management, and other medical personnel, which is an important skill of the OEC technician.

This chapter opens with a brief history of the NSP and Charles Minot "Minnie" Dole, its founder. It then discusses the history of OEC and of Dr. Warren Bowman, the man who is credited with its inception. The last portion of the chapter gives a brief overview of the medical-legal and ethical issues OEC technicians may encounter.

NSP'S EARLY YEARS

Over New Year's 1936, **Charles Minot "Minnie" Dole**, a 36-year-old insurance broker from Greenwich, Connecticut, experienced the need for emergency care and rescue services during a personal skiing mishap at Stowe, Vermont. Minnie, who was skiing with his wife, Jane, and their friends Frank and Jean Edson, took a serious fall partway up the Toll Road. From the nasty angle at which his ankle lay, he knew he had injured himself badly. Frank stayed with Minnie while Jane and Jean searched for help. Although a rudimentary ski patrol was already in existence, it was not set up to "spot" accidents. Jane and Jean eventually located two men and a piece of corrugated tin roofing material, on which they half-carried, half-slid the traumatized patient, bumping down the trail without the benefit of immobilization. X-ray images later showed the injury to be a severely displaced ankle fracture. Because such injuries were difficult to treat in the 1930s, Minnie's doctor told him he might never walk again, let alone ski. But Minnie was determined to recover.

Far more devastating than his own injury was the fatal accident of Minnie's friend, Frank Edson,

CASE Presentation

A call comes in for a motor vehicle accident in the parking lot of a resort where a mountain bike race is occurring. One of the racers had just unloaded his bike. As he was riding to the starting area, a car hit him and left the scene. Upon your arrival, you find a 16-year-old boy lying on the ground holding his shoulder. He is tangled in his bicycle. Quite angry and yelling, he also is bleeding from his forehead. A small crowd has gathered.

What should you do?

KEY POINT

The NSP's Mission and Vision Statement (2020)

Mission: To help keep people safe on the mountain and during other outdoor activities.

Vision 2020: Our curriculum-based programs, such as OEC, achieved the level of an industry leader. We met the changing needs of our principal customers and reached a point of financial, staffing, and systems stability.

in a ski race 2 months later, an event that planted the seed for what would become the NSP. Recommended by Roland Palmedo, president of the New York Amateur Ski Club, who had originally "discovered" ski terrain at Stowe, Minnie was put in charge of a ski safety committee for the National Ski Association (or NSA, now US Ski and Snowboard). In March 1938, he organized a volunteer ski patrol for the first National Downhill Races, to be held at Stowe. NSA President Roger Langley was so impressed with the setup that he asked Dole on the spot to organize a similar patrol on a national basis. This occasion marked the birth of the NSP, which originated as a subcommittee of the NSA. Dole continued to chair the **National Ski Patrol System, Inc. (NSP)**, as it was then known, until 1950 (**Figure 1-2**).

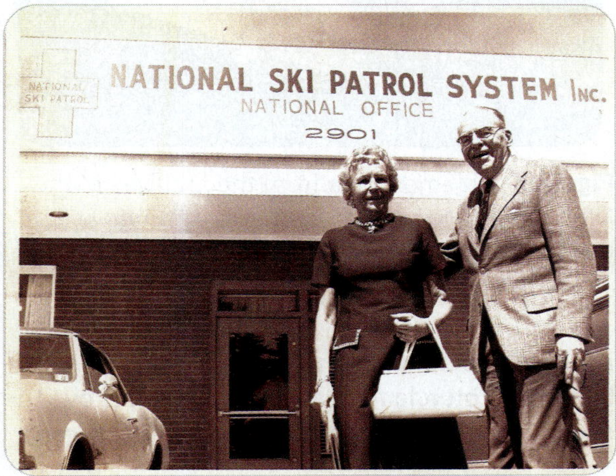

Figure 1-2 Charles Minot "Minnie" Dole, founder and creator of the NSP, and his wife outside the national office of the NSP.

Separating from the NSA in 1953, the NSP became an independent entity, incorporated in New York and Colorado. In 1980, Congress recognized its distinguished legacy of altruistic service by granting a federal charter to the NSP (**Figure 1-3**). Relatively few other institutions, such as the American Red Cross, the Veterans of Foreign Wars, and Boy Scouts of America have earned this coveted endorsement.

As a leading authority on recreational outdoor safety and patient care, the NSP is dedicated to serving the public and the outdoor recreation industry by providing education and accreditation to emergency care and safety-service providers. The organization is composed of more than 30,000 members, serving more than 650 patrols. The

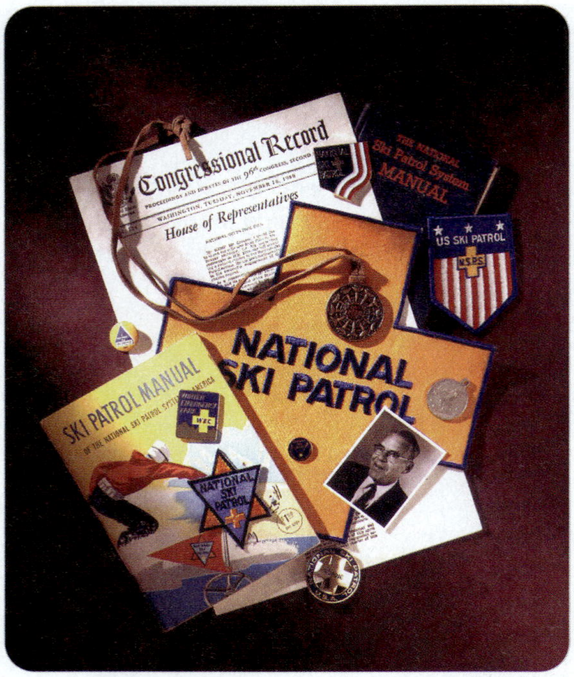

Figure 1-3 Memorabilia from the archives of the NSP, including the federal charter granted by the US Congress of 1980.

© Caleb Hund.

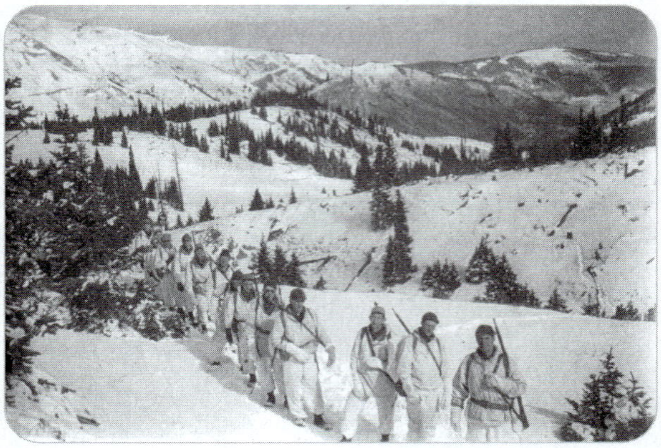

Figure 1-4 The members of the 10th Mountain Division, which specialized in winter warfare during World War II, included many ski patrollers.

Courtesy of Denver Public Library.

NSP's members work on behalf of local ski, snowboard, and bicycle recreation areas to improve the overall experience for outdoor recreation guests.

The NSP Goes to War

By December 1941, the year the first NSP manual was printed, the United States was at war with both Germany and Japan. In 3 years, the NSP had grown to include 180 registered patrols with more than 4,000 personnel trained in first aid, including women for the first time. In addition to mobilizing for winter defense, and since the ski patrol was so successful in locating downed aircraft in the Cascades and Rockies, the NSP was invited to collaborate with the Second and Fourth Air Force, even after the war. Meanwhile, impressed by the stories of Finnish ski troopers against superior Russian forces in the winter of 1939–1940, Minnie Dole contacted and ultimately convinced Army Chief of Staff General George C. Marshall of the value of winter warfare troops.

In early 1942, the 87th Mountain Infantry Regiment was activated at Fort Lewis, Washington, with training on Mt. Rainier. Transferred to newly built Camp Hale, Colorado, in 1943, the 87th was joined by the 85th and 86th regiments to become the famed 10th Mountain Division. The NSP, the only civilian organization ever authorized to recruit for the armed forces, processed the applications of 10,000 volunteers.

In 1944, the "Tenth" was shipped overseas to Italy, where it performed heroically in combat, capturing impregnable mountain strongholds before spearheading a drive to the Po River (**Figure 1-4**). The men who participated in the surprise attack on Riva Ridge, the first of these battles, are memorialized by the Vail ski run of the same name. General Mark Clark called the Tenth the finest division he had ever seen. Following the war's end in 1945, many 10th Mountain Division veterans who had been ski patrollers before the war returned home to become leaders—ski area owners and managers, ski school directors, ski equipment manufacturers—in the growing US ski industry.

The Birth of OEC

Since its founding, the NSP has evolved from a handful of ski patrollers into the world's largest nonurban medical rescue organization. In 1939, NSP established an affiliation with the American Red Cross. Out of this relationship came the publication "Ski Safety and First Aid," which was written by an American Red Cross officer, L. M. Thompson, who became the first chairman of the NSP's Medical Advisory Committee. This position later became the **National Medical Advisor**.

For many years the American Red Cross First Aid Course proved very useful as a basic tool for ski patrollers. However, it became clear in the early 1980s that patrollers required additional prehospital medical care training to care for patients during cold weather and at high altitude. As a result, in 1985 Dr. Warren Bowman, an internist from Billings, Montana, created an emergency responder textbook exclusively for ski patrollers, titled *Winter Emergency Care*. Three years later, this textbook was revised and renamed *Outdoor Emergency Care*. The new text was expanded to include information about a variety of illnesses and injuries in outdoor enthusiasts and for the first time included information about nonwinter emergencies and care for the sick and injured during sporting activities other than skiing. Those changes were made to better reflect the expanding role of OEC technicians in providing year-round emergency care in a variety of settings.

In *Outdoor Emergency Care*, Dr. Bowman created the concept of "intermediate" outdoor medical care. OEC was positioned between the urban and wilderness curricula while emphasizing both. His idea—that OEC technicians would begin the care of a patient in a wilderness situation, would continue care during transport (usually using a toboggan in a ski area), and would further continue care in a first-aid room or ski-area clinic—was unique to the prehospital emergency services community. The concept was widely successful, and the OEC text/curriculum was awarded the year's "Best Educational Program Based on the Needs of Industry or Professional Associations" by the American Society of Association Executives (ASAE) in 1989. Truly, Warren Bowman, MD, is the father of Outdoor Emergency Care (**Figure 1-5**).

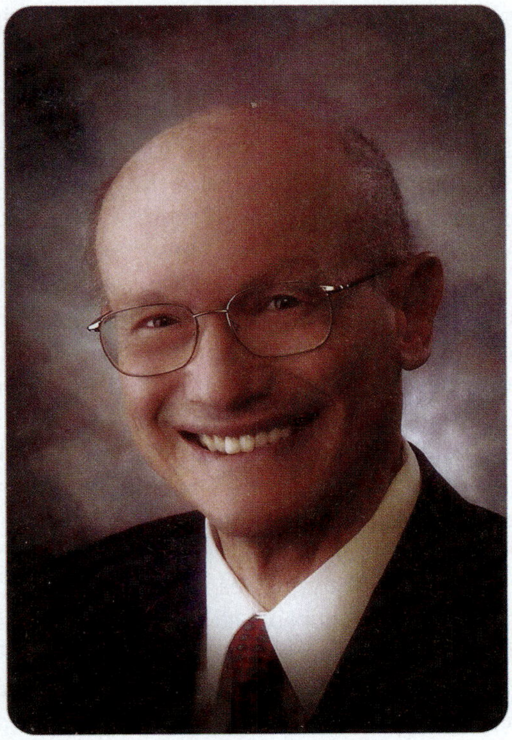

Figure 1-5 Dr. Warren Bowman, the father of Outdoor Emergency Care, developed the concept of "intermediate" outdoor medical care.

Courtesy of Dorothy Bowman.

OEC TODAY

The field of prehospital emergency medical care is ever changing. As a result, the OEC curriculum has improved to meet the needs of patrollers and other outdoor emergency medical care responders. Today, OEC and the NSP's Outdoor First Care (OFC) programs are the primary curricula taught to ski and bicycle patrollers in the United States and patrollers in other countries. They also are used by other prehospital medical responders who may need to provide emergency care in an outdoor setting, such as mountain guides and river guides, law enforcement personnel, and various government agency personnel (**Figure 1-6**).

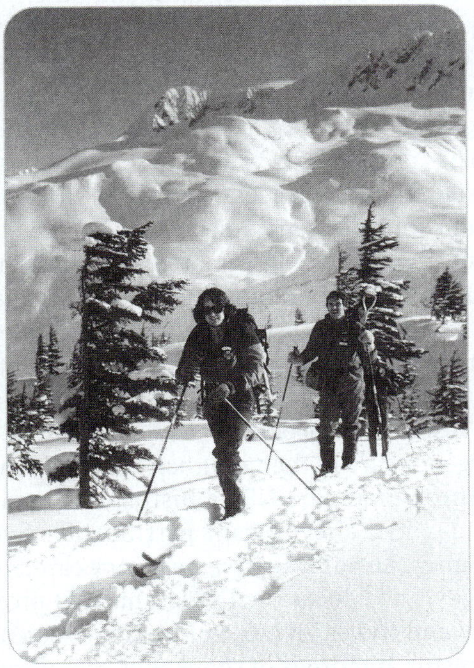

Figure 1-6 For over 80 years the NSP has trained people throughout the world to provide emergency medical care for outdoor enthusiasts.

© National Ski Patrol.

Many older emergency medical publications based training on personal observation, also known as anecdotal information. For instance, the American Red Cross publication *First Aid*

Textbook (1957, page 117) described "A Technique for Administering Manual Artificial Respiration" in which the emergency responder would place the patient on the stomach and push on the upper back with both hands (allowing inhalation), followed by pulling up on the elbows to let the air out of the lungs at a rate of 12 times a minute! This procedure was based purely on past observation and had no scientific basis. The NSP has come a long way since then, improving its course curricula as new medical information becomes available. This sixth edition of *OEC* is written following the principle of *evidence-based medicine*. Reviews of published, scientifically controlled studies plus retrospective evaluations of the outcomes enable us to formulate appropriate care for future patients. These peer-reviewed studies and publications are now the gold standard for prehospital training.

Many of the concepts of splinting, bandaging, and basic soft-tissue first aid presented in *OEC's* first edition (1988) are still appropriate today. Much of the current information in *OEC* on prehospital first-aid treatment comes from scientifically reviewing research from warfare and urban trauma. The equipment ski patrollers use today results from years of work by seasoned OEC technicians who have made their tasks easier by creating different splints, toboggans, and other rescue equipment that work in outdoor environments. This edition of the text contains new information, discusses new equipment, and presents the terminology used by the prehospital community in 2020.

The present OEC curriculum contains the knowledge and skills identified in the NHTSA Curriculum for emergency medical responder training, plus additional information and training for patrollers. The training of OEC technicians has been accepted and used by ski areas and in other outdoor environments throughout the country to meet the evolving training needs of individuals who respond to accidents and deliver essential emergency care in the nonurban environment.

Throughout the NSP's history, its members have devoted a significant part of their lives to providing the public with emergency care, rescue services, and educational programs that promote safety and the enjoyment of outdoor recreation. As a result, hundreds of thousands of injured and ill persons have received prompt, skillful emergency care, and countless lives have been saved.

KEY POINT

The Creed of Service and Safety

The NSP adheres to the creed of "Service and Safety," which was established more than 80 years ago. As the outdoor sports industry has evolved, so too has the NSP. The emergence of new sports such as snow-skating, mountain biking, and downhill bicycle racing, has introduced new equipment and has involved new terrain, which has required that new safety and rescue techniques and new emergency care methods be developed and taught. In addition, greater access to the backcountry has required new training and new regimens for NSP members.

Training: The Focus of the OEC Program

To become proficient as an OEC technician, you must first master the basic concepts of human anatomy and physiology. Without this background, you will be unable to "speak the language" of prehospital providers or understand the concepts of body functions that are so important to providing emergency care (**Figure 1-7**).

The next step is learning how to assess patients. This process requires much diligence and practice. Another important task to be mastered is documentation, using simple time-proven methods that are common to all prehospital and hospital providers. Only after these basics are mastered are you ready to begin learning specific medical interventions.

Learning to intervene when a patient's condition is critical is the next step in the process of becoming an OEC technician. In every encounter with a critical patient, it is important that prehospital providers address the basic principles of making sure the patient has an airway, is breathing, has effective circulation, and does not have a significant neurologic disability, and that they understand their responsibility to intervene when one or more of these conditions has not been met.

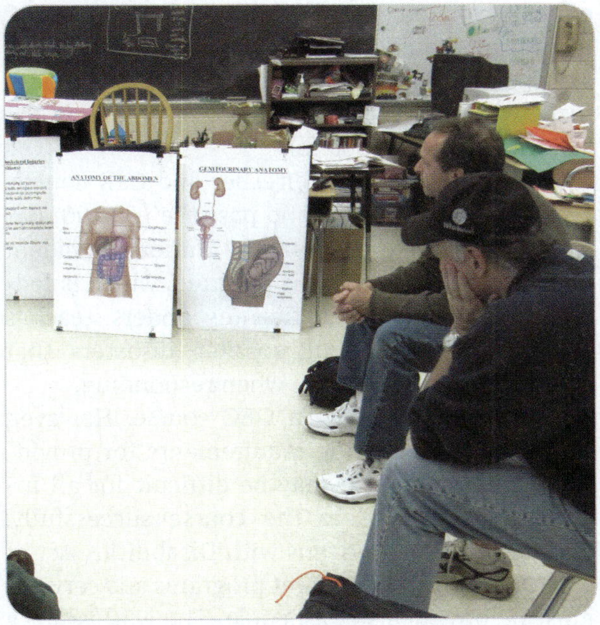

Figure 1-7 An OEC class learning abdominal and pelvic anatomy and physiology.

© Edward McNamara.

The concept of shock also must be understood. Repeated training in evaluation, intervention, and continued care for critical patients is the best method to become proficient in helping very sick or severely traumatized patients.

Learning the normal functions of the body's various systems enables OEC technicians to provide care in both medical and traumatic emergencies. They can apply their knowledge of the body's systems when caring for a patient who has injured a specific body part or who has an illness affecting one or more body systems. From a broken arm to a cardiac event requiring cardiopulmonary resuscitation (CPR), OEC technicians must be able to respond consistently to any emergency, even though the care provided will vary in different situations.

It is important that OEC technicians learn the concepts and the procedures for patient care in special conditions related to high altitude, extremes of temperature, and bodies of water. Members of special populations—children, the elderly, the psychologically impaired, and individuals with special needs—have unique problems. As a certified OEC technician, you will have the tools to care for all of these people in all of these special situations.

In most teaching systems, practice is an effective way to master technical skills. This principle is no different in outdoor emergency care. By learning concepts and then applying those concepts during training, OEC technicians are able to perform effectively in real-life situations outdoors.

As part of your OEC training, instructors will use performance-based objectives to evaluate your progress in becoming an OEC technician. These objectives are learned through repeated practice in a variety of situations and settings.

KEY POINT

Becoming an OEC Technician

To become proficient as an OEC technician, you need to "speak the language" of prehospital providers or understand the concepts important to providing emergency care. Learn the vocabulary or medical words to communicate effectively.

You must learn the objectives found in the beginning of each chapter. These objectives are both knowledge-based and skills-based, so your experience will include learning content and developing hands-on skills. As part of your training, instructors will teach and evaluate your progress based on these objectives learned through reading and discussion, and through repeated practice in a variety of situations and settings.

In most teaching systems, practice is an effective way to master technical skills. This principle is no different in outdoor emergency care. By learning concepts and then applying those concepts during training, OEC technicians are able to perform effectively in real-life situations outdoors.

If a candidate masters the vocabulary, objectives, and skills during the OEC course, he or she will have the tools necessary to pass the OEC course and, with mentoring, become an effective patroller.

Certification and Recertification Requirements

The OEC program is a prehospital emergency care course that has been developed and continuously improved by the NSP, in conjunction with the OEC Program Director, the **National OEC Program Committee**, and the National Education Committee, with input and advice from the **National Medical Committee**. One may complete the course without having the ability to ski, snowboard, or ride a bicycle. To become an "on the hill" OEC technician, you will be required to demonstrate a level of skiing and toboggan handling proficiency to care for and transport an injured skier at a ski area. If you are involved in other sports, you will need to meet their special requirements for transportation. You also will need to be able to perform other duties as required by the area where you patrol.

To receive an OEC certificate of completion, OEC candidates must successfully complete the OEC course. As part of this process, OEC technicians must successfully complete a written examination developed under the direction of the National OEC Program Director and distributed by the NSP's national office. In addition, prospective OEC technicians must successfully complete a practical examination, which is also developed under the direction of the National OEC Program Director and provided by the NSP national office. The test is conducted by trained OEC instructors who function under the supervision and direction of a certified OEC Instructor/Trainer.

Each year, the NSP develops a continuing education program that enables OEC technicians to "refresh" their knowledge and skills. One-third of the total OEC curriculum is reviewed each year. A **refresher** is primarily a "hands-on" learning experience, enabling OEC technicians to demonstrate proficiency in the skills needed to care for a patient. The refresher course may be provided by any currently certified OEC instructor. The refresher is developed by the **National OEC Refresher Committee**, under the direction of the **National OEC Program Director**, and the curriculum is provided to NSP instructors.

Every other year, or as required by the approved CPR certifying agency, each active member of the NSP must successfully complete a course given by one of the NSP-recognized organizations that teaches professional-level CPR and the use of an automated external defibrillator (AED). OEC technicians must also annually demonstrate the skill portion of this CPR curriculum to a recognized CPR instructor, regardless of how long the CPR certificate is good for.

In addition to the refresher and CPR course, all patrollers must take and pass the ICS 100: Basics of ICS course given by the National Incident Management System. This program, which is federally mandated for all first responders, teaches OEC technicians about possible disasters that could occur and their role when responding.

Anyone may take an OEC course. However, because of the specific requirements for providing hands-on care, it may be difficult for all individuals to complete the course successfully. Because of the Americans with Disabilities Act of 1990, state and government programs and services must be provided to all people. The NSP is not a state or government agency and is not regulated by laws regarding public accommodations. However, the NSP encourages its patrols to attempt to provide reasonable accommodations to students with disabilities, based on time and financial considerations. If an OEC instructor judges that students cannot complete the course with reasonable accommodations or could harm themselves or others while participating, that instructor has sole discretion in limiting those students to all or part of the course. These limitations may be necessary if others in the class are hindered in learning in a timely fashion.

Working in Outdoor Environments

As an OEC technician, you will have to master many roles. Your responsibilities will include that of scene manager, caregiver, patient advocate, and role model for the management who has trusted you to care for recreational enthusiasts. Your training will give you the tools to assess and help many people in outdoor environments. Each time you respond to an incident, others will be assessing you: your appearance, presentation, demeanor, and interaction with members of the public. Their assessments will reflect on you, your local ski area or responder agency, and the NSP.

As an OEC technician, you will provide guidance to others in nonmedical ways as well. The family of a patient, a scared child with a painful broken leg, or an autistic teen who is separated

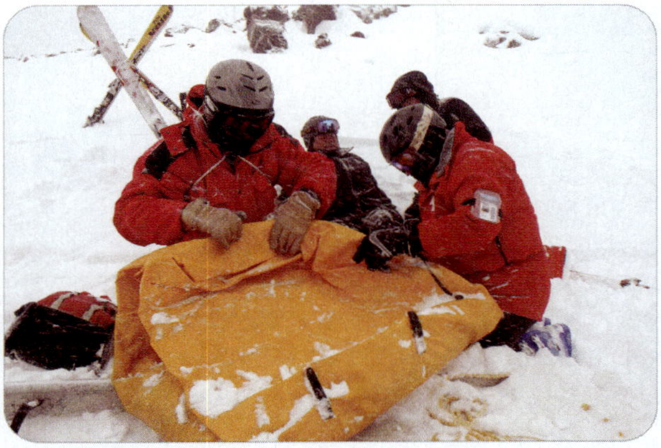

Figure 1-8 You might be challenged both physically and mentally at some accident scenes.

© Studio 404.

from his caregiver will all look to you for guidance. Someone may ask you a simple question about where the restroom is located. Act professionally in a kind and helpful way at all times.

There will be times as an OEC technician when you will be stressed, both physically and mentally (**Figure 1-8**). You must cope with this stress during and after providing care to severely ill or injured patients. The well-being of each OEC technician is the responsibility of everyone in your patrol or rescue agency. Working as a team, your group will provide help to each member during stressful situations. When a rescue has been unsuccessful—as some will be, even though everything possible was done to help the patient—you may be needed to assist a peer cope with the aftermath. At other times, you will need others to help you cope with an unfortunate situation.

You will have the unique opportunity, as an OEC technician, to be the first person to help someone with a severe medical problem. Following your initial evaluation, stabilization, and transport, you will deliver patients to members of the EMS community, such as an ambulance crew, who take over the patient's care. You will learn how to communicate with other members of the prehospital team to speed the patient's entry into the next phase of care. The more knowledge you have of the complete package of prehospital care, the better you will be in providing your part of the patient's care.

After giving a higher-level medical person (such as an EMT or paramedic) a concise report that includes what the patient's problem is, what treatment you have provided, and what your concerns are, you will then see the patient being transported to the hospital for definitive care (**Figure 1-9**). It is at that point that you realize all the effort and OEC training was worth it.

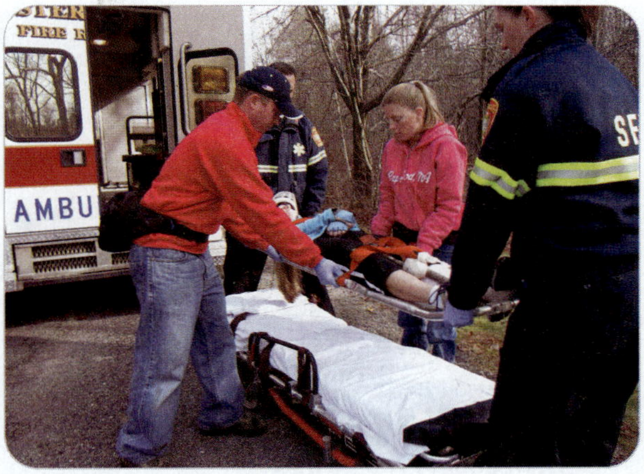

Figure 1-9 Patrollers will need to interact with the EMS responders as the patient care is transferred to a higher level of care.

© Edward McNamara.

ETHICAL AND LEGAL ISSUES

Just as you must learn to manage an accident scene or the medical aspects of patient care, you also must learn to manage the legal aspects of rendering emergency care. Understanding how to reduce legal risk arising out of an accident situation is an important part of patrolling. The pertinent legal principles, when properly applied, will help you function as an OEC technician as you render care to patients and will reduce the legal risk inherent in any accident.

This section discusses and explains several legal terms and concepts in order to familiarize OEC technicians with them generally. This is not a comprehensive reference for legal issues that OEC technicians may encounter. Further, it does not constitute provision of legal advice and should not be relied upon as legal guidance. Any legal questions should be directed to a competent legal authority, duly licensed by the jurisdiction in which the matter may arise.

Throughout the history of the NSP—since Minnie Dole started ski patrolling over 80 years ago—ski patrollers have developed a good image with the skiing public. Minnie was the ultimate role model in his approach to patrolling. This

CASE Update

You immediately assess the situation and make sure the scene is safe by instructing bystanders to stop any traffic. The injured teen is still yelling, so you calm him down. You stop the bleeding on his forehead. Following your initial assessment, having found no evidence of head or spinal injury, you call for help and EMS transport on the radio and ask a responsible bystander to keep the crowd back. One bystander says he got the license plate number of the car, so you ask him to stay. Another OEC technician arrives, and you instruct him to splint the boy's shoulder. Area management and the police are called.

What should you do now?

"good image," which patrollers have earned over the NSP's long history, is a significant protection for the patroller. Being considered the Good Samaritans of the slopes has historically meant that patrollers are rarely sued. Therefore, maintaining the good image and friendly attitude toward the skiing, snowboarding, and bicycling public remains an important goal of your education as an OEC technician.

Ethical Issues Facing OEC Technicians

As an OEC technician, you should hold yourself to a high ethical standard. Historically, NSP patrollers and OEC technicians have always maintained a high standard of ethical conduct with the public and with fellow OEC technicians. Maintaining high **ethics** and the public's respect for OEC technicians is one of the duties and privileges of the job.

The ethical principles used in resolving dilemmas in our daily lives also apply when helping a stranger who is a patient. Those principles are applied to all interpersonal relationships. OEC technicians should follow the following five ethical principles (Beauchamp & Childress, 1994):

- *Respect autonomy (independence).* An individual has the right to act as a free agent. All are free to decide how they live their lives as long as their decisions do not harm the lives of others. Everyone has the right to exercise freedom of thought or choice. Under certain circumstances, people have the right to refuse care.
- *Do no harm (nonmaleficence).* OEC technicians should not engage in any activities with the public that harm others. Any intervention provided should not cause further harm to the patient.
- *Benefit others (beneficence).* Our actions should actively promote the health and well-being of others. This principle is expressed in the NSP's federal charter: ski OEC technicians have a responsibility to promote skier safety.
- *Be just (justice).* Being just and fair balances the rights of one individual against those of others. This principle assumes three standards: impartiality, equality, and reciprocity. These standards are based on the Golden Rule, which states, "Treat others as you wish to be treated."
- *Be faithful (fidelity).* This principle involves loyalty, truthfulness, promise keeping, and respect of others.

Good Samaritan Laws and Duty to Act

As previously discussed, the public has long viewed OEC technicians as "Good Samaritans," people who help other people but expect nothing in return. But what protects such Good Samaritans from legal harm when they help someone who could suffer irreversible physical harm or death, but a bad outcome ensues?

Over time, a group of laws—known as the **Good Samaritan laws**—have been enacted throughout the United States. These laws may protect voluntary OEC technicians in providing first-aid care. In general, they state that a volunteer rescuer is not civilly liable for any act or omission in giving any assistance or medical care if (1) the act or omission is not one of gross negligence, (2) the assistance or medical care is provided without fee or other compensation, and (3) the assistance or medical care is provided at the scene of an emergency, in transit to a medical facility, or through communications with personnel providing emergency assistance.

Good Samaritan laws may protect volunteer rescuers from negligent actions, but not from acts of gross negligence. **Gross negligence** has been defined as an intentional failure to perform a manifest duty in reckless disregard of the consequences as affecting the life or property of another, and it also implies a thoughtless disregard of the consequences without the exertion of any effort to avoid them. Gross negligence can also be considered a wanton or reckless disregard of the injured person by the rescuer. Consider, for example, the Colorado Good Samaritan law:

> 13-21-108. Persons rendering emergency assistance exempt from liability:
>
> (1) Any person licensed as a physician and surgeon under the laws of the state of Colorado, or any other person, who in good faith renders emergency care or emergency assistance to a person not presently his patient without compensation at the place of an emergency or accident, including a health care institution as defined in section 13-64-202 (3), shall not be liable for any civil damages for acts or omissions made in good faith as a result of the rendering of such emergency care or emergency assistance during the emergency, unless the acts or omissions were grossly negligent or willful and wanton. This section shall not apply to any person who renders such emergency care or emergency assistance to a patient he is otherwise obligated to cover.
>
> (2) Any person while acting as a volunteer member of a rescue unit, as defined in section 25-3.5-103 (II), C.R.S., notwithstanding the fact that such organization may recover actual costs incurred in the rendering of emergency care or assistance without compensation at the place of an emergency or accident shall not be liable for any civil damages for acts or omissions in good faith.
>
> (3) Any person, including a licensed physician, surgeon, or other medical personnel while acting as a volunteer member of a ski patrol or ski area rescue unit, notwithstanding the fact that such person may receive free skiing privileges or other benefits as the result of his volunteer status, who in good faith renders emergency care or assistance without other compensation at the place of an emergency or accident shall not be liable for any civil damages for acts or omissions in good faith.

Clearly, paragraph 3 of Colorado's law is intended to apply to ski patrollers specifically. Many other states have similar laws specifically worded to protect volunteer ski patrollers; however, OEC technicians should be familiar with the laws of their own state because Good Samaritan laws vary from to state to state.

Good Samaritan laws are designed to encourage volunteers to provide first-aid care without the worry of being sued for negligence. These laws reflect the good work that voluntary rescuers provide the public. However, it is important that OEC technicians make sure that the ski area or resort where they work or volunteer has adequate insurance protection and that they have adequate personal insurance. Good Samaritan laws are not legislated in all states. Your area management can inform you what impact the laws may have on you as an OEC technician in your state.

A second important concept regarding an OEC technician's legal obligation to provide care involves the "duty to rescue" (or "duty to act"). In general, an average citizen has no legal duty to rescue another individual who needs medical care. However, once OEC technicians or other rescuers have put on a uniform, whether they are on duty or off, the public has a reasonable expectation that a rescuer will provide care to an injured person. The **doctrine of public reliance** is created whenever a rescuer may have a legal obligation to render first-aid care to an injured person in need of such care. The primary exception to this rule is when performing such care may place the safety of a rescuer or others at risk.

The legal issue as to whether an OEC technician is required to provide first-aid care when not on duty is primarily governed by individual state or provincial laws. Most states and provinces do not require OEC technicians to provide such first-aid care. However, some states or provinces require individuals who are licensed by the state or province to render emergency care anytime they are present at an accident scene. Reviewing and understanding the relevant laws and codes concerning this legal point are important for an OEC technician's own legal protection.

Anything that gives members of the public a reasonable expectation that an OEC technician has the ability to provide first-aid services—for example, the wearing of a patrol jacket or other OEC insignia, even while off duty—may trigger the doctrine of public reliance. Therefore, even off-duty but identifiable OEC technicians are representing to the general public that they have the ability to provide first-aid care, and thus those OEC technicians should provide such first-aid care as required (**Figure 1-10**).

OEC technicians have both a moral duty and a legal duty to act. If you find someone who is injured or sick while you are off duty but are the only one around, you may have a *moral* duty to act, and you should be helped by the Good Samaritan laws. However, if you are on duty, you may have a *legal* duty to act, and you should follow the guidelines established by your management and state emergency medical system.

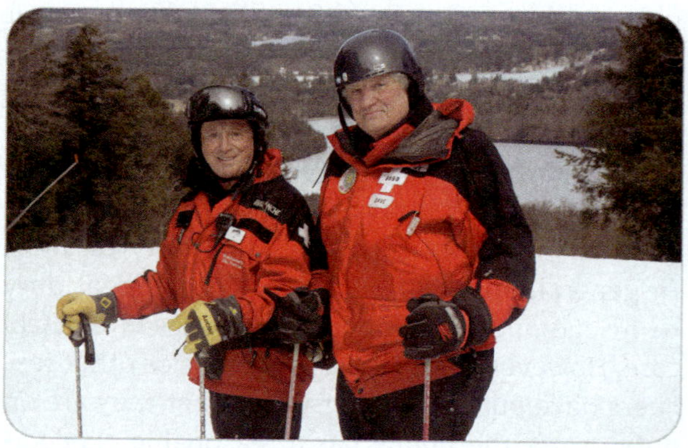

Figure 1-10 When skiing in your NSP uniform, you must act professional and ready to assist an injured patron.

Abandonment

An OEC technician who inappropriately terminates first-aid care once begun could be liable under the legal doctrine of **abandonment**. Once an OEC technician has started providing first-aid care in an emergency situation, he or she should continue providing such care until one of the following conditions has been met:

- All the care that is required has been given.
- The injured person has been transferred to another caregiver of equal or higher training and certification.
- The injured person has specifically informed the rescuer that he or she no longer wants the rescuer to provide such emergency care.
- The patient is transported safely to a medical treatment facility.
- Continuing such emergency medical care threatens the rescuer's safety.

Examples of abandonment include initiating care on an injured child and then leaving the child alone while you handle another accident or leaving a patient who is awaiting ambulance transport alone in the aid room while the patient goes into shock. Once again, exceptions to the doctrine of abandonment are when providing such care could threaten a rescuer's own safety or when competent patients have informed a rescuer that they no longer want first-aid care.

Negligence and Breach of Duty

Negligence can occur when an OEC technician harms an individual by not performing up to the technician's standard of training. Failure to provide care within the standard of training that a reasonable and prudent OEC technician is expected to provide under the circumstances can also be negligence. For example, an improperly placed splint that results in further harm to the patient could be considered negligence. Therefore, it is important that a patroller exercise care and meet the standard of training when performing first-aid activities in order to avoid legal negligence.

Once a **duty to act** is established, you are legally required to render appropriate care after you approach a patient. This duty of care is an obligation imposed on you as an OEC technician that requires you to be reasonable in providing any care that could foreseeably harm the patient. The failure to perform a promised act or obligation of due care is considered a **breach of duty**.

In many states, it is important to document evidence of any *contributory negligence* by the patient involved in an accident. In this situation, the patient actually contributes to his or her own harm. In such states, if the injured person was negligent in a manner that contributed to the cause of the accident, then the injured skier may not recover monetary damages as a result of the accident. A skier's statement that he or she was "going too fast" or "wasn't looking ahead" could be considered an admission by the skier of contributory negligence and could prevent the skier from receiving a monetary recovery in court.

States that do not recognize the concept of contributory negligence might recognize the legal concept of *comparative negligence*. In such states, the legal system determines the degree or percentage of fault attributable to the patient and to other parties and then adjusts any monetary award for damages resulting from the accident based on those degrees of comparative fault.

In addressing either of these two legal principles, OEC technicians should fully document the circumstances surrounding the accident and any care rendered. The OEC technician should be familiar with the materials published by the National Ski Areas Association on documenting and investigating accidents and should perform these functions as directed by their area management.

Assumption of Risk

A legal principle that protects patrollers is the doctrine of the *assumption of risk*. This doctrine means that when skiers or snowboarders choose to participate in these sports, they assume that the sport has inherent risks.

OEC technicians should record the details of such accidents with great attention to "how" the accident was caused. Many of the accidents that occur as skiers or snowboarders go up the mountain occur because skiers do not properly follow directions. If a skier or snowboarder does not follow the proper procedures, make sure such information is recorded on the accident forms.

The same principle also applies to accidents that involve equipment such as snowmobiles. Collisions with such objects should be carefully documented because encountering this type of equipment might not be considered part of the "inherent risk" of skiing.

Preparing Documentation

As part of your OEC training, you will learn to document what occurred at the accident scene. This documentation is extremely important because it might be the only reliable source of information for reconstructing in court what happened at the accident scene many years earlier. Doing a good job in preparing such documents and accident forms is a vital part of your training and a critical part of the risk management of an accident scene (**Figure 1-11**).

Proper documentation includes a detailed description of the accident situation; pictures, when appropriate; names of all OEC technicians involved in working at the accident scene; and names, addresses, and phone numbers of all witnesses. It is very important to document any statement the injured person makes concerning the accident. Proper documentation and preservation of all evidence are the best legal protections for OEC technicians and thus are skills that must be learned. However, to the extent permitted by the circumstances, OEC technicians should always

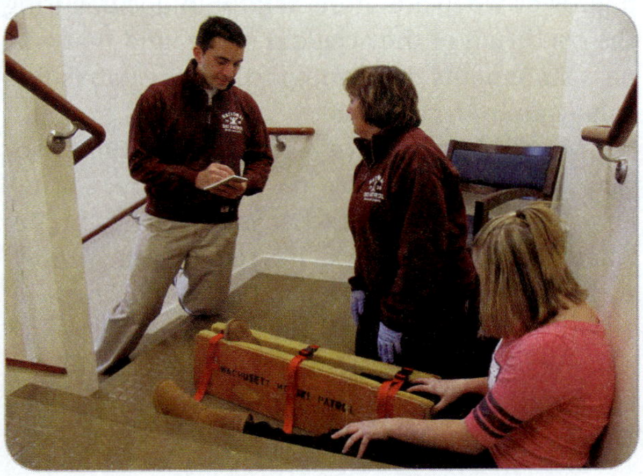

Figure 1-11 When filling out a report, you must thoroughly document the care and treatment rendered at the time of the accident. You may be called to testify several years after the event, and the report will be all that you have to go on.

record completely and accurately all of the facts involved in the accident as those facts are presented to them.

It is part of an OEC technician's learned skills in the risk management of accidents to preserve statements by the injured person or any witnesses concerning either the good job performed by OEC technicians or any admissions of fault made by the injured person. Writing down these types of statements is known as *preservation of evidence*. Should an accident attended by an OEC technician proceed to litigation, both the technician and the snow sports resort will appreciate that the accident forms preserved the evidence.

OEC technicians should understand that evidence that is vital to their protection can be destroyed by such events as changing snow conditions or replacement of signage; therefore, it is important that they preserve all of the evidence and accounts of the events involving an accident in a timely way. Preserving evidence is vital not only to winning legal cases, but also in preventing such cases from ever being filed.

Preserving all evidence requires good sense, judgment, and lots of patience, so it is important to take the time to do a thorough job of completing the accident form documentation. Write everything down on the accident form neatly, completely, and with careful attention to preserving evidence that supports the fact that the patrollers did a good job. Remember that media such as photos or video are often helpful in documenting the condition of the accident scene, and that witness statements can be important in establishing what caused the accident.

Most ski areas have a risk-management program to preserve this type of evidence. Patrollers should understand what is expected of them when a serious accident that requires the preservation of evidence and additional investigation occurs at their ski area. Understanding the area's risk-management system is a vital part of the teamwork a patrol and patrollers have with the area's management.

Scope of Training

As previously indicated, OEC technicians are trained in the NSP Outdoor Emergency Care curriculum, in the local protocols for emergency care required in their areas, and in the requirements of the state laws and regulations that govern first-aid care. Some training, such as use of special equipment, may be unique to the local rescue unit or patrol. This scope of training will combine with what you have learned in the OEC curriculum class to become part of the level of training you are expected to perform in your local area.

The scope of training may be different for different members of a medical response team. Emergency medical responders and OEC technicians usually assess the patient, provide emergency lifesaving care, and perform noninvasive interventions. Other medical providers may perform invasive or advanced medical procedures. It is important for members of the medical response team to understand their roles and the limitations that are placed on them pursuant to their level of training.

Standard of Training Versus Standard of Care

When providing first-aid services, OEC technicians must remember that they are trained in the NSP's Outdoor Emergency Care curriculum. OEC technicians and emergency medical responders are not physicians and are not trained to provide advanced life-support techniques, such as administering drugs. OEC technicians are taught to use their judgment and, when the accident situation requires it, to request additional medical support from someone with a higher level of training. By exercising sound judgment and acting within their **standard of training**, OEC technicians reduce their legal risk. It is when OEC technicians perform procedures they are not trained to do that legal issues arise.

Understanding the limits of the standard of training is important in reducing your legal risk as an OEC technician. Simply put, you must know your limitations. It is important to understand that the information set forth in this textbook does *not* define the **standard of care** of an OEC technician; the information sets forth only the standard of training that is taught by the NSP's Outdoor Emergency Care program.

The standard of care an OEC technician might be required to perform includes the training set forth in this textbook, but it also includes the local area's protocols; the state's emergency medical services restrictions, laws, and procedures; and circumstances within the geographic area in which the rescuer works. It is each OEC technician's responsibility to understand these additional elements, which, in conjunction with the training set forth in this textbook, define the standard of care that OEC technicians should provide.

In addition to the training OEC technicians receive in the NSP's Outdoor Emergency Care, patrollers need to be familiar with the local first-aid protocols established by the ski area or land management area in which they serve. Those protocols, which become part of the OEC technician's standard of care, vary. They are important because OEC technicians who do not perform under both the OEC standard of training and the local protocol standards might be placing themselves at legal risk.

There may be an exception when working either professionally or voluntarily as an OEC technician with OEC training. In most states when an OEC technician is a physician, nurse, or individual who is trained at a higher level of medical care than an OEC technician, the OEC technician must provide first aid at the higher standard of care, being the standard of care created by training.

Joint Statement of Understanding

When you work as an OEC technician at a ski area, you should be aware that you are patrolling as an "agent" of the ski area, not on behalf of the NSP. This distinction conforms to an agreement between the NSP and the National Ski Areas Association in a document titled "The Joint Statement of Understanding." This agreement states that it "is specifically agreed and understood that the NSP does not control the patrol activities of patrollers while they are patrolling at their respective ski areas." As such, it is understood, and may be asserted, that the ski area bears legal responsibility for patrolling activities that fall within the scope of duties of OEC technicians. It is also understood and agreed that the NSP provides educational training to individual OEC technicians in the classroom and on the slopes, including toboggan handling training, and OEC certification.

Patient's Consent

Before providing first-aid care, OEC technicians should obtain permission from the patient for that care. The same is true for any other medical provider. When you approach the patient, simply ask, "May I help you?" If the answer is yes, then you have permission, or **consent**, to provide care. OEC technicians should be familiar with several concepts relating to consent, including informed consent, expressed consent, implied consent, and minor consent.

To give **informed consent**, the injured person must understand what actions the responder plans to take and agree to them. As a general rule, it is important that OEC technicians tell the injured person what they plan to do. When you arrive on scene and approach the patient, simply say, "I'm David with the ski patrol. May I help you?" Once you have collected the history, ask, "May I examine you, care for you, and transport you?" If the patient is competent and says yes, then you have obtained **expressed consent** to treat the patient. *Competent* in this context means the person sufficiently understands what first aid will be rendered to make an independent decision. Before rendering first aid, and if the circumstances permit, inform the injured person of the first-aid procedures you will perform, such as, "I am going to put your leg in a quick splint," so the injured person can continue to provide expressed consent as you proceed.

The concept of expressed consent can become complex at an accident scene. For example, an injured skier might provide a ski patroller with expressed consent to provide basic first aid; however, the injured skier might refuse to allow a patroller to transport him or her down the mountain. This situation involves both expressed consent and a refusal of care. If there is a refusal of care and the patroller, using a patroller's good judgment, believes that the refusal places the injured skier at risk, then the patroller should create an accident form, and the injured skier's refusal should be carefully documented.

Another type of consent is **implied consent**, which means the patient is not capable of providing expressed consent but would request first-aid care if he or she could (**Figure 1-12**). In general when an injured individual is not capable of providing expressed consent, implied consent may apply. A classic example of such a situation is when an OEC technician arrives at an accident scene and finds an unresponsive injured skier. In such situations, the general law allows the OEC technician to assume the skier has consented to receive first aid. Other examples of situations in which implied consent applies are when the injured skier is delusional or unresponsive as a result of taking alcohol

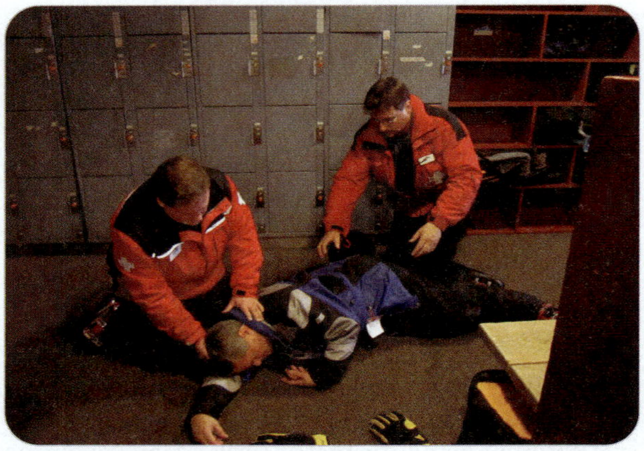

Figure 1-12 Implied consent gives health care providers permission to treat some patients, even if the patient's verbal authorization has not been given.

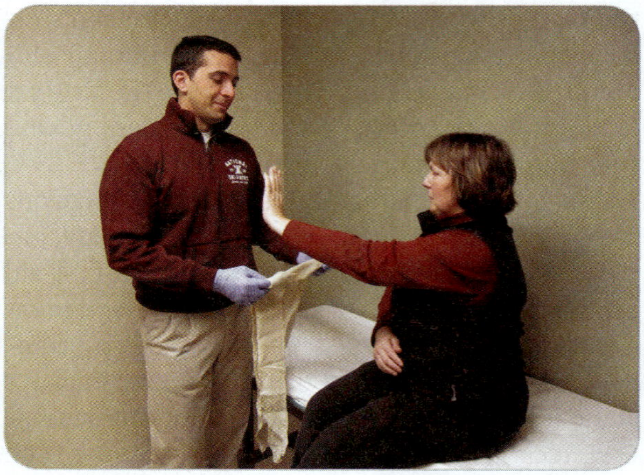

Figure 1-13 If the patient refuses care, you need to document the refusal.

or drugs and when the injured skier is otherwise physically unable to give expressed consent. In some situations, consent can be given by a spouse or a parent of an injured skier who is unable to provide such consent.

Consent Involving Minors

Some states have determined that minors do not have the judgment necessary to provide expressed consent. In those instances, OEC technicians should attempt to obtain **minor consent** from a parent or legal guardian. However, if a parent or legal guardian is not available, implied consent typically allows OEC technicians to conduct first aid and provide transportation. In addition, in many ski areas, groups of minors provide group leaders or chaperones written consent-to-treatment forms. Therefore, if a parent or guardian is not available, OEC technicians should look to the group leader or chaperone to obtain expressed consent after ascertaining that the group leader or chaperone has the authority to provide such consent. Even though there may be no legal obligation to do so, OEC technicians should use their good judgment and try to contact the parent or the legal guardian by telephone to keep that parent or legal guardian informed as to the minor's immediate first-aid needs.

Refusal

Allowing an injured skier the opportunity to refuse first aid is important. If the injured skier denies an OEC technician's offer to provide first-aid assistance, this denial should be carefully documented. It is important to document that you have explained the risks the patient is taking by refusing care. Without proper documentation, OEC technicians may be exposing themselves to risk according to the doctrine of abandonment. Therefore, if a skier refuses first aid, OEC technicians should document the refusal in writing, signed by the injured skier and, if possible, witnessed by another OEC technician (**Figure 1-13**).

If a patient refuses first-aid treatment, attach a *written* refusal of first aid to an accident form in which all the required basic information has been entered. If the injured skier refuses to cooperate in preparing a written refusal of care form, the OEC technicians involved should carefully document that refusal and complete an accident form that includes the circumstances surrounding the injured skier's refusal of first aid. Having another OEC technician as a witness on the completed form verifies that the injured skier refused first aid. In such circumstances, OEC technicians should consider notifying the ski area's risk-management personnel.

When an injured skier is competent to provide consent but refuses despite a risk of serious injury or death if treatment is not provided, it is usually best to provide the treatment. The legal risk of not providing treatment outweighs the legal risk of not complying with the directions of the injured skier, who might later be found incompetent to have provided such directions.

Assault and Battery

OEC technicians who continue to provide care after receiving a competent refusal of such first aid are placing themselves at legal risk of being accused of assault and battery. This situation could lead to both civil and criminal offenses. Touching someone who does not desire to be touched is known as **battery**, whereas placing a person in a position in which he or she reasonably fears that battery will occur is known as **assault**.

The use of physical force is very rarely justified. An example in which some force is justified is restraining an injured skier who has a head injury and is thrashing around on the ground in order to protect the individual from further trauma.

If a skier threatens you with the use of force, back away and call for more patrollers and area security staff. If possible, isolate the individual from the rest of the skiing public and, if appropriate, request assistance from local authorities who are authorized to forcibly restrain the individual, if necessary.

OEC technicians are trained to avoid scenarios in which they could be accused of assault or battery. When they do find themselves in such circumstances, they are trained to request assistance from management and from the local police. All OEC technicians should become familiar with their ski area's policies on the forcible restraint of individuals.

Judgment

One of the core skills of OEC technicians is learning to use proper judgment. OEC technicians are trained to rely on their "judgment" because each accident situation is different. If an OEC technician sees that the people at an accident scene are escalating emotionally, or if an adversarial relationship is developing between the injured skier and witnesses concerning the accident, the OEC technician should immediately request additional help. Additional OEC technicians can help calm such situations and serve as excellent witnesses. Obtaining additional help to control the skiing traffic near the accident scene is only good judgment.

Using good judgment to manage an accident scene both helps provide the proper emergency medical care required and reduces legal risk. As an OEC technician, you should remember to (1) provide the care within your standard of training, (2) practice and maintain your skills so you can remain proficient in providing first-aid care, and (3) use good judgment and planning to manage the medical and legal aspects of the accident scene in a safe manner.

Training

Training OEC technicians poses its own legal risks. By the very nature of training, trainers must challenge the skills of their trainees so that each trainee's skills grow and improve. Since ski patrolling can be inherently dangerous, training OEC technicians can be dangerous. Controlling that danger through risk management and proper supervision is part of what a trainer must do. But the legal obligations and responsibilities go both ways; trainees must recognize that they have limited skills and should not place themselves in situations that, beyond stretching their own skills, endanger themselves and other trainees. Trainees must accept the responsibility for their own risks, and trainers must be skilled enough to train trainees properly, without exposing them and others to unnecessary risk.

EMS System Regulations

Each state has its own emergency medical services (EMS) system. Different states prohibit the use of different types of medical procedures unless the provider has obtained proper training and certification from the state or province. The NSP has not designed the information in *Outdoor Emergency Care, Sixth Edition* for any particular state or province but has, instead, designed the text to provide the best outdoor emergency care training for OEC technicians everywhere. Therefore, it is important that OEC technicians understand the level of care they can provide to patients based on their particular state's or province's EMS laws, rules, and regulations (**Figure 1-14**).

Privacy Laws

The general trend of current laws is to keep medical information about injured persons private. To that end, the US Congress passed the **Health Insurance Portability and Accountability Act (HIPAA)** of 1996. HIPAA was enacted to protect the privacy of an individual's medical information. The act specifically pertains to care providers who are compensated for the care they provide when the patient's information is transferred electronically.

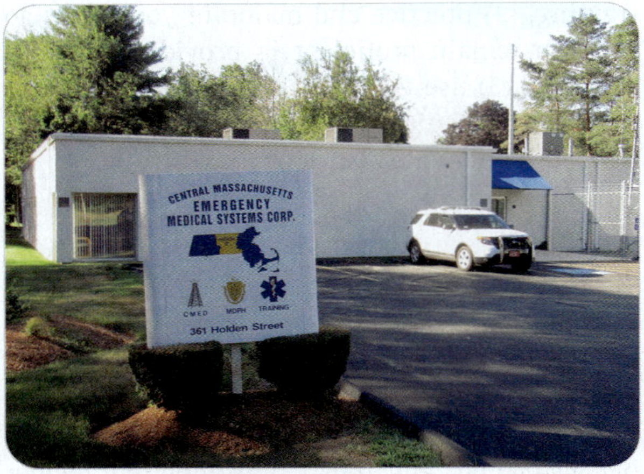

Figure 1-14 Know your state's or province's EMS laws, rules, and regulations.

Central Massachusetts Emergency Medical System Corp., © Edward McNamara.

HIPAA likely does not apply to volunteer patrolling activities because patrollers do not receive direct compensation for the medical services they render to injured skiers, and patrollers generally do not bill for medical services electronically or transfer medical information electronically.

However, the application of HIPAA could vary from ski area to ski area. For example, some ski areas operate a medical clinic as part of the ski area's medical facility. Because the clinic might be governed by HIPAA regulations, a patrol should ensure that its base of operations is physically separate from the clinic, so that the public can distinguish between patrol operations and clinic operations.

Additionally, some paid patrols might be subject to HIPAA requirements. Failure to comply with HIPAA laws may result in serious consequences, including fines and criminal prosecution. The determination of whether HIPAA applies to your patrolling activities must be made by your ski area. It is not an NSP decision. Check with your area management to find out whether HIPAA laws apply to you.

Even though most volunteer patrols are exempt from HIPAA laws, that exemption does not mean there should be no attempt to keep private the medical information obtained from an injured skier. Health care privacy laws do apply, and all patient information must be kept confidential. Simply put, OEC technicians should always be conscious of the privacy of injured skiers and should not use their names or provide any information that could identify them, unless absolutely necessary.

Teamwork

One of the best ways to manage the legal aspects of an accident scene is for OEC technicians to remember that they are part of a team of fellow OEC technicians. Making the decision to call for additional help is one important way to manage an accident situation properly. Additional OEC technicians assisting at an accident scene not only help OEC technicians with the first-aid needs of the patient but also act as witnesses, preventing the situation in which it is a skier's word against a single OEC technician's word. This team's ability to support an OEC technician's account of events at the accident scene reduces that OEC technician's legal risks.

CASE Outcome

Another OEC technician arrives, and you instruct him to find the boy's parents. You care for the boy, rendering first aid until the ambulance arrives. Management arrives, as do the police, and you direct them to the witness so that his statement may be obtained. The boy's parents are found in their condominium and come to the scene. You explain to them what happened. While the mother accompanies her son to the hospital, you go back to the aid room and complete your paperwork. The next day, the mother calls the patrol room to tell you her son dislocated his shoulder, had it reduced, and will be all right. Management informs you that the police found the driver who hit the boy.

CHAPTER REVIEW

In Summary

- Charles Minot "Minnie" Dole was the founder of the National Ski Patrol (NSP).
- The textbook *Winter Emergency Care*, now titled *Outdoor Emergency Care*, was designed by Warren Bowman, MD, to give OEC technicians the skills to begin the care of a patient in a wilderness situation, continue care during transport (usually using a toboggan in a ski area), and continue care in a first-aid room or ski-area clinic.
- To receive an Outdoor Emergency Care (OEC) certificate of completion, OEC candidates must successfully complete the OEC course. The course includes a written and a practical examination.
- After completion of the basic OEC class, the technician must take a refresher course annually to maintain the certification. The refresher course covers one-third of the total curriculum each year. In addition, technicians must maintain responder-level CPR and demonstrate the skill annually to a CPR instructor.
- OEC technicians should always maintain a high standard of ethical behavior.
- Good Samaritan laws protect a person from legal liability when the person volunteers to perform an act to help someone else. They are not in effect in all states!
- OEC technicians have a moral and legal duty to act.
- Documentation is an important component of patient care and a critical part of risk management.
- It is important for OEC technicians to understand their roles and limitations and to understand the level of care they can provide to patients based on their particular state's or province's EMS laws, rules, and regulations.
- Whenever possible, obtain consent before caring for a patient.

Key Terms

Abandonment The act of withdrawing one's support or help from, especially in spite of duty, allegiance, or responsibility.

Assault The act of making a person reasonably fear that battery will occur.

Battery The act of touching someone without his or her consent.

Breach of duty The failure to perform a promised act or obligation of due care.

Charles Minot "Minnie" Dole The founder and creator of the National Ski Patrol.

Consent Permission or approval to perform a proposed or requested action.

Doctrine of public reliance A reasonable expectation held by the general public that an OEC technician can and will provide first-aid services.

Duty to act A person's legal obligation to perform an action.

Ethics The science (study) of morality or behavior that defines what is "good" or "right."

Expressed consent Consent given when a competent injured person gives permission to provide first-aid treatment and transport.

Good Samaritan laws Laws that protect a person from legal liability when the person volunteers to perform an act to help someone else.

Gross negligence An intentional failure to perform a manifest duty in reckless disregard of the consequences as affecting the life or property of another. It also implies a thoughtless disregard of the consequences without the exertion of any effort to avoid them.

Health Insurance Portability and Accountability Act (HIPAA) A law requiring that medical personnel who are compensated for the services they provide maintain patient confidentiality during the electronic transmission of medical records, among other requirements.

Implied consent A form of consent that is not expressly granted by a person, but instead is inferred from a person's actions and the facts and circumstances of a particular situation.

Informed consent Consent a person gives based on an appreciation and understanding of the facts, implications, and possible future consequences of an action.

Minor consent Consent a parent or legal guardian gives for the treatment of a minor, because legally the minor is not competent to give consent to medical treatment. The ability to provide such consent varies among states.

National Medical Advisor A licensed physician with an interest in outdoor/wilderness medicine and ski patrolling who is appointed by the National Ski Patrol's chairman and approved by the National Ski Patrols board of directors to advise the NSP in all matters of medical concern; chairs the National Medical Committee.

National Medical Committee A group of physicians that includes the Division Medical Advisor from each division of the National Ski Patrol, the National OEC Program Director, and other physicians selected at large as approved by the National Board and the National Medical Advisor.

National OEC Program Committee A committee composed of all Division OEC Supervisors and the National Medical Advisor, and chaired by the National OEC Program Director; provides insight and guidance to the board of directors annually on matters related to the functioning of the OEC program.

National OEC Program Director A National Ski Patrol (NSP) member who is responsible to the board for the effective management and operation of the national OEC program. This individual is an active specialist in the field of outdoor medicine and is appointed by the NSP chairman and confirmed by the NSP board of directors. The National OEC Program Director also chairs the national OEC Program Committee and serves as a member of the National Education Committee and the National Medical Committee.

National OEC Refresher Committee A committee responsible for developing the annual OEC Refresher program. It is appointed and supervised by the National OEC Program Director.

National Ski Patrol System, Inc. (NSP) The largest winter rescue group in the world, as recognized by the US Congress under Title 36 of the US Code; the premier snow sports rescue organization in the United States.

Negligence The failure to exercise the care that a reasonably prudent person with similar training would exercise in a similar circumstance.

Outdoor Emergency Care (OEC) A course of medical instruction developed and taught by the National Ski Patrol.

Prehospital care Any medical care rendered by trained personnel prior to arrival at a hospital.

Refresher Annual required continuing education training, usually given each year in the fall, that covers one-third of topics taught in the OEC curriculum.

Standard of care A level of care an OEC technician must render based on OEC training, local medical protocols, and the requirements of a state's EMS system.

Standard of training The training of National Ski Patrol OEC technicians as set forth in the OEC course, using this text as a reference.

Winter Emergency Care A textbook, developed by Dr. Warren Bowman, that was the precursor to the *Outdoor Emergency Care* text.

Chapter Questions

1. The Outdoor Emergency Care course was created by the National Ski Patrol to:
   a. establish a standard of care for ski patrollers and others involved in outdoor emergency care.
   b. be the primary resource in becoming a ski patroller, bike patroller, or prehospital provider responding to outdoor emergencies.
   c. respond to a request from Minnie Dole to develop training for patrollers working at ski resorts.
   d. create a worldwide standard of care for anyone providing outdoor emergency care.
2. The first emergency responder textbook created exclusively for ski patrollers was titled:
   a. *Winter Emergency Care.*
   b. *Outdoor Emergency Care.*
   c. *Ski Safety and First Aid.*
   d. *Safety on the Snow.*
3. Who created and founded the National Ski Patrol?
   a. Roger Langely
   b. Roland Palmedo
   c. Minnie Dole
   d. Warren Bowman
4. To maintain OEC certification, you must:
   a. complete a refresher course that covers one-third of the curriculum every year.
   b. complete a refresher course that covers the key objectives of the entire curriculum every year.
   c. complete a refresher course that covers the key objectives of the entire curriculum every 3 years.
   d. demonstrate CPR and AED skills every 2 years.
5. Although regulations may differ from state to state, the general laws that may protect OEC technicians from liability while providing emergency care to a patient are known as:
   a. emergency rescue protection laws.
   b. Good Samaritan laws.
   c. volunteer rescue liability laws.
   d. first rescuer liability laws.
6. Which of the following statements concerning *standard of training* is true?
   a. Acting within the standard of training is fundamental to reducing an OEC technician's legal risk.
   b. Standard of training is the same thing as standard of care.
   c. Standard of training includes the mountain area's protocols.
   d. Standard of training includes specific state laws and procedures.
7. Failure to exercise the care that a reasonably prudent person with similar training would exercise in a similar circumstance is known as:
   a. negligence.
   b. assault.
   c. gross negligence.
   d. standard of care breach.
8. Which of the following is *not* a concept relating to patient consent?
   a. Informed consent
   b. Minor consent
   c. Implied consent
   d. Absolute consent
9. Consent that is based on an appreciation and understanding of the facts, implications, and possible future consequences of an action is known as:
   a. implied consent.
   b. educated consent.
   c. expressed consent.
   d. informed consent.

10. An OEC technician who leaves a patient before the patient's care is transferred to the next level of care could most accurately be accused of:
    a. negligence.
    b. breach of duty.
    c. abandonment.
    d. assault.

Reference

Beauchamp, Tom L., and James F. Childress. 1994. *Principles of Biomedical Ethics*, Fourth Edition. New York, New York: Oxford University Press.

Answers: 1. b, Objective: 1-1, p. 2; 2. a, Objective: 1-1, p. 2; 3. c, Objective: 1-2, p. 2; 4. a, Objective: 1-3, p. 8; 5. b, Objective: 1-4, p. 10; 6. a, Objective 1-5, p. 14; 7. a, Objective 1-6, p. 12; 8. d, Objective 1-7, p. 15; 9. d, Objective 1-7, p. 15; 10. c, Objective 1-6, p. 12

CHAPTER 2

EMERGENCY MEDICAL CARE SYSTEMS

OBJECTIVES

Upon completion of this chapter, the OEC technician will be able to:

2-1 List several attributes of an emergency care system.

2-2 List four nationally recognized prehospital emergency care provider levels.

2-3 Compare and contrast direct medical oversight and indirect medical oversight.

2-4 Describe the purpose of quality improvement.

KEY TERMS

Advanced emergency medical technician (AEMT), p. 27
Advanced life support (ALS), p. 29
Basic life support (BLS), p. 28
Emergency medical care system, p. 24
Emergency medical dispatcher (EMD), p. 30
Emergency medical responder (EMR), p. 27
Emergency medical services (EMS), p. 26
Emergency medical technician (EMT), p. 27
Medical director, p. 30
Medical oversight, p. 32
National Highway Traffic Safety Administration (NHTSA), p. 26
Outdoor Emergency Care (OEC) technician, p. 24
Outdoor First Care (OFC) provider, p. 24
Paramedic, p. 27
Prehospital providers, p. 27
Protocols, p. 34
Scope of practice, p. 27

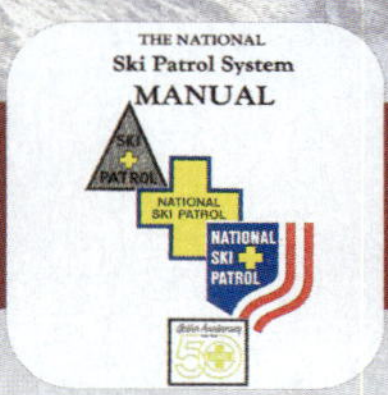

HISTORICAL TIMELINE **1941.** First NSP Ski Patroller's Manual published. Women are allowed to join the NSP.

CHAPTER OVERVIEW

Each day, tens of thousands of people around the world are involved in an emergency medical situation. Often these individuals require treatment before reaching a medical facility. In the past, people who became acutely ill or injured had to rely on friends, relatives, or strangers to come to their aid and transport them to a hospital. As a result, victims often suffered permanent, debilitating problems or died. Today, patient outcomes are significantly better, thanks to the advent of modern **emergency medical care systems**, which bring specifically trained personnel and resources to the scene of an emergency shortly after the situation occurs or symptoms become apparent. This coordinated response is part of an organized continuum of care that begins the moment the emergency care system is activated and continues long after the patient reaches the hospital.

Emergency medical care systems have been in use around the world since before the Pharaohs. Most early systems were conceived and implemented by the military, but they provided little more than the transport of wounded soldiers from battlefields to nearby doctors. Today, modern emergency care systems are complex networks designed primarily for civilian use, and they bring a broad range of medical services and resources directly to the patient on scene and during transport to a designated critical care facility.

An emergency care system is a formal, organized network of specially trained personnel, equipment, and facilities that responds to medical emergencies, regardless of cause, location, or the patient's ability to pay. It is a portion of the overall public health system. Its purpose is to bring specialized resources to the scene of both natural and human-caused medical emergencies as soon as possible so that potential lifesaving procedures can be implemented.

In the United States, emergency care systems came from federal legislation enacted in the 1960s in response to the large number of highway fatalities. Later, these systems were expanded to decrease the number of out-of-hospital cardiac arrest and stroke-related deaths. All aspects of health care, including emergency medical care systems, are constantly changing to meet the needs of the communities they serve and to reflect changes in medical knowledge, procedures, and technology. Regular monitoring helps to ensure that emergency care systems are in a constant state of readiness and will function as designed. An emergency care system requires considerable coordination and oversight to ensure that services are delivered to the highest level of quality possible and are provided in accordance with local, area, and state practices.

In many parts of the world, **Outdoor First Care (OFC) providers** and **Outdoor Emergency Care (OEC) technicians** interface with the local emergency system. These responders provide emergency assistance and transportation services to patients located in outdoor, nonurban settings typically not served by traditional 9-1-1 providers. Having a basic understanding of what makes an emergency care system effective will help OEC technicians operate more effectively and better serve their patients (**Figure 2-1**).

CASE Presentation

You find a woman lying in the snow after a skiing accident. She says she cannot move her legs. After making the scene safe, you rapidly assess her, finding no movement or feeling below the waist. You call dispatch and tell them what you have found.

What is the first thing you and dispatch should do?

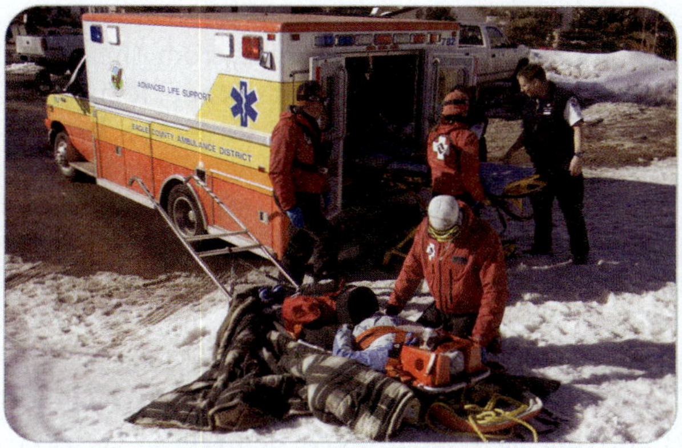

Figure 2-1 An emergency care system is a formal, organized network of specifically trained personnel, equipment, and facilities. Here, two patrollers work together to provide aid to a patient.

© Scott Smith.

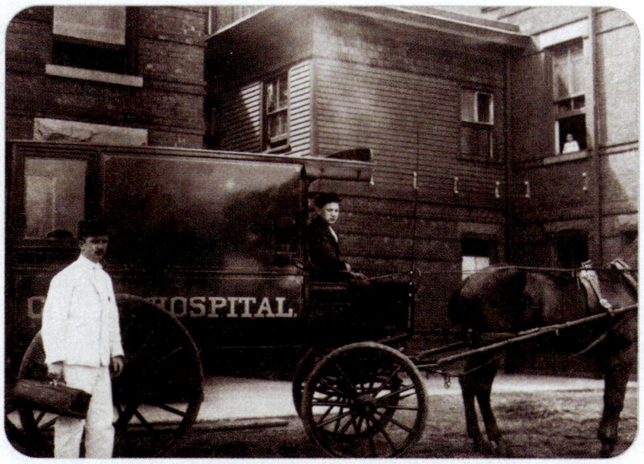

Figure 2-2 Modern-day ambulances evolved from primitive vehicles.

© Bettman/Getty Images.

THE HISTORY OF EMERGENCY CARE

Rendering first aid to a critically ill or injured patient before the person reaches a hospital or transporting a patient from the field to a medical facility are not new concepts, as history yields numerous examples of such practices:

- *Crusades (the 11th century).* The Knights of St. John provided basic first aid to injured soldiers from both sides of the conflict and transported them on horse litters to hospital tents for treatment. It is during this period that the concept of ambulances was first introduced.
- *Napoleonic Wars (1799–1815).* The French physician Baron Dominique Jean Larrey created the first army medical corps and sent trained attendants with medical equipment onto the battlefield to treat injured soldiers and to bring them to doctors.
- *American Civil War (1861–1865).* Clara Barton distributed medical supplies to injured soldiers on the battlefields and nursed wounded soldiers. She later became the head of the Union Army's field hospitals and founded the American Red Cross.
- *World War I (1914–1918).* Ambulances used during the "Great War" had trained attendants who transported wounded soldiers from the front lines, a practice that greatly reduced the mortality rate among wartime casualties (**Figure 2-2**). The Thomas half-ring traction splint was first used in the field and saved the lives of many soldiers with broken femurs.
- *Royal Flying Doctors of Australia (1928).* Using fixed-wing aircraft, physicians were flown into remote locations in the Australian outback to treat patients with serious illnesses and injuries.
- *World War II (1941–1945).* In 1943, large fixed-wing multipatient ambulance airplanes were developed to transport wounded soldiers back to the United States following initial care abroad.
- *Korean War (1950–1953).* Air evacuation using helicopters, or "air ambulances," was introduced. This innovation significantly reduced the time a soldier spent between being wounded and receiving treatment at a mobile army surgical hospital, or MASH unit (**Figure 2-3**). Air evacuation dramatically increased survival rates and was later perfected during the Vietnam War. It served as the blueprint for modern civilian-based aeromedical transportation services accessible by patrols in many parts of the United States.

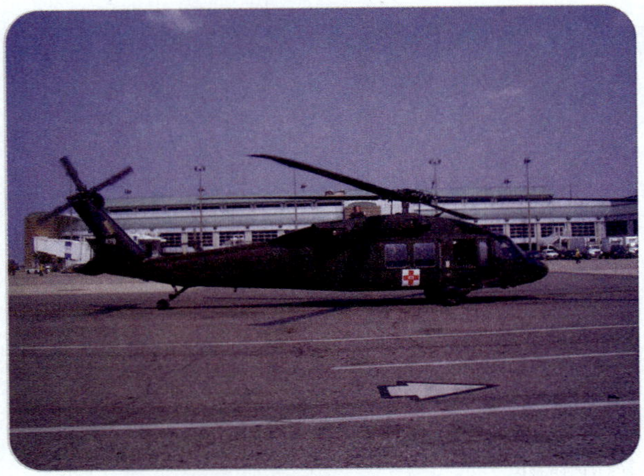

Figure 2-3 Evacuation using helicopters, or air ambulances, was introduced during the Korean War and is still used today.

Today's emergency care systems reflect the lessons learned from historical milestones in medicine. Although civilian-based ambulance services have existed in the United States since the early 1900s, it was not until 1966 when the National Academy of Sciences released its landmark report "Accidental Death and Disability: The Neglected Disease of Modern Society" (the "White Paper") that the groundwork for the modern emergency care system was laid. This paper exposed the causes, inherent problems, and high costs associated with highway crash–related deaths and pressed public officials to take action to mitigate the problem. Until that time, prehospital emergency transportation was provided primarily by funeral homes and volunteer rescue squads using laypersons with little or no formal medical training.

Later that same year, the newly enacted Highway Safety Act required states to adopt formal highway safety programs to decrease the number of traffic fatalities. This act provided funding for the development of state **emergency medical services (EMS)** offices and directed the creation of national education curricula for EMS providers. It also permitted the **National Highway Traffic Safety Administration (NHTSA)**, the federal agency tasked with overseeing the development of emergency care systems in the United States, to withhold highway funds from those states that did not comply. Modern ambulance and rescue services and prehospital practitioners emerged from the Highway Safety Act. Over the next decade, legislators passed additional federal and state laws, including the Emergency Medical Services Act of 1973, to address the need for the standardization of training, ambulance equipment, and emergency medical practices. The EMS Act identified 15 essential components for EMS systems. In 1996, the NHTSA released a report titled *EMS Agenda for the Future*, which modified the list to include 14 attributes of an effective emergency care system and provided strategies for fully integrating prehospital activities with the overall health care system.

In January 2019 the National Highway Traffic Safety Administration (NHTSA) enacted *EMS Agenda 2050* as a multidisciplinary, national review of all aspects of EMS delivery. The goal is to develop a more cohesive and consistent system across the country.

The vision of *EMS Agenda 2050* is that a people-centered EMS system is one in which people receive comprehensive, quality care in the place most comfortable and convenient. This care is based on sound research focused on producing the right outcomes. In this people-centered system, patients who need it will receive transport that is safe and efficient (not necessarily at a high rate of speed and with lights and sirens). Care in a people-centered system will focus not only on lifesaving interventions, but also on reducing physical, emotional, and psychological suffering. Such EMS systems will be an integrated part of a larger healthcare system focused on proactively preventing injuries and illnesses rather than reactively responding to treat them. EMS clinicians will have access to and be able to contribute to a patient's comprehensive medical record, allowing not only improvements of treatment for individual patients, but also updates in prevention, diagnosis, and treatments as our understanding and technology advance.

The EMS Agenda 2050 guiding principles, include an EMS system design that is:

- Inherently safe and effective so the entire system from start to finish is designed to minimize exposure to injury, infections, illness, or stress.
- Integrated and seamless, where EMS is fully integrated with all other aspects of healthcare

and is engaged with other emergency services and within the communities in which they operate.
- Reliable and prepared, ensuring EMS care is delivered consistently and compassionately and is guided by sound research at all times, by all EMS providers, at all levels, or from all agencies.
- Socially equitable, so that access to care and the quality of care are not determined by a patient's age, socioeconomic status, gender, ethnicity, or where they live.
- Sustainable and efficient, meaning systems must be fiscally responsible, providing value to the community with a minimum of waste and a maximum of accountability.
- Adaptable and innovative, evolving to meet the changing needs of the people whom they serve by continuously evaluating new tools and techniques, education programs, and system designs.

In order to retain our role in the emergency medical responder field the National Ski Patrol will need to become educated on the new EMS agenda and determine what our role is going to be as we move forward toward 2050.

LEVELS OF EMERGENCY PERSONNEL

In the United States, emergency care systems utilize specially trained **prehospital providers** to deliver on-scene medical care. These providers are divided into four nationally recognized categories: **emergency medical responder (EMR)**, **emergency medical technician (EMT)**, **advanced emergency medical technician (AEMT)**, and **paramedic**. Each category has different training requirements, scopes of practice, and recertification requirements. EMTs, AEMTs, and paramedics must complete an approved state EMS or other authorized agency training program and be certified or licensed by the state or province in which they work. In 2006, a consensus document was developed titled the "National EMS Scope of Practice Model," or "Scope of Practice." A **scope of practice** is a set of rules, regulations, and ethical considerations that define the extent, boundaries, and limitations of a prehospital provider's duties.

Emergency Medical Responder

An EMR serves as the first responder of an emergency care system and is often the first formally trained health care provider to reach the patient. EMRs are trained to provide immediate lifesaving treatment and stabilization to critically ill or injured patients while awaiting additional emergency response. Treatment is generally rendered using minimal equipment. EMR-level personnel also assist higher-level EMS providers, both at the scene and during transport. The most common EMR-level personnel are police officers, firefighters, lifeguards, and ski/bike patrollers (**Figure 2-4**).

The training requirements for an EMR vary depending on subsequent certification and may or may not include minimum course or examination requirements. EMR-level training generally does include hands-on training but not in a clinical environment. Whether EMR-level personnel do or do not function under medical oversight depends on the emergency care system design, although such oversight is recommended. OEC technician training and qualifications meet or exceed the training requirements of NHTSA.

Emergency Medical Technician

An EMT is an individual who has completed an NHTSA-approved EMT National Standard training course or its equivalent. EMT courses must meet minimum national training standards, which

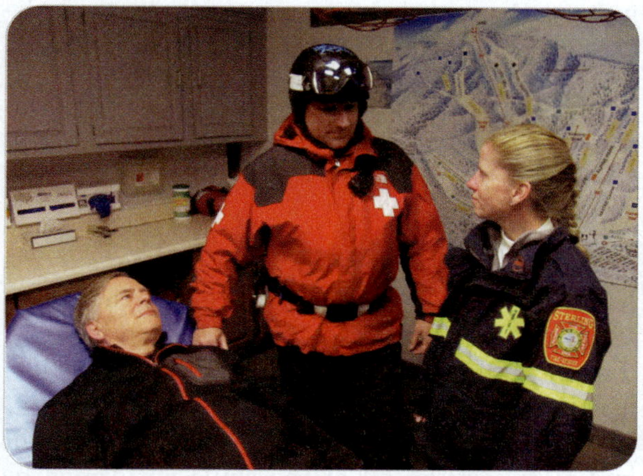

Figure 2-4 A ski patroller a patient over to an EMS provider.

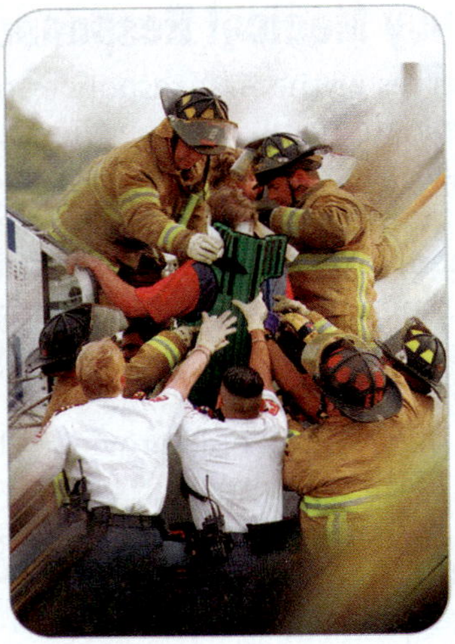

Figure 2-5 EMTs must meet certain education requirements and maintain their certification through additional training and testing.

consist of a minimum number of hours of didactic and practical instruction as well as clinical experience in an acute care setting (e.g., an emergency department, an ambulance, an intensive care unit). EMTs function with medical oversight to provide **basic life support (BLS)** interventions, such as assessing clinical status, splinting fractures, administering certain medications, using an automated external defibrillator, performing CPR, and transporting patients to a medical facility (**Figure 2-5**). With additional training in specific modules, EMTs may be authorized to use certain diagnostic devices or to perform more advanced therapeutic interventions, such as inserting an advanced airway. EMTs may also be involved in injury or illness prevention initiatives.

Advanced Emergency Medical Technician

An AEMT is a person who has completed a NHTSA-approved AEMT National Standard training course or its equivalent, which includes didactic and practical instruction as well as clinical internships in one or more acute care settings. AEMTs function under medical oversight and may perform all of the skills performed by EMTs, as well as other intermediate therapeutic interventions using basic and advanced equipment and medications typically found on an ambulance. Equipment may vary by county, state, or province.

Paramedic

A paramedic is an allied health care professional who has successfully completed a NHTSA-approved paramedic course, which includes extensive didactic, practical, and clinical training requirements. Paramedics operate under medical oversight and provide a higher level of prehospital care than all EMTs using a variety of basic and advanced equipment and medications, including narcotics (**Figure 2-6**).

Other EMS Personnel

Other members of the emergency care system include physicians (MD and DO), physician assistants (PAs), nurse practitioners (NPs), registered nurses (RNs), licensed practical nurses (LPNs), and allied health care professionals (such as respiratory therapists, phlebotomists, laboratory technicians, radiology technicians, and electrocardiography technicians) who provide definitive health care services within a hospital or medical facility. Under special circumstances (such as natural or human-caused disasters), these providers may assist prehospital personnel in the field. For this reason, resources within a local emergency care system must be fully integrated and coordinated, so that they may be quickly mobilized when needed.

Most emergency care systems deploy personnel to emergencies using a stratified, or tiered,

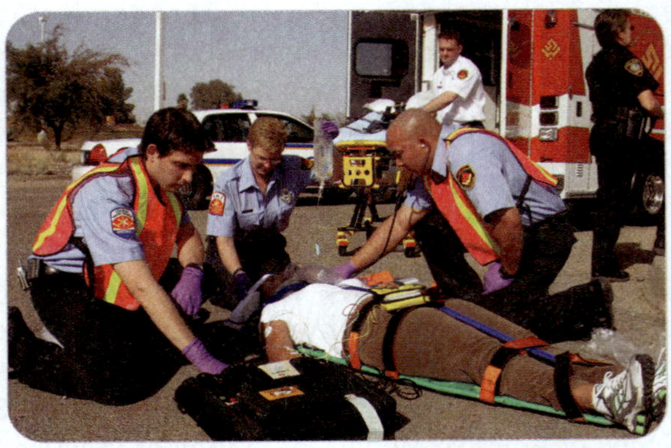

Figure 2-6 Paramedics can perform additional duties and provide a higher level of care than EMTs or AEMTs.

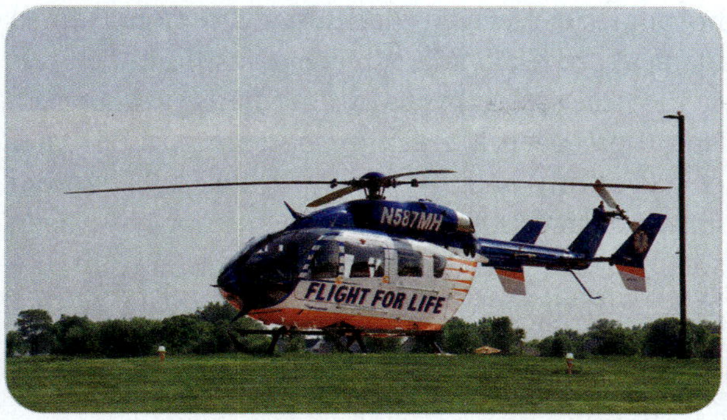

Figure 2-7 A life-flight air ambulance.

approach based on the patient's current condition or anticipated needs. This approach helps to ensure that adequate system resources are available should other emergencies arise.

- *Tier 1.* EMRs arrive quickly at the scene and initiate basic emergency care while awaiting the arrival of higher-level emergency providers. In certain settings, EMRs (e.g., ski/bike patrols, search-and-rescue teams, wilderness first responders) may transport the patient to a location that is more accessible to rescue vehicles.
- *Tier 2.* EMTs arrive shortly after EMRs and provide BLS measures. If the situation warrants, EMTs may either await the arrival of **advanced life support (ALS)** providers or transport the patient to a definitive care facility.
- *Tier 3.* AEMTs and/or paramedics arrive after EMRs/EMTs. They provide ALS measures and transport the patient to a definitive care facility.
- *Tier 4.* Critical care providers (e.g., critical care paramedics, nurses, physicians) bring to the scene additional ALS equipment, therapies, and interventions that are beyond the traditional paramedic scope of practice. They transport the patient to a specialized hospital via helicopter, fixed-wing aircraft, critical care ambulance, or other means (**Figure 2-7**).

EMERGENCY FACILITIES

Medical facilities such as hospitals or acute care clinics are important parts of the emergency care system where definitive patient treatment is delivered. Most remote facilities are now integrated with larger facilities in the public health system.

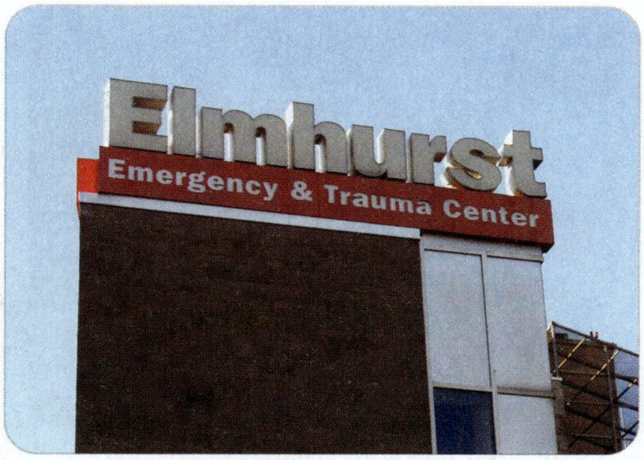

Figure 2-8 A Level I trauma center can provide a higher level of care for critically injured patients.

Depending on the types of acute care services provided, facilities may be accredited or designated to provide either the full range of treatment to acutely ill and injured patients or the management of specific types of patients or medical conditions. Examples include designation as a trauma center (Levels I–IV), acute pediatric care facility, burn center, stroke center, or toxicology center (**Figure 2-8**). Facility designations may be local, regional, or state level. A ski patrol may use the closest medical facility for less urgent medical care or stabilization of a patient, while critical patients are transferred to a trauma center.

CONTINUITY OF CARE

Continuity of care is the seamless delivery of high-quality emergency medical care that occurs from a patient's initial contact with an EMR through definitive treatment. Consider the following situation, which illustrates how continuity of care might occur in an outdoor, nonurban setting:

> A middle-aged patient is cross-country skiing with friends in the backcountry and collapses. She complains of having severe chest pain. Thinking the patient could be having a heart attack, one friend stays with the woman while two others go to summon help. They encounter a Forest Service employee who calls 9-1-1 for assistance.

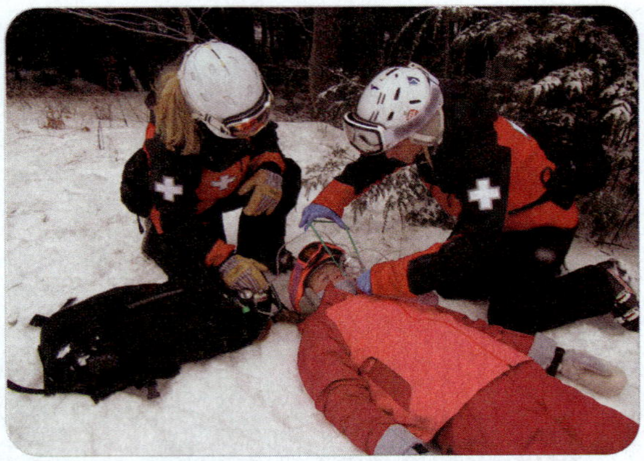

Figure 2-9 An alpine patroller assists a patient by providing additional oxygen.

The **emergency medical dispatcher (EMD)** notifies nearby patrollers, who reach the patient, assess her, and place her on oxygen (**Figure 2-9**). Believing the woman is having a heart attack, they request that a toboggan be brought to the scene and that an ALS ambulance meet them at the trailhead.

They transport the woman to the trailhead where a paramedic establishes intravenous access and administers medication to lessen the damage to the heart. The team transfers the patient to the ambulance crew, and paramedics monitor her heart while en route to a regional cardiac center.

During the trip to the hospital, the woman's symptoms worsen. The paramedic notifies a **medical director** (doctor) at the hospital by radio, who orders other medicines to be administered. The woman's symptoms stabilize. At the hospital, she is taken to the emergency department, where her condition is further stabilized by physicians and nurses before she is transferred to the heart catheterization lab. Following the procedure to open a clogged blood vessel, the woman stays in the critical care unit before being sent home to recuperate. She makes a complete recovery.

From the moment the woman was initially contacted by ski patrollers to her discharge from the hospital, she received continuous care from trained medical professionals. At each transition, the level of medical care provided to the patient increased. Had there been a break in the continuity of care or had at any time the care provided not followed local practices, the outcome might not have been so favorable. This team approach is one of the hallmarks of an effective emergency care system (**Figure 2-10**).

THE IMPORTANCE OF COMMONALITY IN EMERGENCY CARE SYSTEMS

Emergency care systems require a team approach. People and resources provide the framework for an emergency care system, but the glue that holds everything together and ensures the team's effectiveness is commonality—specifically, *having common goals, using a common language, and following common practices and procedures*.

Having a common language is essential for any profession. Using a shared vocabulary ensures

> **KEY POINT**
>
> **Precision *Does* Matter!**
>
> Consider these examples involving commonality of language:
>
> *"The patient is complaining of pain in his arm."*
>
> Do you know *which* arm is sore?
>
> *"The patient has pain in his left arm."*
>
> Do you know *where* on the arm the pain is located?
>
> *"The patient has midshaft pain of the left forearm."*
>
> Can you now locate the exact site of the injury?
>
> **Which description is most precise? Which one sounds most professional?**

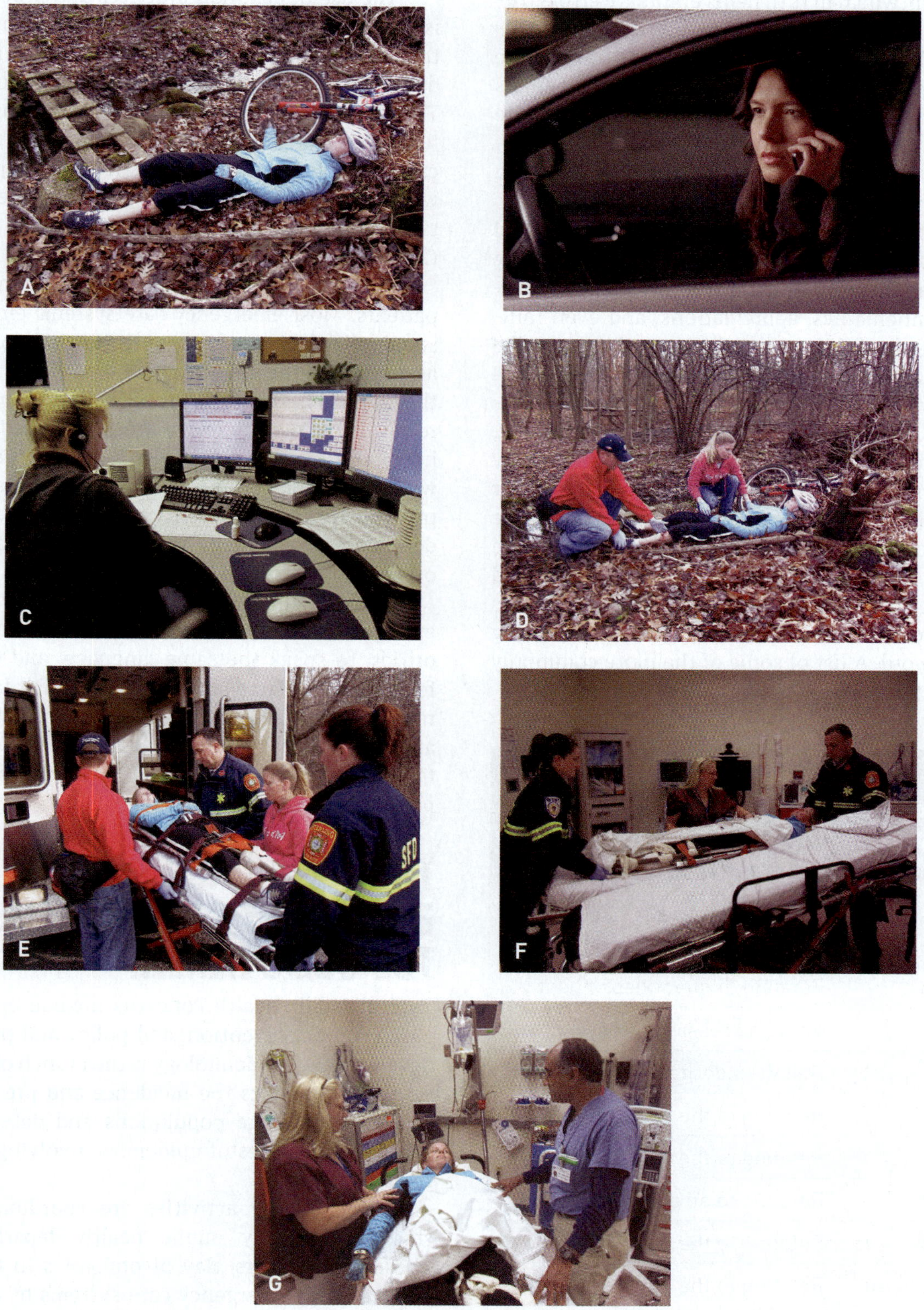

Figure 2-10 A. A mountain biker is injured on the trail. **B.** A passing motorist sees an accident and calls 9-1-1 on her cell phone. **C.** An emergency medical dispatcher receives a call and allocates resources. **D.** OEC technicians provide medical care to the injured mountain biker. **E.** OEC technicians hand off a patient to a local EMS provider. **F.** A local EMS provider hands off the patient for further treatment at the hospital. **G.** The chain of care continues at the hospital.

precision, which in turn helps eliminate errors. Toward this end, the OEC curriculum contains medical and rescue terms and phrases to reflect the language spoken universally by different members of the emergency care system. In addition, these terms convey professionalism, enabling OEC technicians to communicate with other providers with greater precision.

Medical and rescue terminology is derived from numerous sources and is constantly growing and changing. Much is derived from Latin, acronyms, mnemonics, abbreviations, and even military jargon. "Medical-speak" is used to describe human anatomy and physiology, assessment findings, treatments, equipment, and rescue operations. As new practices, procedures, equipment, and medications come into use, new terminology is put into use. When you encounter an unfamiliar term, look at the parts of each word. Typically, the center of a word contains the stem, or root. There may be a prefix at the beginning of the word and a suffix at the end of the word. Each of these parts helps you determine and remember the meaning of the word. A list of some of the more commonly encountered prefixes is provided in **Table 2-1**.

Table 2-1 Prefixes Commonly Used in Medical Terminology

Prefix	Meaning
Brady-	Slow
Tachy-	Rapid or swift
Therm-	Relating to quantities of heat
Hyper-	Above, excessive, or beyond
Hypo-	Below, underneath, or deficient
Naso-	Relating to the nose
Oro-	Relating to the mouth
Arterio-	Relating to an artery
Cardio-	Relating to the heart
Hem-, hema-, hemo-	Relating to the blood
Neuro-	Relating to nerves, the nervous system, or nervous tissue
Vaso-	Relating to vessels, as in a blood vessel

The use of common practices and procedures is as important as a common language, because they help to streamline processes, reduce redundancy and waste, and facilitate continuity of care. This is especially important when dealing with life-threatening emergencies. Imagine the ramifications if OEC technicians began CPR on a patient with cardiac arrest only to have other rescuers take over with a different technique. This is why CPR has become standardized.

Consider another situation involving multiple patients. Most emergency care systems employ a standardized approach that prioritizes patients according to the severity of their injuries. Using this approach, the most seriously injured patients receive treatment first and are transported to the hospital before those with less serious injuries. But what might happen if rescuers used different approaches or used different criteria to make these decisions? How might this affect the patients' outcomes?

Commonality enables rescuers within an emergency care system to focus on the same priorities, to speak the same language, and to perform rescue-related activities in a similar fashion, regardless of training level or clinical setting. This approach to teamwork enables rescuers to work together more effectively and to provide the best possible outcome for patients.

THE RELATIONSHIP OF EMERGENCY CARE SYSTEMS TO PUBLIC HEALTH

Typical public health concerns include epidemiology, injury prevention, and policy and program development. Epidemiology is the branch of medicine that monitors the incidence and prevalence of disease in large populations and detects the sources and causes of epidemics involving infectious diseases.

Public health activities are coordinated by state and county public health departments. These departments play pivotal roles in the development of emergency care systems by coordinating system activities and resources, offering specialized training, and in some states providing **medical oversight** and a host of other services to rescue personnel. As members of an emergency care system, OEC technicians have an obligation to assist public health officials in such

CASE Update

The patrol dispatcher activates the emergency care system by calling 9-1-1. He explains that the patient has no movement or feeling below the waist and requests ALS and air transport since there is a probable spinal cord injury.

You get additional information from the patient and keep the woman calm and warm while awaiting assistance. You are careful not to move her. Once ski patrollers arrive, they assist you in placing the patient on a long spine board. The patient is transported to an awaiting ambulance crew, who transport the patient to a helicopter landing zone and then a definitive care facility.

What is your next responsibility?

department-sponsored activities, such as helping in disaster relief efforts, identifying outdoor safety issues, promoting safety in outdoor recreation, and conducting mass immunizations.

THE ROLE OF RESEARCH IN EMERGENCY CARE SYSTEMS

Research plays an essential role in health care and serves many purposes. It is used to identify epidemiological and pathological trends, to report clinically relevant findings, and to introduce new technologies, practices, and techniques.

In the past, new techniques, equipment, and medications were often introduced or adopted for field use without a clear understanding of the clinical benefits. As a result, so-called technological advancements were either no better than what they replaced or failed to achieve desired results. Some were even harmful. Today, *evidenced-based* research is the driving force behind the latest innovations in emergency medicine technology. Such research has helped reshape how prehospital care is delivered, the types of equipment and procedures used by field providers, and the training requirements of emergency care system personnel.

Medical research directly affects OEC technicians and other prehospital providers, who increasingly will be called upon to help collect data, identify potential areas of study, and even manage research projects. The information gained from these activities will be used to develop safety policies and safer equipment, injury prevention programs, and clinical procedures that reduce snow sport–related injuries. It will also enable OEC personnel to provide high-quality care that has been scientifically proven to benefit patients.

COMMUNICATION SYSTEMS IN EMERGENCY CARE SYSTEMS

Communication systems are the vital links that connect all the components of the emergency care system and enable them to work together in a coordinated fashion. A typical EMS communication system consists of hardware (e.g., telephones, cell phones, radio communications equipment, computers), software, and specialized professionals who manage these resources. Effective communications improve patient outcomes and are essential for successful rescue operations.

In the United States, radio communications systems are regulated by two agencies: the Interdepartment Radio Advisory Committee of the Department of Commerce, which regulates radio use by federal agencies, and the Federal Communications Commission (FCC), which regulates radio use by nonfederal entities. Radio frequencies used by ski patrols must be licensed by the FCC. Unauthorized communications or unlicensed operation can result in substantial fines. The NSP has volunteer telecommunications advisors who will assist ski patrols in complying with FCC licensing requirements. If you are a rescuer for another

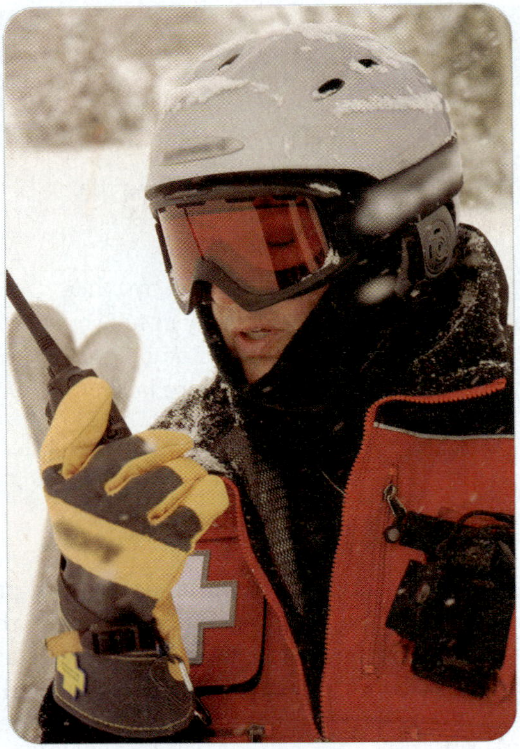

Figure 2-11 Patrollers use radios to communicate with each other as well as with area management or local EMS.

© Studio 404.

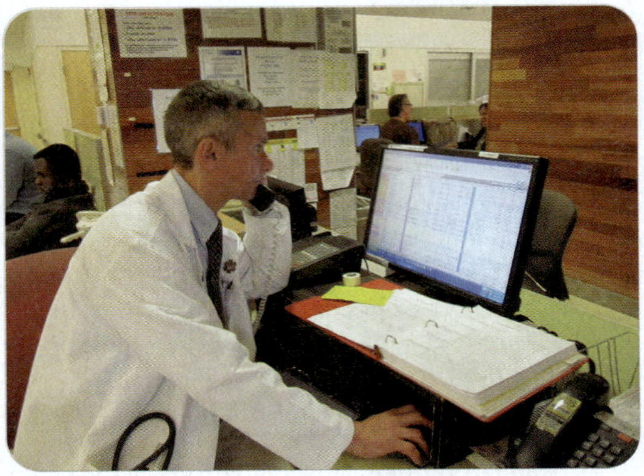

Figure 2-12 This physician is in communication with emergency personnel in the field providing direct medical oversight.

© Edward McNamara.

nonfederal agency, contact the FCC (www.fcc.gov) for licensing information.

OEC technicians communicate with each other and with other members of the emergency care system by various means, including two-way radios, landline telephones, and cell phones. Of these, portable radios are the daily workhorses for OEC technicians (**Figure 2-11**). However, because of topography, portable radios used in direct, unit-to-unit communications have a limited range. This limitation can be overcome by using base stations, repeaters, or other infrastructure. NSP's volunteer telecommunications advisors can assist patrols by recommending ways to improve signal coverage.

MEDICAL OVERSIGHT IN EMERGENCY CARE SYSTEMS

In the United States and many other countries, a licensed physician assumes legal responsibility for a patient's care throughout an emergency, from the time an EMR begins care through discharge from the emergency care system. Such medical oversight by a physician ensures continuity of care and that the patient receives proper treatment in accordance with local care guidelines (**Figure 2-12**).

There are two types of medical oversight: direct oversight and indirect oversight. Both types of medical oversight use preestablished medical orders, known as **protocols**, which have been approved by the local medical authority.

Direct oversight, or online medical control, involves real-time voice contact with a licensed physician who helps guide decisions concerning patient care. Direct oversight is usually conducted via telephone or radio, but it may also occur using video conferencing or other communication devices. The presence of a physician who oversees a patient's treatment at the scene is yet another form of direct medical oversight. Direct oversight is used primarily to oversee the provision of advanced care procedures or medications. It also serves as a means by which prehospital providers may consult with a physician to discuss complex cases or to obtain specific clinical, technical, or procedural information.

Indirect oversight uses standing orders (protocols) developed by a local medical authority. Also called offline medical control, prehospital providers are not required to directly contact a physician before initiating specific treatments. This form of medical oversight is designed to expedite patient care and is commonly used for "preauthorizing" both routine procedures, such as oxygen administration, and advanced lifesaving procedures or medications given by advanced providers that must be urgently administered.

EMERGENCY CARE PROTOCOLS

Protocols are written instructions describing what should be done in a given situation. They serve as guidelines that identify the assessment and treatment considerations for commonly encountered emergencies. Protocols are developed on a local level by emergency care professionals who are familiar with the area's medical needs, available resources, system capabilities, and local standard of care. In the case of ski/bike patrols, protocols can be developed by the local patrol's medical director, in concert with management, and may include practices and procedures that are not included in the OEC text. They should be reviewed annually and revised as needed to reflect changes in policies, procedures, equipment, medications, or other key system-related factors.

Given the complexities and variables associated with outdoor emergency medicine, protocols should be considered fluid instruments; they cannot be expected to address *every* situation that one might face. OEC technicians will likely confront situations for which no specific protocol exists. When these situations—known as "gray areas"—occur, use good judgment to ensure the patient receives the best possible medical care. Should there ever be doubt as to the proper course of action or treatment to follow, consultation with online medical control, if available, is recommended.

THE IMPORTANCE OF DOCUMENTATION IN EMERGENCY CARE

Good documentation is one of the hallmarks of a true medical professional, and it serves many purposes that go well beyond simply providing a record of events (**Figure 2-13**). Documentation provides pertinent clinical details that improve the continuity of care. It also can be used as a research tool; to provide legal protection for care providers, patrols, and ski areas; and to improve the quality of care. A full discussion of documentation is presented in Chapter 8, *Communications and Documentation*.

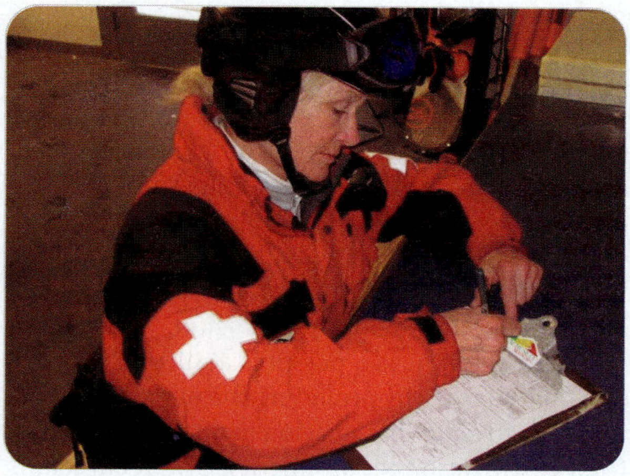

Figure 2-13 Adequate documentation is essential when filling out a patient care report.

QUALITY IMPROVEMENT IN EMERGENCY CARE SYSTEMS

Providing the best patient care possible is a common goal among emergency care personnel, a goal that is best achieved through the implementation of a quality improvement program. Quality improvement, often abbreviated QI, is an ongoing process designed to ensure that the products and services provided meet or exceed customer expectations. In health care, quality improvement may involve careful examination of each step in the case, from initial entry into the emergency care system through definitive care. After review, changes, if needed, will ensure the future care a patient receives is delivered in accordance with local protocols and guidelines.

CONTINUING EDUCATION IN EMERGENCY CARE

Continuing education, often abbreviated CE, is an essential requirement of any professional license or certification (**Figure 2-14**). It is the additional, ongoing training that individuals receive following their initial schooling to increase their knowledge about a given topic or skill. Continuing education enhances a person's ability to perform job-related tasks by providing the person with the most up-to-date information available. As part of their certification requirements, OEC technicians must receive continuing education through required annual OEC refresher coursework.

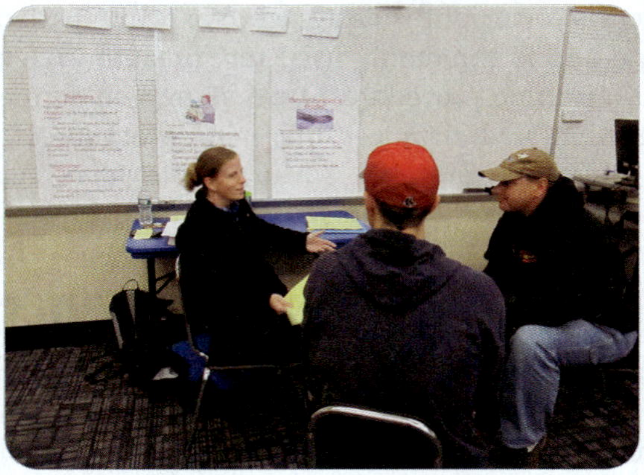

Figure 2-14 Every patroller is required to complete an annual review of OEC skills.

CASE Outcome

The patient survives the spinal cord injury. Your risk manager and medical director discuss the case for educational purposes with the patrollers involved. Care given was exceptional. After much therapy, the patient learns to walk again. She returns a year later, thanking you for getting her to definitive care.

CHAPTER REVIEW

In Summary

- An emergency care system is a network of specially trained personnel, equipment, facilities, and other resources that respond to emergencies.
- Ski/bike patrols and ski/bike patrollers are part of the emergency care system.
- An effective emergency care system has 14 distinct attributes.
- In the United States, there are four types of prehospital emergency care providers: emergency medical responders (EMRs), emergency medical technicians (EMTs), advanced EMTs (AEMTs), and paramedics.
- Emergency care system resources are deployed using a tiered approach based on specific needs.
- Common goals, a common language, and common practices enable the components of an emergency care system to function as a team.
- Public health departments play pivotal roles in the development of emergency care systems by coordinating system activities and resources, offering specialized training, and in some states providing medical oversight and a host of other services to rescue personnel.
- Research is used to identify epidemiological and pathological trends, to report clinically relevant findings, and to introduce new technologies, practices, and techniques.
- Effective communications allow emergency care systems to operate in a coordinated manner.
- Medical oversight and quality improvement ensure that the care patients receive is in accordance with area medical guidelines.
- Quality improvement is an ongoing process designed to ensure that the products and services provided meet or exceed customer expectations.
- Continuing education is an essential requirement of any professional license or certification.

Key Terms

Advanced emergency medical technician (AEMT) An intermediate-level technician who has successfully completed an NHTSA-approved Advanced EMT course or its equivalent and is authorized to provide both basic and intermediate life support.

Advanced life support (ALS) A level of EMS care for which providers are trained and authorized to insert advanced airway devices, initiate intravenous lines, and give medications.

Basic life support (BLS) A basic level of EMS care for which providers are trained and authorized to provide basic interventions, including noninvasive airway devices, application of oxygen, CPR, and basic first aid.

Emergency medical care system A network of specially trained personnel, equipment, facilities, and other resources that respond to medical emergencies. See EMS.

Emergency medical dispatcher (EMD) A person who has been trained to provide emergency medical advice and instructions over the telephone.

Emergency medical responder (EMR) A prehospital provider who is specially trained to provide medical care to patients in prehospital settings. There are many types of EMRs, each with various training requirements and scopes of practice. OEC technicians are trained at EMR level.

Emergency medical services (EMS) A network of services, including rescue operations, prehospital emergency care, ambulance transportation, emergency department services, and public education, for treating victims of illness or injury.

Emergency medical technician (EMT) A basic-level technician who has successfully completed an NHTSA-approved EMT course or its equivalent and is authorized to provide basic life support.

Medical director A physician who is responsible for ensuring and evaluating the appropriate level and quality of care throughout an emergency care system. Also referred to as a medical advisor or physician supervisor.

Medical oversight The process by which a physician monitors the quality of medical care rendered to patients and provides assistance and guidance to prehospital providers and emergency care systems.

National Highway Traffic Safety Administration (NHTSA) The federal agency tasked with overseeing the development of emergency care systems in the United States. It is an agency of the executive branch of the US government and is part of the Department of Transportation. Its mission is "Save lives, prevent injuries, reduce vehicle-related crashes."

Outdoor Emergency Care (OEC) technician A provider who has successfully completed the NSP's OEC course and met the annual refresher requirement. This person must complete CPR training, including AED training.

Outdoor First Care (OFC) provider A person who has completed the NSP's Outdoor First Care course and is trained to render basic first aid in outdoor, nonurban environments.

Paramedic An allied health care professional who has successfully completed an NHTSA-approved paramedic course or its equivalent and is trained to deliver both basic and advanced life support.

Prehospital providers People who are specifically trained to render medical care to patients outside of a hospital or medical care facility.

Protocols Written procedures for assessing, treating, and transporting a patient. Protocols are generally written by a team of emergency care professionals and managed by a medical director.

Scope of practice A set of rules, regulations, and ethical considerations that define the extent, boundaries, and limitations of a prehospital provider's duties.

Chapter Questions

1. A network of specially trained personnel, equipment, facilities, and other resources that respond to medical *emergencies*, regardless of cause, location, or the patient's ability to pay, is called a(n):
   a. health care system.
   b. ambulance care system.
   c. emergency care system.
   d. public health system.
2. Which of the following describes the level of training for an OEC technician?
   a. Completed a first-aid course and professional CPR/AED course
   b. Has had training that includes paramedic instruction
   c. Has training at the emergency medical responder level, plus additional information for a patroller
   d. Has training in all aspects of emergency medical care
3. Which of the following attributes is *not* one of the 14 essential components of an effective EMS system?
   a. Legislation and regulation
   b. Research
   c. Public access
   d. Public acceptance
4. Most emergency care systems deploy personnel to emergencies using a stratified approach based on the patient's condition or anticipated needs. Which of the following lists presents the normal order of deployment of responders?
   a. EMR, AEMT, EMT, paramedic
   b. EMR, EMT, AEMT, paramedic
   c. EMT, AEMT, EMR, paramedic
   d. EMT, EMR, AEMT, paramedic

5. Which of the following choices is an example of indirect medical oversight?
   a. Telephone communication with a doctor
   b. Use of written protocols
   c. Physical presence of a physician
   d. Video conferencing with a doctor
6. Medical guidelines developed at the local level by a medical director, area management, and patrol leadership that include an area's medical needs, available resources, system capabilities, and local standard of care are:
   a. policies.
   b. proceedings.
   c. protocols.
   d. records.
7. Providing the best patient care possible is a common goal among emergency care personnel. This goal is best achieved by:
   a. reading other EMS books.
   b. implementing a quality improvement program.
   c. not following local protocols if you think another method is better.
   d. allowing other personnel to care for the patient.
8. Why is it important that OEC technicians participate in quality improvement programs?
   a. To guarantee the public gets care equivalent to the same care as the local hospital
   b. To identify problems in care delivery and develop a plan to prevent their recurrence
   c. To ensure that professional appearance and manner are maintained at all times
   d. To identify problem employees and create a corrective action plan for them

Reference

National Highway Transportation Safety Administration (NHTSA). *EMS Agenda for the Future: Implementation Guide*, 2010. https://www.ems.gov/pdf/advancing-ems-systems/Provider-Resources/EMS_Agenda_For_The_Future_2010.pdf. Accessed September 19, 2019.

Answers: 1. c, Objective: 2-1, p. 24; 2. c, Objective 2-2, p. 27; 3. d, Objective 2-1, p. 26; 4. b, Objective 2-2, p. 29; 5. b, Objective 2-3, p. 34; 6. c, Objective 2-3, p. 34; 7. b, Objective 2-4, p. 35; 8. b, Objective 2-4, p. 35

CHAPTER 3

RESCUE BASICS

OBJECTIVES

Upon completion of this chapter, the OEC technician will be able to:

3-1 Describe the steps an OEC technician can take to be prepared when responding to a request for assistance.

3-2 Describe how layering clothing can help preserve body heat.

3-3 Describe the five modes of disease transmission.

3-4 Define the following terms:
- Pathogen
- Standard precautions
- Body substance isolation
- Hazardous material

3-5 List common personal protective equipment used by OEC technicians.

3-6 Demonstrate how to safely remove contaminated medical gloves.

3-7 Describe chain of custody.

KEY TERMS

Body substance isolation (BSI), p. 53
Contamination, p. 50
Decontamination, p. 57
Disease transmission, p. 57
Hazardous materials, p. 59
Metabolism, p. 44
Nutrition, p. 44
Occupational exposure, p. 56
Pathogen, p. 49
Personal protective equipment (PPE), p. 53
Safety data sheet (MSDS), p. 59
Standard precautions, p. 53
Ultraviolet radiation (UVR), p. 46

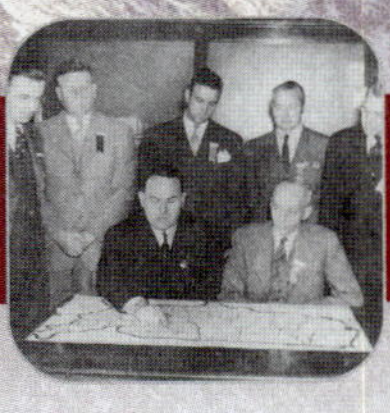

HISTORICAL TIMELINE **1943.** Minnie Dole recruits 3,500 men to join the 10th Mountain Division.

CHAPTER OVERVIEW

OEC technicians must be prepared to respond to a wide variety of situations. Some situations will involve assessment and basic treatment of a single patient in mild weather. Others will be complicated by such factors as darkness, rain, snow, and steep terrain. Because of this potential, it is essential that you have an awareness of your overall well-being, can adapt to environmental changes, and are conscious of scene dynamics. You must also have a basic understanding of infectious diseases and hazardous materials.

One of the most important skills that you must master as an OEC technician is taking care of yourself. Many responders have been injured or killed during rescue operations, further complicating rescue efforts and endangering others. Often, such tragedies result from inadequate preparation and/or failure to ensure one's personal safety. As an OEC technician, you will be exposed to many dangers. To perform your duties safely, you must learn how to adapt safely to your environment. Adjustments include functioning in temperature extremes and identifying and mitigating potential hazards. Managing personal stress during and after a rescue operation is important.

Contagious disease is another hazard you will face routinely. You need to learn how communicable diseases are transmitted and how to protect yourself from becoming infected. Adopting a standardized approach to all patients by wearing appropriate protective equipment and properly decontaminating equipment after each patient encounter will reduce the risk of occupational exposures.

This chapter emphasizes the importance of scene safety. Always make the scene safe before approaching the patient. It is your responsibility to protect yourself and others when approaching each patient. If you or others become injured or exposed to a disease, the rescue may become more complicated.

The end of this chapter addresses hazardous materials and crime scenes. Although the details of these topics are beyond the scope of this text, it is important that you understand your role should you encounter them.

PREPARING TO WORK OUTDOORS

Proper preparation prevents poor performance. This section addresses several factors that can either enhance or impair your abilities to function as an effective rescuer in outdoor environments.

CASE Presentation

It is a chilly afternoon with moderate cloud cover. You have just entered the mid-mountain lodge and are looking forward to a well-earned bowl of hot soup when you are called to respond to a skier who has fallen approximately 30 feet from a chairlift. The skier reportedly landed on a rock pile and is unresponsive. You notify dispatch that you are responding.

Upon arrival, you see that the patient has fallen into a ravine and that extrication will require specialized equipment and other rescuers. Two other OEC technicians are already on scene and have initiated care of the patient. One of the technicians is Peter, the newest member of your patrol, who has been assigned to you for mentoring. He is at the patient's head while the other technician is assessing the patient for injuries. You note that Peter is wearing only a sweater and a lightweight outer shell.

As you approach, Peter, who is shivering, looks up, smiles nervously, and then gives you a brief report on the patient's condition. Peter is not wearing a hat and his gloves appear to be soaked. A light, freezing rain begins to fall.

Do you have one patient to address, or two?

Environmental Considerations

OEC technicians frequently work outdoors, where they are exposed to all types of conditions. It is essential that you continually monitor the weather. There is a major difference between providing care on a warm summer day and providing the same care during a blizzard (**Figure 3-1**). Excessive exposure to heat can lead to heat cramps, heat exhaustion, and heatstroke. Exposure to cold can cause frostnip, frostbite, and hypothermia. Be prepared by taking proactive measures during changing weather.

Mental Preparedness

Mental preparedness is important to maintain well-being. It begins by having a positive attitude. OEC technicians should always be prepared to encounter the worst-case scenario, including inclement weather, interference by bystanders, equipment failure, and emotionally disturbing situations. As you adapt to changing conditions and stress, you will be better able to concentrate on making critical decisions and providing lifesaving treatment.

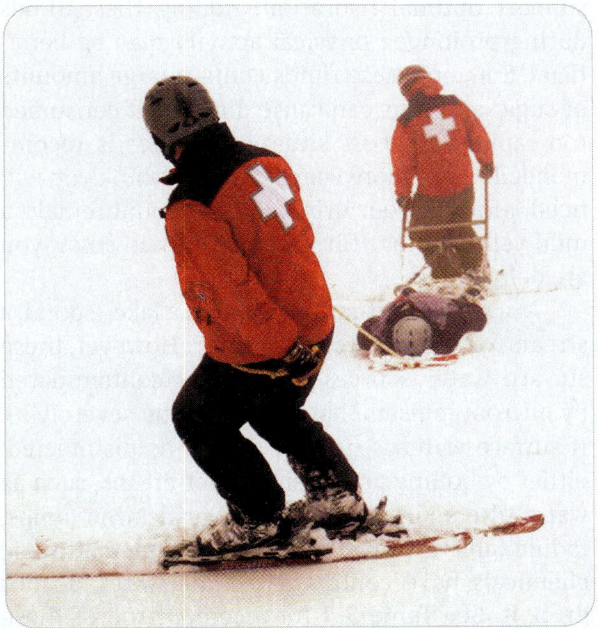

Figure 3-1 Environmental conditions may expose OEC technicians to dangerous situations, including low visibility.

Stress is not intrinsically harmful, but when it begins to affect a person's cognitive, emotional, or behavioral well-being, that person may need help. Abnormal stress responses may be immediate (acute), delayed, or cumulative, meaning the responses grow increasingly severe with repeated stressful exposures. During an abnormal acute stress response, a person may experience chest pain, breathe rapidly, cry, scream, or lose the ability to think rationally. Rescuers who have become overwhelmed by difficult circumstances and cannot adapt to the situation should be removed from the scene and receive care from appropriate personnel.

OEC technicians must be able to recognize abnormal reactions to stress in themselves and in coworkers, so that medical help can be obtained. These issues are presented in more detail in Chapter 33, *Behavioral Emergencies and Crisis Response.*

Physical Fitness

Being physically fit will improve your performance during a rescue. Physical fitness benefits overall well-being by reducing stress, improving cardiovascular and respiratory function, reducing blood pressure, enhancing physical endurance, strengthening muscles and bones, and reducing and controlling weight (**Figure 3-2**). To prepare yourself for the mental and physical rigors associated with rescue work, develop an exercise routine. The routine can involve such activities as

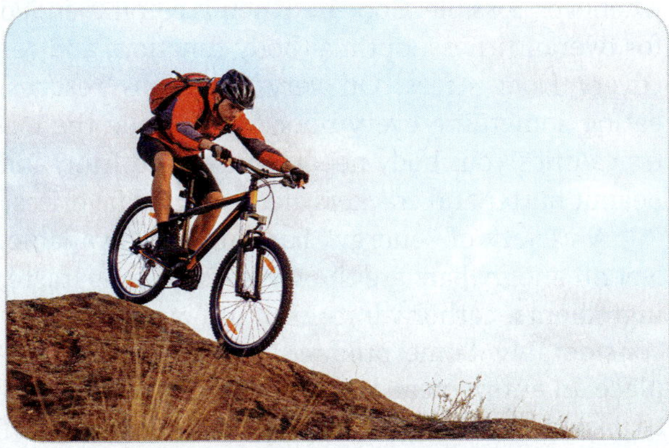

Figure 3-2 Being physically fit will help prepare you to respond to an accident scene.

swimming, walking, hiking, or cycling. If you are starting a new exercise routine, begin slowly to avoid injury. Depending on your age and overall health, you may decide to consult a physician before beginning a workout routine. As progress is made, you can add new activities and include variations in your routine.

Sleep and Fatigue

A lack of proper rest can cause a host of health-related problems. Sleep deprivation and fatigue will reduce both mental and physical capability. Maintain a regular sleep schedule of 7 to 9 hours of uninterrupted sleep each night. Fatigue can affect mood, reduce the ability to adjust to new environments, and impair judgment, which can lead to errors in caring for patients.

Food and Nutrition

The body must have energy to function. Energy is obtained from carbohydrates, fats, and proteins in the diet. The body uses carbohydrates or sugars first. During periods of increased activity and reduced dietary carbohydrate intake, stored fats sustain us, but peak performance during prolonged activity requires carbohydrate supplementation. In times of starvation, once fat is depleted, metabolic pathways use proteins from our tissues for energy. When our tissues' proteins are used, the body becomes weaker.

Being well nourished makes a significant difference in your ability to participate in strenuous outdoor activities and rescue operations. OEC technicians should try to eat healthful, nutritious foods whenever possible. Good **nutrition** is recommended for overall fitness, optimal body function, and recovery from stress. On very strenuous rescues, eating something every hour will provide the extra calories your body needs. Nuts, dried fruit, and peanut butter and crackers are perennial favorites.

A variety of "energy" bars are also available. Not all energy bars are the same. Packaging, taste, ingredients, carbohydrate content, and price vary considerably. Some products are intended to replace an entire meal, whereas others are intended to provide an energy boost until your next meal. If you decide to include energy bars as part of your routine, sample them ahead of time to ensure the products you select are satisfactory.

Hydration

Dehydration is a major concern in any outdoor activity, not only in survival situations. Given an ambient temperature of about 70°F and an average rate of **metabolism**, each day your body loses an average of 1 liter of water through respiration, 0.5 liter through perspiration, and about 1 liter through urination. During exercise or physical activity, especially when performed in a warm environment, you can lose up to 2 liters of fluid per hour. At high altitude, you can lose much more than 1 liter per day through the lungs, just from an increased respiratory rate. To maintain homeostasis and peak performance, you must remain well hydrated.

The organs primarily responsible for maintaining normal fluid balance are the kidneys, which respond to dehydration by reducing urine production. Fluid excesses are handled by increasing urine output. Prolonged and severe dehydration can lead to kidney failure.

To remain properly hydrated, OEC technicians should drink enough nonalcoholic fluids, and when on extended rescues, they should carry replacement fluids. Several commercial "sport" beverages contain electrolytes and other essential components that are specifically intended to support optimal hydration. Adding these fluids during prolonged physical activity may be beneficial. Some of these fluids contain large amounts of sugar and thus can cause diarrhea if consumed too rapidly. In most situations, water is recommended. Carry more water than you think you will need. Monitor your urine, which should remain a mild yellow color. If it becomes dark in color, you are dehydrated.

In a survival situation, water in a lake, a pond, a stream, or snow can be consumed. However, these surface water sources are usually contaminated by microorganisms that can make you severely ill. If surface water is used, it should be disinfected, either by boiling or by using other means, such as water filters, ultraviolet water purification lamps, iodine tablets, or chlorine dioxide tablets. If toxic chemicals have contaminated the water, do not drink it. See **Table 3-1** for a comparison of these various water purification methods.

Overhydration can also be a problem, especially for marathon runners. The electrolyte changes can cause significant heart issues.

Table 3-1 Water Disinfection Methods

Method	Advantages	Disadvantages
Heat (boiling water)	Reliable, simple	Limited by fuel source
Filtration (water filters)	Simple, no added taste, immediate	Heavy, somewhat expensive, bulky; will gradually clog
Disinfectant/ chemicals	Inexpensive, lightweight	Unpleasant taste; must follow directions carefully; must wait defined time before drinking
Chlorine	Readily available	Requires knowledge and experience to use safely
Iodine	Very cheap for large number of tablets	Very short shelf life, especially once bottle is opened
Chlorine dioxide	Individually wrapped tablets	None
Ultraviolet light devices	Eliminates all pathogens, easy and quick to use	Expensive, somewhat heavy and bulky; can fail (use batteries and can be broken); are technique sensitive

Alcohol and Substance Abuse

Avoid any substance that may compromise your ability to think clearly. Alcohol and marijuana, for example, can impair your thought processes, judgment, coordination, and decision-making abilities. Illegal drugs do the same thing. Resulting errors can place you, the patient, and others in immediate danger. Chronic substance abuse can injure organs such as the kidneys or liver and suppress your immune system. Providing care while under the influence of any substance is unethical, dangerous, and fraught with medical and legal risks.

Clothing

Select proper clothing for the work you will be performing, taking into account temperature, possible weather changes, and precipitation. It is important to have additional layers of clothing in your backpack available should the air temperature suddenly drop, you become wet, or you need to share clothing with patients or others. Proper clothing includes items that protect your feet, hands, head, and face. It is surprising how cold you can become due to a soaking rain or cool breeze. Because environmental conditions can change rapidly, consider carrying extra clothing in case those you are wearing become wet or unusable, or in case you need to provide additional clothing to the patient. A lightweight "survival blanket" carried in your backpack might be useful in some situations. They are small, light, and good at trapping heat.

Many synthetic fabrics have been engineered to protect the body from the elements. These materials can wick perspiration away from the body, provide lightweight insulation, repel water, block the wind, or do a combination of all four. Wool is probably the best natural material used in winter clothing because it is an excellent insulator even when wet, although it does take a long time to dry. Cotton is one of the worst materials for cold-weather use outdoors; it breathes well but is a poor insulator. In addition, wet cotton has almost no insulating value and takes a long time to dry. Cotton may be appropriate in hot, dry environments but is a poor choice for cold, windy, and wet conditions.

In cold weather, an OEC technician's wardrobe should include warm, waterproof gloves and glove liners, synthetic or wool socks, a neck gaiter or balaclava, goggles, and a hat or helmet. In the winter, think in terms of three layers: base, middle, and outer (**Figure 3-3**).

- *Base layer.* The base layer usually lies tight against the skin, helping to retain heat while allowing moisture to be transferred toward the exterior, a process known as wicking. Ideally, base layers should be made of silk or a synthetic material such as polyester.

- *Middle layer.* The middle layer serves as the insulating layer by trapping warm air. Common insulating materials are fleece, wool, and down.
- *Outer layer.* The outer layer is designed to be water repellant and wind repellant and should provide protection from sharp objects such as sticks or thorns.

Zippers should be waterproof and have an attached "pull" so that they can be manipulated easily with a gloved hand. A hood that can be folded into the jacket's collar and opened as needed offers additional neck and head protection. Detachable sleeves may be useful in converting a coat into a vest. External and internal pockets and cargo pockets may be useful for carrying smaller rescue equipment.

In warm, sunny weather, wear white lightweight clothing that covers the skin. This approach prevents sunburn and keeps you cool. Clothing is rated using the sun protection factor (SPF) scale. Most summer-weight clothing provides an SPF of 6.5. Sun-protective clothing can have an SPF as high as 30, which is the recommended SPF to prevent sunburn. Synthetic materials (e.g., polyester, nylon) and cotton are best for warm-weather clothing. A hat with a broad brim protects the face and back of the neck from the sun.

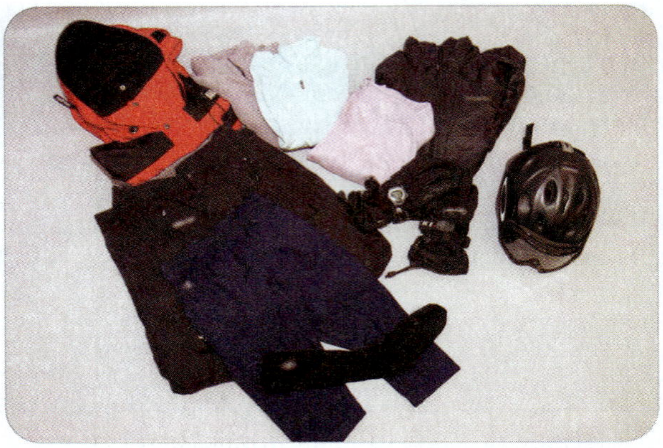

Figure 3-3 An example of the layers of clothing you might wear to keep yourself warm and dry. Your choice will always depend on the ambient temperatures and the level of the activity you will be participating in.

Skin and Eye Protection

Most rescues occur during daylight hours. A small amount (an hour) of daily direct sunlight on skin not covered by clothing is beneficial in promoting the production of vitamin D. Too much sun exposure puts your skin and eyes at risk from **ultraviolet radiation (UVR)**. Excessive exposure to UVR can cause sunburn, skin damage, cataracts, and skin cancer. You can take measures to protect your eyes and skin.

A variety of products are available for protecting the skin from the sun's harmful rays. Sunscreen comes as a lotion, spray, gel, or paste that absorbs or reflects UVR. Most products include an SPF rating; higher numbers provide greater protection. Consider using a sunscreen with a minimum SPF of 50. Follow all manufacturer recommendations when using sunscreen, paying close attention to reapplication recommendations. Adverse skin reactions, such as burning, itching, and rash, can occur from sunscreens.

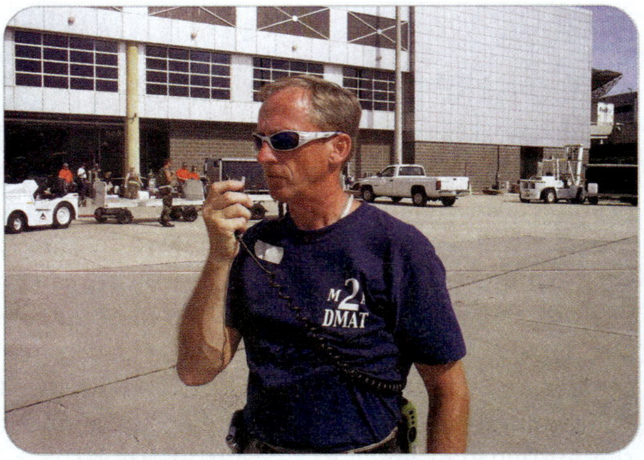

Figure 3-4 You must protect your eyes when out in the sun.

Proper eye protection is easily overlooked, but it is essential. Long-term exposure to sunlight can cause cataracts and damage your retinas and corneas, so reducing the amount of UVR that reaches the eyes helps prevent ocular damage. Wearing sunglasses or goggles with UVR protection is an easy way to reduce UVR exposure. The "wraparound" style of sunglasses or those with side panels provide the greatest protection against solar UVR (**Figure 3-4**). It should be noted that UVR is present even on overcast days.

Unprotected eyes are at risk for a kind of damage to the cornea called ultraviolet keratitis. A common risk factor for this disorder is spending time on highly reflective surfaces such as water and snow, which is why this disorder is commonly called "snow blindness." Just as for sunburn of the skin, you remain unaware of this condition until you experience eye pain hours after exposure.

If you wear contact lenses, you should consider keeping an extra set of contacts or a pair of glasses with you at all times in the event a contact lens is lost. You might also consider carrying small vials of saline solution to help keep your eyes and contacts moist.

Helmets

The National Ski Patrol strongly recommends that OEC technicians wear a helmet when engaging in such activities as skiing, snowboarding, snow machine riding, rafting, kayaking, biking, and technical climbing (**Figure 3-5**). In addition to protecting the head and keeping it warm, wearing a helmet sends a strong safety message to members of the public, who often adopt the equipment and philosophies they see professional rescuers using. Advances in technology have enabled helmets to offer the combination of protection, comfort, and ventilation.

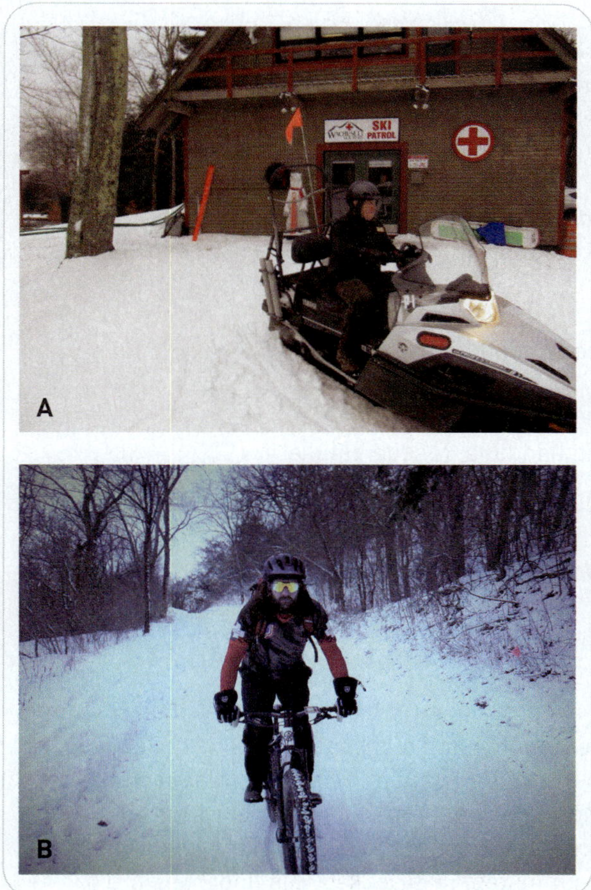

Figure 3-5 A. Helmets are strongly encouraged during certain outdoor activities. **B.** A bike patroller wearing a helmet.

A: © Edward McNamara; **B:** © Deb Endly.

Backcountry Equipment

In outdoor rescue work, you need to carry gear in a first-aid pack for providing patient care plus personal gear for maintaining your own well-being, especially if a long rescue is possible. If you are going into the backcountry, pack a small survival kit that includes items to help with fire starting, navigation, and signaling. Consider packing waterproof matches or a magnesium fire block, because they are more reliable than a lighter. Take a flashlight, a carabiner, a high-quality multipurpose tool, and sunblock. Although GPS units are popular, these devices can fail; therefore a map, a compass, and good navigation skills are still necessary. Additionally, many cell phone GPS apps now exist and can be powerful tools when combined with a portable cell phone charger. Carrying water and compact nutritious packaged food is important.

Your kit should also include a high-quality whistle. Three short blasts are the international sign of distress. Other methods of signaling include radios, cell phones, and signaling mirrors (a compact disk works well at reflecting light). Cell phone service may be limited in many wilderness

KEY POINT

Survival—The "Rule of Threes"

- Three minutes: you can die if you are severely bleeding, if you are without oxygen, or if you are in icy water for 3 minutes.
- Three hours: you may die from exposure within 3 hours without proper shelter.
- Three days: you may die within 3 days without a water supply.
- Three weeks: you can survive up to 3 weeks without food.

locations. However, there has been a significant increase in search-and-rescue calls using cell phones. Other useful items are listed in **Table 3-2**.

Prolonged Rescue Response Preparation

Unlike a response within the boundaries of a ski area ("in bounds"), a response to a request for assistance in the backcountry can take a long time. It can be as brief as an hour or may span several hours or even days. You should always be prepared for the possibility of a prolonged response. Preparation may include carrying a water purification device and a supply of nonperishable food. A lightweight stove may be useful. As mentioned previously, always sample the foods before taking them on a response. Make sure ahead of time that your body tolerates the foods you choose, especially energy bars, which can cause gastrointestinal problems in some people.

Table 3-2 Survival Kit Checklist
• Avalanche tools (beacon, probe, shovel; consider an avalanche airbag) • Large heavy-duty trash bag (50-gallon plastic drum liner works great) • 50 feet of parachute cord or nylon rope (serves multiple purposes) • Insect repellent • Water • Water disinfection supplies • Sunscreen • Consider a few granola bars, dried fruit, bouillon cubes, honey packets (prepackaged) • Knowledge of how to procure food from the environment • Magnesium fire starter (most reliable tool, works when wet) • Waterproof matches (easy to run out of) • Lighter (difficult to use when windy or cold) • Map and compass, and knowledge of how to use them • A portable GPS or GPS cell phone app (can be helpful, but use only in addition to a map and compass) • High-quality survival whistle • Signaling mirror • Head lamp, or at least a flashlight (include spare batteries and bulbs) • Eight-hour candle • High-quality multitool • Safety pins, sewing needles and thread, aluminum foil, bandana, rescue blanket (all useful in a variety of situations)

CASE Update

Reaching into your pack, you hand Peter your spare wool hat and a dry set of waterproof gloves. You then assist the other technician in attending to the injured patient. Still other rescuers arrive to help with the rescue. As you continue to work, the weather becomes more severe as a mixture of rain and snow begins to fall. The temperature starts to drop and the wind increases. Peter's coat is not waterproof, and within minutes he is soaked. His fingertips are becoming numb and he repeatedly takes off his gloves to blow on his hands. You are about to say something to him when his stomach growls loudly. Embarrassed, he looks at you and says, "It was a late night last night, and I skipped breakfast."

What is the best way to help Peter?

Consider including an emergency shelter and bedding among your gear. A compact, single-person tent and ground tarp may be sufficient. In the event that the weather becomes extreme, you may seek shelter in an existing structure, such as within a cave entrance or under rock formations, or you may need to construct a shelter using available materials found in the immediate area. Digging a snow cave or building a snow shelter can be lifesaving.

PROTECTING YOURSELF FROM DISEASE

When you are working as an OEC technician, it is always possible that you will be exposed to an infectious, communicable disease. A *communicable disease* is an illness that can be transmitted from one individual to another. *Infectious diseases* are caused by a microorganism called a **pathogen**, which invade the body. This section focuses on pathogens that cause the most common infectious diseases that OEC technicians may encounter.

Infectious diseases are transmitted in five ways: by direct contact, by indirect contact, via airborne transmission, through ingestion, and via vector-borne transmission:

- *Direct contact* involves close person-to-person contact. Examples of diseases spread by direct contact are hepatitis B, HIV, herpes simplex, gonorrhea, and mononucleosis.
- *Indirect contact* involves physical contact with an object contaminated with pathogens, including clothing, dressings, towels, soil, and bedding. Examples of diseases that may be contracted through indirect contact are athlete's foot (from shower stalls) and lice (from bed linens).
- *Airborne transmission* occurs from inhaling droplets containing infectious pathogens propelled into the air by coughing or sneezing, or by acts of bioterrorism (**Figure 3-6**). Examples of diseases that may be contracted through airborne transmission are the common cold, influenza, meningitis, chicken pox, and tuberculosis.
- *Ingestion* typically involves consumption of food or water that has been contaminated with feces (the fecal–oral route). There are two primary scenarios that could lead a person to ingest feces-contaminated food or water: (1) The person eats food that either was handled by an infected individual, likely because the person did not wash his or her hands after defecating, or was grown in soil contaminated with feces. (2) The person drinks from a water source contaminated with feces. One can also become ill from ingesting food or water contaminated by substances other than feces. Common diseases that are contracted through ingestion are gastroenteritis or severe diarrhea (caused by *Salmonella*, *Shigella*, or *Giardia*) and hepatitis A.
- *Vector-borne transmission* involves the transmission of pathogens to humans by other animals such as ticks and mosquitoes. Bites from infected ticks can cause many disorders, including Lyme disease and Rocky Mountain spotted fever. Mosquitoes transmit malaria, West Nile virus, encephalitis, and a host of other illnesses worldwide. Rabies is transmitted through the bite of a rabid mammal.

Figure 3-6 Sneezing releases thousands of germ-laden droplets into the environment.

KEY POINT

Common Ways of Contracting Diseases

The two most common ways OEC technicians can contract a communicable disease are direct contact with a patient's bodily fluids and inhaling pathogens from someone who is coughing.

Contamination

Contamination occurs once an individual comes in contact with enough organisms to cause symptoms. After the individual becomes exposed and the disease has been acquired, there is a highly variable incubation period. During this time, the offending pathogens multiply until the individual manifests symptoms. In many cases, the person can infect others during the incubation period. Consider the following situation:

> While you are taking care of a skier who has broken her arm but does not otherwise seem ill, she sneezes. Unknown to you, the patient is in the early phase of influenza (the flu). When she sneezed, thousands of virus particles filled the air, which you then inhaled with your next breath. For the next several days, you are in an incubation period during which the virus particles multiply. During this time, you are unwittingly contagious and expose others, including your family, friends, coworkers, and patients, to the virus. A few days later, you start to manifest symptoms. Once you start to feel better, your ability to contaminate others declines. However, because you infected others, illness spreads quickly. In a close work setting such as that of patrols and rescue teams, the disease can infect nearly everyone.

Infectious Diseases

In this section we consider some infectious diseases that OEC technicians may be exposed to.

Upper Respiratory Infections and Pneumonia

Common colds are caused by many different viruses. Simply inhaling enough viruses following someone's sneeze or cough is all it takes to become infected. Pneumonia involves infection of the lung by bacteria, viruses, or fungi. The individuals most at risk are those older than 65 years, younger than 2 years, and having other health problems.

Common colds are characterized by runny or stuffy nose, sore throat, cough, and transient fever. Pneumonia also presents with cough and fever but is more likely to produce chest pain, shortness of breath, weakness, and persistent fever.

Influenza

Influenza, or the seasonal "flu," is caused by a virus that infects the respiratory tract. It is easily transmitted among humans and each year results in many deaths worldwide. Transmission most commonly occurs via the airborne route but also can occur indirectly following contact with a contaminated surface. The viruses can survive for up to 2 days on a hard, nonporous surface such as a doorknob.

Herpes Infections

Herpes is a virus that causes the formation of small blisters, most often around the mouth (**Figure 3-7**). Also known as "fever blisters" or "cold-sores," this condition is transmitted through direct contact with the bodily fluids of an infected individual. The most common method of transmission among outdoor rescuers is the sharing of lip balm or water bottles. For this reason, such sharing is strongly discouraged. There is no known cure for herpes and no vaccine to prevent its transmission. Once an individual becomes infected, blisters may break out several times a year and can be both painful and unsightly. The genitals can also be infected with herpes.

Hepatitis

Infectious hepatitis is an acute viral illness that causes inflammation of the liver. There are several common forms of hepatitis. Hepatitis A is acquired by the fecal–oral route, usually by the

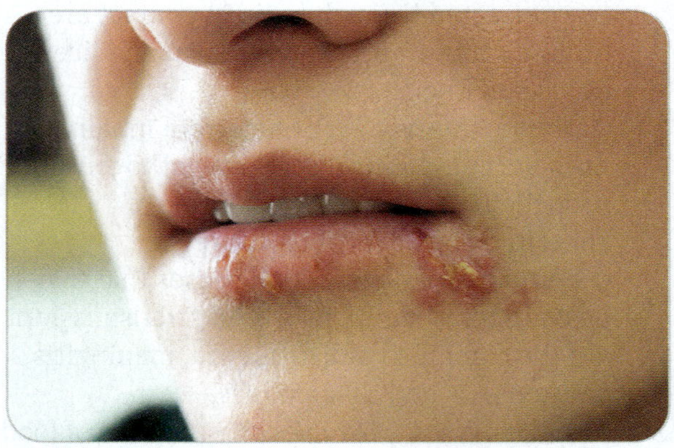

Figure 3-7 Cold sores can be transmitted by sharing lip balm or water bottles.

ingestion of contaminated food or water. Hepatitis B and C are transmitted by exposure to blood, semen, or other bodily fluids; contaminated needles; or sexual contact. Conditions that can develop following hepatitis include liver failure, a chronic form of liver disease called cirrhosis, and liver cancer.

Hepatitis can cause fever, weakness, loss of appetite, nausea, vomiting, jaundice, dark-colored urine, and light-colored stools. Administration of a hepatitis B vaccine is recommended for all health care workers, including OEC technicians. No vaccine is available for hepatitis C. Review your local protocols regarding receiving your hepatitis B vaccine series.

Chicken Pox and Shingles

Chicken pox and shingles are highly contagious viral diseases caused by the varicella-zoster virus. Chicken pox is spread by airborne transmission and direct contact with an infected individual. Shingles is transmitted by contact with an open and oozing blister. Red and itchy blisters that burst, dry out, and crust over appear within a few days. The condition lasts approximately 5 to 10 days, during which new crops of blisters continue to form. Patients remain contagious until all lesions have developed crusts. Shingles occurs in a band or single superficial skin nerve distribution, while chicken pox covers the entire body. Both conditions are very painful. A vaccine is recommended for adults to prevent shingles (**Figure 3-8**).

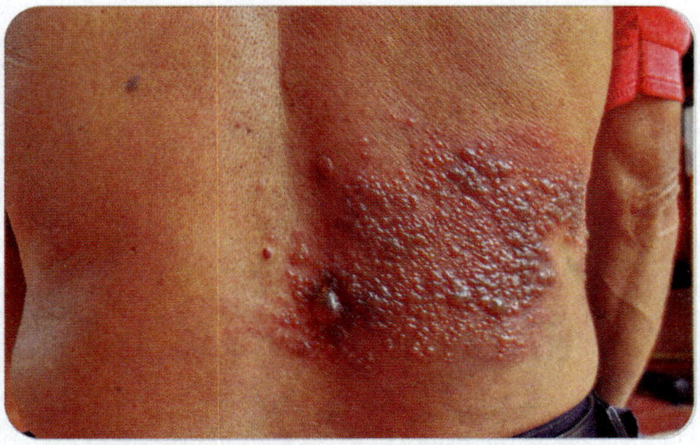

Figure 3-8 Shingles is very painful and highly contagious. It is highly recommended that adults obtain the vaccine.

Tetanus

Tetanus is a serious disease caused by a toxin produced by bacteria that enter the body through a laceration or puncture wound. The disease results in painful tightening of muscles, including jaw spasms. The lay term for this condition is "lockjaw." Due to an effective vaccine program, tetanus is very uncommon except in underdeveloped countries. Once an individual has been vaccinated as a child, a booster is recommended every 10 years. For certain high-risk wounds, your doctor may update your vaccination if it has been more than 5 years since you received your last tetanus vaccine. If you sustain a wound and have not had a tetanus vaccine within the past 5 years, consult your physician.

Whooping Cough (Pertussis)

Whooping cough (pertussis) is a highly contagious bacterial disease seen predominantly in children; however, recently it is being seen in adults more frequently because fewer were vaccinated for it. It is a highly contagious illness that spreads easily from person to person through airborne germs from the nose and throat. Whooping cough starts off like a common cold. Symptoms can include runny nose, low-grade fever, tiredness, and a mild or occasional cough. Over time, coughing spells become more severe. Cough medication does not help. In children, the disease causes uncontrollable, violent coughing spells that make it hard to breathe, eat, or sleep. The classic "whoop" symptom is a high-pitched wheezing sound made when a person gasps for breath after a severe coughing attack. This symptom may be absent in adults with whooping cough. Symptoms of pertussis in adults may include prolonged, severe coughing fits, followed by gasping for breath and vomiting. Coughing may last for several weeks, sometimes 10 weeks or longer.

Whooping cough is prevented through administration of a combination vaccination that also immunizes the person against tetanus and diphtheria.

Human Immunodeficiency Virus and Acquired Immunodeficiency Syndrome

Human immunodeficiency virus (HIV) is a pathogen that is transmitted either through direct contact with bodily fluids containing the virus or through the transfusion of blood containing the virus. It may take up to 6 months following exposure until HIV infection can be detected by blood tests. HIV frequently impairs the immune system, resulting in acquired immunodeficiency syndrome (AIDS).

AIDS patients are susceptible to opportunistic infections such as pneumonia, meningitis, and encephalitis, and to some cancers. Although some antiviral therapies can dramatically help individuals infected with this virus, there is still no effective vaccine to prevent HIV infection or effective cure for AIDS. Prevention of infection is of paramount importance. Effective use of body substance isolation lowers your risk of catching this virus.

Tuberculosis

Tuberculosis (TB) is a bacterial infection most commonly spread by the airborne route. The disease usually involves the lungs but can affect many other body systems as well. Signs and symptoms include cough, fever, night sweats, weight loss, fatigue, and coughing up blood. TB is detectable and treatable, but the active phase of the infection can be difficult to treat and often requires lengthy antibiotic therapy. A resurgence of TB in recent years has coincided with the emergence of strains that are resistant to commonly used antibiotics. Many health care facilities provide annual skin testing to detect exposure or early illness. Refer to your local protocols regarding recommendations for TB testing.

Meningitis

Meningitis, an inflammation of the membranes that surround the spinal cord and brain, can be caused by bacteria or viruses. Signs and symptoms can include headache, nausea and vomiting, stiff neck, chills, fever, confusion, rash, altered mental status, and irritability. Seizure and coma also may occur.

Viral meningitis is usually self-limited, but bacterial meningitis can be a devastating illness that requires early recognition and aggressive treatment. Certain types of bacterial meningitis are highly contagious, and individuals who have had close contact with patients, including exposed but unprotected health care workers, may need to take prophylactic antibiotics.

Rabies

Rabies is a serious viral disease transmitted through the bite of a diseased animal. Bats, raccoons, skunks, foxes, dogs, cats, groundhogs, wolves, weasels, and other animals can be infected with the rabies virus (**Figure 3-9**). Once symptoms of rabies develop, usually 30 to 50 days after infection, the disease is uniformly fatal. Fortunately, a highly effective vaccine is available and should be given immediately to anyone bitten by a rabid animal. It is essential that you contact a physician immediately after any animal bite in order to manage the wound and to determine if rabies vaccination is indicated.

Measles

Measles is a disease caused by an infrequently encountered virus that infects the respiratory system and produces a characteristic rash. It is highly contagious and is spread through airborne transmission. Death can occur in some people. Previously, due to effective immunization programs, measles was rare in the United States. However, in 2019, there were several localized outbreaks of this disease in parts of the United States where nonvaccination rates are high.

Most adults were vaccinated as children. Many people born between 1957 and 1989 received one dose of the MMR (measles, mumps, rubella) vaccine because that is what was recommended at the time. In 1989, however, the CDC updated its guidelines, recommending two doses. Only people who received two doses of the measles vaccine as

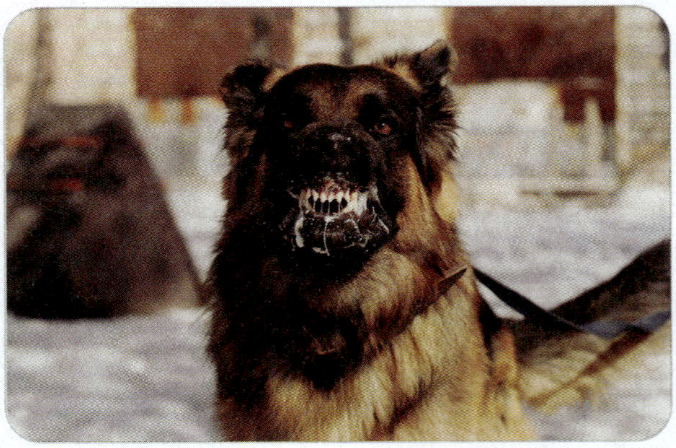

Figure 3-9 Be aware that rabies can be transmitted from any animal.

children are protected for life, according to the CDC. If you are not sure if you had two doses, a blood test can determine if you have established immunity. An adult booster vaccination is recommended if you do not have immunity.

Vaccination Recommendations

Because of the potential exposure to communicable diseases, it is recommended that OEC technicians be properly vaccinated against the diseases in **Table 3-3**. In the United States, Canada, and Europe, most children are vaccinated for common communicable diseases as part of a childhood immunization program. OEC technicians should undergo hepatitis B vaccination and should consider receiving an annual seasonal influenza vaccine. A valuable resource on vaccinations can be found at the Centers for Disease Control and Prevention (CDC) website: www.cdc.gov.

Standard Precautions and Body Substance Isolation

To reduce the number of health care workers acquiring illness from patients, the CDC has developed guidelines called **standard precautions**. *Following these guidelines, health care workers treat every patient as potentially infectious.* Central to this approach is the concept of **body substance isolation (BSI)**, in which measures are taken to prevent the patient's bodily fluids from contacting any unprotected portions of the rescuer's person. Standard precautions and BSI are designed to prevent the transmission of pathogens. It is essential that OEC technicians be protected from patients' bodily fluids (**Table 3-4**).

Be wary of any objects that may be contaminated with bodily fluids, including bandages, equipment, towels, blankets, clothing, paper products, and a patient's other belongings. It is your responsibility to practice standard precautions on every patient that you encounter, regardless of the patient's clinical signs, condition, age, or background. Do not succumb to the temptation of assuming the patient is "safe."

Personal Protective Equipment

Using the concept of standard precautions ensures that all patients are treated as though they harbor potentially contagious pathogens. Because many patients with a communicable disease have no obvious signs of illness, it is important that a protective barrier be placed between you and each patient. This protective barrier prevents the transmission of disease using specialized protective medical equipment known as **personal protective equipment (PPE)**.

PPE is designed to safeguard rescuers from exposure to infectious agents in the patient's bodily

Table 3-3 Vaccine Recommendations

Vaccine	Schedule	Indication
Hep B (hepatitis B)	Three doses	Advisable due to risk of exposure to blood and other bodily fluids
Seasonal influenza ("the flu")	Annual	All health care workers, especially those with high-risk medical conditions or who are older than 65 years
Meningococcal (meningitis)	——	Not routinely indicated for health care personnel, but prophylaxis after exposure may be recommended
Tdap (tetanus, diphtheria, and pertussis)	One-time dose for adults	Considered in lieu of the Td vaccine due to a resurgence of pertussis in some areas
Pneumococcal (pneumonia)	One dose; revaccination considered more than 5 years after first dose	Certain adults at risk due to underlying medical conditions or age greater than 65 years
Shingles (Shingrix)	Two doses, 2 to 6 months apart	Age 50 or older

Table 3-4 Body Fluids

- Blood
- Saliva and sputum
- Vomit
- Tears
- Nasal secretions
- Urine
- Cerebrospinal fluid
- Feces
- Menstrual blood or vaginal secretions
- Placental fluid
- Synovial (joint) fluid
- Pericardial fluid (from within the heart sac)
- Peritoneal (abdominal) fluid
- Pleural (lung) fluid
- Semen

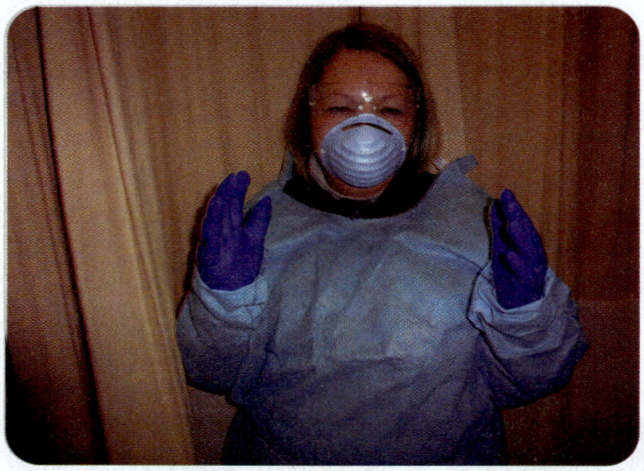

Figure 3-10 Protecting yourself from pathogens is extremely important to keep yourself safe.

fluids (**Figure 3-10**). Although intact skin acts as a good barrier to infection, skin is vulnerable to damage and to dermatologic conditions that can weaken this barrier. Additionally, your mucous membranes (eyes, nose, and mouth) are particularly susceptible to the entry of pathogens. As an OEC technician, you will need to determine what level of personal protection is appropriate for each specific circumstance.

Disposable Medical Gloves

Before touching any patient, you should first put on a pair of disposable gloves. Always carry several pairs of gloves with you when you are away from the first-aid area. Because many people are allergic to natural latex rubber, use gloves made from latex-free materials such as polyvinyl chloride, nitrile, or other synthetic materials. Any item you touch is potentially contaminated and must be thoroughly cleaned at the end of an incident. Anyone who touches potentially contaminated equipment with an ungloved hand is also potentially contaminated and might become infected or spread the disease.

Use the following procedure to put on a pair of disposable medical gloves:

1. Whenever possible, wash your hands before donning gloves. Use antimicrobial gel if soap and water are not available.
2. Grasp one glove using your nondominant hand.
3. Slide your dominant hand into the glove, with fingers slightly spread apart. Wiggle your fingers to ensure a snug fit with no air pockets.
4. With the gloved hand, pick up a second glove.
5. Place the remaining hand into the glove as described in step 3.
6. You may wish to interlock the fingers of both gloved hands to ensure a snug fit and to remove any remaining air pockets.

It is imperative to change gloves after every encounter with a patient, and before touching another patient, to prevent the transmission of pathogens from one patient to another, a condition known as cross-contamination. Make sure all contaminated items, including medical gloves, do not come into contact with anything else. Any item touched, such as a cell phone, should be considered contaminated.

To prevent self-contamination, you must remove your gloves properly and dispose of them with other contaminated waste. Do not place contaminated gloves into your pocket or medical kit! The time-tested key to removing gloves is "dirty to dirty and clean to clean." That is, a contaminated surface (gloved hand) should only touch another contaminated surface (the external surface of the glove), whereas a clean surface (ungloved hand) should only touch another clean surface (the interior surface of the glove).

Follow the steps in **OEC Skill 3-1** to remove disposable gloves after use:

OEC SKILL 3-1 Removing Contaminated Gloves

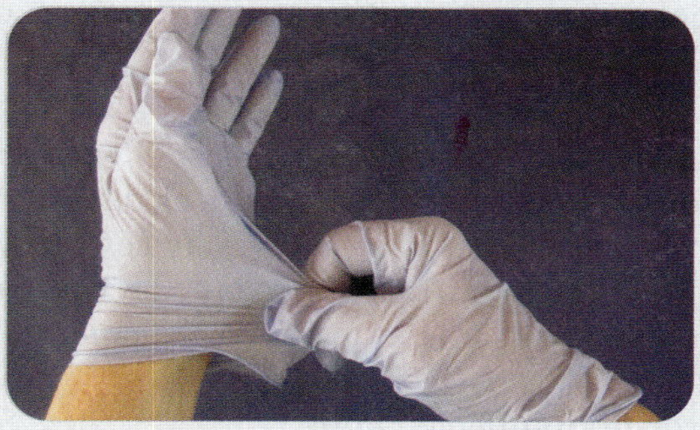

1 Using your dominant hand, grasp the exterior of the opposite glove at the wrist.

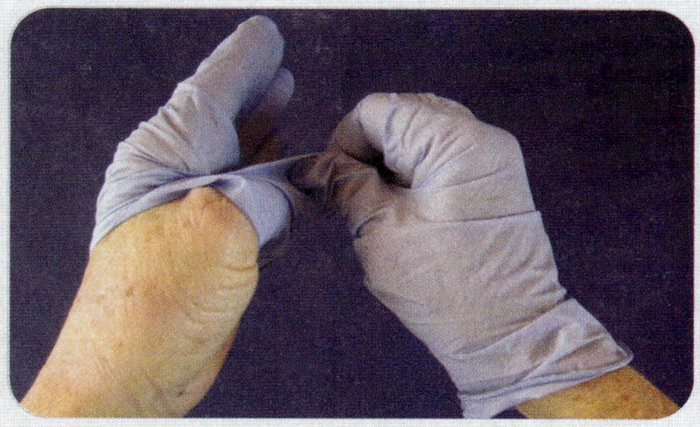

2 Carefully fold the glove over and peel it back, turning it inside out.

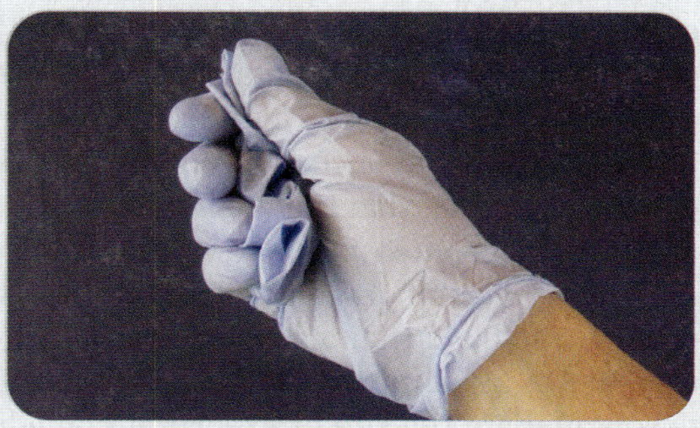

3 Once removed, hold the glove in your gloved dominant hand.

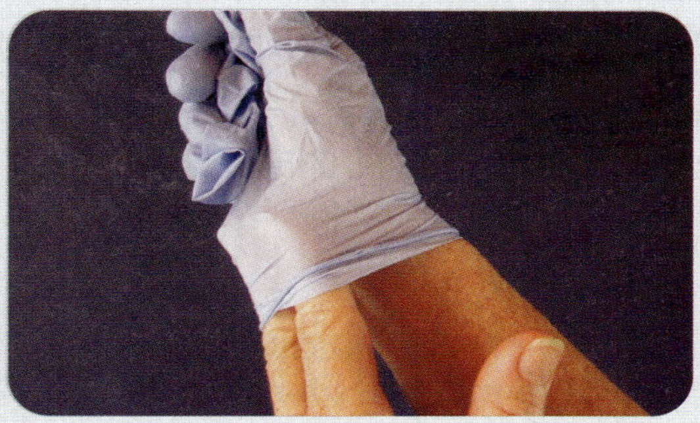

4 Place your ungloved fingers inside the cuff of the glove on your dominant hand, being careful not to touch the exterior.

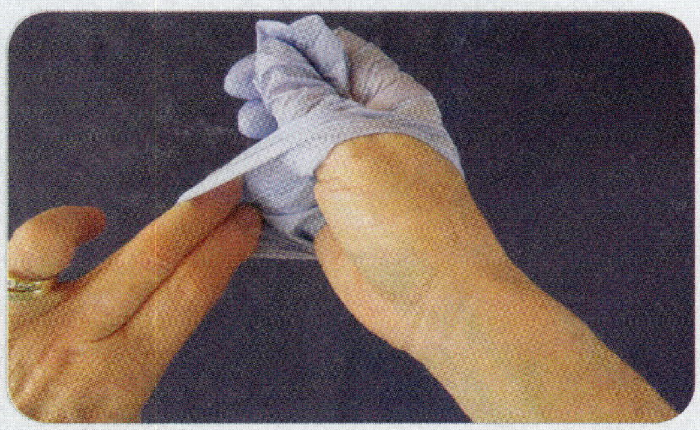

5 Carefully peel the glove off the hand, turning the glove inside out as you remove it. When finished, both gloves should be turned inside out, with the second glove serving as a container for the first glove.

Eye Protection

Eye protection should be worn during every encounter with a patient. Wearing eye protection is especially important when there is a risk of bodily fluids getting splashed or splattered into your eyes. For skiers, ski goggles may serve as an emergency substitute for safety glasses, but they may be difficult to clean if they become contaminated. Sunglasses and prescription glasses also offer some protection, they but provide a less effective barrier than safety glasses. To provide better protection, sunglasses and prescription glasses should have attached side shields.

Surgical masks provide an effective barrier to airborne droplets and protect your nose and mouth from exposure to bodily fluids (**Figure 3-11**). Some masks have attached shields that protect the eyes. Masks also protect the patient from any pathogens that you may have. Use of a mask is especially important if you are suffering from a cold, influenza, or other airborne-transmitted disease. Additionally, you should place a mask on any patient who has, or is suspected of having, an airborne-transmitted disease, especially influenza.

Medical Gown

To complete your PPE, you should consider wearing a medical gown. Although not all situations warrant the use of a gown, you should wear one if there is a risk of bodily fluids being splashed or sprayed (such as a nosebleed or arterial bleed). For ski patrollers, most ski parkas and pants are waterproof and should suffice in protecting you while on patrol. However, if your clothing becomes exposed, you should thoroughly decontaminate it immediately after the incident.

Hand Washing

Hand washing is one of the most effective methods for preventing the spread of disease. Wash your hands *before and after* every contact with a patient (**Figure 3-12**). Use soap and water or a waterless alcohol-based antimicrobial product.

Occupational Exposure

Despite your best efforts to follow standard precautions using proper BSI and PPE, you may still sustain an **occupational exposure**. The risk of becoming infected depends on many factors, including the type of pathogen, type of bodily fluid involved, and route of exposure. Injection of blood confers the highest risk, followed by a contaminated needlestick (**Figure 3-13**). Exposure of mucous membranes and broken skin is still a concern but entails less risk, and exposure to intact skin is a minimal risk. You must report all exposure incidents to your supervisor.

Local protocols should be in place to assist any rescuer who has sustained an occupational exposure. In the meantime, you should immediately decontaminate the site of exposure. Immediately rinse the affected area with water. If the exposure site is your eyes, flush them copiously with water. If the exposure site is your skin, use soap and rinse thoroughly with water.

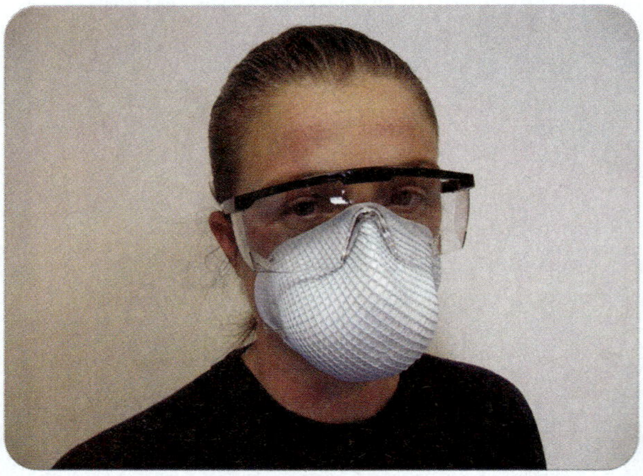

Figure 3-11 Wraparound eye protection or glasses with side shields will protect your eyes. The mask protects your nose and mouth from any potential pathogens.

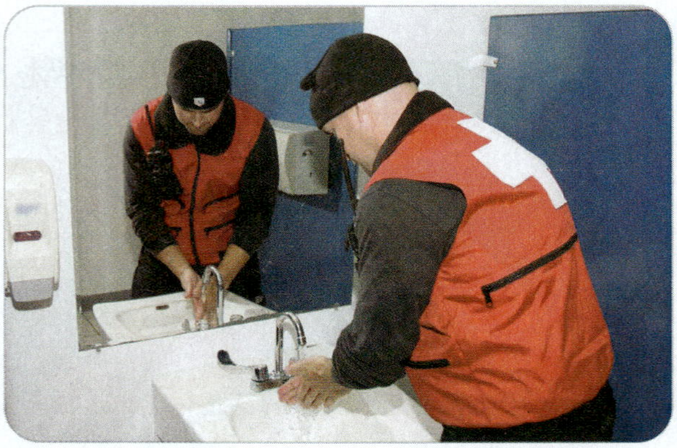

Figure 3-12 Always remember to wash your hands before and after removing gloves to protect yourself.

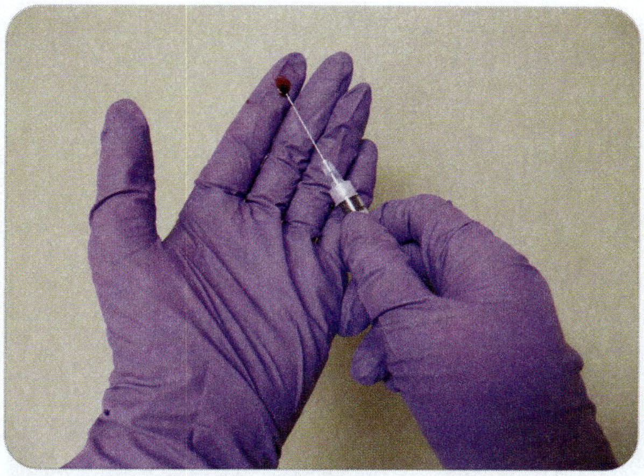

Figure 3-13 An accidental needlestick.

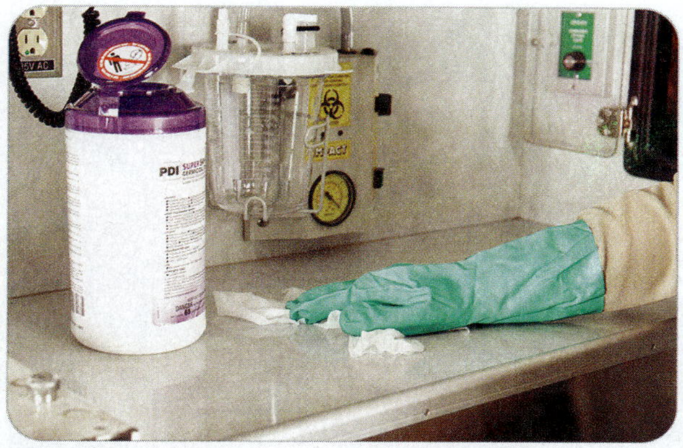

Figure 3-14 When processing medical equipment used during patient care, you will need to follow manufacturer recommendations for the solution that is being used. Allow the solution adequate contact time for disinfecting per label directions.

Postexposure prophylaxis is any preventive treatment that is started immediately after exposure to a pathogen to prevent infection and the development of disease. Decisions surrounding postexposure prophylaxis are complex and involve the nature of the exposure as well as the medical history of the source patient. The source patient may be asked to provide blood for testing for HIV infection and hepatitis, and you also may be asked to be tested to provide a baseline. Your medical provider will determine appropriate treatment. Effective prevention is time sensitive and, if indicated, should be initiated promptly.

Proper Care of Equipment After Use

Medical equipment used during patient care will have come into contact with dirt and microorganisms; that is, it has become contaminated. Before this equipment can be used again, it needs to be processed (**Figure 3-14**). Dirt can be removed by cleaning, usually with soap and water. **Decontamination** is the process of removing disease-producing organisms, such as bacteria, and other harmful substances, such as poison, gas, and radiation. Disinfection destroys disease-producing organisms using special chemicals.

Decisions to clean and/or to disinfect vary and are based on a review of the activities that occurred during the call. Before cleaning or decontaminating equipment, consult with your local protocols and guidelines regarding the recommended procedure.

When cleaning or disinfecting equipment, use appropriate PPE. This is especially important if you have any open wounds on your hands. The use of heavier and more durable utility gloves, such as household rubber gloves, may be considered as well. In addition, to avoid accidental exposure through the mouth or nose, as well as splashes to the eyes, use a mask with an eye shield. The amount of PPE to be worn when cleaning equipment should be guided by the amount of cleaning that will be needed and the potential for splashing. Durable goods should be cleaned and disinfected following manufacturer recommendations.

In the following sections we consider the procedures recommended by the National Institute for Occupational Safety and Health (NIOSH), in collaboration with the National Center for Infectious Diseases, for dealing with contaminated objects.

Disposable Items

Many items that rescuers use are disposable, including gloves, bandages, cardboard splints, cervical collars, and paper sheets. Dispose of them appropriately in biohazard (red) containers or in bags (**Figure 3-15**). Double bag if there is any possibility of leakage.

Infectious Waste

The procedures for disposal of infectious waste are determined by the relative risk of **disease transmission** and by local regulations, which vary widely. In all cases, local regulations should be

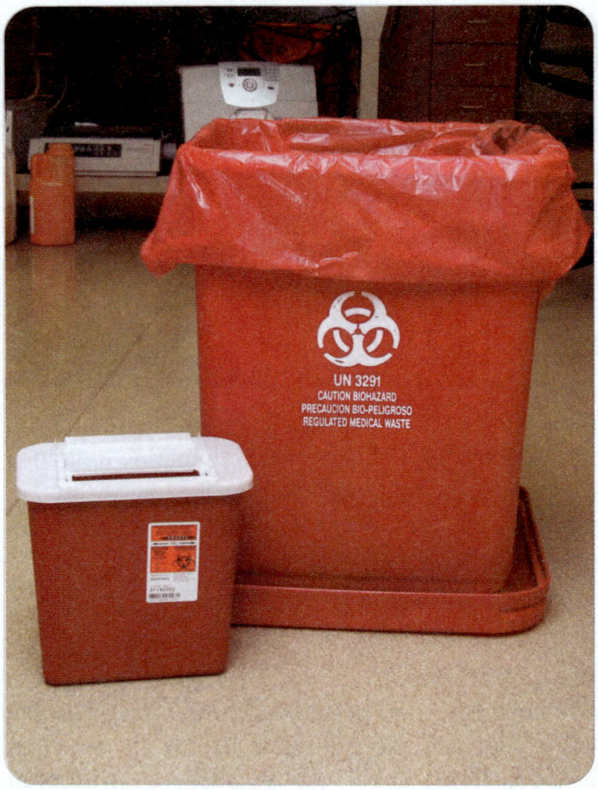

Figure 3-15 Contaminated items and other wastes should be bagged appropriately and disposed of according to your local protocols.

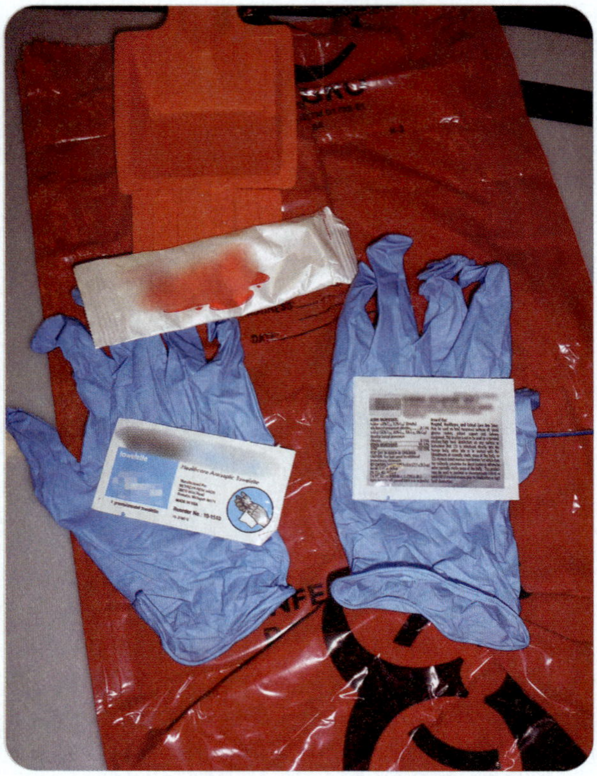

Figure 3-16 This spill kit has everything you will need, and it changes a liquid to a solid for easy cleanup.

consulted before you follow disposal procedures. In general, infectious waste should either be incinerated or decontaminated before disposal in a sanitary landfill. Where it is permitted, bulk blood, suctioned fluids, excretions, secretions, and infectious wastes that can be ground up may be carefully poured down a drain connected to a sanitary sewer.

Bed Linens, Blankets, and Contaminated Clothing

Any nondisposable linen or clothing that is contaminated with blood or other bodily fluids should be placed into and transported in red hazard bags or containers that prevent leakage. Personnel involved in the bagging, transport, and laundering of contaminated clothing should use PPE. The clothing should be washed and dried according to manufacturer instructions. Boots and leather goods may be brush-scrubbed with soap and hot water using standard precautions. Most items can simply be laundered, but use caution with certain specialty items, such as ski jackets. Follow the clothing label instructions to avoid damage to these items.

Spills

While observing standard precautions and using PPE, first remove visible spilled material using disposable towels or other appropriate means. Then decontaminate the spill area using a germicide approved by the Environmental Protection Agency or a 1:10 solution of household bleach, and decontaminate your equipment and supplies as well. Wash your hands following the removal of gloves. Where snow is contaminated with blood or other bodily fluids, remove the contaminated snow by shovel to an area away from the public and treat it with one of the previously mentioned solutions; then treat the shovel with the same solution. As an alternative, you may use one of the commercially available "spill kits" to assist with the cleanup process (**Figure 3-16**). Most kits convert the spilled liquid into a solid for easy pickup and have been shown to be effective even on some porous surfaces such as snow.

Sharps

Handle all sharp objects, or "sharps," with extreme caution. Being stuck or cut by a sharp object that is contaminated by bodily fluid carries a significant risk for HIV infection and hepatitis. Commonly encountered sharps include needles and broken glass. Place the sharp objects into an approved sharps container, which should include a lid and rigid walls to prevent accidental punctures and spills (**Figure 3-17**).

Needles usually have a safety cap. Because many needlesticks occur when attempting to replace the caps, it is preferable to place used needles directly into a "sharps container" without recapping them. Safer needle caps, which recover the needle without risk, are now in use and have significantly reduced exposures by needlestick. Never touch the needle itself. Instead, handle the syringe only.

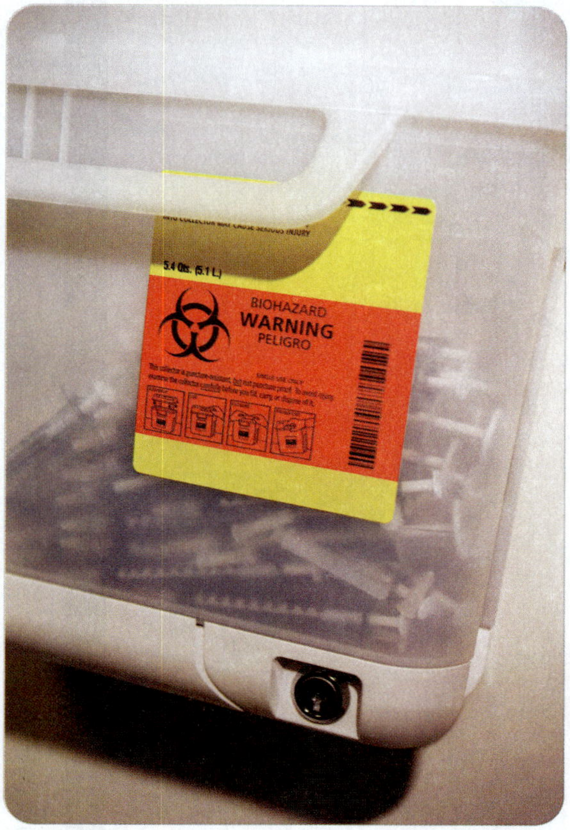

Figure 3-17 Sharps containers come in a variety of sizes depending on location needed and anticipated volume of sharps.

DEALING WITH HAZARDOUS MATERIALS

As part of the scene size-up and assessment for dangers, you may encounter **hazardous materials**. (Note that in this text, *hazmat* is used as an adjective—for example, "hazmat incident.") A hazardous material is any solid, liquid, or gas that has the potential to cause harm to humans, animals, or the environment, either by itself or through interaction with other factors. Hazardous materials include materials that are radioactive, flammable, explosive, or corrosive, as well as pathogens, allergens, and other biohazardous substances. Examples of hazardous materials are avalanche explosives, chlorine, cleaning chemicals, gasoline, and propane. Some hazardous materials can cause health problems if ingested or inhaled; others can be dangerous upon contact with intact skin or the eyes. Many chemicals cause immediate health problems, such as respiratory distress and loss of vision; others are more insidious and may take years to manifest, as is the case with asbestos, which poses a long-term risk of lung cancer.

It is your job to recognize any material that may be hazardous. If you identify a potential hazmat situation, call 9-1-1 and report the incident. Most locales have hazmat teams that are trained to manage these scenes safely. Your job is to prevent yourself and others from becoming contaminated by the substance. As a general rule, you should stay uphill and upwind from any potentially hazardous material.

Most resort facilities utilize and store hazardous substances, including cleaning solvents, fertilizers, petroleum-based products, and explosives. Hazardous materials stored at your facility may be identified by safety placards (**Figure 3-18**). Your facility also should have readily available information concerning any hazardous materials that are on site. In the United States, this information is available on the manufacturer's **safety data sheet (SDS)**. The SDS for a given substance describes known health risks and provides information on the safe handling of the substance. When you respond to a scene involving hazardous

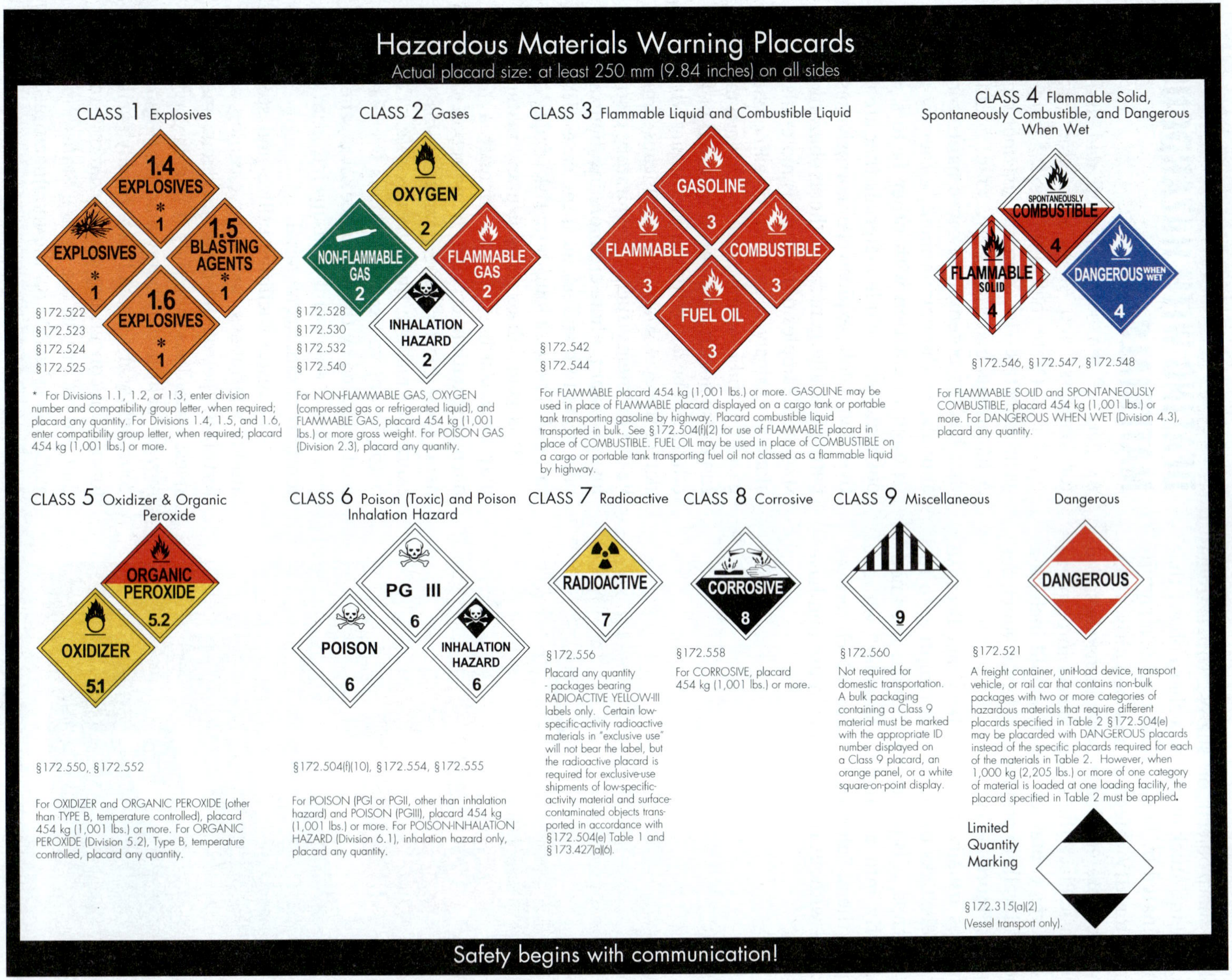

Figure 3-18 The Department of Transportation requires the use of placards to identify materials as flammable, radioactive, explosive, and/or poisonous.

U.S. Department of Transportation, Pipeline and Hazardous Materials Safety Administration.

materials, first ensure your own personal safety. In major hazmat situations, it is recommended that you stay at least 250 feet from the scene. If you are downwind, it is recommended you stay 500 feet away. You may need to delay care of patients until the scene is secured by trained hazmat personnel. Delaying the care of patients is difficult to do and against our instincts, but it is the best option in a hazmat incident.

SDSs provide an overview of the materials, including instructions for handling, storage, decontamination, and emergency care. If you work in an area that has a high potential for a hazmat situation, consider taking additional specialized training. For more information about hazardous materials, refer to Chapter 34, *Special Operations and Ambulance Operations*.

CRIME SCENE MANAGEMENT

OEC technicians may occasionally encounter crime scenes (**Figure 3-19**). If you discover a potential crime scene, notify law enforcement immediately. The responding law enforcement officer is in charge of the crime scene. If no law enforcement personnel are present, do not assume that the scene is safe to enter. If a law enforcement officer is present, do not approach the scene until the officer notifies you that it is safe to do so.

Take care to follow instructions so that you do not disturb the scene. Make sure the area is cordoned off and that members of the public do not enter the scene. Take precautions not to remove, move, or otherwise disturb anything in the environment, except as is absolutely necessary to provide critical care to patients. Any mishandling of evidence can make it inadmissible in court. To avoid this problem, it is important to create an accurate "paper trail," or "chain of custody," accounting for the location of the evidence at each step, from the time of its discovery to its presentation in court. Let law enforcement personnel handle any materials that could be used as evidence.

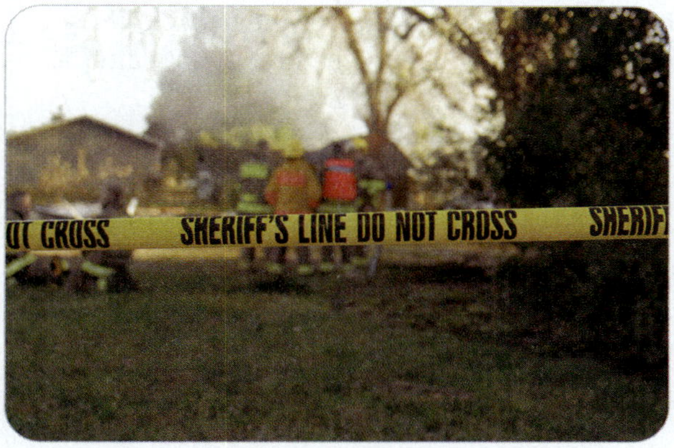

Figure 3-19 Do not interfere with a crime scene.

Examples of crime scenes include sites of homicides, hostage situations, domestic violence, or assaults. If you have any doubt about how to proceed, consult with the law enforcement officer in charge of the scene. For more information about crime scenes, refer to Chapter 34, *Special Operations and Ambulance Operations*. See **Table 3-5** for additional tips concerning crime scene preservation.

Relations with the Media

Any incident to which you respond may involve the media. Reports can be generated and subsequently appear on media outlets even if no "official" media personnel are at the scene. Given today's technology, *anyone* can become an "on-scene reporter" and begin transmitting reports on events, including text, pictures, audio, and streaming video.

While working at the scene, always be careful what you say and how you say it. Statements or comments spoken while on scene, your actions while caring for patients, your interactions with bystanders, and the overall scene dynamics all can be broadcast to a wide audience within minutes. As a health care provider, you must respect the privacy of patients, treating all information regarding their care as confidential. You may need to insist that bystanders and media personnel relocate. Mountain hosts (mountain safety personnel), safety patrollers, and law enforcement officials may be able to assist with keeping media away from the scene. Take every possible measure to ensure that scene safety and patient care remain the top priority. Media relations are a secondary concern.

Always consult management before speaking to the media. Many organizations have a designated, formally trained public information officer who is authorized to speak to the media (**Figure 3-20**).

Table 3-5 Crime Scene Preservation Tips

Table 3-5 Crime Scene Preservation Tips
Approaching the Scene: • Identify the minimum number of rescuers needed. (Consider whether one rescuer is sufficient.) • Send in the most trained rescuer. • Take the minimum amount of needed equipment to the scene. • Minimize contact to only what is needed to care for the patient.
Entering the Scene: • Minimize disturbance of the scene. • While coming into the scene, pay attention to where you put your feet. (Do not kick or step in anything.) • Do not wander around the scene. • Unless necessary in caring for a patient, do not change the lighting, position of the drapes, TV or radio settings, furniture position, and so on. • While in the scene, do not smoke, eat, drink, or use the bathroom.
Weapons and Ropes: • Assume that all guns are loaded. • If a weapon must be moved in order to care for a patient, only one *gloved* person (preferably a law enforcement officer) should handle the grip of the weapon. • Before moving a weapon, mark or outline its location. • If a rope needs to be removed to care for a patient, make sure that in doing so no knots are either cut or untied.
Clothing: • Do not shake or turn clothing inside out. • Minimize destruction of clothing. • Cut around (not through) any bullet hole, puncture, or other damaged areas. • Leave all removed clothing with law enforcement personnel.
Providing Care: • Use gloves. • Keep medical equipment close to the patient. • Stay close to the victim. • Keep your hands out of pooled blood. • Collect and remove all packaging, wrappers, and used bandages.
Treating the Patient: • If the person is deceased, do not disturb any belongings, and do not clean or cover the body. • Advise victims of sexual assault to not wash, clean, change clothes, or use the bathroom until after a medical/forensic examination. • If resuscitation is required, transfer the victim from the scene to an ambulance as soon as possible. • Remind EMS that any sheets used under the victim for transport should be "bagged" because they may contain evidence.

Remember: Although crime scene preservation and patient care occur in tandem, patient care takes priority.

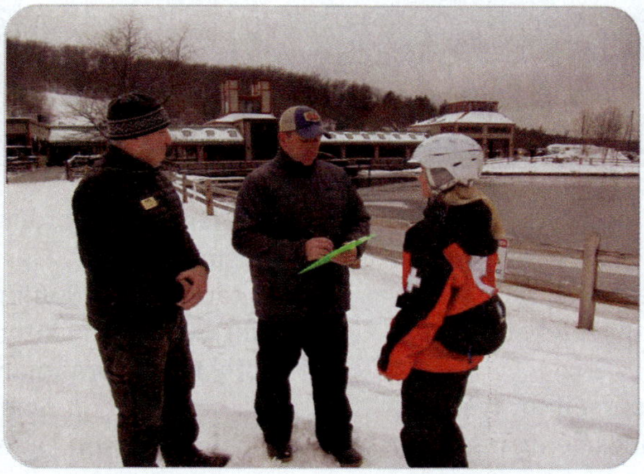

Figure 3-20 It is best to have management present if interviewed.

CASE Outcome

Pulling Peter aside, you instruct him to remove his wet jacket, and you give him your backup waterproof jacket. You also hand him two of your energy bars. As the rescue efforts continue, Peter realizes that he was not prepared for the scene. You instruct another rescuer to take Peter back to the ski area first-aid station so that he can be checked and warmed up. A few minutes later, Peter is heading to the first-aid room on the back of a snowmobile, covered with a wool blanket. Although Peter survived this event without any major complications, he learned some valuable lessons about being appropriately prepared, both physically and mentally.

CHAPTER REVIEW

In Summary

- To perform your duties safely, you must learn how to adapt safely to your environment.
- Adequately prepare yourself for rescue operations. This includes being mentally prepared, being physically fit, getting enough sleep, eating right, hydrating, avoiding substances that may compromise your ability to think clearly, wearing the appropriate clothing and personal protective equipment, and having the appropriate equipment available.
- Your personal pack should include appropriate first-aid gear and personal gear.
- Learning the *Rule of Threes* may save your life.
- Infectious diseases are transmitted in five ways: by direct contact, by indirect contact, via airborne transmission, through ingestion, and via vector-borne transmission.
- It is recommended that OEC technicians be properly vaccinated against certain diseases.
- Standard precautions, body substance isolation, and personal protective equipment are essential for preventing the transmission of disease.
- Hand washing is one of the most effective methods for preventing the spread of disease.
- The risk of becoming infected depends on many factors, including the type of pathogen, type of bodily fluid involved, and route of exposure.
- Request assistance in hazmat and crime-scene situations.

Key Terms

Body substance isolation (BSI) The practice of isolating all bodily substances (blood, urine, tears, feces, and so on) of patients from rescuers in order to decrease disease transmission.

Contamination Soiling of an object, water, or air by foreign material such as dirt, debris, bodily fluids, or radiation.

Decontamination The process of rendering an object, person, or area free of harmful substances such as bacteria, poison, gas, and radiation.

Disease transmission The transfer of illness from an infected individual to a healthy individual.

Hazardous materials Substances that have the potential to harm people, animals, or the environment. The term hazmat is often used adjectively (e.g., "hazmat incident").

Metabolism The chemical processes occurring within a living cell or organism that are necessary for the maintenance of life.

Nutrition The body's process of utilizing food substances needed for growth and the maintenance of life.

Occupational exposure An event in which a worker comes into contact with a bodily fluid or hazardous material while on the job.

Pathogen An infectious agent that can cause disease or illness.

Personal protective equipment (PPE) Items worn by medical providers, including gloves, mask, safety eyeglasses (or mask with shield), and gown, to protect them from bodily fluids.

Safety data sheet (SDS) A form that contains relevant information pertaining to a specific substance, with a focus on the hazards it poses to workers.

Standard precautions Practices used by health care workers to protect themselves from exposure to bodily fluids based on the assumption that all patients are potentially infectious.

Ultraviolet radiation (UVR) Waves of solar energy that are beneficial in small amounts but harmful to the skin and eyes upon overexposure.

Chapter Questions

1. To be prepared to respond to incidents, OEC technicians should strive to:
   a. get 7 to 9 hours of sleep each night.
   b. maintain a positive attitude.
   c. ensure proper hydration and nutrition.
   d. All of the above
2. In cold weather, it is important to dress in layers to preserve body heat. Which layer is the insulating layer that traps warm air?
   a. Sublayer
   b. Base layer
   c. Middle layer
   d. Outer layer
3. Bites from infected ticks can cause Lyme disease and Rocky Mountain spotted fever. These infectious diseases are said to be caused by:
   a. direct contact.
   b. indirect contact.
   c. airborne transmission.
   d. vector-borne transmission.
4. An OEC technician does not put on gloves while caring for a bleeding patient who has been injured. Her reasoning for not putting on gloves is she will not touch the blood. You tell her that she should be practicing infection prevention practices, called:
   a. standard precautions.
   b. standards of care.
   c. standard operations.
   d. standard of training.
5. Your patient is a groundskeeper at your resort. He has sustained burns on his hands as a result of touching a chemical. The chemical would be considered a(n):
   a. hazardous material.
   b. infectious material.
   c. environmental contaminant.
   d. pathogen.
6. Microorganisms that transmit infectious diseases are called:
   a. hazardous materials.
   b. infections.
   c. environmental contaminants.
   d. pathogens.
7. Which of the following is an example of PPE that an OEC technician would use to prevent exposure to infectious agents in the patient's bodily fluids?
   a. Disposable medical gloves and surgical mask
   b. Hand washing and equipment decontamination procedures
   c. Sharps container and biohazard waste bags
   d. Blood tests and vaccinations
8. There has been a crime at your resort. Law enforcement has arrived and secured the scene. They indicate that you may enter the scene to provide care to a victim. During your patient assessment, you discover a knife that was used to injure your patient. You begin a careful account for the location of the knife. This accounting is called:
   a. crime scene precautions.
   b. chain of custody.
   c. standard precautions.
   d. weapon accounting.

Answers: 1. d, Objective 3-1, p. 44; 2. c, Objective 3-2, p. 46; 3. d, Objective 3-3, p. 49; 4. a, Objective 3-4, p. 53; 5. a, Objective 3-4, p. 59; 6. d, Objective 3-4, p. 49; 7. a, Objective 3-5, p. 54; 8. b, Objective 3-7, p. 61

CHAPTER 4

INCIDENT COMMAND AND TRIAGE

OBJECTIVES

Upon completion of this chapter, the OEC technician will be able to:

4-1 Define incident command system.
4-2 Describe the primary responsibilities of each of the five functional areas of the incident command system.
4-3 Describe the mnemonic ID-ME.
4-4 Describe and demonstrate how to use the SALT triage system.
4-5 Describe and demonstrate how to use the START triage system.
4-6 Describe the mnemonic 30–2-Can Do.

KEY TERMS

30–2-Can Do, p. 80
Chain of command, p. 69
Facility, p. 73
Incident, p. 68
Incident commander (IC), p. 70
Incident command system (ICS), p. 69
Multiagency coordination system (MACS), p. 69
Multiple-casualty incident (MCI), p. 77
National Incident Management System (NIMS), p. 68
Personnel accountability system, p. 69
Resource management, p. 69
SALT triage system, p. 78
Section chiefs, p. 71
Span of control, p. 69
START triage system, p. 80
Strike team, p. 72
Task force, p. 72
Triage, p. 80

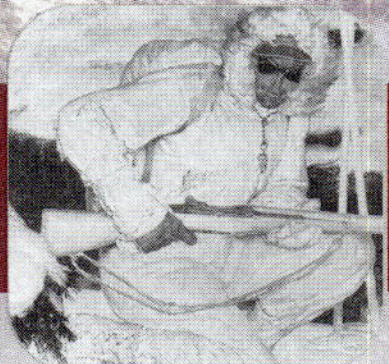

HISTORICAL TIMELINE **1944.** 10th Mountain Division soldier near Camp Hale, Colorado.

CHAPTER OVERVIEW

Emergencies can happen at any time, in any place, and under a variety of circumstances. Each emergency is unique and presents rescue personnel with countless challenges, so OEC technicians must be prepared to respond to and manage a wide variety of situations, whether they are natural or human-made, small or large, simple or complex (**Figure 4-1**). Fortunately, in managing any type of emergency, patrollers can use the federally mandated **National Incident Management System (NIMS)**.

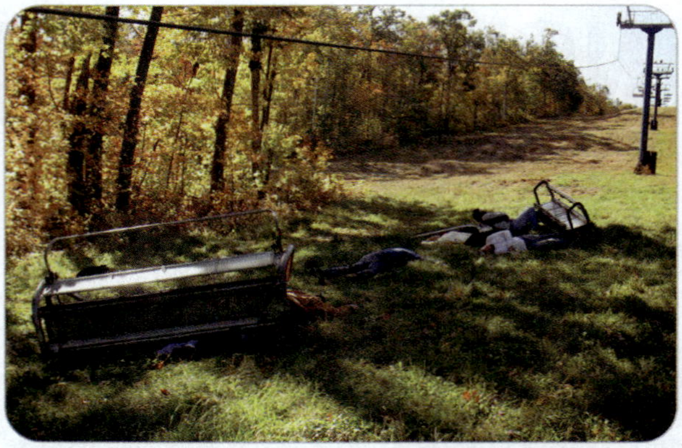

Figure 4-1 Chairlift accident where chairs have fallen off of the cable.

THE NATIONAL INCIDENT MANAGEMENT SYSTEM

NIMS is a standardized framework for responding to, and managing, emergencies or situations involving multiple jurisdictions. NIMS was established in 2003 by President George W. Bush, who signed Homeland Security Presidential Directive 5 in response to the terrorist attacks of September 11, 2001. NIMS is a national "all-hazards" model for incident management that provides "a consistent nationwide approach for federal, state, tribal, and local governments to work effectively and efficiently together to prepare for, prevent, respond to, and recover from domestic incidents, regardless of cause, size, or complexity" (US Department of Homeland Security, n.d.). An **incident** is defined as "anything out of ordinary day-to-day activities that necessitates a response" and includes medical emergencies, search-and-rescue missions, natural disasters, fires, terrorist and weapons of mass destruction events, disease outbreaks, public vaccination programs, and such planned events as important meetings, conferences, or large public events.

NIMS is designed to improve overall incident management interoperability, integration, and coordination. It is federally mandated for use by all government and civilian organizations and personnel whose duties include responding to and managing emergency situations. This mandate extends to ski/bike patrols and OEC technicians,

CASE Presentation

You and three other patrollers are eating lunch in the mid-mountain cafeteria when you are dispatched to respond to "a skier who has fallen from a lift and may be hurt." As you walk out of the lodge, you see a large group of people standing at the top of the slope. You observe that many individuals are hastily removing their skis and then running over to the edge. As you ski over to their location, you quickly see the source of their concern. Looking downhill, the scene before you is pure chaos. All the way down the lift line, people are frantically clinging to lift chairs. Several appear to have fallen from the lift, some as far as 40 feet. Small groups of bystanders have gathered around some of the patients and appear to be rendering aid. People are frantically waving both upslope and downslope, trying to get help. You hear muffled yells for help and screaming in the distance.

What is the first thing you and the other patrollers should do?

who may be called upon to take the lead in managing an incident involving external public safety organizations or to assist other public safety agencies during an incident.

NIMS provides numerous benefits that enable rescuers from different agencies to work together effectively at an incident. Among these benefits are the standardization of roles, functions, processes, terms, and forms; modularization, which allows rescuers to use only those components they need; and, flexibility, which permits rescue leaders to create special solutions to resolve unique incident-related challenges. Additionally, NIMS provides the following managerial benefits:

- A formal **chain of command** (a rank structure for management)
- Management by objectives
- **Span of control** (the total number of individuals or resources supervised by a single person)
- **Personnel accountability system** (a system that readily identifies both the locations and the functions of all members operating at an incident scene)
- Integrated communications
- **Resource management** (includes mutual-aid agreements; the use of special federal, state, local, and tribal teams; and resource mobilization protocols)

NIMS activities consist of four major components:

- *Command and management* focuses on managing incidents using standardized processes, the **multiagency coordination system (MACS)**, and public information systems (**Figure 4-2**).
- *Preparedness* emphasizes planning, training, practical exercises, standards and certification, mutual aid, and information and publications (**Figure 4-3**).
- *Resource management* used to identify and categorize incident resources; to certify and credential personnel; and to acquire, inventory, mobilize, track, recover, and rehabilitate incident resources.
- *Communications and information management* deals with interoperability and the flow and use of NIMS and incident-related information.

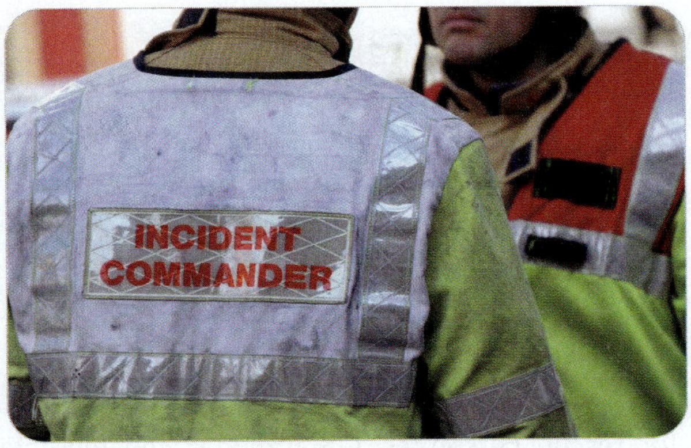

Figure 4-2 The incident commander is responsible for directing the response and coordinates the resources at MCIs.

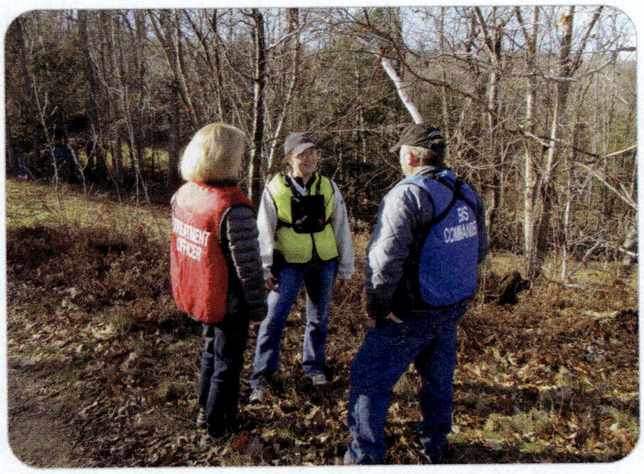

Figure 4-3 Team members discussing their coordinated response to the MCI.

As part of NIMS's federal mandate, all rescue organizations within the United States must adopt the **incident command system (ICS)**.

INCIDENT COMMAND SYSTEM

The ICS provides a method for managing any incident, regardless of its cause, size, scope, or complexity. Developed in the 1970s as a method for managing California wildfires, ICS has evolved into an all-hazards management plan that provides a core set of doctrines, concepts, principles, terminology, and organizational processes that help responding organizations operate in a standardized fashion. The system improves efficiency, reduces confusion, and provides a safer work environment

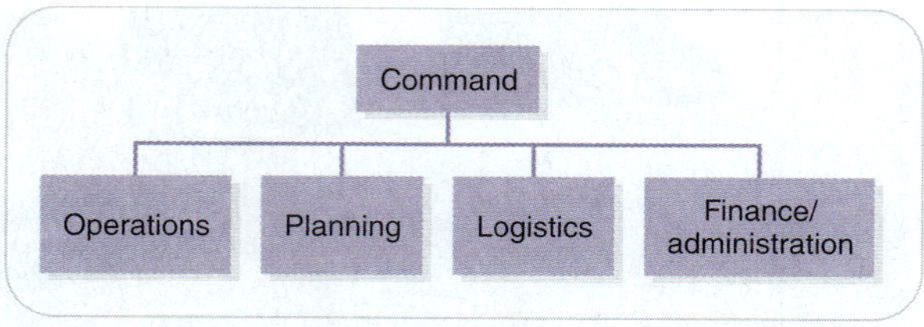

Figure 4-4 The major functional components, or sections, of the ICS structure.

for rescue personnel. ICS provides considerable flexibility in that it can grow or shrink to accommodate the needs of each incident.

The ICS structure consists of five functional areas, each of which has specific responsibilities. The areas are interdependent and, depending on the size of the incident, may either be combined and managed by a single person or expanded and managed individually. The functional areas are as follows (**Figure 4-4**):

- Incident command
- Operations section
- Planning section
- Logistics section
- Finance/administration section

Incident Command

Of the five functional areas, incident command is the first to be established at any incident and is managed by an **incident commander (IC)**. Identification of the IC is essential, as this person provides overall leadership and direction for managing the incident. The role of IC is typically assumed by the most senior person among the initial responders arriving at the scene (**Figure 4-5**).

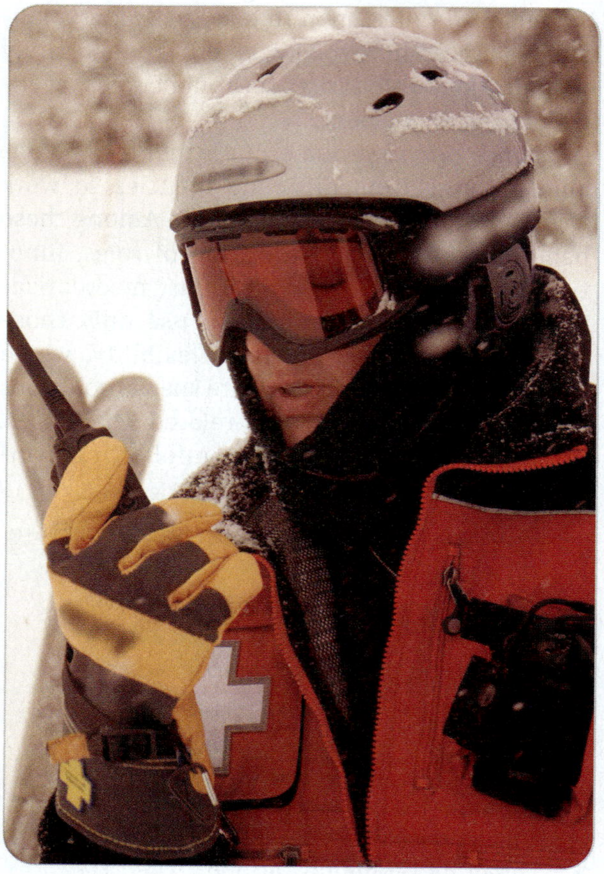

Figure 4-5 A patroller acting as an IC of an incident uses the radio to communicate pertinent information from a safe distance.

After conducting an initial assessment of the scene, the IC establishes an incident command post, or ICP, which serves as the IC's base of operations while managing the incident. The ICP must be established in a safe, secure location that is near the incident but is away from any hazards. The IC serves in this capacity until one of the following occurs: the incident is over, the IC is relieved by another qualified IC, or, the IC's operational period (specified amount of work time) is complete. Ideally, an operational period should not exceed 12 hours, and it can be much shorter depending on the nature of the incident and the task to be performed. To avoid confusion, there is only one IC at a time per incident. The IC's several key responsibilities include the following tasks:

- Assume command of the incident.
- Establish an ICP.
- Provide overall incident management.
- Determine incident objectives and strategies.
- Determine/develop the organizational structure needed to manage the incident.

If needed, incident command can be expanded to include one or more of the following three additional positions that can assist the IC:

- *Public information officer*, who serves as the primary source for incident-related information and media relations.
- *Incident safety officer*, who is responsible for the health and safety of all incident workers and for assessing incident hazards.

- *Liaison officer*, who serves as the primary contact with all rescue organizations assisting on the incident. This person's responsibilities include coordinating efforts with local, state, and federal organizations and officials.

Collectively, the IC and these three officers are known as the command staff (**Table 4-1**).

The command staff is responsible for overall incident management and for developing the incident action plan, or IAP, which outlines the objectives and strategies for the operational period. The objectives identify the goal(s), or what must be accomplished, whereas the strategies specify the tasks that must be performed to achieve the objectives. Depending on the size of the incident, the IAP may be communicated orally or in writing. For small incidents, the IC typically provides this information orally to subordinates; for large incidents, this information is given to the chief of each of the four sections—operations, planning, logistics, and finance/administration—orally and in writing to execute their specific section-related tasks. **Section chiefs** constitute the general staff and report directly to the IC.

Large incidents involving multiple jurisdictions or multiple agencies may need to be organized under a "unified command" structure in which the commanders from each on-scene agency work together to achieve the overall incident goals and objectives while simultaneously carrying out their respective jurisdictional activities.

Operations Section

Operations is the next section to be established at an incident and is the functional area responsible for executing the strategies of the IAP. This functional area is managed by an operations section chief who oversees the following responsibilities:

- Participating in the planning process (to create the IAP)
- Reducing immediate hazard(s)
- Saving lives and property
- Establishing situational control
- Restoring the scene to normalcy

The operations section chief achieves these goals by constantly assessing the nature and scope of the incident, as well as the hazards present, and by determining the resources needed to achieve the IAP. A resource is defined as "an individual, a piece of equipment and its complement, or a crew or team of individuals with an identified work supervisor that can be used at an incident." Resources are the assets, both physical and human, that are used to execute incident-related

Table 4-1 Titles and Organization of ICS Personnel

Organizational Level	Supervisory Title	Reports To	Support Position (if needed)
Command staff	Incident commander (IC)	—	Deputy IC
	Staff officers: • Information officer • Incident safety officer • Liaison officer	 IC IC IC	 Assistant information officer Assistant incident safety officer Assistant liaison officer
General staff	Section chiefs: • Operations section chief • Planning section chief • Logistics section chief • Finance section chief	 IC IC IC IC	 Deputy operations chief Deputy planning chief Deputy logistics chief Deputy finance chief
Branches	Branch directors	Section chief	Deputy branch director
Groups/divisions	Group officers	Branch director	—
	Division supervisors	Branch director	—
Units	Unit leaders	Section chief	Unit manager/coordinator

tasks. Depending on incident size, the operations section chief may create one or more branches to perform specific tasks (see Table 4-1). Branches can be named using specific predesignated ICS names (e.g., medical branch, police branch, fire branch, air operations branch) or can be named for a specific operational need (e.g., search branch, avalanche branch). Branches are managed by a director who reports directly to the operations section chief.

If needed, branches can be expanded to include one or more groups or divisions (**Figure 4-6**). For instance, under the medical branch, groups are often created for triage, treatment, and transportation of patients. Given their medical expertise, OEC technicians are commonly assigned to these groups. Groups are managed by an officer, whereas divisions are managed by a supervisor. Both roles report directly to the branch director (see Table 4-1). If needed, resources may be formed into strike teams or task forces to perform specific operational tasks. A **strike team** consists of resources of the same type (e.g., a group of Nordic patrollers or river guides) and is managed by a strike team leader, whereas a **task force** includes a combination of different resources (e.g., a sheriff's deputy, an NSP Alpine patrol, and a search-and-rescue team) with common communications and is managed by a task force leader. The leaders from both groups report directly to the branch director under which they are operating (**Figure 4-7**).

Command and operations sections are established on every incident, although they may be managed by a single individual on small, isolated incidents. The next three functional areas—planning, logistics, and finance/administration sections—are usually established only on large incidents that last days, weeks, or even months (e.g., natural disasters, human-caused incidents).

Planning Section

The planning section collects, assesses, distributes, and uses incident-related data. It also

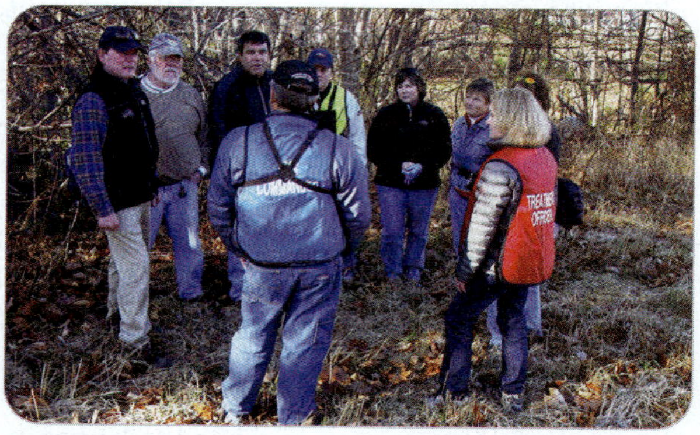

Figure 4-7 Ski patrollers confer with a branch director at the scene of an MCI.

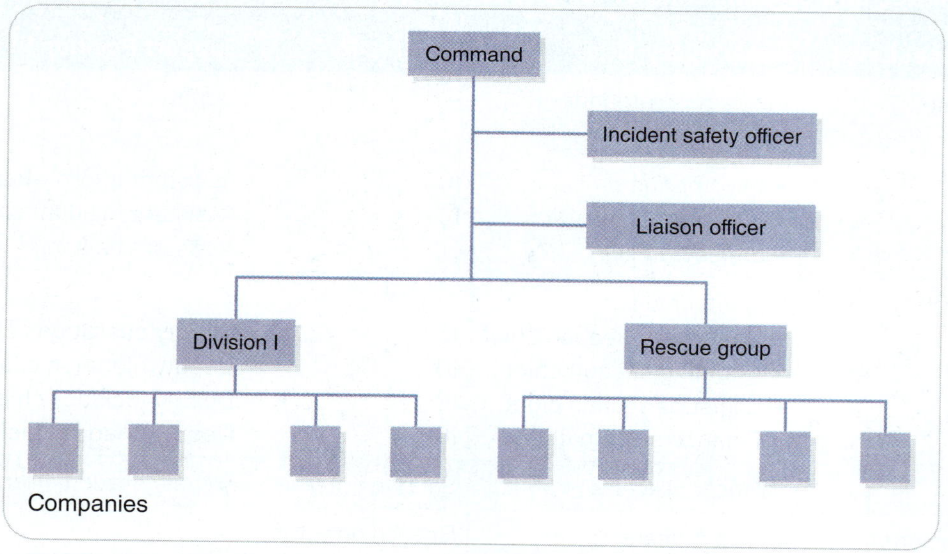

Figure 4-6 Divisions and groups are organized to manage the span of control and to supervise and coordinate units working together.

coordinates the preparation of the IAP and other incident documents. This section achieves its goals by performing the following activities:

- Determine incident resource needs.
- Gather and analyze incident-related data.
- Create probability projections (e.g., incident needs, outcomes).
- Prepare contingencies and alternative strategies.
- Assist in the preparation of incident documents and maps.
- Maintain incident records (except financial records).

The planning section is managed by the planning section chief, who chairs all planning meetings. If needed, the planning section chief may activate one or more of the following units:

- *Resources unit* is responsible for maintaining the status of every resource at the incident.
- *Situation unit* is responsible for obtaining up-to-date information about the incident and providing that information to the public information officer.
- *Documentation unit* is responsible for providing ICS paperwork, clerical support, and incident documentation (except financial documentation) to incident personnel.
- *Demobilization unit* is responsible for rehabilitating equipment, personnel, and the environment, and for overall incident cleanup efforts.

Each unit is managed by a unit leader who reports directly to the planning section chief. If needed, the planning section chief may also request assistance from technical specialists to help gather information, evaluate the situation, or prepare projections and forecasts.

Logistics Section

The logistics section provides support for all the functional areas and has the following responsibilities:

- Acquire resources (e.g., personnel, equipment, services).
- Order/obtain supplies (e.g., food, water).
- Manage internal communications equipment.
- Maintain equipment.
- Develop a transportation system or supply line (to support operational needs).

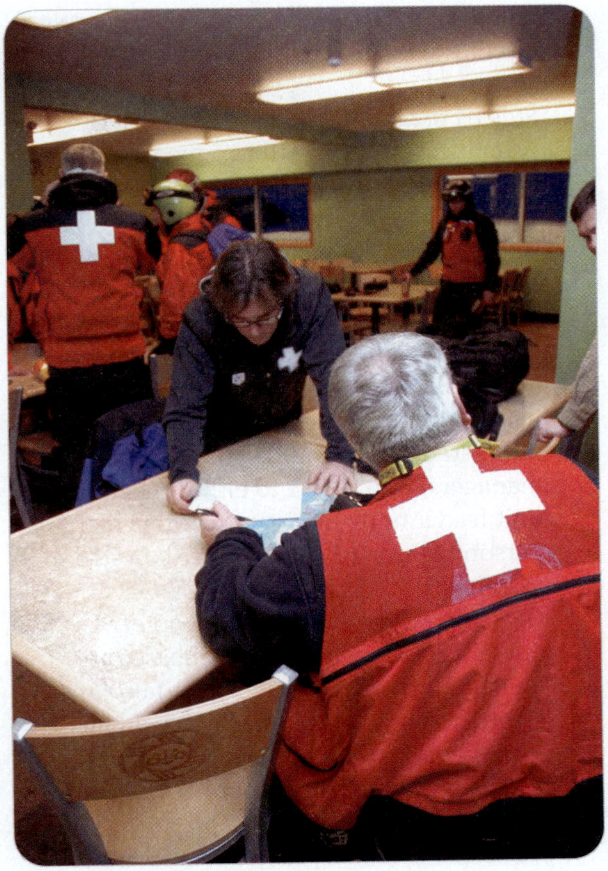

Figure 4-8 The base center is where patrollers come for their assignments in an MCI.

The logistics section is managed by the logistics section chief, who, in addition to these duties, is also responsible for ensuring that all incident facilities meet specified needs. A **facility** is any primary work area in or around the incident in which incident-related activities are planned, organized, directed, or conducted (**Figure 4-8**). Depending on the nature of the incident, one or more of the following facilities may be established:

- *Incident command post (ICP).* Site where all command functions are undertaken. Every incident must have an ICP. The ICP is the first incident facility created and is named after the incident (e.g., Bridger Command).
- *Base.* Site where logistics functions are coordinated/administered. There is only one base per incident, and it is often adjacent to the command post. The base is named after the incident (e.g., Hayman Base) and is

managed by a base manager, who reports to either the facilities unit leader or the logistics section chief.

- *Staging areas.* One or more sites where resources are kept until assigned. Staging areas may be near or remote from the incident and are numbered (e.g., Staging Area 1). They are managed by a staging area manager, who reports to the operations section chief. Resources in a staging area are considered out of service until assigned.
- *Camps.* Sites where incident personnel may eat, sleep, and rehabilitate. Camps are numbered (e.g., Camp 1) and are run by camp managers, who report to either the facilities unit leader or the logistics section chief. Personnel located in camps are considered assigned.
- *Helibase.* Site from which helicopter operations are conducted. Helibases are named for the incident (e.g., Buffalo Creek Helibase) and are managed by the helibase manager, who reports to either the air operations branch director or the operations section chief.
- *Helispot and landing zones.* Temporary or permanent sites where helicopters can safely land and take off. Helispots and landing zones are numbered (e.g., H1, LZ1) and are managed by a helispot manager, who reports to the helibase manager.

Note that not every facility must be established at every incident. Some incidents may require only a command post, whereas others may require each type of facility. Other facilities that may be found at an incident include the following:

- *Communications center.* The primary site at which all incident-related communications are coordinated
- *Rehabilitation center.* The site where the physical condition of incident personnel is monitored
- *Demobilization center.* The site where incident resources are discharged from the incident

Regardless of the type of facility established, all incident facilities share several key characteristics:

- They must be located in a secure, safe area that is free from hazards.
- They should be located out of public view.
- They must be able to grow in size as needed.
- They must be accessible to incident personnel.

The logistics section is managed by a logistics section chief, who may activate any of the following branches and units:

- Service branch
    - *Communication unit.* Responsible for installing, testing, maintaining, and repairing incident communications equipment
    - *Medical unit.* Responsible for developing a medical plan that provides for the treatment and transportation of ill or injured incident personnel
    - *Food unit.* Responsible for (1) assessing, ordering, and preparing food to support incident personnel and (2) maintaining and securing all food service areas
    - *Security unit.* Responsible for assessing and mitigating security risks to incident personnel and facilities and for establishing a secure perimeter around the incident
- Support branch
    - *Supply unit.* Responsible for ordering, receiving, storing, and processing all incident resources (personnel and supplies
    - *Facilities unit.* Responsible for setting up, maintaining, and demobilizing all incident support facilities
    - *Ground support unit.* Responsible for monitoring, fueling, maintaining, and repairing incident equipment and for providing support transportation for incident operations

Finance/Administration Section

The finance/administration section is responsible for providing financial management, accountability, and administrative services to support incident management activities. This section is responsible for the following activities:

- Authorize expenditures.
- Negotiate contracts with vendors.
- Maintain reimbursement records.
- Maintain injury, death, and damage documentation.
- Track costs associated with mutual-aid agreements.

The information gathered and documented is required to ensure that all incident-related expenses are tracked and paid, and it is crucial for incidents related to a president-declared disaster because these expenses are reimbursed under the federal Robert T. Stafford Disaster Relief and Emergency Assistance Act, also known as the Stafford Act (Public Law 100-707).

The finance/administration section is managed by the finance section chief, who may activate any of the following units:

- *Time unit*. Responsible for recording the amount of time that resources are used at the incident
- *Procurement unit*. Responsible for administering all financial and vendor contracts and leases
- *Compensation/claims unit*. Responsible for processing all incident-related claims and injury compensation
- *Cost unit*. Responsible for collecting and analyzing incident cost data and for providing cost estimates

The planning, logistics, and finance/administration sections are most commonly activated on large incidents, especially those involving multiple jurisdictions or spanning a large geographic area. Such incidents include natural disasters such as wildfires, floods, tornadoes, and hurricanes, as well as human-caused events such as building collapses, fires, civil unrest, and acts of violence.

As a scalable framework, ICS allows users to create additional organizational levels within the functional areas to perform specific tasks whenever the span of control—the total number of individuals or resources supervised by a single person—becomes greater than one person can manage effectively. Under ICS, span of control is limited to three to seven resources, with five being the average. Span of control ensures that each individual at the incident reports to only one supervisor. This system greatly improves communications and the overall effectiveness of managing incident resources.

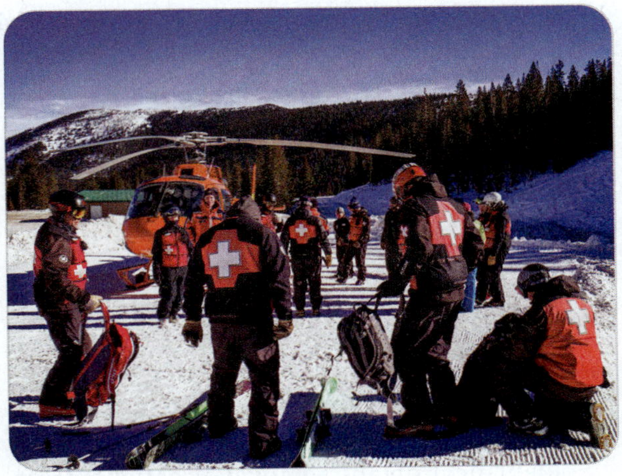

Figure 4-9 Patrollers preparing to search for avalanche victims.

ICS AND THE OEC TECHNICIAN

When an incident occurs at a ski slope or other outdoor venue, OEC technicians are generally the first rescuers to arrive on scene (**Figure 4-9**). As a result, they will likely serve in a variety of key ICS roles. Roles that an OEC technician may assume or be assigned include:

- IC
- Operations chief
- Medical branch director
- Triage, treatment, and/or transportation group officers

Depending on the nature and scope of the incident, these roles may be combined as necessary. As IC or operations section chief, an OEC technician is responsible for performing all section-related tasks, as previously described. The first task of the IC is to assume command of the incident by notifying dispatch. The second task is to assess the scene and develop an understanding of what resources will be needed. The third task is to establish a command post. For ski patrollers, the ICP is often located at the bottom of a ski lift, especially if the incident involves a lift. Once the ICP is established, the IC identifies key tasks to be performed, assigns resources to complete the tasks, and manages the overall incident. When serving as the operations section chief, OEC technicians perform and/or oversee all rescue and patient treatment activities. On large or complex incidents, the operations section chief may wish to establish a medical branch, which is managed by a medical branch director who, if desired, can expand this branch into three groups: triage, treatment, and transportation groups.

- *Triage group.* The triage group is responsible for identifying, collecting, and sorting patients. It is managed by a triage officer, who may perform the group's tasks personally or delegate them to others. Depending on the nature of the incident and available resources, the triage officer may establish near the greatest concentration of patients a "triage funnel," which serves as the entry point to the EMS branch and is designed to speed the identification and removal of patients from the incident. OEC technicians who are assigned to the triage group are tasked with the following duties:
  - Prioritize patients for treatment according to injury severity and likelihood of survival (primary triage).
  - Provide minimal care (open the airway, control life-threatening bleeding).
  - Move patients to the treatment area.

  Triage is covered in more detail in the next section.
- *Treatment group.* The treatment group is responsible for providing on-scene care to patients who have been triaged by the triage group. The group is managed by a treatment officer, who oversees the group's activities. OEC technicians who are assigned to the treatment group perform one or more of the following tasks:
  - Establish an easily identifiable treatment area that has been approved by the IC. This task may include individual color-coded areas for each triage category.
  - Reassess each patient's triage status (secondary triage).
  - Provide emergency care to patients in accordance with state and local protocols.
  - Provide an updated casualty report to the EMS branch officer.
  - Prepare patients for transport.
  - Move patients to the transport area.
  - Maintain a written record of activities.
- *Transportation group.* The transportation group oversees the movement of patients from the incident to one or more medical facilities. Depending on the size of the incident, the total number of patients, the severity of patients' injuries, and the resources available, these facilities may include the patrol's mountain aid station. The transportation group is managed by a transportation officer who, like other group officers, may perform the group's tasks personally or delegate them to others. The transportation group is responsible for determining the number of patients in each triage category that each facility within the emergency care system can receive. This report, known as a hospital capacity status report, helps to ensure that patients are properly distributed, and it lessens the chance that any one facility will become overwhelmed by too many patients. The group's other responsibilities include the following:
  - Identify transport needs. This task involves determining how many toboggans, all-terrain vehicles, ambulances, helicopters, and so on are needed.
  - Coordinate the transport and distribution of patients to medical facilities. This task involves determining the mode of transport for each patient and sending patients according to the hospital capacity report and/or in accordance with state, regional, or local protocols.
  - Track patients. This task involves obtaining key patient data and recording which facility each patient was sent to.
  - Provide updates to the EMS branch director, informing the director of current transport needs, how many patients remain on scene, and so on.

  On a large incident, the transportation officer may wish to have an individual serve as a transport coordinator. This person helps ensure the smooth departure of patients from the scene.

In addition to their primary duties, each group is responsible for maintaining a written record of its activities and for submitting individual group reports to the medical branch director, as requested. Once a group has completed all of its assigned tasks, group personnel and resources may be reassigned to perform other incident-related tasks.

CASE Update

You contact patrol dispatch to declare a major MCI, give a brief situation report, and call for additional resources. You also identify yourself as the IC. As IC, you start to determine the nature and extent of the incident by sending your fellow patrollers downhill to assess the situation. At the same time, you establish an ICP in the lift operator's booth, which gives you a sweeping view of the scene. Given the number of patients you can see, you decide that an operations section should be created, and you inform dispatch that you need additional resources, both from the ski area and from the local emergency care system.

A patroller calls you on the radio and tells you there are "at least 30 patients on the ground and at least 120 trapped on the lifts." With this information you begin to formulate your IAP.

A few minutes later, the patrol director enters the ICP and assumes the role of IC. You give her a quick verbal report of the situation and what you have done so far. The transfer of incident command to the patrol director is announced over the radio so that everyone is aware of the change. She then designates you as the operations section chief and directs you to go to the scene to lead the rescue efforts. Upon your arrival, a patroller informs you that the lift has collapsed and that "there are patients all the way down to the bottom!" Before you can catch your breath, a person approaches you and identifies himself as a doctor. He tells you that he is one of several emergency physicians who have come to help.

What should you do now?

TRIAGE

OEC technicians occasionally encounter incidents involving more than one patient, or even large numbers of patients. Such a situation is known as a **multiple-casualty incident (MCI)**—an incident involving two or more patients in which the number of patients exceeds the capability of immediately available resources. When such an incident occurs, rescuers must quickly assess the patients to determine the severity of their conditions and to rapidly identify specific resources that will be needed. The resources available on scene are often not sufficient to meet immediate needs, forcing rescuers to make difficult decisions regarding how to best allocate personnel, equipment, and supplies to maximize their benefit. These decisions, while fraught with emotions, can be made objectively by using a technique known as triage.

Triage is a process of prioritizing patients for treatment and transportation based on specific criteria, depending on the triage method that is being followed. This information serves as a guide for determining the severity of a patient's overall medical condition and provides a basis for determining which patients receive medical care and transportation first. Using this systematic approach, rescuers can assess large numbers of patients in a relatively short period of time. This approach facilitates decision making so that precious resources can be allocated to "do the most good for the most people."

The word *triage* originates from the French verb *trier*, which means "to sort." The concept was first introduced by Baron Dominique Jean Larrey, chief surgeon of Napoleon's Grande Armée, who developed the practice during the Peninsular Wars of the early 19th century as a means of prioritizing the medical needs of battlefield casualties. The practice enabled French physicians to rapidly identify soldiers whose injuries were survivable and who could be made fit to return to active duty in a relatively short period of time. Today, triage is the preferred method for evaluating large numbers of casualties and is a fundamental rescue skill that all OEC technicians must master.

Triage is implemented only when the sheer volume of patients, the severity of injuries, or on-scene problems overwhelm emergency care personnel or outstrip available resources. On small incidents (fewer than 5–10 patients), the IC may elect to perform triage personally. The process provides a means of organizing patients into categories based on their medical needs and moving them out of the immediate (danger) area as expeditiously as possible. There are four common triage categories, which you can remember by using the mnemonic ID-ME (pronounced "I.D. Me"):

- I Immediate (red)
- D Delayed (yellow)
- M Minimal (green)
- E Expectant (black/gray)

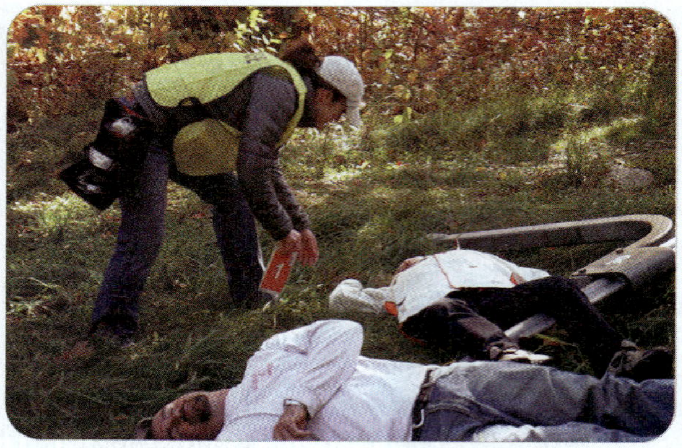

Figure 4-10 Triage tagging at a chairlift MCI scene.

© Mike Halloran.

Triage Methods

There are many different types of triage systems used by EMS agencies and military personnel around the world (**Figure 4-10**). Following is a description of two systems that have gained popularity in the United States, SALT and START. Additionally, comprehensive MCI systems such as SMART are available. The SMART triage system, or pack, offers a full range of ICS and triage resources, including triage tags, triage personnel vests, and the START triage protocol, in one comprehensive package.

Check with your state to determine which triage system you should use. Some states require all emergency care systems to use a single system, whereas others are less stringent.

> **KEY POINT**
>
> **The Teller Lift Collapse**
>
> In December 1985, a faulty weld caused the bullwheel on the Teller Lift at Keystone Resort in Colorado to fall 8 to 10 feet, sending a violent shock wave down the lift cable.
>
> Of the 370 people on the lift at the time of the accident, 50 to 60 were thrown to the ground. It is not known how many people did not have their safety bar down.
>
> Coincidentally, a medical conference was being held at the resort at the time of the accident. As a result, more than 30 emergency physicians were on hand within 15 minutes to help NSP personnel treat the patients.
>
> Two people later died as a result of their injuries.

SALT Triage

The **SALT triage system** is the widely accepted system now highly recommended by EMS agencies in the United States. SALT is an acronym for *s*ort, *a*ssess, *l*ifesaving interventions, and *t*reatment and/or *t*ransport. This system was developed as an all-hazards method of triaging all patients regardless of age or special needs (**Figure 4-11**). It is endorsed by the American College of Emergency Physicians, American Trauma Society, National Association of EMS Physicians, National Disaster Life Support Education Consortium, and State and Territorial Injury Prevention Directors Association.

SALT is essentially a four-step process that allows the responder to quickly triage, tag, and move patients to a location where treatment can safely take place.

Step 1: Sort

The triage officer makes the announcement that all individuals who can *walk* should move immediately to a designated location and will be further triaged and treated later. Those left should be asked to make some purposeful movement, such as waving a hand or moving a leg, which indicates they are

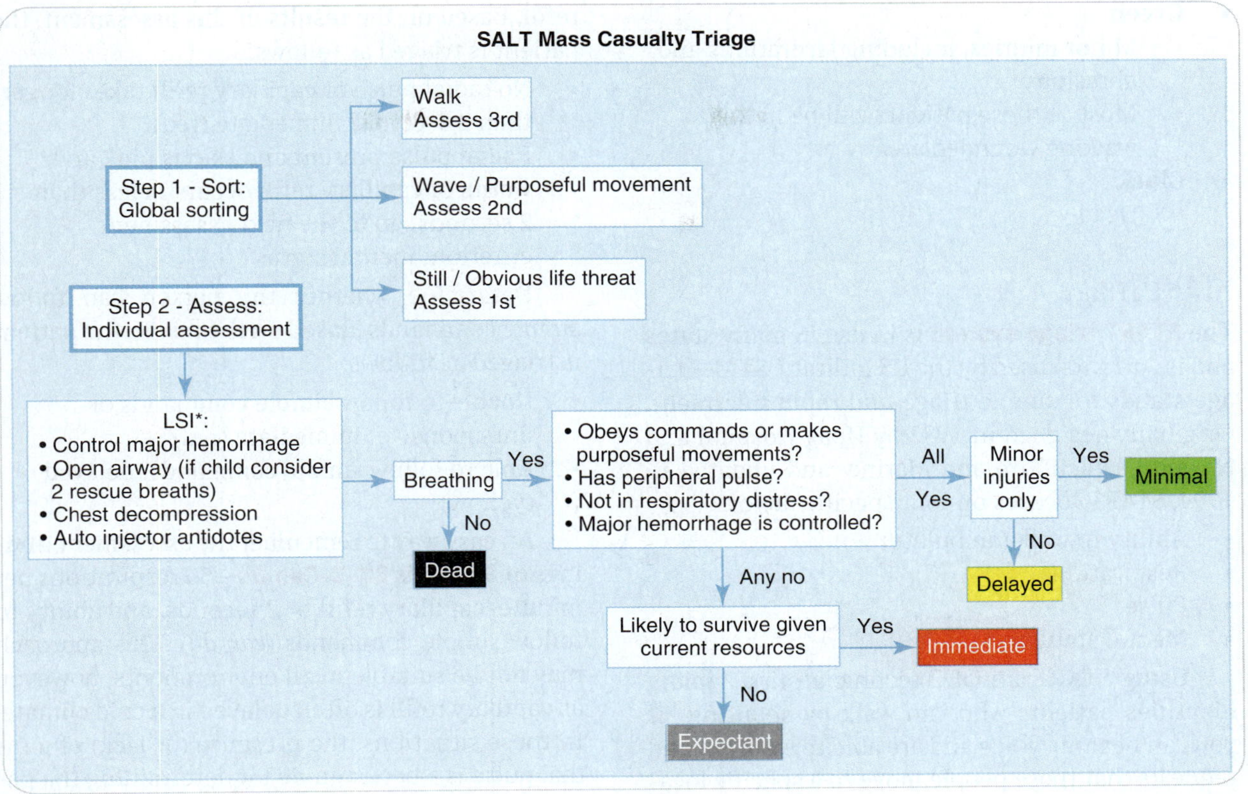

Figure 4-11 The SALT triage flowchart.

Chemical Hazards Emergency Medical Management, U.S. Department of Health and Human Services. http://chemm.nlm.nih.gov/chemmimages/salt.png. Accessed October 16, 2017.

able to follow a command. Those who do not move are considered to have a severe or life-threatening injury and would be triaged first because they may need immediate lifesaving treatment.

Step 2: Assess

This phase begins with assessing each patient and providing immediate lifesaving interventions to those who were unable to walk or wave.

Step 3: Perform Lifesaving Interventions

The lifesaving interventions would include:

- Control major bleeding by using a tourniquet.
- Open the airway by using an oropharyngeal airway or by positioning. No advanced airways are used in this stage. If the patient is a child, two rescue breaths may be given.
- Chest decompression may be conducted if the triage officer is trained in advanced life support and has the equipment on hand.
- Autoinjector antidotes may be given if the triage officer has them on hand since they will take less than a minute to apply and do not require the triage officer to remain with the patient.

Step 4: Provide Treatment and/or Transport

After lifesaving interventions, patients are assigned to a triage category. The SALT triage categories vary slightly from the ID-ME mnemonic. ID-ME presents four *common* triage categories, whereas SALT presents five categories: immediate (red), expectant (gray), delayed (yellow), minimal (green), and black (dead). These categories are described as follows:

- **Red**
  - No peripheral pulse
  - Inability to obey commands
  - Respiratory distress
  - Uncontrolled major hemorrhaging
- **Gray**
  - Injuries that are likely to be fatal based on resources currently available
  - Brain matter showing, burns over 90% of body, or other immediate life-threatening injuries that cannot be resolved
- **Yellow**
  - Fractures, burns, or dislocations
  - Patients who do not fit in other categories

- **Green**
  - Minor injuries, including lacerations and abrasions
  - Most of these patients will be in the walking wounded area
- **Black**
  - Dead

START Triage

The **START triage system** is in use in many states and is currently used by the US military. START triage stands for *s*imple *t*riage *a*nd *r*apid *t*reatment. Originally designed in 1983 by Hoag Hospital and Newport Beach Fire and Marine, and updated in 1994, START focuses on four specific factors:

- Ability to walk (ambulate)
- Respirations
- Pulse
- Mental status

Using START, an OEC technician first rapidly identifies patients who can walk by shouting "If you can hear my voice and are able to walk . . ." and requests that these people move to a specific location, where they are to wait until they can be assessed by other rescuers. This simple tactic allows patients with less-serious injuries to be quickly separated from those with more-serious medical problems. The walking wounded are tentatively triaged as *minimal* (green) but will be reassessed later when more resources become available.

Once the walking wounded have been removed from the area, the remaining patients can generally be triaged into one of the four common triage categories in less than 30 seconds. This categorization centers on assessing the patient's RPMs—that is, their *r*espirations, *p*erfusion, and *m*ental status.

The first step is to assess whether the patient is breathing. If the person is not breathing, attempt to open the airway, using no equipment or medical aids. Obvious foreign bodies or debris should be removed. The patient is then triaged based on the following findings:

- No respirations: expectant or deceased (dead) (black/gray)
- Respirations greater than 30/min: immediate (red)
- Respirations less than 30/min: go to the next assessment criterion: perfusion

Next, check to see if the patient has a heartbeat by assessing the radial pulse or capillary refill. Based on the results of this assessment, the patient is triaged as follows:

- No radial pulse or capillary refill takes longer than 2 seconds: immediate (red)
- Radial pulse present and skin is pink and warm, or capillary refill occurs in less than 2 seconds: go to the next assessment criterion: mental status

Determine whether the person can follow simple commands. Based on the result, the patient is triaged as follows:

- Unable to follow simple commands or unresponsive: immediate (red)
- Able to follow simple commands: delayed (yellow)

An easy way to remember the assessment findings of START is **30-2-Can Do**—*30* respirations per minute, capillary refill of *2* seconds, and ability to follow simple commands (*can do*). This approach may not be suitable in all environments, however, as capillary refill is often delayed in a cold climate. In these situations, the presence (or lack) of a radial pulse is a better guide for determining the patient's perfusion status.

Triage Tags

Triage tags are all-weather cards that are physically attached to the patient or the patient's clothing to indicate the triage category to which the person has been assigned. They enable rescuers to see this information "at a glance," without the need to reassess the patient.

Several types of triage tags are commonly used in the United States, including the Medical Emergency Triage tag, or METTAG, the All-Risk Triage tag, the START triage tag, and the SMART triage tag (**Figure 4-12**). Of these, the METTAG and the SMART tag are the two types that OEC technicians will most likely encounter—unless the incident results in a federal response that includes mobilization of National Guard units, which use a military triage tag known as the Field Medical Card, or FMC. Although all three civilian tags correspond to the four triage categories, both the METTAG and START tags incorporate other universal features that allow them to be used by laypersons during large disasters. All three tags include a unique identifier number, which helps rescuers track patients as they move through the emergency care system. The METTAG and SMART tags also have bar-coding numbers that enable

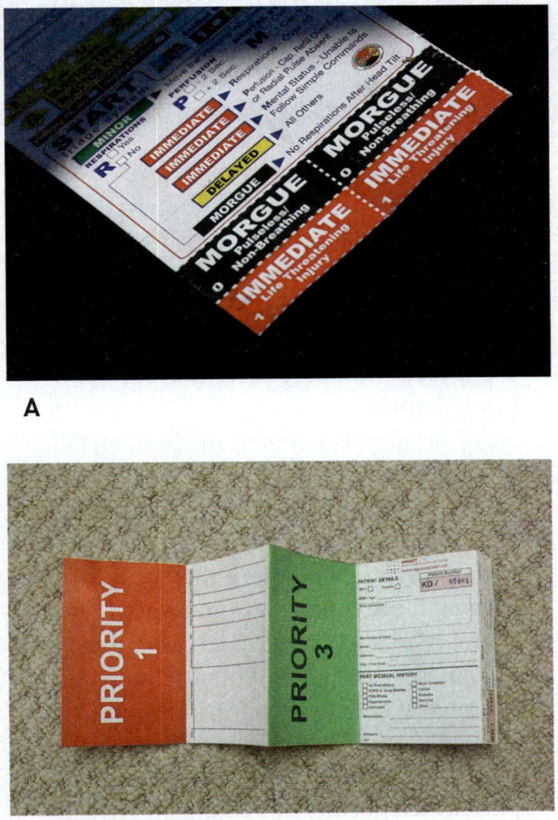

A

B

Figure 4-12 A. A START triage tag is ripped to the level of severity. **B.** A SMART triage tag is folded to the level of severity.

A: © Mike Blake/Reuters; **B:** Courtesy of Richard Pilbery.

new computerized systems to track patients as they move through the medical system.

Triage should be considered a dynamic process that may need to be performed more than once. This is especially true for incidents involving large numbers of patients, because a person's condition can improve or deteriorate over time. For instance, a patient who is found unconscious with a bleeding head wound may initially be triaged as *immediate*, but if the person wakes up and the head wound is found to be a minor laceration that has stopped bleeding, the patient may then be categorized as *delayed* or even as *minimal*. Conversely, a person with apparent anxiety might initially be triaged as *minimal* and subsequently be triaged as *immediate* if the signs and symptoms begin to suggest that the patient is experiencing a heart attack.

Triage may also need to be performed again as additional resources or more-highly trained personnel arrive, or as patients are transported to definitive care facilities, thereby allowing on-scene personnel to assume additional duties. An increase in available resources may allow living patients previously categorized as *expectant* to be reevaluated. For instance, once all other *immediate* patients have been removed from the scene, which increases the resources available, a living patient with a massive head injury who was previously categorized as *expectant* might be automatically upgraded to *immediate*.

CASE Outcome

You soon have several patrollers and ski resort staff members on scene. To maintain a proper span of control, you inform the IC that you are creating two operations branches: a rescue and evacuation branch and a medical branch. You assign a director to each. The rescue branch is tasked with evacuating stranded skiers from the lift, and the medical branch is tasked with assessing, treating, and transporting the patients. The medical branch is expanded into three divisions: triage, treatment, and transportation. A supervisor is assigned to manage each division. Physicians are assigned to the triage and treatment divisions to help care for the patients. Primary triage reveals the following distribution of patients: 11 immediate (red), 18 delayed (yellow), 21 minimal (green), 0 expectant (black/gray). As more resources arrive, they are assigned to one of the two branches.

This incident took more than 4 hours to manage, during which time the operations section evacuated 220 people from the lift and treated or transported more than 100 patients, including 50 who had fallen from the lift.

CHAPTER REVIEW

In Summary

- All rescue organizations and personnel are federally mandated to use the National Incident Management System (NIMS).
- NIMS is a standardized framework for responding to, and managing, emergencies or situations involving multiple jurisdictions.
- NIMS provides numerous benefits that enable rescuers from different agencies to work together effectively at an incident.
- As part of NIMS's federal mandate, all rescue organizations within the United States must adopt the incident command system (ICS).
- The ICS provides a method for managing any incident, regardless of its cause, size, scope, or complexity.
- The ICS structure consists of five functional areas: incident command, operations, planning, logistics, and finance/administration.
- Incident command is the first functional area to be established at any incident and is managed by an incident commander (IC).
- If needed, incident command can be expanded to include a public information officer, an incident safety officer, and a liaison officer. The IC and these three officers are known as the command staff.
- Every incident must have an IC.
- The operations section is responsible for executing the strategies of the incident action plan (IAP).
- The planning section collects, assesses, distributes, and uses incident-related data. It also coordinates the preparation of the IAP and other incident documents.
- The logistics section provides support for all the functional areas.
- The finance/administration section is responsible for providing financial management, accountability, and administrative services to support incident management activities.
- When an incident occurs at a ski slope or other outdoor venue, OEC technicians are generally the first rescuers to arrive on scene and will likely serve in a variety of key ICS roles.
- As IC or operations section chief, an OEC technician is responsible for performing all section-related tasks.
- OEC technicians occasionally encounter incidents involving more than one patient, or even large numbers of patients. When such an incident occurs, rescuers must quickly assess the patients to determine the severity of their conditions and to rapidly identify specific resources that will be needed. This process includes patient triage, or prioritizing patients for treatment and transportation based on specific criteria.
- The four common triage categories can be remembered using the acronym ID-ME: *i*mmediate (red), *d*elayed (yellow), *m*inimal (green), or *e*xpectant (black/gray).
- Several methods of triage are used throughout the world, including SALT and START.
    - SALT is an acronym for *s*ort, *a*ssess, *l*ifesaving interventions, and *t*reatment and/or *t*ransport.
    - START is an acronym for *s*imple *t*riage *a*nd *r*apid *t*reatment.
- Triage tags are all-weather cards that are physically attached to the patient or the patient's clothing to indicate the triage category to which the person has been assigned. Several types of triage tags are commonly used in the United States.
- Triage is a dynamic process that may need to be performed more than once.

Key Terms

30–2-Can Do A mnemonic for remembering the assessment findings of the START triage system: *30* respirations per minute, capillary refill of *2* seconds, and ability to follow simple commands (*can do*).

Chain of command A rank structure for management.

Facility Any primary work area in or around an incident in which incident-related activities are planned, organized, directed, or conducted.

Incident Anything out of ordinary day-to-day activities that necessitates a response (e.g., emergencies, disasters, outbreaks, vaccination programs, important meetings or conferences).

Incident commander (IC) The person who provides overall leadership at an incident.

Incident command system (ICS) A formal, organized method for managing an incident, regardless of its cause, size, scope, or complexity.

Multiagency coordination system (MACS) A process for managing an incident in which multiple agencies that have different command structures and communication capabilities are participating.

Multiple-casualty incident (MCI) An incident involving two or more patients and in which the number of patients exceeds the capability of local resources.

National Incident Management System (NIMS) A federally mandated "all-hazards" approach for responding to and managing an incident. It was created as a result of Homeland Security Presidential Directive 5.

Personnel accountability system A system that readily identifies both the locations and the functions of all members operating at an incident scene.

Resource management Under NIMS, a response component that includes mutual-aid agreements; the use of special federal, state, local, and tribal teams; and resource mobilization protocols.

SALT triage system A triage system developed as an all-hazards method of triaging all patients regardless of age or special need. The acronym SALT stands for *s*ort, *a*ssess, *l*ifesaving interventions, and *t*reatment and/or *t*ransport.

Section chiefs The heads of the functional areas within the incident command system.

Span of control The total number of individuals or resources supervised by a single person; usually three to seven individuals or resources. The optimal number is considered to be five.

START triage system A triage system commonly used by public safety personnel. The acronym START stands for *s*imple *t*riage *a*nd *r*apid *t*reatment.

Strike team A group of resources of the same size or type that is managed by a strike team leader (e.g., a group of Nordic patrollers).

Task force A combination of different resources with common communications that is managed by a task force leader (e.g., a sheriff's deputy, an NSP Alpine patrol, and a search-and-rescue team).

Triage A process of prioritizing patients for treatment and transportation based on their clinical signs and symptoms. It operates under the philosophy of "Do the most good for the most people."

Chapter Questions

1. The incident command system has:
   a. three functional layers.
   b. four functional layers.
   c. five functional layers.
   d. six functional layers.
2. The incident command system is used for:
   a. mass-casualty incidents only.
   b. small-casualty incidents only.
   c. mass-casualty incidents and wildfires only.
   d. all-hazards management plans.

3. The incident commander always needs to appoint a(n):
   a. public information officer.
   b. incident safety officer.
   c. liaison officer.
   d. None of the above
4. The planning section is responsible for all of the following *except*:
   a. determining incident resource needs.
   b. developing a transportation system or supply line.
   c. gathering and analyzing incident-related data.
   d. preparing contingencies and alternative strategies.
5. START focuses on all of the following *except*:
   a. ability to walk.
   b. respirations.
   c. pulse.
   d. pain level.
6. What color tag should be used for a START patient who has capillary refill greater than 2 seconds?
   a. Black
   b. Red
   c. Yellow
   d. Green
7. SALT uses gray tags for patients:
   a. who have no visible injuries.
   b. who appear to have lost some mental functions.
   c. who are likely to die.
   d. All of the above
8. SALT uses yellow tags for patients:
   a. who are not expected to survive.
   b. who can walk to a safe area.
   c. with respiratory distress.
   d. with injuries that do not fit in other categories.

Reference

US Department of Homeland Security. n.d. NIMS Frequently Asked Questions. https://www.fema.gov/pdf/emergency/nims/nimsfaqs.pdf. Accessed October 3, 2019.

Answers: 1. c, Objective 4-1, p. 70; 2. d, Objective 4-1, p. 69; 3. d, Objective 4-2, p. 70; 4. b, Objective 4-2, p. 73; 5. d, Objective 4-5, p. 80; 6. b, Objective 4-5, p. 79; 7. c, Objective 4-4, p. 79; 8. d, Objective 4-4, p. 79

CHAPTER 5

MOVING, LIFTING, AND TRANSPORTING PATIENTS

OBJECTIVES

Upon completion of this chapter, the OEC technician will be able to:

5-1 Explain how to use good body mechanics.

5-2 Demonstrate the following:
- Power grip
- Power lift

5-3 Demonstrate the moves that can be used when there is not a spinal injury:
- Extremity lift
- Direct ground lift
- BEAN/bridge lift

5-4 Demonstrate the moves that can be used when you suspect a spinal injury:
- Draw-sheet, plastic slider, or flat transfer lift
- Logroll

5-5 Demonstrate the following urgent moves:
- Shoulder drag
- Feet drag
- Blanket drag
- Underarm-wrist drag

5-6 Demonstrate the following nonurgent moves:
- Human crutch
- Two-person assist
- Chair carry
- Fore-and-aft carry

5-7 Describe and demonstrate the use of the following devices for lifting and moving patients:
- Backboard
- Portable stretcher
- Scoop stretcher
- Basket/Stokes stretcher
- Sitting lifting device

5-8 Discuss how you place a patient in a toboggan while protecting the injury.

5-9 Explain the purpose and correct steps of packaging a patient.

5-10 Explain a landing zone and proper helicopter safety.

KEY TERMS

Body mechanics, p. 86
Carry, p. 88
Drag, p. 88
Landing zone (LZ), p. 108
Lift, p. 88
Move, p. 87
Spinal motion restriction, p. 87

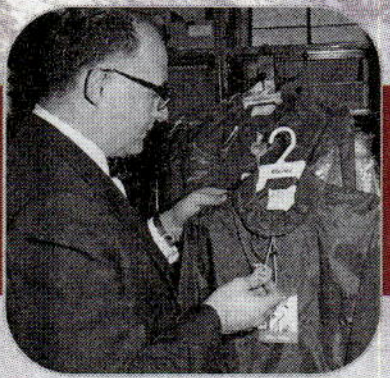

HISTORICAL TIMELINE

1946. NSP adopts "Rainier red"–colored jackets from the White Stag company as the official patroller jacket.

CHAPTER OVERVIEW

As an OEC technician you will care for backcountry, bike path, ski slope, and indoor patients who need to be lifted, moved, or positioned for care. Sometimes you will perform these tasks under difficult conditions, often with limited resources. In addition to moving or lifting patients from awkward positions, OEC technicians may need to carry, lift, or transport a patient package weighing more than 300 pounds. Even when sharing this weight between other rescuers, it can be extremely difficult on ice, snow, or uneven terrain.

Transporting a patient is a role an OEC technician performs on a regular basis. Transport can be performed on foot with the patient walking with assistance, by skiing down a slope with the patient in a toboggan, by carrying the patient strapped to a backboard or litter, or by using motorized ground vehicles. Transport can be a complex task with decisions based on numerous factors, including manpower, safety, weather, equipment, and specific patient needs that require advanced care. Rapid packaging and transport of a patient to definitive care are important.

This chapter will help OEC technicians learn how to lift, move, and transport a patient in a safe and efficient manner. It also describes body mechanics and proper lifting techniques (**Figure 5-1**). Urgent and nonurgent moves are covered, as are various moving and transporting devices. The chapter concludes with a discussion about final transport of the patient and basic helicopter operations and safety.

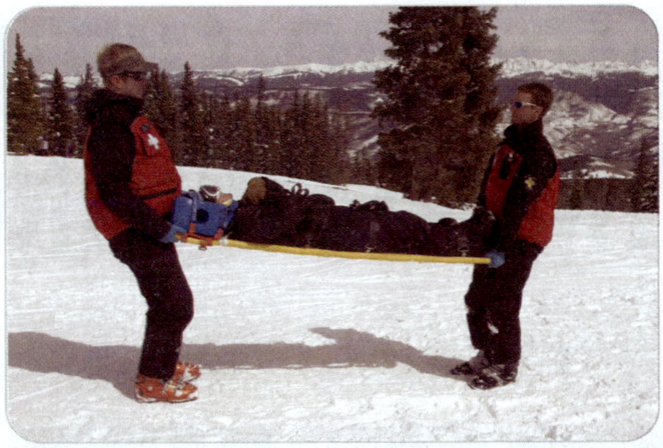

Figure 5-1 When lifting a patient on a backboard or to a gurney, you must use good body mechanics to protect your back.

BODY MECHANICS

When moving or transporting a patient, the top priority is your own safety. Many injuries sustained by OEC technicians can be prevented by understanding the **body mechanics** of lifting and practicing good lifting techniques. Statistics from national EMS organizations report that as many as 50% of emergency medical responders have sustained a back injury that resulted in loss of time at work. Make sure you are not one of these statistics. When lifting a heavy patient, use your strong leg muscles, not your back muscles. The upper thigh leg muscles are well suited for lifting. They are among the strongest muscles in the body.

The use of good body mechanics distributes the weight evenly down the entire spinal column, through the pelvis, and to the bones of the legs. The shoulders need to be aligned over the spine, not in front of or behind the upright spine. When a person exhibits poor body mechanics and lifts improperly, the vertebrae are misaligned (**Figure 5-2A**). This misalignment causes the load to be unevenly distributed, and the resulting force can damage discs, spinal nerves, and/or adjacent muscles and ligaments. In some cases, this damage

CASE Presentation

Having arrived at the bottom of a chairlift that has malfunctioned and stopped, you make sure the chairlift is "locked" and will not move. You find the patient unresponsive on the ground with a chair still hanging above him at the loading area. Helping this person is very difficult, because the chair is obstructing your ability to perform a patient assessment.

What are the first steps you should take?

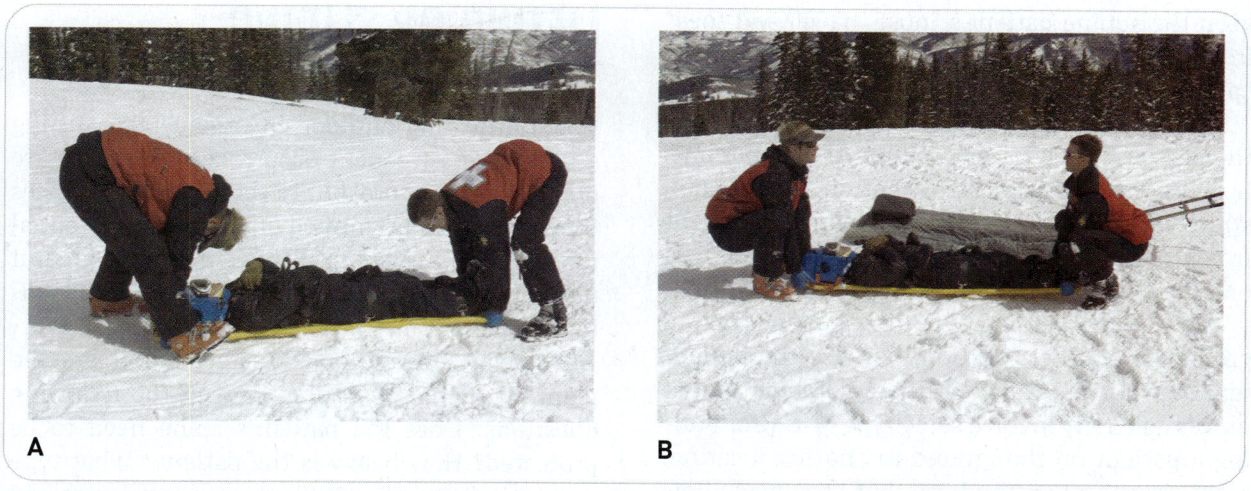

Figure 5-2 Reduce your risk of sustaining a lift-related back injury. **A.** Using improper lifting/body mechanics could result in an injury to your back. **B.** Use the proper position when preparing to lift.

can be long-term or even permanent. Protect your back! Stay as close to the patient as possible, keeping your back straight.

Follow these back-smart tips to reduce your risk of sustaining a lift-related back injury (Figure 5-2B):

1. Know your physical limitations.
2. Plan the move and/or lift.
3. Get help! Do not try to move or lift an object that is too heavy to handle by yourself.
4. Keep your feet at shoulders' width.
5. Keep your back straight. (Do not bend at the waist.)
6. Get a good grip on the object being lifted.
7. Bend your knees.
8. Lift with your legs, not with your back.
9. Keep your shoulders centered over the upright, aligned spine.
10. Keep the object close to your body.
11. Keep your head up as you lift.
12. Turn moving your feet, not your hips or back. (Avoid twisting your back.)
13. When lifting, make sure you communicate clearly with other people lifting.

MOVING A PATIENT

A **move** is the transport of a patient from one location to another. A move may be just a few inches, or it can be many feet. It may be performed in an urgent way using one or two rescuers or in a more controlled manner using multiple rescuers. Some patients require minimal assistance in moving, whereas others cannot move at all on their own. Once a patient is under your care, you are responsible for their safety. Dropping a patient is one of the greatest areas of liability in emergency medical care. It may be appropriate to allow a patient to assist in a move, but don't allow the patient to move unassisted.

Using the right method and the right equipment for the situation is important for reducing the risk of injury to the patient and yourself. A wheelchair, stair chair, or military-type stretcher kept in the aid room can be used to move many patients. Keep in mind that when caring for patients, we often move them at least three times.

1. From the ground to a toboggan or stretcher
2. From the toboggan or stretcher to the exam table
3. From the exam table to the ambulance stretcher or other means of transport

A patient can be lifted, dragged, or carried. For a patient in great pain due to illness or physical injury, a move can be traumatic. Each move may further aggravate the patient's condition. Plan for any problems that could occur before moving a patient. When performing any move with multiple helpers, a command such as "Lift on three" is given by the lead rescuer.

Some trauma situations require protecting the injured person's spine, or restricting the spine from motion. This is referred to as **spinal motion restriction**. Moves for patients needing spinal motion restriction observe two basic principles: keep the patient's spine in the best anatomic alignment possible, and minimize spinal movement. An easy way to remember these principles is to always keep the supine patient's "nose, navel, and toes" in a straight line, which keeps the long axis of the spine in proper alignment.

A **lift** is a way of moving the patient by raising the person from a lower position to a higher one. It is used for putting the patient on a backboard, stretcher, litter, or toboggan; removing the patient from a vehicle; or simply moving the person from one surface to another.

A **drag** is a method of pulling a patient on the ground to another location. Because the patient may be unresponsive or incapacitated, urgent moves generally involve some type of drag or pulling a patient on the ground to another location. Most drags protect the head, but they may allow the spine to flex or move, which can aggravate any spinal injury that is present. In an emergency, if there is no better way possible to move the patient, always drag the unresponsive patient in a straight line, reducing sideways movement of the spine. The winter environment and snow can be used to your advantage. Use the frozen surface to slide the patient in a rescue sled rather than attempting a carry.

A **carry** is the act of lifting and moving the patient, usually a short distance. When outside, a backboard with straps can be used as a litter for carrying the patient short distances. Longer distances require special litters or carrying methods.

LIFTING OR SLIDING THE PATIENT

When providing outdoor emergency care, lifting a patient is a frequent occurrence. Most lifts are nonurgent in nature, but in certain circumstances they need to be performed urgently. The potential for rescuer injury when lifting a patient is great if not performed correctly. When appropriate, sliding the patient may be easier than lifting.

Lifting a heavy object safely requires some planning. Begin by asking yourself the following questions: Does the patient's spine need to be protected? How heavy is the patient? What type of terrain is involved? Which carrying device will work best for the situation? Is there risk of further harm to the patient?

Power Grip

The power grip maximizes the force of the hands and enables you to firmly grip and hold on to an object. This technique can be used with the power lift (described next) when lifting or moving a patient. The power grip provides the tightest grip possible by ensuring that the palms and fingers are in constant contact with the object.

To perform the power grip, follow the steps in **OEC Skill 5-1**.

OEC SKILL 5-1 Performing the Power Grip

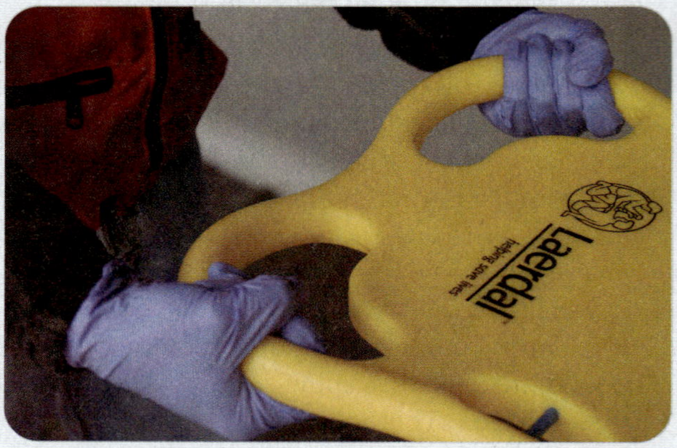

1. Place your hands, palms up, approximately 10 inches apart.
2. Reach underneath the object that is being lifted and firmly grasp the object, closing your hands.
3. If possible, loop your thumb over your index and middle fingers.

Power Lift

Weight lifters have long known the importance of proper form, enabling them to lift heavy weight without becoming injured. This technique, the power lift, uses good body mechanics and the power of the leg muscles. The power lift is a good method of lifting because it aligns the spine and evenly distributes the weight to be lifted.

To perform a power lift, follow the steps in **OEC Skill 5-2**.

Patient Moves Without Spinal Protection

The Extremity Lift

The extremity lift is a commonly used lift in rescue operations. The responsive patient may be lying at ground level or sitting. A word of caution: this lifting method places pressure on the patient's chest and thus may not be tolerated by all patients, especially elderly patients and patients with breathing disorders. It is specifically indicated for any patient who does not have a spine injury and must be moved quickly from one location to another. This lift is often used to move a patient onto a transport device. It is not recommended for patients who are very heavy or obese.

To perform an extremity lift, follow the steps in **OEC Skill 5-3**.

Direct Ground Lift

A direct ground lift is used to raise a patient lying on his or her back and place the patient onto a flat surface such as a stretcher, bed, or backboard

OEC SKILL 5-2 Performing the Power Lift

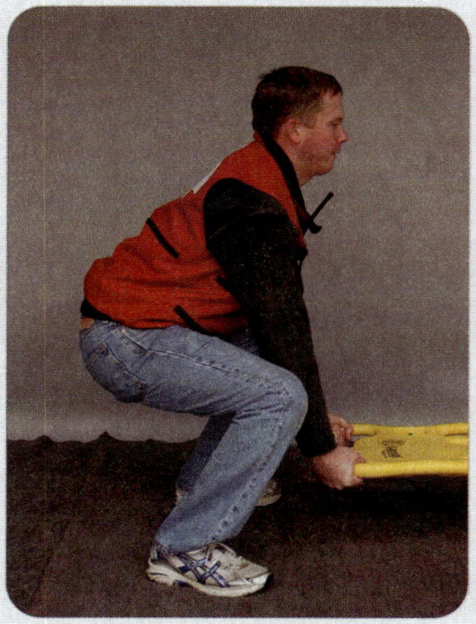

1 Maintain a wide stance by placing your feet shoulder-width apart (approximately 15 inches apart). Bend your knees and squat, keeping your back straight and your shoulders over the spine. Firmly grasp the item to be lifted with your palms up (power grip).

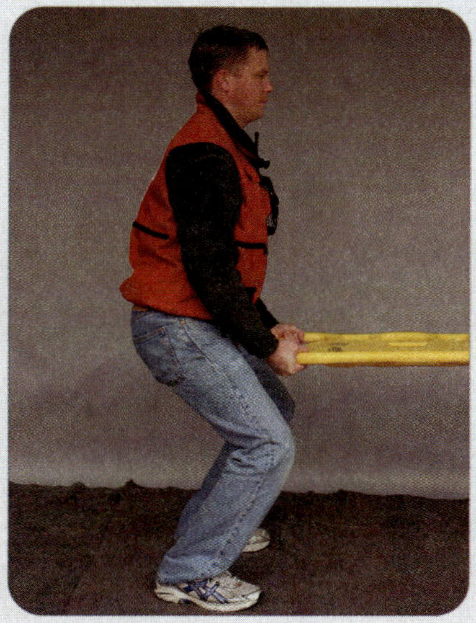

2 Keep your back straight and your head up.

(continues)

OEC SKILL 5-2 Performing the Power Lift (*continued*)

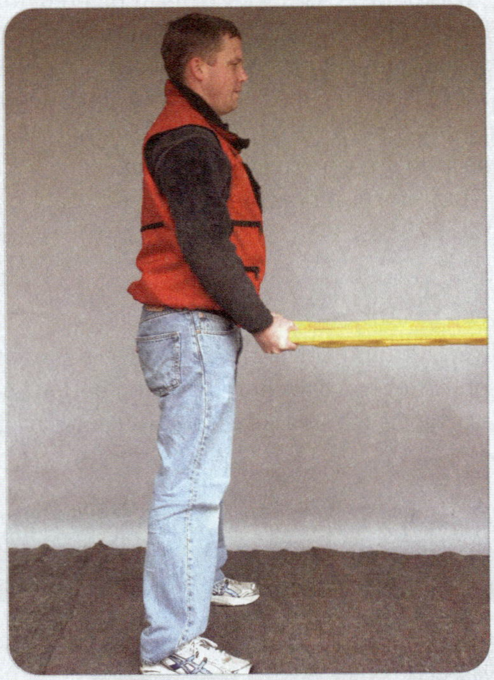

© Mike Halloran.

3 Straighten your legs to lift the object.

OEC SKILL 5-3 Performing the Extremity Lift

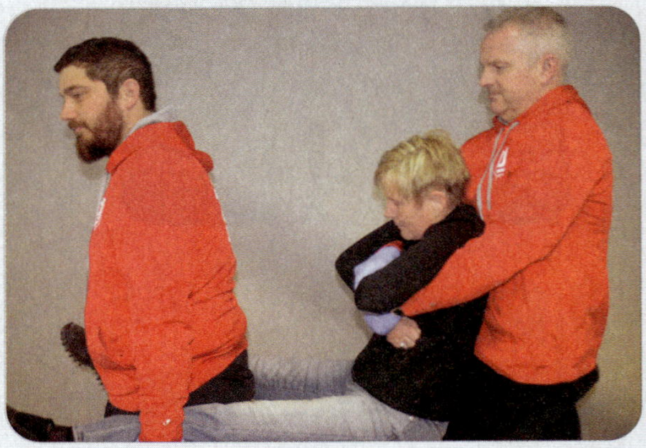

1 The rescuers place the patient in a sitting position with the arms crossed on the chest. Rescuer 1 reaches under the armpits, grabbing the patient's wrists.

2 Rescuer 2 holds and supports the patient's legs at the knees.

3 When a command is given, both rescuers move into a crouching position, keeping their spines straight and heads up, and then lift the patient at the same time.

4 Once both rescuers are standing, they may carry the patient.

used as a litter. This lift is only for patients who do not have a suspected spinal injury. It may be performed with as few as two rescuers, but ideally it is performed using four rescuers. The patient is placed supine (on the back) and then is lifted with all rescuers maintaining a safe back position.

To perform a direct ground lift, follow the steps in **OEC Skill 5-4**.

BEAN/Bridge Lift

Like a direct ground lift, a BEAN, or bridge, lift is used to raise a patient who is lying on his or her

OEC SKILL 5-4 Performing the Direct Ground Lift

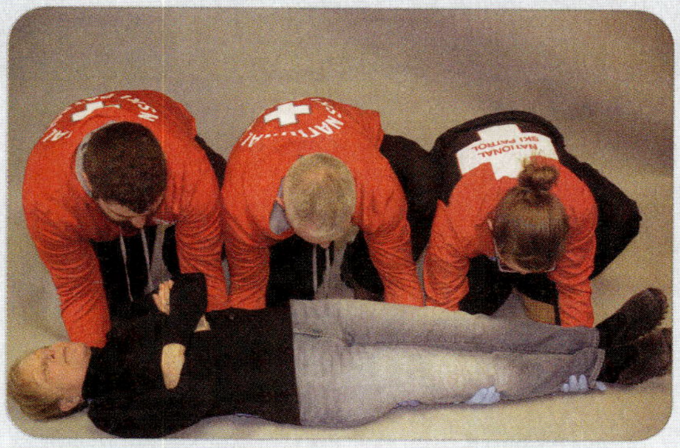

1 All the rescuers kneel along the same side of the patient.

- If there are two rescuers, one should be at the patient's head and chest and the other should be at the patient's pelvis and knees.
- If there are three rescuers, they should be at the patient's head, chest/waist, and buttocks/knees.
- If there are four rescuers, they should be at the patient's head, chest, waist, and knees.

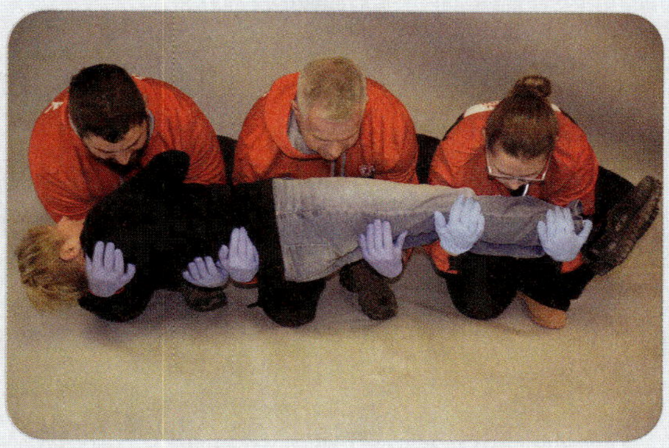

2 The rescuers place their arms under the patient, with one rescuer holding the head. The rescuer at the patient's head usually directs the lift. When the person in charge gives the command, the rescuers roll the patient toward their chests.

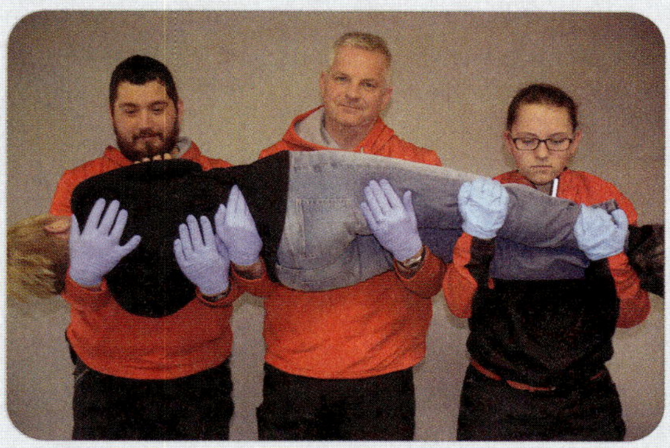

3 On command, the rescuers all stand in unison. On command, the rescuers lower the patient onto the equipment in unison.

back. There should be no suspicion of spinal injury. BEAN is an acronym for *b*ody *e*levation *a*nd *n*onmovement. The BEAN technique uses four to six rescuers and involves keeping the patient in proper anatomic alignment and raising the patient from the ground while a backboard is slid under the patient.

To perform a BEAN or bridge lift, follow the steps in **OEC Skill 5-5**.

Patient Moves with Spinal Motion Restriction/Protection

Draw-Sheet, Plastic Slider, or Flat Transfer Lift

The draw-sheet, plastic slider, or flat transfer lift technique can lift a patient a few inches or can be used to transfer a patient a very short distance. It

OEC SKILL 5-5 Performing the BEAN/Bridge Lift

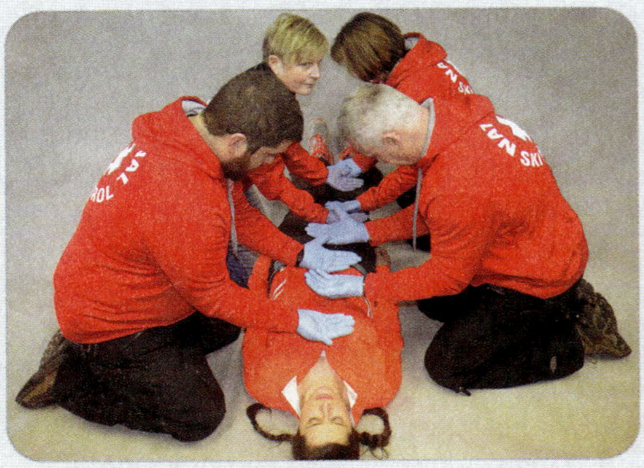

1 Two or three rescuers kneel on either side of the patient, staggering their positions. An additional rescuer or bystander will be required to move the backboard into position at the appropriate time.

- If there are four rescuers, they should be at the patient's head, chest, waist, and knees. An additional rescuer or bystander will be required to move the backboard into position at the appropriate time.
- If there are five rescuers, they should be at the patient's head, chest, waist, thighs, and knees. An additional rescuer or bystander will be required to move the backboard into position at the appropriate time.
- It is recommended that rescuers rehearse the lift by placing their hands on top of the patient to determine where their hands will be placed under the patient. The hands are alternately sequenced to ensure sufficient coverage.

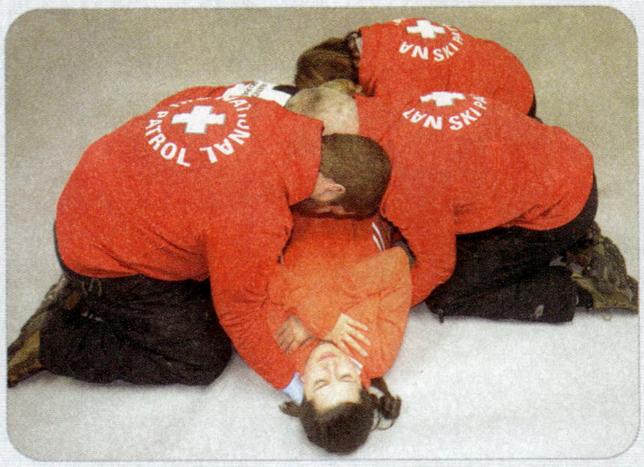

2 Rescuers then place their arms under the patient, following the same pattern as rehearsed. Ideally, the rescuers' arms should be nearly touching.

OEC SKILL 5-5 Performing the BEAN/Bridge Lift (*continued*)

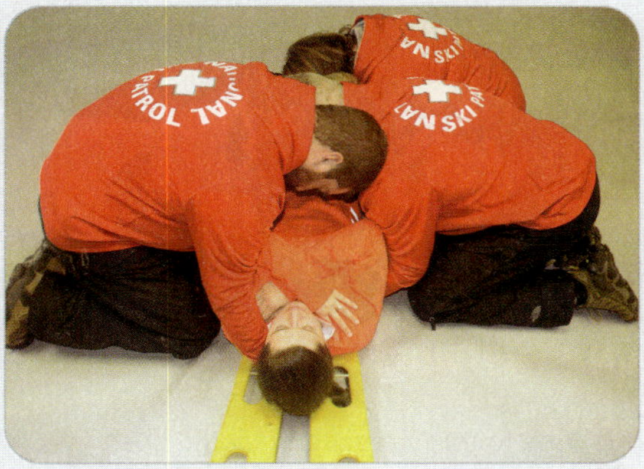

3 One rescuer prepares the backboard or other device. The rescuer closest to the patient's head directs the lift. On command, rescuers raise the patient about 5 to 6 inches.

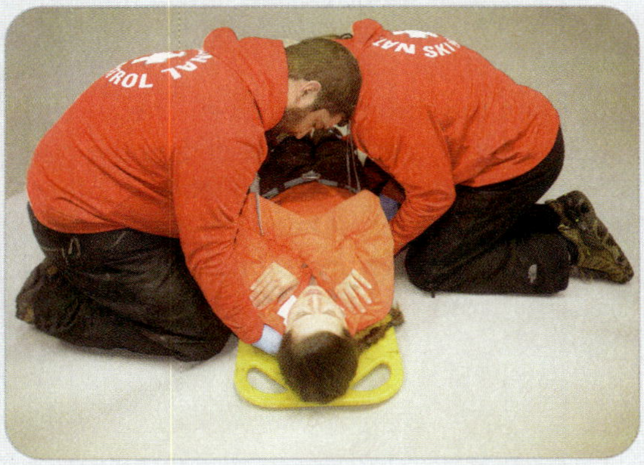

4 The backboard is positioned under the patient, sliding it up from the patient's feet. To lower the patient, the steps are reversed.

may be used when transferring a patient from an elevated ski toboggan onto a cart or an examination table, or to an ambulance stretcher from an examination table. A draw-sheet lift, or flat transfer, is accomplished with a sheet of plastic or fabric that is placed under a patient and then used to slightly raise the patient or slide him or her from one surface to another. A draw sheet may be improvised using a standard bed sheet or blanket, or it may be commercially produced. Commercial products are favored because they generally have handles, which facilitate the lift. One of these products is the SKED, which is a heavy sheet of plastic that rolls up for storage and transport. When folded around the patient, the SKED becomes semi-rigid, also allowing transport of the patient by lifting horizontally or vertically (when the patient is strapped in securely) or by sliding on the smooth bottom surface.

Of the four lifting/sliding techniques described, this method has the lowest risk of back injury to rescuers. It involves pulling the patient once the sliding device is placed under the patient. Great caution must be used when transferring a large or heavy patient using a sheet because the fabric can rip.

To perform a draw-sheet, plastic slider, or flat transfer lift, follow the steps in **OEC Skill 5-6**.

Logrolling a Patient

One way of placing a patient onto a backboard or assessing the patient's spine is by using a logroll. When properly done, the spine is kept in

OEC SKILL 5-6 Performing the Draw-Sheet, Plastic Slider, or Flat Transfer Lift

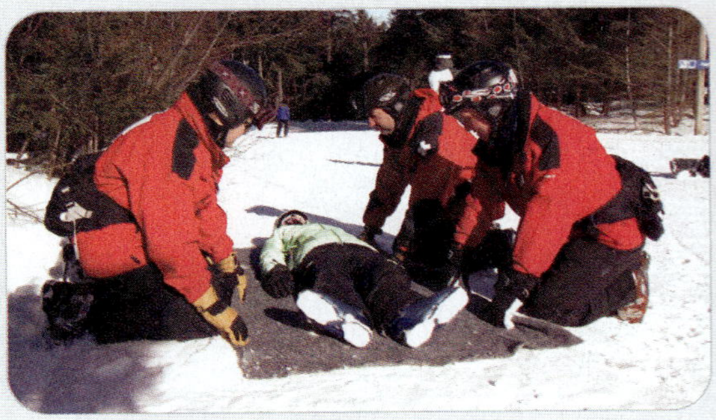

1 The rescuers place a sheet, blanket, or plastic device under the patient, using a logroll in both directions to protect the spine if necessary.

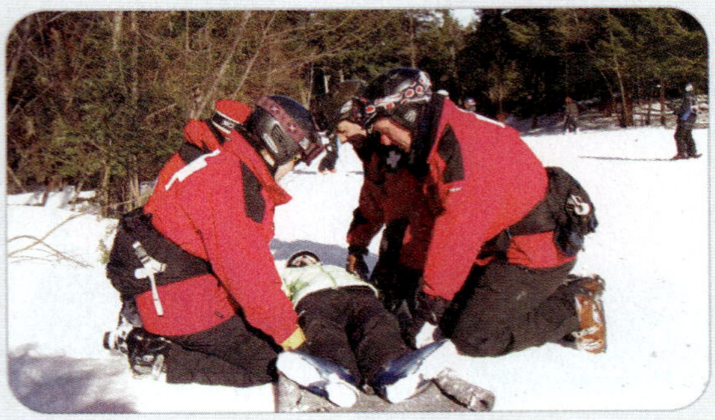

2 One to three rescuers should position themselves on each side of the patient and should roll the edges of the sheet up to the patient's sides.

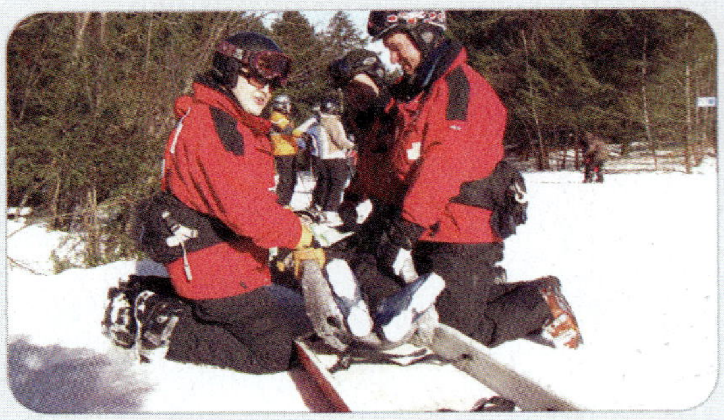

3 When the command is given, the rescuers gently lift while sliding the patient to the destination bed, table, or other flat surface. They must keep the patient's body in alignment when transferring.

KEY POINT

Pelvis Fractures: Using a Lift is the Preferred Method

People with pelvic fractures should not be logrolled unless absolutely necessary. Pelvic fractures are unstable, and the blood that has clotted around each fracture site will be disturbed by logrolling, causing increased internal bleeding and possibly shock. After applying the pelvic binder, it is best to gently use the BEAN lift for patients with a suspected pelvic fracture. One way to apply the pelvic binder would be to slide it under the knees or behind the middle of the back and then slowly inch it into place using one person on each side of the patient. If there also is a suspected spinal column injury, protect the spine by keeping it straight as you minimally lift, and be gentle with the pelvis. Follow the spinal motion restriction assessment, discussed in Chapter 21, *Spine, Brain, and Nervous System Injuries*, to determine possible spinal injury. In the event that there is not enough help available, another technique may need to be considered for the move to include sliding the patient onto the board lengthwise.

alignment. This method can be used when you suspect a spinal injury.

To perform a logroll, follow the steps in **OEC Skill 5-7**.

URGENT AND NONURGENT MOVES

Depending on the situation, OEC technicians perform two types of moves: urgent moves and nonurgent moves. Regardless of the type of move, one principle must be observed: the patient cannot be dropped or allowed to fall. Remember, the first principle of medicine is "Do no harm." If during your assessment a spinal injury is suspected, protect the patient's spine.

Urgent Moves

As the name implies, an urgent move is reserved for situations in which the patient and/or rescuer must move quickly to safety or the patient's medical condition is life threatening and requires

OEC SKILL 5-7 Logrolling a Supine Patient onto a Backboard

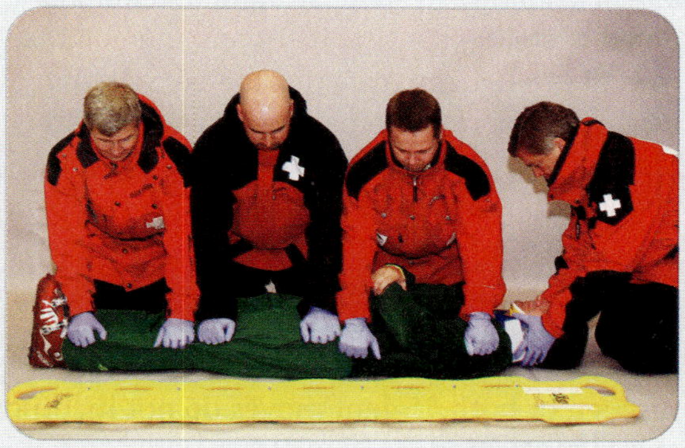

1 Three or four rescuers kneel on the side of the patient away from the backboard, staggering their positions. These rescuers have their knees up against the patient. An additional rescuer needs to maintain proper head and neck position of the patient.

- If the patient is unresponsive, it may help to tie the patient's ankles and feet together with a cravat first.
- If there are three rescuers, they should be at the patient's head, chest, and thighs. If there are four rescuers, they should be at the patient's head, chest, waist, and knees.
- It is recommended that rescuers first place their hands on the top of the patient to determine where their hands will be placed under the patient. The hands are alternately sequenced (may be crisscrossed) to ensure sufficient coverage.

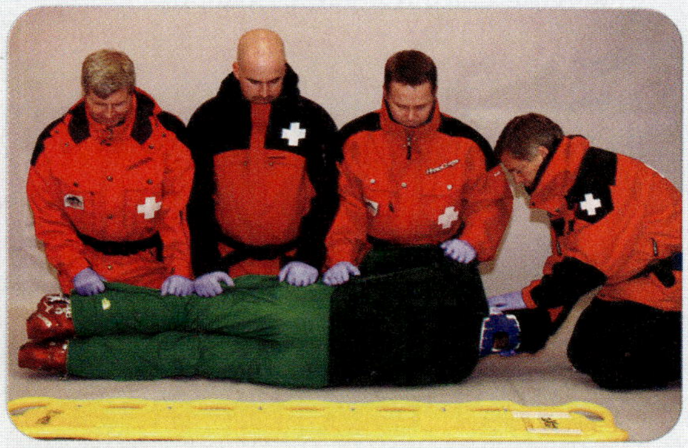

2 Usually the rescuer at the head is the lead. While maintaining the head in axial alignment, the lead calls the roll. Rescuers reach across the patient and grab the clothing firmly, following the same pattern as rehearsed. Ideally, the rescuers' arms should be nearly touching. When the lead rescuer gives the command, the rescuers roll the patient onto the side, toward themselves and up against their thighs, keeping the spine straight. The rescuer at the head keeps the head and neck in alignment with the rest of the spine.

(continues)

OEC SKILL 5-7 Logrolling a Supine Patient onto a Backboard (*continued*)

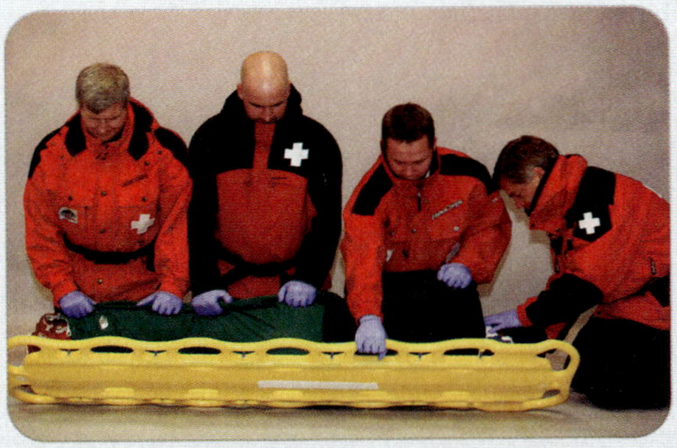

3 On another command, rescuers roll the patient back onto the backboard or stretcher, keeping the spine straight.

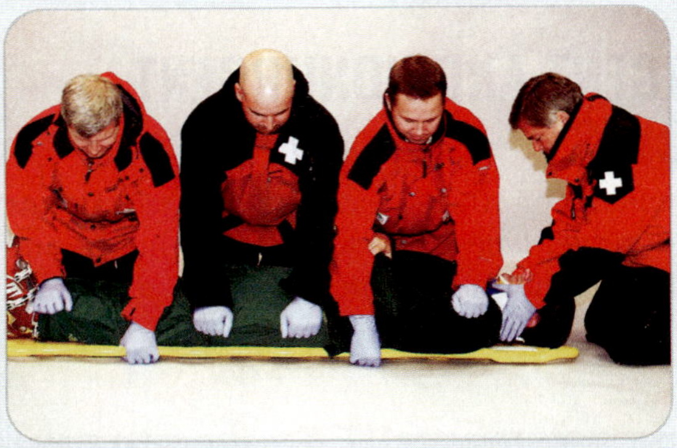

4 If the patient is not centered on the backboard, long-axis drags (described later), keeping the spine straight and pulling under the patient's shoulders and then on the feet, are then used to center the patient. A side slide, moving the patient in a coordinated fashion so that the spine remains in alignment, is acceptable.

KEY POINT

Situations Requiring Urgent Moves

Some situations requiring urgent moves include:

- Risk of avalanche
- Fire, explosion, or structural collapse
- Hazardous materials
- Risk of rock fall
- Rising water
- Wild animals present
- Very bad weather that makes care impossible
- Patient with cardiac arrest who needs CPR

immediate transport. The primary indication for an urgent move is the presence of a hazard that could prove life threatening to the patient, the rescuer, or both. Urgent moves do not incorporate spinal protection.

In most instances, an urgent move is performed before the patient is assessed. However, because the dynamics of a scene can change quickly, an urgent move may be performed at any time when the patient must be moved quickly and there is insufficient time or resources to perform the move in a more controlled or leisurely fashion. Among the many factors that determine the difficulty of an urgent move are the terrain, the patient's size and weight, and the number of rescuers available to assist. Most urgent moves are short distances. The greatest risks when performing an urgent move are delaying lifesaving interventions (e.g., opening the airway, controlling external bleeding), aggravating an existing injury, or injuring a rescuer.

Long-axis drags are commonly used for urgent moves. There are four types of long-axis drags:

1. Shoulder (or clothes) drag (**Figure 5-3**)
   - Bend down on one knee and grab the patient's clothing at the shoulders.

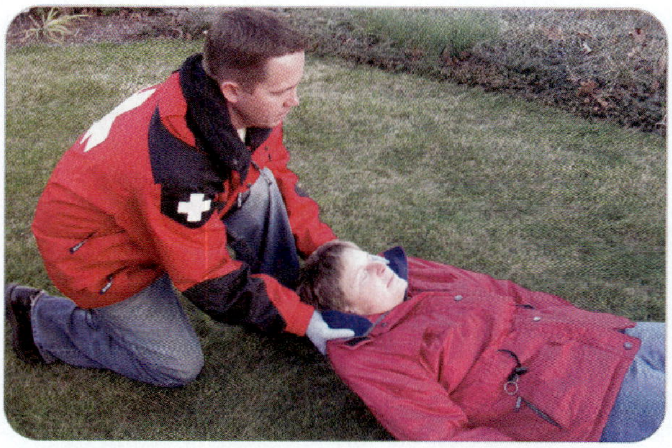

Figure 5-3 A one-rescuer shoulder drag.

© Edward McNamara.

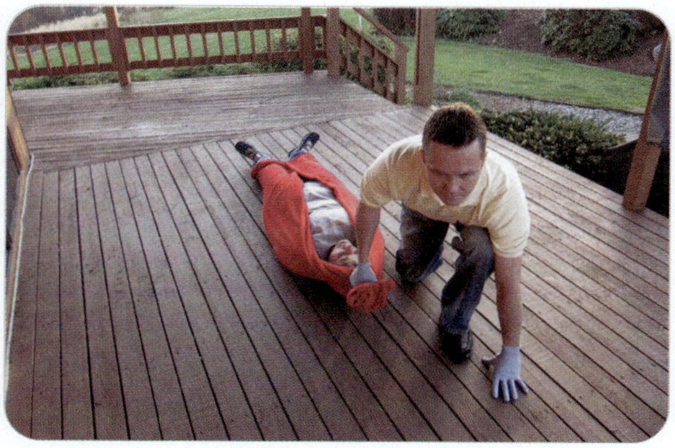

Figure 5-5 The one-rescuer blanket drag.

© Edward McNamara.

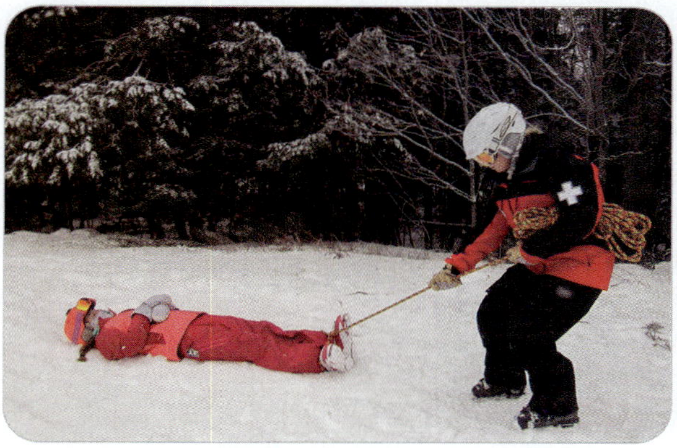

Figure 5-4 The feet drag.

© Edward McNamara.

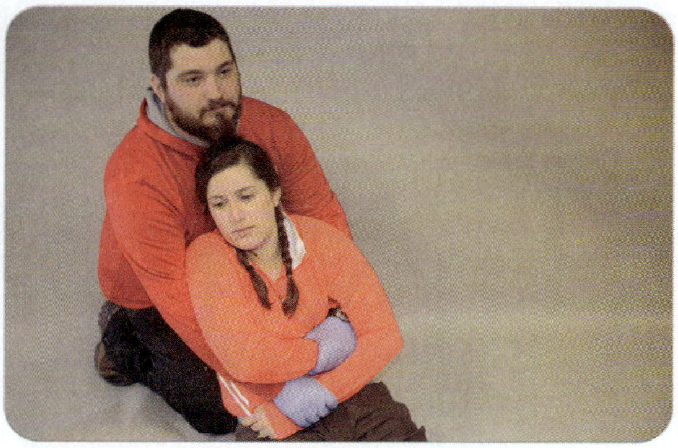

Figure 5-6 The underarm-wrist drag.

- Support the patient's head with both of your forearms.
- Raise your head while moving from kneeling to standing.
- Drag the patient to the desired location.

2. Feet drag (Figure 5-4)
   - Bend down on one knee and grasp the patient's feet/ankles.
   - Raise your head while moving from kneeling to standing.
   - Drag the patient to the desired location.
   - An alternative method is to pull on a rope or sheet that is tied around the ankles.
   - This method should be used only if you cannot get to the patient's head and shoulders.
3. Blanket drag (Figure 5-5)
   - Move the patient onto a blanket.
   - Bend down on one knee and firmly grasp the blanket either with one or both hands.
   - Raise your head while moving from kneeling to standing.
   - Drag the patient, pulling the blanket to the desired location.
4. Underarm-wrist drag (Figure 5-6)
   - Place the patient in seated position.
   - Bend down on one knee, reach under the patient's armpits, and grasp the wrists.
   - Raise your head while moving from kneeling to standing.
   - Drag the patient to the desired location.

Nonurgent Moves

When a patient is moved in a controlled fashion, it is a nonurgent move. One or more rescuers either *assist* the patient in relocating or *carry* the patient by physically lifting and relocating the patient. Depending on available resources, a nonurgent move may be performed with little or no equipment or using specialized equipment designed specifically

CASE Update

Because the patient needs a rapid primary assessment and the lift chair is in the way, you perform an urgent shoulder drag, protecting the patient's head and neck. You firmly grab the unresponsive patient's jacket on top of the shoulders with both hands, cradle the head between your forearms, and drag him 10 feet from the chair on flat ground, where you immediately perform a primary assessment.

What are the next steps you should take?

OEC SKILL 5-8 Performing the Human Crutch

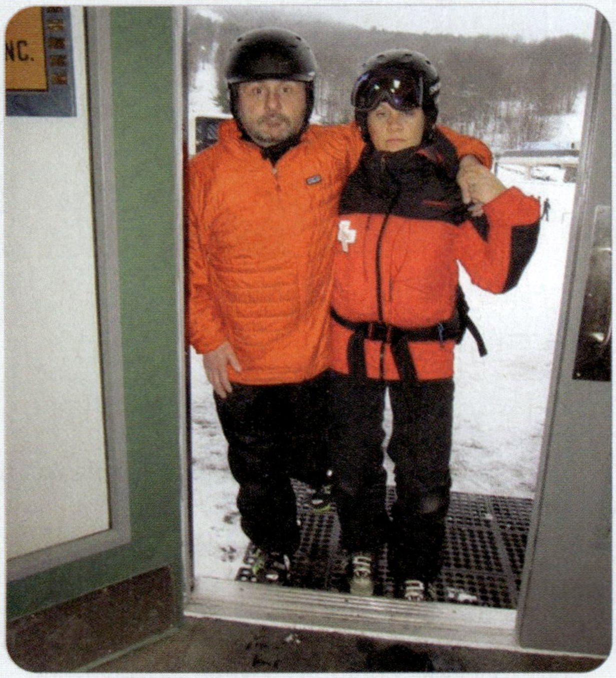

© Edward McNamara.

1. The rescuer assists the patient to stand on the good leg.
2. The patient places an arm over the rescuer's shoulder on the *same* side as the injured leg.
3. The rescuer grasps the patient's wrist with one hand while simultaneously wrapping the opposite hand around the patient's waist, providing support. The rescuer also may hold onto the patient's belt or pants.

for transport. A backboard with straps can be used as a transport device.

Human Crutch

Also known as a one-person assist, the human crutch is one of the most common methods used for moving a patient. This can be used to help a patient move from the aid room to a vehicle or from a vehicle to a stretcher. When performing this technique, the rescuer acts as a crutch by taking the weight off an injured leg, thereby helping the patient walk with assistance.

To perform a human crutch, follow the steps in **OEC Skill 5-8**.

Two-Person Assist

The two-person assist is similar to the human crutch except two rescuers are available, one on each side of the patient. It is preferable to the human crutch in that it provides greater stability, which lessens the risk of falling.

To perform a two-person assist, follow the steps in **OEC Skill 5-9**.

Chair Carry

A chair carry may be used to move a patient who is able to sit up unassisted. This technique requires two rescuers. Depending on the strength of the rescuers and the size of the patient, this technique is effective for carrying a person over short-to-moderate distances.

To perform a chair carry, follow the steps in **OEC Skill 5-10**.

OEC SKILL 5-9 Performing the Two-Person Assist

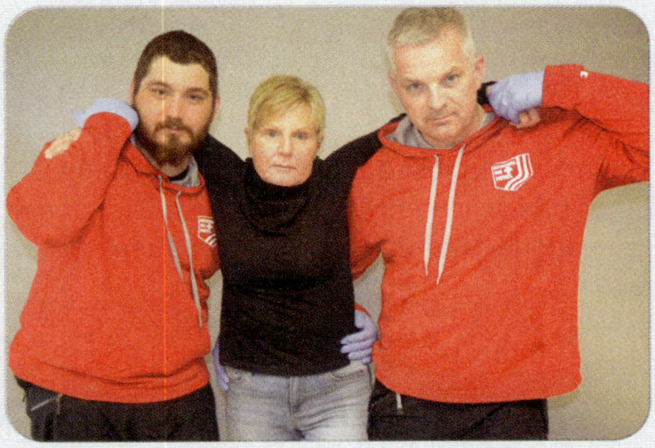

1 The rescuers assist the patient to stand on the good leg.

2 The rescuers stand on either side of the patient. The patient places an arm over each rescuer's shoulder.

3 Each rescuer grasps the patient's wrist on their side. The rescuers then wrap their opposite hand around the patient's waist, or the two rescuers can hold onto the patient's belt or pants on each side.

OEC SKILL 5-10 Performing the Chair Carry

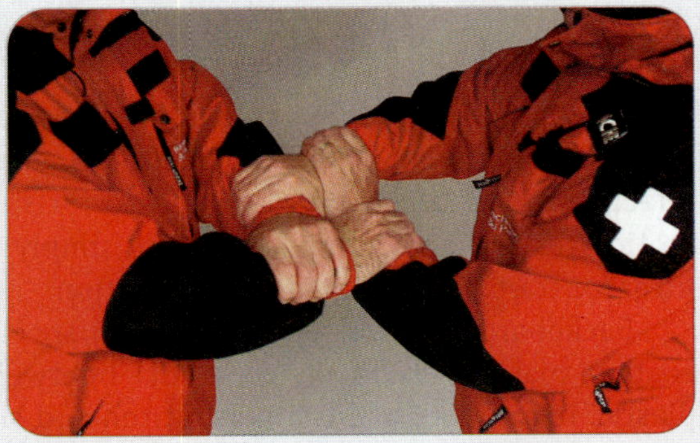

1 Two rescuers stand to either side of the patient; they should be facing each other. This carry is easier if both rescuers are close to same height.

(continues)

OEC SKILL 5-10 Performing the Chair Carry (*continued*)

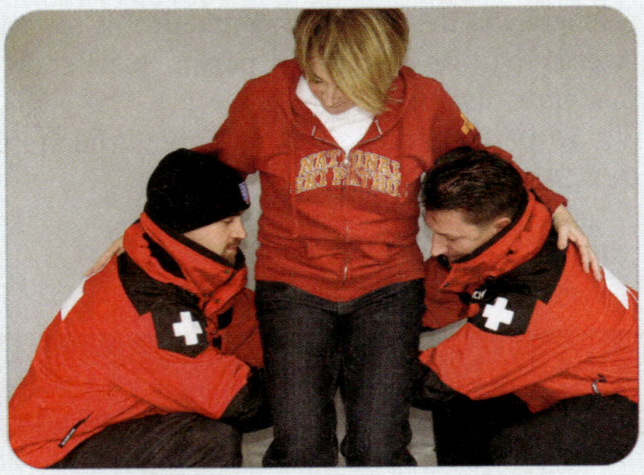

2 The rescuers squat down next to the patient, using good body mechanics, and the patient places his or her arms around the rescuers' shoulders and necks.

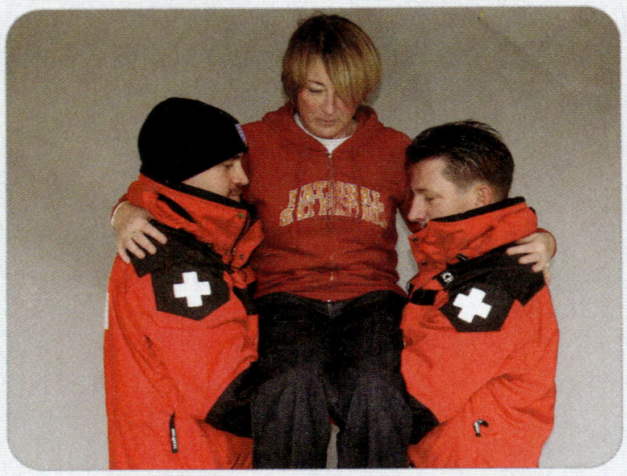

3 The rescuers extend their dominant arm out in front of their body. They grasp their extended arm just below the elbow with their other hand then slowly bring the "chair" under the patient. The rescuers lift the patient off the ground.

Fore-and-Aft Carry

The fore-and-aft carry, used in conjunction with the extremity lift, is performed by two rescuers to carry a patient over a short-to-moderate distance.

To perform a fore-and-aft carry, follow the steps in **OEC Skill 5-11**.

TRANSPORT EQUIPMENT

Many commercial devices are available to aid in moving, lifting, or carrying a patient. Used properly, this equipment facilitates good body mechanics and lessens one's risk of injury. Additionally, the transport equipment listed in **Table 5-1** is very useful in handling patients.

Backboard

A backboard, or long spine board, is usually readily available and can be used to transport patients effectively. The backboard can be used for spinal motion restriction when necessary, or simply as a litter for transport from a difficult location.

Backboards are manufactured from specially coated marine-grade plywood or lightweight plastic. It is blood, bodily fluids, water, and snow resistant.

OEC SKILL 5-11 Performing the Fore-and-Aft Carry

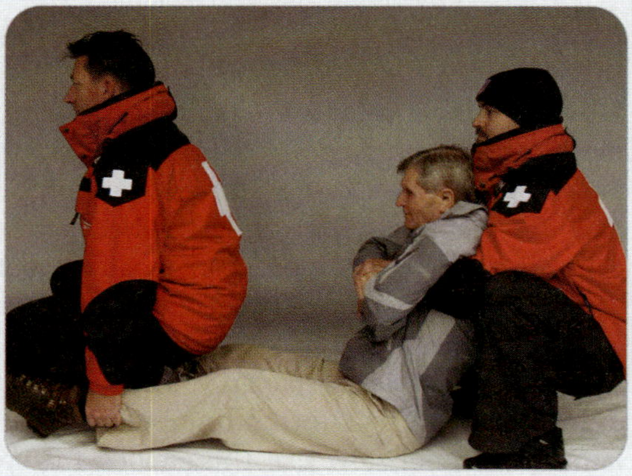

© Mike Halloran.

1. The rescuers place the patient in a sitting position.
2. Rescuer 1 (the taller of the two rescuers, located at the patient's head) folds the patient's arms across the patient's chest, reaches under the armpits, and grabs the wrists.
3. Facing away from the patient, Rescuer 2 kneels between the patient's legs and either grasps behind the patient's knees or grasps the patient's lower legs.
4. On a command, both rescuers crouch, keeping their backs straight, and then stand, lifting the patient in unison.
5. Once both rescuers are standing, they may carry the patient.

Table 5-1 Common Equipment to Move, Lift, or Carry a Patient
• Backboard or long spine board
• Portable stretcher
• Scoop stretcher
• Wheeled ambulance stretcher
• Basket/Stokes stretcher
• Sitting lifting device
• Improvised litters
• Toboggan or sled

Backboards are used for a variety of purposes, including immobilization of suspected fractures of the spine, hip, pelvis, or femur; carrying a patient over short distances outside; or for transferring a patient between a bed and transport device. It also

KEY POINT

Backboards and Patient Care

Prolonged contact with any hard surface can cause back pain and increase the risk of skin ulcers/pressure sores, which will develop in just a few hours. This is especially important in a backcountry rescue operation in which a patient will be placed on a backboard for an extended time. OEC technicians are encouraged to pad the backboard with a closed cell foam pad or blanket, if available. Additionally, all gaps in the backboard should be filled with towels, shirts, or other padding to reduce the incidence of pressure sores.

is an excellent tool for extrication because of the ease of sliding patients without suspected spine injuries onto it. The patient should be placed onto a backboard using one of the proper lifting methods previously described or, in cases involving suspected spine injury, using a logroll. For extrication or spinal protection, strap the patient on the backboard, so they do not slip off.

Portable Stretcher

A portable stretcher consists of an aluminum frame and a vinyl-coated platform (**Figure 5-7**). Slightly wider than a standard backboard, the device has cut-outs for rescuers' hands at each corner and along each side to facilitate carrying using multiple rescuers with the power grip. This device is available as either a one-piece stretcher or as a folding stretcher. Both devices are lightweight and are resistant to blood, bodily fluids, and water. A patient is moved onto the device using one of the techniques described in the *Lifting or Sliding a Patient* section in this chapter.

Scoop Stretcher

A scoop stretcher is a two-piece aluminum or high-density thermoplastic device that is slightly concave and has an open center section, allowing it to conform to the patient's body. The wide end of the device is used to support the head and torso, whereas the narrow end is used to support the lower legs and feet. It can be adjusted to match the patient's height.

To use a scoop stretcher, follow the steps in **OEC Skill 5-12**.

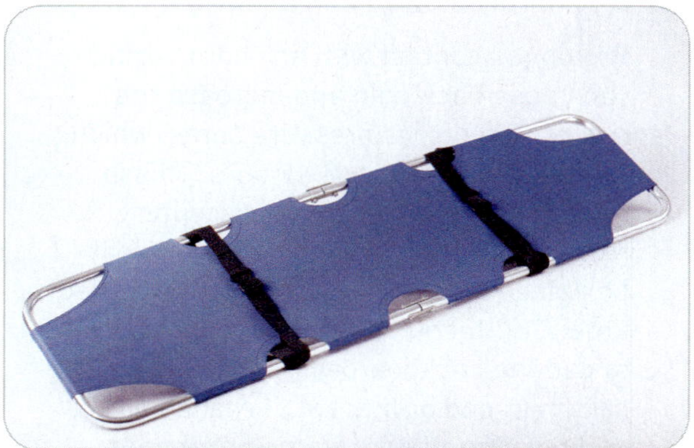

Figure 5-7 Portable stretcher/flexible stretcher.

Wheeled Ambulance Stretcher

Wheeled ambulance stretchers, or cots, are the most commonly used stretchers in EMS ambulances (**Figure 5-8**). They have levers and controls for raising and lowering the bed parts and can raise or lower the patient's head or feet. In some cases they are battery-operated. Because of their adaptability, they make transport of patients much easier, especially when loading or unloading a patient into an ambulance. Ambulance personnel now use this device for spinal motion restriction.

This stretcher can be modified for use in an aid room, so a toboggan can be placed on it. The toboggan can then be raised, allowing easier transfer of a patient to fixed exam table

Basket Stretcher

The basket stretcher, or Stokes stretcher, was initially used by the military for transferring patients between ships (**Figure 5-9**). Originally constructed of metal and wire mesh, today's basket stretchers are constructed from high-impact plastics and ultra-light materials. Some can even be disassembled into two parts, making them easy to carry and reassemble at the point of use. It is great for backcountry operations or rescues requiring a great distance of travel.

Sitting Lifting Device

Made from 3/4-inch or 1-inch plywood, a sitting lifting device allows a patient to sit on a board with an injured leg extended (**Figure 5-10A**). Handholds cut into the wood enable two rescuers to carry the patient for a short distance. A third rescuer may be needed to hold the leg on the board. This device is used to carry a patient from an aid room to a car when an ambulance is not needed. It is especially useful for leg injuries that have been immobilized in a splint (**Figure 5-10B**). It is not used for spinal motion restriction.

OEC SKILL 5-12 Using a Scoop Stretcher

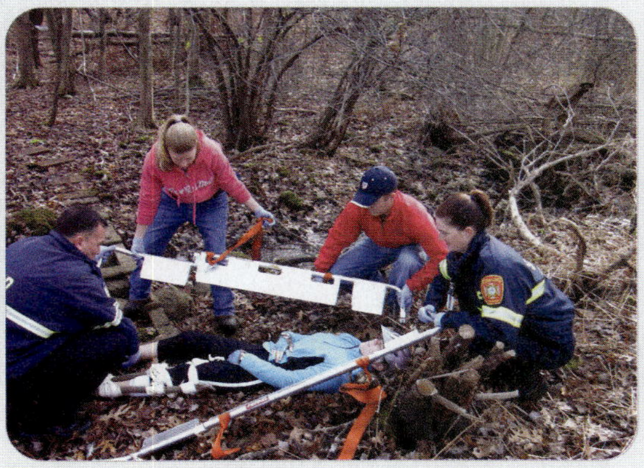

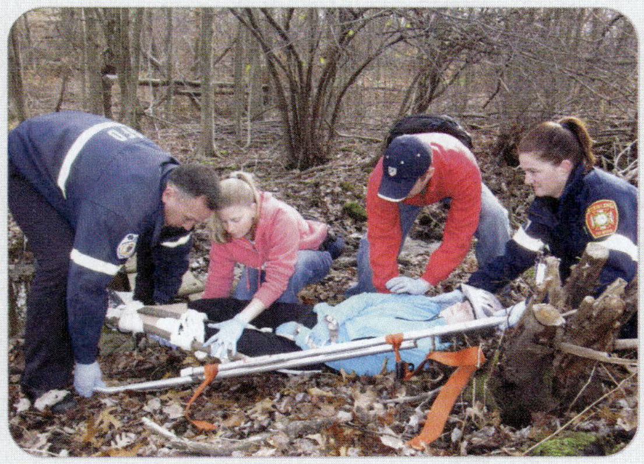

1 Disconnect the two sides of the stretcher. Place the two parts of the stretcher beside the patient and adjust for length, 1 to 3 inches longer than the patient.

2 Ensure that both sides are the same length by checking that the number of exposed holes in the tubing is the same on both sides. Slide both parts of the stretcher beneath the patient until the mechanical fittings at each end touch. Slightly lift the patient to avoid pinching the patient's backside or your fingers.

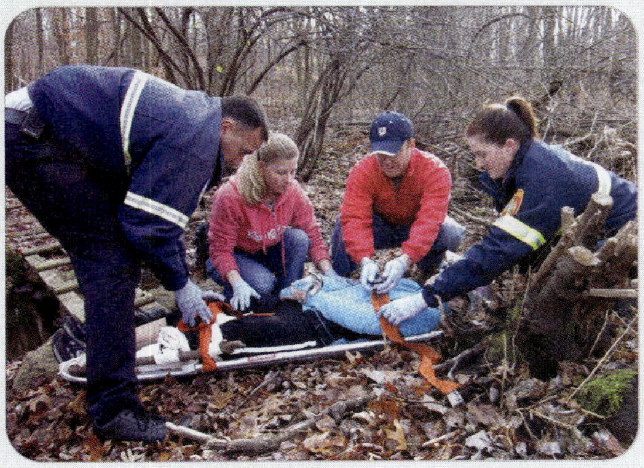

3 Connect the two sides of the stretcher by firmly pressing the two ends back together until you hear a loud "click" at each end. Secure the patient to the device using straps or a commercial device. To remove the stretcher, reverse the procedure.

Improvised Litters

When a patient in the backcountry must be evacuated using only the equipment available, an OEC technician may need to make a litter. Step one is the construction of a rigid frame for dragging or carrying. Skis, paddles, or available wood can be lashed together to make this frame. Next the patient is placed in a sleeping bag, and a closed-cell foam pad is placed between the patient and the frame. Another simple technique for a lighter patient is to thread two poles through the arm holes

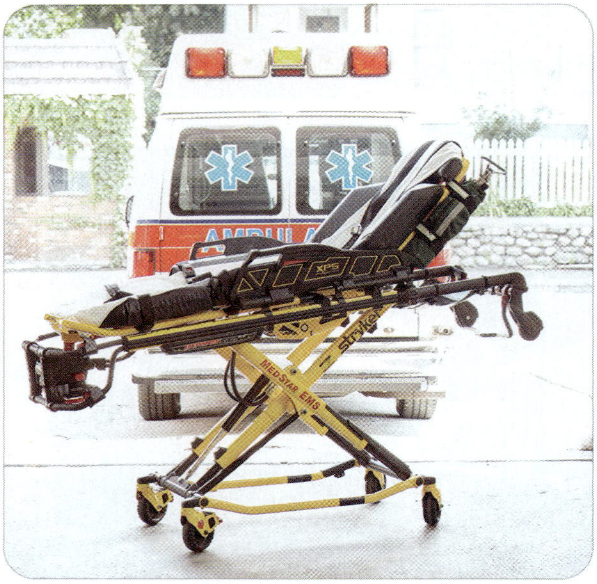

Figure 5-8 A wheeled ambulance stretcher.

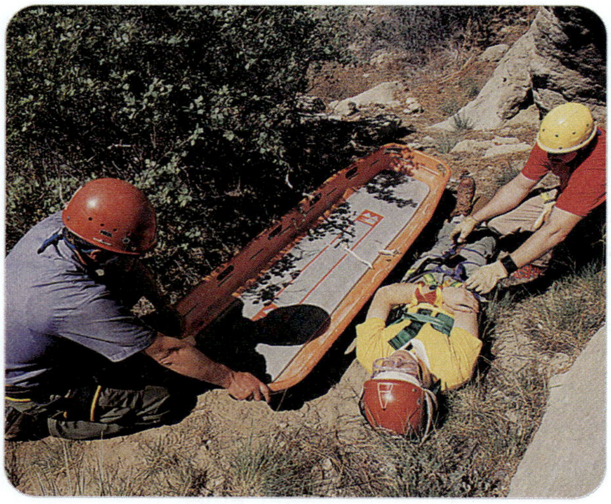

Figure 5-9 A basket stretcher.

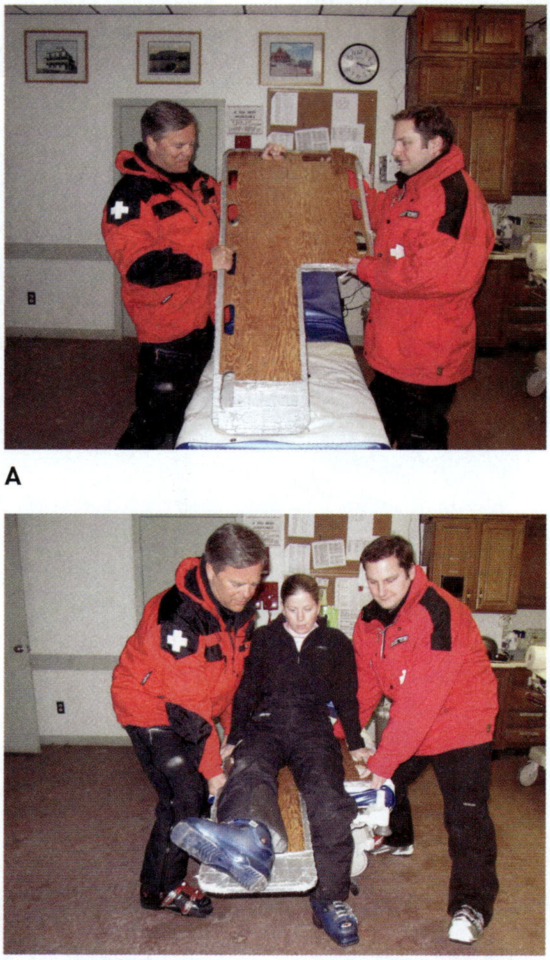

Figure 5-10 A sitting lifting device is useful when transferring a patient from the aid room to a car. **A.** A sitting lifting device. **B.** A patient using the sitting lifting device.

of several jackets and use the resulting litter to carry the patient (**Figure 5-11**).

Toboggan

The toboggan is used as the primary device for transporting patients by ski patrollers (**Figure 5-12**). Toboggans are made of reinforced fiberglass, aluminum, and steel. They are used to move a patient down a hill by a rescuer on skis, or, using a special adapter, the rescuer can drag the toboggan behind a snowmobile. When not on snow, OEC technicians may use a stretcher or other device to transport patients.

Most ski patrol rescue toboggans are equipped with a basic "sled pack," which contains blankets, splinting materials, a backboard, straps, cervical collars, and other items necessary for routine operations. In addition, many patrols have a specialized emergency pack that includes oxygen and an automated external defibrillator to handle major emergencies.

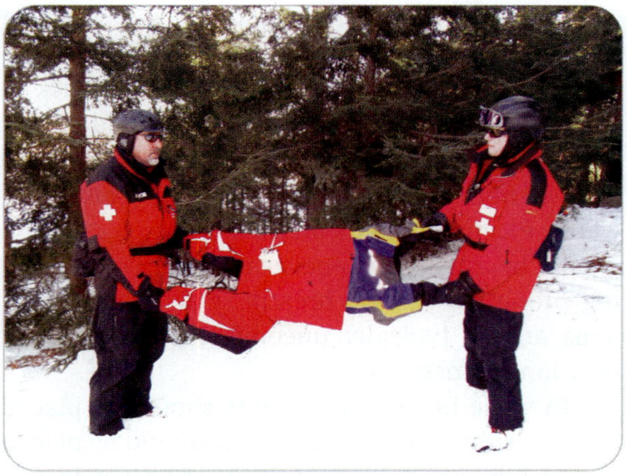

Figure 5-11 Improvised litter using two poles and jackets.

© Edward McNamara.

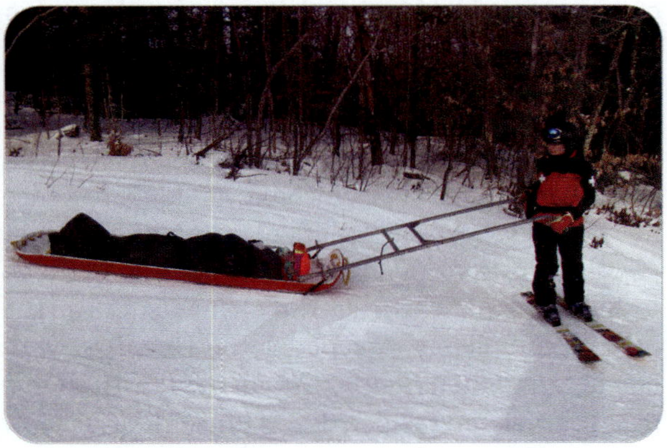

Figure 5-12 A toboggan is used to transport patients from the accident scene to the aid room.

© Edward McNamara.

KEY POINT

Improvised Litters

Equipment that can be used to make a litter includes:

- Climbing rope
- Closed-cell foam pad used for sleeping
- Trekking poles
- Skis
- Pack frames
- Raft oars or paddles
- Sleeping bag

The toboggan must be prepared before the patient is loaded into it. When on a slope, it is usually easier for the rescuers to lift the patient uphill into the toboggan, with the toboggan perpendicular to the hill. The patient is placed into the toboggan using a lifting or moving technique that best suits the injury or illness involved. A pad or blanket may be placed under the patient to improve overall comfort. If the patient is on a backboard, the backboard is loaded into the toboggan.

A toboggan can be used as a spinal protection device. Proper loading of the patient into the toboggan is important, keeping the spine straight to avoid further injury.

PACKAGING A PATIENT

Packaging is a process in which the patient is adequately prepared for transport, reducing the risk of further injury or worsening of symptoms. Packaging needs vary depending on the patient's injuries or illness and environmental conditions. For instance, when packaging a patient during a winter rescue, it is important that the patient remain warm during transport. Likewise, if the patient has a broken leg, it is important that the leg is properly splinted and secured to prevent unnecessary movement during transport. If any special equipment is used, it must be packaged with the patient.

In general, proper patient packaging consists of four steps:

1. The patient is properly positioned on the transport device, usually a toboggan or litter.
2. The patient is made as comfortable as possible.
3. The patient is securely fastened on the transport device.
4. All necessary medical equipment is transported with the patient.

Positioning a Patient in a Toboggan

Judgment is always needed when placing a patient in a toboggan. Bike/Nordic patrollers should follow similar rules when transporting patients using their specific devices. When using a toboggan, the first step in packaging the patient is deciding whether the patient's head should be positioned uphill or downhill. This decision is based on the patient's injuries or illness and the care that has been rendered. Generally, the most comfortable way to transport the patient is to place the injury uphill because on steep terrain, gravity will cause increased weight on the injured part, possibly causing problems.

Consider a patient whose broken upper leg has been placed in a traction splint. If the patient is placed in a head-uphill position, it is harder to maintain traction on the injured leg because gravity is working against maintaining traction. Additionally, the patient will tend to slide downhill, toward the front of the toboggan, making traction less effective. For this reason, patients with lower-extremity injuries are placed in a head-downhill position.

Patients with multiple injuries present unique challenges. In these cases, prioritize and place the more significant injury uphill (**Figure 5-13**). For example, if a patient has a possible broken wrist and a broken femur, the leg injury is placed uphill.

There can be important *medical* reasons to place an injured arm or leg downhill. Patients with breathing difficulty should be placed in a head-uphill position. Doing so makes breathing easier because there is less pressure from the abdominal contents pushing upward on the chest cavity. Propping the chest up with a pack or blanket behind the patient's back may be helpful. Putting a second person in the sled to hold the patient's upper body up is difficult and can be extremely dangerous. Patients with a serious head injury should generally be transported in a head-uphill position.

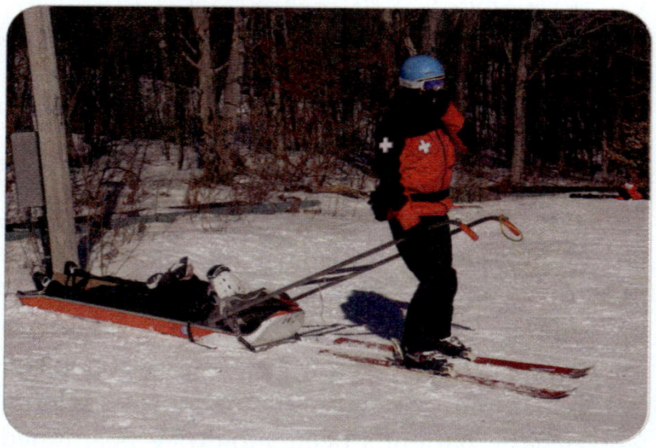

Figure 5-13 A patient in the toboggan with the injury (leg) uphill.

In nearly all injury situations, it is best to place patients on their back (supine). Rarely, a patient may not be able to lie on his or her back in the toboggan. It is difficult to place individuals on their back if they have an anterior dislocated hip and will not move the leg that is sticking out backwards. Placing patients on their stomach or prone should be avoided whenever possible because lying prone may create breathing or airway problems and is typically uncomfortable, especially over long transports.

In some instances, patients should be placed on their side. A pregnant woman should be placed on her left side. In this position, the vena cava is not compressed by the baby, allowing blood to return to the heart. For a patient who cannot stop vomiting, use the recovery position, which involves placing the patient on his or her side. For comfort, consider placing the patient on his or her "good" uninjured side in the toboggan. When the patient needs spinal protection with a backboard, place the patient supine with a collar.

Being transported during an emergency can be a nerve-wracking, uncomfortable experience for patients. Make the patient as comfortable as possible. In freezing conditions, it is important to insulate the patient from the elements. Cover the patient completely, except for the face, first with blankets and then (if used in your area) with a large plastic sheet, or wrapper, that is impervious to snow and rain. Conversely, in warm or hot climates it may be necessary to provide some shade for the patient. Use padding to lessen the effects of the inevitable bumps that occur during transport. If neck, back, or spine injuries are not suspected, a pillow may be placed under the patient's head or knees to provide additional comfort for the ride down the mountain.

Use the attached straps to secure the patient to the toboggan or transport device to keep the patient from falling out. Extremities that are splinted must remain securely in place and must not be allowed to move around. Straps across the chest should be snug but not so tight as to restrict the patient's breathing. Whenever possible, avoid placing straps directly over known injuries, as doing so may cause pain.

When packaging the patient, it is important that essential medical equipment remain with the patient. If the patient is receiving oxygen, the oxygen tank should accompany the patient. Other medical equipment is placed in the toboggan or transport device between the patient's legs or to the outside of an uninjured leg. Avoid placing any equipment near the patient's head. Equipment must be secured within the toboggan with appropriate straps, without putting pressure on an injured body part. Some oxygen delivery systems can be attached to the handlebars of a toboggan. It is best not to place unused rescue or personal equipment in the toboggan with the patient. Instead, have another patroller perform "cleanup" and carry or ski these items to the aid room.

Ski patrollers learn how to drive a ski toboggan in the transport portion of their training. The patroller at the front handles "drives" the sled and determines the route down the hill while the patroller on the tail rope acts as a backup if the driver falls.

FINAL TRANSPORT OF PATIENTS

Patients may need additional transport to an aid room or to a waiting ambulance at a road. Dragging patients in a toboggan is difficult. OEC technicians may have access to various engine-powered transport vehicles such as a snow machine or an all-terrain vehicle (ATV). Transport vehicles enable patients to be transported over relatively long distances faster. These ATVs have special racks or decks to which a backboard or litter can be attached. The use of transport vehicles requires additional training. Patients who need further advanced care can be transported by one of two means: ground or air.

Ground Transport

Once a patient arrives at a road or patrol room, additional ground transportation options, such as ambulances or private vehicles, are available. Most patients can leave in a car for follow-up care, if needed. Some patients need EMS transport by ambulance to a definitive medical facility following transport into the aid room.

Air Transport

Air transport is an effective mode for transporting a patient out of a backcountry setting. This transport method is used for patients with serious injuries or illness, for patients who require immediate evacuation to a specialized definitive care facility, or when using ground transport would be too slow, overly complex, or hazardous. It also is used when roadways are impassable or unavailable. There may be weather limitations for air transport.

Patients can be transported by air in two ways: helicopter or airplane (**Figure 5-14**). Planes need to land and take off on a runway or a similar long flat surface. The length of the runway required varies, depending on the type of aircraft used. Because of this need for a runway, planes are used less frequently in backcountry rescue operations than are helicopters.

Helicopters have revolutionized mountain rescue operations. Their ability to land in tight spaces makes them logical rescue and transport vehicles. However, helicopters have limitations regarding their use, including factors relating to weather, altitude, weight, time of day, and need of a flat unobstructed area for landing.

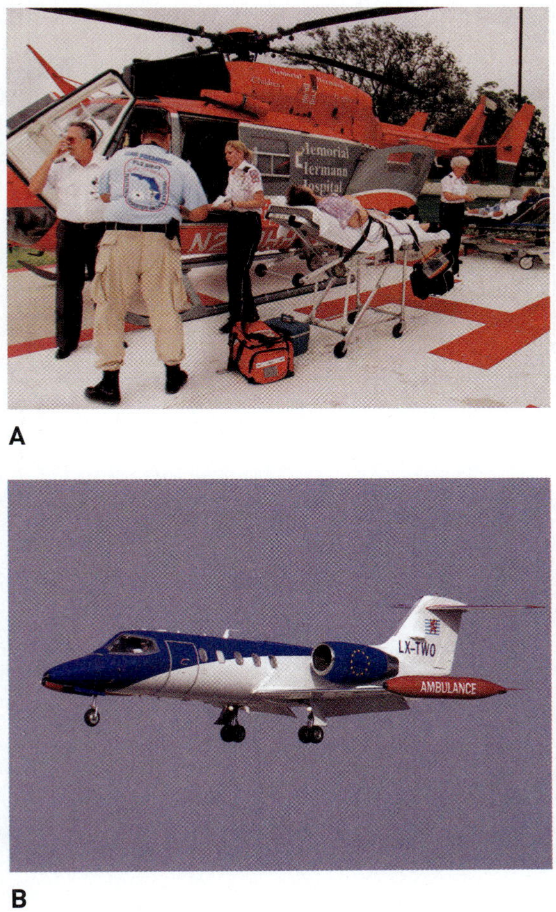

Figure 5-14 **A.** A rotary wing-aircraft (helicopter). **B.** A fixed-wing aircraft (airplane).

A: Courtesy of Ed Edahl/FEMA; B: © InsectWorld/Shutterstock.

Landing Zone Selection

Most helicopter crashes occur during takeoff or landing. For this reason, the **landing zone (LZ)** should be an area of at least 100 feet by 100 feet and should be flat with no more than an 8-degree slope (**Figure 5-15** and **Table 5-2**). The area should be free of overhead obstructions, such as wires and power lines, even if visibility is excellent. If overhead obstructions are present near the LZ, notify the pilot of their locations over the radio well before the helicopter's arrival.

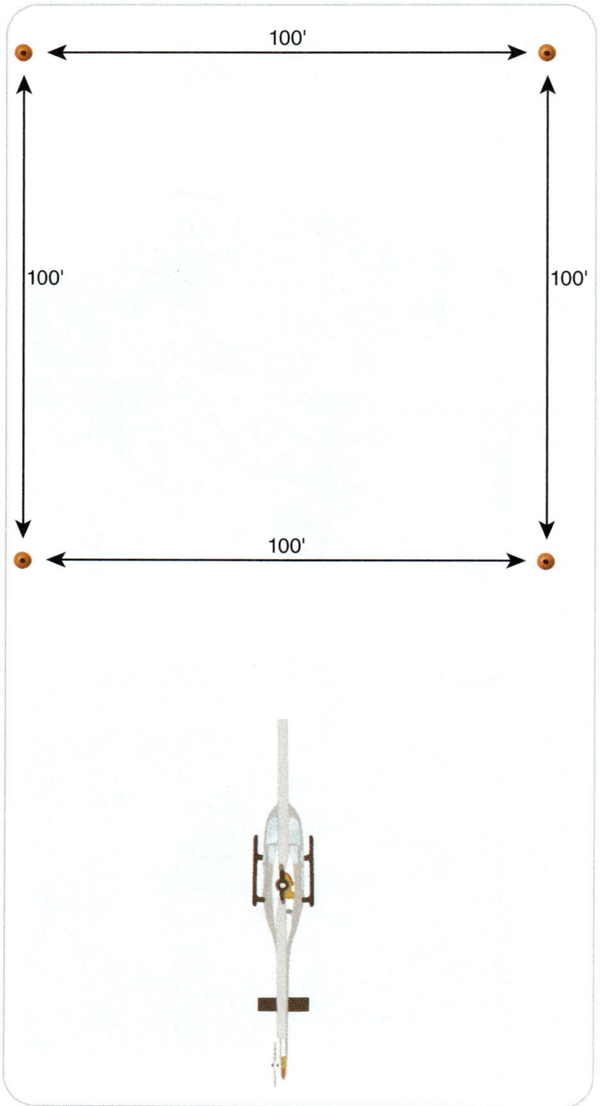

Figure 5-15 Some characteristics of a helicopter landing zone.

Table 5-2 Landing Zone Guidelines
• The LZ must be a minimum of 100 feet by 100 feet.
• The site must be free from overhead obstructions and wires.
• The site should be on firm ground (avoid areas with loose debris).
• The site should be well lit.
• Keep emergency lights on, but do not point any lights toward the aircraft, because they could temporarily blind the pilot.
• Keep pedestrians and vehicles at least 100 feet from the LZ.

Likewise, loose objects in the LZ can create a dangerous situation, both for the helicopter crew and for rescuers on the ground. A helicopter's rotors can generate winds of more than 100 miles per hour. Small stones, loose clothing, and lightweight gear should be removed from the LZ or secured to prevent them from being blown away or into the rotors.

The LZ should be well lit. Headlights from cars can light the ground up to 100 feet outside the zone, allowing the pilot to see the ground. Place chemical light sticks or small strobe lights on all four corners of the LZ, securing them in place with tent stakes or by other means. Do not shine any lights toward the helicopter, because they can temporally blind the pilot.

The LZ must be secured. No pedestrians, animals, or traffic should be within 100 feet of the aircraft. No one other than the landing coordinator is allowed within the LZ area during takeoff or landing.

Ground-to-Air Communications

Effective communication between the pilot and the ground crew is an essential component of safe rescue operations involving aircraft. As a rule, participation in helicopter landings and takeoffs should involve only personnel formally trained in these procedures.

Before the helicopter arrives, the landing coordinator should contact the pilot to obtain both an estimated time of arrival, often abbreviated ETA, and the direction of arrival. This information should be conveyed to other rescuers on the ground to ensure that the LZ remains clear of personnel, gear, and any potential obstructions. In return, the landing coordinator should provide the pilot with the LZ coordinates and current weather conditions, including wind direction, if known. As the helicopter makes its final approach to the LZ, the landing coordinator should use universal ground-to-air signals.

Ground Operations

Once the helicopter is safely on the ground, do not approach the aircraft until signaled to do so by the pilot or crew chief (**Table 5-3**). Often, a crew member will exit the aircraft to escort you to it. If signaled to approach the helicopter unescorted, maintain eye contact with the pilot or crew chief, and approach only from the front of the craft so that you remain in the pilot's field of vision.

Never approach a helicopter from the rear, and approach from the downhill side (**Figure 5-16**). The tail rotor spins so fast that it is nearly invisible and is lethal if inadvertently walked into. Stay low and avoid holding anything above your head because the main rotor may be lower than you think. Depending on the grade of the LZ, the overhead rotor blades may be no more than a few feet above the ground. Avoid wearing anything loose or long (like a scarf) that can be blown away or pulled into the blades by the rotor wash. Take off a loose hat.

Table 5-3 Basic Helicopter Safety
• Do not approach a helicopter unless signaled to do so or escorted by a crew member.
• Always approach a helicopter from the front. Never approach the helicopter from the rear, where tail rotor is located.
• Always remain in sight of the pilot.
• Stay low.
• Do not hold anything above your head.
• Take off your hat.
• Remove any loose clothing (e.g., hats, scarves, lightweight items) when in or near the LZ.

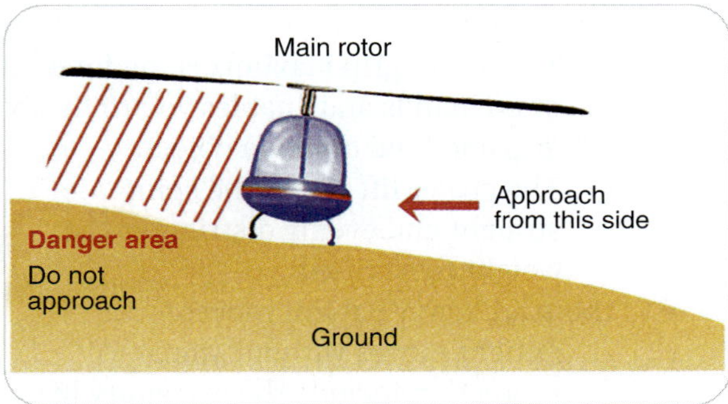

Figure 5-16 Approach a helicopter only when directed by the flight crew and always from the downhill side.

CASE Outcome

The patient becomes responsive. He is now fully alert and complains of arm pain. Following your full evaluation, you find the patient has had a concussion and a possible broken forearm. Since he is now alert, you take a history. There is no evidence of spinal injury, either by history or exam. You splint the arm, place him securely in a toboggan, and transport him to the aid room. Because of his previous unresponsiveness, you recommend transport to the hospital. Later you learn he had a mild concussion that resolved and was placed in a cast for a forearm fracture.

CHAPTER REVIEW

In Summary

- Transporting a patient is a role an OEC technician performs on a regular basis. To do so, OEC technicians will need to move patients, whether by lifting, dragging, or carrying. Plan each move carefully; get help when lifting.
- Use good body mechanics. The use of good body mechanics distributes the weight evenly down the entire spinal column, through the pelvis, and to the bones of the legs. Keep your back straight and lift with your legs.
- The power lift and the power grip can be used together.
    - The power grip maximizes the force of the hands and enables you to firmly grip and hold on to an object.
    - The power lift aligns the spine straight and evenly distributes the weight to be lifted.
- There are many patient moves.
    - Patient moves without spinal protection include the extremity lift, the direct ground lift, and the BEAN/bridge lift.
    - Patient moves with spinal restriction include the draw-sheet, plastic slider, or flat transfer lift and the logroll.
- There are urgent and nonurgent moves. Urgent moves do not incorporate spinal protection.
- Urgent moves include the long-axis drags. There are four types of long-axis drags:
    - Shoulder drag
    - Feet drag
    - Blanket drag
    - Underarm-wrist drag
- Nonurgent moves include the human crutch, two-person assist, chair carry, and fore-and-aft carry.
- Know and use the common equipment that can help you move, lift, or carry a patient:
    - Backboard or long spine board
    - Portable stretcher
    - "Scoop" stretcher
    - Wheeled ambulance stretcher
    - Basket/Stokes stretcher
    - Sitting lifting device
    - Improvised litters
    - Toboggan or sled
- In general, proper patient packaging consists of four steps:
    - The patient is properly positioned on the transport device, usually a toboggan or litter.
    - The patient is made as comfortable as possible.
    - The patient is securely fastened on the transport device.
    - All necessary medical equipment is transported with the patient.
- Patients may need additional transport to an aid room or to a waiting ambulance at a road. Ground or air transport may be used.
- Patients can be transported by air in two ways: airplane or helicopter. It is important to follow all guidelines regarding air transport.

Key Terms

Body mechanics The relationship between the body's anatomic structures and the physical forces associated with lifting, moving, and carrying; the ways the body moves to achieve an action.

Carry The act of lifting and moving the patient, usually a short distance.

Drag A method of pulling a patient on the ground to another location.

Landing zone (LZ) An area picked for the landing of aircraft that meets specific size and safety requirements.

Lift A way of moving the patient by raising the person from a lower position to a higher one.

Move The transport of a patient from one location to another.

Spinal motion restriction Restricting the entire spine to limit spinal motion, protecting the spinal cord from injury.

Chapter Questions

1. When lifting, good body mechanics include:
   a. bending from the back to pick up a loaded backboard.
   b. bending at the knees and back to pick up a loaded backboard.
   c. bending the knees and squatting, keeping your back straight and shoulders over your spine.
   d. refusing to pick up a loaded backboard, because it may hurt your back.
2. A power grip is when you:
   a. grab someone's shirt to perform an urgent move, getting the patient out of danger.
   b. place your hands, palms down, approximately 10 inches apart.
   c. place your hands, palms up, approximately 10 inches apart.
   d. bend your knees and squat, keeping your back straight and your shoulders over the spine.
3. A direct ground lift is used only when you do not suspect a spinal injury. Performing this lift would include:
   a. using two to four rescuers.
   b. the patient lying on his or her back.
   c. all rescuers kneeling along the same side of the patient.
   d. All of the above
4. What moves can be used when there is a suspected spinal injury and spinal motion restriction/protection is necessary?
   a. Extremity lift, direct ground lift, bridge lift
   b. Draw-sheet/plastic slider/flat transfer lift, logroll, BEAN lift
   c. Draw-sheet/plastic slider/flat transfer lift, bridge lift
   d. Draw-sheet/plastic slider/flat transfer lift, logroll
5. A shoulder drag is what type of move?
   a. An urgent move
   b. A nonurgent
   c. A move that requires three to four rescuers
   d. A move used to relocate a patient more than 10 feet
6. A chair carry is what kind of move?
   a. An extremity lift move
   b. A move used when the scene is not safe
   c. An urgent move
   d. A nonurgent move
7. A backboard can be used:
   a. only for immobilization of suspected fractures of the spine, hip, pelvis, or femur.
   b. only as a transport device.
   c. only for femur fractures.
   d. for immobilization, carrying a patient over short distances, and as a transport device.

8. What are the four steps to packaging a patient?
   a. Properly position the patient, make the patient as comfortable as possible, securely fasten the patient, and transport necessary medical equipment with the patient.
   b. Properly position the patient, use an ATV or snow machine, securely fasten the patient, and always keep the patient's head up.
   c. Properly position the patient, securely fasten the patient, use a toboggan, and always keep the patient's head down.
   d. Properly position the patient, transport necessary medical equipment with the patient, let the patient choose a comfortable position, and always keep the patient's head up.

9. Generally, the patient is most comfortable when transported:
   a. lying supine, always with the injury facing downhill.
   b. lying on the injured side to keep the injury warm.
   c. with frequent adjustments from front to back.
   d. with the injury directed uphill.

10. Which of the following options includes all of the steps to basic helicopter safety?
   a. Always approach from the front, remain in sight of the pilot, remove any loose clothing, and stay low.
   b. Do not approach unless signaled to do so, always approach from the front, remain in sight of the pilot, stay low, do not hold anything above your head, and take off your hat and remove any loose clothing.
   c. Approach from any side, remain in sight of the pilot, stay low, and take off your hat.
   d. Remain in sight of the pilot, stay low, do not approach unless signaled to do so, remove any loose clothing, and always approach from the front.

Answers: 1. c, Objective 5-1, p. 89; 2. c, Objective 5-2, p. 88; 3. d, Objective 5-3, p. 91; 4. d, Objective 5-4, p. 92; 5. a, Objective 5-5, p. 96; 6. d, Objective 5-6, p. 99; 7. d, Objective 5-7, p. 101; 8. a, Objective 5-9, p. 105; 9. d, Objective 5-8, p. 106; 10. b, Objective 5-10, p. 109

CHAPTER 6

ANATOMY AND PHYSIOLOGY

OBJECTIVES

Upon completion of this chapter, the OEC technician will be able to:

6-1 Identify and properly use each anatomic term for body direction, movement, and position.

6-2 Identify the location and function of each of the body's organs.

6-3 Describe the anatomy (structure) and physiology (functioning) of each body system.

6-4 Explain how blood flows through the heart.

6-5 Explain how tissue in the body gets oxygen and nourishment.

6-6 Name and describe the location of the major bones in the body.

6-7 Define and explain the three types of muscles.

KEY TERMS

Abduction, p. 115
Adduction, p. 115
Artery, p. 118
Blood pressure, p. 125
Body system, p. 117
Brain, p. 125
Capillaries, p. 122
Cardiovascular system, p. 120
Cells, p. 117
Central nervous system, p. 125
Diaphragm, p. 119
Digestive system, p. 129
Endocrine system, p. 131
Extension, p. 115
Flexion, p. 115
Human anatomy, p. 114
Human physiology, p. 114
Immune response, p. 138
Immunity, p. 138
Integumentary system, p. 132
Ligaments, p. 132
Lymphatic system, p. 137
Muscular system, p. 134
Nervous system, p. 125
Neuron, p. 127
Organs, p. 114
Peripheral nervous system, p. 125
Reproductive system, p. 135
Respiratory system, p. 117
Skeletal system, p. 132
Tendon, p. 134
Tissue, p. 117
Urinary system, p. 130
Vein, p. 118

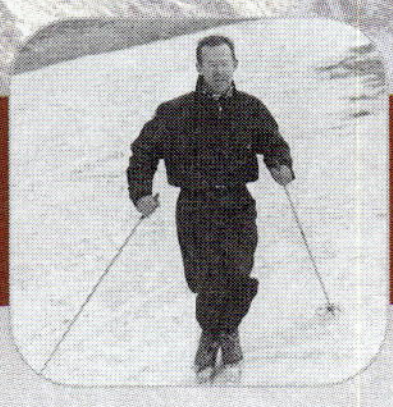

HISTORICAL TIMELINE **1949.** Edward Taylor accepts appointment as the second National Director of the NSP.

CHAPTER OVERVIEW

The human body is complex, containing body systems that work together to keep it functioning properly. These systems circulate nutrients and oxygen to body tissues, control movement, provide structure, allow complex thought, provide reproduction, and perform many other functions to maintain life.

To assess and manage a patient, you must have a basic understanding of anatomy (structure) and physiology (function). Each of the body systems interacts with other systems to function properly. Injury or illness to one system will cause problems in other systems. Understanding the anatomy and physiology of the body systems, and how they interact with each other, will help you recognize and understand injuries and illnesses. Further, it is important to learn the body's systems and anatomic terminology so that you can communicate with other prehospital providers.

HOMEOSTASIS

Homeostasis is the process by which an organism maintains a stable internal environment by adjusting its physiological processes. In humans, the body systems interact with each other. For example, the integumentary and cardiovascular systems help to preserve a steady internal body temperature, and the nervous system works with the cardiovascular system to maintain a steady blood pressure. The endocrine system also works with the cardiovascular system to maintain a normal level of glucose in the blood.

Illnesses and injuries that alter normal body physiology or damage organs or organ systems can adversely affect homeostasis. Uncorrected, these disruptions can cause organs and organ systems to fail, leading to a host of medical disorders and even death. It is therefore essential that OEC technicians have a basic understanding of human anatomy and physiology and be able to use this information when assessing and caring for patients.

ANATOMY AND PHYSIOLOGY

Human anatomy is the study of the structure of the body. It includes gross anatomy, which focuses on structures that can be seen with the unaided eye, and microscopic anatomy, which focuses on structures that can be seen only under a microscope. **Human physiology** is the study of the mechanical, physical, bioelectric, and biochemical functions of humans.

The human body has many **organs** that are included in the body's systems. As we explain each system, the organs of that system will be discussed. Organs can be solid, like the liver, or hollow, like the large intestine. It is important to remember that solid organs usually contain significant amounts of blood and if ruptured can cause severe internal bleeding and shock. You need to know the location of the body's organs.

Terms for Body Planes and Directions

Terms universally used to communicate with other emergency medical personnel refer to planes and direction (**Figure 6-1**).

- *Anterior/posterior*. The term *anterior* refers to the front of the body, whereas *posterior* refers to the back of the body. (Example: The eyes are anterior to the ears; the ears are posterior to the eyes.)
- *Superior/inferior*. *Superior* describes any part nearer the patient's head, whereas *inferior*

CASE Presentation

During an off-road bicycle race, two riders collided. The first patient has obvious abrasions and a deformed wrist. The second appears dazed, and his leg below the knee is crooked.

What should you do? What body systems and structures might be involved?

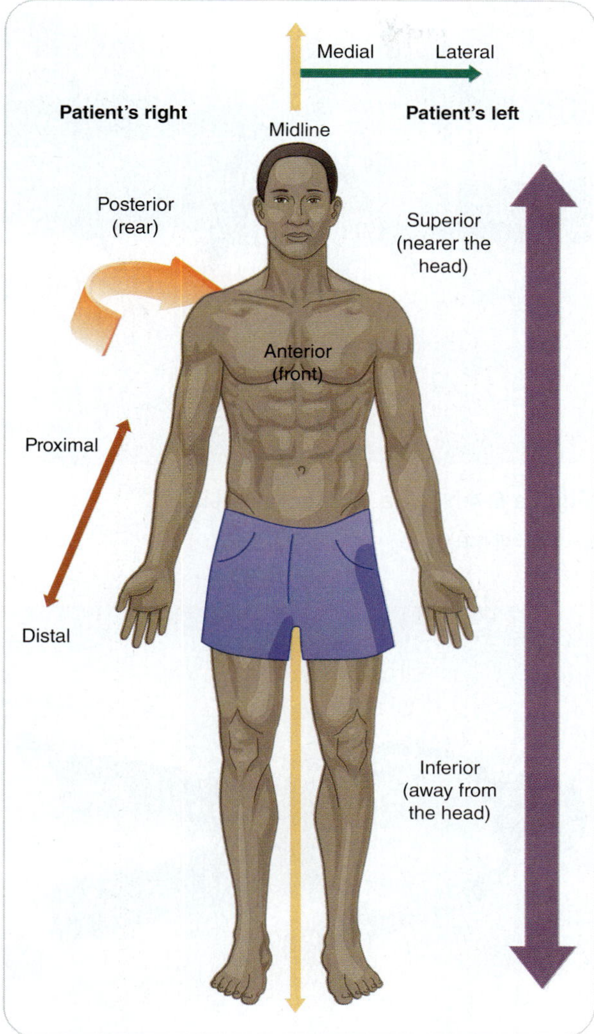

Figure 6-1 Directional and anatomic terms are used to describe locations on the body, body direction, and body movement.

describes any part nearer the patient's feet. (Example: The knee is superior to the foot; the foot is inferior to the knee.)

- *Medial/lateral.* The terms *medial* and *lateral* are based on the body's midline, an imaginary line that runs down the middle of the body from the head to the ground and creates right and left halves. Any part closer to the midline is *medial*, whereas any part away from the midline is *lateral*. (Example: The navel is medial to the hip; the hip is lateral to the navel.)
- *Proximal/distal. Proximal* refers to any part close to the trunk (chest, abdomen, and pelvis), and *distal* refers to any part away from the trunk and nearer to the extremities (arms and legs). (Example: The hip is proximal to the knee; the knee is distal to the hip.)
- *Superficial/deep. Superficial* refers to any part near the surface of the body, whereas *deep* refers to any part away from the surface. (Example: The skin is superficial to the bones; the bones are deep to the skin.)
- *Internal/external. Internal* refers to the inside, whereas *external* refers to the outside. (Example: The liver is an internal organ; the skin is an external organ.)
- *Right/left. Right* and *left* always refer to the *patient's* right and left, not your own.

Terms for Movements

Flexion is the term used to describe a bending or flexing movement, such as bending at the knee or making a fist. **Extension** is the opposite of flexion, or a straightening movement, such as making the arm straight at the elbow (**Figure 6-2**). The prefix *hyper* used in front of either term describes movement *beyond* the normal range of movement (e.g., hyperflexion, hyperextension).

Abduction describes taking an extremity away from the midline of the body, such as moving the arm out to the side. The prefix *ab* means away from. **Adduction** is the opposite of abduction; it occurs when an extremity is moved toward the midline of the body, such as moving legs that are spread apart together so that they touch each other (**Figure 6-3**). The prefix *ad* means toward.

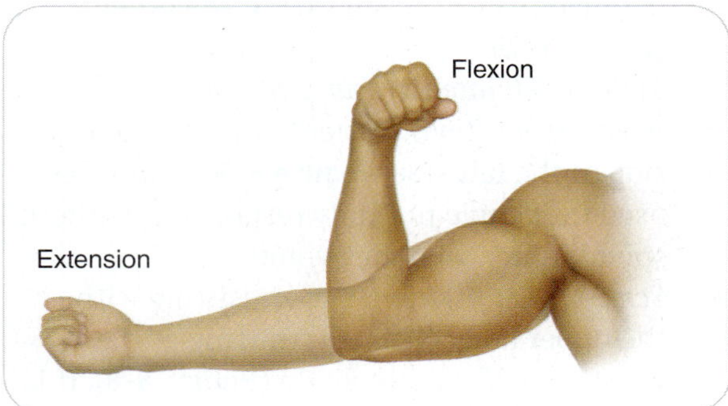

Figure 6-2 Flexion and extension at the elbow.

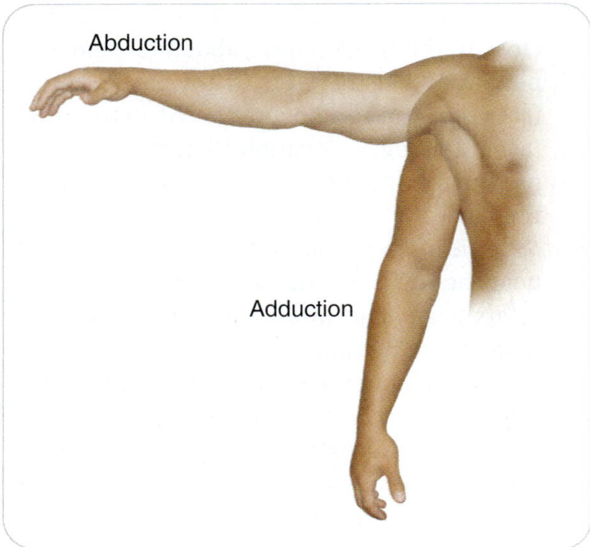

Figure 6-3 Adduction and abduction at the shoulder.

Terms of Position

As a rescuer, you often will need to describe a patient's position to other emergency response personnel and health care providers. Using correct terms will help you communicate the nature and extent of a patient's injury quickly and accurately. Terms of position include the following:

- *Normal anatomic position.* Patient standing with body erect, arms down at the sides, and palms facing forward (**Figure 6-4**). This position is the basis for all medical terms that refer to the body.
- *Supine position.* Patient lying flat on the back, faceup (**Figure 6-5**).
- *Prone position.* Patient lying on the abdomen (stomach), face to one side or the other (**Figure 6-6**).
- *Right or left lateral recumbent position (recovery position).* Patient lying on the right side or the left side (**Figure 6-7**). It may be used for people not fully responsive, without spinal injury, who may vomit.
- *Semi-Fowler position.* Patient sitting with the upper body elevated, starting at the waist, to a 45-degree angle (**Figure 6-8**). It is commonly used for patients who are awake and are not suspected of having a severe injury or illness.

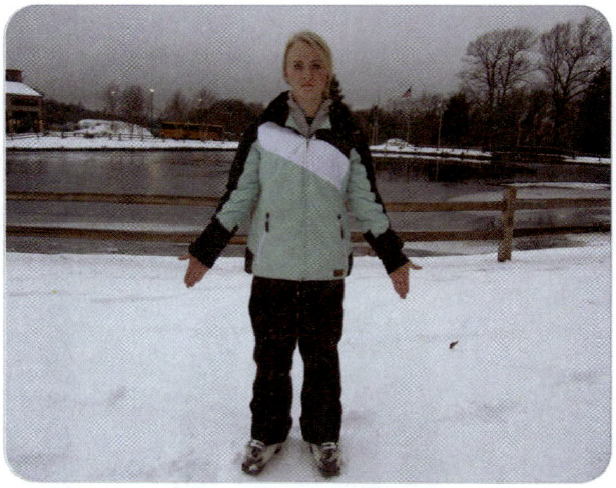

Figure 6-4 Normal anatomic position.

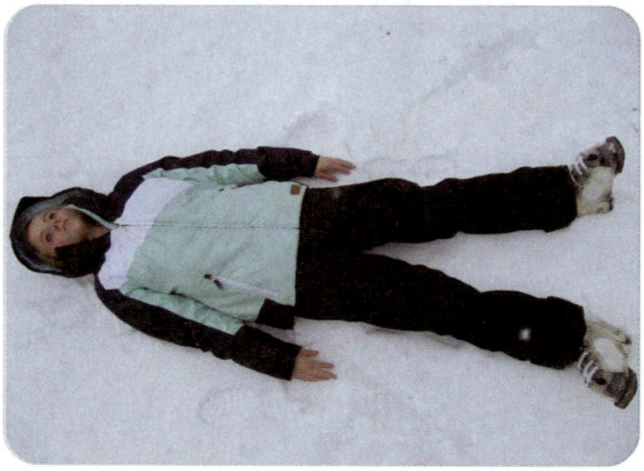

Figure 6-5 Supine position.

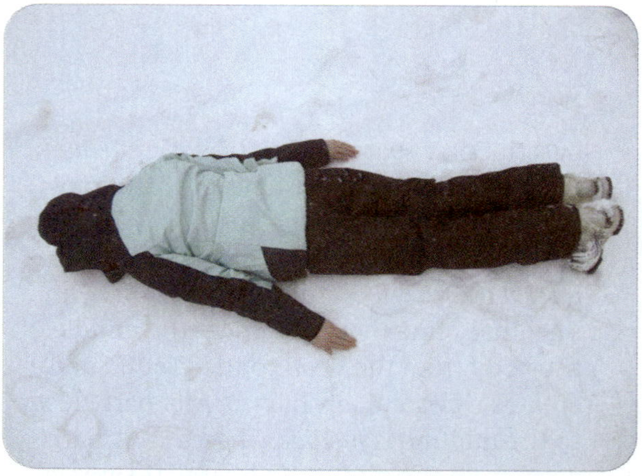

Figure 6-6 Prone position.

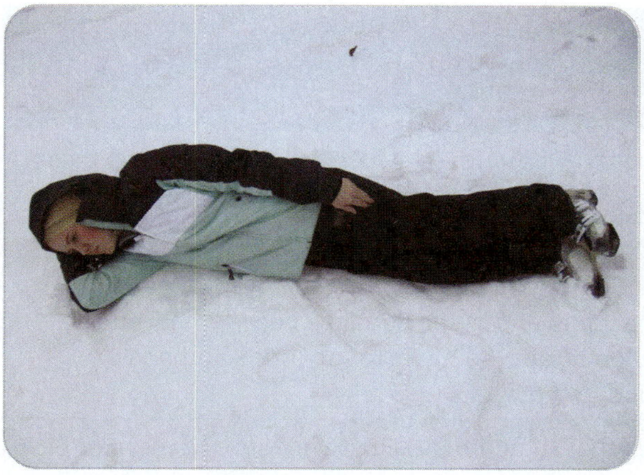

Figure 6-7 Lateral recumbent position.

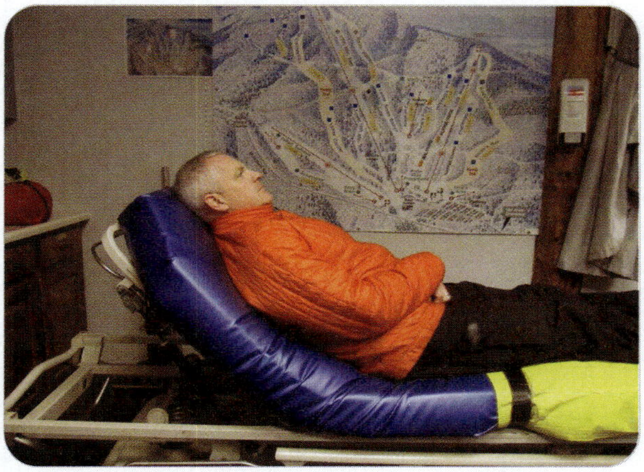

Figure 6-8 Semi-Fowler position.

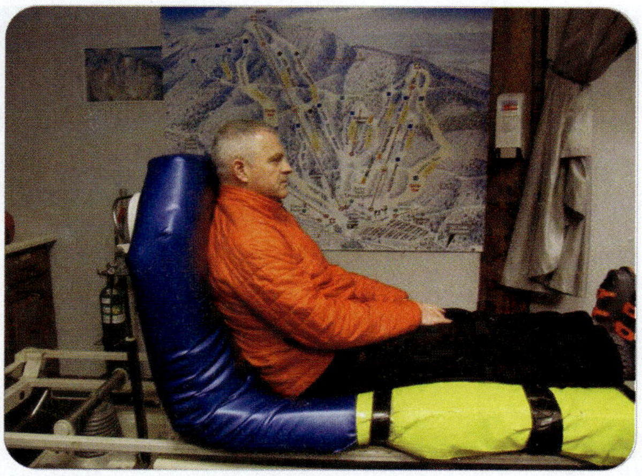

Figure 6-9 High-Fowler position.

- *High-Fowler position.* Patient sitting fully upright with the knees straight or slightly bent (**Figure 6-9**). It is typically used for patients who are experiencing severe breathing problems.

BODY SYSTEMS

The human body performs many complicated functions. The human body is made up of billions of different **cells** that contribute in special ways to keep the body functioning normally. Cells form **tissue**, which in turn forms organs. A group of organs work together to form a **body system**, performing a specific body function needed for life (**Table 6-1**). For example, the cardiovascular system consists of the heart, blood vessels, and blood, with its main function to transport nutrients needed for life, including oxygen.

The Respiratory System

The **respiratory system** consists of organs that move air into (inhalation) and out of (exhalation) the body, delivering oxygen to and removing carbon dioxide from the blood in a process called respiration (**Figure 6-10**). This process helps balance the body's internal pH (the amount of acid in the blood).

The respiratory system is divided into the upper and lower airways by the epiglottis, a leaf-shaped flapper valve that folds down over the top of the trachea (windpipe) to prevent food or liquid from entering the trachea during swallowing. While eating, if the epiglottis does not close properly, the food may "go down the wrong pipe," causing the person to start coughing. Similarly, when an unresponsive person vomits, the epiglottis may not be closed, allowing stomach contents into the lungs. Because stomach contents are highly acidic, if regurgitated, they can cause significant damage to lung tissue.

Upper Airway

The upper airway includes the nose, mouth, tongue and jaw, pharynx (throat), larynx (vocal cords), and epiglottis. During inspiration, air enters the body through the nose and mouth, where it is warmed and moistened. Large particles are filtered by hairs within the nose. Air travels through or by each structure into the lower airway.

Table 6-1 Main Body Systems

Body System	Body Function
Respiratory system	Organs and structures that bring air containing oxygen into the body and eliminate carbon dioxide to the environment through the process of breathing, or ventilation.
Cardiovascular system	Organs and structures that circulate blood around the body using the heart, arteries, and veins, delivering oxygen and nutrients to organs and cells. This system carries chemical waste products away from the cells and helps equalize body temperature. • **Artery**: tubular vessel that carries blood from the heart to the lungs and body. • **Vein**: tubular vessel that carries blood to the heart.
Nervous system	A group of organs and other structures that regulate all body functions. This system collects and processes information, with the brain acting as the central computer of the body, sending and receiving information to and from all organs through a complicated wiring system.
Digestive system	A group of organs and other structures that use mechanical and chemical processes to break down food and absorb nutrients into the body. This system also eliminates waste or unused food.
Urinary system	Organs and structures that remove wastes and toxins from the blood and excrete them as urine. This system maintains the body's water and electrolyte balance.
Endocrine system	A collection of glands that produce chemical substances, called hormones, that travel through the bloodstream influencing target organs.
Integumentary (skin) system	Specialized tissues covering and protecting the body. The skin helps retain fluids, regulates temperature, transmits information from the environment to the brain, and protects the body from the outside environment.
Skeletal system	The bones and other supporting tissues that provide structure to the body, provide attachment points for muscles, protect internal organs, allow movement, store minerals, and constitute the major site where blood cells are made.
Muscular system	Tissues that allow movement of the body, beating of the heart, and movement within the organs of the digestive system and other tubular structures (e.g., helping move food through the intestines, allowing blood vessels to contract to raise blood pressure).
Reproductive system	Organs and other structures responsible for human reproduction.
Lymphatic system	Organs and other structures that remove extra fluid from tissues, absorb and transport fats from the cardiovascular system, and produce white blood cells and transport them from the lymph nodes.

Lower Airway

Just below the epiglottis, the lower airway consists of the trachea, bronchi, and lungs, which contain the bronchioles and alveoli. Air passes through the larynx and travels down the trachea through the tubes within the lungs. The trachea contains rings of cartilage and can be felt in the anterior neck. Air moving down the trachea passes into the right and left bronchi to enter each lung. These hollow tubes carrying air, called bronchi, continue to divide into smaller and smaller passages, called bronchioles, like the branches of a tree. The bronchioles have muscular walls that can constrict. When cold air, chemical irritants, or other factors are encountered, the bronchiole tubes get smaller to decrease airflow.

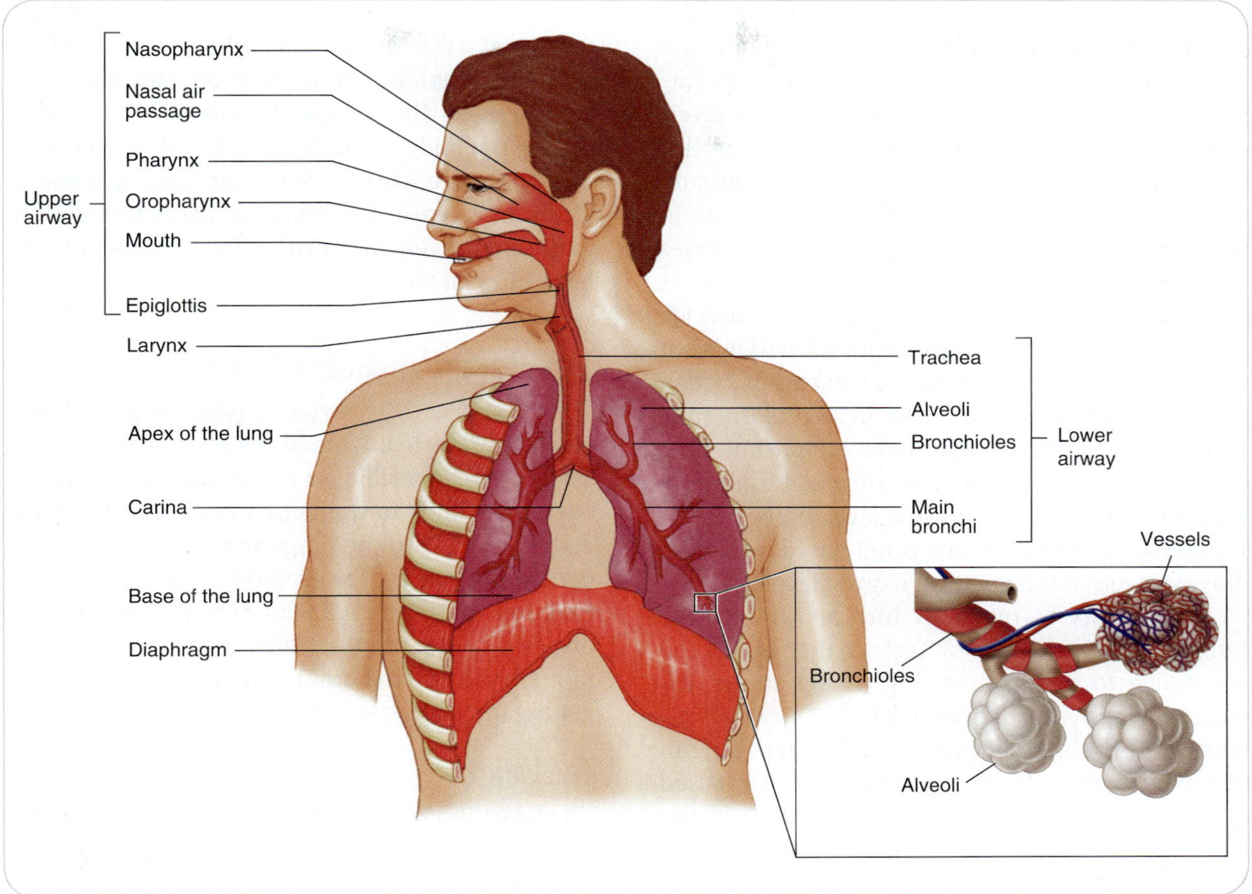

Figure 6-10 The respiratory system.

At the ends of each bronchiole are small air collection sacs called alveoli. Each alveolus is surrounded by tiny blood-containing, thin-walled tubes, known as capillaries. The alveoli allow carbon dioxide and oxygen exchange between the inhaled air in the sacs and the blood in these capillary tubes. Thousands of alveoli are responsible for gas exchange. The capillaries then feed bigger blood vessels, taking oxygen-rich blood through the heart and then to the body.

Ventilation, the act of breathing, is the mechanical process of moving air into and out of the lungs, bringing in oxygen from the environment and then sending a waste product, carbon dioxide, back out. The flow of air into the lungs is caused primarily by contraction of the **diaphragm**, the large, thick, flat muscle that separates the chest and abdomen.

Contraction of the diaphragm results in the expansion of the lungs by creating negative pressure within the thoracic cavity, drawing air into the lungs. Air then flows out of the lungs in a passive process resulting from the combination of relaxation of the diaphragm and recoil of the chest wall, which together decrease the lung size. Accessory muscles between the ribs and in the neck can expand the chest directly, aiding inspiration, especially during labored or rapid breathing. The diaphragm is controlled automatically from nerves that come out of the spinal cord in the neck. If the spinal cord is injured above where these "phrenic" nerves come out of the cervical spine (C3 to C5), the person stops breathing.

The amount of air pulled into and removed from the lungs in one minute is called minute ventilation (or minute volume). This amount is based on the volume of each breath and the breathing rate. Deeper breaths and a faster rate of breathing increase the minute volume, and thus affect the amount of oxygen that goes into the lungs.

Although one may think that breathing is dependent on the amount of oxygen in the blood, it is controlled by the level of carbon dioxide, as carbonic acid, in the blood. If carbon dioxide levels increase (either due to increased production of carbon dioxide by the body or due to decreased minute ventilation causing carbon dioxide to build up in the lungs and blood), the respiration rate increases automatically so that an increased volume of air is moved each minute until the excess carbon dioxide is eliminated. Therefore, in most individuals it is not the lack of oxygen, but instead the excess of carbon dioxide, that causes an increase in respiratory rate. In certain individuals who have significant lung disease, usually from smoking, the blood contains a chronically high carbon dioxide level. In these individuals, the drive to breathe is not based on carbon dioxide levels, but instead on oxygen levels.

The ability to move air into and out of the lungs is often affected by factors that affect the resistance to airflow, slowing it. Resistance increases when the diameter of the airways decreases. If the tube becomes smaller, less air can move through it. In the upper airway, decreased diameter can be due to swelling or injury. In the lower airway, resistance to airflow is most often due to constriction of the small muscles in the walls of the bronchioles (from irritants, cold air, or asthma). It can also occur when the airways are inflamed from infection, plugged with mucus, or compressed. The increased resistance to airflow causes the body to move less air with each breath or to do more work to move the same volume of air. In most cases the body increases the work to maintain movement of the same volume of air by breathing faster.

The Cardiovascular System

The **cardiovascular system** (circulatory system) consists of the heart, blood vessels, and blood. This system is responsible for delivering oxygen, nutrients, and fluids to the body's cells and for taking carbon dioxide to the lungs and other waste products to the kidneys for excretion. The bloodstream functions both as a nutrient provider and a waste disposal route for the body. It also carries hormones made by the brain and other organs to target organs when needed.

The Heart

The heart is a highly efficient muscular organ that pumps blood throughout the body. It is about the size of a closed fist (**Figure 6-11**). The heart is

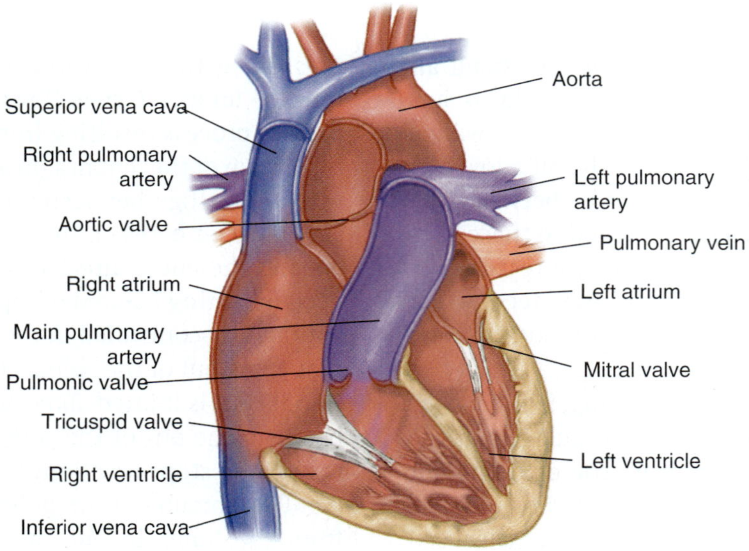

Figure 6-11 The heart is a four-chambered muscle that pumps blood to all parts of the body.

located in the chest cavity between the two lungs, posterior to the sternum and slightly to the left of the midline.

The heart is divided into four compartments, called chambers. The right and left upper chambers are called atria, and the right and left lower chambers are called ventricles. The two chambers on the right side of the heart are separated from the two chambers on the left side by a wall. Blood in the heart does not travel from the right side to the left side. There are four valves in the heart, two on each side. These valves allow blood to flow only in one direction when the heart muscle squeezes and moves the blood.

The heart functions as two pumps: right and left. The right side of the heart pumps blood to the lungs; the left side pumps blood to the rest of the body, including the muscles of the heart (**Figure 6-12** and **Figure 6-13**). All the blood from the left side of the heart going to the body goes through the aorta, which is the big artery on top of the heart. Arteries that supply blood to the heart muscle, called coronary arteries, arise from the first part of the aorta.

The heart's coordination of pumping is regulated through a specialized electrical network of cells that "pace" the heart. These "pacemaker" cells create an electric current that is conducted through the heart and causes the heart's muscle to contract in a coordinated way. In actuality, all muscle cells in the heart can generate their own electric current, but under normal conditions more dominant pacemaker cells provide the electric impulse for coordinated contractions. The electric impulse begins in the muscle of the right atrium and spreads through both atria, causing contraction of both atria. The impulse then spreads to cells in the right and left ventricles, leading to a coordinated contraction of both ventricles. This electrical system causes the heart muscle to contract in such a way that blood is pumped out of the heart, with the right side supplying blood to the lungs so that the lungs can oxygenate it and the left side supplying oxygenated blood to the rest of the body.

The heart's pacemaker cells fire at a basic rate that can be changed when needed by input from autonomic nerves (described later in this chapter). For example, during exercise, the body senses that more blood needs to be pumped, so the heart works harder automatically, providing more blood to the muscles.

In a diseased heart, if one group of pacemaker cells fails, the next one in the chain can take over, but this results in a slower heart rate and often less-coordinated contractions. In addition,

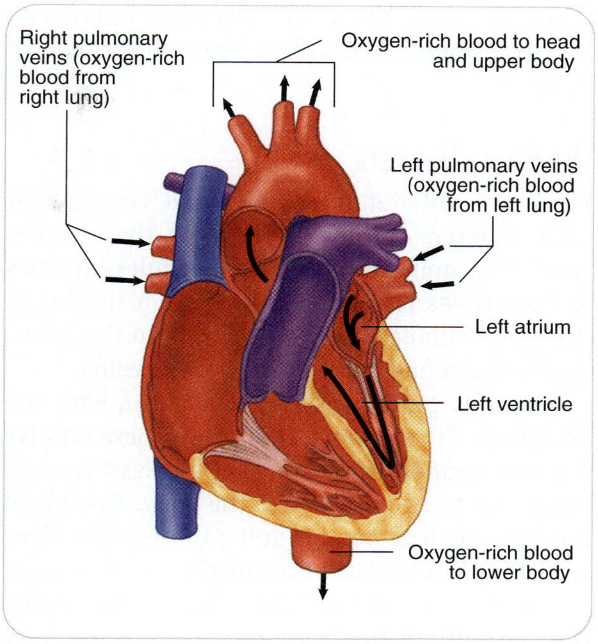

Figure 6-13 The left side of the heart receives oxygen-rich blood from the lungs through the pulmonary veins.

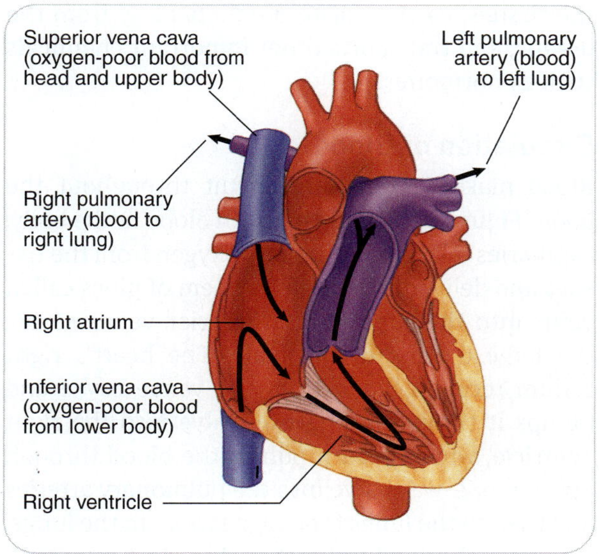

Figure 6-12 The right side of the heart receives oxygen-poor blood from the venous circulation.

abnormalities in the heart's electrical system can lead to an abnormal heartbeat or rhythm, called an arrhythmia.

The Blood Vessels

There are different types of blood vessels that serve different purposes. They are the arteries, arterioles, capillaries, veins, and venules. Arteries and arterioles carry blood away from the heart. Veins and venules bring blood back to the heart. Capillaries connect the arteries to the veins.

Arteries contain oxygen-rich blood, with the exception of the pulmonary arteries. These arteries that come out of the right side of the heart contain blood that has gone through the body. This blood is oxygen depleted and is going through the right side of the heart back to the lungs for more oxygen.

Capillaries connect the arterial side of the vascular system to the venous side. These very small tubes near all of the body's cells provide nutrients, oxygen, and other substances to the cells. The capillaries exchange these needed substances for waste materials, including carbon dioxide. Through the capillaries, the waste products enter the bloodstream and are carried to the kidneys and lungs to be excreted.

The venous system carries blood from the tissues back to the heart. Venous blood still has some oxygen in it, but less than arterial blood, as oxygen has been given to the body's tissues. The exception is the pulmonary veins, which carry oxygenated blood from the lungs to the heart.

On the venous side, venules on the other side of the capillaries are the smallest tubes that carry the blood back to the heart. These venules merge into larger veins, which merge into still larger veins as they get nearer to the heart. The superior and inferior venae cavae, the largest veins, act as reservoirs, supplying oxygen-depleted blood to the heart. Thus, the blood goes through a closed circular system.

The Blood

There are four main components of blood: red blood cells, white blood cells, platelets, and the straw-colored liquid in which they are suspended, called plasma (**Figure 6-14**). The function of the red blood cells is to carry oxygen to the body's cells and assist in removing carbon dioxide from them. Oxygen is carried primarily by hemoglobin in the red blood cells, with a small amount of oxygen dissolved in

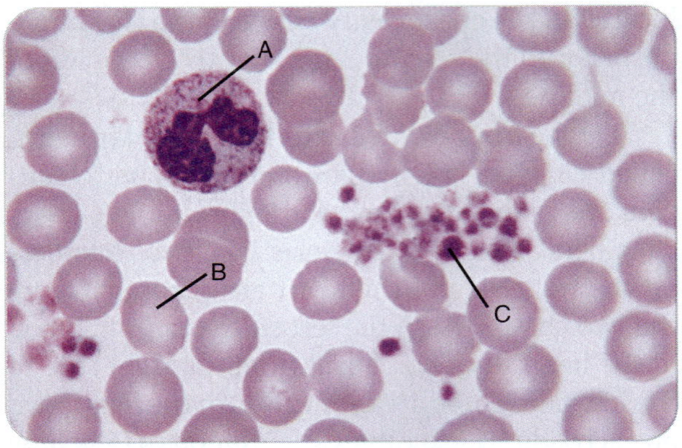

Figure 6-14 The main components of blood are white blood cells **(A)**, red blood cells **(B)**, platelets **(C)**, and straw-colored liquid called plasma.

the plasma. Carbon dioxide is dissolved primarily in the plasma as carbonic acid, with a small amount carried by the red blood cells. The iron in the hemoglobin of red blood cells gives blood its red color and is necessary for oxygen transport.

White blood cells are part of the body's immune system, helping the body defend itself against infection. There are several types of white blood cells, each providing defense against different microorganisms.

Platelets are the component of blood (along with specialized proteins from the liver in the plasma) that forms blood clots to stop bleeding.

Plasma carries the blood cells and nutrients to the tissues, carries waste products away from the organs, and transports other important chemicals such as hormones.

Circulation of Blood

Blood makes a complete circuit throughout the body (**Figure 6-15**). Starting with blood in the body, capillaries take blood with less oxygen from the tissues and deliver it through a system of pipes called veins into the superior and inferior venae cavae, the largest veins in the body. The heart's right atrium receives blood from the venae cavae and pumps it through a one-way valve into the right ventricle, which in turn pumps the blood through another one-way valve into the pulmonary arteries and then to the lungs for oxygenation. In the lungs, oxygen is obtained and carbon dioxide is released.

Through veins from the lungs back to the heart, the left atrium receives this oxygen-rich blood and delivers it through a valve to the left

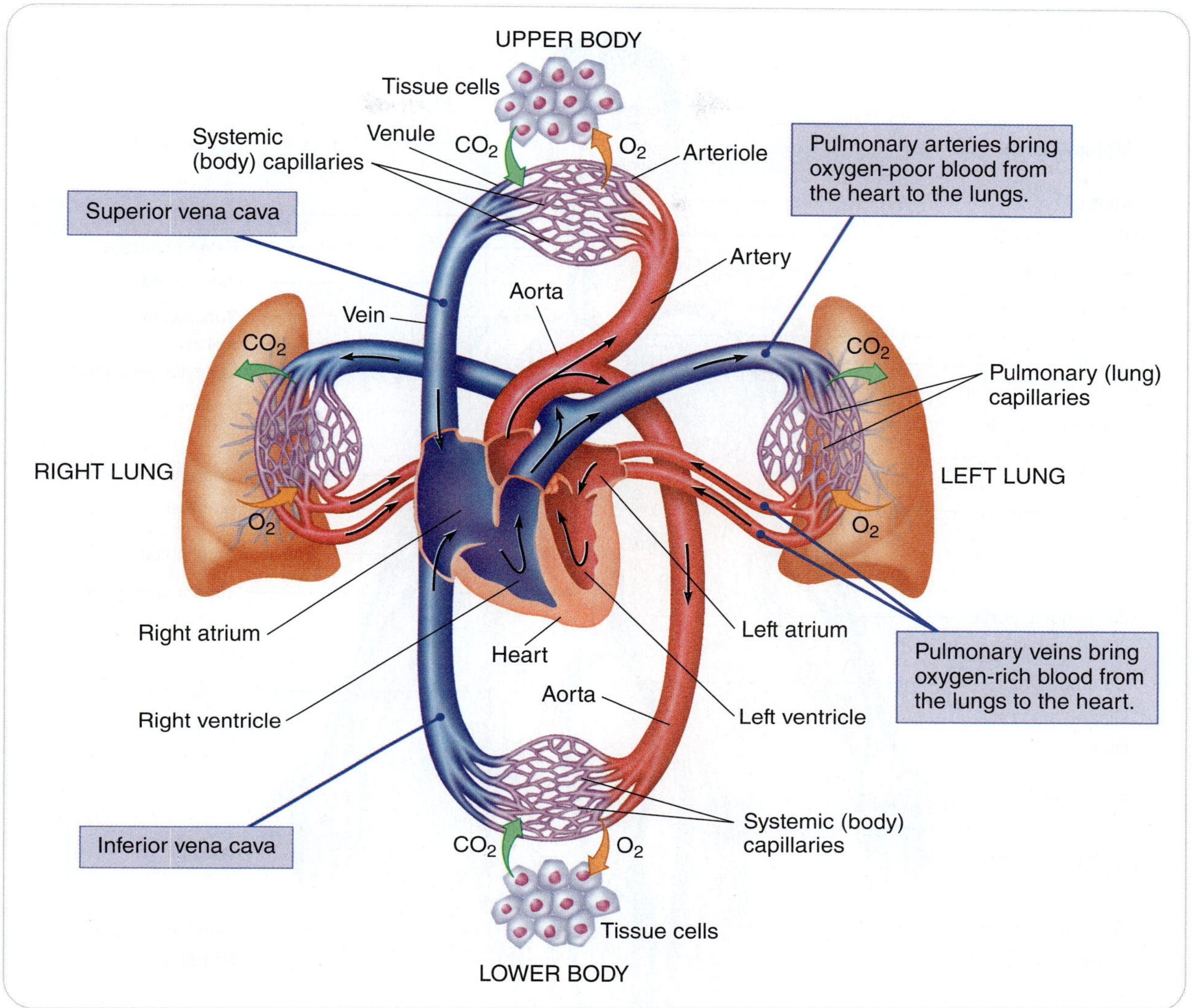

Figure 6-15 Blood flows throughout the entire cardiovascular system.

ventricle. The oxygen-rich blood is then pumped through another one-way valve into the aorta and then on to the arteries. The aorta, the major artery that leaves the left side of the heart, supplies all other arteries with blood. The arteries travel throughout the body, carrying blood with increased oxygen to the tissues. As arteries travel farther from the heart, they branch into increasingly smaller vessels, called arterioles. These narrow arterial vessels carry blood into the smallest blood vessels, the capillaries.

Once in the capillaries, nutrients in the blood from the digestive system's vascular supply and oxygen from the lungs pass through the thin capillary walls to the cells, while waste from the cells pass into the capillaries. The blood then travels through veins of increasing sizes during its return to the heart.

When the blood reaches the capillaries, there is not enough pressure to get the blood back to the heart through the veins. Although there is not a specific pump that forces blood through the veins back to the heart, movement in some organs and the tightening of muscles in the arms and legs squeeze the veins and thus send blood back to the heart. The veins have small one-way valves in their tubes, allowing blood to go only toward the heart (**Figure 6-16**).

There is a large artery and vein that enter each kidney off the lower aorta and vena cava. These vessels carry blood into and out of each kidney, where waste is filtered into the urine. Thus, blood is cleaned after filtering through the kidneys.

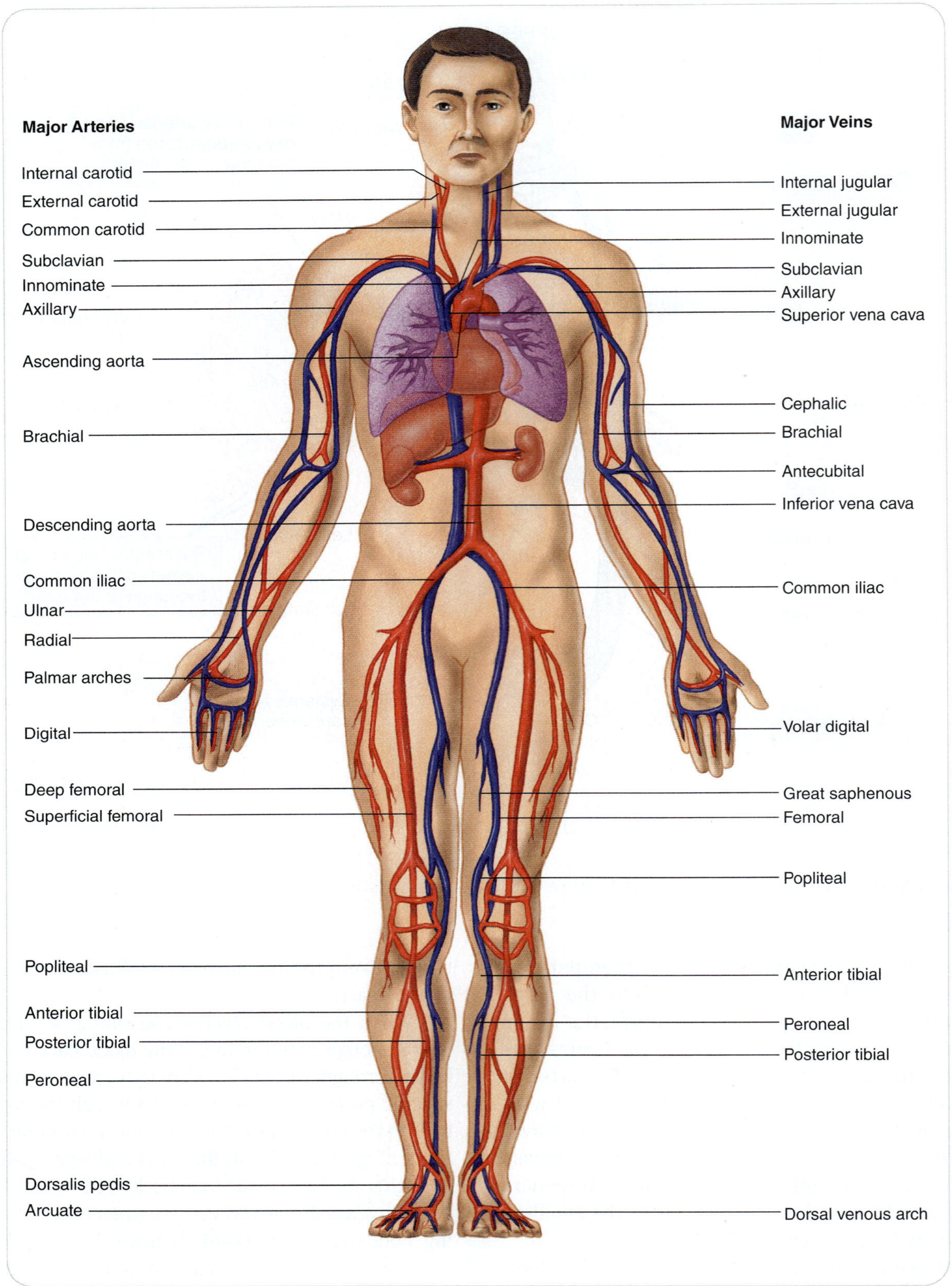

Figure 6-16 The cardiovascular system, also known as the circulatory system, consists of the heart, blood vessles, and blood.

Blood Pressure and Pulse

As the heart pumps blood from the left ventricle to the body, a wave of pressure, called **blood pressure**, can be felt by palpating arterial pulse points. There are five main arteries close to the skin, where a pulse may be taken: carotid, brachial, radial, dorsalis pedis, and femoral (**Figure 6-17**). Blood pressure consists of two measures: the systolic pressure (when the left ventricle maximally squeezes blood into the aorta) and the diastolic pressure (when the left ventricle is at rest).

The blood pressure is measured in millimeters of mercury (mm Hg), or the amount of pressure needed to raise a column of mercury in a glass tube a certain height in millimeters. New blood pressure cuffs are calibrated for this measurement and do not use mercury in a glass tube as they did in the past. Blood pressure is expressed as "systolic pressure over diastolic pressure"—for example, 120 over 80, written as 120/80 mm Hg. Normally, there is always some pressure in the arteries. The diastolic pressure represents the lowest pressure *maintained* in the arteries.

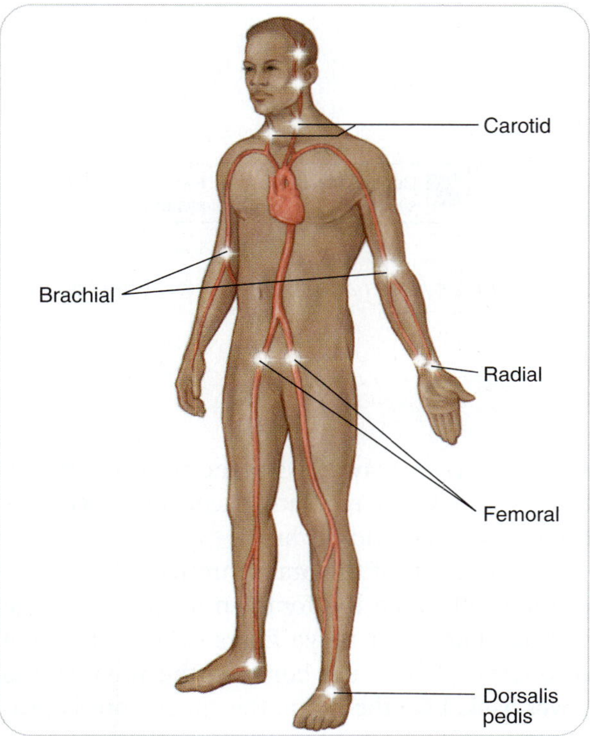

Figure 6-17 There are five main arteries close to the skin, where a pulse may be taken: carotid, brachial, radial, dorsalis pedis, and femoral.

The difference between the systolic blood pressure and the diastolic blood pressure is known as the pulse pressure. The factors that affect blood pressure are the cardiac output (the volume of blood pumped per minute) and the resistance in the blood vessels. The resistance in the blood vessels is determined by the amount of constriction or dilation in the arterioles. Small automatically controlled muscles surround the arterioles and make them bigger or smaller.

The Nervous System

The **nervous system** is the most complex of all the body systems. The computer of the nervous system, the **brain**, is responsible for the control of all the body systems. The brain coordinates the function of sensation, controls muscles, keeps body organs functioning automatically, and integrates consciousness, memory, emotions, and the use of language.

The nervous system can be divided into two main *anatomic* parts: the **central nervous system**, often abbreviated CNS, and the **peripheral nervous system**, often abbreviated PNS (**Figure 6-18**). The central nervous system consists of the brain and spinal cord. The peripheral nerves connect to the spinal cord just inside the spine bones, or vertebrae, and go to the body.

The brain can be divided into three major portions: the cerebrum, the cerebellum, and the brainstem (**Figure 6-19**). The top of the brain, the cerebrum, is the largest part (approximately 75%) and is responsible for higher functions such as sense perception, voluntary movement, speech, thought, and memory. It is divided in the middle into left and right halves, called cerebral hemispheres. Interestingly, the right side of the brain controls the left side of the body, and left side of the brain controls the right side of the body.

The cerebellum is in the middle of the brain, below the posterior aspect of the cerebrum and above the brainstem. It controls balance and coordination. Below the cerebellum is the brainstem. The pons and the medulla oblongata are parts of the brainstem. The brainstem controls the most fundamental life-support functions of the body, such as heart rate and breathing. The brainstem gives rise to 12 specialized "cranial" nerves that support important functions, such as smell, sight, facial movement, and hearing. The spinal cord comes out of the bottom of the brainstem.

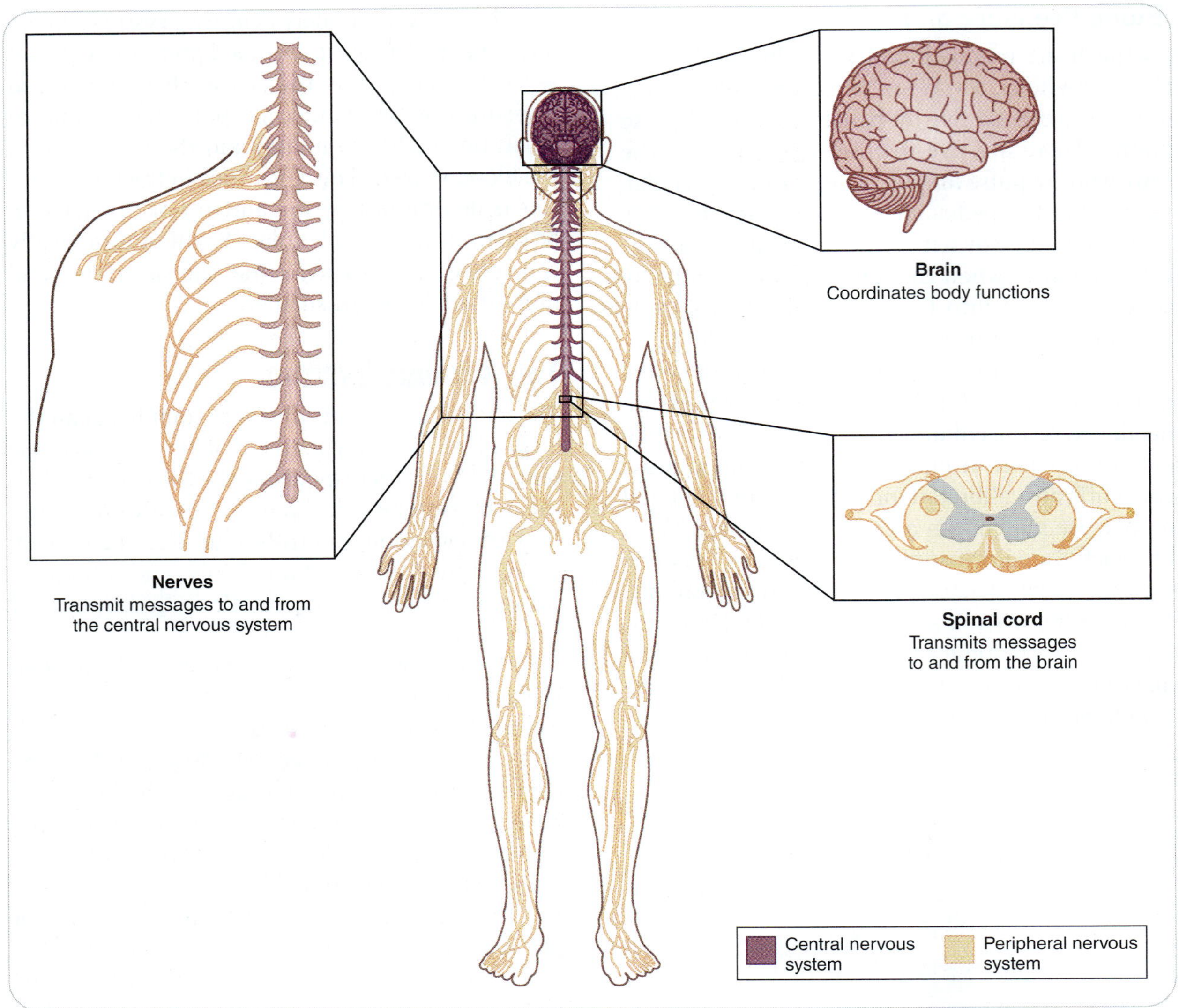

Figure 6-18 The nervous system is composed of the central nervous system and the peripheral nervous system.

The brain and spinal cord are covered by three protective layers, collectively known as the meninges, which are in turn protected by the bones of the skull, the vertebrae, and soft tissues (**Figure 6-20**). Circulating within these layers, bathing the brain and spinal cord and providing further protection, is cerebrospinal fluid.

Cerebrospinal fluid (CSF) is a clear fluid that is produced inside the brain and circulates throughout the central nervous system in a network of canals within the meninges. The brain is suspended in the CSF, protecting the brain from striking the inside of the skull. The flow of CSF carries metabolic wastes away from the nervous system tissues and helps regulate chemical concentrations and pH around the brain.

Coming out of the brain through a large hole in the skull called the foramen magnum, a large ropelike bundle of nerve fibers called the spinal cord travels inside the bones of the spine to the lower back. Like the brain, the spinal cord is protected by CSF and the three layers of the meninges, and it is also protected by the vertebral bodies. In the lower back, at the level of the first lumbar vertebra, the nerve fibers of the spinal cord fan out in a structure known as the cauda equina (Latin for

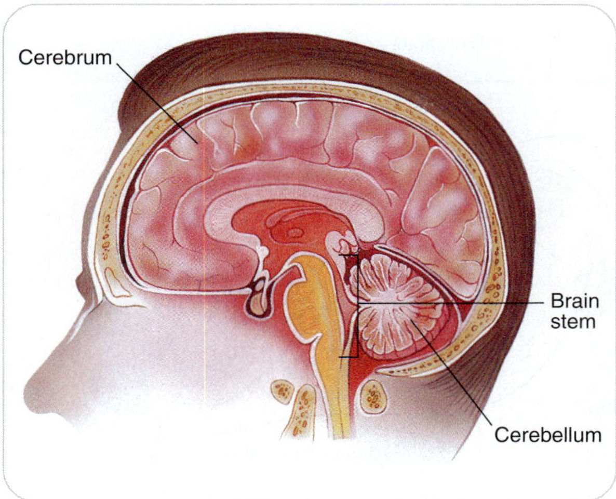

Figure 6-19 The brain has three major subdivisions: the cerebrum, the cerebellum, and the brainstem.

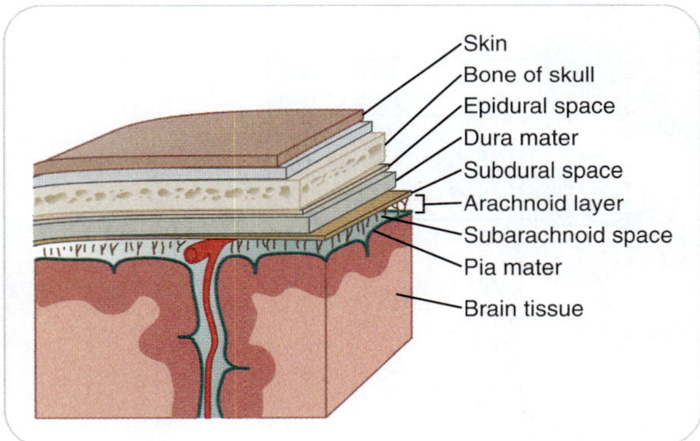

Figure 6-20 Meninges are the layers of protective membranes covering the brain and spinal cord.

"horse's tail"), which represents the distal portion of the spinal cord.

The peripheral nervous system is the portion of the nervous system located outside the brain and spinal cord. These nerves attach to the spinal cord. The **neuron**, the fundamental functional unit of the nervous system, is the cell that conducts information.

The nervous system functions as a well-trained and highly efficient command center. Information such as sensation, temperature, and position of the body is transmitted from nerve endings in the body by the peripheral nervous system to the brain through the spinal cord. Motor instructions from the brain by way of the spinal cord travel through the peripheral nerves to the muscles.

The nervous system also can be divided into two *functional* systems: the voluntary and autonomic systems. The voluntary system controls movement of the muscles and transmits sensations from the sensory organs to the brain and spinal cord. The autonomic (or automatic) system is involuntary and controls the involuntary actions of the organs and glands.

Information from the body's internal organs is transmitted by the autonomic nervous system to the central nervous system, where it is processed, and a response is generated. This response is then transmitted from the brain, through nerves in the spinal cord, to target organs such as the heart, adrenal glands (where special hormones are made), and skeletal muscles. The body reacts accordingly. For example, in response to a threat, a person's brain tells the adrenal glands to release adrenaline, increasing the heart rate and the tensing of muscles for flight.

The autonomic nervous system can be divided into two subsystems: the sympathetic and parasympathetic divisions (**Figure 6-21**). The sympathetic division controls the body's response to stressors such as pain, fear, and a sudden loss of blood. These actions are sometimes referred to as the fight-or-flight response, discussed in the next section. The effects of the parasympathetic division are the opposite of those of the sympathetic division.

Fight, Flight or Freeze Response

It is important that OEC technicians are aware of how the body responds to stressful situations. A stress response is stimulated by one or more of the body's five senses: sight, smell, hearing, taste, or touch. Seeing a grossly deformed body part, smelling the stench of a decaying animal, hearing someone retch, tasting foul water, or feeling broken bones move are all sensory cues that can make an OEC technician feel physically ill.

Stress responses are controlled by the nervous system. When stressed, the body exhibits numerous physical signs and symptoms, such as nausea, diarrhea, dry mouth, sweaty palms, increased heart rate, rapid breathing, and dilated pupils.

The fight-or-flight response (sometimes called the "fight, flight, or freeze" response) is a

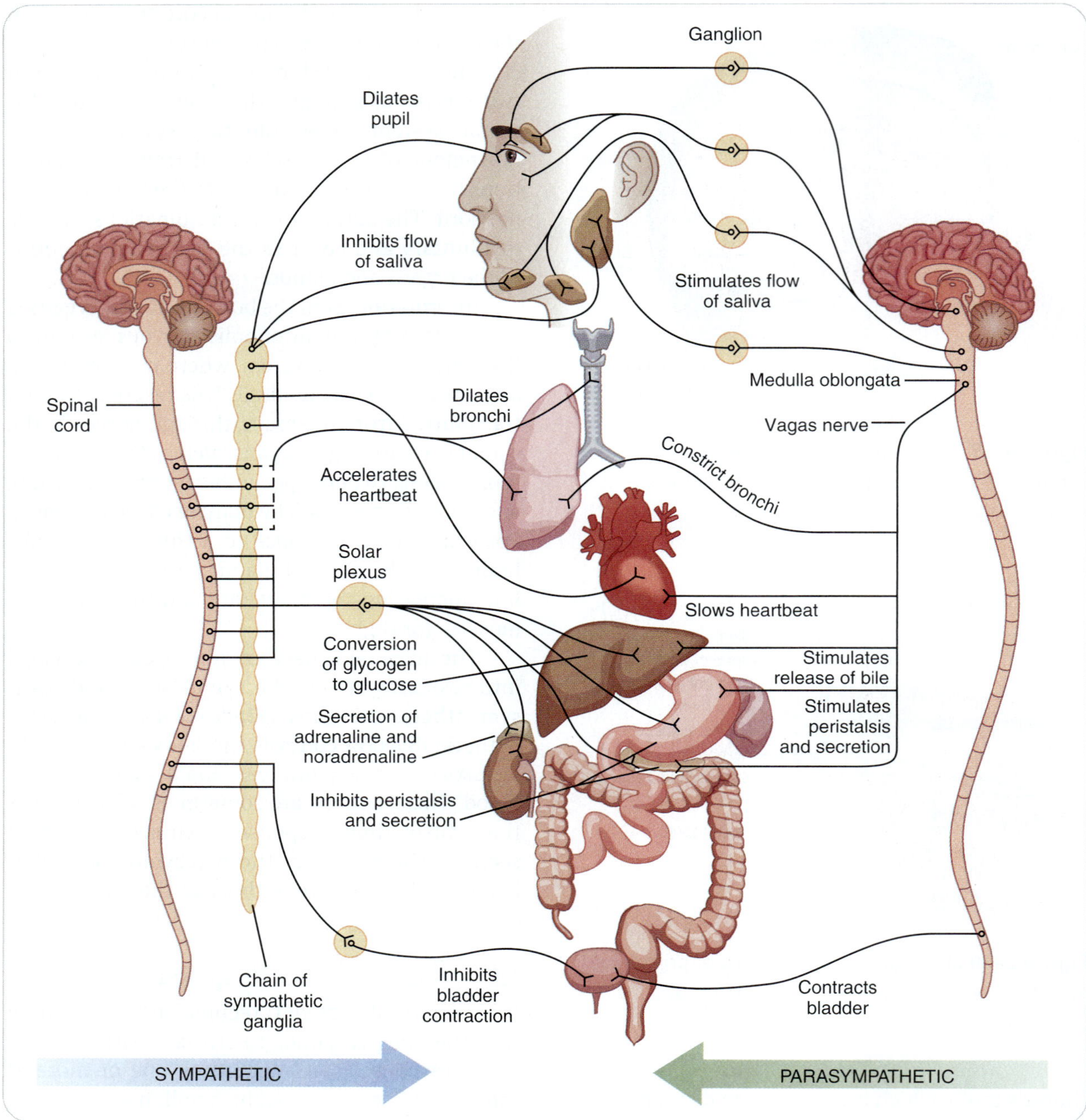

Figure 6-21 The autonomic nervous system can be divided into two subsystems: the sympathetic and parasympathetic divisions.

function of the autonomic nervous system, the part of the central nervous system that we do not control voluntarily. Breathing, heart rate, and digestion are a few of the functions the autonomic nervous system controls. The release of chemicals such as epinephrine (adrenaline) by the adrenal glands during stress affects the autonomic nervous system, causing elevated heart rate and blood pressure, pupil dilation, increased respiratory rate and airway capacity, and increased blood flow to the muscles of the arms and legs. The extra blood flow to muscles provides the additional oxygen and nutrients needed for rapid skeletal movement in the fight, flight, or freeze response.

The Digestive System

The **digestive system**, also known as the gastrointestinal system, consists of the organs that work together to process food and absorb water (**Figure 6-22**). The digestive system is composed of the alimentary tract (food passageway) and several accessory organs that contribute to the digestive process. Together, the organs of the digestive system break down food, absorb nutrients, and eliminate indigestible food components and some wastes. The simplest and most common method of describing portions of the abdomen is by quadrants. The quadrants are four equal areas formed by two imaginary lines that intersect at right angles at the umbilicus (**Figure 6-23**).

Digestion occurs both mechanically and chemically. Mechanical digestion refers to the physical breaking down of food that begins with chewing, swallowing, and moving the food through the digestive tract. Chemical digestion refers to the process whereby chemicals break foods down into components the body can absorb, such as fatty acids and amino acids. Some of these chemicals come from accessory organs that drain into the digestive system: the pancreas and gallbladder.

Food enters the digestive system through the mouth, where it is chewed and mixed with saliva,

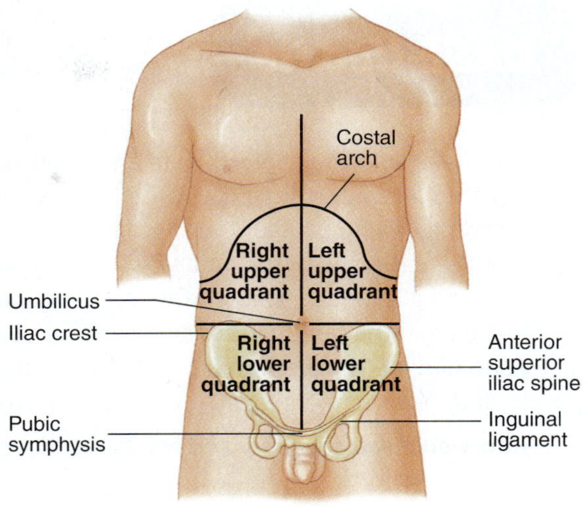

Figure 6-23 The quadrants of the abdomen—right upper, right lower, left upper, and left lower.

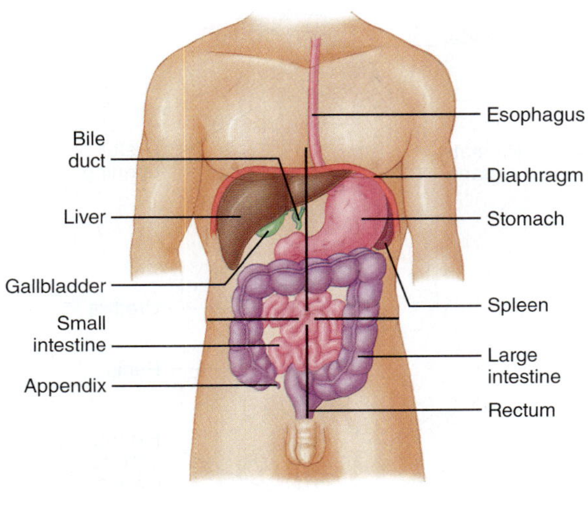

Figure 6-22 The organs of the digestive system. This system helps to break down food, absorb water and nutrients, and eliminate waste.

which breaks down starch into sugar. Particles of food then pass down the esophagus, the passageway to the stomach. The inside layer of tissue of the stomach releases hydrochloric acid, which breaks up the food into smaller pieces. Food travels from the stomach into the small intestine. The small intestine consists of three parts: the duodenum, jejunum, and ileum. Each of these parts functions differently in nutrient absorption.

The pancreas secretes pancreatic juices, or enzymes, into the upper small intestine that aid in the digestion of fats, starches, and proteins. Also, the pancreas has specialized cells that make the sugar-regulating hormones insulin and glucagon, which are released into the bloodstream. These hormones are discussed in this chapter as part of the endocrine system.

The liver, the largest organ in the abdomen, aids in the digestion of fats by making bile. The gallbladder stores and releases bile into the upper small intestine. The liver is responsible also for breaking down many toxic substances absorbed through the intestines and for producing many of the major proteins released into the bloodstream needed by the body.

Following the digestion of food into a liquid, tiny nutrients are absorbed through the small intestine's wall into a group of venous blood vessels in the intestines. The nutrients then go to the liver

CASE Update

You make sure the scene is safe and apply body substance isolation prior to evaluating both patients. After checking the ABCs (airway, breathing, and circulation), looking for serious bleeding, taking a history, and performing a physical exam on each patient, you determine that the patient with the deformed wrist has no other apparent injuries except scrapes. As you perform a full head-to-toe exam on the patient with the deformed lower leg, you find he also has pain in the left upper quadrant of his abdomen. When you gently palpate this part of his abdomen, he winces with pain. Had you not done the full-body exam, you may have missed this finding. You contact dispatch to request immediate assistance.

How would you precisely and accurately describe these injuries to dispatch?

(for absorption and processing) before continuing in the blood to the heart through the inferior vena cava. Then the heart pumps the nutrients to the body.

Unused food and some wastes from the liver (including old red blood cells) end up in the large intestine or colon. Stool, also called feces, gets its characteristic brown color from the breakdown of old red blood cells. The material passing through the small intestines is liquid, so the large intestine absorbs water from this material, making it solid, formed stool. Gas-forming bacteria that are normal residents in the intestines aid in the digestion of the food, and they also create noxious gases, primarily methane. Both the stool and the gas are expelled from the anus. If the colon does not absorb water properly, diarrhea results.

The Urinary System

The **urinary system** consists of organs and other structures involved in the elimination of waste products that are filtered from the blood by the kidneys and excreted in urine (**Figure 6-24**). These waste products include the normal by-products of the body's metabolism and some toxins that may have been introduced into the blood.

The urinary system in men and women consists of the kidneys, ureters, urinary bladder, and urethra. The kidneys are in the lower back outside the abdominal cavity at the lower margin of the rib cage, one on each side. The ureters are tubes coming out of each kidney that carry urine to the bladder. The bladder is a muscular bag that stores

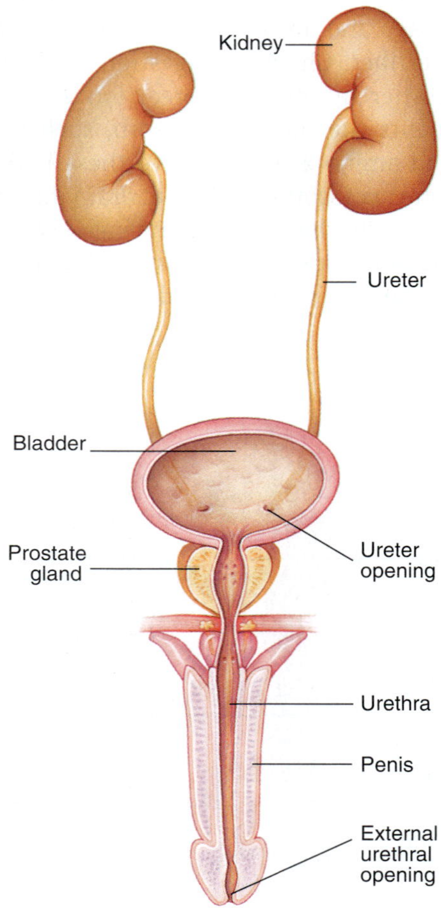

Figure 6-24 The kidneys, ureters, bladder, and urethra make up the urinary system in the male anatomy.

the urine until it is excreted. The urethra is a tube that carries the urine from the bladder to the point of exit from the body. Muscle at the top of the urethra controlled by the automatic nervous system controls urine continence. The muscle can be released voluntarily when urination occurs.

One large artery and vein attach to each kidney, allowing blood to flow through the kidneys. The kidneys produce urine by filtering metabolic wastes into the ureters from the blood. They are selective, as they keep nutrients in and excrete waste.

Water in the body is controlled by the kidneys. Several endocrine hormones in the blood regulate water balance by either increasing or decreasing the amount of sodium chloride (salt) that is excreted by the kidneys. If salt is retained, water is retained. If salt is excreted in the urine, water also is excreted. Also, the urinary system functions in maintaining the balance of other electrolytes and in controlling the pH of the blood.

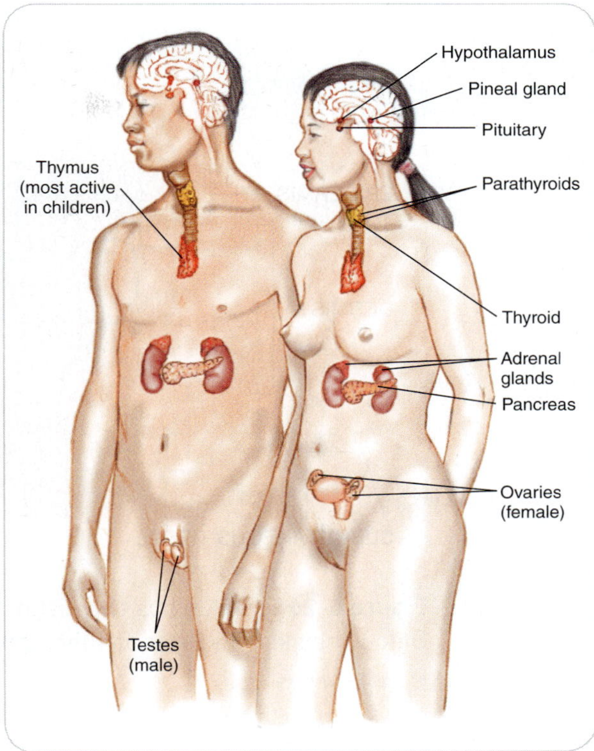

Figure 6-25 Structures of the endocrine system secrete chemicals and hormones that influence activity in different parts of the body.

The Endocrine System

The **endocrine system** is made up of ductless glands that secrete hormones, which are chemical substances that enter the bloodstream and influence a variety of functions in distinct parts of the body.

The major endocrine glands include the pituitary, hypothalamus, thyroid, adrenals, pancreas, gonads (ovaries, testes), parathyroid, pancreas, and pineal (**Figure 6-25**).

The pituitary gland, also known as the "master gland," secretes different chemicals into the bloodstream that regulate growth in children and the activities of many other glands. It also affects kidney function. It is in the center of the brain.

The hypothalamus secretes hormones that act on the pituitary gland. The hypothalamus helps control the regulation of water excretion by the kidneys. This gland is also inside the brain.

The thyroid gland, located in the anterior neck, regulates metabolism, growth, and development. It also partially regulates nervous system activity. Inside the thyroid are the parathyroids, which regulate calcium metabolism.

The adrenal glands are located on top of the kidneys and secrete several hormones, including epinephrine (adrenalin), which functions in the fight-or-flight response and affects heart rate, digestive and kidney function, and the contraction of smooth muscles, including those in the lungs and blood vessels. These glands also secrete cortisol (cortisone), which helps regulate the body's response to stress and is necessary for life.

The pancreas, located in the middle of the abdomen, has both an endocrine function (the secretion of hormones that regulate blood glucose) and a non-endocrine function, making enzymes for digestion. The hormones insulin and glucagon regulate blood sugar in the bloodstream. Insulin lowers blood sugar, while glucagon raises it.

The gonads (ovaries in females and testes in males) produce hormones that control reproduction and sex characteristics. They produce sperm in males and eggs in females.

The pineal gland is a tiny gland in the brain that helps regulate daily wake/sleep patterns by secreting melatonin.

Although all hormones are important, insulin, glucagon, and epinephrine affect the body rapidly. As prehospital responders, OEC technicians must know what they do.

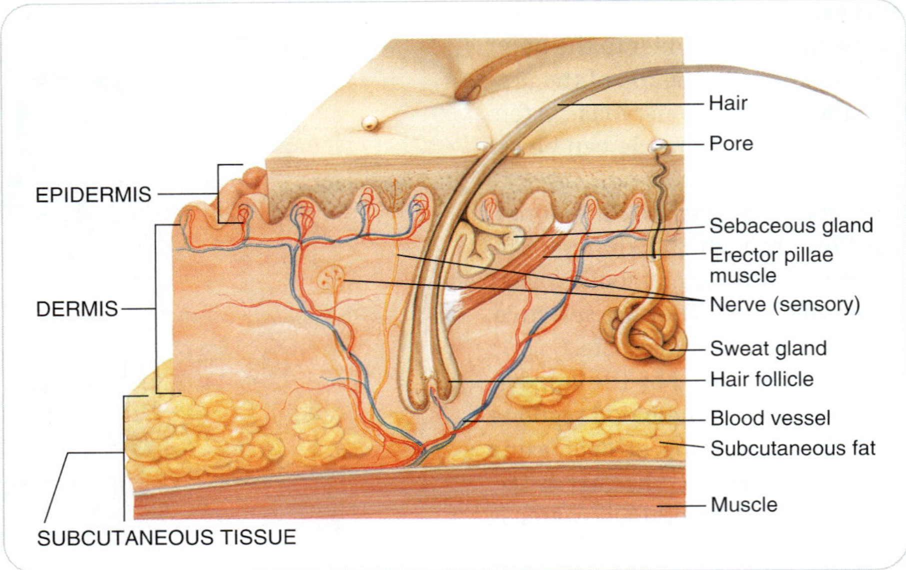

Figure 6-26 The skin has two distinct layers, the epidermis and the dermis. Below the skin is a layer of subcutaneous tissue.

The Integumentary System

The **integumentary system** consists of the skin, hair, nails, sweat glands, and oil glands. The skin provides a protective barrier that separates our tissues, organs, and other systems from the outside world.

The skin is the body's largest organ. It has two major layers, the epidermis and the dermis (**Figure 6-26**). The superficial epidermis contains the skin's pigmentation and protects us from the environment. The dermis contains blood vessels, nerve endings, glands, and hair and is the primary source of the skin's elasticity and strength. Under these layers is the deep subcutaneous layer, which is composed of fatty tissue.

The skin not only is the largest organ system in the body, it also serves several major functions, including protection of the body from injury and invasion by bacteria and other disease-producing pathogens. The skin serves as one of the major organs in the regulation of body temperature and fluid balance. When blood vessels in the dermis dilate, the blood circulates close to the skin's surface, allowing for the release of heat. When those blood vessels constrict, less blood flows to the skin's surface, causing the skin to appear pale or ashen and feel cool. This function helps to conserve heat in the body by keeping the blood closer to the body's core. The evaporation of sweat produced by sweat glands in the skin also helps control body temperature. Glands in the skin produce an oily substance that keeps it from drying out.

The Skeletal System

The **skeletal system** includes bones and ligaments that support the body's structure (**Figure 6-27**). The adult skeleton has over 200 bones. Bone is a hard, dense tissue that forms the skeleton. The outer region of a bone is called the cortex, and the inner region contains porous tissue called marrow.

Bones have varied sizes and shapes, enabling them to perform specific functions. Long bones form the arms and legs, whereas flat bones form the skull and pelvis. Spinal bones have a unique shape of their own.

Where two or more bones join, they form a joint. Strong, tough, fibrous bands called **ligaments** hold the bones at a joint together. Ligaments restrict joint movement based on their location. Most joints allow movement, but some (those in the skull) are immovable, and others (those in the pelvis) allow only slight movement.

Movable joints have a normal range of motion—a distance they can move freely without

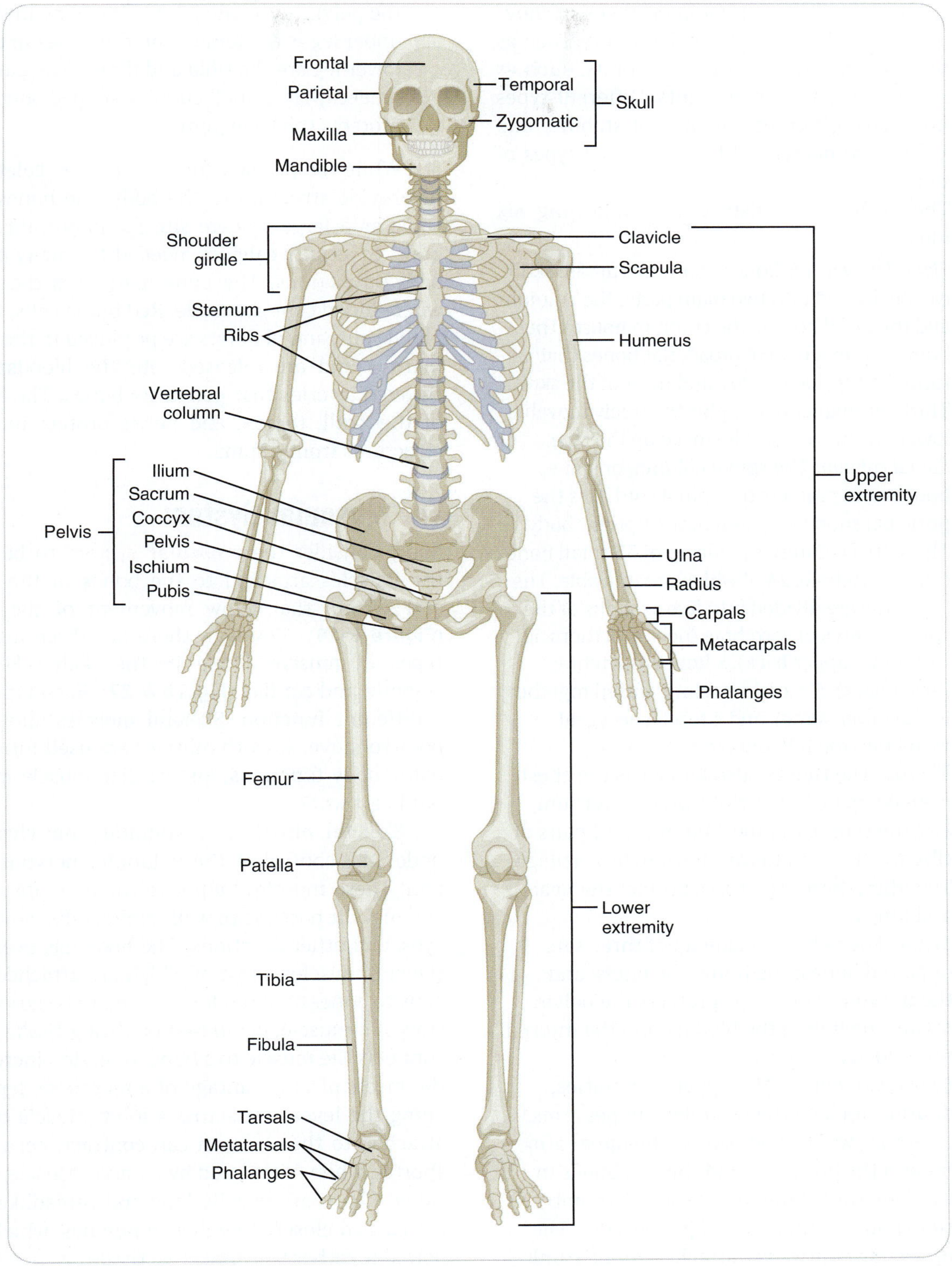

Figure 6-27 The skeletal system supports the body's structure, giving shape and form to the body.

causing injury. The most common types of movable joints are the ball-and-socket joints, such as the hip and shoulder, and hinged joints, such as the elbow, knee, and finger joints. Different types of joints have different amounts of stability and allow different degrees of flexibility and types of movement.

The skeleton consists of the following six sections:

- *Skull.* The various bones that make up the skull can be divided into two main parts: the cranium and the facial bones. The cranium houses the brain. It is made up of broad, flat bones that form the top, back, sides, and front of the skull. Thirteen smaller bones plus the freely movable lower jaw (the mandible) make up the face.
- *Spinal column.* The spinal column, or spine, houses and protects the spinal cord. It is the principal support system of the upright body. The spinal column is made up of 33 small bones called vertebrae, 24 of which are movable. The vertebrae are divided into five sections of the spine: 7 cervical vertebrae (neck), 12 thoracic vertebrae (upper back), 5 lumbar vertebrae (lower back), 5 sacral vertebrae (fused together in the lower spine), and 4 fused coccygeal vertebrae (the tailbone, or coccyx).
- *Thorax.* The thorax, also known as the chest, is made up of 12 pairs of ribs, the sternum, and the thoracic spine. Ten of the 12 pairs of ribs are attached to the sternum by cartilage. Together, these structures protect the heart and lungs.
- *Pelvis.* The pelvis is made up of three sets of paired bones: the ilium, the pubis, and the ischium. The pelvis protects the pelvic organs, including the bladder and the internal reproductive organs.
- *Upper extremities.* The upper extremities, or arms, include the shoulders, upper arms, forearms, wrists, and hands. The upper arm bone is the humerus, and the two bones in the forearm are the radius (on the thumb side) and the ulna (on the pinkie side). The upper extremities are attached to the trunk at the shoulder girdle, made up of the clavicle (collarbone) and the scapula (shoulder blade).
- *Lower extremities.* The lower extremities, or legs, consist of the hips, upper and lower legs, ankles, and feet. They are attached to the pelvis at the hip joints. The bone in the upper leg is the femur, and the bones in the lower leg are the tibia and fibula. The patella (kneecap) is a small circular-shaped bone that protects the knee joint.

While the primary function of the skeleton is to provide structure to the body, the bones also serve as a large storage site for important minerals, especially calcium, needed for many of the body's functions. The bone marrow is the place where blood cells are made. Red blood cells, white blood cells, and platelets are produced in the bone marrow and are released into the bloodstream through arteries that penetrate bones. The bones of the skull, thorax, and pelvis protect internal structures from trauma.

The Muscular System

Many consider the **muscular system** to be only the muscles attached to the bones of the skeletal system that allow movement of the body (**Figure 6-28**). However, there are three distinct types of muscle tissue in the body—skeletal, smooth, and cardiac (**Figure 6-29**). Each type has a different function. Skeletal muscles allow the body to move, smooth muscles are used for automatic body functions, and cardiac muscle makes our heart work.

Skeletal muscles, or voluntary muscles, are under the control of the voluntary nervous system. These muscles help give the body its shape and make it possible to walk, smile, talk, move the eyes, and other functions. The body has over 600 skeletal muscles, most of which are attached directly to bones or to tendons. A **tendon** is the extension of a muscle, composed of strong tissue, that connects the muscle to a bone. A tendon increases the mechanical advantage of a muscle by lengthening the lever arm across a joint. Muscle tissue attached to the skeleton can contract, becoming shorter, when stimulated by a nerve. Muscle cells, called fibers, are usually long and threadlike and are packed closely together in bundles, which are bound together by connective tissue.

Contraction of a skeletal muscle results in movement of a joint, so a person is able to walk or pick up a glass. Skeletal muscles are typically paired such that one muscle produces flexion of a joint and an opposing muscle produces extension

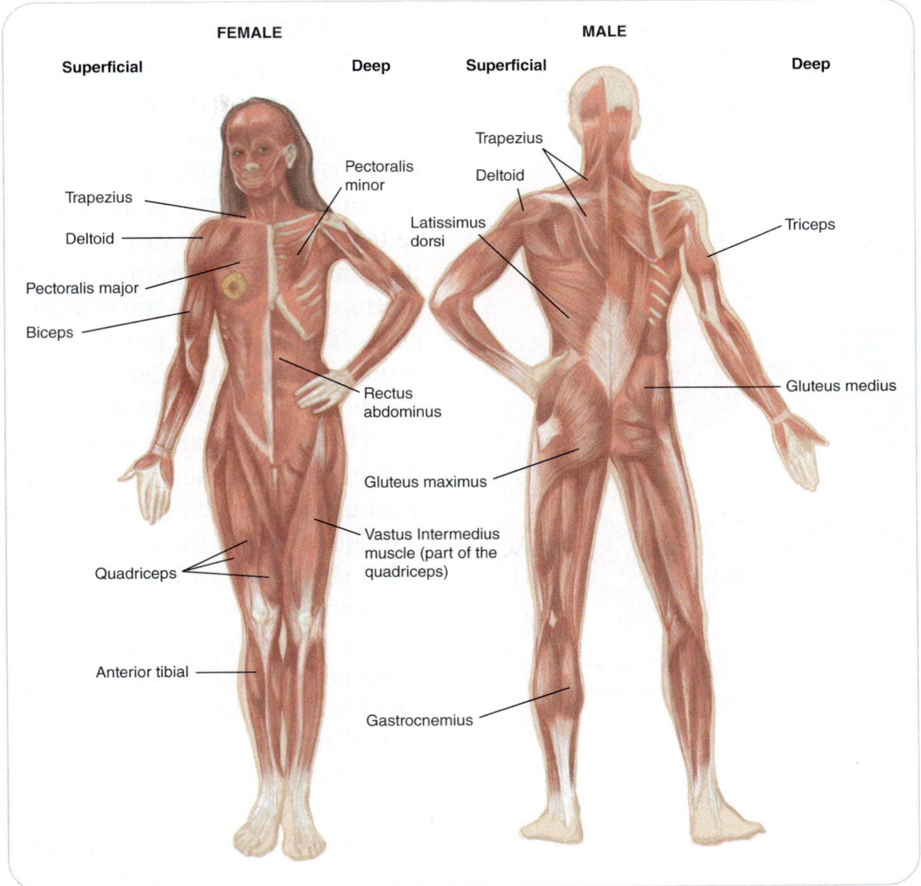

Figure 6-28 Major skeletal muscles of the muscular system.

of a joint. For example, contraction of one set of muscles on the palm side of the forearm will produce flexion and allow for grasping a glass of water, whereas contraction of another set of muscles on the back of the forearm will produce extension and release the glass.

Smooth muscles, also called involuntary muscles, are found in the walls of tubelike organs, ducts, and blood vessels. They also form much of the intestinal wall. These muscles are involuntarily controlled for normal body functions. Contraction of smooth muscle helps with movement of urine or blood. Smooth muscle inside the wall of the intestines moves the food being digested along the gastrointestinal tract toward the anus.

Cardiac muscle is found only in the walls of the heart and shares some of the properties of skeletal and smooth muscle. Cardiac muscle has the unique property of being able to generate its own electrical impulses independent of the nervous system. Contraction of cardiac muscle causes the pumping action of the heart that moves blood through the cardiovascular system.

The Reproductive System

In both men and women, the **reproductive system** includes the organs for sexual reproduction. Puberty usually begins between the ages of 10 and 14 years and is controlled by hormones secreted by the pituitary gland, or "master gland," in the brain. Hormones secreted by the pineal gland in the brain influence the secretion of male or female sex hormones, which leads to the maturation of reproductive organs. These hormones also control what are called secondary sex characteristics, such as facial hair in males, breast development in females, and pubic hair in both sexes.

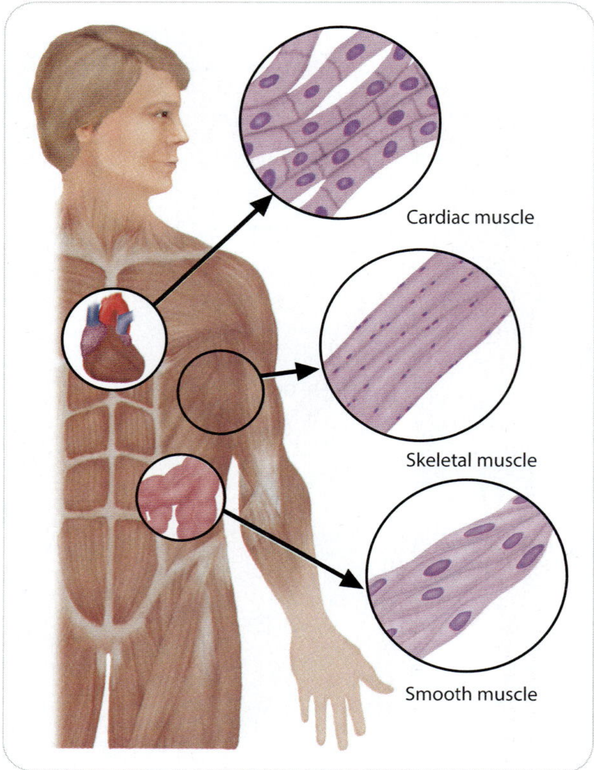

Figure 6-29 The three basic types of muscles: skeletal, smooth, and cardiac.

Male Reproductive System

Many of the male reproductive structures are located outside of the pelvic cavity and thus are more vulnerable to injury than are those of females (**Figure 6-30**). The two testes hang from the underside of the penis in a sac-like structure called the scrotum. Inside the pelvic cavity are the prostate gland and the seminal vesicles. The urethra extends from the bladder to the tip of the penis. The penis, the prominent external phallus, is the terminal part of both the urinary and the reproductive systems in males.

The testes produce sperm and testosterone, the primary male sex hormone. The prostate and seminal vesicles make and store the seminal fluid, the liquid part of the man's ejaculate. Sperm are small structures with a whiplike tail and a head that contains the genetic material needed to fertilize a woman's egg. Sperm made in the testes combine with the seminal fluid to form semen, which is ejaculated during intercourse. Most of the male's urethra is part of the urinary system and transports urine from the bladder. The last part of the urethra also is part of the reproductive system through which semen is ejaculated. The sperm contributes half the genetic material to offspring.

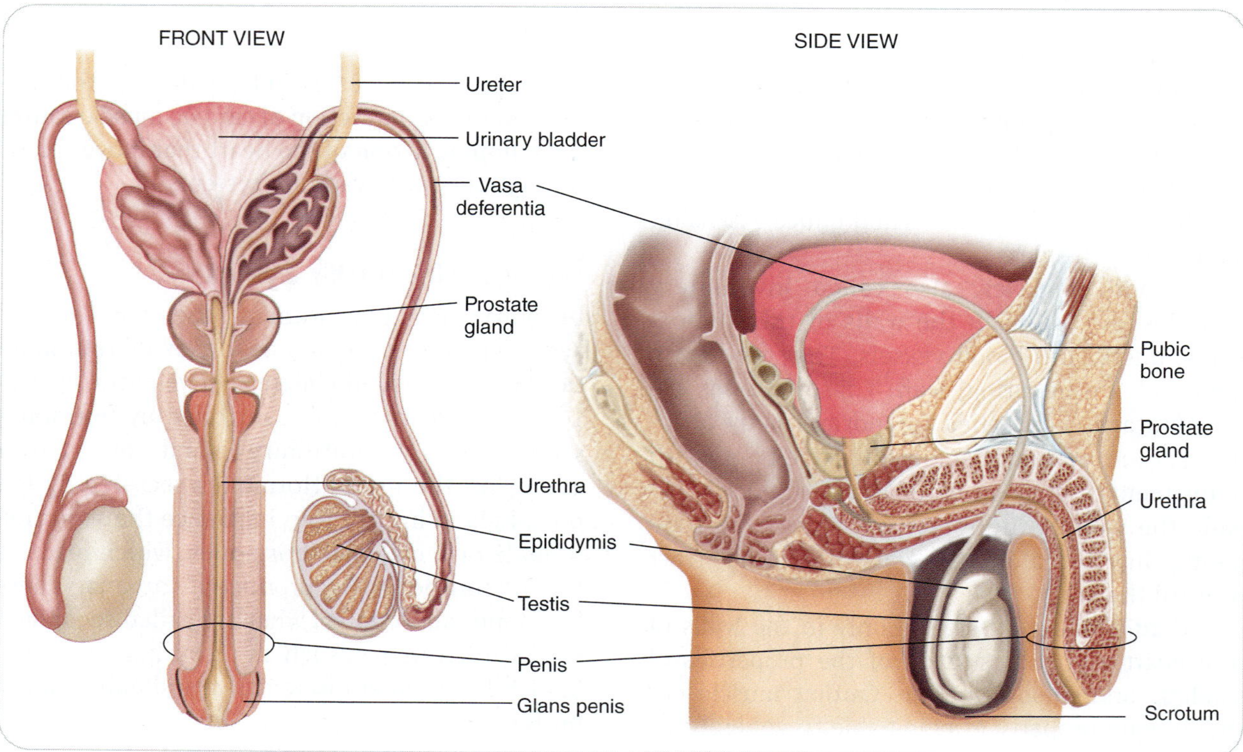

Figure 6-30 Male reproductive system.

Female Reproductive System

The female reproductive system consists of the ovaries, fallopian tubes, uterus, cervix, and vagina, and it is protected by the pelvic bones (**Figure 6-31**). The external structures consist of two vertical lips called the labia, as well as the vulva and the clitoris. The breasts, or mammary glands, of a woman are sometimes included in this system. They produce milk for the newborn.

Endocrine glands in the body, including the hypothalamus and pituitary glands, interact with the reproductive system by releasing hormones that control and coordinate the development and functioning of the female reproductive system.

From the onset of a woman's first menstrual cycle to the time of menopause (when the woman no longer has menstrual cycles), a woman is in the time window known as "child-bearing age." The average age for the onset of the menstrual cycle is 12 years, and the average age for the onset of menopause is approximately 52 years.

The menstrual cycle is approximately 28 days in length. About midway through the cycle, typically a single egg is released from one of the ovaries. This egg travels through the fallopian tube to the uterus. If united with a sperm, the fertilized egg may attach to the lining of the uterus to initiate pregnancy. If two eggs are released and both are fertilized, fraternal twins may be conceived. The female's ovum contributes half the genetic material to the offspring.

The Lymphatic System

The **lymphatic system** returns excess interstitial fluid located around cells to the bloodstream, transports particulate materials such as molecular proteins and bacteria from the tissues, absorbs fats and fat-soluble vitamins from the intestines, and produces lymphocytes (along with the bone marrow), which are white blood cells that are a primary weapon against microorganisms invading the body.

The lymphatic system consists of various organs, a network of vessels that carry lymphatic fluid, and numerous lymph nodes located throughout the body (**Figure 6-32**). The spleen, located in the left upper abdomen, is the largest organ of the lymphatic system. Other parts of the lymphatic system include the tonsils and adenoids in the throat, and the thymus gland located in the anterior neck.

When pathogens from a nearby infection reach the lymph nodes through lymph vessels, the lymph nodes become enlarged and painful from producing additional white blood cells, called lymphocytes, to fight the infection. The spleen filters the blood, removing bacteria, dead tissue, and foreign matter from it, and produces white blood cells that fight infection. The tonsils and adenoids and the thymus help fight infection. The lymphatic system helps with the immune response.

The Immune Response

The immune system consists of a network of specialized cells and organs from several other

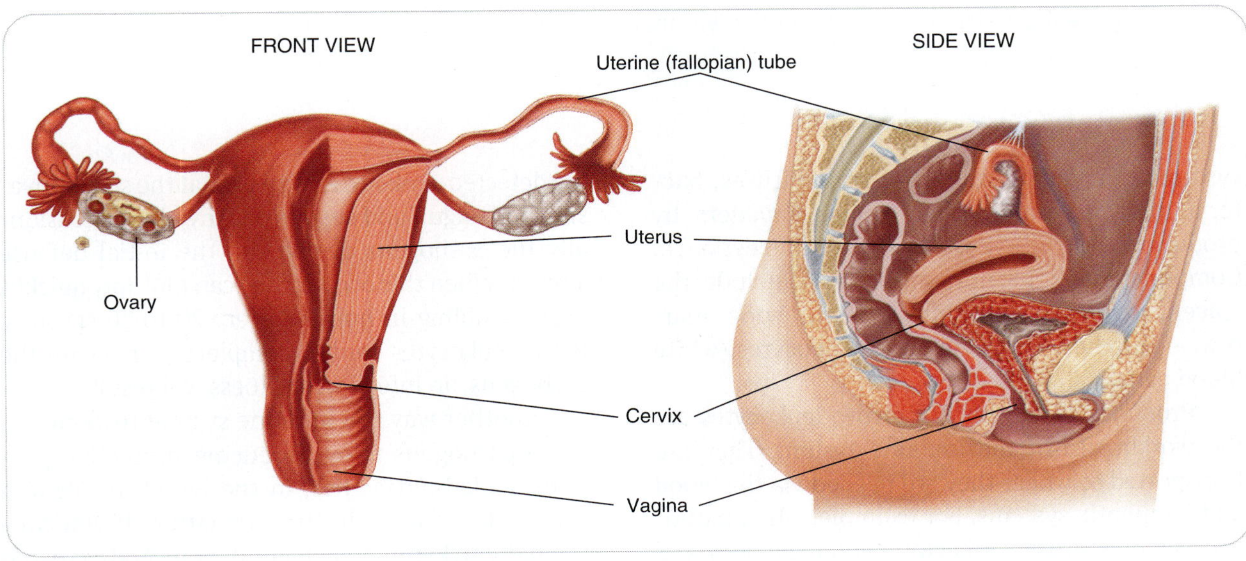

Figure 6-31 Female reproductive system.

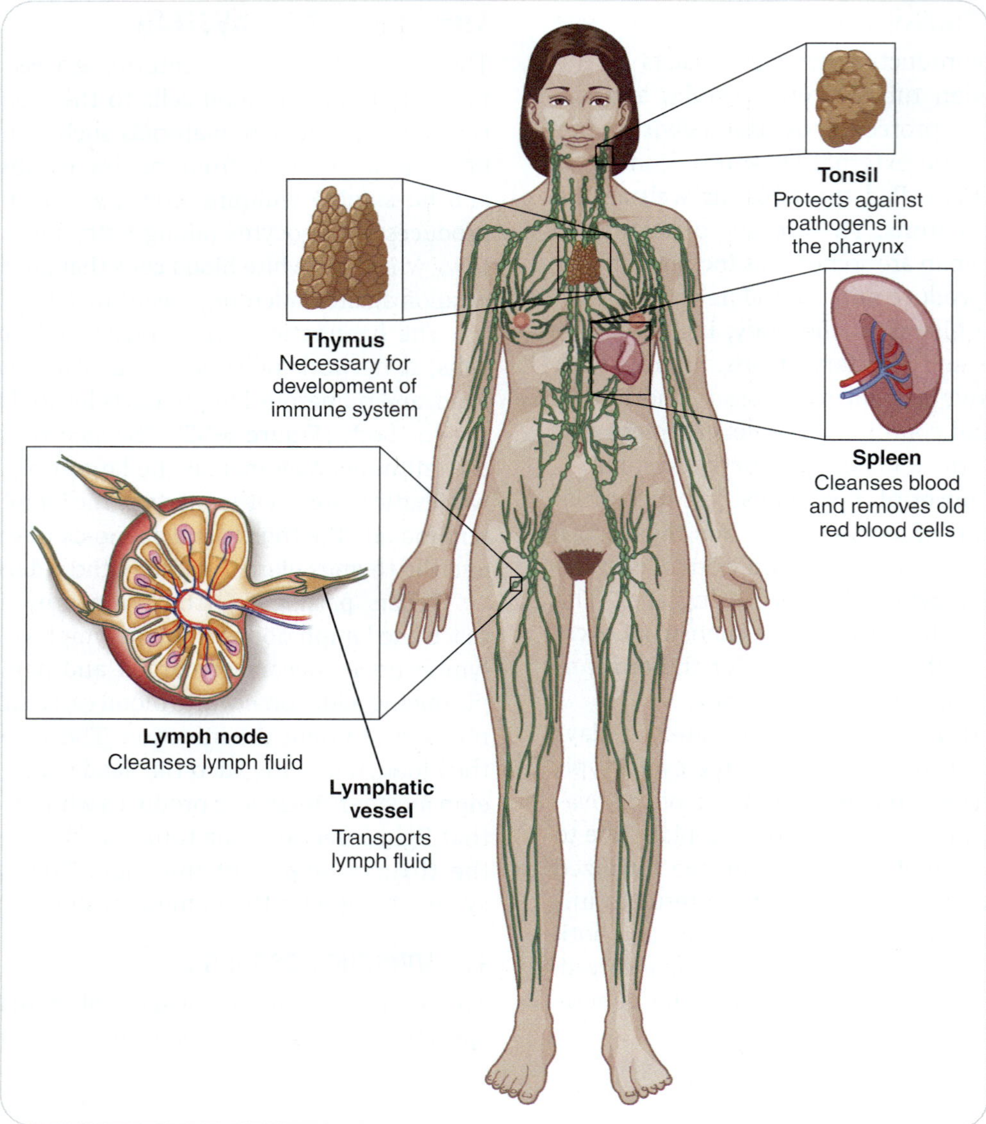

Figure 6-32 The components of the lymphatic system.

systems that defend the body from viruses, bacteria, parasites, and other foreign invaders by producing **immunity**, or an **immune response**. Components of the immune system include the spleen, thymus, lymphatic system, bone marrow, antibodies, hormones, and leukocytes (white blood cells).

Produced in the bone marrow, leukocytes are the workhorses of the immune system. They are transported to where they are needed via the blood and lymphatic systems. For example, when pathogens such as viruses or bacteria enter the body and are detected, leukocytes converge at the site of invasion and engulf and destroy the invaders. Occasionally the pathogens overwhelm the initial defense system. When this occurs, they can multiply quickly, often doubling in number every 20 to 30 seconds. If the leukocytes cannot completely eradicate the pathogens, an infection or illness will result.

Another way the immune system responds to some pathogens is by producing protective proteins, called antibodies, in the lymph nodes and spleen that remain in the circulation. If you contracted chicken pox as a child, your body created antibodies specifically against the chicken pox virus. Those antibodies remain in your body, protecting you from future attacks by the chicken pox virus for many years.

Many government health authorities have instituted aggressive vaccination programs to prevent the spread of such diseases as influenza, mumps, measles, polio, and tetanus. Smallpox has been essentially eradicated from the world by the most extensive and successful immunization campaign in history. Massive immunization programs have helped reduce the spread of influenza.

CASE Outcome

You notify dispatch that you have two patients, one with a deformed lower leg who had decreased mental status but is now alert. He also has left upper quadrant pain near the spleen. The second patient has a deformed wrist and abrasions. Both have normal distal pulses and neurologic function in their injured extremities. Vital signs are stable. You request additional patrollers and call for an ambulance. You request advanced life support (ALS), as the one patient may have a ruptured spleen. You now begin caring for the injured patients.

Other OEC technicians soon arrive. You inform them of the injuries you have found. Working together, you and the other OEC technicians treat and package the two patients.

After transport to the aid room, the patient with the tibial injury and possible ruptured spleen goes to the hospital with ALS providers, and later you learn he had a ruptured spleen and broken tibia. The other patient goes by car to the hospital and is treated for a broken wrist.

CHAPTER REVIEW

In Summary

- Human anatomy is the study of the *structure* of the human body.
- Human physiology is the study of the *function* of the human body.
- It is essential that OEC technicians have a basic understanding of human anatomy and physiology and be able to use this information when assessing and caring for patients.
- Emergency medical personnel use directional and anatomic terms that refer to the locations on the body, body direction, and body movement.
- A group of organs work together to form a body system, performing a specific body function. There are 11 body systems that interact to allow the body to function and maintain homeostasis:
    - Respiratory system
    - Cardiovascular system
    - Nervous system
    - Digestive system
    - Urinary system
    - Endocrine system
    - Integumentary (skin) system
    - Skeletal system
    - Muscular system
    - Reproductive system
    - Lymphatic system
- The organs and systems of all humans are the same.
- Understanding the normal anatomy and physiology of the body's organs and systems will assist you in determining illness or trauma in a patient.
- An injury or illness in one system can and often will affect other systems, causing the human body to quickly lose its ability to function normally.

Key Terms

Abduction Motion of a limb away from the midline.

Adduction Motion of a limb toward the midline.

Artery A tubular vessel that carries blood from the heart to the lungs and body.

Blood pressure Pressure or force inside the walls of the body's arteries.

Body system A group of organs and other structures that work together to perform specific functions.

Brain The organ in the nervous system responsible for the control of all the body systems. The brain coordinates the function of sensation, controls muscles, keeps body organs functioning automatically, and integrates consciousness, memory, emotions, and the use of language.

Capillaries Tiny blood vessels that connect arteries to veins. They provide nutrients and oxygen to and remove waste from cells.

Cardiovascular system Organs and structures that circulate blood around the body using the heart, arteries, and veins, delivering oxygen and nutrients to organs and cells. This system carries chemical waste products away from the cells and helps equalize body temperature. May also be referred to as the circulatory system.

Cells The basic units of all living tissue.

Central nervous system The part of the nervous system that includes the brain and spinal cord.

Diaphragm The large, thick, flat muscle between the chest and abdomen that is used for breathing.

Digestive system Also known as the gastrointestinal system, a group of organs and other structures that use mechanical and chemical processes to break down food and absorb nutrients into the body. This system also eliminates waste or unused material that is eaten.

Endocrine system A collection of glands that produce chemical substances, called hormones, that travel through the bloodstream influencing target organs.

Extension The straightening of a joint.

Flexion The bending of a joint.

Human anatomy The study of structures that can be seen with the unaided eye and structures visible only through a microscope in humans.

Human physiology The study of the mechanical, physical, bioelectric, and biochemical functions of humans.

Immune response The body's response to a substance foreign to the body, such as bacteria.

Immunity The state of being protected from a disease, especially an infectious disease.

Integumentary (skin) system Specialized tissues covering and protecting the body. The skin helps retain fluids, regulates temperature, transmits information from the environment to the brain, and protects the body from the outside environment.

Ligaments Fibrous tissues that connect a bone to another bone.

Lymphatic system Organs and other structures that remove extra fluid from tissues, absorb and transport fats from the cardiovascular system, and make white blood cells and transport them from the lymph nodes.

Muscular system Tissues that allow movement of the body, beating of the heart, and movement within the organs of the digestive system and other tubular structures (e.g., helping move food through the intestines, allowing blood vessels to contract to raise blood pressure).

Nervous system A group of organs and other structures that regulate all body functions by collecting and processing information, using the brain and a complicated wiring system to all organs.

Neuron A specialized cell that conducts electrical impulses; a nerve cell.

Organs Structures containing similar tissues that act together to perform specific body functions.

Peripheral nervous system The part of the nervous system outside the central nervous system.

Reproductive system Organs and other structures responsible for human reproduction.

Respiratory system Organs and structures that bring air containing oxygen into the body and eliminate carbon dioxide to the environment through the process of breathing, or ventilation.

Skeletal system The bones and other supporting tissues that provide structure to the body, provide attachment points for muscles, protect internal organs, allow movement, store minerals, and constitute the major site where blood cells are made.

Tendon An extension of a muscle that attaches to a bone.

Tissue A collection of cells acting together to perform a specific body function.

Urinary system Organs and structures that remove wastes and toxins from the blood and excretes them as urine. This system maintains the body's water and electrolyte balance.

Vein A tubular vessel that carries blood to the heart.

Chapter Questions

1. A patient who has severe breathing problems but no other symptoms should be placed in what position?
   a. Supine (flat on the back)
   b. Recovery (on the side)
   c. High-Fowler (sitting upright)
   d. Semi-Fowler (upright, but leaning back)
2. The spleen is part of the lymphatic system. Name one other organ of that system.
   a. Gallbladder
   b. Tonsils
   c. Liver
   d. Kidney

3. The skeletal system includes bones and _______ that support the body's structure.
   a. tendons
   b. muscles
   c. joints
   d. ligaments
4. Blood travels from the right side of the heart to the:
   a. left side of the heart.
   b. lungs.
   c. lower body.
   d. coronary artery.
5. Nutrients in the blood come from the __________system.
   a. urinary
   b. gastrointestinal/digestive
   c. respiratory
   d. lymphatic
6. The sternum is located in which body section?
   a. Thoracic
   b. Lumbar
   c. Spinal
   d. Pelvic
7. Involuntary or smooth muscles are found in which of the following structures?
   a. Muscles of the arms and legs
   b. Blood vessels and intestines
   c. The central nervous system
   d. The heart and blood vessels

Answers: 1. c, Objective 6-1, p. 117; 2. b, Objective 6-2, p. 137; 3. d, Objective 6-3, p. 132; 4. b, Objective 6-4, p. 121; 5. b, Objective 6-5, p. 129; 6. a, Objective 6-6, p. 134; 7. b, Objective 6-7, p. 135

CHAPTER 7

PATIENT ASSESSMENT

OBJECTIVES

Upon completion of this chapter, the OEC technician will be able to:

7-1 Explain and demonstrate the following five parts of a patient assessment:
- Scene size-up
- Primary patient assessment
- History taking
- Secondary patient assessment
- Reassessment

7-2 Describe the importance of controlling major bleeding as a first step during the primary patient assessment.

7-3 Describe the first steps you take when you encounter a patient who is responsive.

7-4 Explain how the ABCDs are used in assessing a patient.

7-5 Describe the difference between a sign and a symptom.

7-6 Demonstrate how to assess the pupils.

7-7 Demonstrate how to assess eye movement.

7-8 List the normal vital signs for an infant, child, and adult.

7-9 Demonstrate where you can take five pulses in five different locations on the body.

7-10 Describe and demonstrate how to assess the following vital signs:
- Level of responsiveness
- Pulse
- Respiratory rate
- Blood pressure
- Oxygen saturation

KEY TERMS

Allergy, p. 156
AVPU scale, p. 149
Blood pressure, p. 168
Breath sounds, p. 166
Chief complaint, p. 155
DCAP-BTLS, p. 159
Decerebrate posturing, p. 154
Decorticate posturing, p. 154
General impression, p. 148
Level of responsiveness, p. 149
Mechanism of injury, p. 147
Nature of illness, p. 147
OPQRST, p. 157
Palpate, p. 159
Paresthesia, p. 154
Patient assessment, p. 144
PERRL, p. 161
Primary patient assessment, p. 148
Pulse, p. 152
Pulse oximeter, p. 171
SAMPLE, p. 156
Scene safety, p. 147
Scene size-up, p. 146
Secondary patient assessment, p. 158
Sign, p. 156
Symptom, p. 156
Vital signs, p. 165

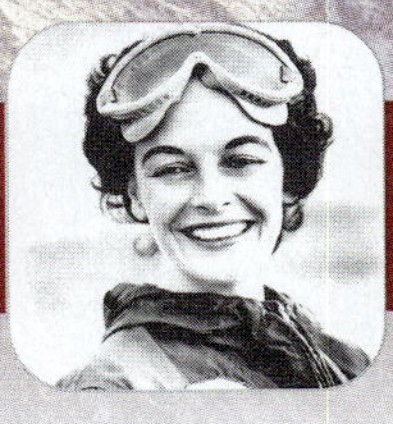

HISTORICAL TIMELINE 1952. Jerry Nunn, NSP patroller and the first US Forest Service Snow Ranger.

CHAPTER OVERVIEW

The human body has many organs and systems that interact, keeping us healthy. When we are ill or experience trauma, our organs can fail and body functions may be compromised or stop working completely. By understanding normal human anatomy and physiology and completing a thorough patient assessment, you can identify obvious or sometimes subtle abnormal findings to determine the cause of a patient's problem and then formulate an appropriate treatment plan.

You will use an assessment process to gather information about the scene, the events leading up to the incident, and the patient's history and physical condition. This information can be collected from a variety of sources, including the patient, the patient's family and friends, bystanders, the scene, and even other rescuers.

PATIENT ASSESSMENT

As part of **patient assessment**, you should first do a scene size-up, taking in a general overview of the incident and the surrounding area. This size-up is followed by a primary patient assessment to identify any life-threatening issues that require immediate intervention. Next take a history from the patient of what happened, and obtain the patient's past medical history. After gathering this information, you will perform a secondary patient assessment, which includes conducting a head-to-toe physical examination and monitoring the patient's vital signs. While performing a patient assessment, some problems may need immediate attention, so patient assessment and patient management often occur simultaneously. Reassessment is the final step and is necessary to detect and respond to any changes in the patient's condition. The overall patient assessment process consists of five parts (**Figure 7-1**) (**OEC Skill 7-1**):

- Scene size-up
- Primary patient assessment
- History taking
- Secondary patient assessment
- Reassessment

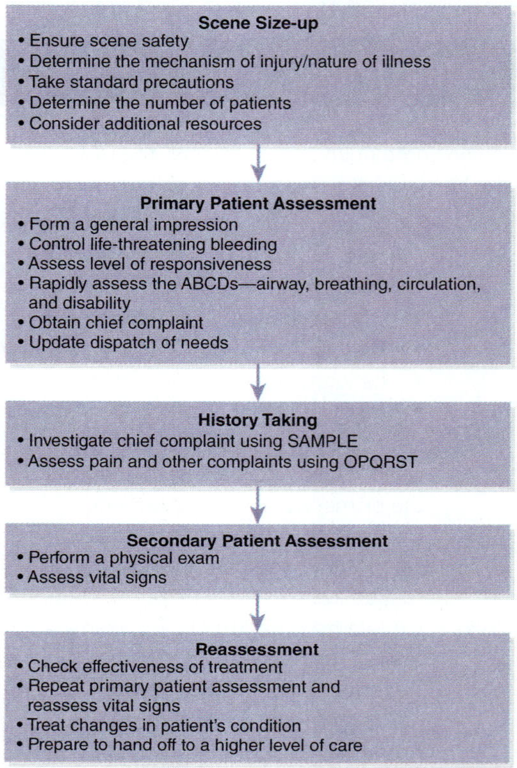

Figure 7-1 The patient assessment process.

CASE Presentation

You respond to a call to assist a patient who has fallen in the lodge. When you arrive on scene, you find a male in his mid-50s sitting on the floor beside a table. His wife reports that her husband was eating a burger, complained of chest pain, then fell to the floor, injuring his wrist. He did not lose responsiveness. After making sure the area is clear of hazards and quickly managing the crowd that has gathered, you begin assessing the man. He appears to be having difficulty breathing and is complaining of chest pain, saying, "I feel like an elephant is sitting on my chest." The wife insists you look at his wrist.

What should you do?

OEC SKILL 7-1 Performing a Patient Assessment

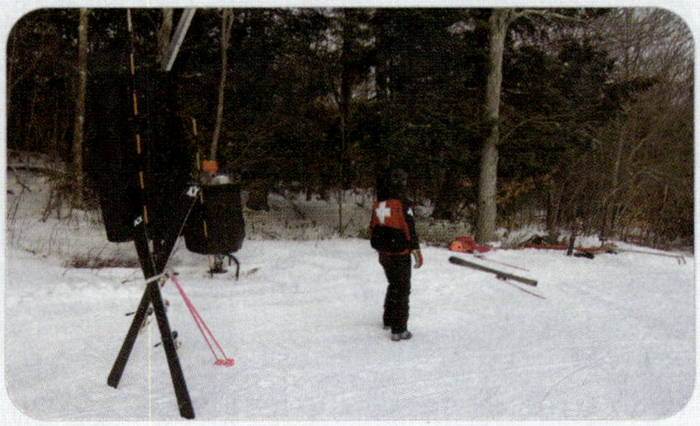

1 Perform a scene size-up. The scene size-up is performed by ensuring scene safety, determining the mechanism of injury or nature of illness, taking standard precautions, determining the number of patients, and considering whether additional resources are needed. At this point, the patroller must also make an initial assessment of the need for spinal motion restriction.

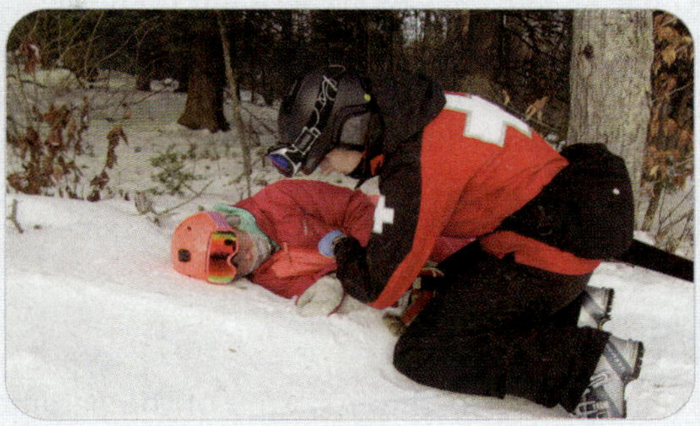

2 Perform a primary patient assessment. The primary patient assessment includes forming a general impression of the patient; controlling life-threatening bleeding; assessing level of responsiveness; rapidly assessing airway, breathing, circulation, and disability; obtaining the chief complaint; and updating dispatch of needs.

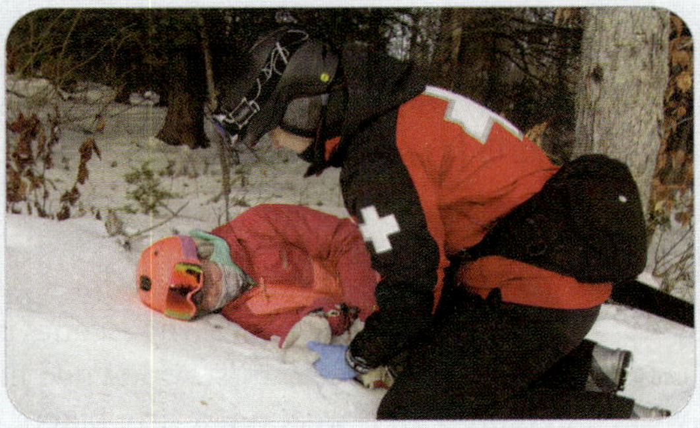

3 Obtain a complete history from the patient. History taking includes using SAMPLE to investigate the chief complaint and OPQRST to assess pain and other complaints.

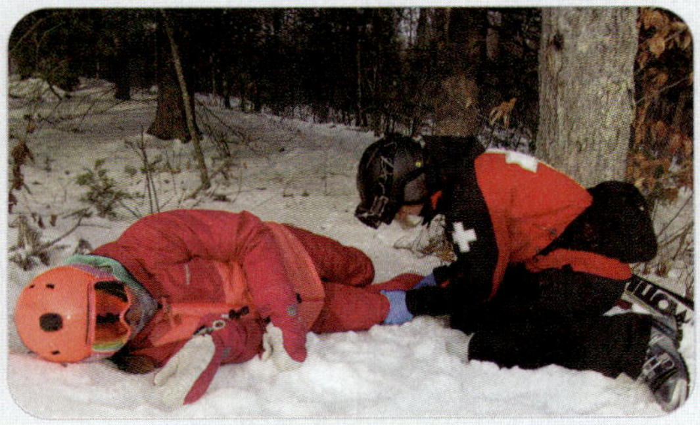

4 Perform a secondary patient assessment. The secondary patient assessment includes performing a physical exam of the patient and assessing vital signs.

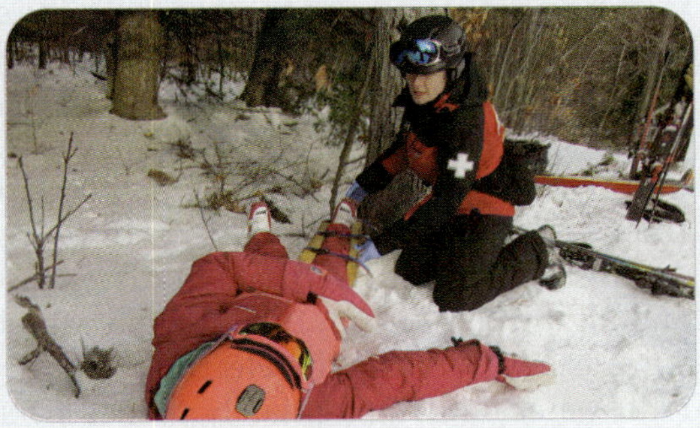

5 Perform a reassessment. The reassessment includes checking the effectiveness of treatment provided, repeating the primary patient assessment and reassessing vital signs, treating changes in the patient's condition, and preparing to hand off the patient to a higher level of care.

Performing a patient assessment may seem overwhelming at first. The key is to use a systematic, standardized approach for every patient evaluation to make sure key medical information is not overlooked. Patient assessment is an essential and fundamental skill that you will use in each patient encounter; therefore you must master this skill. As you take an initial OEC course and participate in annual refreshers, practice helps you improve your ability to perform a good assessment.

SCENE SIZE-UP

The **scene size-up** is the first step of the patient assessment process and is best defined as a general overview of the incident and its surroundings. This information will help you determine the safety of the scene, the type of incident, use of standard precautions, the mechanism of injury or nature of illness, and the need for additional resources. In addition, at this point consider the need for spinal motion restriction of the patient (Figure 7-2).

Ensure Scene Safety

Some resorts and other agencies want to know when you arrive on scene at a rescue. If local protocol requires that you report your arrival,

Scene Size-up
- Ensure scene safety
- Determine the mechanism of injury or nature of illness
- Take standard precautions
- Determine the number of patients
- Consider additional resources

↓

Primary Patient Assessment

↓

History Taking

↓

Secondary Patient Assessment

↓

Reassessment

Figure 7-2 Scene size-up.

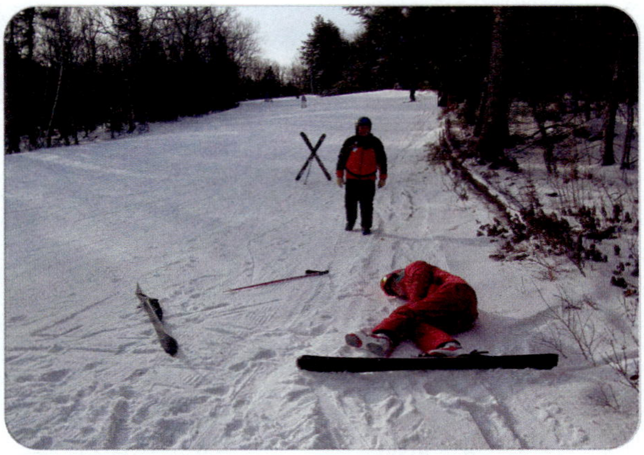

Figure 7-3 Scene size-up helps determine the safety of the scene, the type of incident, the mechanism of injury or nature of illness, and the need for additional resources.

notify your dispatch when you reach the scene. If the base did not put out the call for you to respond, they are now aware there is a possible rescue. Make sure you provide the necessary information based on your local communications protocols.

Scene size-up involves scanning the area to determine what needs to be done (Figure 7-3). This scan establishes a first impression. Is there a chair derailment, a fire, or one patient sitting on the snow holding his wrist? If a call was sent out, was this what dispatch described, or is the situation different? Get mentally prepared for the rescue.

Before you enter a scene to care for a patient, your *priority* is to make sure the scene is safe (Figure 7-4). Look for hazards. A downed electric wire, a person with a weapon, a fire, bikers riding toward you on an off-road path, or skiers coming down a slope above you could harm the rescuer or patients. Always mitigate dangers before proceeding to help the victim. Allowing another person, or yourself, to become a second victim will complicate matters.

There are many ways to make the scene safe. If on a ski slope, place crossed skis well above you on the hill (Figure 7-5). If in a blind spot on a bike path or ski slope, have another person help you by waving off bikers or skiers who could collide with you. Drag a person near a fire away to a safe location. Avoid someone with a weapon until police arrive and disarm the person. Do not approach electric wires until you know the electricity is off. Avoid swift water until appropriately trained personnel

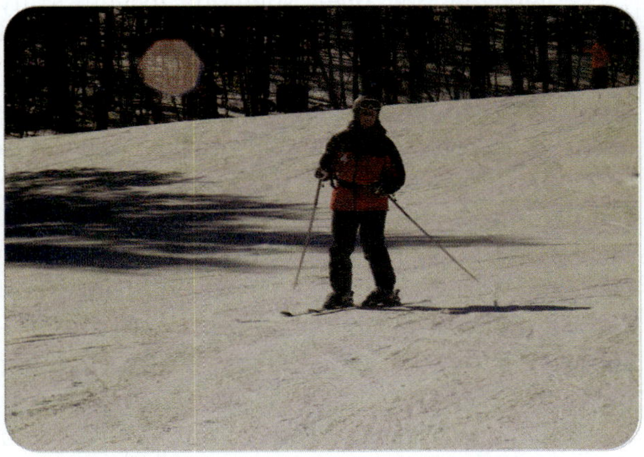

Figure 7-4 As you approach the scene, evaluate the area for scene safety and look for clues as to what may have happened.

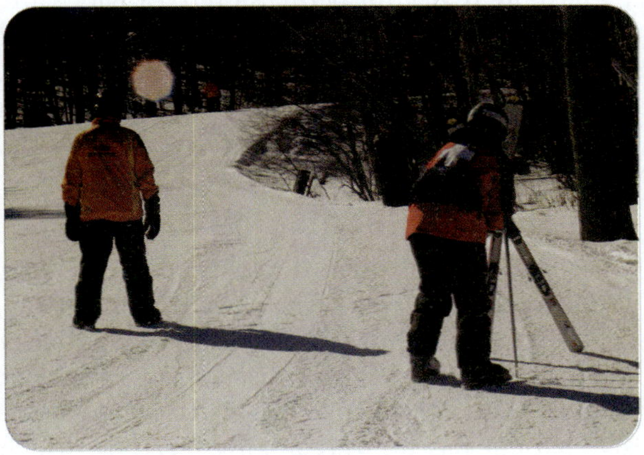

Figure 7-5 Mark the scene by placing your skis above the accident site or having a mountain host or reliable person stand above the accident site to prevent others from approaching the accident scene.

arrive. In short, remove potential hazards or have law enforcement or special rescue teams make the scene safe first. **Scene safety** is always the first step when you approach a patient.

Determine the Mechanism of Injury or Nature of Illness

After making the scene safe, you need to determine the events that caused the situation (**Figure 7-6**). In trauma, a force has acted on the body, causing injury. This trauma is called the **mechanism of injury** (sometimes abbreviated MOI). If the patient

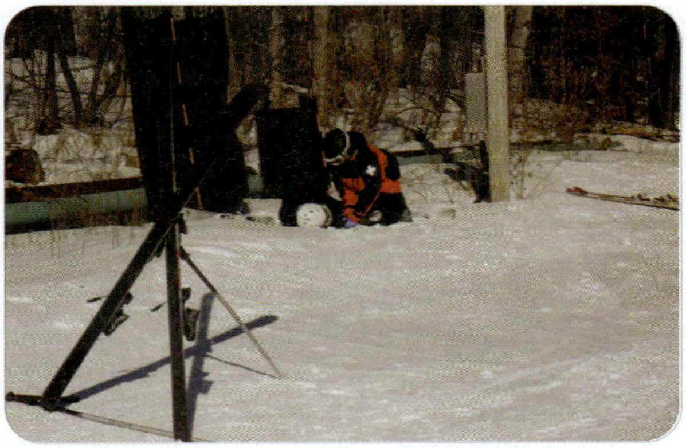

Figure 7-6 The patroller needs to determine the mechanism of injury or the nature of illness.

is sick or ill from a medical condition, you need to determine the **nature of illness** (sometimes abbreviated NOI).

Take Standard Precautions

OEC technicians must protect themselves from hazardous materials and bloodborne pathogens. Use any necessary personal protective equipment, applying gloves and other protective equipment before touching the patient.

Determine the Number of Patients

During scene size-up, you should determine how many patients there are. At most scenes, there is one patient. If there are multiple patients, rapidly determine the severity of each patient's problems and triage the patients (for more information on triage, see Chapter 4, *Incident Command and Triage*). Life-threatening problems take priority.

Consider Additional Resources

The incident may require additional personnel or special equipment. Special equipment may be needed for someone who has fallen over a cliff or for a chairlift accident. Law enforcement personnel may be needed for someone with a weapon. If there is a fire or spilled fuel, fire department units are needed. If power lines are down, the utility company needs to be called. Even though you do not know the condition of the patient(s) at this point, call for additional resources immediately, because requesting specialized help may take time. Later, as you look at each patient, you can call for more equipment or resources as needed.

PRIMARY PATIENT ASSESSMENT

The second part of the patient assessment sequence is the **primary patient assessment** (**Figure 7-7**). The purpose of the primary patient assessment is to form a general impression and identify and immediately treat life threats. Life threats may be excessive bleeding or problems with the patient's airway, breathing, circulation, and/or disability. If you find a life threat, it must be corrected immediately. If there is more than one life threat, such as excessive bleeding and an obstructed airway, correct these problems before moving on in the patient assessment process.

Form a General Impression

You have acquired quite a lot of information quickly, having performed a scene size-up. As you approach the patient, you have an idea of the mechanism of injury or nature of illness, possible hazards, and specialized personnel and equipment needed. You should have a general idea of what has occurred. Now form a **general impression** about the patient's condition.

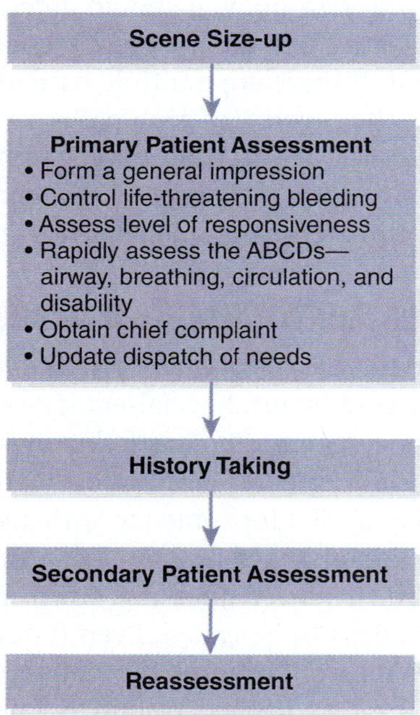

Figure 7-7 Primary patient assessment.

When you first meet someone in your daily life, you look at the person and form an initial general impression. Assessment of a patient is a similar process, but your focus is on rapidly identifying any life-threatening problems, which will help you determine your priority of care. You will note the patient's approximate age, sex, race, level of distress, and overall appearance. Using the knowledge obtained from OEC and past experience, you will begin to decide what steps to take first. Unresponsive patients usually have a life-threatening problem.

This overall view of the patient will give you an impression of his or her needs. Is the person conscious? Talking? Moving? Stable? Is immediate intervention needed?

If the patient is responsive when you approach, let the person know who you are and that you are there to help. Ask for permission to provide care, and show respect during your evaluation. Do not stand over patients. Make them feel comfortable. Address them by name, which reassures them you have been listening to what they say.

Control Life-Threatening Bleeding

In most cases, identifying and correcting life-threatening issues begins with the airway, followed by breathing, circulation, and disability (ABCD). This sequence is discussed in the next section. However, when a responsive or unresponsive patient has life-threatening bleeding, which can be considered a circulation issue, it is more appropriate to address this life threat first, following a sequence of circulation, airway, breathing, and disability (CABD). In these cases, controlling life-threatening bleeding takes priority over airway and breathing concerns.

As you approach the patient, look for and immediately control life-threatening bleeding. As mentioned, this step should occur before addressing airway or breathing concerns. In some cases, blood loss can be very rapid and can quickly result in shock or even death. Without blood in the vascular system, death will occur in less than 5 minutes. Signs of blood loss include active bleeding from wounds and/or evidence of bleeding such as blood on the clothes or near the patient. Serious bleeding from a large vein may be characterized by steady blood flow. Bleeding from an artery is characterized by a spurting flow of blood. When you evaluate an unconscious patient, do a sweep for

> **KEY POINT**
>
> **Stop the Bleed**
>
> Stop the Bleed, a national program started in 2015 by various federal agencies, teaches people how to control bleeding. When a patient has significant bleeding, stopping it is the most important thing that can be done to save the person's life. The program shows how to apply pressure to a traumatic wound, how to pack a wound, and, if bleeding is not controlled, how to apply a tourniquet.

blood by quickly and lightly running your gloved hands from head to toe, pausing periodically to see if your gloves are bloody.

Initially, direct pressure with your gloved hand and soon thereafter a sterile bandage over the wound will control bleeding in most cases. Direct pressure stops the bleeding and helps the blood to coagulate, or clot, naturally. Most minor bleeding can be adequately controlled by using direct pressure. When direct pressure is not quickly successful or whenever you encounter obvious arterial hemorrhage of an extremity, apply a pressure dressing. If you are unable to control bleeding from an extremity, apply a tourniquet. For deep wounds with excessive bleeding where a tourniquet cannot be applied, like the buttock, pack the wound with gauze and then apply pressure. More information about bleeding and applying a tourniquet can be found in Chapter 19, *Soft-Tissue Injuries and Burns*.

Assess Level of Responsiveness

It is important to determine the patient's level of responsiveness. Is the person alert and able to communicate? If a person can speak normally and there is no major bleeding, the airway, breathing, and circulation are intact. Simply saying, "Are you OK?" and receiving the response "I need help" reveals that the patient has a pulse and airway, is breathing, and understands you (ABCD).

Most patients will be fully responsive, so always introduce yourself to the patient and ask for permission to help. If the patient is an adult who is alert and oriented, simply say, "Hi, I'm Paul with the ski patrol. May I help you?" If caring for a minor, ask a parent or guardian who is present for permission to care for the child. If a child is alone or you have an unresponsive patient, you should care for this patient using implied consent.

Put the patient at ease by talking in a calm, reassuring manner. At this point you do not fully know the patient's condition, so avoid telling the person he or she will be all right.

If the patient tells you he or she does not want help, respect the person's wishes. However, if you truly think the patient has a problem, stay nearby, watching to determine that the person is OK. Patients may initially refuse care, only to later decide they need help.

While introducing yourself, make eye contact and try to get down to the patient's level. A patient's initial appearance will help you decide whether the problem is serious or minor. Ask the patient's name and speak calmly, using the person's name. Consider simultaneously assessing the patient's pulse, using the radial pulse for an adult and the brachial pulse for a child. The assessment of the pulse is for quality—fast or slow, strong or weak, regular or irregular. This finding will help you make an initial assessment about the patient's condition, especially if the patient is unresponsive. Even if the patient is fully responsive, you will have valuable information by taking a pulse.

For patients who are not completely responsive, assess the **level of responsiveness**, a measure of the patient's awareness and responsiveness to you and the surrounding environment. Level of responsiveness is a continuum that ranges from the patient being fully alert and oriented to various levels of unresponsiveness.

Patients should be questioned about their name, their physical location, the approximate time of day, the day of the week, and the events leading up to the situation. When patients can answer all these questions correctly, they are said to be awake, alert, and oriented to person, place, time, and event. The inability to correctly answer even one of these questions suggests a potential neurologic problem and is considered abnormal. An abnormal level of responsiveness can result from brain injury, lack of oxygen, or a wide range of medical conditions.

The easiest way to assess level of responsiveness is to use the **AVPU scale** (**Table 7-1**). This

KEY POINT

Is the Patient Awake, Alert, and Oriented to Person, Place, Time, and Event?

Patients should be questioned about their name, their physical location, the approximate time of day, the day of the week, and the events leading up to the situation. The inability to correctly answer even one of these questions suggests a potential neurologic problem and is considered abnormal. It is not appropriate to ask the name of the president, the date, or other questions that patients may not know.

Table 7-1 AVPU Scale

A—Alert: The patient is fully awake, opens his or her eyes without prompting, and can speak to you; the patient is aware and responsive to the surroundings.
V—Verbal: The patient does not open his or her eyes spontaneously, but responds to your voice or a loud sound by opening the eyes, making some type of vocal sound, or moving an extremity slightly.
P—Pain: The patient responds only to painful stimuli.
U—Unresponsive: The patient does not respond to any type of stimulus.

simple mnemonic stands for alert, verbal, pain, and unresponsive. Another method to assess neurologic function is the Glasgow Coma Scale (GCS). The GCS is more difficult to use than the AVPU scale and takes longer to perform. Some first responders in the EMS system use the GCS.

To assess the patient using the AVPU scale, first observe whether the patient appears to be awake and alert. A patient who is awake and alert and answers questions appropriately is scored as *A* on the AVPU scale. If the patient does not appear to be alert or has closed eyes, loudly talk to the person or clap your hands. A patient who looks at you or opens his or her eyes is scored a *V* on the AVPU scale. If the patient does not respond to verbal stimuli, attempt to illicit a pain response in the patient. Pinch the earlobe or the muscle between the neck and shoulder (trapezius pinch), or press on the base of the fingernail with a hard object. A patient who responds to pain is noted as *P* on the AVPU scale. A patient who does not respond to pain is scored as *U* for unresponsive. Any score less than *A* is considered abnormal. Obviously, a patient who is deaf will not respond to a verbal stimulus.

Glasgow Coma Scale

The GCS is based on three observations: the patient's best eye response, the patient's best verbal response, and the patient's best motor response. Each component consists of a range of physical responses, and each response is assigned a numerical value. The patient is assessed for the best response for each component, and the sum of the assigned values represents the GCS score. Originally, the GCS was used to predict neurologic outcomes by using it repeatedly over time, but this scale has been adopted for assessing neurologic function by some prehospital systems. Use of the AVPU scale is easier and recommended.

Rapidly Assess Airway, Breathing, Circulation, and Disability

After controlling severe bleeding, correcting life-threatening issues begins with the airway, followed by breathing, circulation, and disability (ABCD). Assess the ABCDs rapidly. These elements are assessed almost simultaneously for any patient.

Airway

If no airway problems exist, the airway is said to be open, or "patent." If an airway problem is discovered, it must be corrected immediately. The most common cause of airway obstruction in the unresponsive patient is the tongue falling back and either partially or completely blocking the oropharynx (throat). Other common causes of airway compromise or blockage include vomit, bleeding, broken teeth or loose dentures, food, gum, candy, chewing tobacco, small toys, other foreign bodies, or structural damage or swelling involving the face, nose, mouth, or neck. Methods for clearing the airway of a foreign body obstruction, including finger sweep, abdominal thrust, gravity and positioning, and suction, are described in Chapter 9, *Airway Management*.

KEY POINT

Assess the ABCDs

A—Airway: Patient has a patent airway that will remain open.

B—Breathing: Patient can breathe, so that oxygen is reaching the body's tissues effectively and carbon dioxide is being removed.

C—Circulation: Patient has blood circulating effectively through the vessels and perfusing the tissues, without significant blood loss.

D—Disability: Patient does not have an injury to the nervous system that causes unresponsiveness, paralysis, or neurologic compromise.

The head tilt–chin lift maneuver is used to open an airway if there is no concern for cervical spine injury (**Figure 7-8A**). The jaw-thrust method is used for a patient with a suspected cervical spine injury, as it avoids aggravating a spine injury (**Figure 7-8B**). It can also be used for someone who does not have a cervical spine injury. Always open the airway using the jaw-thrust maneuver in an unresponsive patient with a traumatic injury.

To perform the jaw-thrust maneuver:

1. Kneel above the patient's head, with your knees straddling the head. (You can use your knees to gently stabilize the head and cervical spine.)
2. Using the fingers of both hands, grasp the angle of the mandible on each side of the jaw.
3. Place your thumbs on the maxilla.
4. Use the thumbs as a lever to lift the mandible upward.

Once the airway is open, using the jaw-thrust method, if possible, hold the jaw to keep the airway open. Both methods for opening the airway are demonstrated in Chapter 9, *Airway Management*. Remember, in the unresponsive patient, always insert an airway adjunct after opening an airway. Also, placing an unresponsive *nontrauma* patient with a pulse who is breathing in the recovery position will help prevent an airway obstruction from vomit or blood (**Figure 7-9**).

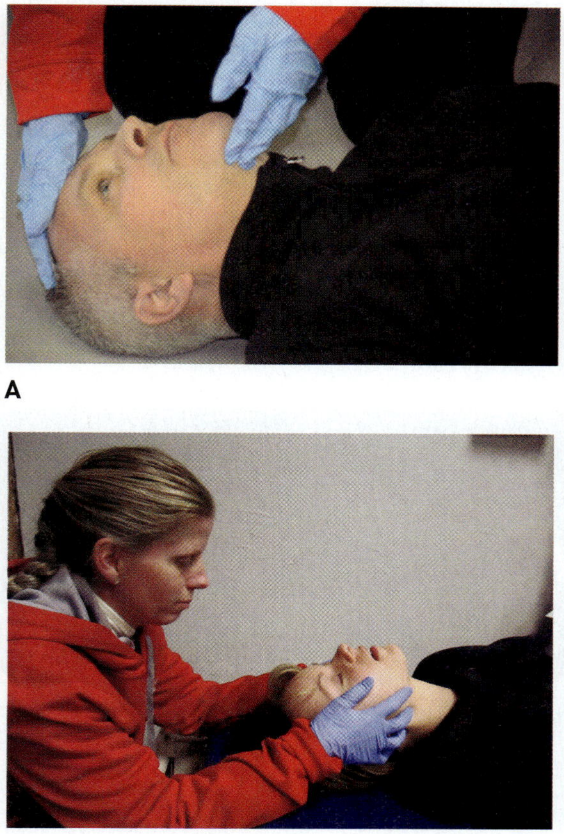

A

B

Figure 7-8 A. The head tilt–chin lift maneuver. **B.** The jaw-thrust maneuver.

KEY POINT

Airway Adjunct

Always insert an airway adjunct in the unresponsive patient after opening an airway.

In the rare situation you are unable to open the airway with the jaw-thrust maneuver, even if there could be a potential for a spine injury, use the head tilt–chin lift maneuver. Without an airway, death will occur. Both these techniques lift the tongue off the back of the throat to open the patient's airway.

KEY POINT

Cardiac Arrest

When a patient is in cardiac arrest, the ABCDs should be assessed simultaneously and in the interest of minimizing the time to first compression.

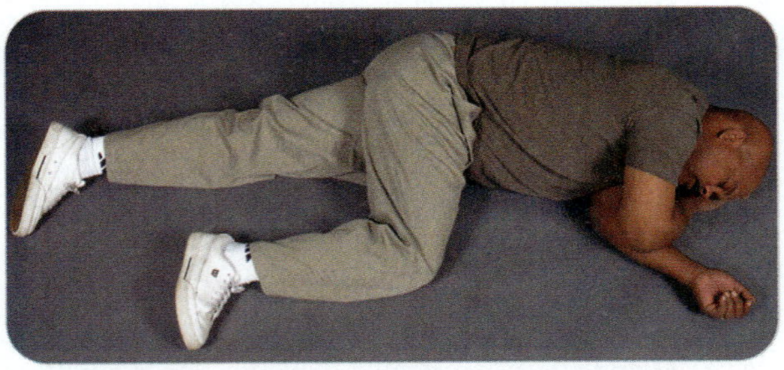

Figure 7-9 The recovery position.

Breathing

As you determine if the patient's airway is open, assess the patient's breathing using a process known as "look, listen, and feel." *Look* to see if the chest rises and falls with each breath. Place your ear near the patient's open mouth and *listen* for the sound of air moving in and out. *Feel* for air on your cheek during exhalation, and place your hand on the patient's chest to *feel* for chest wall movements. If breathing is not present and a carotid pulse was found, begin assisting ventilations. If oxygen is available, immediately administer it to the patient.

Assess the respiratory rate by counting the breaths for 30 seconds, then multiply by 2 to determine the number of breaths per minute (**Figure 7-10**). If the patient is breathing, ask yourself the following questions: Is the respiratory rate fast or slow? Normal respiratory rate for an adult or an adolescent is 12 to 20 breaths per minute, whereas normal respiratory rate for an infant is 20 to 60 breaths per minute. Are the patient's respirations deep (fully expanding the chest), shallow (barely moving the chest), or labored (indicating breathing difficulty)?

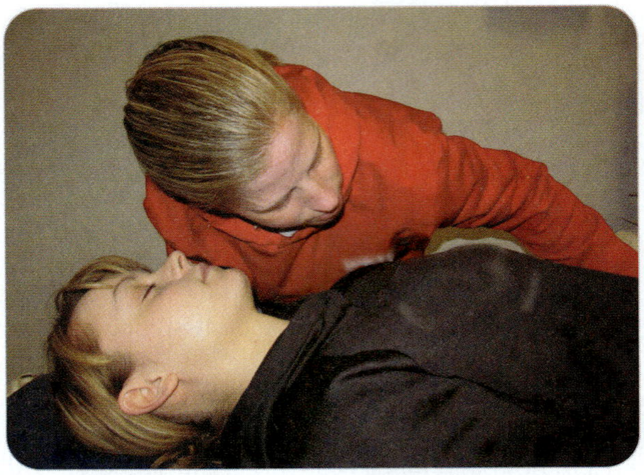

Figure 7-10 It is essential to get an accurate respiratory rate for the patient initially and then at least every 5 to 15 minutes, depending on the patient's condition.

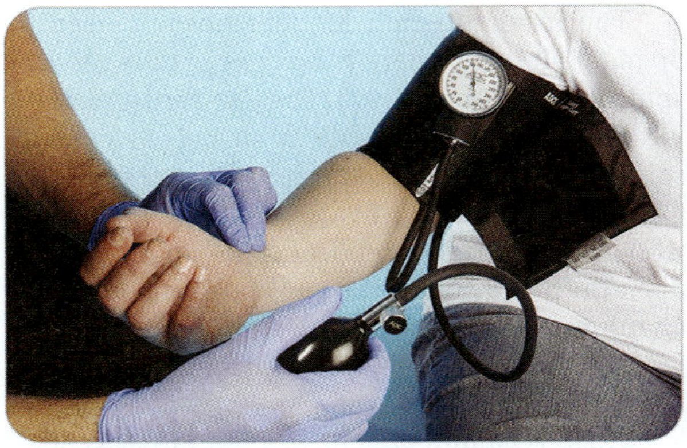

Figure 7-11 Assessing the radial pulse.

Circulation

Make sure the patient has effective blood circulation in the body by feeling peripheral pulses, assessing skin color, and evaluating capillary refill. On alert adult patients, the **pulse** is most often checked first at the wrist over the radial artery (**Figure 7-11**). This check should not occur on an arm that is injured or has a tourniquet. In all children younger than 8 years of age, assess circulation by checking the brachial pulse, above the elbow (**Figure 7-12**).

In 2018, the American Heart Association recommended the sequence of assessment and care

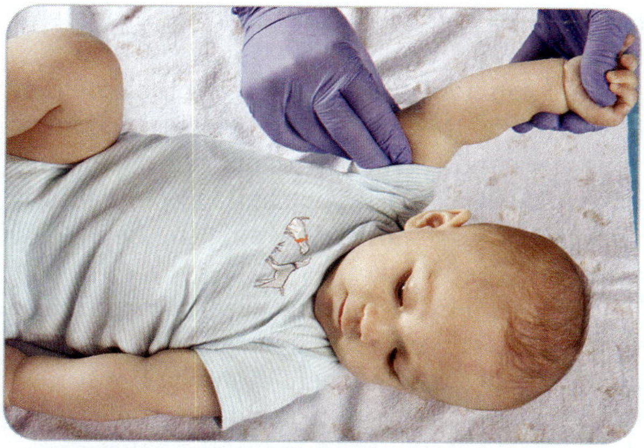

Figure 7-12 Assessing the brachial pulse.

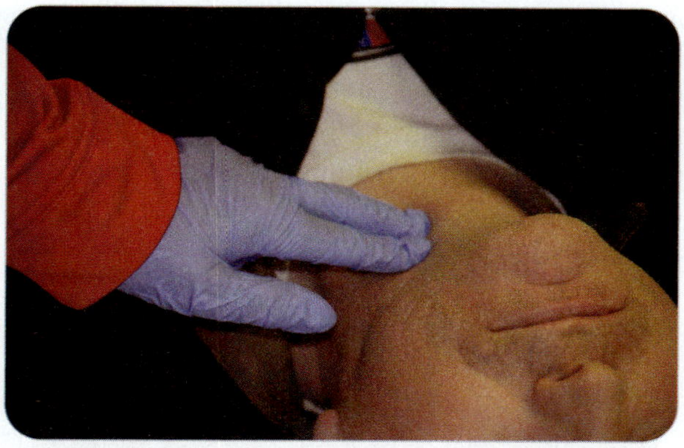

Figure 7-13 Use the carotid pulse location for an unresponsive adult.

as circulation, airway, and breathing (CAB) for an unresponsive patient in cardiac arrest who has not sustained trauma. For a rescuer trained in cardiopulmonary resuscitation (CPR), the circulation, airway, and breathing are assessed simultaneously. To assess circulation (heartbeat) in an unresponsive adult, check for a pulse over the carotid artery (**Figure 7-13**). Place your index and long fingers together on the larynx (Adam's apple) in the neck. Then slide your fingers toward the ear, on the side closest to you, until they drop into a groove. Press your fingers into this groove to feel the carotid artery pulse. Always use your index and middle fingers to assess a pulse, not your thumb. You may feel your own pulse if you use your thumb. The most important thing an OEC technician can do for an unresponsive patient with a pulse is open and maintain the airway. Simultaneously check the pulse, open the airway, and check breathing, taking no longer than 10 to 15 seconds. If a pulse is present, but the patient is not breathing, you need to check the airway to make sure it is open. If there is still no breathing, begin rescue breaths. If the patient is pulseless in cardiac arrest, call for additional help and an automated external defibrillator, and start CPR as soon as possible.

If a pulse is present, determine what it feels like. It should be strong and regular. A pulse that is irregular or faint indicates an underlying medical or traumatic disorder. An irregular pulse has a different time interval between beats (skips beats). Determine the pulse rate by holding your index finger on the pulse, looking at your watch, and counting the beats for 30 seconds. Multiply this number by 2 to determine the number of beats per minute.

If a pulse is present, evaluate the patient's skin color. Skin that is pale, gray, or blue (cyanosis) indicates that circulation is compromised. Under normal conditions, the skin should have a pink or dark tone, depending on the person's race. Cyanosis also may be detected in the lips, mucous membranes, and earlobes. Assess oral (inner lip) color in patients with dark skin.

Assess capillary refill by pressing on the nail bed of one of the patient's fingers and then quickly releasing the pressure (**Figure 7-14**). Under normal conditions, the nail bed will turn white when pressed and then return to its normal pink color in less than 2 seconds once the pressure is released. A nail bed that is cyanotic or does not return to a pink color within 2 seconds indicates that circulation is not normal. An abnormal capillary refill exam (one in which refill takes longer than 2 seconds) should prompt you to investigate the underlying causes more thoroughly. Keep in mind that cold environmental conditions cause the capillaries in the nail bed to be pale, blue, or slow to refill, because peripheral blood vessels are narrowed in response to the cold.

Disability

Many prehospital responders add "D" for disability to the primary patient assessment process. Disability here means an injury to the nervous system, indicated by a finding such as unresponsiveness, paralysis, or neurologic compromise. Patients who can move all their extremities when asked to do so do not have a gross disability (D).

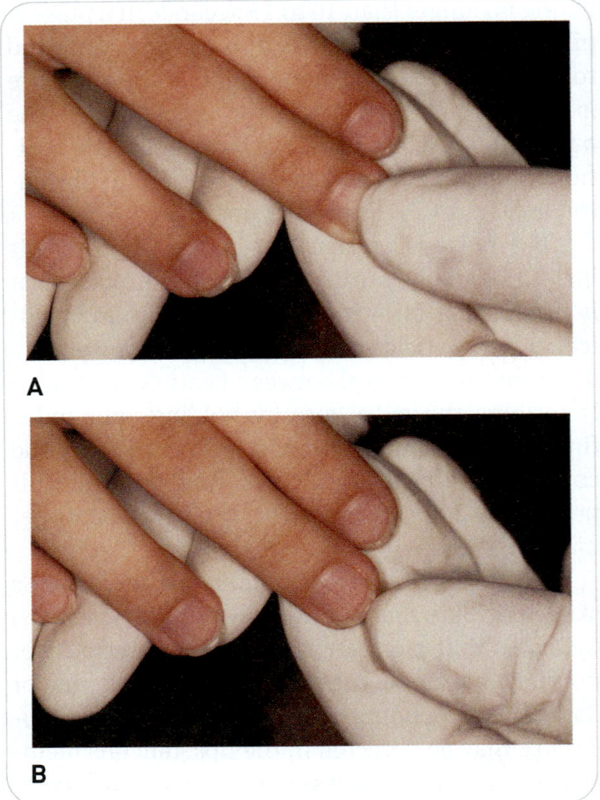

Figure 7-14 A. When checking capillary refill, squeeze the fingertip until the nail turns white. **B.** Then release the pressure and determine the amount of time it takes to return to the normal pink color.

Assess the patient for any life-threatening neurologic disorders, including any problems affecting the brain or spinal cord. You have already assessed the patient's level of responsiveness, a measure of the patient's awareness and responsiveness to the surrounding environment. Level of responsiveness is a continuum that ranges from fully alert to various levels of unresponsiveness. Under normal conditions, a patient is awake and fully oriented.

Neurologic problems can stem from the central nervous system, the peripheral nervous system, or both. Central nervous system problems can be life threatening, while peripheral nervous system problems affect just the nerves involved in the arm or leg from trauma to that extremity. Rarely, you may encounter damage to both systems affecting the body distally. The person may complain of tingling or numbness in the arms or legs, a condition known as **paraesthesia**, or may complain of muscle weakness of one or more of the extremities.

You can assess for neurologic problems rapidly by asking the patient, "Can you feel and move your arms and legs?" If patients can do so, they have understood what you said and purposefully moved their extremities, showing the neurologic system is grossly intact.

In situations involving severe compromise to the central nervous system, you may observe abnormal posturing. There are two "postures" that a patient with a neurologic problem can demonstrate. Both are ominous signs that something is very wrong with the patient. **Decorticate posturing** is abnormal flexing of the arms, clenching of the fists, and extending of the legs due to an injury along the nerve pathway between the brain and spinal cord (**Figure 7-15A**). **Decerebrate posturing** is abnormal extending of the arms and legs, downward pointing of the toes, and arching of the head due to an injury to the brain at the level of the brainstem (**Figure 7-15B**).

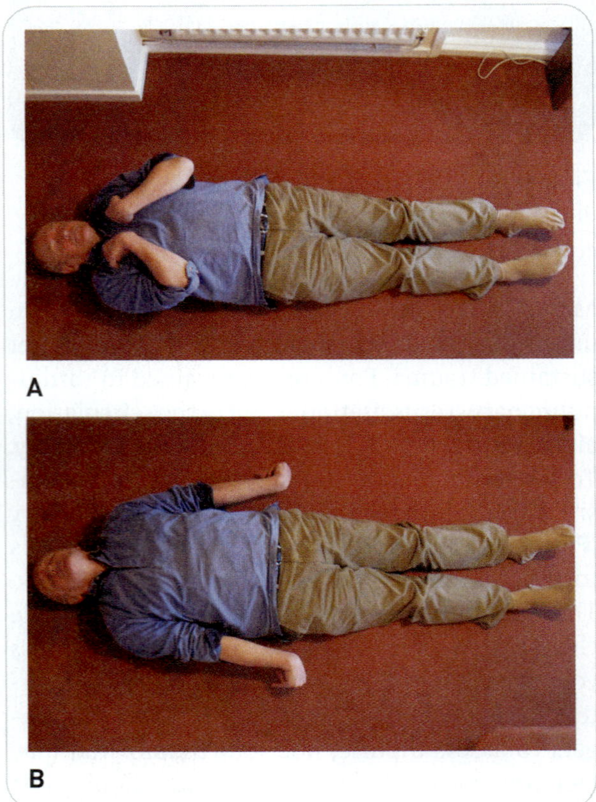

Figure 7-15 A. Decorticate posturing. **B.** Decerebrate posturing.

Patients who have experienced spinal injury or head trauma affecting mental status should remain in spinal motion restriction during the exam. Spinal motion restriction means keeping the spine in a straight line. When a spinal injury is possible and the patient is responsive, alert, and oriented, tell the person not to move his or her head during your examination. These patients should remain in spinal alignment during the exam.

In an unresponsive patient, even if the person has a pulse, has an open airway, and is breathing, you will be unable to obtain a medical history or valuable feedback. If a relative or friend is present, some history may be available. Unless a reliable witness says the patient became unresponsive without any trauma, you must assume that the patient has a cervical spine injury until proven otherwise.

If enough help is available and it is practical to do so, have another rescuer maintain spinal motion restriction of the neck, and logroll the person to the supine position (if not already on the back). If prone, prior to logrolling, examine (palpate) the midline of the spine. You will learn how to assess the spine to see if spinal motion restriction is needed in Chapter 21, *Spine, Brain, and Nervous System Injuries*. Following your assessment, if spinal motion restriction is not needed, you no longer need to protect the neck and back.

Other trauma patients may be examined in the position found or, if it is practical and safe to do so based on the injury, may be placed in a sitting position only after examination of the spine reveals no evidence of injury.

> **KEY POINT**
>
> **Responsive Trauma Patients**
>
> If the patient with trauma is responsive and can speak normally, the airway is open, breathing is present, and there is a pulse. Simply saying, "Are you OK?" and receiving the response "I need help" reveals that the patient has a pulse and an open airway, is breathing, and understands you. However, you still need to control all external bleeding and assess disability as you do for the unresponsive patient.

Obtain Chief Complaint

In a responsive patient, ask the patient what is wrong. The patient's answer is called the **chief complaint** (**Figure 7-16**). The chief complaint is the main reason the person needs your help. Sometimes there is more than one chief complaint that could be from trauma or a medical problem, or both. When a patient is unresponsive, the complaint is "unresponsive." When the patient is unresponsive and you cannot get a chief complaint, look for clues about what the problem could be. Bleeding, a crooked leg, burns, a penetrating object, or a medical alert bracelet could help you understand what has happened (**Figure 7-17**). If other people are present, ask them what happened.

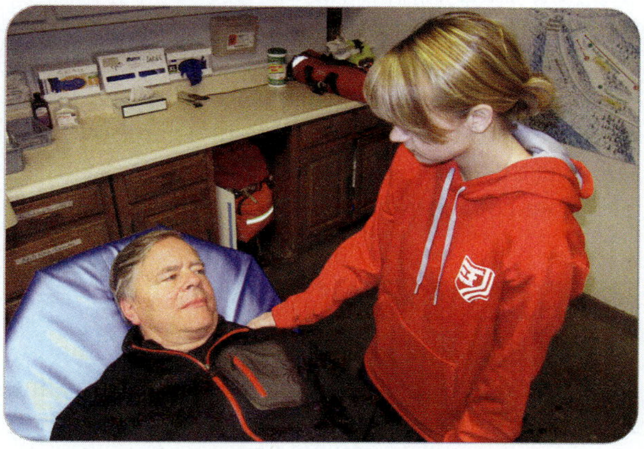

Figure 7-16 Listen to your patient, who will give you clues as to what is wrong.

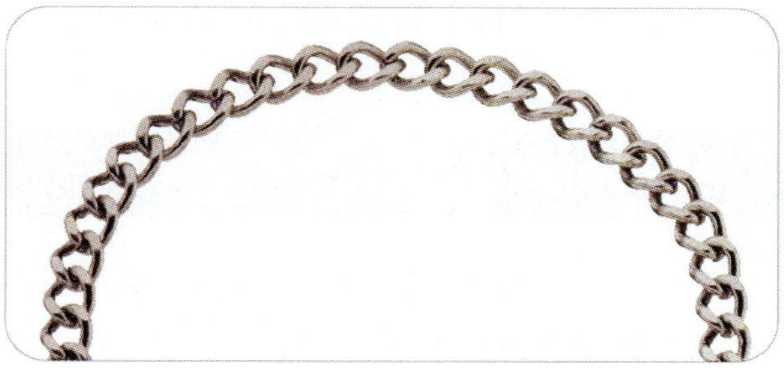

Figure 7-17 Medical alert bracelets can be decorative pieces of jewelry that patients can wear around the neck, wrist, or ankle.

KEY POINT

Examples of Chief Complaints

"My wrist hurts."

"I can't breathe."

"I hit my head and have a headache."

"I twisted my knee and can't stand up."

"My shoulder hurts."

"I have chest pain."

Update Dispatch of Needs

Call dispatch and give them more details. Provide the patient's sex and age (approximate if unresponsive), the chief complaint, the level of responsiveness, and the status of the ABCDs. If more resources are needed, request them immediately. If rapid transport is needed to a medical facility, request it at this time. Do not give the patient's name over the radio, as this is not important, and anyone who has a scanner could possibly hear your transmission.

HISTORY TAKING

Further medical history is used to collect important historical information about the patient and the events surrounding his or her current condition (**Figure 7-18**). When taking a history from the patient, if there is a positive finding, follow-up questions may be needed. For example, if a patient has chest pain, ask: Have you had this before? Have you had a heart attack? Do you take medications for your heart? Does the pain go down your arm?

KEY POINT

The OEC Technician and Diagnosis

OEC technicians do not "diagnose" medical problems; rather, they evaluate the patient, form an impression of what is wrong, and then take appropriate actions to help the patient.

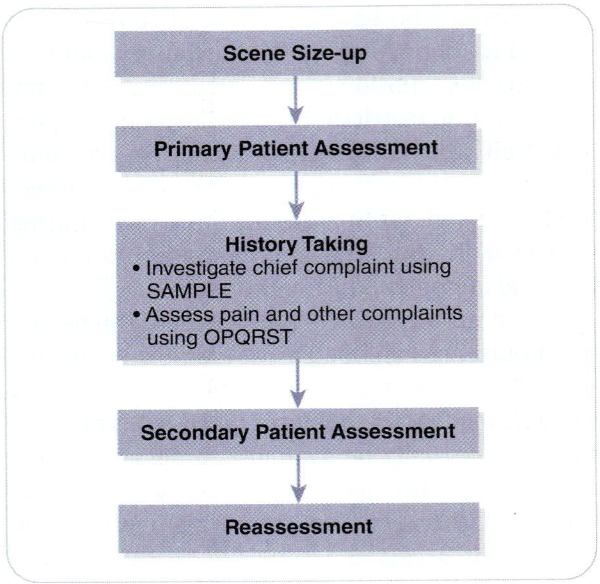

Figure 7-18 History taking.

Investigate the Chief Complaint Using SAMPLE

As part of the history taking, ask the patient about other medical information, such as what medical problems the patient may have, what medications the patient is taking, or whether the patient has any known allergies. To facilitate the organized collection of this information, use the mnemonic **SAMPLE**, which represents signs and symptoms, allergies and adverse reactions, medications, pertinent past medical history, last time the patient ate or drank, and events leading up to the incident (**Table 7-2**).

The patient's presenting signs and symptoms are important. A **symptom**, or *subjective* complaint, is qualitative in nature. Symptoms are typically provided by the patient, the patient's family, friends, or bystanders and are emotion-based descriptions. Examples of symptoms include descriptions of pain, weakness, fatigue, nausea, blurred vision, and/or impending doom.

A **sign** is any *objective* finding or evidence of disease that you can detect using your senses (see, feel, hear, smell) or that you can quantify. Examples of signs are dilated pupils, a deformed arm, audible respiratory wheezing, a foul odor, elevated blood pressure, and low pulse oximeter reading.

Ask the patient if he or she has an **allergy** or has had an allergic reaction in the past, and what occurred. This includes allergies to medications,

Table 7-2 SAMPLE

S—Signs and symptoms
A—Allergies
M—Medications presently taken (prescription, over-the-counter, and illegal drugs)
P—Past medical history: illnesses, surgeries, or other medical problems
L—Last oral intake: last time the patient ate or drank something
E—Events that led up to the present medical problem (what happened?)

foods, materials, insects, or animals. It is helpful to tell medical personnel, who continue care, about medication allergies.

Find out if the patient is taking any medications or is supposed to be taking any medications, including prescription medications, over-the-counter medications, herbs, vitamin supplements, homeopathic remedies, or illicit drugs or alcohol. This information is very important because many of these substances can mask symptoms or react with one another. If the patient is taking a prescription medication, ask if he or she is taking it as prescribed. If you don't know what the medication is being taken for, ask the patient. The patient will usually know. Certain medications are used for blood clots or cardiac problems that can make a person bleed excessively. If someone is bleeding, it is good to know if they are on one of these medications.

Determine the patient's past medical history, including any previous medical problems such as heart disease, a breathing problem, diabetes, or high blood pressure, and any previous surgeries. Although these problems may have been resolved or are seemingly under control, this information may help you anticipate problems. For instance, knowing that a patient has a history of a previous heart attack is important if the person is complaining of chest pain or shortness of breath.

Be direct. Ask the patient, "Do you have any significant medical problems?" or "Do you have any medical conditions for which you are seeing a physician or are supposed to be seeing a physician?" For example, when talking to a patient experiencing knee pain after a fall, it is helpful to know if the person has hurt the knee before or has had knee surgery.

Find out when the patient last ate or drank something, including any alcoholic beverages. For diabetic patients who are not fully responsive, this information is very important, as their blood sugar could be low if they have not eaten and taken their diabetic medication. It also will be helpful should the patient require surgery in the immediate future.

Ask the patient about the events leading up to the medical problem, especially what the patient was doing when the symptoms first occurred. Simply put, you are trying to determine what happened. This information helps bring the pieces of the assessment puzzle together and helps you to treat the patient's injuries and/or illness more effectively. For example, if the patient has abdominal pain, ask about nausea or vomiting. If the patient reports vomiting, ask how many times the patient has vomited, for how long the vomiting has occurred, whether the vomit was clear or had blood in it, and when the patient vomited last. This information helps you determine if the vomiting is a life threat. For example, blood in the vomit could be life threatening, and repeated vomiting within a brief period is also a serious situation.

Assess Pain and Other Complaints Using OPQRST

In addition to gathering the SAMPLE history, the **OPQRST** mnemonic can be helpful in gathering additional information about a patient's pain (**Table 7-3**). OPQRST represents onset, provocation, quality, radiation, severity, and time. Although

Table 7-3 OPQRST

O—Onset: When did the symptoms begin?
P—Provocation and palliation: Does anything make the symptoms better or worse?
Q—Quality: Describe the nature of the symptoms. Is it sharp, dull, or throbbing?
R—Radiation: Determine whether the symptoms move from one area to another location or remain in one spot. "I have pain in my chest that radiates to my jaw."
S—Severity: Describe the severity of the symptoms, using a 0–10 scale, with 0 being no pain and 10 being the worst pain they have ever felt.
T—Time: How long has the patient had the problem?

originally designed for assessing pain, the OPQRST mnemonic works equally well for assessing other complaints and symptoms. It can be used to assess both traumatic and medical complaints.

- *Onset.* Ask the patient about when the symptoms began. What was the patient doing when the complaint was first noticed? Depending on the circumstances, this may be obvious or not so clear. Attempt to find out if the pain came on suddenly or gradually. Determine whether the patient was at rest or engaged in a physical activity when the symptoms began. If the patient has a history of medical problems, ask if the onset feels like any previously experienced condition. Also, ask whether the current symptoms have been constant or intermittent (come and go). Although questions of this nature may have been asked as part of the SAMPLE review, they provide an opportunity to gather additional relevant information.
- *Provocation and palliation.* Ask if the patient has any idea what might have caused the problem. If, for instance, the patient has been on a strenuous hike and has experienced progressive difficulties in breathing, the patient's condition may be connected to the hike. Additionally, ask if anything makes the problem either worse (is a provocation) or better (is a palliation). Attempt to determine if rest provides any relief from the problem, even if only slightly or momentarily. Our hiking patient may indicate that when he stopped hiking, his breathing became much easier.
- *Quality.* Ask the patient to describe the nature of the symptoms. For instance, if the patient presents with pain, ask him or her to describe the pain. Is it sharp, dull, or throbbing? Attempt to determine whether the symptoms have changed in any way since they were first noticed. For instance, the patient may initially have experienced only abdominal pain that has now resolved, only to be replaced by severe nausea.
- *Radiation.* Ask the patient to locate the source of the problem by pointing to where the symptoms are most intense. If the problem involves a large area, ask the patient to draw a circle around the site using his or her fingers. Attempt to determine whether the symptoms move from this area to another location or remain in one spot. If the problem is pain, ask if pressing on the site of the discomfort causes pain in another part of the body.
- *Severity.* Ask the patient to describe the severity of the symptoms. You may find it helpful to ask the patient to rate the severity using a scale of 0 to 10, with 0 being problem-free and 10 being the worst pain the person has ever felt. Repeat the question to monitor changes in the patient's perception of the severity over time.
- *Time.* Ask how long the patient has had the problem. Also ask if the same problem has occurred previously.

The SAMPLE and OPQRST techniques are tools that may help you collect the patient's history. It is very important that you collect all the information on the patient's history that is outlined by the SAMPLE and OPQRST procedures.

SECONDARY PATIENT ASSESSMENT

The purpose of a **secondary patient assessment** is to obtain more information about the specific problem or to perform a more thorough physical assessment of the patient to ensure that no medical or traumatic problem was overlooked during the exam that took place during the primary patient assessment (**Figure 7-19**). Now that the life

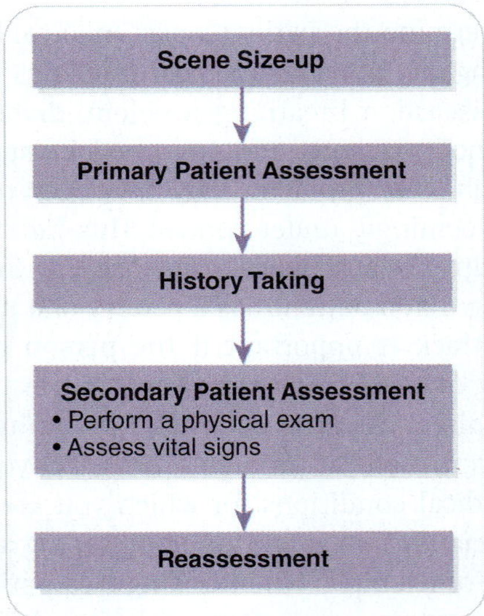

Figure 7-19 Secondary patient assessment.

threats have been addressed, a secondary patient assessment could help you identify hidden injuries or a secondary problem. This new finding may be as simple as a sprained knee or could be a life-threatening problem such as a ruptured spleen. Always look for a medical alert bracelet or necklace, as this can provide important medical information; for example, it may tell you that the patient has diabetes or known allergies.

A secondary patient assessment consists of performing a hands-on physical exam and assessing vital signs. The entire secondary assessment should take 2 to 5 minutes to complete.

Perform a Physical Exam

A physical exam is a systematic head-to-toe, hands-on assessment of the patient. Ask the patient for permission to perform this exam. As with other treatments, if the patient is a competent adult and refuses, you should not proceed.

When touching a patient, always use gloves and other appropriate personal protective equipment. The exam is performed to identify specific clinical findings that will aid in determining the source of the patient's current medical problem or traumatic injury. As part of the physical exam, you will note the patient's *signs*—any objective findings or evidence of a disease that you can detect using your senses (i.e., that you can see, feel, hear, smell) or that you can quantify. First look at the body part, then touch or **palpate** it (**Figure 7-20**).

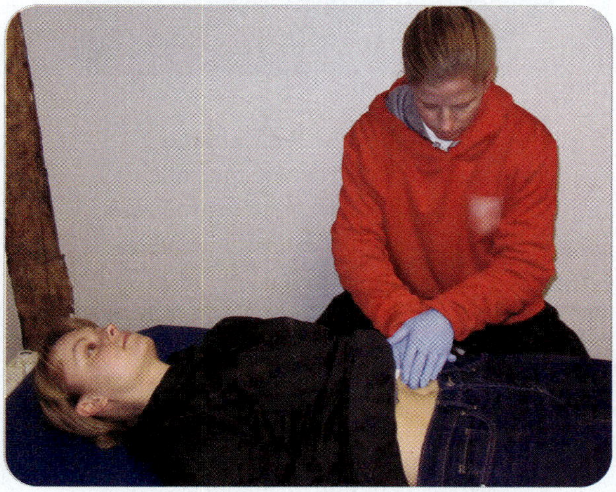

Figure 7-20 This patroller is examining the area of the patient's chief complaint.

You should open or remove clothes to examine each area of the body and then redress the patient, especially during inclement or cold weather. Use common sense when removing clothing, protecting the patient's privacy.

If necessary, you can cut the person's clothes to get a better view of the injury. Cut clothing only if necessary, such as when treating a critical patient or when you cannot otherwise directly examine a body part that appears injured or is painful. If the patient has normal responsiveness, it is best to ask permission to cut clothing.

Patients with certain medical conditions will typically assume a position of comfort. When short of breath, they will sit upright; when abdominal pain is present, they will want to bend their knees. The exam can be done in any position, but it is easier when the patient is made comfortable.

The physical exam is performed in a systematic manner and should take only a few minutes to complete. If a severe problem needing immediate attention is found, take the necessary steps to remedy that issue. Do not be afraid to palpate the patient; touching is an essential part of the exam process. Be thorough, or potential problems might go undetected. Most rescuers start at the head and work down during the exam. Throughout this text, as you read about each body system, a more detailed or focused physical exam will be presented.

When you palpate areas that are tender or swollen, this may cause the patient some physical discomfort. You may want to warn the patient this could hurt. In children it is best to palpate possible painful areas of the body *last* when doing your exam, or they will not let you examine other body parts. Have a child "point to where it hurts," and palpate that body part last.

You may find it helpful to use the **DCAP-BTLS** mnemonic to identify abnormalities as you examine the body (**Table 7-4**).

Examining the Skin

Examine the exposed skin for color, temperature, and moisture. The skin may be bluish from cold weather. Normal skin is "warm, pink, and dry." Certain medical conditions cause sweating or flushed (hot) skin.

Examining the Head

Begin the exam of the head by looking at and palpating the patient's entire head, scalp, and face,

Table 7-4 DCAP-BTLS

D—Deformity	**B**—Burns/bleeding/bruises
C—Contusions	**T**—Tenderness
A—Abrasions/avulsions	**L**—Lacerations
P—Punctures/penetrations	**S**—Swelling

examining from back to front (posterior to anterior). Look for blood or clear fluid draining from the ears or nose. Check the area behind the ears for discoloration (Battle sign).

Next, examine the eyes. Is the white part of the eye yellow, indicating possible hepatitis or liver disease? Look for symmetry and to see if the pupils are constricted, dilated, or unequal (**Figure 7-21**).

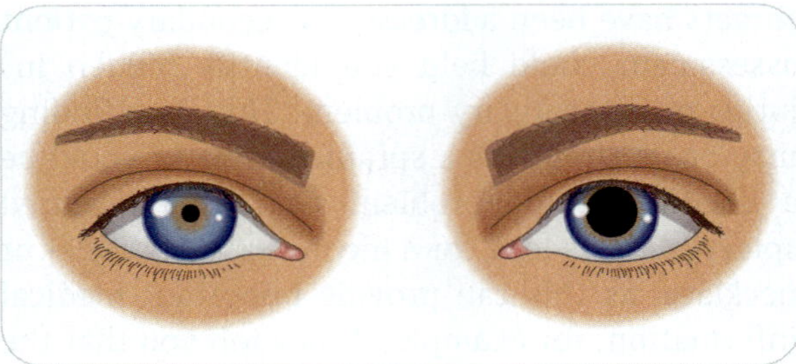

Figure 7-21 Unequal pupils, or anisocoria, can be a normal condition for some patients, and in others a sign of serious head trauma. Be sure to ask your patient what their pupils are normally like.

To assess the pupils' reactions to light, using a small flashlight, follow the steps in **OEC Skill 7-2**. Do not use an LED light, which can injure the eye, unless it is medically approved.

OEC SKILL 7-2 Assessing Pupils

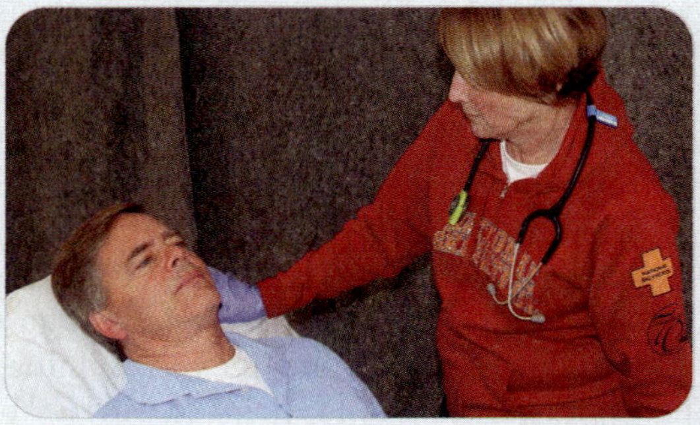

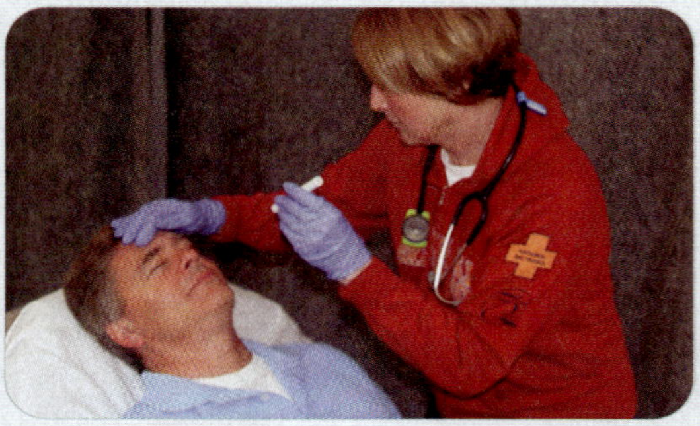

1 Tell the patient to stare at your nose or the center of your forehead. Look at the pupils. Are they the same size? If not, the pupils are said to be asymmetrical. Asymmetry may be caused by an underlying medical or traumatic condition, or rarely it may be normal.

2 Moving from the lateral side of the patient's face, briefly shine the light into the patient's left pupil. Note the reaction of both pupils to the light. *Both* should get smaller, or constrict, when the light is shined into the left pupil. In some cases, you may need to perform this step more than once. Move the light away from the left eye. Repeat this step by shining the light into the patient's right pupil. You should get the same response with the right eye; that is, both pupils should constrict.

If the light conditions are too bright to use a penlight, you can still assess the pupils by shading each of the patient's eyes during the exam. Repeat this process of shading then unshading the eyes several times until you have assessed both pupils. If the pupils are the same size, are both round, and both get smaller when a light is shined into each eye, they are noted as "Pupils are Equal, Round, and Reactive to Light," which can be remembered as **PERRL**.

When assessing eye movement, the eyes should move in unison, unless the patient has an eye injury or a preexisting condition. Medically, such eye movement is called extraocular movement (EOM). If the eyes move correctly, then extraocular movement is intact, or EOMI. To assess eye movement, follow the steps in **OEC Skill 7-3**.

As you are examining the eyes, note whether the light causes the patient any apparent discomfort. Look for any bleeding or fluid leaking from the eye. If the pupil appears elongated or the pupils are not symmetrical, this may indicate an injury to the eye itself, injury to the brain, or previous eye surgery.

Next, look at and palpate the patient's face. Is the face symmetrical, or is one side different from the other? Are the muscles on one side of the face not working, making that side droop? Does the patient's overall color appear normal, or is it pale, yellow, or slightly blue? Check the stability of the facial bones by applying equal but gentle pressure, first on the cheekbones, then on the bone beneath the nose. Check the mouth for evidence of broken or loose teeth, cuts on the inside of the cheeks, swelling, or bleeding. Instruct the patient to clench his or her teeth, and ask whether the teeth feel like they align normally. Ask the patient to stick out his or her tongue. The tongue should come straight out.

Examining the Neck

If you suspect a cervical spine injury, begin by limiting any motion to the neck and spine. If you do not suspect a cervical spine injury, proceed without the need for spinal motion restriction

OEC SKILL 7-3 Assessing Eye Movement

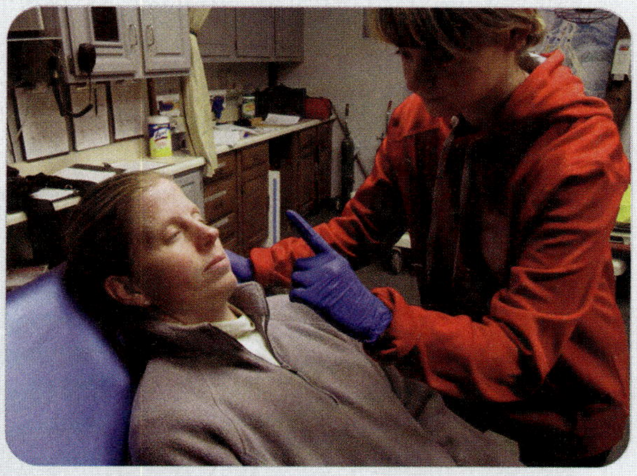

1. Ask the patient to stare at your nose.
2. Hold up your index finger approximately 6 to 8 inches away from the patient's face. Instruct the patient to follow the tip of your finger with his or her eyes without moving his or her head.
3. Slowly move your index finger from the center to the right, then back to center, then over to the left, and then back to center. Next, slowly move your finger from the center upward, then downward past center, and then back up to the center. Finally, slowly move your finger toward you a few inches and then toward the patient's nose. Throughout this step, the patient's eyes should follow your finger and move in sync with one another.

(Figure 7-22). When looking at the neck, can you see any bleeding or deformity? Palpate for tenderness at the base of the skull and down the back of the neck. Make sure you palpate the midline over the spinous processes of the entire neck. Pain over a spinous process could indicate a significant spinal injury. Then, moving from the middle, palpate toward the sides. Look at the neck for symmetry, any deformity, swelling, lacerations, contusions, or other signs of trauma. Gently palpate the front of the neck, noting any tenderness or crackling.

Examining the Chest

First consider modesty, especially in a female patient (Figure 7-23). Tell the person you will examine the chest. Expose and look at the chest wall, both front and back. Note the general color of the skin. Are there any signs of trauma, such as bruising or bleeding? Watch the patient breathe in and out. Does the chest movement appear equal on both sides? Ask the patient to breathe deeply. Does this cause the patient any discomfort? If not, place your hands on each side of the patient's chest, beneath the armpits, and squeeze firmly as the patient breathes in deeply. Does this cause any pain? If not, place one hand on the patient's sternum and the other on the patient's spine between the shoulder blades, squeezing gently. Ask the patient to breathe deeply. Again, does this cause any pain? If a stethoscope is available, listen to the breath sounds. Note the presence and equality of breath sounds on both sides of the chest.

In inclement weather, if there is no suspected chest injury, your examination of the chest may be limited to palpation to avoid unnecessary exposure.

Examining the Abdomen

Again, consider modesty. Expose and look at the abdomen. Does it appear flat or distended? Does it appear pale or otherwise discolored? Ask the patient where it hurts, and then palpate each of four quadrants in turn, always palpating the painful quadrant last (Figure 7-24). Palpate firmly, but not too hard. Note any tenderness, rigidity, or masses.

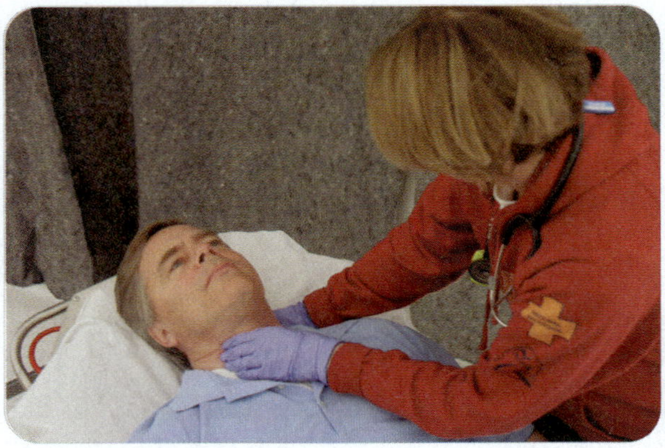

Figure 7-22 A detailed examination of the neck can reveal potential issues with the patient.

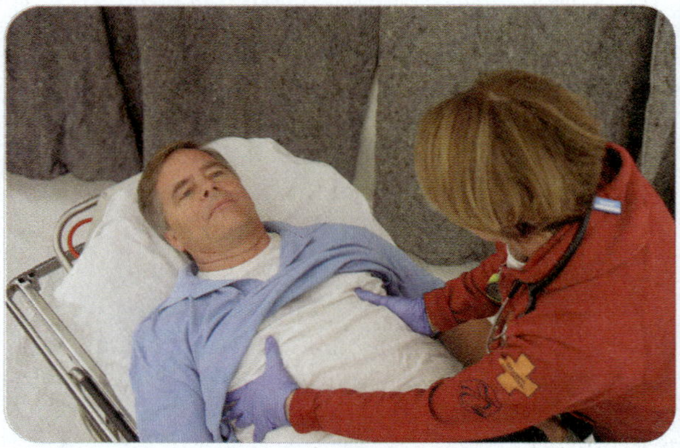

Figure 7-23 When examining a patient's chest, be cognizant of the patient's modesty. Check for equal movement and pain when taking deep breaths.

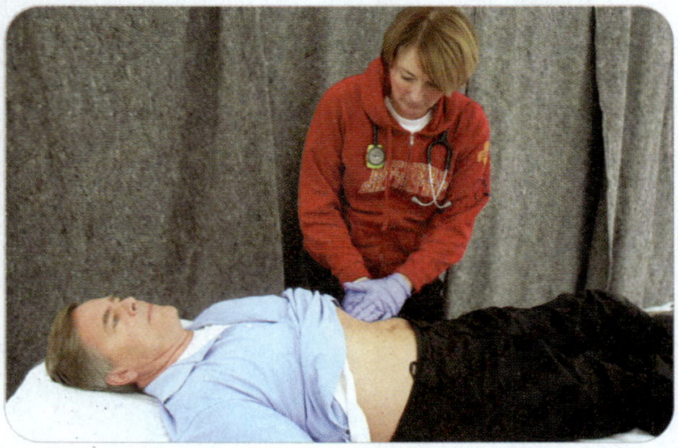

Figure 7-24 Check all four quadrants of the abdomen, feeling for any masses, rigidity, or tenderness.

Examining the Back

If the patient must be examined in a lying position, logroll the patient onto a side to access the back, keeping the neck and spine in alignment if you suspect a spinal injury (**Figure 7-25**). Look at the patient's back, noting the general color of the skin and any abnormalities that may be present. Using a flat, open hand, examine the entire back. Palpate the entire midline length of the spine (over the spinous processes) with the tips of several fingers from the neck to the tailbone. Palpate each side of the back.

Examining the Pelvis

Palpate the bones of the pelvis by placing one hand on each of the iliac crests—that is, on each of the large pelvic bones just above the patient's hips (**Figure 7-26**). Firmly but gently squeeze the bones inward (medially). This test should be performed only *once* because excessive manipulation of an unstable pelvis injury could cause potentially life-threatening bleeding. Note any instability or movement. If external bleeding is apparent, visually inspect the source of bleeding. Preserve the patient's modesty by covering the person with a blanket or jacket. The pelvis, groin, and genital area should be visually examined only if bleeding or other major injury to the area is suspected, and then, if possible, by someone of the same sex.

If you suspect an injury to the anterior pelvis, place the patient's hand over the bones (symphysis pubis) above the genitalia and gently press on the patient's hand, looking for pain (**Figure 7-27**). This technique protects the patient's modesty but allows you to examine the pubic bones.

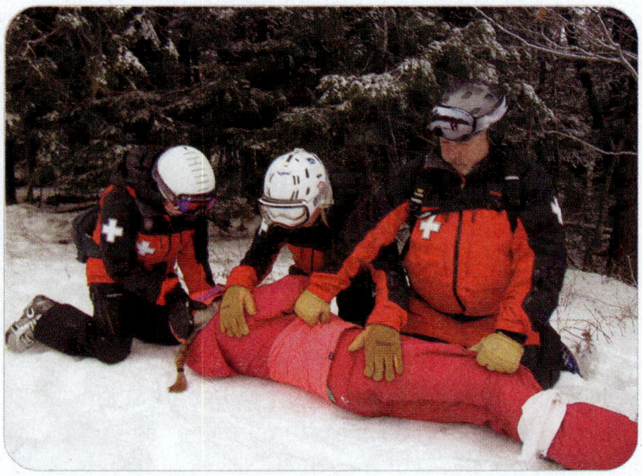

Figure 7-25 Logrolling a supine patient will allow you to adequately examine the back and spine for any deformities.

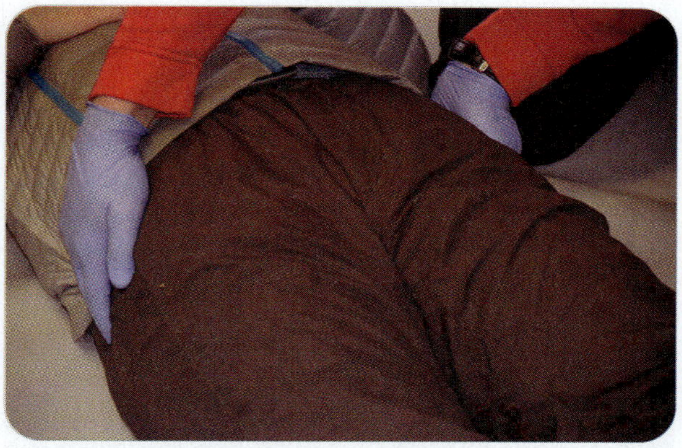

Figure 7-26 Push in gently on the iliac crests when examining the pelvis.

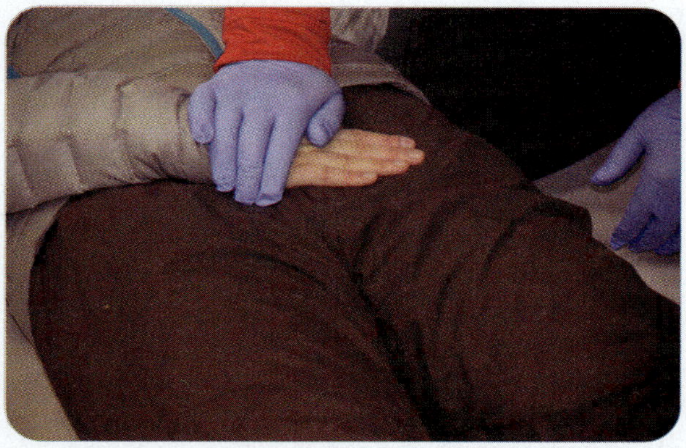

Figure 7-27 You can use the patient's own hand as part of the exam.

Examining the Extremities

Look at the arms and legs. Do they appear normal, or is one bent at an unnatural angle? Is visible bleeding apparent? Ask if the patient has a wet and warm feeling under the clothes, indicating bleeding. When assessing either the arms or the legs, do each side separately.

If the patient complains of arm or leg pain, ask the patient to point to where it hurts. Palpate the *noninjured* part of that extremity first, and then examine the painful part (**Figure 7-28**). Otherwise, the patient may pull away and not let you examine the rest of that extremity. This is especially true in children.

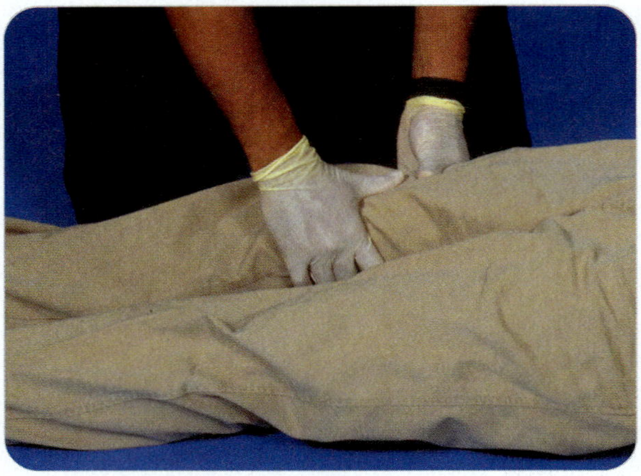

Figure 7-28 Inspect each extremity for cuts, bruises, swelling, obvious injuries, and bleeding.

To assess the entire arm, begin at the shoulder and move distally. First palpate the shoulder blade and clavicle (collarbone), then wrap your hands around the upper arm and with some pressure palpate the entire arm down to the hand. Note any palpable deformities or complaints of pain. Feel the bones of the hand. Do they feel intact? Note the color of the skin. Press on one of the nail beds; does the color immediately return? Ask the patient to make a fist, and then to straighten out the fingers and spread them apart. Check sensation on the palm side of the thumb and fifth (pinkie) finger as well as the back of the thumb.

Repeat this entire exam for the other arm. When complete, feel for equality of pulses by checking both radial pulses at the same time. Do they feel the same? Ask the patient to grip and squeeze the middle and index fingers of both your hands simultaneously. Is the patient's grip equal and strong on both sides?

Now examine the legs. Do they appear normal, or does one or both look deformed? Is there any evidence of bleeding or trauma? Feel for deformities and other signs of injury by palpating the entire length of one leg with one hand on either side of the leg. If conditions permit, inspect the patient's foot, noting the color, overall skin temperature, and presence or absence of a pedal pulse. Repeat the exam on the other leg. Next, place one hand against the bottom of each of the patient's feet and ask the patient to push against your hands with each foot. Strength should be equal on

CASE Update

After ensuring that the scene is safe, you introduce yourself and ask permission to assess, examine, and treat the patient. The patient says, "Yes," so you perform a primary patient assessment while using spinal motion restriction because of the mechanism of injury of falling. The patient is awake and speaks to you in two- or three-word sentences. You determine that his airway is open, but you are concerned that he appears to be having trouble breathing. You check his radial pulse, which is rapid (100 beats per minute) and weak. The patient is alert and oriented to person, place, time, and event. He opens his eyes spontaneously, speaks coherently, and can follow your commands.

In assessing his AVPU score, you assign him an *A* for alert. The patient complains of a persistent pain on the left side of his chest. The history you take reveals that the patient was eating lunch when he had chest pain and fell off his chair onto the floor. He remembers falling on his wrist and does not believe that he lost consciousness. He describes the pain in his chest as "heavy." The pain radiates into the left arm. He also reports being short of breath. He says his wrist hurts some. He reports no allergies to any medications. He states that he takes aspirin on a daily basis because he had a heart attack 10 years ago but has been doing quite well since then. You obtain additional information using the OPQRST mnemonic.

What should you do now?

both sides of the patient's body. Touch the patient on both legs at the lateral and medial side of the ankle. The sensation felt by the patient should be equal. If outdoor weather conditions do not permit a visual exam of the foot, have the patient wiggle his or her toes inside the boot; note whether the patient can feel the toes wiggle. Although not ideal, this method of assessment may have to suffice until later, when the boot may be taken off in a more controlled environment.

Assess Vital Signs

Obtaining **vital signs** is an essential step of the overall assessment process for every patient. Also known as "vitals," vital signs are key objective findings used to evaluate a patient's overall condition. They are used in conjunction with the information gathered from the medical history and during the physical exam to evaluate how well the patient is doing. By repeating the vital signs at intervals, you can see if the patient is improving or getting worse. Check vital signs every 5 minutes for critical or unstable patients and every 15 minutes for stable patients. Whether they are normal or abnormal, vital signs provide valuable information about your patient. It is important for you to learn the normal and abnormal vital signs for all age groups (**Table 7-5**).

In most instances, a complete set of vital signs—consisting of level of responsiveness, pulse rate, respiratory rate, blood pressure, and body temperature—is obtained both at the beginning and at the end of the secondary assessment. Temperature and blood pressure may be difficult to obtain outdoors if appropriate equipment is not available. When outdoors, you should obtain data on level of responsiveness, pulse rate, and respiratory rate. The first set of vital signs, known as "baseline vitals," establishes a reference point against which all other sets of vital signs are compared. First responders should assess vital signs in the following order: level of responsiveness, pulse rate, respiratory rate, blood pressure, and finally temperature. Additionally, oxygen saturation, taken with a pulse oximeter, is now considered a vital sign by many.

Pulse

Assess the rate, quality, and rhythm of the pulse—that is, the number of times the heart beats in a minute, the strength of the heartbeat, and whether the rhythm is regular or irregular. The normal range of pulse rate for an adult is 60 to 100 beats per minute. A rate of less than 60 or greater than 100 beats per minute is abnormal but may not mean there is a significant problem. In fact, trained athletes frequently have a normal resting pulse rate less than 60 beats per minute, whereas high pulse rates can result from exercise, pain, or fear. Nevertheless, the presence of an abnormal pulse rate should raise your suspicion for a potentially serious problem.

Always use the tip of your index and middle fingers, not your thumb, when assessing a pulse. When checking for a pulse, press gently. If you press too hard, you will close off the flow of blood through the artery and will not be able to feel the pulse. Assess pulse quality by determining whether it is strong, bounding, very strong or forceful, or weak. There are five places where an artery is close to the skin, allowing a pulse to be taken easily.

- *Radial pulse.* The radial artery is the most common site used to assess pulse rate in a responsive patient. To feel for the radial pulse, place your index and middle fingers on the bony prominence of the thumb or radial side of the wrist, then slide them toward the

Table 7-5 Normal Vital Signs

	Adult	Child (1–8 years)	Infant (Birth–1 year)
Pulse (beats/min)	60–100	70–150	90–180
Respirations (breaths/min)	12–20	15–30	20–60
Systolic blood pressure (mm Hg)	90–140	80–110	50–95
Temperature	36.1–38.0°C (97.0–100.4°F)	36.1–38.0°C	36.1–38.0°C

palm side of the wrist until they fall into a groove (**Figure 7-29**).

- *Carotid pulse.* To locate the carotid pulse, place your index and middle fingers on the thyroid cartilage (also known as the Adam's apple) and then slide them laterally into the first groove (**Figure 7-30**). Due to the proximity of this site to the heart, the carotid pulse is usually the strongest arterial pulse and is frequently used first when assessing the pulse of an unresponsive patient.
- *Brachial pulse.* To locate the brachial pulse, place your hand at the bony prominence at the ulnar side (medial side) of the elbow and then slide your fingers into the groove at the base of the biceps muscle in the medial aspect of the elbow (**Figure 7-31**). This is the pulse used when assessing a child.
- *Femoral pulse.* To locate the femoral pulse, draw an imaginary line on the patient from the middle of the groin to the hip bone, or iliac crest, and then slide your fingers along this line about one-third of the way from the groin endpoint (**Figure 7-32**). The pulse can be detected along the crease between the leg and the lower abdomen.
- *Dorsalis pedis pulse.* This pulse is located in the middle of the top of the foot between the ankle and the toes (**Figure 7-33**).

Follow the steps in **OEC Skill 7-4** to assess the pulse rate.

Breathing

Assessment of **breath sounds** consists of evaluating the rate and the quality of breaths. Begin by calculating the patient's respiratory rate, an objective

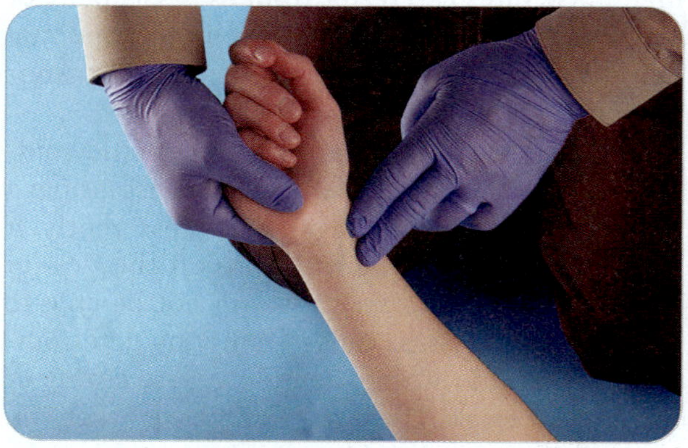

Figure 7-29 The radial pulse is found on the thumb side of the wrist.

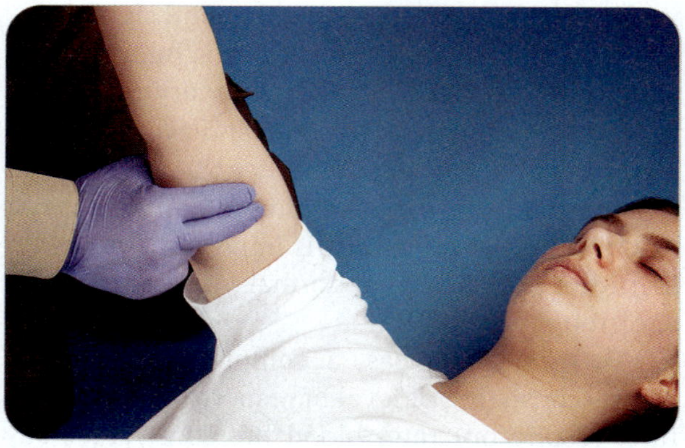

Figure 7-31 The brachial pulse is felt on the inside of the upper arm.

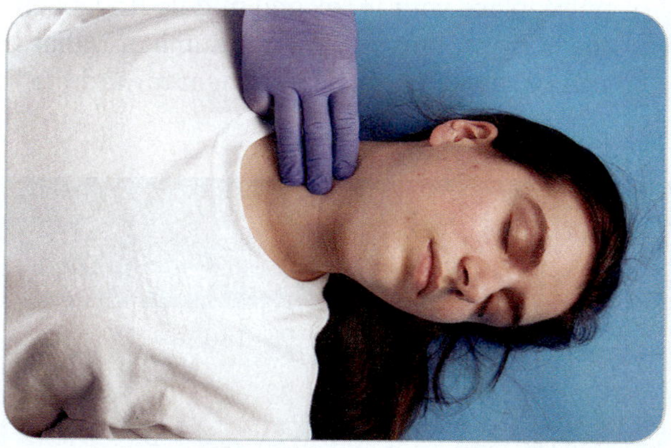

Figure 7-30 The carotid pulse is felt in the neck.

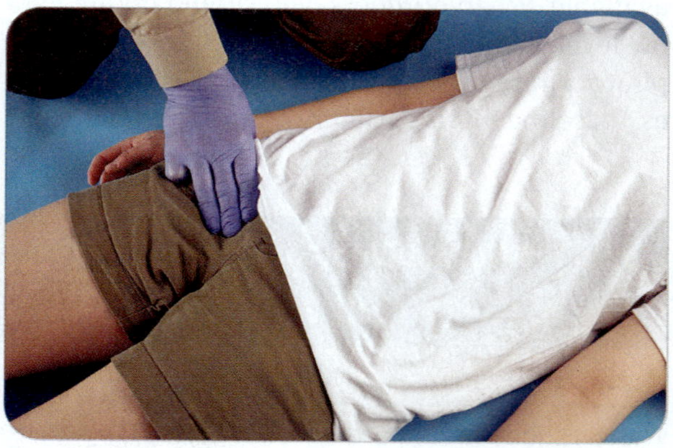

Figure 7-32 The femoral pulse is felt in the groin area.

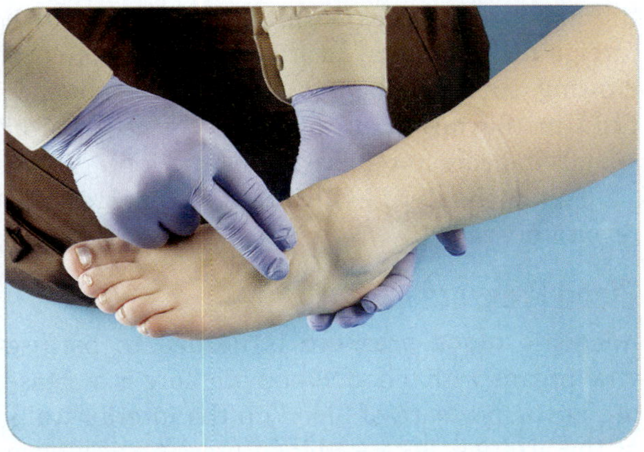

Figure 7-33 The dorsalis pedis pulse is felt on the top of the foot.

measure of the number of times the patient takes a breath in a minute. One breath consists of one inhalation and one exhalation. The normal respiratory rate of an adult is 12 to 20 breaths per minute. A rate less than 12 or greater than 20 breaths per minute is abnormal and may indicate either a current problem directly related to the pulmonary system or a chronic serious medical disorder.

To count the number of breaths in 1 minute, watch the patient breathe for 30 seconds, counting each time the patient inhales. Multiplying this number by 2 provides the respiratory rate. For instance, if the patient breathes 8 times in 30 seconds, the rate is 16 breaths per minute.

If the patient is unresponsive or is wearing heavy clothing, you may have to be more creative

OEC SKILL 7-4 Assessing Pulse

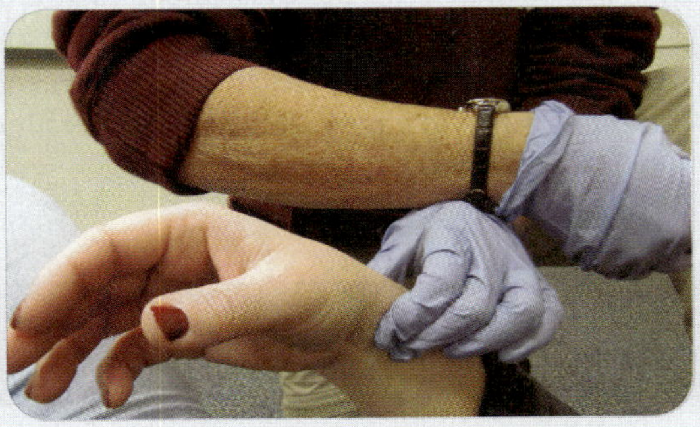

1 Locate the radial pulse on a responsive adult and assess the pulse rate and quality.

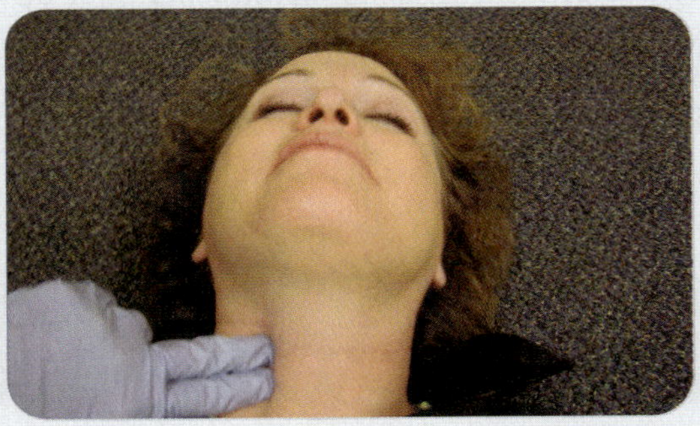

2 Locate the carotid pulse on an unresponsive adult and assess the pulse rate and quality.

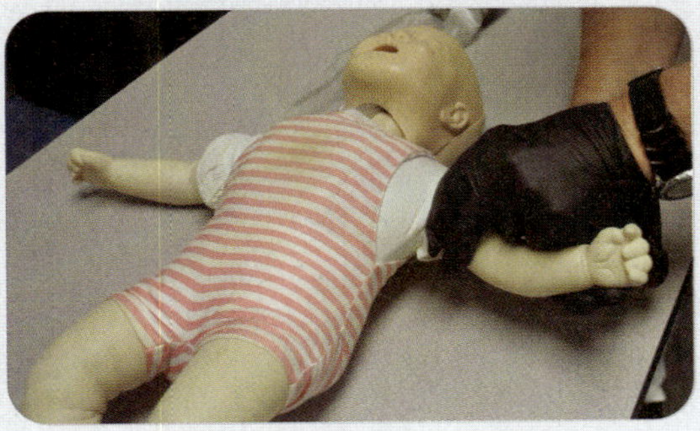

3 Locate the brachial pulse on an infant and assess the pulse rate and quality.

to count breaths. In these instances, count by watching or palpating the rise and fall of the patient's chest, or count breath sounds using your stethoscope. Assess the quality of breaths by determining if they are normal, deep, or shallow.

You may even need to put a small mirror (which fogs during each breath) to the patient's mouth to count the number of exhalations. A conscious patient who knows that you are evaluating the respiratory rate will often override the automatic rate and depth by breathing more slowly and deeply. It may be best to count breaths without the person's knowledge. To do so, place your fingers on the patient's wrist as if you were checking the pulse; at the same time, tip your head slightly downward while moving your eyes upward to subtly watch the chest. Calculate the respiratory rate in the manner previously described. You may want to check the pulse first for 15 seconds and then count the number of breaths for 30 seconds with your fingers still on the wrist. Remember not to ask the patient questions while you are counting the number of breaths, as the count will not be accurate if the patient is talking.

Normal breathing is almost silent. Snoring may indicate an upper airway obstruction. When the upper airway has a partial obstruction by a foreign body, you may hear a harsh, high-pitched crowing sound. Bubbling or gurgling indicates fluid in the upper airway. Wheezes or musical sounds indicate lower airway obstruction.

Follow the steps in **OEC Skill 7-5** to assess the respiratory rate.

Blood Pressure

Adequate **blood pressure** is needed to perfuse vital organs with blood. Blood pressure is a measure of the pressure of blood on the interior walls of the arteries. Because blood pressure was once commonly measured by the movement of mercury up or down in a thin tube, the unit used for blood pressure is millimeters of mercury, abbreviated mm Hg. Old-fashioned mercury blood pressure machines are rarely seen today, as modern electronic devices or cuffs with a gauge are used.

A blood pressure reading consists of two values: the systolic pressure, which is the pressure within the arteries just after the left ventricle maximally contracts, and the diastolic pressure, which is a measure of the pressure within the arteries while the heart is at rest. A blood pressure that is too high or too low may indicate serious illness. A

OEC SKILL 7-5 Assessing Respiratory Rate

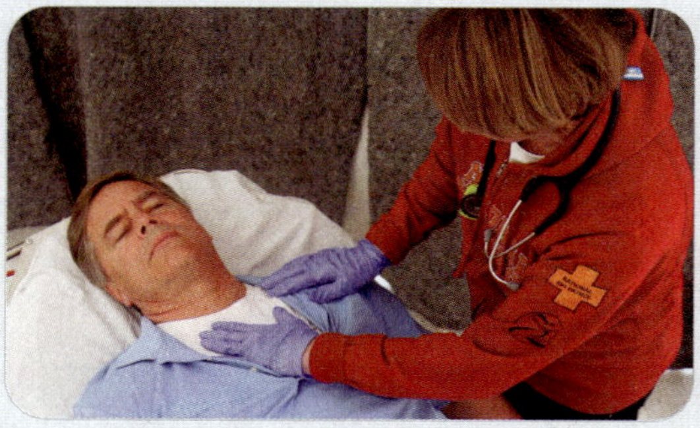

1 Look and feel for the patient's chest to rise and fall.

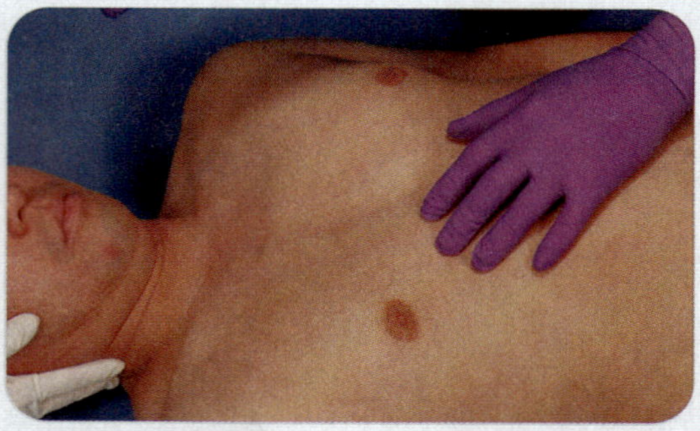

2 Assess the patient's breathing for rhythm, depth, effort, and noise to determine if the patient is breathing within normal limits.

normal blood pressure for a healthy adult is 120/80, which is read as "one hundred twenty over eighty." In this case, the systolic pressure is 120 mm Hg, and the diastolic pressure is 80 mm Hg.

The most common place to check a blood pressure is over the brachial artery in the arm (**Figure 7-34**). To listen to (auscultate) the blood pressure, you will need a blood pressure cuff and a stethoscope. A blood pressure cuff consists of four parts: a flexible rubber bulb with an attached thumbscrew valve, a rubber bladder (cuff) with hoses, a sphygmomanometer (blood pressure gauge), and a nylon or cloth bladder covering.

To obtain a blood pressure reading, follow the steps in **OEC Skill 7-6**.

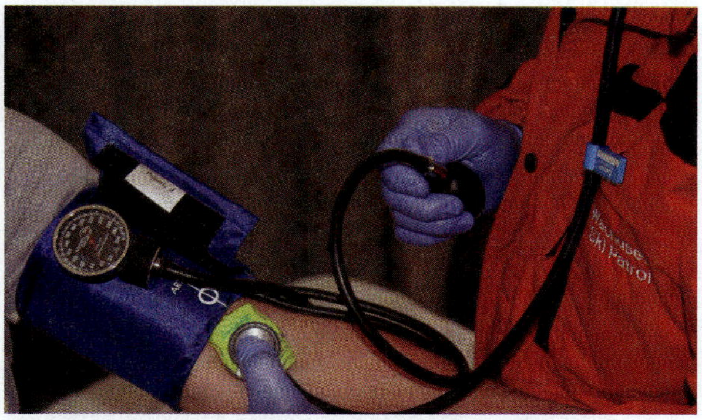

Figure 7-34 Taking a blood pressure at regular intervals will help you determine if your patient is stable.

OEC SKILL 7-6 Obtaining a Blood Pressure Reading

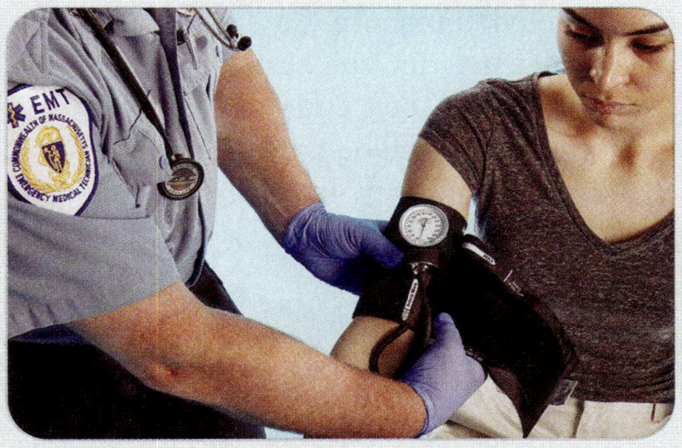

1 Ensure that you have the correct size cuff. (Size options include regular, large adult, and pediatric.) Unscrew the thumbscrew valve on the flexible bulb and deflate the bladder of the cuff. Place the cuff on the patient's upper arm with the cuff 1 to 2 inches above the crease of the elbow. The arrow on the cuff should point to the brachial artery, which is located on the medial side of the arm at the crease of the elbow. The cuff should be placed directly on the patient's skin because you will get a false reading if the cuff is placed over bulky clothing. The cuff should be snug, but not too tight.

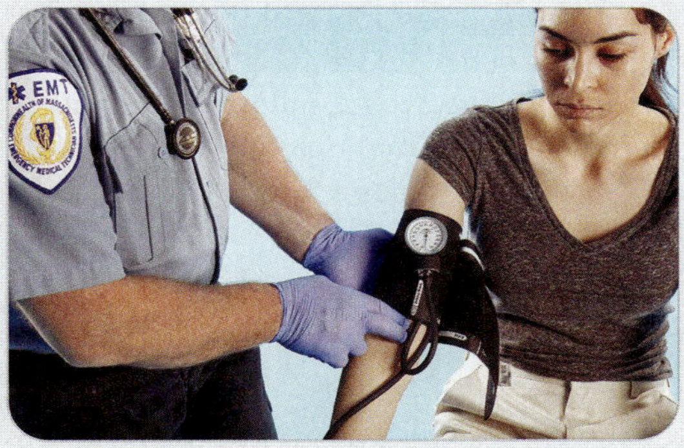

2 Place the sphygmomanometer in a location that is easy for you to read without having to hold it. (Some cuffs have a clip on the sphygmomanometer that enables you to attach it to the patient's clothing or to a loop on the cuff while you are taking the pressure reading.) Place the ear tips of the stethoscope in your ears. The tips should point forward. Palpate the pulse of the brachial artery below the cuff at the crease of the elbow and then place the diaphragm of the stethoscope over the pulse point. (You will not hear a pulse at this time.) Hold the stethoscope in place lightly on the skin as you measure the pressure.

(continues)

OEC SKILL 7-6 Obtaining a Blood Pressure Reading (*continued*)

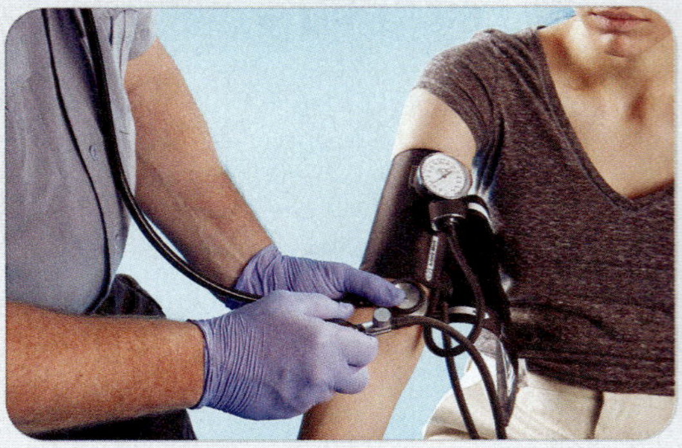

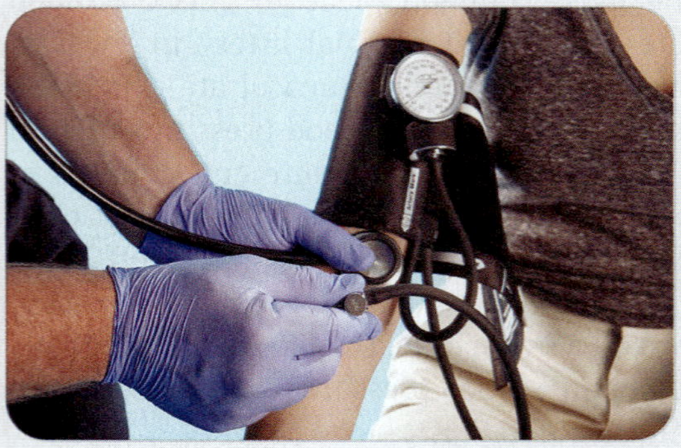

3 Using your other hand, tighten the thumbscrew valve on the sphygmomanometer and inflate the cuff by repeatedly pumping the flexible bulb. Inflate the cuff to a pressure of 160 mm Hg. If you can hear the pulse sound at this pressure, inflate the cuff to 200 mm Hg. If you still can hear the heartbeat, inflate the cuff in increments of 20 mm Hg until you can no longer hear the pulse sound.

4 Gently open the thumbscrew valve and *slowly* release the air from the cuff. As you slowly release the air, listen for the first pulse sound (first "thump"). The reading on the dial at the time of this sound is the systolic blood pressure. Continue to slowly release the air from the cuff. The sound will become very soft and will eventually disappear. The reading on the dial when the sound disappears is the diastolic blood pressure.

If you inadvertently deflate the blood pressure cuff too quickly, fail to detect the systolic or diastolic pressure, or simply forget one of the two numbers, do not reinflate the cuff immediately. Instead, deflate the cuff completely and wait a few seconds before reinflating it. These steps will help ensure accurate readings when you repeat the procedure.

In rare instances, you may continue to hear the pulse sound as you deflate the cuff down to a reading of 0 mm Hg. Should this occur, wait a few seconds, reinflate the cuff, and slowly release the pressure again. This time, after noting the systolic blood pressure, continue to deflate the cuff and listen *carefully*. At some point, you should detect a subtle change in the sound of the pulse sound. The number at which this change occurs is the diastolic blood pressure.

Once you are finished measuring the blood pressure, you may remove the cuff, or you may leave it on the arm *deflated* if you anticipate taking additional readings in a potentially unstable patient. Do not leave an inflated blood pressure cuff on the arm for more than a few minutes because doing so can cut off blood flow to the distal arm and hand, which is painful.

If you do not have a stethoscope, or if it is too noisy to hear the pulse sound using the stethoscope, you can obtain an approximate measure of the systolic pressure with just the blood pressure cuff and your fingers. Although not as accurate as an auscultated blood pressure, this method—known as a palpated blood pressure—provides a useful estimate of the patient's blood pressure. This blood pressure reading would be verbally stated as, "The patient's blood pressure is ninety over palpation," documented as "90/P."

To obtain a palpated blood pressure, follow these steps:

1. Apply the blood pressure cuff above the elbow in the fashion previously described.
2. Find the patient's radial pulse.
3. Inflate the blood pressure cuff until you can no longer feel the radial pulse.

4. Open the thumbscrew and slowly release air from the cuff.
5. The pressure at which you can again feel the radial pulse is the *systolic* blood pressure.

Even if you do not have a blood pressure cuff or are outside, you can still estimate the blood pressure by feeling the presence of an arterial pulse at various locations. The presence of a radial pulse correlates to a minimum systolic pressure of approximately 80 mm Hg. A femoral pulse is equivalent to a systolic pressure of about 70 mm Hg. A carotid pulse is equivalent to a systolic pressure of approximately 60 mm Hg. Although these estimates are roughly accurate, you should not necessarily be reassured by a strong radial pulse. In the setting of trauma or suspected acute internal blood loss, a systolic blood pressure less than 90 mm Hg can be life threatening.

In 2019, the American Medical Association, the American Heart Association, and Johns Hopkins University determined that taking simple steps, such as having the patient empty his or her bladder and having the patient sit with the feet supported, can help obtain an accurate blood pressure reading (**Table 7-6**). Realizing that not all conditions can be controlled prior to taking a blood pressure reading, consider how these factors could affect a blood pressure reading.

Table 7-6 Tips for Measuring Blood Pressure Accurately

1. Have the patient empty his or her bladder. A full bladder can add 10 to 15 mm Hg to the systolic blood pressure.
2. Make sure the patient's feet are on the floor/ground. Failure to support the feet can add 10 to 15 mm Hg to the systolic blood pressure.
3. Make sure the patient's back is supported. Failure to support the back can add 10 to 15 mm Hg to the systolic blood pressure.
4. Don't allow the patient to cross his or her legs. Crossing the legs can add 2 to 8 mm Hg to the systolic blood pressure.
5. Don't talk with the patient during the reading. Talking can add 10 to 15 mm Hg to the systolic blood pressure.
6. Place the cuff on the patient's bare arm. Taking the reading over clothes can add 10 to 40 mm Hg to the systolic blood pressure.
7. Support the arm level with the patient's heart. Failure to do so can add 10 mm Hg to the systolic blood pressure.

Modified from Pickering TG, Hall JE, Appel LJ, et al. Recommendations for blood pressure measurement in humans and experimental animals: part 1: blood pressure measurement in humans: a statement for professionals_x000B_from the Subcommittee of Professional and Public Education of the American Heart Association Council on High Blood Pressure Research. Circulation. Feb 8 2005;111(5):697-716._x000B_O'Brien E, Asmar R, Beilin L, et al. European Society of Hypertension recommendations for conventional, ambulatory and home blood pressure measurement. J Hypertens 2003; 21: 821-848. Retrived from https://www.ama-assn.org/delivering-care/hypertension/ama-johns-hopkins-blood-pressure-control-resources

Temperature

Because of the potentially harsh conditions of outdoor environments, obtaining an accurate reading of a patient's body temperature in the field can be extremely difficult. The most accurate body temperature is a "core" temperature, which requires using a special thermometer. Other methods of assessing temperature, such as placing a thermometer in the patient's armpit or on the forehead, are not accurate.

A battery-operated oral thermometer can give reasonably accurate body temperature readings and is the type of thermometer most often used by OEC technicians. Assessing body temperature in the field beyond classifying the skin as hot, warm, cool, or cold has limited usefulness for OEC technicians.

Normal body temperature ranges from 36°C to 38°C (97–100.4°F) (**Table 7-7**). Most people have a normal temperature near 37°C (98.6°F). Body temperatures below 35°C (95.0°F) are considered hypothermic, whereas temperatures above 39°C (102.2°F) are considered hyperthermic. A significantly abnormal temperature in either direction is harmful to the patient.

Oxygen Saturation Level

Recent medical literature has named another important vital sign. Oxygen saturation levels are measured using a device known as a **pulse oximeter** (**Figure 7-35**). This device measures the percentage of oxygen in the blood using a probe that is attached to a patient's finger or earlobe. A pulse oximetry reading of less than 94% is abnormal and may indicate serious illness or injury. Chronic smokers may live with a low percentage of oxygen in the blood, with an oxygen saturation level much lower than 94%. Higher altitudes will lower the normal oxygen saturation reading.

Table 7-7 Fahrenheit and Celsius Body Temperature Conversions

Fahrenheit	Celsius	
90°	32.2°	
91°	32.7°	
92°	33.3°	
93°	33.8°	
94°	34.4°	
95°	35°	Abnormally low body temperature (hypothermia)
96°	35.5°	
97°	36.1°	
98.6°	37°	Normal body temperature (normothermia)
100.4°	38°	
101°	38.3°	
102°	38.8°	
103°	39.4°	Abnormally high body temperature (hyperthermia)
104°	40°	
105°	40.5°	
106°	41.1°	

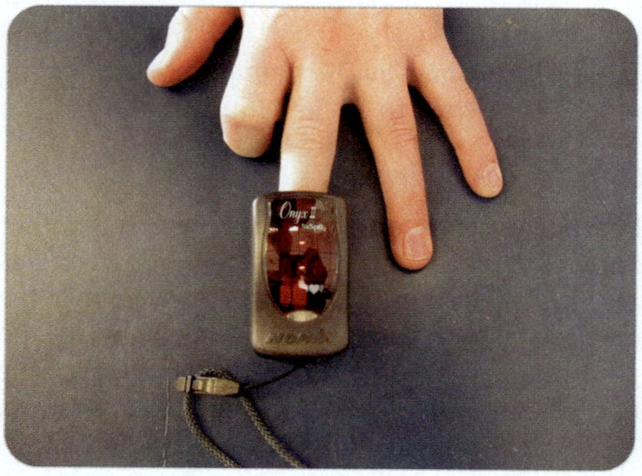

Figure 7-35 Use a pulse oximeter to determine the oxygen saturation of your patient's blood.

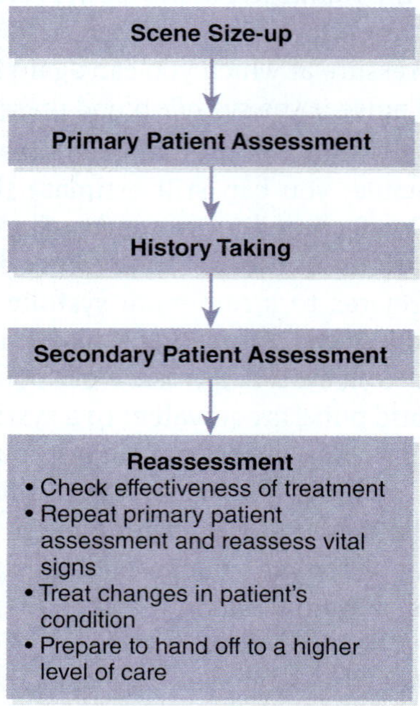

Figure 7-36 Reassessment

The device is simple to use, but caution must be taken, as some less expensive pulse oximeters are not accurate. If the patient's skin looks ashen or gray and the pulse oximeter's reading is normal, trust your eyes and not the device.

Neurologic Assessment

Assess the patient for any life-threatening neurologic disorders, including any problems affecting the brain or spinal cord. You have already assessed the patient's level of responsiveness, a measure of the patient's awareness and responsiveness to the surrounding environment. Level of responsiveness is a continuum that ranges from the patient being fully alert to various levels of unresponsiveness. Under normal conditions, a patient is awake and fully oriented. Look for abnormal posturing (decorticate or decerebrate posturing).

REASSESSMENT

A patient's condition can change over time. During the reassessment, check the effectiveness of your treatment (Figure 7-36). If you need to continue to care for the patient, you must regularly repeat

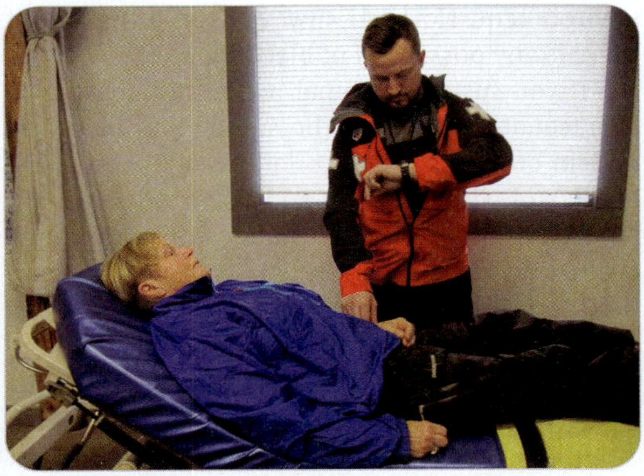

Figure 7-37 Continuous reassessment of your patient is necessary to keep the patient stable until the patient is transferred to a higher level of care.

some parts of the patient assessment. For example, if a patient has bleeding that has been controlled, make sure bleeding does not start again. A patient who is having a heart attack can get worse if the process causing the problem is not helped by giving oxygen.

Check vital signs every 5 minutes for critical or unstable patients and every 15 minutes for stable patients. Continually monitor the ABCDs and repeat the vital signs regularly (Figure 7-37).

If the patient is getting worse, consider what you can do to improve the situation. For example, if the respiratory rate is increasing, check the patient's oxygen saturation with a pulse oximeter and provide oxygen if indicated.

Based on local protocol, have all the necessary paperwork ready to give to the transport personnel. This preparation is especially important for someone who needs rapid transport.

OTHER ASSESSMENT SITUATIONS

Communication Problems

Sometimes the assessment process is complicated by one or more of a variety of factors. These factors include a communication barrier such as deafness or differences in language, very young age, cultural differences, aggressive behavior by the patient, or inability to answer questions because the brain is not getting enough oxygen or glucose.

When confronted with a communication challenge, begin by staying calm. Getting frustrated and agitated will not help the situation. Always assume communication difficulties are the result of an illness or injury until proven otherwise. Look for companions of the patient who may be able to assist you in communicating with the patient. Smile at the patient to demonstrate that you are there to help; a smile is universally understood. Despite your best efforts, there will be times when the patient will not be able to understand you or communicate. In these cases, assess the patient to the best of your ability, and always act with the patient's best interests in mind. If the patient appears to be critically ill or injured but resists your assessment efforts, you may need to care for the patient under implied consent.

Children can be especially difficult to assess and are often scared by the presence of a stranger. Depending on age, the child may not understand that you are there to help. The problem may be compounded if the child is not with the parents. The child may be in pain. Be patient. Explain what is happening, using age-appropriate words the child can understand. Speak slowly and calmly, directly to the child. Fully explain what you are doing, and why, before you begin your assessment. Encourage the child to participate in the assessment process. Never stand over a child; instead, get down to the child's level during the assessment. Allow the child to examine your penlight or stethoscope before you use it.

You may encounter a patient who is combative or aggressive. Never place yourself or others at risk of harm. Combative or aggressive behavior can be a sign of significant illness or injury resulting from a lack of oxygen, decreased blood sugar, an intoxicating substance, or a brain injury. If you think the patient may harm himself or others, request assistance from other rescuers, area security, or law enforcement. Continue to talk to the person and maintain a calm demeanor until additional help arrives. Follow your area, state, or provincial protocols for managing this type of situation.

Cultural Diversity

As you are performing your assessment, be sensitive to differences in cultural norms among your patients. Whereas some patients will feel quite comfortable with your examining them, others may not feel so comfortable. Be respectful. Ask permission before touching the patient or performing your exam. Be prepared to fully explain what you are doing and the need for each step of the physical exam. Depending on the patient's culture, you may need to seek permission, support, or advice from the patient's family or friends before making physical contact with the patient. Women of certain religions may request privacy from men. In this case, a female OEC technician, if available, should perform the exam.

Environmental Considerations

Performing a patient assessment in outdoor environments can be quite challenging and complex. Environmental conditions may prevent you from performing a physical examination of your patient. In addition, harsh environmental conditions may have contributed to your patient's injury and/or illness.

Consider the outside temperature during the assessment process. If the weather is cold, the patient will likely be reluctant to let you remove any clothing. As a result, you may need to perform a secondary patient assessment over bulky clothes, or perhaps you can unzip them, rapidly perform your assessment, and then zip them back up. If you suspect an injury that is associated with bleeding, expose the skin to the elements only as much as is needed to adequately assess and manage the injury. Cover the area with clothes or a blanket as soon as possible.

If you do not suspect bleeding, it may be more beneficial to expose the injury only after the patient has been moved to a more controlled environment. However, always expose the area if there is any possibility of bleeding.

If you suspect a spinal injury and are unable to adequately examine the spine and neurologic system outdoors, use a collar, head blocks, and a backboard with straps as a transportation device, restricting motion of the spine until a thorough evaluation can be performed. Transport the patient to a controlled environment where you can perform a spinal exam. If this exam indicates there is no need for spinal motion restriction, take the patient off of the transportation device. This situation should be rare, occurring in very bad weather or in conditions such as on the side of a cliff. This issue will be discussed in Chapter 21, *Spine, Brain, and Nervous System Injuries*.

In a windy, dusty, rainy, or dark environment, it may be very difficult to even see your patient clearly, let alone perform a thorough assessment. Regardless of the environmental conditions, at a minimum you should assess the patient's ABCDs before attempting to move the patient to a location that is better suited for a secondary assessment.

When faced with difficult conditions, you can do several things to make the assessment process easier. You can protect your patient from the elements: shade the patient's face with your hand while examining his or her face, cover the patient with a blanket when it is cold, or create a temporary cover or shelter to block the sun when it is hot. If the patient is located on a slope or steep incline, you may be able to cut a flat step into the slope or slide the patient down a bit to a more level spot. On the ski slope, kick your boots into the snow, or anchor yourself, your patient, and your equipment with ropes or skis.

No one approach works in every situation. Decide what to do by balancing how urgently you need information to assess the situation adequately and prepare for safe transport against the length of time you must keep the patient exposed to a harsh environment.

CASE Outcome

Suspecting the man has a serious medical condition, possibly having suffered a heart attack, you call for additional OEC technicians and advanced life support. You then perform a physical exam on the patient. During the exam, you notice some discoloration of the patient's wrist. He has equal sensation and movement in all his extremities. Pulses in both the upper and lower extremities are equal and strong. Pulse rate and breathing are abnormally high. Other OEC technicians arrive to assist you. Working together, you package the patient and send him by ambulance to a nearby hospital. You later learn that the patient had a mild heart attack, which the doctors think may have caused him to become dizzy and fall. He also had a broken wrist.

CHAPTER REVIEW

In Summary

- The overall patient assessment process consists of five parts:
  - Scene size-up
  - Primary patient assessment
  - History taking
  - Secondary patient assessment
  - Reassessment
- Patient assessment is a very important skill that you will use in each patient encounter.
- The scene size-up determines the safety of the scene, the type of incident, standard precautions, the mechanism of injury or nature of illness, and the need for additional resources. Your first priority is scene safety.
- The purpose of the primary patient assessment is to form a general impression of the patient and identify and immediately treat life threats. Life threats may be excessive bleeding or problems with the patient's airway, breathing, circulation, and/or disability.
  - Identifying and correcting life-threatening issues begins with the airway, followed by breathing, circulation, and disability (ABCD).
  - However, if the patient has life-threatening bleeding (a circulation issue), follow the sequence of circulation, airway, breathing, and disability (CABD).
- History taking involves collecting important historical information about the patient and the events surrounding the patient's current condition. Use SAMPLE to investigate the chief complaint and OPQRST to assess the level of pain.
- The secondary patient assessment consists of performing a hands-on physical exam and assessing vital signs.
  - During the secondary patient assessment, use the DCAP-BTLS mnemonic to identify abnormalities as you examine the body.
  - Know the normal values of vital signs. Check vital signs every 5 minutes for critical or unstable patients and every 15 minutes for stable patients.
- Reassess the patient frequently.

Key Terms

Allergy An exaggerated immune response to a substance that does not normally cause a reaction.

AVPU scale A mnemonic for assessing neurologic function; represents awake and alert, responds to verbal stimuli or pain, or unresponsive.

Blood pressure The pressure of the blood on the interior walls of the arteries.

Breath sounds An indication of air movement in the lungs, usually assessed with a stethoscope.

Chief complaint The symptom or group of symptoms about which the patient is concerned.

DCAP-BTLS A mnemonic for assessing trauma-related injuries; represents deformity; contusions; abrasions and avulsions; punctures and penetrations; burns, bleeding, and bruises; tenderness; lacerations; and swelling.

Decerebrate posturing Abnormal extension of the arms and legs, downward pointing of the toes, and arching of the head due to an injury to the brain at the level of the brainstem.

Decorticate posturing Abnormal flexing of the arms, clenching of the fists, and extending of the legs; due to an injury along the nerve pathway between the brain and spinal cord.

General impression Initial findings based on the patient's chief complaint, the scene size-up, the mechanism of injury or nature of illness, and the patient's initial appearance.

Level of responsiveness The degree of cognitive function and arousal of the brain; ranges from fully alert to unresponsive.

Mechanism of injury The type of force that acts on the body to cause injury; the method of trauma causing an injury.

Nature of illness The type of medical illness present.

OPQRST A mnemonic that is used in the assessment of a patient's chief complaint; represents onset, provocation and palliation, quality, radiation, severity, and time.

Palpation The act of touching a patient during an examination to feel for any abnormality.

Paraesthesia A sensation of tingling, pricking, or numbness of the skin, or the feeling of "pins and needles" or a limb being "asleep."

Patient assessment The procedure performed to determine a patient's condition, especially any immediate life-threatening injuries or conditions; forms the basis for decision about emergency medical care and transport.

PERRL A mnemonic for assessing the eyes; represents pupils equal, round, reactive to light.

Primary patient assessment A step within the patient assessment process that identifies and initiates treatment of immediate and potential life threats.

Pulse A rhythmic throbbing of the artery caused by the movement of blood.

Pulse oximeter A medical device that measures oxygen saturation level (the oxygen levels in the blood) noninvasively and painlessly.

SAMPLE A mnemonic used to obtain medical history information during the patient assessment process; represents signs/symptoms, allergies, medications, past medical history, last oral intake, and events leading up to the present incident.

Scene safety The process of identifying any hazards or possible hazards that could harm you or others and mitigating them prior to attending to the patient.

Scene size-up A general overview of the incident and its surroundings.

Secondary patient assessment The thorough, systematic physical examination that follows primary patient assessment, any immediate resuscitation, and history taking; includes taking the patient's vital signs.

Sign Any objective finding that can be seen, heard, smelled, or measured (e.g., a bruise, the patient's blood pressure); typically discovered during a physical exam.

Symptom A subjective finding or a departure from normal function or feeling that is noticed by a patient (e.g., pain, blurred vision), reflecting the presence of a medical problem.

Vital signs The key objective findings used to evaluate a patient's overall condition; includes pulse rate, respiratory rate, blood pressure, temperature, and level of responsiveness.

Chapter Questions

1. During the scene size-up, you will need to determine:
   a. the mechanism of injury or nature of illness.
   b. the level of responsiveness.
   c. standard precautions.
   d. the chief complaint.
2. When checking for level of responsiveness, you can use the mnemonic AVPU. The *P* in AVPU stands for:
   a. past medical history.
   b. pain response.
   c. pulse.
   d. pupils.
3. During the patient assessment process, when taking a patient history, which mnemonic can you use to assess pain?
   a. SAMPLE
   b. OPQRST
   c. DCAP-BTLS
   d. AVPU

4. You approach an adult patient who has fallen on a mogul trail. The patient is sitting up and holding her arm against her chest. After ensuring that the scene is safe, you should:
   a. introduce yourself and ask permission to assess, examine, and treat the patient.
   b. call for advanced life support.
   c. complete a secondary patient assessment.
   d. take a SAMPLE history.
5. During the primary patient assessment, when identifying life-threatening issues, which mnemonic should you use?
   a. AVPU
   b. ABCD
   c. CPR
   d. GCS
6. The normal range for a pulse rate in an adult is:
   a. 60 to 100 beats per minute.
   b. 70 to 140 beats per minute.
   c. 80 to 160 beats per minute.
   d. None of the above
7. The normal range for a respiratory rate in a child is:
   a. 12 to 20 respirations per minute.
   b. 15 to 30 respirations per minute.
   c. 25 to 60 respirations per minute.
   d. None of the above
8. Your adult patient has a systolic blood pressure of 70 mm Hg. This is:
   a. within the normal range for an adult.
   b. above the normal range for an adult.
   c. an indication of possible serious illness.
   d. a measure of the pressure within the arteries while the heart is at rest.
9. When assessing breathing, the terms normal, deep, and shallow are used to describe the:
   a. timing of breaths.
   b. rate of breaths.
   c. quality of breaths.
   d. accuracy of breaths.
10. When taking a pulse, you should press gently against the artery with your:
    a. thumb.
    b. ring finger.
    c. palm.
    d. index and middle fingers.
11. Your patient complains of abdominal pain and nausea. These subjective complaints are called:
    a. signs.
    b. symptoms.
    c. vitals.
    d. past medical history.
12. Which of the following is considered a sign?
    a. Dilated pupils
    b. Dizziness
    c. Ringing in the ears
    d. Weakness

Answers: 1. a, Objective 7-1, p. 146; 2. b, Objective 7-1, p. 150; 3. b, Objective 7-1, p. 157; 4. a, Objective 7-3, p. 149; 5. b, Objective 7-4, p. 150; 6. a, Objective 7-8, p. 165; 7. b, Objective 7-8, p. 165; 8. c, Objective 7-8, p. 165; 9. c, Objective 7-10, p. 168; 10. d, Objective 7-10, p. 153; 11. b, Objective 7-5, p. 156; 12. a, Objective 7-5, p. 156

CHAPTER 8

COMMUNICATIONS AND DOCUMENTATION

OBJECTIVES

Upon completion of this chapter, the OEC technician will be able to:

8-1 Define patient privacy.

8-2 Explain the types of medical communication and how they are used.

8-3 List the content that should be included in all verbal communications using the acronym SAILER.

8-4 Explain what a handoff report is used for and what information it contains.

8-5 Explain what field care notes are for and what information would be placed in them.

8-6 Explain the parts of an incident report form.

8-7 Explain the parts of a patient care report.

8-8 Define the purpose of an incident investigation team.

8-9 Describe how to correct a written report.

8-10 Define the parts of a "clinical picture."

KEY TERMS

Communication, p. 180
Field care notes, p. 187
Handoff report, p. 185
Incident investigation (II) team, p. 191
Incident report form, p. 187
Patient care report (PCR), p. 187
Patient privacy, p. 181

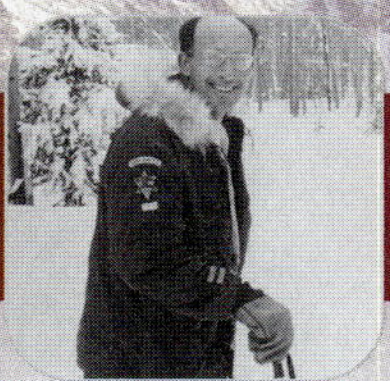

HISTORICAL TIMELINE **1956.** William R. Judd becomes the first-elected National Director of NSP.

CHAPTER OVERVIEW

OEC technicians evaluate patients whose injuries or illnesses range from a scratch on the arm to a life-threatening ruptured spleen. After assessing and collecting information about the patient, you will communicate both orally and in written form your findings and interventions to other medical personnel. During "handoff" of a patient, you must tell the next prehospital provider the information you have gathered, the care rendered, and the patient's response. As a patient is handed off to each provider from the first responder at the original scene to the treating doctor at a hospital, medical communication needs to be consistent. The information that is passed along the chain may be critical in the patient's diagnosis and treatment at the definitive care center and may be used in the future to determine the outcome of any legal case related to the patient's situation. It is important that all medical personnel, from the OEC technician to the physician, use the same "language" when discussing a patient's condition.

To be successful, an OEC technician must first learn the vocabulary used by medical personnel. Throughout this text, you will be introduced to words commonly used by prehospital providers. These same words will be used for verbal and written forms of communication.

Communication is a process whereby information is transmitted from one person to another. In a health care setting, *mis*communication can adversely affect the patient's outcome. This chapter discusses the principles and practices OEC technicians use to collect, record, and communicate essential medical and legal data, both during and after rescue operations. Because complete, accurate, and timely documentation support excellent patient care, this chapter shows you common reports and forms that OEC technicians may be expected to complete and the essential information required for each.

The ability to effectively communicate with others and properly document the interaction with the patient is one of the essential skills that every OEC technician must possess (**Figure 8-1**). This skill, when mastered, is a symbol of a highly trained OEC technician.

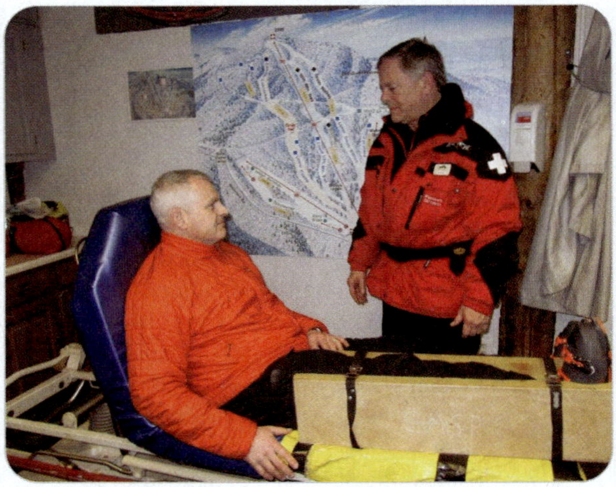

Figure 8-1 Good communication skills are necessary for adequate documentation of the patient assessment and the care rendered.

CASE Presentation

You are directed to respond to a snowboarder who fell while attempting a large jump. Upon arrival, you find a teenage male complaining of right thigh pain. The scene is safe. After introducing yourself and obtaining permission to care for him, you quickly do a primary patient assessment, finding no life-threatening problems. You next obtain a SAMPLE medical history, perform a secondary patient assessment with physical exam, and check vital signs. Only midthigh pain is found.

What should you do now?

COMMUNICATION BASICS

Communication is a process by which a message is transmitted from a sender to a receiver. The goal of communication is to deliver the message in a manner that is understood by the recipient.

Miscommunication occurs when the receiver does not understand the message originally intended by the sender. When using a radio to communicate, factors affecting the transmission of the message, such as gaps in radio or cell phone transmission, can cause miscommunication. Even face-to-face conversations can have communication problems. Stress, information overload, noise, and a host of other factors can adversely affect how a message is understood. Because errors can arise anywhere along the communication process, it is important that senders obtain ongoing feedback from receivers to ensure that the intended message was received and accurately understood.

MEDICAL COMMUNICATION

Medical communication is a specialized form of communication used to transmit health care information. OEC technicians use medical communication primarily to transmit information about an incident and a patient from one person to another. Because health care data typically contain personal protected information, medical communications are generally considered "privileged communications."

As discussed in Chapter 2, *Emergency Medical Care Systems*, all medical personnel, including OEC technicians, need to respect the patient's confidentiality at all times. A patient's personal and medical information is private. Patient information should be shared only with authorized personnel who have a direct need for the information. OEC technicians must safeguard medical communications and prevent unauthorized access to these sensitive data. Basic rules of **patient privacy** are applicable to OEC technicians (**Figure 8-2**).

OEC technicians must be familiar with and demonstrate proficiency in two types of medical communication: oral communication and written documentation. Depending on your role at the scene of an emergency, you will likely use one or both types of medical communication at every incident to which you respond.

> **KEY POINT**
>
> **Medical Communications**
>
> Medical communication continues throughout the entire patient care process. To ensure continuity and efficiency in the care of patients and to avoid misunderstanding, medical communications must be clear, concise, and accurate.

During assessment of a patient, nonverbal communications are also important. During a conversation, you can pick up clues by watching the other person's actions. This nonverbal communication includes behaviors such as facial expressions, eye movements, hand gestures, touch, vocal tone, body posture, positioning, and movement. "Eyeballing" the patient can help you determine whether or not a patient is "sick or not sick."

Oral Communication

Oral communication is the transmission of information verbally, whether by phone, by radio, or in person. This rescuer-to-patient communication begins when you first talk to a patient on scene. Use clear, concise sentences a patient can understand. Children or those with a disability may need a simpler explanation of what you intend to do. Someone with a hearing disability may require a different communication method (**Figure 8-3**). You will need to adapt to the situation.

When talking to another prehospital provider, speak in simple, well-organized, short sentences, using appropriate medical terminology and plain English, not codes. Some EMS agencies may still use codes; however, if the code is misunderstood, problems could result during patient care. Understand the level of medical training of the people with whom you are speaking. OEC technicians use oral communication to convey information to dispatchers, fellow OEC technicians, and other first responders and health care providers, such as when transferring the care of a patient to an EMT or paramedic.

As an OEC technician, your communication with the aid room and the radio dispatcher is very

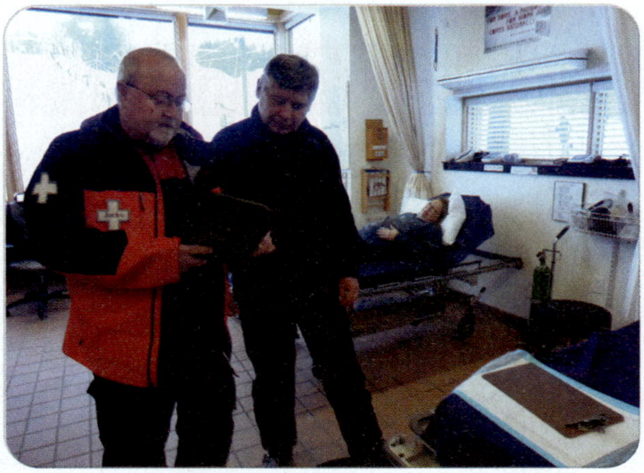

Figure 8-2 When providing sensitive updates to another patroller, it is often best do to this away from the patient and other patients or bystanders.

© Deborah Endly.

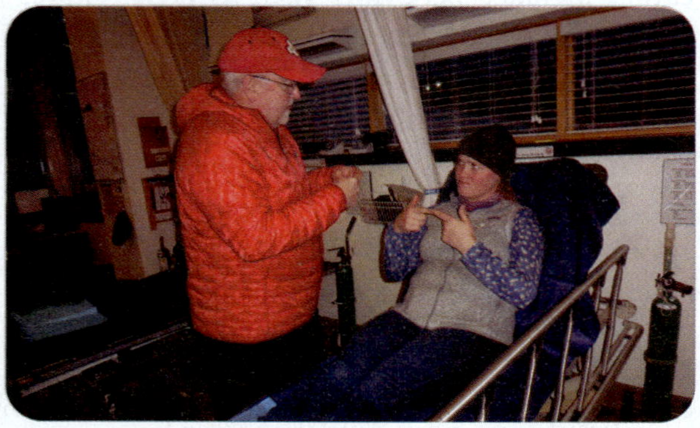

Figure 8-3 Having a person sign for a patient who is deaf is one way to ensure good communication.

© Deborah Endly

important. After a general dispatch call has gone out to all rescuers that there is a possible accident on Fiddler's Elbow and you respond, it is best to radio back to dispatch that you are on scene: "This is Paul, on scene at Fiddler's Elbow. Standby for further information." This lets the dispatcher know someone has arrived at the patient's side, is conducting a patient assessment, and will be assisting the patient shortly. In many cases, management wants dispatchers to record the time when a call is dispatched and when the first rescuer arrives on scene.

After performing the primary patient assessment, you need to tell dispatch what your patient's condition is and what equipment or assistance you need. An easy way to remember the important

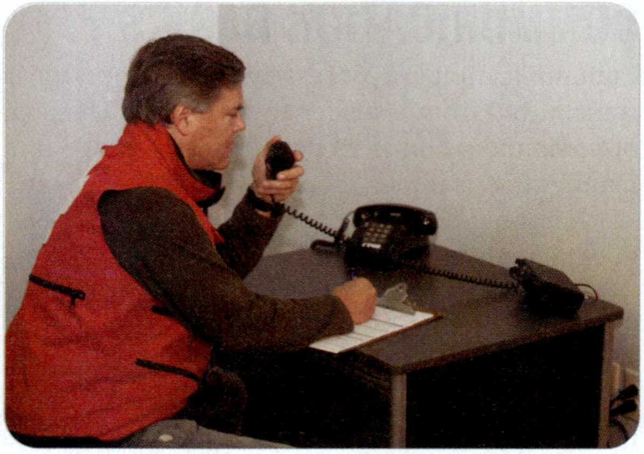

Figure 8-4 Dispatch should be told where you are located so they can send additional resources.

© Mike Halloran.

pieces of information that dispatch needs is to use the acronym SAILER:

- **S** Sex of the patient
- **A** Age of the patient
- **I** Incident, chief complaint
- **L** Location of incident/patient (**Figure 8-4**)
- **E** Equipment needed (e.g., splints, backboards, toboggans)
- **R** Resources needed (e.g., extra help, security personnel, management, BLS or ALS ambulance)

Depending on your local protocols, this information may or may not be presented in this order. With few exceptions, you should be able to convey the information in 30 seconds or less.

Always make sure dispatch acknowledges your message. Ideally, the dispatcher should repeat the

KEY POINT

Patient Privacy

In order to protect a patient's privacy, do not use the patient's name during two-way radio transmissions, unless absolutely necessary. Use a landline or cell phone when a patient's name is given. This prevents the patient's name being heard by someone with a radio scanner.

CASE Update

You notify dispatch of the incident:

You: "Ski Patrol to base."

Dispatch: "Go ahead, Patrol."

You: "I have a 19-year-old male, who fell on the back side of a jump midway down Fiddler's Elbow. Patient has midthigh pain on his right leg. Vital signs are stable. He is fully responsive. Send a toboggan with backboard and traction splint, and extra help. I need an ALS ambulance. Notify management."

At this point, dispatch would radio back the same information to the patroller, confirming that the communication was clear:

Dispatch: "Received, Patrol. You are on scene with a 19-year-old male on Fiddler's Elbow. Requesting toboggan, backboard with traction splint, additional manpower, ALS ambulance, and management."

Ski Patrol would then acknowledge:

You: "That is correct."

Other patrollers arrive to assist you. One patroller helps you care for the injured teenager. You ask another patroller to provide scene safety. Another patroller interviews the patient's friend and witnesses to the incident, recording their names, brief statements, and phone numbers. These field care notes will be added to the patient care report. The bystanders are asked to come to the patrol aid room to continue the interview.

On a small preprinted field-incident form, you record the patient's information. Following care and packaging, which includes a femoral traction splint, you help load the patient into a toboggan, take and record his vital signs again, and transport him to the aid room. Once inside, you help move the patient to a stretcher.

With the assistance of your field care notes, you give an OEC technician or the medical provider on duty in the aid room an oral report about the patient. This report includes a complete description of your initial general impression of the patient, the nature of the patient's injury, the patient's level of responsiveness, vital signs, results from the primary and secondary patient assessments, and the basic care you provided.

What should you and the aid room medical provider do now?

key portion of your message back to you so that miscommunication is less likely, although local protocols will dictate the actual process to be followed.

Most radio protocols do not include the patient's name, unless there is a specific reason for that information, such as a need to find a lost child. Remember, anyone can listen to your transmissions using a scanner, and each patient's privacy should be protected.

Radio Etiquette

Communicating with others by radio entails great responsibility and must be done clearly, concisely, and accurately. This is best accomplished by observing basic radio etiquette and universally accepted terms and practices. OEC technicians must keep in mind that emergency radio transmissions are often monitored and recorded by other rescuers, public safety organizations, and civilian organizations such as news media. Additionally, any recordings made may be subpoenaed during legal proceedings. Thus, it is essential that OEC technicians maintain a professional demeanor when communicating via radio. Common radio etiquette tips include the following:

- Listen before beginning to transmit a message (to prevent inadvertently cutting off another rescuer's transmission).
- Know what you want to say prior to beginning transmission.
- Press the transmit key firmly and hold it for 1 to 2 seconds before speaking (to prevent inadvertently cutting off the beginning of your transmission).
- Speak directly into the microphone but not too close. Approximately 2 to 3 inches is a good distance for clarity. (Shield the microphone from wind to improve communications.)
- Speak clearly and slowly, with a normal voice. Do not shout.
- Use clear terminology, not codes.
- Be concise; make each transmission less than 30 seconds long.
- When finished speaking, wait 1 to 2 seconds before releasing the transmit key (to prevent inadvertently cutting off the end of your transmission).
- Confirm receipt of all transmissions.
- When speaking a word that may be misunderstood, you may need to spell it using the phonetic alphabet.
- When saying a number, say the whole number first, then repeat it by each digit: "sixteen, one-six."
- Do not use profanity or offensive terms.
- Do not say the patient's name (doing so may violate privacy laws).
- Limit communications to official business only.

Radio Terminology

The use of common language and terms is especially critical when communicating via radio and is a key factor in improving mutual understanding among rescue personnel (**Table 8-1**). Using universally accepted terms enables information to be conveyed quickly and precisely.

Table 8-1 Common Radio Terms

Term	Meaning
Affirmative	Yes
Received	Message received, understood
Repeat/say again	Please repeat
Go ahead	Proceed with transmission
Negative	No
Stand by	Busy, please wait
Standing by	Awaiting further information or instructions

When speaking to others over the airwaves, plain English is preferred over the use of radio codes such as the "10 codes" that were often used in the 1970s and 1980s. Radio codes have fallen into disfavor because they are not used in a uniform way and are often specific to a single organization. This lack of uniformity can cause significant problems, especially in situations involving multiple public safety agencies.

NATO Phonetic Alphabet

Occasionally, unusual words, acronyms, or critical combinations of letters must be spelled out to others via radio. This is easily accomplished by using the NATO phonetic alphabet, in which each letter is represented by a universally accepted word (**Table 8-2**). To use the phonetic alphabet, simply state the corresponding phonetic word for each letter, pausing briefly between each word. For example, to communicate "Ben" as a lost child's name, say "B as in Bravo, E as in Echo, N as in November."

Civilian Time and Military Time

Ski patrols, like other rescue groups, express time using military, or "universal," time, a precise method for stating the time that is based on a 24-hour clock (**Table 8-3**). This convention is different from civilian, or "regular," time, which is based on a 12-hour clock. Under regular time, any given time occurs twice in a day and is followed by either a.m. or p.m. (e.g., 7:00 a.m., 7:00 p.m.).

Table 8-2 NATO Phonetic Alphabet

Letter	Accepted Word
A	Alpha
B	Bravo
C	Charlie
D	Delta
E	Echo
F	Foxtrot
G	Golf
H	Hotel
I	India
J	Juliet
K	Kilo
L	Lima
M	Mike
N	November
O	Oscar
P	Papa
Q	Quebec
R	Romeo
S	Sierra
T	Tango
U	Uniform
V	Victor
W	Whiskey
X	X-ray
Y	Yankee
Z	Zulu

Under military time, each 24-hour time period begins at 1 minute past midnight and continues until the following midnight. Military time is expressed using four digits to signify the hours and minutes; the first two digits represent the hour, and the second two digits represent the minutes. Accordingly, a given time can occur only once each day: 7:00 a.m. is 0700, whereas 7:00 p.m. is 1900.

In military time, the hours from 1:00 a.m. to 12:00 p.m. are the same as they appear on the clock. Morning hours up to 9:59 a.m. are preceded by a zero: 0959. From 1:00 p.m. to midnight, add 12 to the hours displayed on the clock. Both systems calculate minutes and seconds in exactly the same manner. Thus, 6:00 a.m. is expressed as 0600 and is pronounced "zero six hundred," whereas 4:25 p.m. is expressed as 1625 (12 + 4 hours = 16 hours + 25 minutes = 1625) and is pronounced "sixteen twenty-five."

It is important to learn your local ski patrol's radio protocol, and it is recommended that your patrol use universally accepted terms and military time.

Communication with Other Prehospital Responders

As other rescuers arrive on scene, you should give each of them a concise oral report. This report includes a brief description of the patient's problems and instructions about how these rescuers can help you. Direct your assistants in a clear, calm, and professional manner, making sure they understand you. As the "lead patroller" at the scene, continue to provide directions and communicate with all on-scene assistants as care is given and preparation for transport occurs. If there is more than one patient, direct other rescuers to help other patients.

Listen to your helpers' suggestions. When appropriate, use their ideas while maintaining overall management of the incident. Never openly criticize another responder on scene. It is better to listen to their ideas and congenially come to a meeting of the minds. Effective communication increases the efficiency of rescue operations and decreases on-scene problems, especially during incidents involving multiple patients.

If you are alone on scene, a bystander may be willing and able to help. Unless the person identifies himself or herself as a qualified medical provider, become a teacher, using simple words and giving the untrained person step-by-step instructions. Talk at the level of a layperson, not medically.

After the patient has arrived in the first-aid station or medical facility, provide a concise oral **handoff report** to the person now caring for the patient (**Figure 8-5**). The handoff report contains

Table 8-3 Comparison of Civilian to Military Time

Civilian Time	Pronunciation (Civilian)	Military Time	Pronunciation (Military)
12:01 AM	One minute past midnight	0001	zero, zero, zero, one
12:30 AM	Twelve thirty AM	0030	zero, zero, thirty
12:00 PM	Noon	1200	twelve hundred
2:00 PM	Two PM	1400	fourteen hundred
11:00 PM	Eleven PM	2300	twenty-three hundred
12:00 AM	Midnight	2400	twenty-four hundred

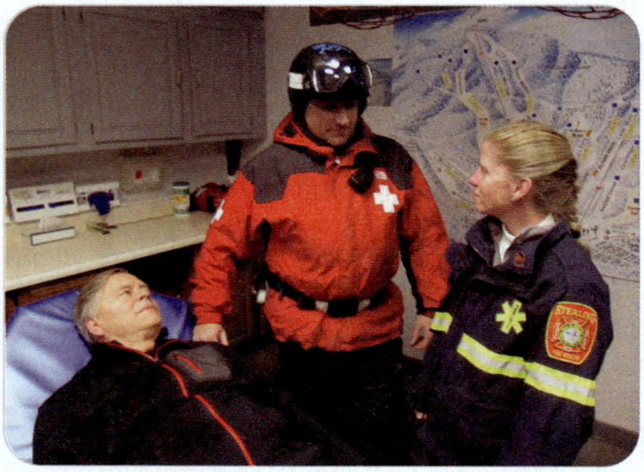

Figure 8-5 Handoff reports are vital when transferring the care of your patient to EMS providers.

KEY POINT

Handoff Report Information

- The patient's name, if known
- The patient's age (approximate if the exact age is unknown)
- The patient's chief complaint
- The patient's injuries or illnesses
- Assessment with pertinent positives and negatives
- All treatment given
- The patient's response to that treatment
- Serial sets of vital signs, including the most current set
- Immediate patient care requirements

more detailed information about the patient than that provided to dispatch. It should emphasize the patient's current condition, treatment, and possible requirements. It may include additional information, such as the patient's name, age, chief complaint, nature of illness or mechanism of injury, assessment findings, vital signs, and response to treatment. After delivering your handoff report, ask the personnel assuming the patient's care if they have any questions. Under normal circumstances, a clear and concise handoff report should take 30 to 60 seconds to complete.

Written Communication

Field care notes and patient care reports are written communications used to document patient encounters and usually are a part of the patient's permanent medical record. Depending on local protocol, this information may be given to the EMT or paramedic who transfers the patient by ambulance as part of a written "handoff report." It may be used for research purposes, to identify or document trends, for quality-improvement reasons, and to assist in risk management. Written reports also are used as medical-legal records. In most ski areas, these written incident reports become the cornerstone of incident risk management.

Learning to properly document and preserve what happened during a patient encounter is vital for OEC technicians and the ski area alike. You

> **KEY POINT**
>
> **Wilderness Tips**
>
> In a wilderness environment where radio communication is not available, you may need to use handwritten field care notes and runners (individuals who will carry the notes between the senders and receivers) to transmit information. These notes will generally include information concerning both patient care, equipment necessary, and your needs for evacuating the patient. They are often retained as part of the rescue documentation and may be considered by management to be a part of the patient's medical record.

may encounter the following three types of written communication: field care notes, incident report forms, and patient care reports.

> **KEY POINT**
>
> **National Ski Areas Association**
>
> The National Ski Areas Association (NSAA) is the trade association for ski area owners and operators in the United States and is one of NSP's most important ski-industry partners. NSP and NSAA have historically worked together to improve skiing safety and have developed incident reporting forms adopted throughout the ski industry.

Field Care Notes

It is common for OEC technicians and other rescue personnel to take notes while they are involved with rescue operations. These notes, known as **field care notes**, generally include essential information about the incident, including the person's name, level of consciousness, serial vital signs, medications, and other relevant data. Witnesses' names and contact information may need to be recorded. Often information such as vital signs is documented along a timeline and is later transferred to, or becomes a part of, a patient care report, depending on your area's local protocol. These notes can be very helpful when handing off a patient to another medical provider.

Incident Report Form

Most OEC technicians use an **incident report form** published by the National Ski Areas Association or a ski area's insurance company. This incident report form contains all the fundamental information needed to document an incident (**Figure 8-6**). Properly completing this form or one like it is a skill OEC technicians must learn. One part of this form asks the patient to describe what happened. Always document and preserve any patient statements, such as, "I knew I was going too fast" or "I should not have been skiing that slope."

Patient Care Reports

When a patient needs *additional medical documentation* because of significant injury or illness, a **patient care report (PCR)** form is used (**Figure 8-7**). A PCR is used to record specific information about the medical care provided to the patient. This report becomes part of the patient's permanent medical record. Your resort's risk manager and local medical adviser should approve any PCR used.

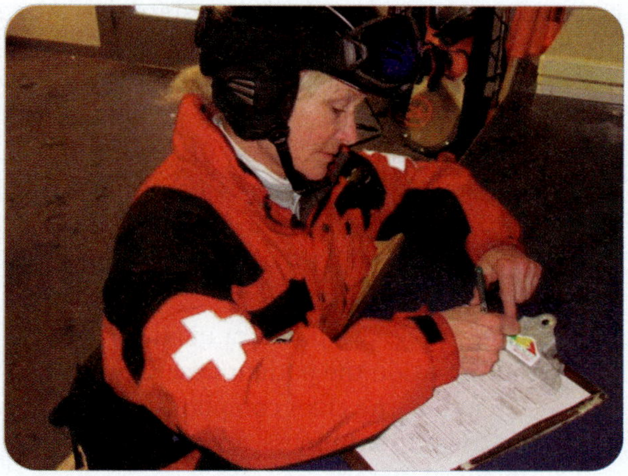

Figure 8-6 Incident report forms may be paper or electronic. Your area may require you to use a different form.

KEY POINT

Incident Report Form Information

- Patient identification information
- Cause of the injury: mechanism of injury (if medical problem, nature of illness)
- Names of individuals at the incident, including OEC technicians and witnesses
- Patient's statement concerning what caused the incident (must be in patient's own words)
- Emergency care given at the incident scene
- Patrollers on scene and in the aid room and what they did to assist
- Emergency care given in the aid room
- Further comments about the incident
- Witness information

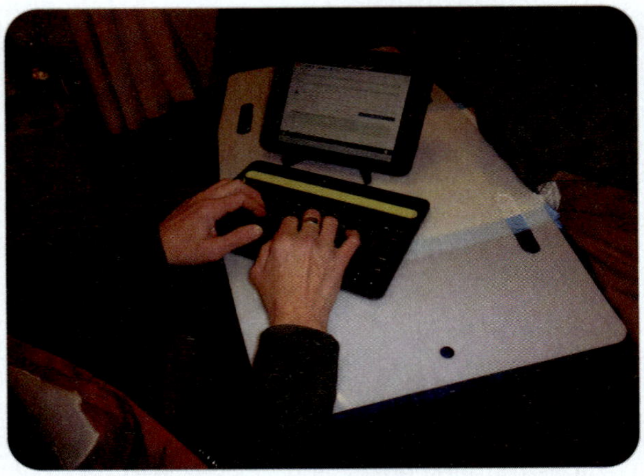

Figure 8-7 The information from your patient care report will be valuable to EMS responders.

© Deborah Endly.

Based on local protocol, a copy of the PCR might be a part of the handoff report to the EMS provider and accompany the patient to a definitive care facility. PCRs have several formats, including closed, open, and mixed.

A *closed-format PCR* has a series of check boxes or limited fill-in-the-blank sections, allowing the PCR to be completed quickly (**Figure 8-8**). This form may be favored by members of a multi-tiered emergency care system in which the field care of the patient is routinely transferred to other providers. Many ambulance carriers use this form.

In contrast, in an *open-format PCR*, information is organized under broad headings such as Patient Information, SOAP or CHEATED notes, SAMPLE, Vital Signs, Patient Condition, Treatment, and Transport (**Figure 8-9**).

SOAP is an acronym that represents four report components:

- **S** Subjective: *Symptoms* or qualitative information the patient describes, including the chief complaint, the history of the present illness, and pertinent past medical history
- **O** Objective: *Signs*, or observable, quantitative findings discovered during the scene size-up and physical exam, including vital signs
- **A** Assessment: The general impression of the medical problem
- **P** Plan: The treatment planned for the patient

The CHEATED acronym for medical documentation represents the primary components of the patient assessment and management process:

- **C** Chief complaint: The patient's primary problem
- **H** History: SAMPLE history of the present illness and past medical history
- **E** Examination: Physical exam
- **A** Assessment: General impression of the patient
- **T** Treatment: All aspects of treatment rendered, including that provided by bystanders
- **E** Evaluation: Changes in the patient's condition over time; the patient's response to treatment
- **D** Disposition: Information indicating whether the patient refused treatment, was treated and released, or was taken to a higher level of care such as a hospital

Beneath each heading is a blank section in which the OEC technician writes in all pertinent findings and incident-related content. Because they are more loosely structured, open-format PCRs generally take more time to complete than either closed- or mixed-format PCRs.

A *mixed-format PCR* combines the two previous styles and includes both check boxes for common

NSAA

INCIDENT REPORT FORM

RESORT____________________

DATE________ DAY OF WK.________ TIME OF INCIDENT________ ☐ AM ☐ PM INCIDENT #________

LOCATION	☐ ON-HILL ☐ LIFT ☐ PREMISE ☐ TUBING HILL DESCRIBE SPECIFIC LOCATION: __________ ☐ EASIER ○ ☐ MORE DIFFICULT ☐ ☐ MOST DIFFICULT ◆ ☐ EXPERTS ONLY◆◆ ☐ FREESTYLE TERRAIN▢ ☐ NOT APPLICABLE
INJURED PERSON	NAME________ ☐ MALE ☐ FEMALE DOB______ ADDRESS________ AGE______ CITY______ STATE____ ZIP____ HT______ HOME PH______ CELL PH______ OCCUPATION______ WT______
SKIING HISTORY	**ABILITY**: ☐BEG ☐N/APP ☐INTERMEDIATE ☐ADV/EXPERT **LESSONS**: ☐ IN LESSON INSTR______ ☐ N/APPLICABLE **NUMBER OF TIMES ON:** ☐TRAIL ☐TODAY____ ☐LIFT ☐PRIOR____ OTHER____ **EQUIPMENT REMOVED BY:** ☐ FALL ☐ PATROL ☐ INJURED ☐ OTHER
PATIENT HISTORY	PRIOR INJURY/ILLNESS- DESCRIBE________ YEAR INJURED______ CORRECTIVE LENSES NEEDED? ☐YES ☐NO WORN? ☐YES ☐NO MEDICAL INSURANCE? ☐YES ☐NO LIST ANY MEDS TAKEN:________ TICKET TYPE______ ALLERGIES/MEDICAL ALERT DESCRIBE________ GROUP NAME______
EQUIPMENT	☐ ALPINE ☐ NORDIC ☐ SNOWBOARD ☐ OTHER EQUIP: ______ ☐ OWNED ☐ AREA RENTAL ☐ OTHER RENTAL ☐ BORROWED ☐ DEMO BINDING MAKE______ MODEL______ SKI/BOARD #______ BOOT #______ SHOP NAME______ ADDRESS______ LEFT DIN: TOE __ HEEL __ RIGHT DIN: TOE __ HEEL __ HELMET WORN? ☐ YES ☐ NO HELMET AREA RENTAL? ☐ YES ☐ NO HELMET RENTAL #______
DESCRIPTION OF INCIDENT (Patient's words)	____________ ____________ ____________ ____________ **THE ABOVE STATEMENT IS TRUE AND CORRECT** INJURED'S SIGNATURE______ **PARENT/GUARDIAN SIGNATURE**______ I REFUSE FIRST AID: INJURED'S SIGNATURE (PARENT/GUARDIAN IF MINOR)______
PROBABLE INJURY	☐ FRACTURE ☐SPRAIN/STRAIN ☐ PUNCTURE/LACERATION ☐ BRUISE/CONTUSION ☐ ABRASION ☐ CONCUSSION ☐DISLOCATION ☐ FROSTBITE ☐ MULTIPLE ☐ OTHER______
INJURY ZONE	☐ LEFT ☐ RIGHT ☐ BOTH ☐ MULTIPLE ☐ HEAD ☐ FACE ☐ EYE ☐ NOSE ☐ MOUTH ☐ TEETH ☐ NECK ☐ SHOULDER ☐ ARM ☐ WRIST ☐ HAND ☐ THUMB ☐ CHEST ☐ BACK ☐ ABDOMEN ☐ HIP ☐ UPPER LEG ☐ KNEE ☐ LOWER LEG ☐ ANKLE ☐ FOOT ☐ OTHER ______
FIRST AID RENDERED	ON HILL:________ ________ AT FIRST AID STATION:________
PATROLLERS INVOLVED	AT SCENE:________ TRANSPORTING:________ AT FIRST AID STATION:________
TRANSPORT & DESTINATION	ARRIVED AT FIRST AID STATION BY: ☐ PATROL/TOBOGGAN ☐ WALK-IN ☐ OTHER ______ LEFT FIRST AID STATION BY: ☐ WALKED OUT ☐ ASSISTED TO CAR/BUS ☐ AMBULANCE **DESTINATION:** ☐ HOME ☐ LODGE ☐ RETURN SKIING ☐ MEDICAL FACILITY:______
SITE CONDITIONS	**SURFACE AT SCENE:** ☐POWDER ☐CORN ☐VARIABLE ☐PACKED POWDER ☐LOOSE GRANULAR ☐FROZ GRAN/HARD PACKED ☐WET ☐OTHER______ **VISIBILITY:** ☐ CLEAR ☐ OVERCAST ☐ FOG ☐ SNOWING ☐ RAINING ☐ SNOW BEING MADE NEAR SCENE **TEMPERATURE:** ☐ BELOW 0 ☐ 0-32 ☐ ABOVE 32 **WIND:** ☐ CALM ☐ MODERATE ☐ HIGH
WITNESSES	NAME______ PHONE______ ADDRESS______ CITY______ STATE____ ZIP____ NAME______ PHONE______ ADDRESS______ CITY______ STATE____ ZIP____

SIGNATURE OF INDIVIDUAL COMPLETING REPORT: ________ DATE REPORT COMPLETED:______

PRINT NAME:________ Rev. 9/06

Figure 8-8 A sample of a closed-format patient care report.

BLUE RIDGE SKI RESORT PATIENT CARE REPORT

Name: Sex: Age:

S: A:

O: M:

A: P:

P: L:

E:

VITAL SIGNS

	Time	Pulse	Blood Pressure	Respirations	LOC
1					
2					
3					
4					

TREATMENT:

PATIENT CONDITION: TRANPORT:

Figure 8-9 A sample of an open-format patient care report.

Courtesy of Dr. David Johe.

types of data and blanks for specific comments (**Figure 8-10**). Many computer-generated PCRs use this method, allowing space for typed comments.

Nearly all PCRs for seriously ill or injured patients include a section for recording vital signs taken throughout the patient's care. Spaces are provided to record serial sets of vital signs, including pulse, blood pressure, respirations, temperature (when appropriate), oxygen saturation, and level of consciousness. The SAMPLE acronym is found on many of these forms.

Remember: "If it isn't documented, it didn't happen." Therefore, make sure you fully document all the medical facts associated with the incident, all the scene facts (day, time, and conditions), and the names of all the patrollers and

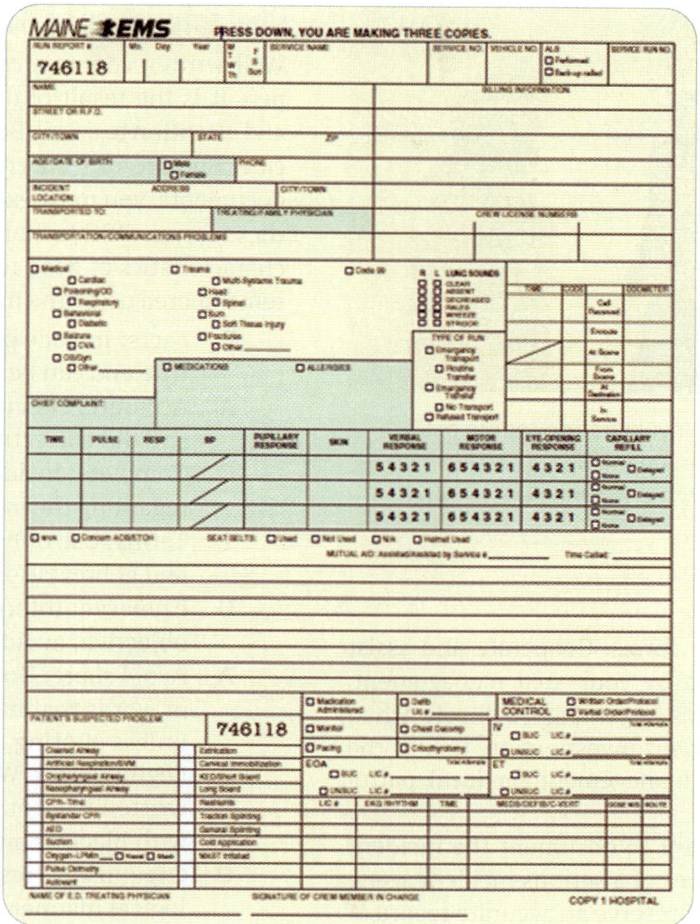
MAINE EMS

PRESS DOWN, YOU ARE MAKING THREE COPIES.

746118

746118

COPY 1 HOSPITAL

Figure 8-10 A sample of a mixed-format patient care report.

Courtesy of Maine EMS.

witnesses involved in the incident. Also include the statements of the patient, the mechanism of injury, vital signs, and anything else that will enable you to review the documents. This documentation may include taking photographs or making diagrams if appropriate. Years later, if legal consequences occur, you may need to accurately reconstruct what happened at the incident. Your notes could prove extremely helpful in such cases.

Further Documentation When Needed

In addition to previously mentioned skills, the OEC technician must know when to ask for help. Most areas have hill captains or area risk managers who are trained in recognizing high-risk situations. These individuals can be invaluable in helping with documentation and managing the legal risks associated with the incident. Some areas may have an incident investigation team. When you need documentation help in a difficult rescue, use the resources available at your area.

Incident Investigation Team

Your ski or recreational area may have an **incident investigation (II) team**. Local protocols from management will dictate when and how this team is activated. The assistance of such a team is recommended for any serious incident (**Figure 8-11**). The II team will investigate any incident involving a life-threatening condition, a death, or an accident in which liability is suspected. An II team also may be required to respond to a lift-related accident or to an injury involving a motorized vehicle or other humanmade object.

II team members gather maps, photos, witness statements, accident reports, PCRs, and other information. You may be asked to assist the team when gathering this information or help the

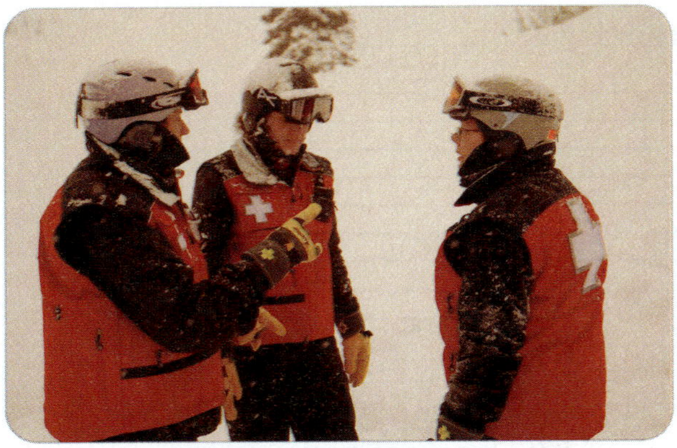

Figure 8-11 Incident investigation teams are often dispatched when an incident involves severe injuries or death, or when the incident involves resort property.

team complete other forms. Cooperate and assist the team as directed by your area management. If you have questions regarding your role when helping with an accident investigation, talk to the II leader, your area management, or local patrol representative.

It is also important to document the incident scene and take pictures of a serious incident scene *as soon as possible* to preserve an accurate record of events. Any delay in documenting important information can result in the loss of that information. For example, a delay in taking photographs when the wind is blowing may result in a lost opportunity to document the skier's tracks before they are blown away. This would be a loss of potentially crucial information indicating what direction the skier was headed prior to the accident. If accomplishing this task promptly requires more help, ask for help from your II team or area's risk manager.

KEY POINT

Emergency Documentation

In most cases, if emergency care is not carefully documented in writing, then it is presumed that the emergency care was not given. An incomplete or messy report can suggest that the emergency care given was lax.

Characteristics of Good Report Writing

Well-written communication does not simply happen. It is the result of determined professionalism and attention to detail. Because both the PCR and incident report form are considered medical and legal documents, you must exercise care when filling out these forms. OEC technicians should adhere to the characteristics of good report writing, which can be remembered using the mnemonic FACTUAL-OEC:

- **F** Facts: Include only information that is true and can be documented.
- **A** Accurate: Describe what you saw, heard, and did correctly.
- **C** Complete: Include all relevant information regarding the incident and the patient.
- **T** Terms: Use only accepted medical terms and abbreviations.
- **U** Unbiased: Information should be objective; avoid opinions.
- **A** Avoid slang: Do not use informal words or words that have multiple meanings, unless quoting the patient.
- **L** Legible/legal: Written reports should be written in clear, easy-to-read language, with black or blue ink.
- **O** Organized: Present information in a logical manner; this is important when using an open-format PCR.
- **E** Error-free: Ensure that all words are spelled correctly and that proper grammar is used.
- **C** Checked: Proofread the document before submitting it.

Correcting Errors and Creating Addendums

When filling out reports and forms, it is only natural that OEC technicians will occasionally make a written error that needs correction. To correct a written mistake, draw a *single* line through the error (**Figure 8-12**). Never scratch out, erase, or otherwise obliterate the error, because doing so can suggest that the OEC technician is attempting to hide something. Next, write in the correct information, either above or next to the error. Finally, place your initials and, ideally, the current date and time next to the corrected error.

Occasionally, important information obtained during patient care may be inadvertently omitted in your written report. To add information to a previously completed report or form, follow your local area's protocol. A standard procedure is to

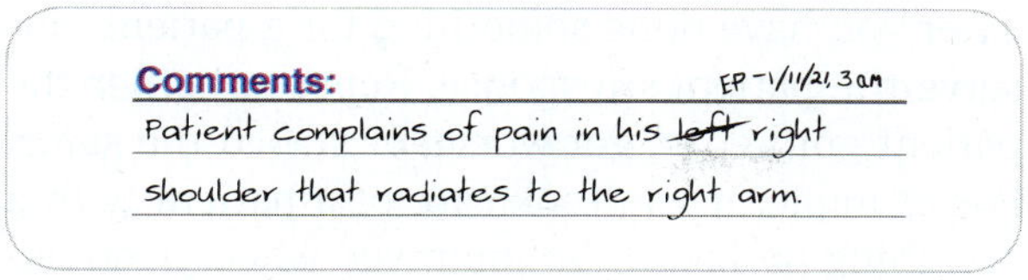
Comments: EP-1/11/21, 3am
Patient complains of pain in his ~~left~~ right
shoulder that radiates to the right arm.

Figure 8-12 To correct a mistake on a written report, draw a single line through the error, enter the correct information, and write your initials and the date and time beside the edit.

complete and sign the *additional* written information and then attach it to the original form. This addendum should be completed as soon as the need for additional information is identified. Any delay in its submission reduces its credibility and potential usefulness. If an addendum is created, the date and time this is done should be noted on the document. Always sign the addendum, and tell your risk manager you added information.

Computer-Generated Forms

Many agencies and some ski areas fill out and submit incident-related forms electronically. The use of electronic devices to prepare forms has the advantage of recording specific information needed to document any patient encounter in an easy-to-read format. These systems allow a risk manager to rapidly organize information about patient encounters. However, these electronic devices often provide limited space to enter additional information. The result is that some critical data may not be included.

OEC technicians may need to supplement electronically prepared forms with additional written documentation. If the computer-generated form allows you to list only two patrollers but four patrollers were involved in the incident, or the form does not provide enough space to properly describe the events, treatment, or handling of the incident, you will need to supplement the electronic form with additional written information. Local management should tell you how to document additional information.

Essential Content of Medical Communication to Higher Medical Personnel

When you communicate medical information to others, it is important that you provide an accurate clinical picture, because the recipient of this communication does not have prior knowledge of the circumstances surrounding the incident. Medical information should be presented clearly and succinctly in an organized manner, whether presented orally or in writing.

Although medical communications and documents vary, the information contained in these communications is standard. A report to EMS personnel should take less than 60 seconds. When transferring a patient, you should communicate to the receiving medical provider a clinical picture that includes these basic points:

- Age and sex
- Chief complaint
- History of present illness
- Past medical history
- Physical exam
- General impression
- Treatment
- Response to treatment

Age and Sex

Report the patient's sex and actual or approximate age.

Chief Complaint

The chief complaint is what the patient tells you is wrong. Whenever possible, this should be recorded in the patient's own words. The patient may say, "My chest hurts," or may tell you, "I ran into a tree." If a patient is found unresponsive, use that as the chief complaint.

History of Present Illness

The history of present illness should provide a description of the circumstances surrounding the events of the incident and include all subjective descriptions presented by the patient. For an illness, this includes the symptoms the patient had before asking for help. For trauma, it is a description of the circumstances before the injury.

Past Medical History

The past medical history includes medical problems related to the chief complaint and any other pertinent medical history. It also includes present medications, allergies, and last oral intake.

Physical Exam

The physical exam includes all the objective findings obtained during the primary and secondary patient assessments. Both positive and negative findings may be important. These findings include the level of responsiveness and all vital signs.

General Impression

A general impression is what you think the medical problem is based on the information that you gathered during the whole patient evaluation. Even though a general impression is not a final "diagnosis," you should formulate a medical impression because this information may be used to make treatment decisions. An example of a general medical impression is "possible right femur fracture."

Treatment

The treatment is a description of everything you have done in caring for the patient. It may include nothing more than "transported in the position of comfort," or it may include the various treatments provided during a full resuscitation. If you administered oxygen, applied a splint, or immobilized the spine, report those actions in the treatment section.

Response to Treatment

One of the most frequently overlooked aspects of medical communications is describing how the patient responded to the treatment rendered. After you have done something for a patient, observe the patient's response. Report whether the patient got better, got worse, or stayed the same. For example, if you took care of a patient with a breathing problem who improved when given oxygen, you might state, "Oxygen was supplied at 15 liters per minute via nonrebreather mask and the patient responded by having a slower respiratory rate and was able to talk in full sentences."

KEY POINT

Clinical Picture Information

OEC technicians must learn how to give a concise, accurate patient clinical picture to the medical personnel assuming care of the patient. The clinical picture includes information about the patient's age and sex, chief complaint, history of present illness, past medical history, physical exam, treatment, and response to treatment. It also includes the OEC technician's general impression of the patient.

CASE Outcome

The OEC technician in the aid room continues care with you as the ambulance arrives. The aid room OEC technician gives the following handoff report to the paramedic who is transferring the patient to the hospital:

> "The patient is Adam Lee, a 19-year-old male who went off a large jump, landing on his right leg. He was wearing a helmet. His friends state that he never lost consciousness. When we arrived on scene, the patient was *A* on the AVPU scale, and this has not changed. He complained of right thigh pain and had tenderness in that location. The thigh was exposed, and there was no bleeding or bone penetration. There was no other obvious trauma. He denies drinking alcohol or taking drugs today. He has no medical problems and no allergies. He had lunch at noon. Vitals have been stable. He was put in the traction splint on the hill, helping the pain, and distal sensation, circulation, and motor remains intact. He appears to have a right midshaft femur fracture. Here is a copy of the PCR, which includes our care and patient information. Do you have any questions?"

Lastly, you complete the incident report form documenting the case and place it in the patrol director's box. You are later informed that the patient was admitted to the hospital with a fractured femur.

CHAPTER REVIEW

In Summary

- Effective medical communications are one of the traits of a highly skilled OEC technician.
- Medical communications include oral communication and written documentation.
    - Oral communication is the transmission of information verbally, whether by phone, by radio, or in person. Use universally accepted terms to convey information quickly and precisely.
    - Field care notes, incident report forms, and patient care reports are examples of written communications.
    - Careful documentation is important both for medical and legal reasons. You must exercise care when filling out these forms.
- Breakdowns in the communication process can create misunderstandings and errors.
- Basic rules of patient privacy are applicable to OEC technicians.
- When transferring a patient, you should communicate to the receiving medical provider a clinical picture of the patient. The clinical picture includes patient age and sex, chief complaint, history of present illness, past medical history, physical exam, general impression, treatment, and response to treatment.
- If it isn't documented, it didn't happen; document reports completely and accurately.

Key Terms

Communication A process whereby information is transmitted from one person to another.

Field care notes Notes written by OEC technicians at the scene of a patient rescue; may include a timeline, vital signs, witnesses' names, and other pertinent information.

Handoff report An oral or written report given at the transfer of a patient from one provider to another.

Incident investigation (II) team A group of personnel, usually including representation of management at a resort, who evaluate and document any accident that needs further legal documentation.

Incident report form A form provided by the National Ski Areas Association, a ski resort, or an insurance carrier, used by OEC technicians to document an incident; the forms include patient information and the circumstances leading to injury.

Patient care report (PCR) A report documenting a patient's complaints and past medical history, plus a chronological (timeline) account of the examination and treatment of the patient, including vital signs. The PCR is a legal document.

Patient privacy The practice of maintaining the security and confidentiality of patient records. It includes the conversational discretion of health care providers and the security of all medical records.

Chapter Questions

1. What is the preferred radio response for saying "yes"?
    a. Okay
    b. Affirmative
    c. Absolutely
    d. Yeah

2. The OEC technician can verbally report to others in a timely method about an incident using the acronym SAILER. The acronym is best represented by which of the following?
   a. The patient's sex and age, the chief complaint, your location, the resources you need
   b. The patient's name, sex, and complaints, your location, need of a toboggan, and airway status
   c. The patient's sex and complaints, your location, and need of oxygen and blankets
   d. The patroller, the patient's sex and complaints, location of the patrol room, and presence of other patrollers
3. You are at the scene of a two-patient incident. Your first patient is ready for transport. The patroller with a toboggan just arrived. Your oral report to this patroller is called a:
   a. trade-off report.
   b. patient report.
   c. handoff report.
   d. tag-out report.
4. What is typically the first type of document an OEC technician will use for recording patient care?
   a. Incident report form
   b. Patient care report
   c. Handoff report
   d. Field care notes
5. An incident report form is developed/provided by:
   a. the National Ski Areas Association.
   b. your area's management.
   c. your area's insurance provider.
   d. Any of the above
6. On which form would you be most likely to use the SOAP or CHEATED acronyms?
   a. Patient care report
   b. Annual report
   c. Handoff report
   d. NSP application
7. When should pictures of a serious incident be taken?
   a. The next day when the safety officer is available
   b. As soon as possible to preserve an accurate record
   c. While the patient is still on scene
   d. When area management gets around to it
8. When making a correction on a report, what is the correct procedure?
   a. Erase the error and write the correct information in.
   b. Totally cross out the incorrect information and write in the correction.
   c. Use Wite-Out (correction fluid) to cover the mistake and write over it.
   d. Make a single line through the error, write the correction nearby, and mark the time and date of the change and your initials.
9. The "clinical picture" of a patient contains information obtained by:
   a. asking the patient SAMPLE questions.
   b. doing a primary survey.
   c. doing a secondary survey.
   d. All of the above

Answers: 1. b, Objective 8-2, p. 184; 2. a, Objective 8-3, p. 182; 3. c, Objective 8-4, p. 185; 4. d, Objective 8-5, p. 186; 5. d, Objective 8-6, p. 187; 6. a, Objective 8-7, p. 188; 7. b, Objective 8-8, p. 192; 8. d, Objective 8-9, p. 192; 9. d, Objective 8-10, p. 193

CHAPTER 9

AIRWAY MANAGEMENT

OBJECTIVES

Upon completion of this chapter, the OEC technician will be able to:

9-1 Describe the function of the epiglottis.

9-2 Describe the mechanism of breathing.

9-3 Describe and demonstrate how to manually open the airway or mouth using the following techniques:
- Cross-finger technique
- Head tilt–chin lift maneuver
- Jaw-thrust maneuver

9-4 Describe and demonstrate the proper way to clear an airway using the methods of finger sweep, suctioning, gravity and positioning, and abdominal thrusts.

9-5 Explain and demonstrate the recovery position.

9-6 Describe the function of the oropharyngeal and nasopharyngeal airway, and demonstrate the sizing and placement of these devices.

9-7 Demonstrate the use of a face shield and a pocket mask.

9-8 Explain the tips for safely using oxygen.

9-9 Explain the indications for and administration of oxygen.

9-10 Demonstrate how to place an oxygen cylinder into service.

9-11 Describe the various devices used for delivering oxygen to a patient.

9-12 Explain what a pulse oximeter is and demonstrate how it is used.

9-13 Explain gastric distention and how to avoid it.

KEY TERMS

Airway, p. 198
Bag-valve mask (BVM), p. 216
Barrier device, p. 210
Epiglottis, p. 198
Exhalation, p. 199
Face shield, p. 210
Finger sweep, p. 201
Flowmeter, p. 212
Gastric distention, p. 219
Head tilt–chin lift maneuver, p. 200
Inhalation, p. 198
Jaw-thrust maneuver, p. 200
Nasal cannula, p. 215
Nasopharyngeal airway (NPA), p. 206
Nonrebreather mask, p. 215
Oropharyngeal airway (OPA), p. 206
Patent, p. 199
Pocket mask, p. 210
Pulse oximeter, p. 218
Suctioning, p. 201

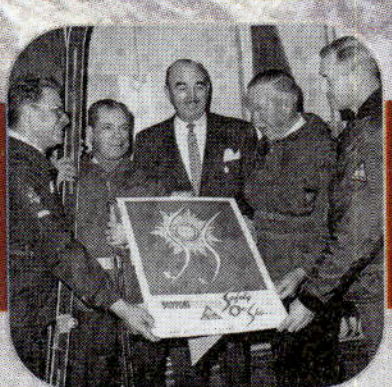

HISTORICAL TIMELINE **1959.** NSP establishes a national advisory committee related to ski safety.

CHAPTER OVERVIEW

Having an open **airway** and adequate breathing are crucial factors for maintaining homeostasis because every cell in the body depends on a constant supply of oxygen. Under normal conditions, the airway is "open and clear," which permits breathing and the exchange of gas between the environment and the lungs. Without a continuous source of oxygen, death occurs rapidly.

OEC technicians need to assess a patient's airway quickly, immediately correcting any airway problems. Be prepared to open, clear, and maintain the airway using a variety of methods. OEC technicians need to deliver supplemental oxygen whenever it is indicated and provide artificial ventilations if either spontaneous breathing is not observed or the patient's breathing efforts are ineffective. Each of these skills can be lifesaving.

ANATOMY AND PHYSIOLOGY

The airway is divided into upper and lower components (**Figure 9-1**). The upper airway begins at the mouth and nose and ends at the larynx next to the **epiglottis**. The nasopharynx, better known as the nasal cavity, warms and humidifies air as it enters the body and the hairs in it remove dust particles. The oropharynx, better known as the oral cavity, also helps to warm inhaled air. Next is the larynx, or voice box, at the top of the trachea. If *either* the nose or the mouth is blocked off, air can still get into the lower airway. If *both* are blocked, air cannot get into the lungs.

The epiglottis is a leaf-shaped structure that allows air into the trachea and lungs when open. When swallowing, it closes and prevents food or liquids from entering the lower airway by covering the top of the airway. Below the epiglottis is the larynx, or voice box, which has two cords that vibrate, making sound when we speak.

The lower airway includes the trachea, bronchi, and lungs, containing the bronchioles and alveoli. The trachea is a tube made of cartilage that splits into two mainstem bronchi, one to each lung. These bronchi continue to branch into many smaller bronchioles and end in tiny alveoli, where gases are exchanged in the lung. For more information about the airway, review the appropriate section in Chapter 6, *Anatomy and Physiology*.

Respiration is the act of breathing, where air enters the body through the airway passage and then is expelled back into the environment. Oxygen in the air enters the lungs, and carbon dioxide, a waste product, leaves the lungs. Breathing is a mechanical process, both active and passive in nature, consisting of two phases: inhalation and exhalation. Both phases are controlled by the nervous system and occur automatically.

Inhalation, also known as inspiration, is an *active* process during which the respiratory muscles contract, creating negative internal pressure in the chest cavity, thereby causing air to flow into the lungs. The diaphragm between the chest and the abdominal cavities is the main breathing muscle.

CASE Presentation

While bike patrolling, you and your partner find a middle-aged bicyclist with a pulse who is not breathing and is unresponsive to painful stimuli. It appears that he fell over a cliff approximately 20 feet from a mountain bike path, striking his head and neck on a rocky outcrop. You note minor bleeding coming from the patient's mouth as well as a deep cut on his chin. His pulse is rapid at 108 beats per minute. The cyclist's left arm appears bent at an unnatural angle. You radio for help, equipment, oxygen, and ALS transport.

What should you do?

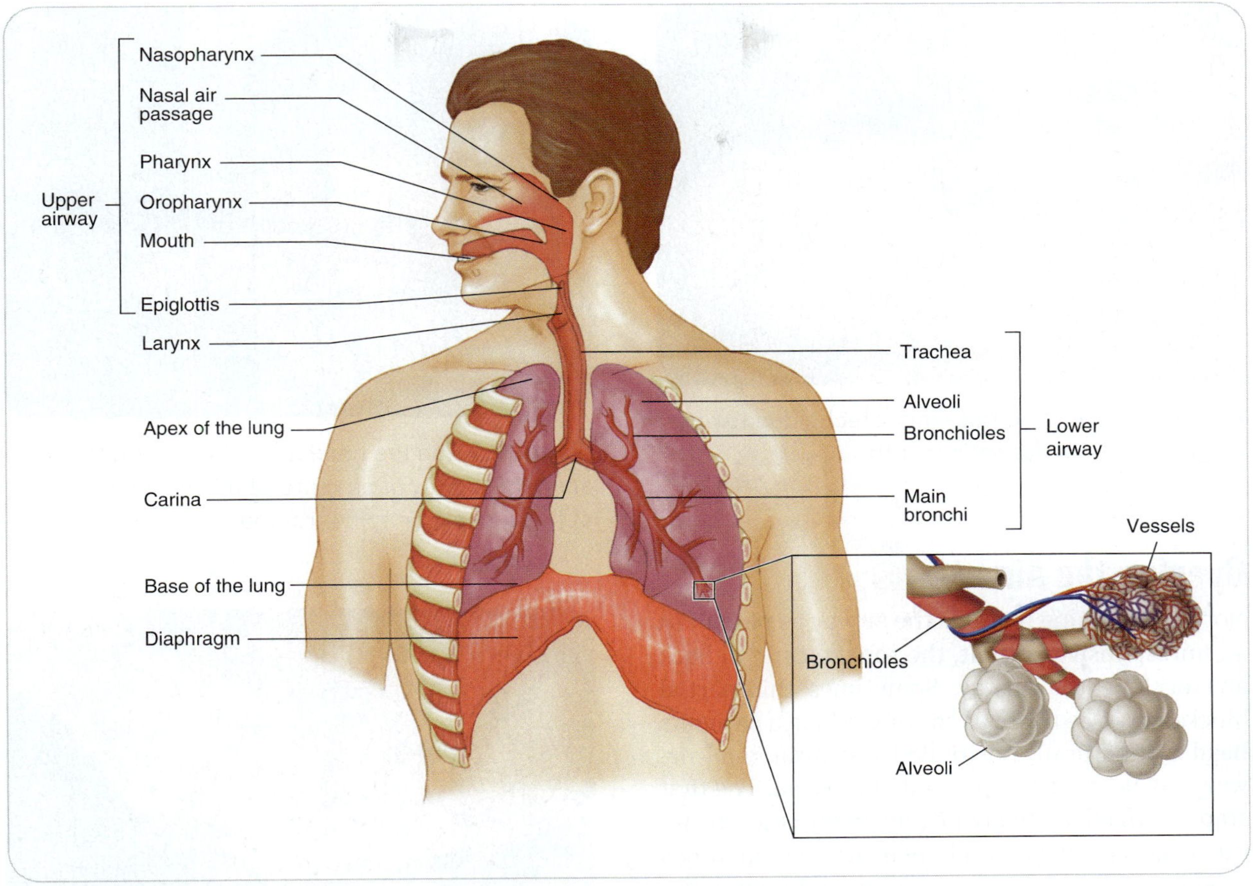

Figure 9-1 Anatomy of the upper and lower airways.

Exhalation, or expiration, is the *passive* phase of respiration. During this phase, the respiratory muscles relax, decreasing pressure within the chest, expelling any unused air and gaseous waste products from the lungs and out of the body. For more detailed information about the mechanics of breathing, refer to Chapter 6, *Anatomy and Physiology*.

AIRWAY MANAGEMENT

Airway management is the physical process that ensures the airway is open and clear, or **patent**. When the airway is obstructed, breathing cannot occur. The most common cause of an obstructed airway is posterior positioning of the tongue. Foreign material can also obstruct the airway. Numerous methods and tools are used to manage a partially or completely occluded airway. By learning the principles of opening and maintaining an airway, you will improve a patient's chances for survival.

Opening the Mouth

One way to open an *unresponsive* patient's mouth is the cross-finger technique (**Figure 9-2**):

1. Follow standard precautions.
2. Using your dominant hand, cross your index finger under your thumb.
3. Place your thumb and index finger against the patient's upper and lower teeth. (Be careful not to insert either finger between the patient's teeth.)
4. Spread your thumb and finger apart to open the patient's mouth.

Do not use the cross-finger technique if someone is responsive, as the person may bite down. Some prehospital responders now just push the chin down to open the mouth, which avoids placing the fingers near the teeth. This approach does not open the airway but allows you to look inside the mouth for an airway obstruction such as hard candy, vomit, or other foreign material.

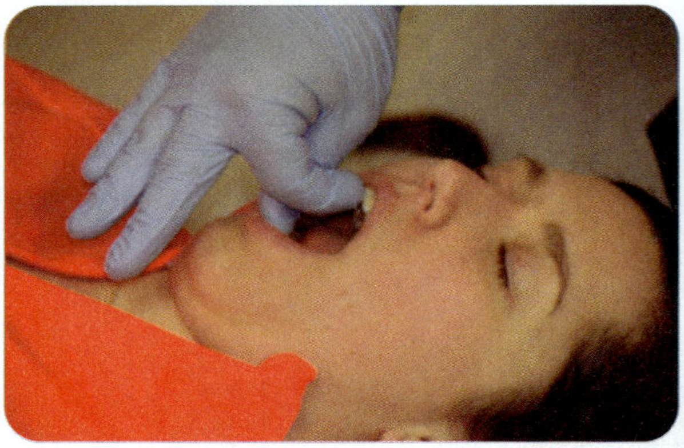

Figure 9-2 Use the cross-finger technique to open an unresponsive patient's mouth.

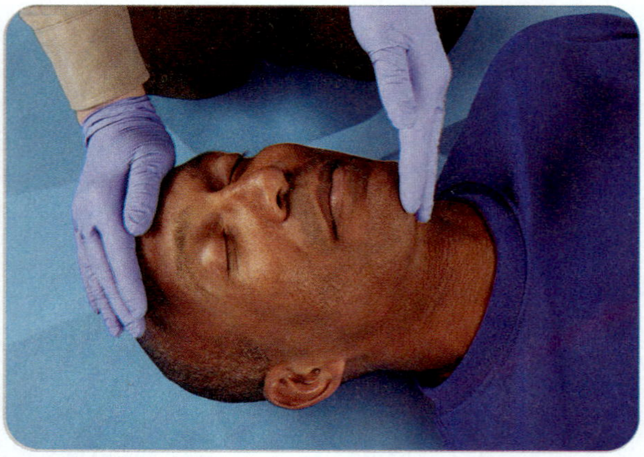

Figure 9-3 Use the head tilt–chin lift maneuver to open the airway of patients who have no possibility of head, neck, or spine trauma.

Opening the Airway

Normal breathing requires the airway be patent. In an unresponsive patient, the tongue can fall back and occlude the airway. Sometimes this partial blockage can be heard as snoring. When a patient's head is unnaturally positioned, the misaligned airway may become compressed or blocked. The first step in effective airway management is to ensure the airway is aligned and open. The two methods used by OEC technicians to align and open a patient's airway are the head tilt–chin lift and the jaw-thrust maneuvers.

The **head tilt–chin lift maneuver** is the primary technique OEC technicians use to open a patient's airway (**Figure 9-3**). Because this procedure manipulates the neck, it should be used only on patients who have no possibility of head, neck, or spine trauma. To perform the head tilt–chin lift maneuver:

1. Kneel beside the patient's head.
2. Place one hand on the patient's forehead.
3. Place two or three fingers of your other hand under the patient's chin.
4. Gently pull the chin up while simultaneously pushing down on the forehead. Do not compress the soft tissue under the chin.
5. Maintain the position to ensure the airway remains open.

If the patient has sustained head, neck, or spine trauma or there is even a *concern* about a potential cervical spine injury, open the airway using the **jaw-thrust maneuver** (**Figure 9-4**). This method opens the airway while allowing only minimal movement of the cervical spine. When performing a jaw thrust, it is essential the neck is not moved and remains in an anatomically neutral position, because any neck movement could result in spinal injury. The jaw-thrust method may also be used to open the airway in someone who does not have a neck injury. To perform the jaw-thrust maneuver:

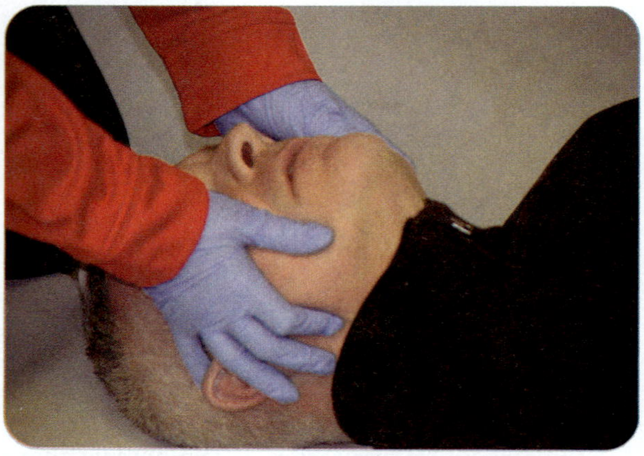

Figure 9-4 If the patient has sustained head, neck, or spine trauma or there is even a *concern* about a potential cervical spine injury, open the airway using the jaw-thrust maneuver.

1. Kneel above the patient's head, with your knees straddling the head. (You can use your knees to gently stabilize the head and cervical spine.)
2. Using the fingers of both hands, grasp the angle of the mandible on each side of the jaw.
3. Place your thumbs on the maxilla.
4. Use the thumbs as a lever to lift the mandible upward.

Clearing the Airway

Foreign material such as blood, mucus, fluids, broken teeth, foreign bodies, dirt, and food can obstruct the airway. Debris must be cleared quickly to ensure adequate oxygen flow and prevent aspiration of fluid or solids into the lungs. OEC technicians can remove mechanical or foreign body obstructions from the airway with the finger sweep, suction, gravity and positioning, or abdominal thrusts.

Finger Sweep

The **finger sweep** is indicated only for patients who are unresponsive when a foreign body is seen in the mouth. Placing a finger into the mouth of a person who is responsive could stimulate the gag reflex, inducing vomiting, or it could cause the person to bite down, injuring the rescuer's finger. Do not do a "blind finger sweep" by inserting your finger farther than you can see, as this might push the object inward, further compromising the patient's airway. To finger sweep an unresponsive patient, follow the steps in **OEC Skill 9-1**.

Suctioning

Another common method for clearing the airway is **suctioning**. This method works well whenever repeated vomiting or active oral bleeding occurs. There are two basic types of suction devices used in the outdoor emergency care field: manually operated devices and mechanical, battery-powered devices (**Figure 9-5**).

Manually operated suction devices are lightweight and compact and can provide adequate suction for short periods of time. They require a continuous manual pumping action by the rescuer. These devices usually have a small container for collecting fluids and debris. The container fills quickly, so these devices do not work well when there is a lot of material to suction.

Battery-powered suction devices provide excellent suctioning capabilities. Some suction devices may be powered by an electric motor using alternating current (AC), while others operate off a vacuum source from a vehicle engine (i.e., the ambulance). Portable motorized units use rechargeable batteries. These devices are usually very reliable, providing suction for extended periods of time. They can be heavy, so they may not be ideal for all circumstances (e.g., patrol backpack).

Regardless of whether it is manually operated, battery powered, or other, all suction devices must be capable of generating a strong vacuum. Suctioning can be done on either a responsive patient or an unresponsive patient, and it can be performed using either a rigid or a flexible suction catheter.

A rigid suction catheter, also known as a tonsil tip or Yankauer catheter, has a wide-diameter tip, is made of clear plastic, and is curved or angled

OEC SKILL 9-1 Performing the Finger Sweep

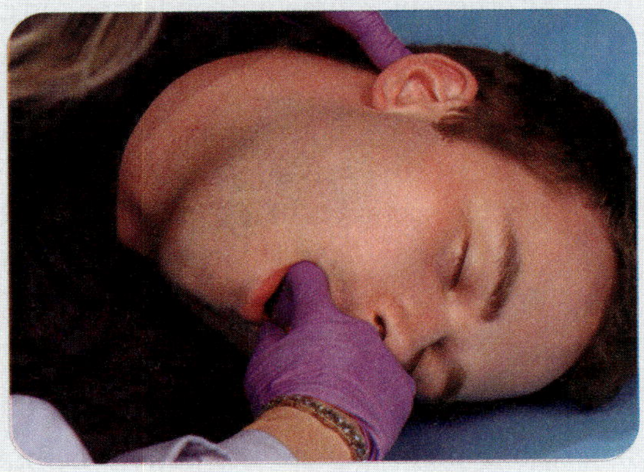

1. Follow standard precautions.
2. Open the unresponsive patient's mouth using the cross-finger technique.
3. Insert your gloved index finger into the patient's mouth so the tip of your finger is behind or beneath the foreign object. (Be careful not to push the foreign object farther into the airway.)
4. Curve your finger into a hook and remove the object. (You may need to repeat this technique more than once to completely clear the airway.)

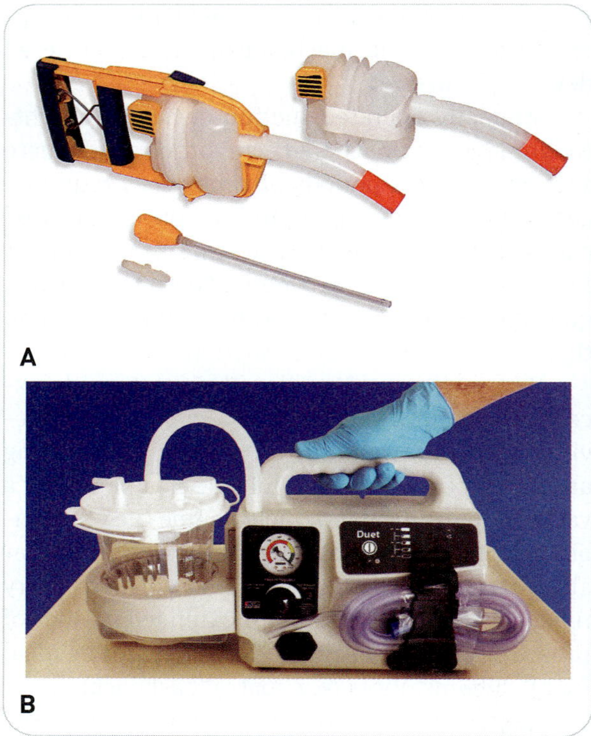

Figure 9-5 A. Most patrollers use the manually operated suction device. **B.** A mechanical battery-powered suction device.

A: Courtesy of Laerdal Medical; **B:** Courtesy of SSCOR Inc.

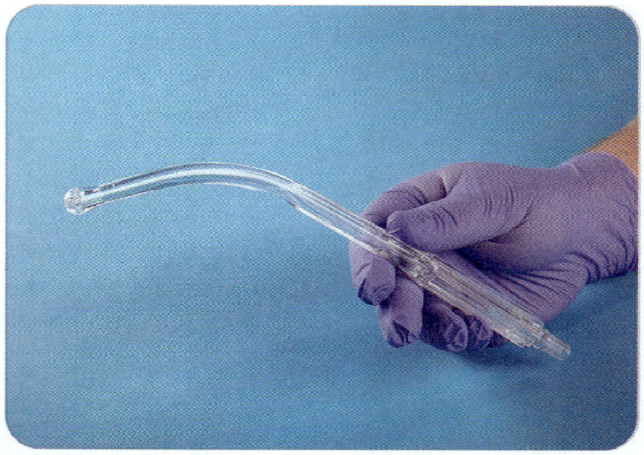

Figure 9-6 A rigid suction catheter.

© Jones & Bartlett Learning.

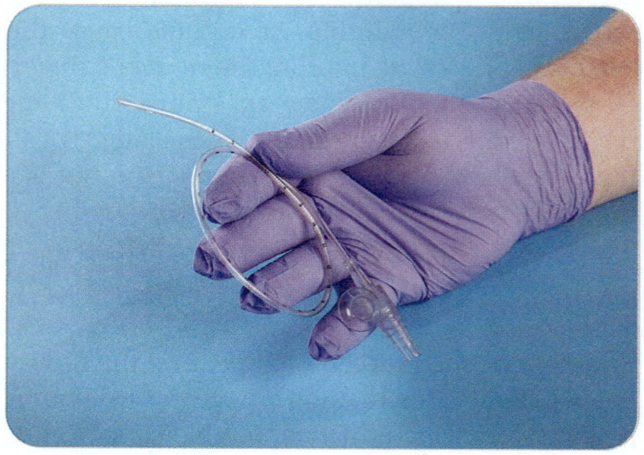

Figure 9-7 A flexible suction catheter.

© Jones & Bartlett Learning.

(**Figure 9-6**). Ideally, it should have a port (hole) in the handle, which enables the OEC technician to control the flow of suction. When the hole is covered with the thumb, suction is applied. Conversely, little or no suction occurs when the hole is left uncovered. On one end, the catheter has a connector to which suction tubing is attached. The other end of the catheter has one or more holes through which fluid and solid matter are removed. Rigid suction catheters are primarily used to suction the oropharynx but also can be used to suction around the external nasal passages.

A flexible suction catheter is a tube constructed of clear silicone or soft plastic (**Figure 9-7**). Its pliable design allows it to enter narrow passageways. For this reason, it is used to suction the nasopharynx, but it also may be used for oropharyngeal suctioning. This device may also be used for suctioning the stoma (surgical hole in the front of the neck) on some patients. As with a rigid catheter, a flexible suction catheter has an adapter on one end that connects to a suction tube; the other end is open.

Of the two types, rigid suction catheters are used more often. These are less affected by temperature and other environmental conditions and can remove large volumes of debris rapidly. ALS personnel use sterile soft, flexible catheters for deep suctioning of the lower airways. Both types of suction catheters are connected to a collection container through a clear, flexible suction tube. Manually powered suction devices usually have an integrated suction catheter directly connected to a disposable collection container, which is replaced following use.

Principles of Suctioning

If possible, preoxygenate the patient before suctioning by giving high-flow oxygen by mask. Once you have prepared the suctioning device for use, open the patient's mouth and look in the oropharynx to locate the fluid or object you need to remove. Insert the tip of the suction catheter into the pharynx *before applying suction*. Be careful not to insert the catheter farther than you can see because doing so may result in trauma to the soft oral tissues, initiate the gag reflex in a responsive or semiresponsive patient, or force a foreign body farther into the airway. Once you have located the foreign material, initiate suction only as deep as you can see to prevent pushing foreign matter farther into the airway. Using either a side-to-side or circular motion, suction the airway as you slowly pull the catheter out from the airway. Remember to always protect the cervical spine if you suspect any spinal trauma. In an airway emergency, preoxygenation is not always possible. The goal of suctioning is to clear the airway as quickly as possible to avoid aspiration of blood, vomit, or other material.

Besides removing fluid and debris, suctioning also removes oxygen. For an adult patient, apply suction for no more than 10 to 15 seconds at a time. In a child, suction the airway for only 5 to 10 seconds. Repeat the procedure as needed until the airway is clear.

If there are large pieces of debris, the holes in the tip of the catheter may be too small to get this material sucked into the tubing, so the catheter tip can be inserted repetitively. The material sticking to the end can be wiped off each time. Remember each time you put the catheter *in*, uncover the thumb hole. With active oral bleeding or repeated vomiting, it may be necessary to use gravity (roll the patient onto the side) and suction concurrently to clear the airway. Report to ambulance personnel what material was suctioned out, especially if it included blood.

After each incident, the suction unit must be thoroughly cleaned and disinfected before being placed back into service. Additionally, all disposable equipment, such as the suction catheter, suction tubing, and collection bag, must be replaced. If the suction unit is battery operated, replace or recharge the batteries as necessary. If the suction unit is manually powered, replace the catheter collection assembly. Always put disposable medical equipment in a biohazard container to dispose of it properly. To suction a patient's airway, follow the steps in **OEC Skill 9-2**.

Gravity and Positioning

Gravity is a time-honored method for quickly removing fluid and solids from the airway, and it requires no special equipment. This technique can be effective regardless of whether the patient is responsive or unresponsive. If the patient is responsive and can follow simple commands, instruct the person to lean forward with the head down (in a dependent position) to allow vomit, blood, and any solids to flow or fall out of the mouth or nose. If the patient is unresponsive, roll the person into the recovery position, discussed in the next section. In the presence of a suspected spinal injury, the patient may be rolled onto the side while another rescuer maintains the patient's head and neck in a neutral position. If foreign material is wedged in the pharynx, gravity may not work.

Abdominal Thrusts

Abdominal thrusting is a maneuver to dislodge a foreign body immediately after someone begins choking. It can be used in any patient older than 1 year. Note that back blows are given to infants. Suspect an airway obstruction if you encounter a person grasping his or her throat, or trying to speak but unable to do so; in this situation, abdominal thrusts can be lifesaving (**Figure 9-8**). Hard candy, a piece of meat, or a small part of a toy can block the airway. If the person can speak, the airway is not obstructed.

This procedure, originally described by Heimlich, is used if the patient is responsive. Stand behind the standing or sitting patient. Reach around and put one fist, thumb toward the patient, between the xiphoid process and the navel. Grasp your fist with the other hand. Begin firm upward *thrusts*, not hugs (**Figure 9-9**). Repeat these thrusts until the foreign object is expelled or the patient becomes unresponsive.

If the patient is unresponsive, begin chest compressions as you would with CPR. These chest compressions will have the same effect as the abdominal thrusts.

For infants with an obstructed airway, deliver five back blows, followed by five chest thrusts. Repeat as necessary.

Keeping the Airway Open and Clear

Recovery Position

Once the airway is opened and cleared, it must remain this way to ensure adequate breathing. The easiest method to achieve this, until other airway equipment or rescue personnel are available, is to

OEC SKILL 9-2 Suctioning a Patient's Airway

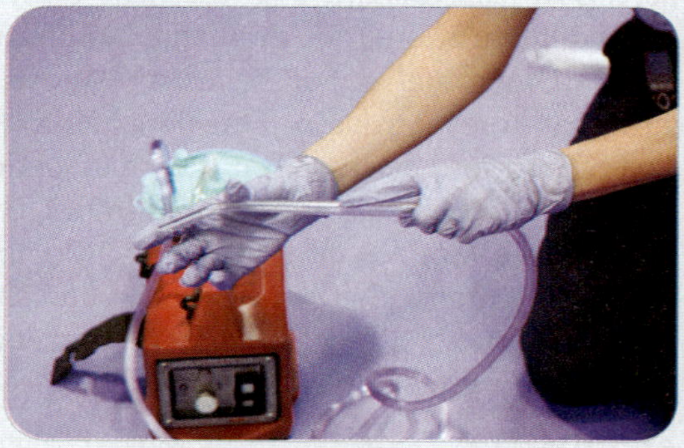

1 Make sure the suctioning unit is properly assembled and turned on. Clamp the tubing, and make sure the unit generates a vacuum of more than 300 mm Hg.

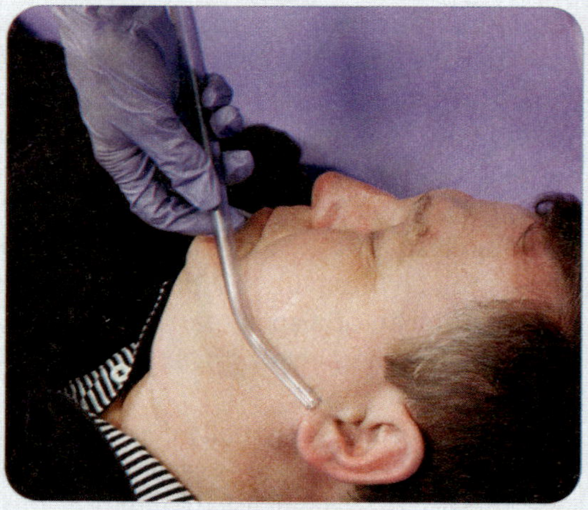

2 Measure the catheter from the corner of the mouth to the earlobe or angle of the jaw.

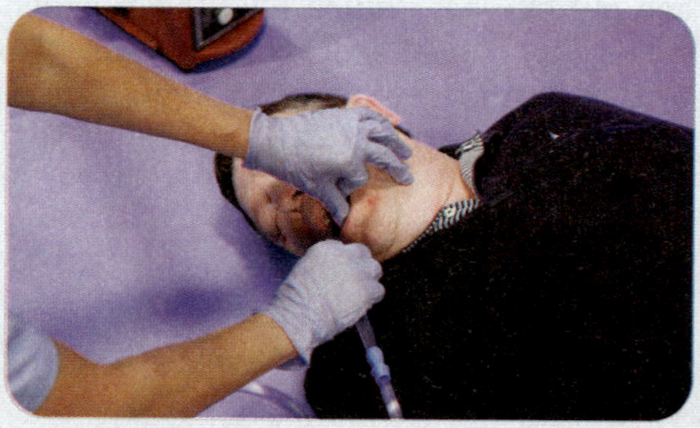

3 Turn the patient's head to the side (unless you suspect cervical spine injury), open the mouth using the cross-finger technique, and insert the catheter to the predetermined depth without suctioning.

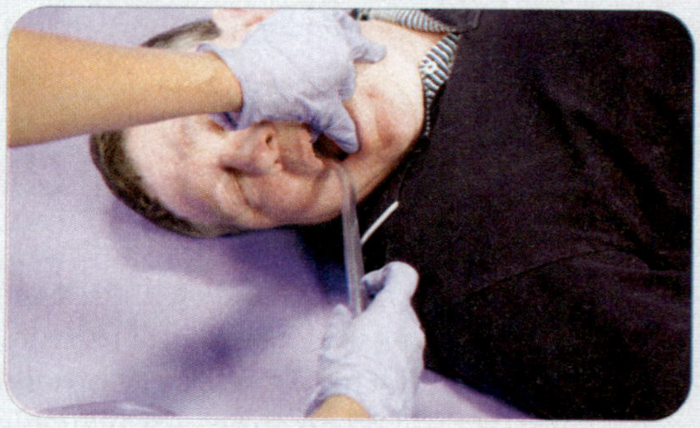

4 Apply suction in a circular motion as you withdraw the catheter. Do not suction an adult for more than 15 sections, a child for more than 10 seconds, and an infant for more than 5 seconds.

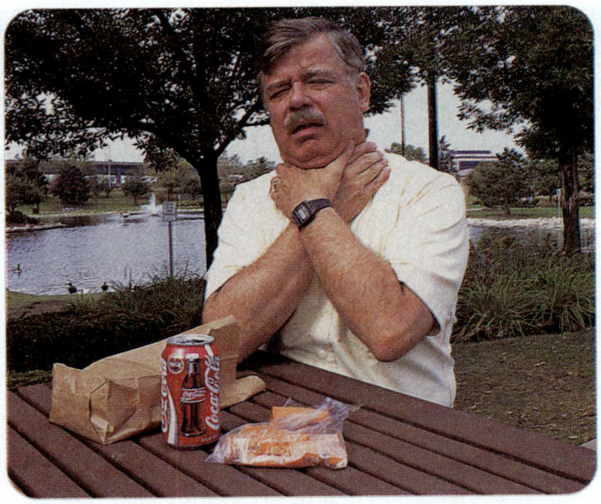

Figure 9-8 The universal sign of choking is a person who grasps his or her throat and has difficulty breathing.

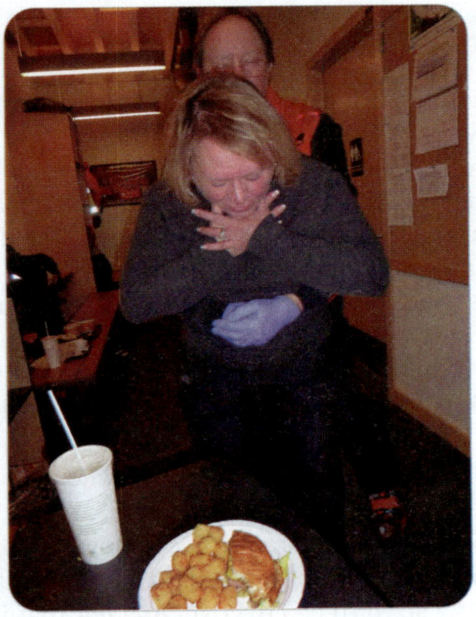

Figure 9-9 You must use forceful abdominal thrusts to remove an obstruction.

place the patient in the recovery (left lateral recumbent) position (**Figure 9-10**). This position can be used for any unresponsive patient where a spine injury is *not* suspected. It also may be used for responsive patients or any patients with an altered level of responsiveness who cannot manage their airway. When alone, rescuers should use this

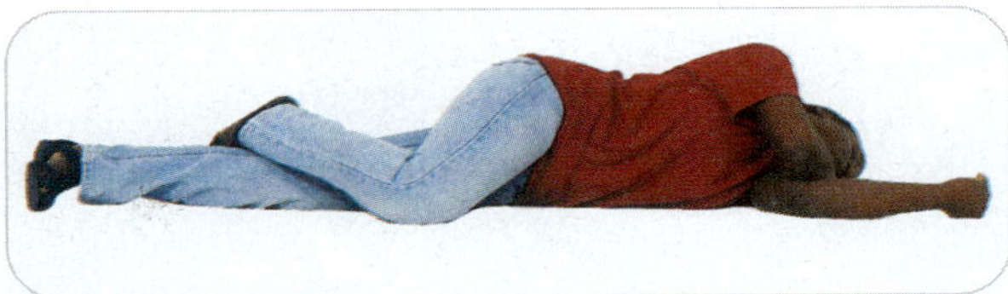

Figure 9-10 Once the airway obstruction has been removed, place your patient in the recovery position and monitor until EMS arrives.

technique to allow them to do other care-related tasks. To place the patient in the recovery position:

1. Kneel at the patient's left side, preferably with your knees near the patient's hips or chest.
2. Extend the patient's left arm so it extends over the person's head.
3. Gently roll the patient toward you onto the left side so the patient's head rests on his or her straightened arm.
4. The patient's head should be tilted at a *slight* downward angle, with the mouth open, to allow secretions to flow out of the mouth.
5. Flex the patient's right knee at a right angle to anchor the patient into this position.
6. Position the patient's right arm so it is in front of the patient and does not block the rescuer's access to the patient's airway.
7. Always make sure the airway remains open.

Airway Devices

Sometimes it is necessary to insert an airway device to keep the airway open. The OEC technician has two options—a nasopharyngeal airway or an oropharyngeal airway (**Figures 9-11** and **9-12**).

KEY POINT

Airway Protection During Transport of Unresponsive Patient

When an unresponsive patient is loaded into a toboggan for transport to the aid station, it is recommended to insert an oral or nasal airway to protect the airway.

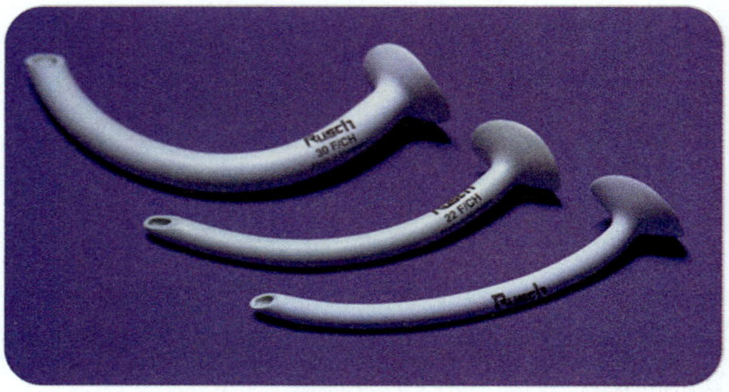

Figure 9-11 A nasopharyngeal (nasal) airway.

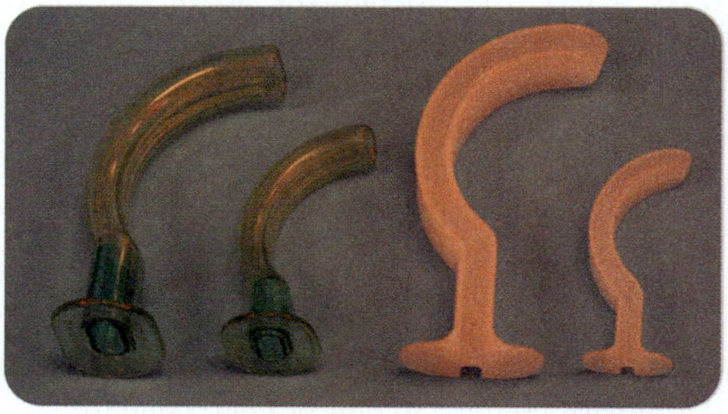

Figure 9-12 An oropharyngeal (oral) airway.

The device used depends on the patient's level of responsiveness (**Table 9-1**). *You should always place an airway device in an unresponsive patient.*

A **nasopharyngeal airway (NPA)** is a flexible tube inserted into the nasopharynx (nose). It is made of soft, latex-free plastic. Also known as a nasal trumpet, this mechanical airway provides an unobstructed pathway from one of the nostrils to the posterior nasopharynx, keeping the passageway open for air exchange. When properly sized, the adjunct is well tolerated, even in responsive patients, as it does not stimulate the gag reflex. NPAs come in a variety of sizes and can be used in all patients, from small children to large adults.

Do not use this airway in patients with massive head or facial injuries due to possible injury pushing the tube into the brain.

For proper insertion of an NPA, follow the steps in **OEC Skill 9-3**. The steps to insert an NPA can be remembered using the acronym SLIC.

If the patient's level of responsiveness improves, you may need to remove the NPA. To do so, simply grasp the NPA by the flange and withdraw the adjunct using a steady downward motion that follows the device's curvature.

Table 9-1 A Comparison of Oropharyngeal and Nasopharyngeal Airway Devices

Oropharyngeal Airway	Nasopharyngeal Airway
Placed in the mouth. Relieves airway obstruction caused by tongue.	Placed in the nose. Relieves airway obstruction caused by the tongue or by mucus and nasal swelling.
Relatively easy to insert.	Easy to insert.
Must not be used in a responsive patient or a person with an intact gag reflex.	Can be safely used in responsive and semiresponsive patients or in a person with an intact gag reflex.
Can be placed in patients who have nasal trauma.	Caution required if used in patients who have facial trauma.

An **oropharyngeal airway (OPA)** is a hard-plastic device inserted into the oropharynx (mouth) to help keep the airway open. The device displaces the relaxed tongue and prevents it from lying across the epiglottis and occluding the airway. When the OPA is in place, the tongue rests within the curvature of the device. An OPA is indicated only for unresponsive patients who do not have a gag reflex and are unable to protect the airway. The device is frequently used when assisting ventilations with a bag-valve mask.

OPAs come in several sizes, ranging from #0 for infants to #6 for large adults. An OPA must be properly sized to be effective. An OPA that is too small will force the tongue downward and block the oropharynx, whereas an OPA that is too large can enter the esophagus or damage the epiglottis or vocal cords.

Attempting to place an OPA into a patient who is either fully or partially responsive will stimulate the gag reflex, which may result in vomiting and possible aspiration of gastric contents. If the soft palate is touched by the OPA and the person gags, remove the OPA and do not reinsert it.

For proper insertion of an OPA, follow the steps in **OEC Skill 9-4**.

OEC SKILL 9-3 Inserting a Nasopharyngeal Airway

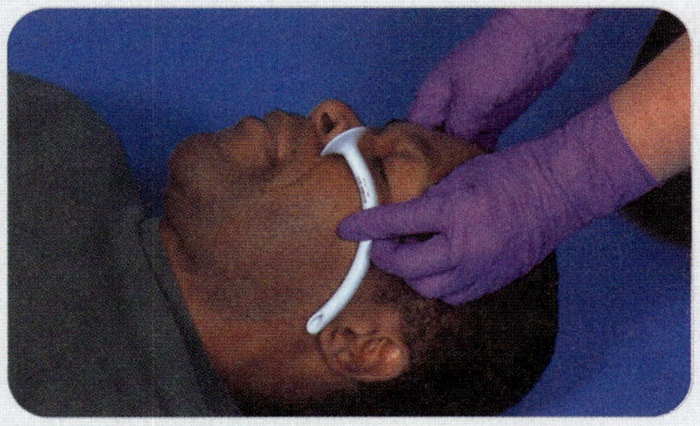

1 **S Size the device.** NPAs come in a variety of sizes. To be effective, the device must be sized appropriately. A tube that is too small may become blocked by the tongue, whereas a tube that is too large may enter the esophagus or stimulate the patient's gag reflex. To size an NPA, hold the tube against the side of the patient's face. The flange should rest against the nostril, the end should just touch the patient's lower earlobe on the same side of the face, and the outside of the tube should be slightly smaller than the nostril into which it will be placed.

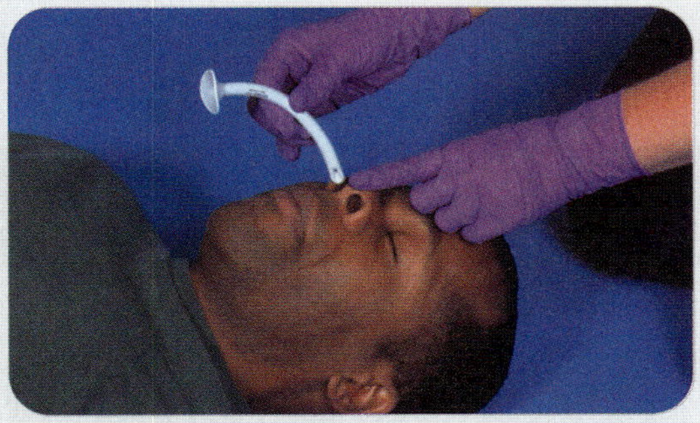

2 **L Lubricate the adjunct.** Apply a small amount of water-based lubricant along the entire length of the NPA tube. Be careful not to apply too much lubricant, which could aggravate an existing airway problem. The goal is to provide a slippery surface, so the tube can slide gently into position as shown.

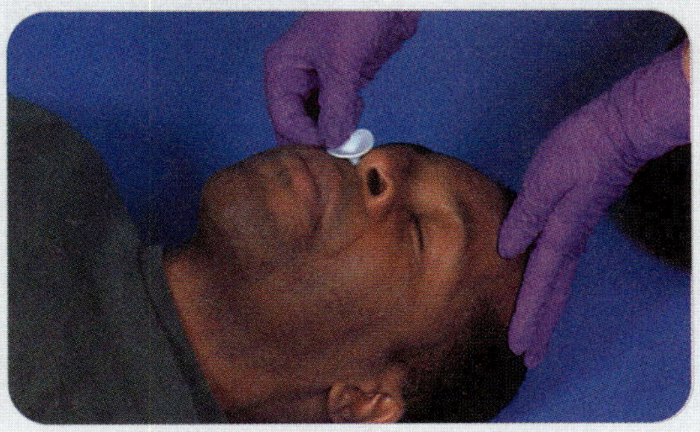

3 **I Insert the device.**

- Hold the tube between your thumb and first two fingers.
- Place the bevel side of the tube toward the nasal septum.
- Gently insert the tube into the nostril while following the curvature of the tube until the flange is flush with the nostril. Do not force the tube into position; doing so can cause a nosebleed, an obstruction, or other injuries. If an obstruction is met, pull the tube back slightly and reinsert, again while rotating the tube between your fingers. Properly placed, the curvature of the tube will follow the natural curve of the nasal passage and lie in the distal portion of the nasopharynx directly above the larynx.

(continues)

OEC SKILL 9-3 Inserting a Nasopharyngeal Airway (*continued*)

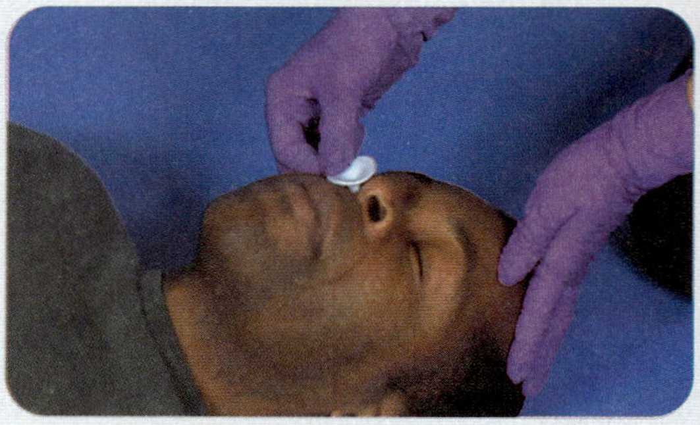

4 C **Check the device.** Confirm proper placement of the tube by listening to the patient breathe. You should be able to hear or feel air movement through the tube. If no air is detected, check to see if the patient is still breathing. If the patient is not, assist the patient's ventilations. If the patient is breathing, the tube may be obstructed, may need to be repositioned, or may need to be removed and resized. Rarely, foreign material inside the nose can obstruct the opening of the NPA.

OEC SKILL 9-4 Inserting an Oropharyngeal Airway

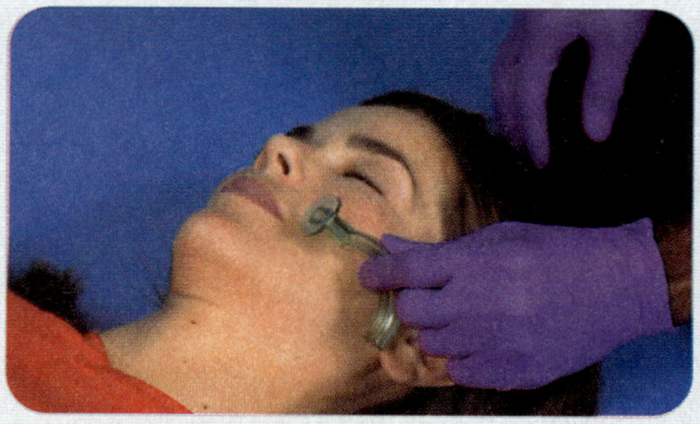

1 To properly size an OPA, hold the adjunct against the side of the patient's face with the flange adjacent to the corner of the patient's mouth. The tip of the adjunct should touch the angle of the jaw on the same side of the face; alternatively, measure from the corner of the mouth to the earlobe on the same side of the face.

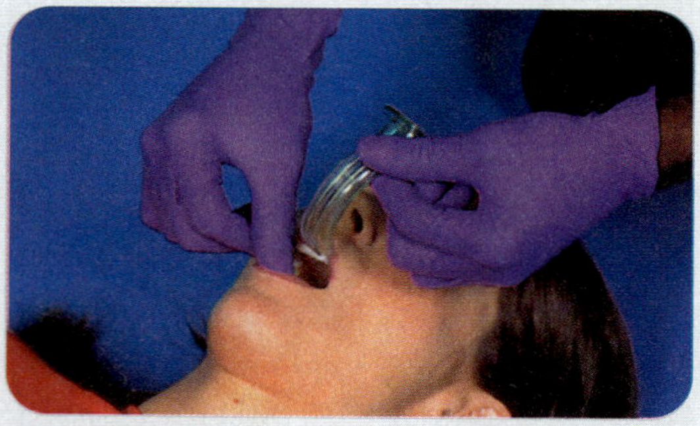

2 To insert an OPA, open the patient's mouth using the cross-finger technique or push down on the chin. Insert the OPA, with the tip pointed up toward the roof of the mouth, until it is halfway into the mouth.

OEC SKILL 9-4 Inserting an Oropharyngeal Airway (*continued*)

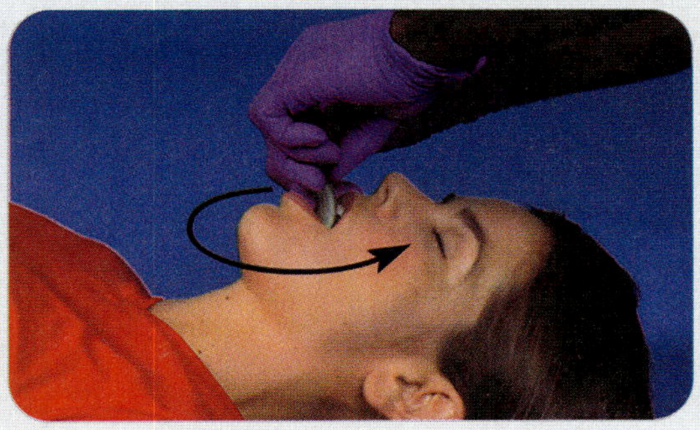

3 Rotate the adjunct 180 degrees so the tip faces toward the patient's tongue. The tongue should now lie along the curve of the OPA, and the external flange should rest against the patient's lips. In children, the device is not rotated 180 degrees before insertion. The tip is pointed toward the tongue, not the roof of the mouth when inserted.

KEY POINT

Oropharyngeal Airway

Medical providers may use an OPA as a bite block to protect the teeth. It may also be used as a spacer between the teeth that will prevent damage to an advanced airway device such as a breathing tube placed in the oral airway.

Confirm proper placement by listening for breaths, watching the chest rise and fall, and feeling air moving in and out of the OPA. Air should be able to move freely in and out of the airway (either spontaneously or when using a ventilation assistance device such as a pocket mask or bag-valve mask). If air does not move freely, the tongue may have been pushed farther back into the posterior pharynx and may be blocking the airway. Remove the OPA, confirm it is properly sized, and then reinsert it.

An alternative method for placing an OPA involves the use of a tongue blade, bite block (a device used to hold the mouth open and prevent the patient from biting the tongue or the oral airway), or another smooth object. Using a tongue blade, depress the tongue toward the floor of the mouth. Then, insert the adjunct along the side of the mouth, with the tip pointing toward the inside cheek, until the OPA is halfway into the mouth. Rotate the OPA 90 degrees until the flange rests on the patient's lips.

An OPA should be left in place until one of two conditions arises: either the patient begins to gag or a more advanced airway device is inserted by an ALS provider. However, if you need to remove an OPA, grasp the adjunct by the flanges and pull it both outward and slightly downward, following the natural contour of the tongue. Removal should be performed in one swift motion to reduce the incidence of vomiting and other complications. Have a suction device ready in case the patient vomits.

KEY POINT

Inserting an Oropharyngeal Airway

The steps to insert an OPA can be remembered using the acronym SIC:

S: Size the airway.

I: Insert the airway.

C: Check the airway for proper placement.

CASE Update

Your partner immediately performs a jaw-thrust maneuver to open the unresponsive patient's airway. The patient begins breathing. As your partner protects the patient's spine, you carefully roll the patient onto his left side in the recovery position to allow blood to flow out of the airway. Noting several broken teeth in the patient's airway, you perform a finger sweep to remove the debris. Upon arrival of a suction device, you suction out the airway. Although the patient's pulse is strong, his respirations are becoming increasingly shallow and erratic. His lips are cyanotic.

What should you do now?

Barrier Devices

If the patient is not breathing, use a barrier device to provide rescue breaths. A **barrier device** is a personal protective device that provides a nonporous layer between you and the patient to prevent the transmission of communicable diseases. It is an effective way to ventilate a patient until more sophisticated airway equipment and oxygen become available.

Barrier devices permit OEC technicians to provide rescue breaths using the residual oxygen in the rescuer's lungs. The mixture of gases in exhaled air contains approximately 15% to 16% oxygen, which is enough to provide initial oxygenation to a patient who is not breathing. Room air is 21% oxygen. The most common barrier devices used for this purpose are face shields and a pocket masks.

A **face shield** is a clear, usually rectangular, plastic sheet that includes a mouthpiece through which rescue breaths are administered. Some face shields also have an integrated one-way valve/bite block that directs airflow into the patient's airway while preventing the rescuer from becoming contaminated. To use a face shield, perform the following procedure:

1. Kneel at either side of the patient's head.
2. Remove the face shield from its protective package and place the shield over the patient's mouth and nose. If the device contains an integrated one-way valve/bite block, place the valve into the patient's mouth, between the teeth.
3. Pinch the patient's nose and seal your lips on the shield around the valve (as if you were performing normal mouth-to-mouth resuscitation) and provide rescue breaths. You should see the chest rise and fall with each breath.

A **pocket mask** is a triangular or pear-shaped mechanical breathing device made from clear, soft plastic or silicone (**Figure 9-13**). Some older styles are circular, or donut shaped. The pocket mask is used to deliver mouth-to-mask rescue breathing.

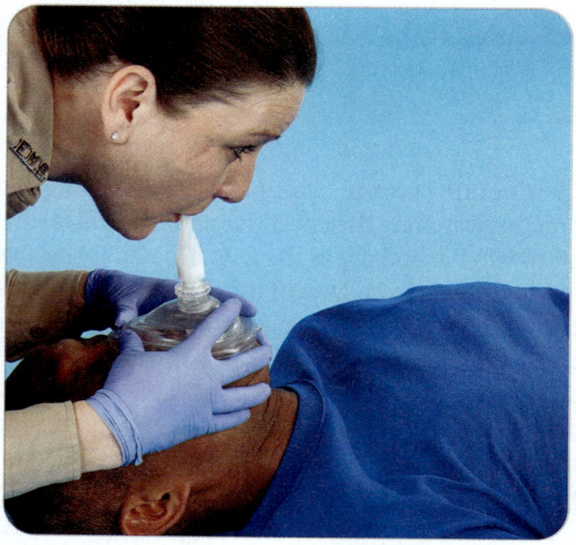

Figure 9-13 A pocket mask offers better protection from blood and secretions than a face shield.

The apex of the mask fits over the bridge of the patient's nose. Some pocket masks include a built-in oxygen port that allows the device to be connected to supplemental oxygen. Used correctly, a pocket mask provides an excellent seal on the patient's face and offers better protection from blood and secretions than a face shield. Creating an adequate seal and delivering appropriate rescue breaths with a pocket mask is an important skill in emergency airway and respiration care. Practice this skill until you are very comfortable with it.

To assemble and use a pocket mask:

1. Remove the device from its protective package or case.
2. Open the mask (by pulling on the connector, if necessary).
3. Connect the one-way valve to the mask. (Follow the manufacturer's instructions to ensure the valve is pointed toward the patient.)
4. Connect the breathing tube to the one-way valve.
5. Kneel at the top of the patient's head, and open the airway using either the head tilt–chin lift or the jaw-thrust maneuver.
6. Fit the mask onto the patient, placing the top of the triangle on the bridge of the patient's nose. The mask should fit in the groove between the patient's lower lip and chin. If the mask does not fit in the groove, the mask may not be the correct size, or it may need to be repositioned on the face.
7. Place your thumbs on the top of the mask, near the bridge of the patient's nose, while simultaneously placing your index fingers on the bottom of the mask, which is over the section between the lower lip and chin.
8. Place the middle, ring, and little fingers of both your hands under the mandible and pull upward, toward the mask (as opposed to pushing the mask down onto the face).
9. Place your lips around the open port and deliver a rescue breath. The patient's chest should rise and fall with each breath. If the patient's chest does not rise or if you hear air escaping between the mask and the patient's face, reposition the device and then deliver another rescue breath. If the chest still does not rise, follow obstructed airway procedures.

A NuMask is an airway device that can be used during CPR for rescue breathing. It has an intraoral seal and a simple grip, making mouth-to-mask ventilation easy. The patient side of the device has a snorkel-like end that fits inside the patient's mouth between the lips and the teeth. The other end (the rescuer's end) has a one-way valve with a filter, allowing protection of the rescuer. Since the patient side is inside the lips, holding it in place is easier. However, this device must be placed between the patient's lips and teeth correctly to be effective.

OXYGEN THERAPY

Oxygen is an odorless, colorless, and tasteless gas essential to human survival. Air consists of 78% nitrogen, 21% oxygen, and 1% other gases. If the body does not receive enough oxygen, cellular or tissue damage, organ failure, shock, or death can occur.

Many OEC technicians give supplemental oxygen as part of their regular care. In some areas, OEC technicians are not legally permitted to administer oxygen. To determine if you are permitted to provide oxygen therapy in your state, province, or area, check with your patrol director, area management, or state EMS office.

Depending on where care is given, a doctor's order to give oxygen may be needed. A patrol's medical advisor may provide this authorization as either an indirect or direct order, or it may be obtained through the local emergency care system's medical control. It is best to develop a local protocol concerning oxygen delivery with input from a local doctor, management, and the patrol's leadership.

Oxygen administered to patients is 100% pure medical oxygen. Unlike industrial oxygen, which should not be administered to patients, medical oxygen contains no impurities. Medical oxygen is stored as a compressed gas in specially marked cylinders that either are solid green or have a large green stripe on top. Medical-grade oxygen may require a doctor's prescription.

Oxygen Equipment

Several pieces of equipment are required to administer supplemental oxygen, including an oxygen cylinder, a pressure regulator/flowmeter, and a nasal cannula or face mask. The characteristics

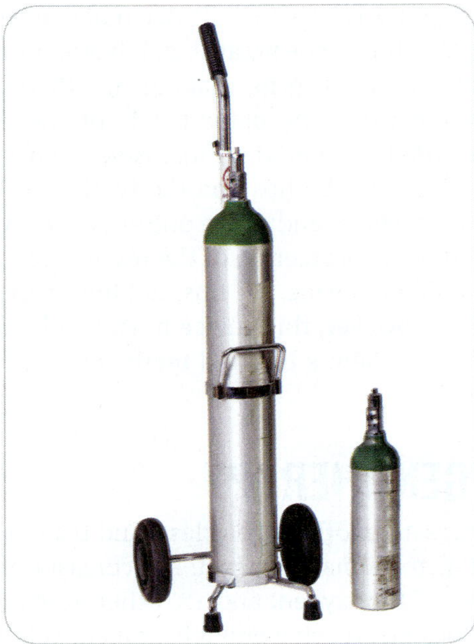

Figure 9-14 Oxygen tanks come in various sizes.

Table 9-2 Oxygen Cylinder Sizes and Volumes

Size	Volume (Liters)
D	350
Super D	500
E	625
M	3,000

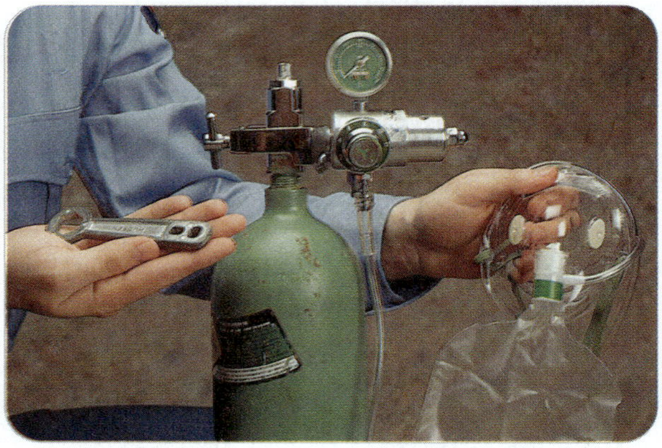

Figure 9-15 Oxygen administration equipment.

and operation of each piece of equipment are described in the following sections.

Oxygen Cylinders

Oxygen is compressed to 2,000 pounds per square inch (psi) and stored in portable cylinders. Many oxygen cylinders are constructed of lightweight aluminum, although older or larger cylinders are made of steel. Oxygen cylinders come in a variety of sizes (**Figure 9-14** and **Table 9-2**). The portable oxygen cylinders used by most ski patrol systems are either size D or E. When full, these cylinders contain 350 to 625 liters of oxygen. At 4 liters per minute (LPM), a full D cylinder lasts about 70 minutes. At 15 LPM, it lasts about 20 minutes. Calculations can be made for other flow rates, but these numbers give a good idea of how much oxygen is available based on the rate given.

Oxygen cylinders must be marked with a green color and be labeled as medical oxygen. A valve at the top of the oxygen cylinder allows you to control the flow of oxygen from the cylinder. Oxygen administration equipment is shown in **Figure 9-15**. Larger oxygen cylinders are usually found on ambulances, in hospitals, and in ski patrol first-aid rooms or base camps.

Pressure Regulator/Flowmeter

Oxygen can be used only when the pressure is regulated down to about 50 psi, which is done by using a pressure regulator. The pressure regulator and the **flowmeter** are a single unit attached to the outlet of the oxygen cylinder (**Figure 9-16**). After the pressure has been reduced, you can adjust the flowmeter to deliver oxygen at a rate of 2 to 15 LPM. Because patients with different medical conditions require different amounts of oxygen, the flowmeter lets you select the proper amount of oxygen to administer. A gasket between the cylinder and the pressure regulator/flowmeter ensures a tight seal and maintains the high pressure inside the cylinder. Always check for this gasket before attaching the regulator.

Nasal Cannulas and Face Masks

The third part of an oxygen-delivery system is a device that ensures the oxygen is delivered to the

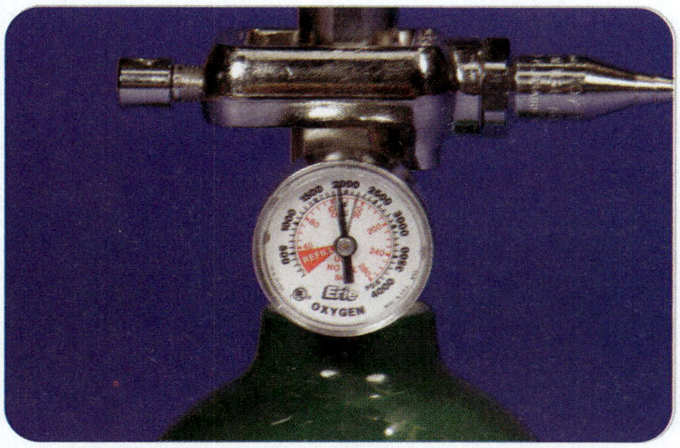

Figure 9-16 The regulator/flowmeter attaches to the outlet of the oxygen cylinder.

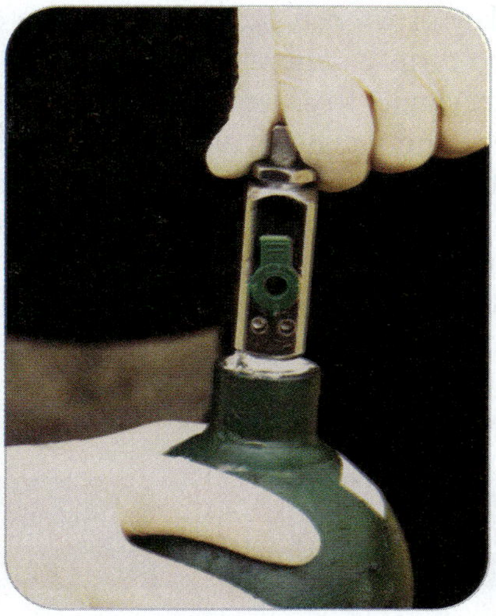

Figure 9-17 A valve stem with pin-index holes.

patient and is not lost in the air. A nasal cannula has two small holes, which fit into the patient's nostrils. A nasal cannula delivers 1–6 LPM and delivers between 35% and 50% oxygen. A face mask is placed over the patient's nose and mouth to deliver oxygen through the patient's mouth and nostrils. Nonrebreather face masks deliver higher concentrations of oxygen (up to 90%) than standard oxygen face masks. For the most part, OEC technicians will use nonrebreather face masks. These two oxygen-delivery devices are discussed more fully in the section on administering supplemental oxygen.

Oxygen Safety

Oxygen actively supports combustion and can quickly turn a small spark or flame into a serious fire. Never use oxygen near a spark or flame such as candles, a campfire, a stove, or a heater. Do not allow a patient or others to smoke when oxygen is being used. Keep oil, grease, or other petroleum-based or combustible materials away from oxygen cylinders and oxygen regulators.

Oxygen cylinders are vessels containing highly compressed gas. They should be laid on their side, kept in a protective carrier, or firmly secured to a wall to prevent them from falling. Turn the oxygen cylinder off when it is not in use.

If the valve stem at the top of the cylinder is damaged, the cylinder can take off like a rocket. Oxygen cylinders should be kept inside sturdy carrying cases that protect the cylinder and regulator/flowmeter.

Indications for Oxygen Therapy

Oxygen should be administered to anyone who is short of breath and patients with suspected cardiac or respiratory arrest, cardiac-related chest pain, stroke, significant blood loss, shock, decreased level of responsiveness, or significant head injury. By administering supplemental oxygen, an OEC technician increases the oxygen saturation of hemoglobin in the blood, providing more oxygen to the body's tissues. Insufficient oxygen to the body's tissues results in hypoxia. When injured, patients who have chronic lung disease (usually from smoking), those whose respiratory rate has been decreased by an overdose of depressant drugs, or those who have a failing heart may be hypoxic and need oxygen. These signs and symptoms, and the conditions with which they are associated, are covered in other chapters.

Administering Supplemental Oxygen

To administer supplemental oxygen, place the regulator/flowmeter over the stem of the oxygen cylinder and line up the pins on the pin-indexing system correctly (**Figure 9-17**). Check for the mandatory gasket and make sure it is not damaged. Tighten the securing screw firmly by hand. With the special key or wrench provided, turn the cylinder valve two turns counterclockwise to allow oxygen from the cylinder to enter the regulator/flowmeter.

Check the gauge on the pressure regulator/flowmeter to see how much oxygen pressure remains in the cylinder. If the cylinder contains less than 500 psi, the amount of oxygen in the cylinder is too low for emergency use and should be replaced with a full cylinder (2,000 psi).

To administer oxygen, you will need to adjust the flowmeter to deliver the desired liter-per-minute flow of oxygen. The patient's condition and the type of oxygen delivery device you use (a face mask or a nasal cannula) dictate the proper flow. When the oxygen flow begins, place the face mask or nasal cannula onto the patient's face.

To place an oxygen cylinder into service, follow the steps in **OEC Skill 9-5**.

OEC SKILL 9-5 Placing an Oxygen Cylinder into Service

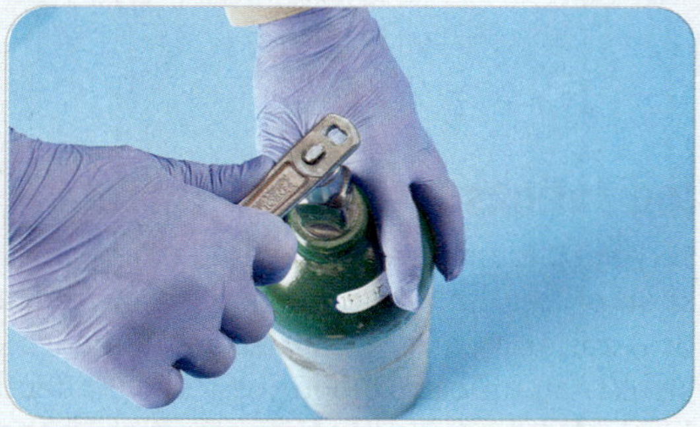

1 Using an oxygen wrench, turn the valve counterclockwise to slowly "crack" the cylinder.

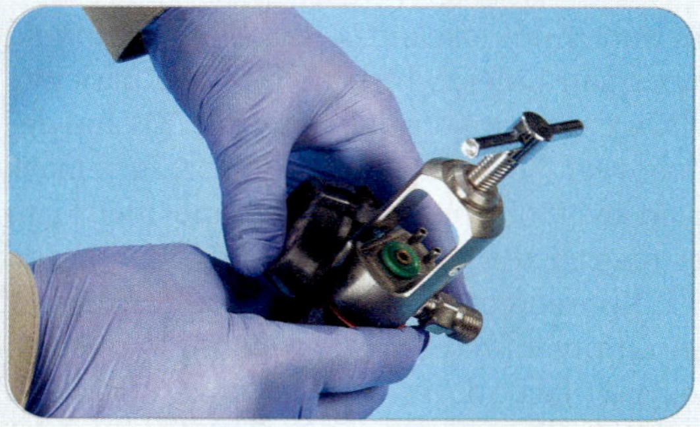

2 Attach the regulator/flowmeter to the valve stem using the two pin-indexing holes and make sure that the washer is in place over the larger hole.

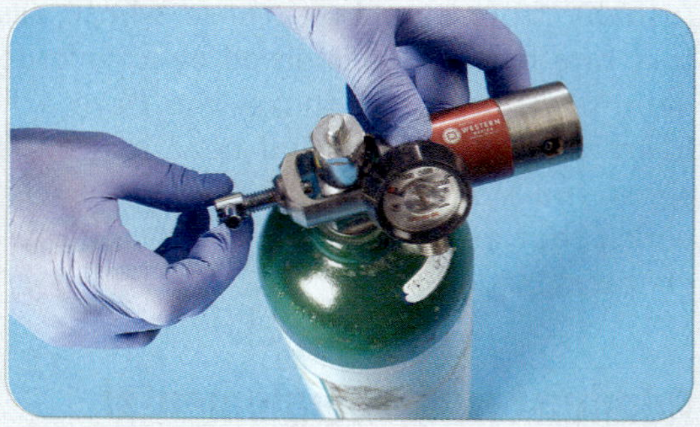

3 Align the regulator so that the pins fit snugly into the correct holes on the valve stem, and hand tighten the regulator.

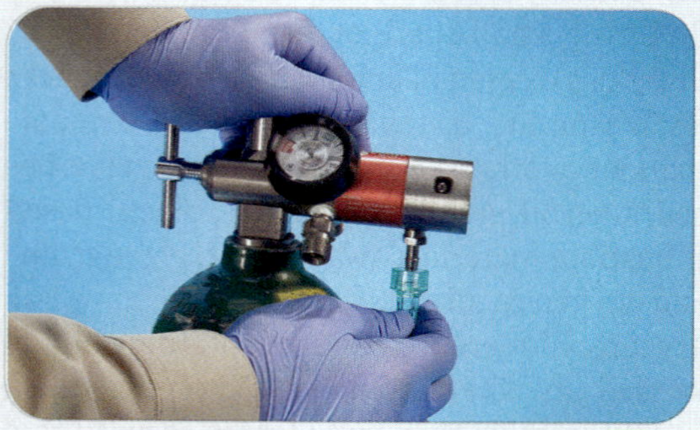

4 Attach the oxygen connective tubing to the flowmeter.

KEY POINT

Adjusting the Flow Rate

When continuous oxygen therapy needs to be delivered in remote settings or during incidents where extrication or transport is prolonged, adjust the flow down, so the oxygen lasts longer, or use multiple cylinders.

Oxygen Delivery/Ventilation Devices

As discussed, different devices are available for giving oxygen to a patient. The delivery method chosen should meet the patient's needs. OEC technicians must be very familiar with the indications, setup, and use of each airway delivery device. The nasal cannula and nonrebreather mask are used only if the patient is breathing. The bag-valve mask is used to assist breathing.

Nasal Cannula

A **nasal cannula** is a flexible, circular tube attached to an oxygen source by a long clear hose (**Figure 9-18**). It has two short, pliable hollow prongs inserted (concave down) into the patient's nostrils for passively delivering smaller amounts of oxygen, or low-flow oxygen. Administration flow rates vary from 1 to 6 LPM, with 2 to 4 LPM being the typical rate (**Table 9-3**). Low-flow oxygen can be used for fairly stable patients, such as those with mild shortness of breath. This delivers an oxygen concentration of 24% to 44%. The actual percentage of oxygen varies according to whether the patient breathes exclusively through the nose or also through the mouth.

Nasal cannulas do have several drawbacks. Prolonged use is associated with drying of the nasal passages. Blowing oxygen into the nose can be irritating. Since only low flow rates can be delivered with a nasal cannula, it is not recommended for use on patients who require high concentrations of oxygen who have signs of respiratory distress, shock, or severe chest pain. For patients who refuse to wear a mask that delivers a higher concentration of oxygen, the use of a nasal cannula at 2 to 4 LPM is better than providing no supplemental oxygen at all.

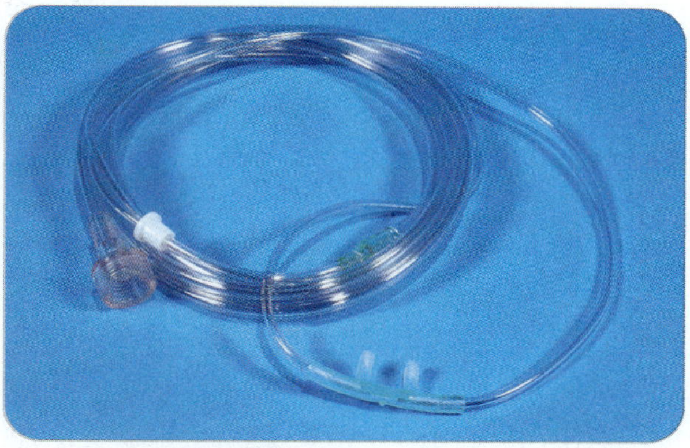

Figure 9-18 The nasal cannula is a good way to provide supplemental oxygen to a responsive patient.

Table 9-3 Oxygen Delivery Through a Nasal Cannula

Flow Rate	Percentage of Oxygen Delivered
1 LPM	24%
2 LPM	28%
3 LPM	32%
4 LPM	36%
5 LPM	40%
6 LPM	44%

To use a nasal cannula, connect the end of the tubing to the regulator and set the oxygen regulator to the desired flow rate in LPM. Put the tubing on the patient's head, usually behind each ear, and tighten it with the prongs upward in the nose. Loosen or tighten for comfort.

Nonrebreather Face Mask

The **nonrebreather mask** is a face mask that covers both the nose and the mouth and attaches with the use of an elastic cord around the patient's head. An attached collapsible reservoir bag, typically 1 liter, connects to an oxygen source (**Figure 9-19**). Before placing the mask on a patient, the reservoir bag is inflated with oxygen. Approximately one-third of the air from the reservoir is depleted each time the patient inhales, and it is then replaced by the flow from the oxygen supply. If the bag becomes completely deflated, the patient will no longer have a

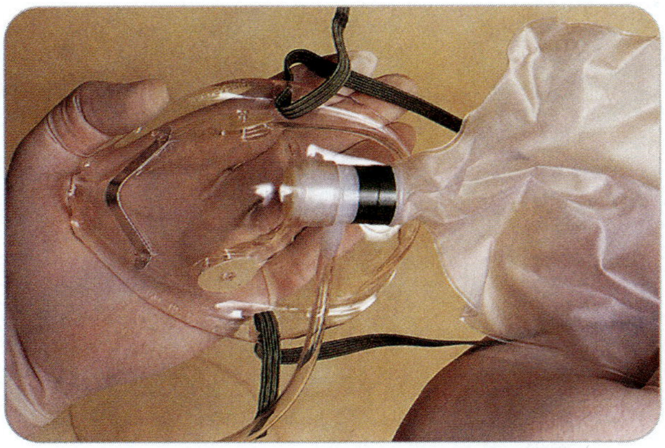

Figure 9-19 A nonrebreather oxygen mask will deliver a higher concentration of oxygen to your patient.

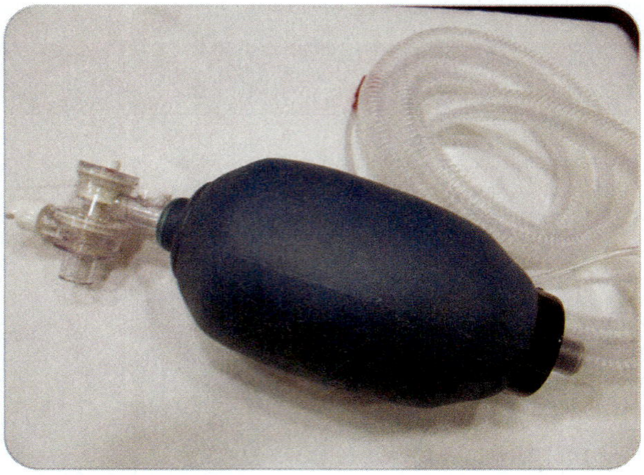

Figure 9-20 A bag-valve mask can deliver the highest percentage of oxygen to a critical patient. Be sure to select the appropriate size of mask and bag for the patient you are treating.

source of air to breathe. Use nonrebreather masks for patients who require a high flow of oxygen, including patients experiencing serious shortness of breath, severe chest pain, carbon monoxide poisoning, and congestive heart failure.

Exhaled air is directed through a one-way valve in the mask, which prevents the inhalation of room air and the reinhalation of exhaled air. The valve, along with a sufficient seal around the patient's nose and mouth, allows for the administration of high concentrations of up to 90% oxygen.

There are disadvantages of a nonrebreather mask. The mask covers both the nose and the mouth, possibly causing anxiety. Reassurance may relieve the patient's anxiety. Communication with the patient may be difficult due to the mask's position over the mouth and the noise of oxygen flow.

To prepare a nonrebreather mask for use, remove the mask from its protective wrapper and connect the attached connecting tubing to the regulator. Set the regulator at the desired flow rate, usually 15 LPM while simultaneously holding down the flap valve located inside the nose piece of the mask until the reservoir completely inflates. After the bag inflates, place the mask on the patient's face, placing the elastic strap behind the patient's head to hold the mask in place.

Once the mask is properly positioned on the patient's face, gently squeeze the aluminum nose piece to help ensure a good seal. Then observe while the patient breathes. Upon each inspiration, the reservoir bag should deflate by about one-third of its total volume. Adjust the flow from the initial 15 LPM downward so oxygen is not wasted, provided the bag stays partially inflated during inspiration. This is very important during a prolonged rescue. A fully deflated bag results in less oxygen for the patient.

Bag-Valve Mask

A **bag-valve mask (BVM)** is a ventilation device OEC technicians use for patients who are not breathing, need assisted ventilation, or are critical. The system consists of an oxygen reservoir, a self-expanding squeezable bag (about the size of a football), a one-way valve, a universal adaptor, and a clear flexible face mask (**Figure 9-20**). The mask is typically constructed from silicone, whereas the reservoir and universal adapter are generally fashioned from plastic. With the mask in place on the patient, when you squeeze the bag, oxygen (when connected) or just air is delivered to the patient. BVMs come in three basic sizes: adult, child, and infant. When the appropriately sized bag is used, the device should automatically deliver the correct volume of oxygen per breath. The unit should be latex-free.

With an oxygen flow rate of 15 LPM and an adequate mask-to-face seal, a BVM with an oxygen reservoir can deliver nearly 100% oxygen. The volume delivered also can vary, depending on bag size and depth of ventilation (**Table 9-4**). Because of its size, it is usually included as part of a large medical backpack.

One-Person BVM Ventilation

The one-person BVM technique should be used only when other rescuers are not available to assist.

Table 9-4 Bag-Valve Mask Ventilation Volumes

Size	Volume
Adult	1,200–1,600 mL
Pediatric	500–700 mL
Infant	150–240 mL

If two rescuers are available, use the two-rescuer method. A properly sized oral or nasal airway should be inserted into the unresponsive patient before using a BVM to help keep the airway open when assisting with ventilation.

First assemble the system. Fully expand the bag. Connect the reservoir. If available, connect oxygen and set the flow rate to 15 LPM. The reservoir should begin to fill immediately. Attach the universal, L-shaped adapter to the other end of the bag. Last, connect the face mask to the universal adapter. The system is now ready to use.

To perform one-rescuer BVM ventilation, follow these steps:

1. Assemble your equipment and kneel next to the top of the patient's head. Open the patient's mouth using the head tilt–chin lift or jaw-thrust maneuver (**Figure 9-21**).
2. Suction as necessary to clear secretions. Insert an oral or nasal airway (**Figure 9-22**).
3. Select the appropriate mask and position it properly on the patient's face. Place the mask on the patient's face with the apex (top) of the mask over the bridge of the patient's nose (**Figure 9-23**). The base of the mask fits in the groove between the patient's lower lip and chin. With your nondominant hand, place your thumb on the mask over the bridge of the patient's nose and your index finger on the mask over the patient's lower lip, forming a "C" shape around the mask-valve opening. With your little, ring, and middle fingers, grasp the underside of the patient's mandible.
4. Pull upward with your fingers on the jaw, opening the airway. To form a tight seal, the mandible should be pulled up toward the mask rather than the mask being pushed onto the patient's face. With your dominant hand, compress the bag, watching for chest rise to deliver a breath. If you become tired, reverse your hands (**Figure 9-24**).

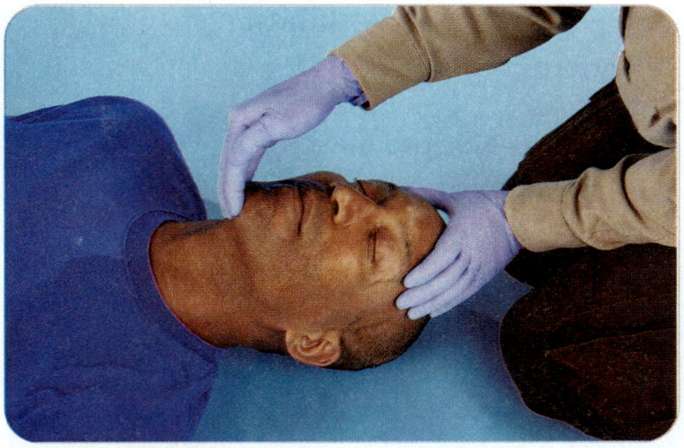

Figure 9-21 Open the airway using the head tilt–chin lift or jaw-thrust maneuver.

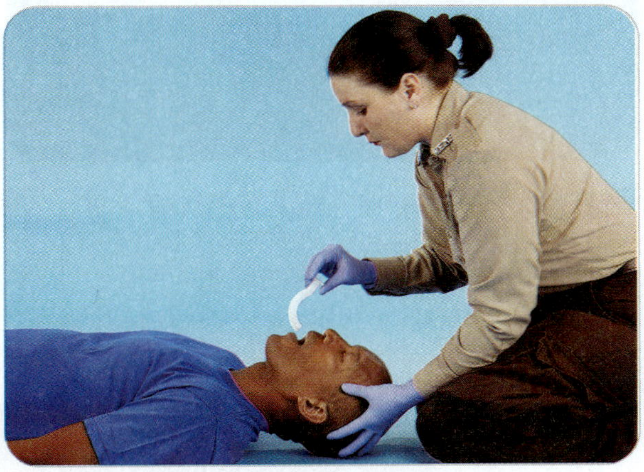

Figure 9-22 Suction as necessary and insert an oropharyngeal or nasopharyngeal airway.

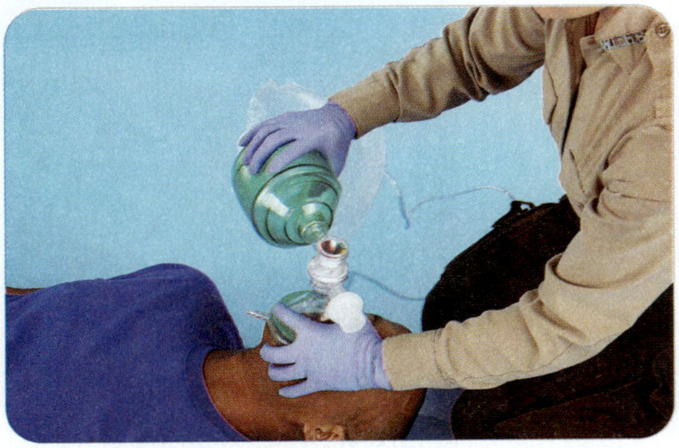

Figure 9-23 Select the appropriate mask and place it on the patient's face.

Two-Person BVM Ventilation

To perform two-person BVM ventilations, follow these steps:

Rescuer 1 (holds the mask):

1. Assemble your equipment and kneel to the side of the patient's head.
2. Place the mask onto the patient's face as described previously in the one-person BVM technique.
3. Place your thumbs alongside the edges of the mask. The thumbs and the padded portions of the palm at the base of each thumb should be in contact with the mask.
4. Using the middle, ring, and little fingers of each hand, grasp the underside of the mandible and pull upward, opening the airway. As before, the mandible should be pulled up toward the mask rather than pushing the mask onto the face.

Rescuer 2 (bagger):

1. Kneel beside Rescuer 1, near the top of the patient's head.
2. Squeeze the bag with both hands while watching for chest rise (**Figure 9-25**).

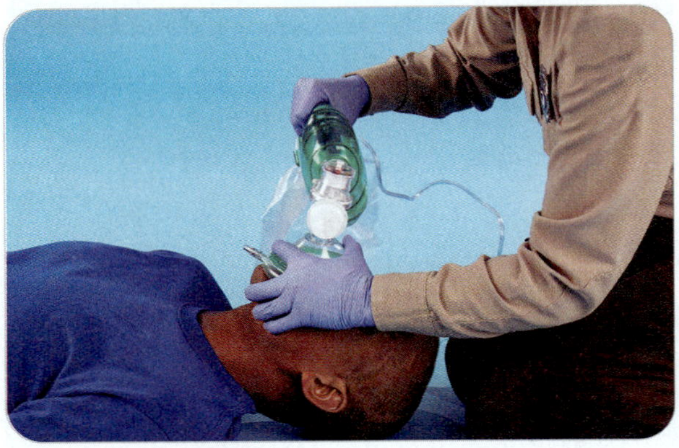

Figure 9-24 Pull upward with your fingers on the jaw, opening the airway. Compress the bag, watching for chest rise to deliver a breath.

Pulse Oximetry

A **pulse oximeter** is a noninvasive device that evaluates oxygenation at the tissue level by measuring oxygen saturation of hemoglobin in red blood cells (**Figure 9-26**). The device has a photoelectric sensing probe and a monitor. The probe is clipped onto a finger, toe, or earlobe, measuring the oxygenation of the blood in the capillaries.

The "pulse ox" gives a reading of % O_2 saturation, or O_2 sat. Normal oxygen saturation is

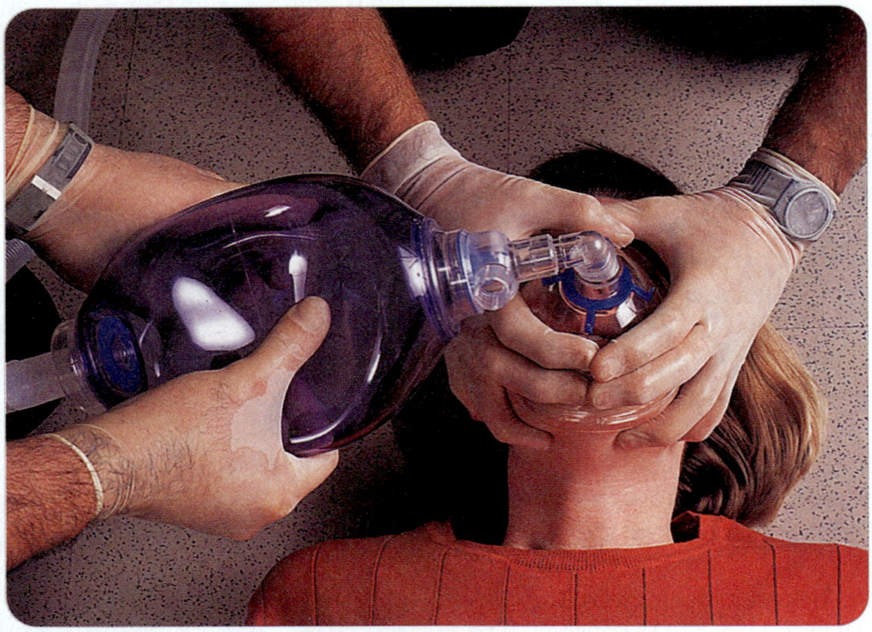

Figure 9-25 With two-person BVM ventilation, you hold the mask in place while your partner squeezes the bag.

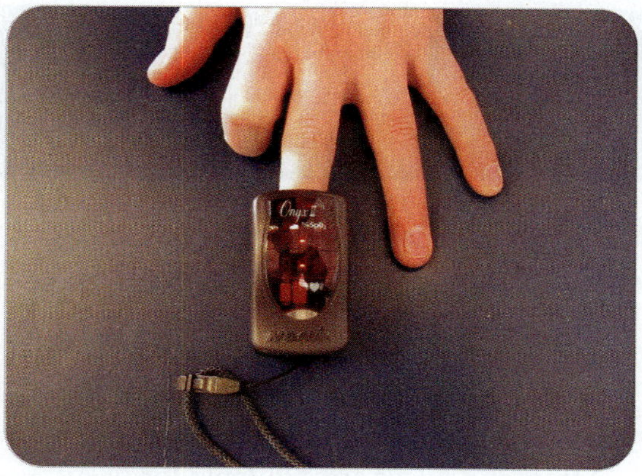

Figure 9-26 Pulse oximeter.

KEY POINT

Pulse Oximetry

When placing a patient on high-flow oxygen, start at 15 LPM. Using a reliable pulse oximeter, adjust the flow, keeping the patient's oxygen saturation between 94% and 99%.

between 94% and 99% when a person is breathing room air normally at sea level. Some people with chronic lung disease may have lower normal levels than this. Patients with an oxygen saturation less than 94% generally require treatment unless they have a chronic condition that causes perpetually low oxygen saturations.

Pulse oximetry, like other diagnostic instruments, is not foolproof and should not be used as the sole method of assessing oxygenation because false readings can occur. Factors that can cause false readings include nail polish, cold weather, shock, carbon monoxide poisoning, a low red blood cell count, and device malfunction. Clinical assessment of the patient generally is more reliable than a pulse oximeter.

Gastric Distention

Whenever artificial ventilations are provided, the patient's stomach can fill with air, causing abdominal bloating, known as **gastric distention**. This condition occurs when the amount of pressure pushing air or oxygen into the upper airway exceeds the pressure keeping the opening of the esophagus closed, causing gas to be directed down the esophagus and into the stomach. Partial or total obstruction of the upper airway can also cause gastric distention to occur. The condition is more common in children than in adults. This can be prevented by administering slow, gentle breaths. *Do not overventilate* the patient by squeezing the bag too fast. CPR teaches to ventilate at a controlled rate. The chest should rise and fall as if the patient were breathing in a normal fashion.

If the stomach becomes distended, make sure the airway is open. Do not push on a distended stomach because the result is nearly always vomiting, which can lead to aspiration of the vomit. If the patient does vomit, place the patient on his or her side in the recovery position, suction the airway, and then resume rescue breathing.

CASE Outcome

As other providers and equipment arrive, you request another OEC technician to assist you in two-person ventilation using a BVM attached to oxygen, and you suction the patient as needed. The patient's arm is splinted. Continuing to immobilize the patient's head and spine, you and the other providers place the patient onto a stretcher and transport him to a waiting ambulance. Later you learn the patient had a severe head injury. The doctor who treated the patient credits your team for effective airway management.

CHAPTER REVIEW

In Summary

- Respiration is the act of breathing, where air enters the body through the airway passage and then is expelled back into the environment.
- Breathing consists of two phases, inhalation and exhalation.
- Airway management is a skill every OEC technician must master. The airway must remain open and clear. PRACTICE OFTEN!
- The head tilt–chin lift maneuver is the preferred technique for opening the airway of medical patients; the jaw-thrust must be used to open the airway of trauma patients with a head or neck injury and may be used on medical patients.
- If foreign bodies can be seen blocking the airway, use a finger sweep to clear the airway.
- Suctioning, gravity and positioning, and abdominal thrusts are alternative methods of clearing the airway.
- Suction for a maximum of 10 to 15 seconds for an adult and 5 to 10 seconds for a child.
- The recovery position can help keep a patient's airway open and clear.
- If it is necessary to insert an airway device to keep the airway open, a nasopharyngeal airway (NPA) or an oropharyngeal airway (OPA) may be used. An OPA should be inserted only in a patient who does not have a gag reflex. Always attempt to place an airway adjunct in a patient who is unresponsive.
- A barrier device should be used to provide rescue breaths until the arrival of a bag-valve mask and oxygen.
- Several pieces of equipment are required to administer supplemental oxygen, including an oxygen cylinder, a pressure regulator/flowmeter, and an oxygen delivery device.
- Oxygen cylinders are vessels containing highly compressed gas. They should be laid on their side, kept in a protective carrier, or firmly secured to a wall to prevent them from falling. Turn the oxygen cylinder off when it is not in use.
- Different devices are available for giving oxygen to a patient, including the nasal canula, face masks such as the nonrebreather mask, and the bag-valve mask.
- If oxygen saturation is between 94 and 99%, oxygen is not needed.

Key Terms

Airway The natural passageway that allows air to enter and exit the lungs.

Bag-valve mask (BVM) A manually operated resuscitator consisting of an oxygen reservoir, a self-expanding squeezable bag, a one-way valve, a universal adaptor, and a face mask; used to assist patient ventilations.

Barrier device A personal protective device that provides a nonporous layer between the provider and the patient to prevent the transmission of communicable diseases.

Epiglottis A thin, leaf-shaped structure posterior to the tongue; covers the larynx when swallowing, preventing food or liquid from entering the airway.

Exhalation The act of expelling breath or air out of the lungs.

Face shield A clear, usually rectangular, plastic sheet that includes a mouthpiece through which rescue breaths are administered.

Finger sweep A method of clearing the airway when a foreign body is seen in the mouth of an unresponsive patient.

Flowmeter A device on oxygen cylinders used to control and measure the flow of oxygen.

Gastric distention Inflation of the stomach with air; can lead to vomiting.

Head tilt–chin lift maneuver A method used to open the airway when there is a possible cervical spine injury. The head is tilted as the chin is lifted.

Inhalation The act of drawing breath or air into the lungs.

Jaw-thrust maneuver The primary technique used to open a patient's airway, where the jaw is thrust forward.

Nasal cannula An oxygen delivery device consisting of plastic tubing with two open prongs that are inserted into the patient's nostrils; provides low-flow oxygen when connected to an oxygen source.

Nasopharyngeal airway (NPA) A trumpet-shaped airway adjunct made from soft rubber or silicone inserted into the nostril to maintain a patent airway.

Nonrebreather mask An oxygen delivery device that has a mask, a one-way flow valve, and a reservoir bag; when connected to an oxygen source, provides a high concentration of supplemental oxygen.

Oropharyngeal airway (OPA) A rigid plastic airway adjunct inserted into the oropharynx to maintain a patent airway.

Patent A descriptive term for an airway that is open and clear.

Pocket mask A triangular or pear-shaped barrier device made from clear, soft plastic or silicone.

Pulse oximeter A device that attaches to a patient's finger, toe, or earlobe and photoelectrically measures blood oxygen content as a percentage of oxygen saturation.

Suctioning The process of creating a vacuum to clear foreign material that is obstructing the airway.

Chapter Questions

1. What is the function of the epiglottis?
   a. Exchanging carbon dioxide and oxygen between the air and the blood
   b. Warming and humidifying air as it enters the body
   c. Preventing food or liquids from entering the lower airway
   d. Removing dust particles that enter the airway
2. The purpose of a pulse oximeter is to:
   a. evaluate oxygenation at the tissue level.
   b. assist with the oxygenation of a patient who is not breathing.
   c. assist with the breathing of a patient who is experiencing dyspnea.
   d. measure breathing and pulse rates.
3. You are called to the lodge and find a woman who is slumped in a chair. Upon assessment, you find that she is unresponsive and breathing normally. Her airway appears to be open and clear. Her friend tells you that she had complained of not feeling well and then "fell asleep." The preferred way to position this patient would be:
   a. supine.
   b. in the recovery position.
   c. in a position of comfort.
   d. in a semi-Fowler position.
4. You are artificially ventilating a patient, and you notice signs of gastric distention. The patient vomits. In order to correct the problem and prevent aspiration, you should:
   a. increase the rate and pressure of the ventilations.
   b. press down on the distended stomach.
   c. perform a blind finger sweep in the oropharynx.
   d. place the patient in the recovery position and suction the airway.
5. When administering supplemental oxygen to a patient, it is important to remember to:
   a. use only petroleum-based lubricants.
   b. secure the tank.
   c. tighten screws and knobs as much as possible.
   d. leave the cylinder on when not in use.
6. When determining whether to use supplemental oxygen, you should consider:
   a. signs of hypoxia.
   b. the patient's illness or injury.
   c. the patient's oxygen saturation levels.
   d. All of the above

7. When performing a finger sweep, it is important to:
    a. ensure the patient is responsive.
    b. perform a "blind" finger sweep.
    c. curve your finger into a hook to remove an object that can be seen.
    d. preoxygenate the patient.

8. You appropriately size a nasopharyngeal airway by measuring the:
    a. distance from the patient's mouth to the angle of the jaw.
    b. diameter of the patient's larger nostril.
    c. distance from the patient's nostril to the earlobe.
    d. diameter of the patient's thumb.

Answers: 1. c, Objective 9-1, p. 198; 2. a, Objective 9-12, p. 218; 3. b, Objective 9-5, p. 203; 4. d, Objective 9-13, p. 219; 5. b, Objective 9-9, p. 212; 6. d, Objective 9-9, p. 213; 7. c, Objective 9-4, p. 201; 8. c, Objective 9-6, p. 207

CHAPTER 10

SHOCK

OBJECTIVES

Upon completion of this chapter, the OEC technician will be able to:

10-1 Define shock.
10-2 Describe the three primary causes of shock.
10-3 Describe how the body compensates for shock.
10-4 Define the two stages of shock.
10-5 List the four major types of shock.
10-6 List the classic signs and symptoms of shock.
10-7 Describe and demonstrate the management of shock.

KEY TERMS

Anaphylactic shock, p. 228
Anticoagulants, p. 231
Cardiogenic shock, p. 228
Distributive shock, p. 228
Fainting, p. 230
Hypovolemic shock, p. 227
Neurogenic shock, p. 229
Obstructive shock, p. 229
Perfusion, p. 224
Peripheral vascular resistance, p. 226
Pulmonary embolism, p. 230
Sepsis, p. 228
Septic shock, p. 228
Shock, p. 224
Stroke volume, p. 226
Tachycardia, p. 226
Tachypnea, p. 226

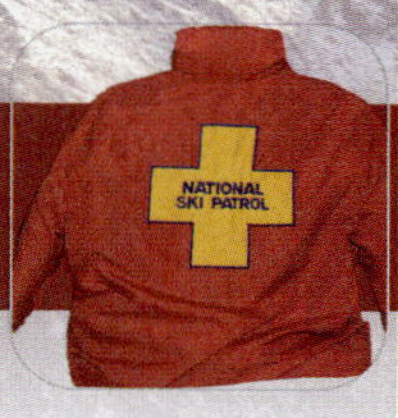

HISTORICAL TIMELINE **1964.** The NSP adopts the gold cross as its official emblem.

CHAPTER OVERVIEW

One of the most serious threats to life is the condition known as shock. **Shock** is defined as inadequate perfusion or flow of blood to the cells, causing cellular and tissue hypoxia due to reduced oxygen delivery. **Perfusion** is the circulation of blood within an organ or tissue in adequate amounts to meet the cells' current needs for oxygen, nutrients, and waste removal. The body is perfused via the cardiovascular (circulatory) system.

Although the potential causes of shock are numerous, shock occurs when one or more components of the cardiovascular system fail. This sets into motion a series of events that, unless corrected, may cause other body systems to fail and death to ensue. Shock is initially reversible but must be recognized and treated immediately to prevent progression to irreversible organ dysfunction.

Shock is one of the most serious problems that OEC technicians will encounter. It is caused by various medical and traumatic conditions. Unfortunately, the signs and symptoms of shock may not be apparent initially because the body compensates, maintaining normal vital signs. The patient's overall health, age, and medications taken may make shock more difficult to recognize at first. OEC technicians must be keenly aware of the causes of shock and the body's responses to it. Using this information, OEC technicians will be better able to recognize shock and initiate appropriate treatment (**Figure 10-1**).

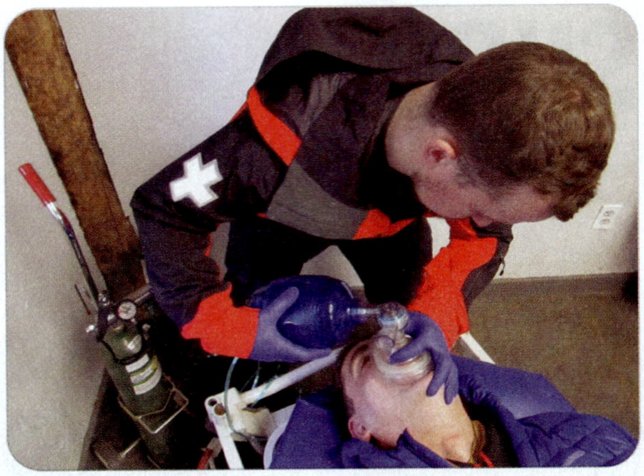

Figure 10-1 A patroller assisting with respirations.

ANATOMY AND PHYSIOLOGY

The cardiovascular (circulatory) system, described in detail in Chapter 6, *Anatomy and Physiology*, includes the heart, blood vessels, and blood. When functioning properly, the heart pumps oxygenated blood through arterial vessels to the capillaries, where oxygen and carbon dioxide are exchanged at a cellular level. Deoxygenated blood travels through venous blood vessels to the heart, which pumps the blood on to the lungs. There, carbon dioxide is excreted into the atmosphere and the blood is oxygenated and returned to the heart, which begins the cycle again.

Problems affecting any part of the circulatory system can disrupt this process, resulting in decreased blood flow, cellular hypoxia, and shock.

CASE Presentation

On a gentle slope, you find an approximately 55-year-old man holding his left side. You identify yourself and ask if you can examine him. While talking to him, you find he fell about 10 minutes ago on his left side. As you begin your assessment, the man says he's fine and really doesn't think any examination is necessary. Although he appears a little pale, his radial pulse seems normal, perhaps a little slow. As you gently touch his left upper abdomen and lower chest, he winces slightly.

What should you do?

Review of the anatomy and physiology of the circulatory system will help you understand shock. If the pump (heart), blood vessels (arteries and veins), or blood is affected, tissue will not receive oxygen and nutrients, resulting in shock.

CAUSES OF SHOCK

There are different types of shock, resulting from three basic causes. Any of these three conditions results in decreased perfusion, with insufficient oxygen or nutrients reaching vital organ tissue. When two or more of these conditions occur together, shock develops rapidly.

1. *Pump failure.* If the heart cannot pump correctly (i.e., the heart fails), then cardiac output decreases and blood is not pumped to the body adequately to sustain life.
2. *Failure of blood vessels to respond properly.* In this condition, the veins and arteries expand too much, pooling blood in them. The smooth muscle in the arteries and veins does not constrict these tubes during some pathological conditions.
3. *Low fluid volume.* In this condition, there is not enough blood to pump through the system. Blood can be lost through internal or external bleeding, or a medical condition can decrease the amount of healthy blood. Also, body fluids can be lost due to dehydration, from causes such as diarrhea or vomiting, burns, or excessive intake of diuretics (fluid pills).

STAGES OF SHOCK

Shock is a progressive disorder that can be divided into two stages: compensated shock and decompensated shock (**Table 10-1**).

Compensated Shock

The human body can compensate to maintain homeostasis even during times of stress or harm. The body's systems have built-in redundancy and flexibility that correct adverse conditions without incurring a total shutdown of body systems or long-term organ damage. In times of increased metabolic demand, the body activates various compensatory mechanisms that help restore homeostasis, but those mechanisms can function only for a while unless the problem is corrected.

Table 10-1 The Progression of Shock

Progression	Signs and Symptoms
Compensated shock	• Agitation • Anxiety • Restlessness • Feeling of impending doom • Altered mental status • Weak, rapid (thready), or absent pulse • Clammy (pale, cool, moist) skin • Pallor, with cyanosis about the lips • Shallow, rapid breathing • Air hunger (shortness of breath), especially if there is a chest injury • Nausea or vomiting • Capillary refill of longer than 2 seconds in infants and children • Marked thirst • Narrowing pulse pressure
Decompensated shock	• Falling blood pressure (systolic blood pressure of 90 mm Hg or lower in an adult) • Labored or irregular breathing • Ashen, mottled, or cyanotic skin • Thready or absent peripheral pulses • Dull eyes, dilated pupils • Poor urinary output

KEY POINT

Blood Pressure and Shock

During the early stages of shock, the patient's blood pressure is maintained.

If the body detects a decrease in the amount of blood being circulated or a sudden decrease in the amount of oxygen reaching the cells, the brain sends signals that stimulate the release of epinephrine, a hormone that causes **tachycardia** (the heart to beat faster) and the ventricles to contract more forcefully. Both changes increase the **stroke volume** (amount of blood pumped out of the left ventricle into the aorta during one heartbeat), which enables more blood, oxygen, and nutrients to reach the body's tissues and organs.

In addition, the central nervous system controls smooth muscles in the blood vessels, contracting the vessels (decreasing their diameter) or dilating them (increasing their diameter). **Peripheral vascular resistance** refers to the tightening of the smaller-diameter blood vessels in the extremities. By increasing resistance of blood flow to the extremities, blood flow to the vital organs increases, a key compensation in the early phases of shock.

At the same time, the brain sends signals to increase the rate and depth of respirations to bring more oxygen into the body and expel more carbon dioxide. This combination of tachycardia, increased stroke volume by the heart, increased peripheral vascular resistance, and increased oxygen, by faster breathing, helps to stabilize the internal environment, at least temporarily.

Compensated shock, therefore, is the body's ability to maintain blood perfusion and oxygenation to vital tissues under adverse conditions. If left uncorrected, shock would inevitably lead to death (**Figure 10-2**). It is important to keep in mind that the body's ability to compensate for shock early can mask a gravely serious uncorrected condition, giving you the false impression that the patient is less sick or less injured than is in fact the case.

The first signs of shock are tachycardia, **tachypnea** (respiratory rate greater than 20 breaths per minute), delayed capillary refill (greater than 2 seconds), cool skin, anxiety or restlessness, and a *normal* blood pressure. Treated early, this form of shock is correctable and generally has no long-term adverse effects. Untreated, however, shock will progress until the body is no longer able to compensate. Treatment involves correcting the condition causing shock.

Decompensated Shock

If the body's compensatory mechanisms are unable to restore blood perfusion to the tissues, cellular hypoxia will worsen, and the body's organs and systems will fail. Heart rate will continue to rise, systolic blood pressure will now begin to fall (to below 90 mm Hg), and respirations may become shallow. The skin will become grossly pale

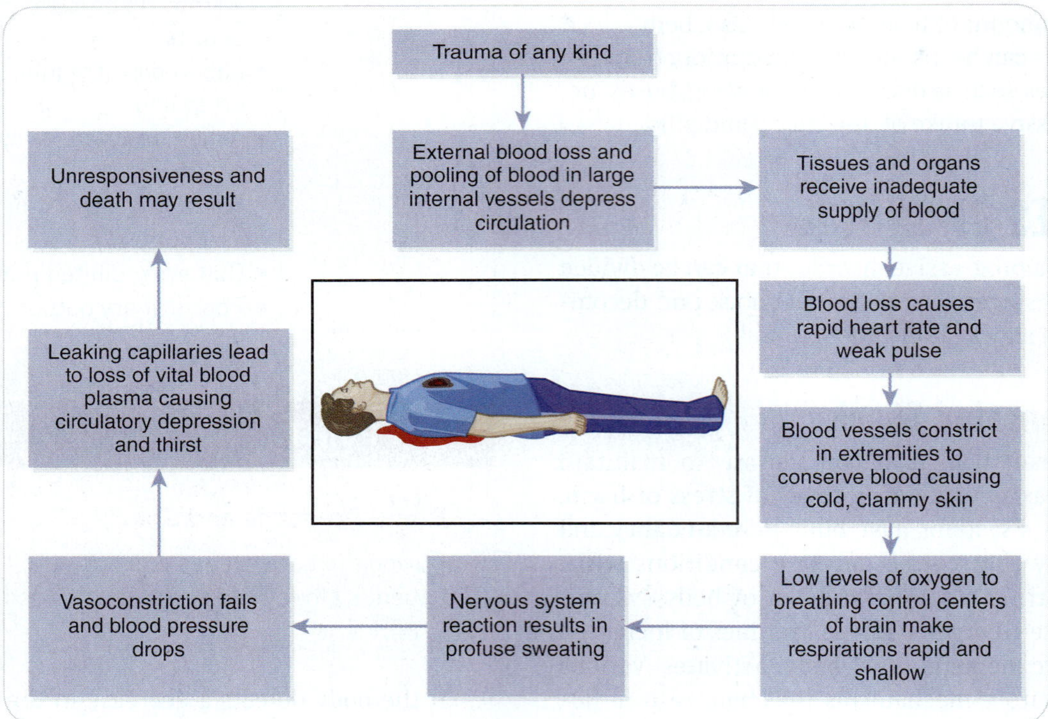

Figure 10-2 The progression of shock.

or cyanotic and will be cool and moist to the touch. Due to severe constriction of the blood vessels in the extremities, capillary refill will be significantly delayed and may become undetectable. The patient's level of responsiveness will decrease (less than *A* on the AVPU scale) due to decreased oxygen in the brain. Treated early, decompensated shock may be corrected, but serious complications can result.

Once the body's compensating mechanisms fail, vital signs deteriorate very rapidly as cells begin to die. This sets into motion a cascading effect that cannot be reversed. As more cells die, the tissues of various organs die, resulting in organ system failure and eventually death. Despite even aggressive treatment, this form of shock is not reversible and is fatal. It is difficult for a first responder to determine when shock can no longer be reversed.

TYPES OF SHOCK

As previously noted, shock occurs when one or more of the circulatory system's components are adversely affected by disease or injury. These problems can be either volume related (e.g., not enough blood), pump related (e.g., heart not pumping correctly), or container related (e.g., dilated blood vessels). With these possible causes firmly in mind, OEC technicians must be familiar with four major types of shock: hypovolemic shock, cardiogenic shock, distributive shock, and obstructive shock. Hypovolemic shock is caused by loss of circulating blood volume or body fluids. Cardiogenic shock is caused by the heart not pumping correctly. Distributive shock is a result of poor vessel function, resulting in the circulating blood pooling in the blood vessels. Obstructive shock is caused by a blockage in the cardiovascular system preventing blood flow.

Hypovolemic Shock

Hypovolemic shock results from a critical decrease in circulating fluid volume from bleeding or a loss of internal body fluid (**Figure 10-3**). This is the most common type of shock an emergency medical responder will see from a patient who has excessive bleeding. There are hemorrhagic and nonhemorrhagic causes of hypovolemic shock. Injuries involving bleeding result in hemorrhagic shock, while severe dehydration from vomiting and diarrhea may result in nonhemorrhagic shock.

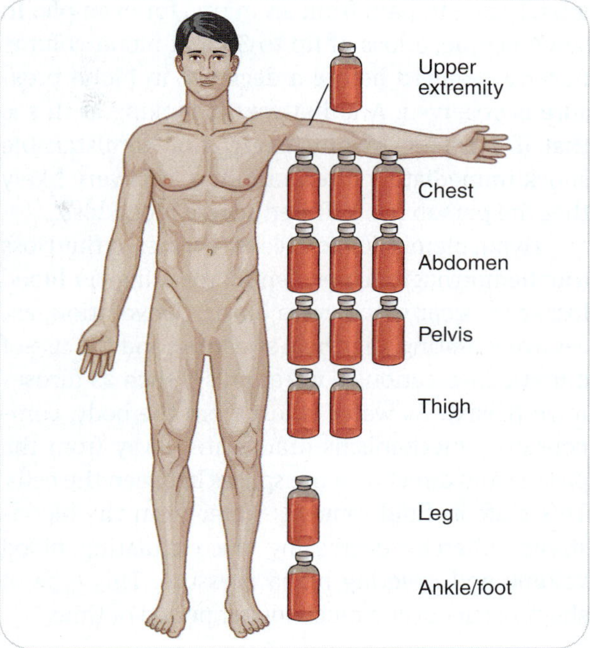

Figure 10-3 Potential blood loss from injuries in various parts of the body. Each bottle equals 1 pint (473 mL).

Of the two, hemorrhagic shock is more common and has more far-reaching effects.

Blood loss that results in hemorrhagic shock can be caused by a variety of problems, including trauma, gastrointestinal bleeding, vascular disruption, vaginal bleeding, and bleeding that is a complication of pregnancy. Bleeding disorders and certain medications (discussed later) may increase the severity of bleeding by preventing blood from clotting normally.

Blood loss can be external and obvious, or it can be internal and hidden. The American College of Surgeons divides blood loss due to hemorrhage into four classes, ranging from class I, mild blood loss (less than 15% of total blood volume, or the equivalent of donating 1.5 units of blood) to class IV, extremely life threatening (blood loss of 40% of total blood volume or greater). Due to the body's compensating mechanisms, a decrease in blood pressure may not be noted until more than 20% to 30% of total blood volume is lost.

The body can typically compensate for blood loss. Only with significant hemorrhage do alterations in blood pressure occur. An early indicator of hemorrhage is a relative tachycardia, but it can be difficult to attribute increased heart rate to shock in the context of someone who may be experiencing anxiety due to pain from an injury, for example. In some people, a loss of up to 30% of blood volume may be required before a decrease in blood pressure is observed. Another way of looking at this is that if a person manifests signs of unmistakable shock immediately after an injury, it is very likely that the person has suffered severe blood loss.

Hypovolemia due to excessive water or fluid loss (nonhemorrhagic hypovolemia, meaning no blood loss) can occur with severe burns, dehydration, excessive vomiting, diarrhea, sweating, and the use of diuretic medications ("water pills") such as furosemide (Lasix). As water is lost from the body, compensatory mechanisms draw water away from the plasma and direct it to the spaces between the cells. This shift in fluid removes water from the bloodstream, thereby decreasing the circulating blood volume and lowering blood pressure. This type of shock occurs over a much longer period of time.

Cardiogenic Shock

Cardiogenic shock is a condition in which the heart cannot adequately pump blood, resulting in poor cardiac output. Although the heart is a robust organ, it may fail for a variety of reasons, including valve problems, which prevent the heart from filling or emptying properly; heart attack, which results from heart muscle damage; slow or fast heart rates, which decrease cardiac output; legal and illegal medications; and trauma to the heart.

Distributive Shock

Distributive shock occurs when blood vessels lose their ability to constrict appropriately. The resulting decrease in arterial vascular resistance causes blood to pool within the capillary beds, producing a sudden drop in blood pressure and cellular hypoxia. Thus, distributive shock is a container-related problem. Under normal conditions, arterial resistance (the diameter of the blood vessels) is regulated by certain body chemicals, the nervous system, and local nerve receptors that help to ensure blood is delivered to where it is needed. Based on the underlying cause, distributive shock (when the blood vessels dilate, pooling blood in the vessels) is subdivided into three subtypes: anaphylactic shock, septic shock, and neurogenic shock.

Anaphylactic Shock

Anaphylactic shock is caused by a severe allergic reaction to a substance (**Figure 10-4**). Common causes of anaphylaxis include insect bites or stings; consumption of shellfish, nuts, or other foods; and use of certain medications (**Table 10-2**). Normally, when an offending source is introduced into the body, the immune system responds by releasing chemicals that aid the immune response to neutralize the foreign substance. In a susceptible person, these chemicals cause generalized dilation of the blood vessels and a host of other pathological problems. Without intervention, anaphylactic shock can quickly lead to respiratory arrest and death. A complete description of anaphylaxis, including causes, assessment, and treatment, is provided in Chapter 14, *Allergies and Anaphylaxis*.

Septic Shock

Septic shock is caused by a severe systemic infection known as **sepsis** and is the most common cause of distributive shock. Normally the immune system's white blood cells are released from the capillaries and attack and destroy pathogens such as invasive bacteria. If the pathogens or their toxins overwhelm the body and get into the

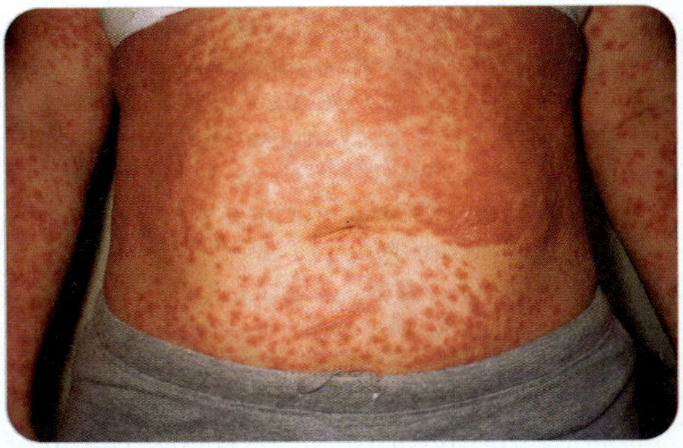

Figure 10-4 This patient is suffering from an anaphylactic reaction.

Courtesy of Carol B. Guerrero.

Table 10-2 Causes of Allergic Reactions

- Foods (peanuts, sesame seeds, tree nuts, soy, milk, eggs, chocolate, shellfish)
- Environmental irritants (smoke, airborne particles)
- Pollen (weeds, grasses, trees)
- Molds (mildew, spores)
- Animal dander (skin flakes, fur)
- Medications (antibiotics, pain medications)
- Chemicals (latex)
- Other causes (blood transfusions, organ transplants, radiographic dyes)

bloodstream, sepsis occurs, resulting in a potentially life-threatening illness that involves severe fever, shaking "chills," and shock.

Although most infections resolve quickly, a variety of factors can increase the likelihood of sepsis, including how resistant the body is to the pathogens, how virulent the pathogens are, how well the immune system is functioning, and the overall health of the individual. Underlying medical conditions may also affect one's ability to fight infection. Additionally, medications can adversely affect the immune system. Unless sepsis is corrected, the pathogens will multiply beyond control, causing profound vasodilation, cellular hypoxia, and death.

Neurogenic Shock

Neurogenic shock, sometimes called spinal shock, is caused by a marked drop in blood pressure resulting from disruptions of the central nervous system, most often from a spinal cord injury. When the spinal cord is damaged, normal neurologic input to the blood vessels is disrupted, causing the vessels to dilate.

Fortunately, this process is not generally seen immediately after a spinal cord injury, usually occurring hours or possibly days later. *OEC technicians should never attribute low blood pressure (hypotension) seen with a recent traumatic spinal cord injury to neurogenic shock only. The most likely cause of shock in any trauma patient presenting with signs and symptoms of shock is hemorrhagic shock due to blood loss.*

Obstructive Shock

Obstructive shock results when a blockage prevents oxygenated blood from reaching vital organs. The cause can be either external pressure being placed on the heart or a blockage within the body's vascular system. Thus, the problem can be pump-related (heart) or container-related (blood vessels). The most common causes of obstructive shock are tension pneumothorax, pericardial tamponade, and pulmonary embolism.

Tension Pneumothorax

Between the membrane on the outside of each lung and the membrane on the inside of the chest cavity is a potential space, called the pleural space. This space is filled with a very small amount of pleural fluid, the lubricating properties of which allow the lungs to move freely while expanding and

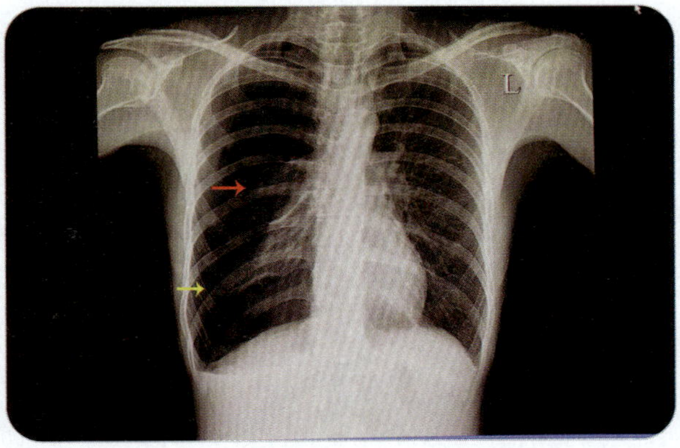

Figure 10-5 A tension pneumothorax is accumulation of air in the space between the inside of the chest cavity and the lung that causes the lung to collapse.

contracting during inhalation and expiration. If the integrity of the chest wall or lung is compromised (most often by trauma), air can seep into the pleural space causing a tension pneumothorax (air in the pleural space compressing the lung) (**Figure 10-5**). Unless the air is given a way to escape, pressure within the chest cavity will rise, causing the lung to collapse and obstruction of venous blood returning to the heart, thus impeding the heart's ability to pump effectively. This obstruction can significantly reduce the amount of blood that enters and exits the heart, causing a corresponding drop in blood pressure and shock. Thus, tension pneumothorax is a pump-related disorder caused by obstruction of blood flow. A complete description of tension pneumothorax, its causes, and treatment are covered in Chapter 23, *Chest Trauma*.

Pericardial Tamponade

Obstructive shock can occur if fluid accumulates within the pericardium, the sac surrounding the heart. This fluid accumulation is called pericardial tamponade (**Figure 10-6**). As a result, the right side of the heart, which pumps blood to the lungs, cannot expand (collapses) from the pressure of the fluid, decreasing cardiac output and causing shock. The right side of the heart is more vulnerable to such collapse than the left side because the walls of the right side are thinner and less muscular than those on the left side. Pericardial tamponade is thus a pump-related problem. Fluid that accumulates in the pericardial space may be free blood caused by penetrating chest trauma, fluid that slowly accumulates from a medical condition, or pus resulting from a massive

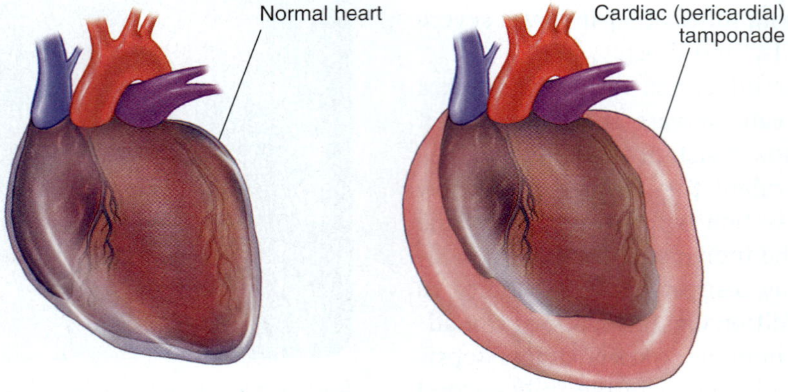

Figure 10-6 Pericardial tamponade.

cardiac infection. Pericardial tamponade is covered in more detail in Chapter 23, *Chest Trauma*.

Pulmonary Embolism

A **pulmonary embolism**, or thromboembolism, is a condition where a blood clot becomes stuck in and blocks a pulmonary artery (**Figure 10-7**). The pulmonary artery connects the heart to the lung, where oxygen enters the blood. When a blood clot, called a thrombus, breaks loose at a distant location, usually a vein in the legs or pelvis, it can travel as an embolism through the right side of the heart and lodge in the pulmonary artery. The resulting blockage disrupts the flow of blood through the lungs and back to the heart and prevents gas exchange in the lungs. Pulmonary embolism is rapidly fatal if it occurs in a large pulmonary artery

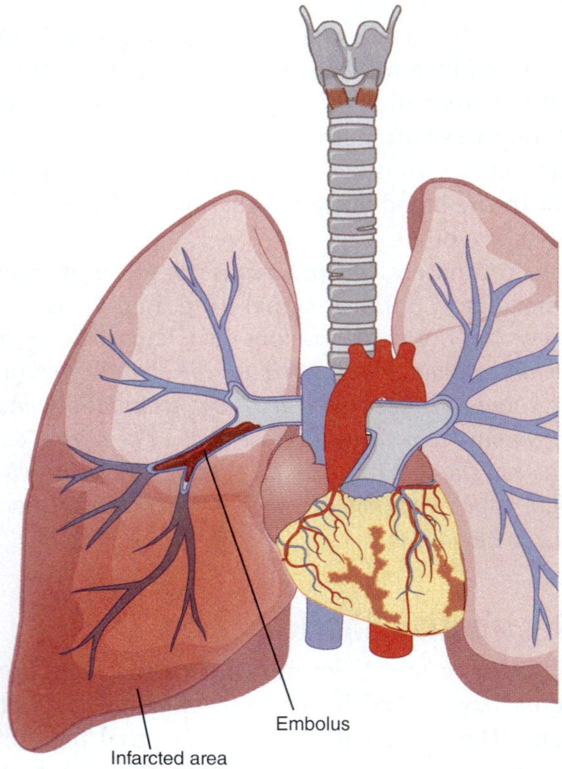

Figure 10-7 A Pulmonary embolism.

KEY POINT

Fainting

Fainting, or syncope, is a loss of consciousness that results from a lack of blood flow to the brain. This condition may occur suddenly, resulting from the temporary dilation of the body's veins and pooling of blood in those vessels. Hypotension or low blood pressure of *brief duration* occurs. Because less blood is getting to the brain, a syncopal episode occurs. Syncope is usually caused by fear, bad news, or an upsetting stimulus such as the sight of blood. It is resolved by placing the patient, or helping the patient to lie, in a supine position with the feet raised 12 inches.

Syncope is not a type of shock. Although usually a benign condition, it can be the result of an arrhythmia or other serious medical condition. The patient should be advised to seek medical care.

CASE Update

You suspect the man may be injured and secure the area by placing both your skis and his in an "X" several yards above your location. When you return, you obtain a more complete history. He tells you that his doctor recently put him on a blood thinner to prevent clots. He also tells you that he is taking a beta-blocker for high blood pressure. As you are talking with him, the man appears slightly confused and says, "I don't feel very well." You radio for help, oxygen, and ALS transport.

What do you think the problem is? What should you do next?

and is not treated immediately. A more detailed description of pulmonary embolism is presented in Chapter 13, *Respiratory Emergencies*.

FACTORS AFFECTING SHOCK

Young and healthy individuals have the greatest capacity to compensate for shock, especially in its early stages, whereas very young and older or chronically ill individuals have less effective compensatory mechanisms and may abruptly decompensate after an initial period of *apparent* stability. Other factors can influence how the body compensates for shock.

Children maintain vital signs even though they are in shock for a while. They have better early compensating mechanisms than adults, with tachycardia and tachypnea present early. However, when they reach a certain point in shock, they "crash" rapidly into irreversible shock. The *symptoms* of shock in children usually appear late or delayed. A reliable indicator to the onset of shock in children is sudden lethargy or fussiness. Do not rely on blood pressure, which is maintained in early shock in children. Hypovolemic shock is the most common type in children, due to blood loss or hypovolemia from vomiting and/or diarrhea.

The presence of injury or illness, for example, can affect the severity of shock and can have cumulative effects. Preexisting medical conditions such as diabetes, heart disease, or anemia (a reduction in the number of circulating red blood cells) can hasten the effects of shock. Mind-altering substances can mask or mimic the signs of shock by altering vital signs and also can eliminate pain from an injury. Even prescribed medications can alter the body's response to shock. OEC technicians must be aware that certain medications can mask the classic signs of shock by preventing the body's compensatory mechanisms from working properly.

One group of prescribed medications that can affect the presentation of shock is the beta-blockers, which are used to treat heart disease and high blood pressure. Because beta-blockers limit the heart's ability to beat faster, users of these medications may not be able to generate a faster heart rate when the body is in shock. If the heart rate cannot increase, then the body's ability to compensate for shock by increasing cardiac output is limited. Among the most widely used beta-blockers are atenolol (Tenormin), metoprolol (Lopressor), and propranolol (Inderal).

Another group of medications of which you should be aware are **anticoagulants**, which inhibit the blood's natural ability to clot (**Table 10-3**). Anticoagulants can prolong bleeding, which can worsen hemorrhagic shock. Thus, even a seemingly minor injury can result in profound shock due to the body's inability to stop bleeding. Any patient who is taking one or more of these medications must be carefully assessed for any evidence of hemorrhaging, both external and internal. Aspirin will also prolong bleeding. You must control bleeding in all patients.

Table 10-3 Anticoagulants
• Warfarin (Coumadin) • Enoxaparin (Lovenox) • Clopidogrel (Plavix) • Dabigatran (Pradaxa) • Rivaroxaban (Xarelto) • Apixaban (Eliquis)

KEY POINT

Beta-Blockers and Shock

Beta-blockers prevent the heart from speeding up, much like a governor on a car motor prevents the engine from over-revving. During shock, the heart cannot respond to pump more blood to the tissues.

Table 10-4 Signs and Symptoms of Shock

- Tachycardia (fast heart rate)
- Hypotension (low blood pressure), occurs *later*
- Tachypnea (shortness of breath)
- Thirst, weakness, and nausea
- Pale, cool, diaphoretic skin
- Restlessness or combativeness
- Altered mental status (occurs *later*)

PATIENT ASSESSMENT FOR SHOCK

Assessment of patients in shock is no different than it is for any other patients. It begins with a scene size-up, during which potential threats to rescuer safety are identified and mitigated. Try to identify the mechanism or injury or nature of illness, including evidence of trauma, heart attack, external or internal bleeding, allergy, or infection.

The scene size-up is followed by a primary patient assessment, looking at the ABCDs (airway, breathing, circulation, and disability). Remember, when a responsive or unresponsive patient has life-threatening bleeding, it is more appropriate to address this life threat first, following a CABD sequence (circulation, airway, breathing, and disability). If there is a life threat, correct it or start CPR if needed. After the ABCDs are addressed, if the patient is in shock, call for help, request ALS if available, and transport immediately.

When obtaining the history, pay close attention to known allergies, as they may have precipitated or contributed to the patient's condition. Determine if the patient is taking any medications that could alter the body's compensatory response to shock. Additionally, consider the patient's age and determine whether the patient has taken any mind-altering drugs.

If you begin to suspect impending shock during your secondary patient assessment of a patient who appears stable initially, immediately shift gears, correcting the ABCDs and arranging transport. Examine the patient carefully for any evidence of injury, both external and internal. Careful consideration of the mechanism of injury, along with your knowledge of the locations of internal organs, could lead you to suspect internal bleeding.

Obtain vital signs and repeat them, noting each value; even subtle changes in the pulse rate, blood pressure, or respiratory rate could indicate an underlying shock state. Be ever vigilant for the "classic" signs and symptoms of shock (**Table 10-4**).

Although it is important to recognize the classic signs and symptoms of shock, remember that shock is a developing condition that may not be obvious when the patient is first examined due to the compensatory mechanisms previously described. Normal age-specific vital signs can be seen in the early stages of shock. It is important to note that hypotension and altered mental status come later in shock. Frequent reassessment of the patient is essential and should include monitoring the vital signs and mental status at regular intervals.

When assessing a patient for shock, keep in mind the types of shock, the conditions with which they are associated, and whether the clinical picture you are seeing fits the situation. Pay close attention to the pulse pressure (the difference between systolic and diastolic pressures) because a narrowing of pulse pressure is an early indicator of shock in cardiac tamponade. Hot, dry skin, especially when combined with fever and low blood pressure, may indicate septic shock. Assess the patient's face and hands for evidence of swelling, which could indicate an anaphylactic reaction. Neurogenic shock typically presents with warm, dry skin as opposed to the more classic presentation.

MANAGEMENT OF SHOCK

Management of a patient in shock centers on returning the patient to a state of homeostasis. Given that shock is caused by inadequate tissue perfusion and oxygenation, initial treatment is focused on correcting any problems causing shock.

Follow the steps in **OEC Skill 10-1** for the treatment of a patient in shock.

OEC SKILL 10-1 Managing Shock

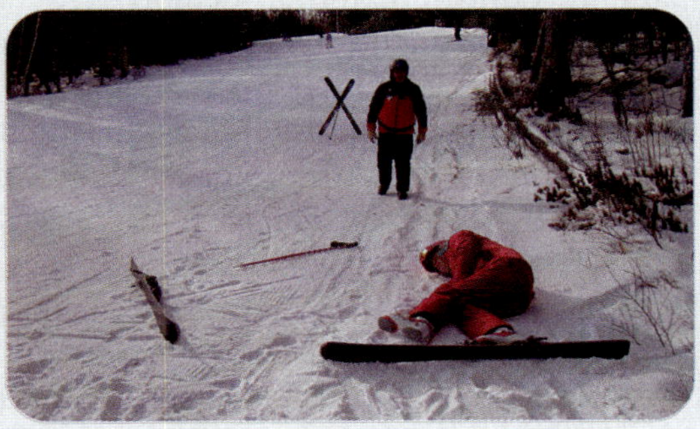

1 Assess scene safety and follow standard precautions.

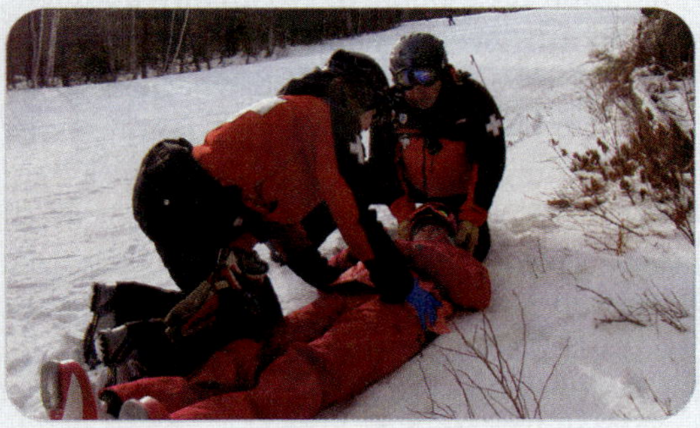

2 Perform a primary patient assessment. Control major bleeding and assess ABCDs. Correct any problems found. If the patient has no pulse, begin CPR.

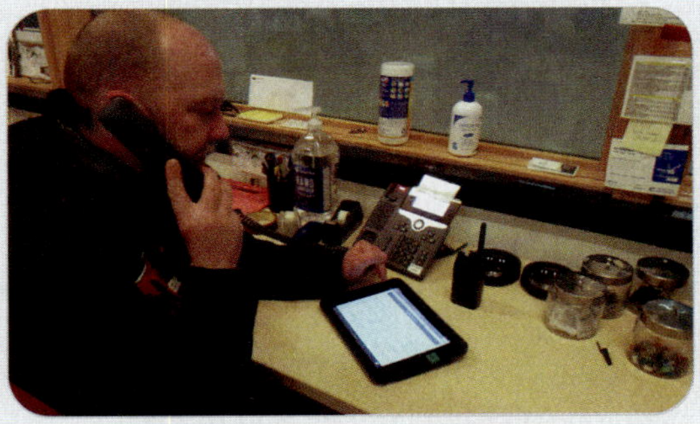

3 Call for help and arrange for transport that includes ALS.

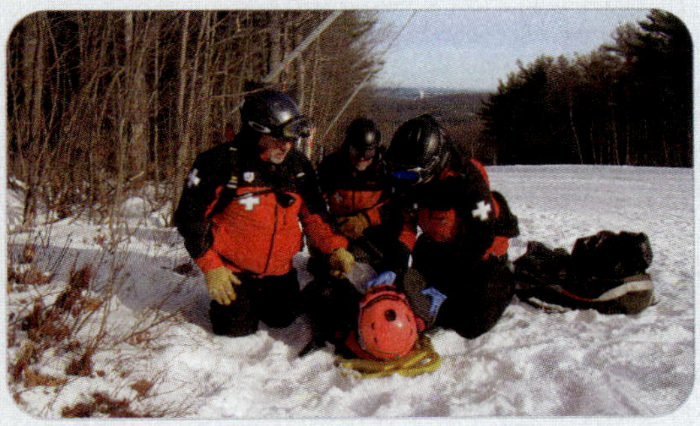

4 Monitor the airway and administer high-flow oxygen.

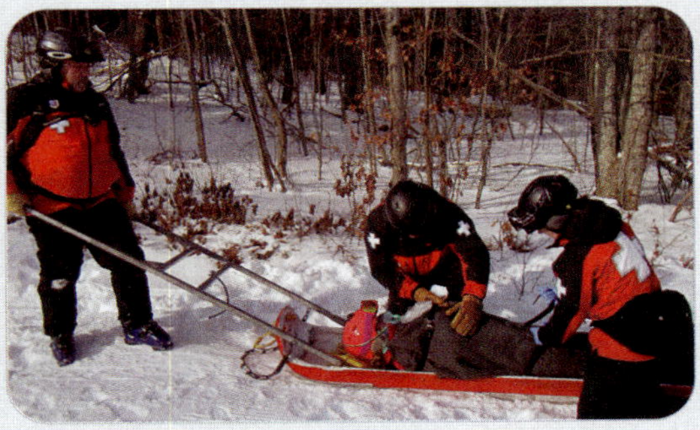

5 To prevent heat loss, keep the patient warm and dry. Provide rapid transport.

Major bleeding and problems affecting the ABCDs identified during the primary assessment must be corrected. If the patient has no pulse, immediately begin CPR. Ensure that the patient's airway is open and clear, using airway adjuncts, and suction as necessary. Support the patient's ventilatory efforts as needed. If the patient is not breathing or if breathing is slow or shallow, assist ventilations using either a pocket mask or a bag-valve mask connected to supplemental oxygen. If the patient is unresponsive, insert a properly sized oropharyngeal airway or a nasopharyngeal airway.

For a patient who is breathing, administer high-flow oxygen at 15 liters per minute via nonrebreather mask to maximize tissue oxygenation. If a pulse oximeter is available and the patient's hand is warm, titrate oxygen so that the reading on the pulse oximeter remains between 94 and 99%. If oxygen is not easily available, do not delay transport of the critical patient. Control external hemorrhage (severe bleeding) using the techniques presented in *Soft-Tissue Injuries and Burns* is Chapter 19 Keep the patient warm and dry. Additional treatment depends on the nature of other problems that are present. If you can, correct the *cause* of shock. The treatments for specific causes of shock, such as anaphylaxis, heart attack, and tension pneumothorax, are covered in other chapters.

Other therapies, such as intravenous therapy, blood, or medications, can be administered by advanced care providers and are often lifesaving.

CASE Outcome

Two other patrollers arrive on scene. You inform them you believe the patient is suffering from shock due to internal injuries from the fall. The situation has been made worse because he takes a beta-blocker and an anticoagulant. Working with the other patrollers, you quickly put the man on high-flow oxygen and place him into a toboggan. You ski down with the toboggan team and help them move the patient into the first-aid hut. Soon after, a helicopter arrives and transports the patient to a local trauma center.

Several months later, you are in the ski area's cafeteria when someone taps you on the shoulder. It's the man and he thanks you for "saving my life" and informs you that your suspicions were confirmed. Lifting his sweater, he shows you an abdominal scar. He tells you that the impact of the crash ruptured his spleen and that had you not stopped and insisted that he be treated, he likely would have died of shock.

CHAPTER REVIEW

In Summary

- Shock is caused by inadequate perfusion, or flow of blood to the cells, causing cellular and tissue hypoxia due to reduced oxygen delivery.
- Review of the anatomy and physiology of the circulatory system will help you understand shock. If the pump (heart), blood vessels (arteries and veins), or blood is affected, tissue will not receive oxygen and nutrients, resulting in shock.
- There are different types of shock, resulting from three basic causes: pump failure, failure of blood vessels to respond properly, and low fluid volume.
- Shock is a progressive disorder that can be divided into two stages: compensated shock and decompensated shock.
- There are four major types of shock:
  - *Hypovolemic* shock results from a critical decrease in circulating fluid volume from bleeding or a loss of internal body fluid. There are hemorrhagic and nonhemorrhagic causes of hypovolemic shock.
  - *Cardiogenic shock* is a condition in which the heart cannot adequately pump blood, resulting in poor cardiac output.
  - *Distributive shock* occurs when blood vessels lose their ability to constrict appropriately.
  - *Obstructive shock* results when a blockage prevents oxygenated blood from reaching vital organs. The most common causes of obstructive shock are tension pneumothorax, pericardial tamponade, and pulmonary embolism.
- Shock is a life-threatening condition.
- It is important to quickly identify the cause of shock and correct it if possible. The longer shock goes uncorrected, the less likely the patient is to recover.
- A patient's blood pressure may be normal during the early phase of shock.
- Elderly patients do not compensate well for shock.
- Children maintain vital signs better than adults, until they go into irreversible shock.

Key Terms

Anaphylactic shock A type of distributive shock that occurs when a person reacts violently to a substance to which he or she has become sensitized.

Anticoagulants Medications that prevent blood from clotting; "blood thinners."

Cardiogenic shock A type of shock caused by inadequate function of the heart, or pump failure, resulting in poor cardiac output.

Distributive shock A type of shock resulting from widespread dilation of the small arterioles, venules, or both.

Fainting A loss of consciousness that results from a lack of blood flow to the brain. This condition may occur suddenly, resulting from the temporary dilation of the body's veins and pooling of blood in those vessels. May also be referred to as syncope.

Hypovolemic shock A type of shock caused by an inadequate amount of fluid or volume in the circulatory system.

Neurogenic shock A type of distributive shock that is caused by disruptions of the central nervous system, most often from a spinal cord injury.

Obstructive shock A type of shock caused by a blockage that prevents oxygenated blood from reaching vital organs.

Perfusion The circulation of blood within an organ or tissue in adequate amounts to meet the cells' current needs for oxygen, nutrients, and waste removal.

Peripheral vascular resistance The tightening of the smaller-diameter blood vessels in the extremities, enabling increased blood flow to the vital organs.

Pulmonary embolism A condition where a blood clot becomes stuck in and blocks a pulmonary artery. May also be referred to as thromboembolism.
Sepsis A serious medical condition caused by the presence of pathogenic organisms or their toxins in the blood, leading to a systemic inflammatory response.
Septic shock A type of distributive shock that is caused by severe systemic infection.
Shock Inadequate perfusion, or flow of blood to the cells, causing cellular and tissue hypoxia due to reduced oxygen delivery.
Stroke volume The amount of blood pumped out of the left ventricle into the aorta during one heartbeat.
Tachycardia A heart rate greater than 100 beats per minute in adults.
Tachypnea A respiratory rate greater than 20 breaths per minute in adults.

Chapter Questions

1. Shock is defined as:
   a. failure of the cardiovascular (circulatory) system to maintain adequate blood flow to tissues.
   b. failure of the kidney to maintain adequate urine output.
   c. failure of the nervous system to send signals to the tissues.
   d. failure of the heart to beat correctly.
2. In order to compensate for shock, the brain sends signals to the body causing:
   a. blood vessels in the extremities to dilate.
   b. blood vessels of the heart to constrict.
   c. rate and force of heart contractions to increase.
   d. rate and depth of respirations to decrease.
3. A patient who is stung by a bee goes into anaphylactic shock. Blood vessels dilate, causing blood to pool in the vessels. What type of shock is this?
   a. Hypovolemic
   b. Cardiogenic
   c. Obstructive
   d. Distributive
4. You have been treating a patient with severe head injuries. His pulse is rising, his systolic blood pressure is falling, his respirations are shallow, his skin is cyanotic, and he has an altered mental status. In which stage of shock is this patient?
   a. Compensated
   b. Decompensated
   c. Irreversible
   d. Neurogenic
5. A man has a laceration on his arm and is bleeding. A woman nearby tells you that she cannot stand the sight of blood and then faints. Her fainting is the result of:
   a. temporary dilation of the body's veins, resulting in the pooling of blood in those vessels.
   b. the heart not adequately pumping blood, resulting in poor cardiac output.
   c. a critical decrease in circulating blood volume from bleeding or a loss of internal body fluid.
   d. blockage within the body's vascular system preventing oxygenated blood from reaching vital organs.
6. Your patient has received a crushing injury to the abdomen. You do not find any external injuries. You notice that your diaphoretic patient's skin has become pale and cool. Your patient is anxious and complains of thirst and nausea. Your emergency care should include:
   a. cooling the patient with damp towels or ice packs to the neck, armpits, and groin.
   b. transporting the patient in the toboggan with the head uphill.
   c. arranging for rapid transport to a medical facility.
   d. providing water.

7. A patient has a possible ruptured spleen, with a fast heart rate and dropping blood pressure. This type of shock is called:
   a. hypovolemic.
   b. cardiogenic.
   c. obstructive.
   d. distributive.

8. A patient with signs of shock attributed to pump failure has:
   a. poor cardiac output.
   b. femoral arterial bleeding.
   c. tension pneumothorax.
   d. sepsis.

Answers: 1. a, Objective 10-1, p. 224; 2. c, Objective 10-3, p. 226; 3. d, Objective 10-5, p. 228; 4. b, Objective 10-4, p. 226; 5. a, Objective 10-6, p. 230; 6. c, Objective 10-7, p. 232; 7. a, Objective 10-5, p. 227; 8. a, Objective 10-2, p. 225

CHAPTER 11

ALTERED MENTAL STATUS

OBJECTIVES

Upon completion of this chapter, the OEC technician will be able to:

11-1 Define altered mental status.

11-2 List causes of altered mental status using the mnemonic AEIOU-TIPS.

11-3 Describe and demonstrate the management of a transient ischemic attack.

11-4 List the signs and symptoms of the following medical conditions:
- Focal (partial) seizure
- Generalized seizure
- Hypoglycemia
- Hyperglycemia

11-5 Describe how to assess a patient with altered mental status.

11-6 Define FAST-ED and explain how this can be used to identify someone who is having a stroke.

11-7 Describe and demonstrate the management of the two types of stroke:
- Hemorrhagic stroke
- Ischemic stroke

11-8 Demonstrate the treatment of a patient with altered mental status.

KEY TERMS

Absence seizure, p. 245
Altered mental status, p. 240
Aura, p. 245
Clonic activity, p. 245
Coma, p. 243
Delirium, p. 242
Dementia, p. 244
Diabetes mellitus, p. 248
Epilepsy, p. 244
Generalized seizure, p. 245
Glucose, p. 240
Hyperglycemia, p. 248
Hypoglycemia, p. 248
Insulin, p. 241
Polydipsia, p. 248
Polyuria, p. 248
Seizure, p. 244
Stroke, p. 248
Tonic activity, p. 245

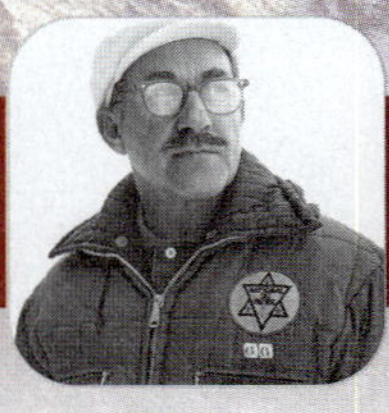

HISTORICAL TIMELINE **1968.** Harry Pollard becomes National Director.

CHAPTER OVERVIEW

The body constantly monitors its internal and external environment and rapidly adapts to changes. This process is controlled by the central nervous system (CNS), which regulates the functions of the other body systems. The CNS consists of the brain and spinal cord. The components of the nervous system were described in Chapter 6, *Anatomy and Physiology*.

To function properly, the CNS requires a steady stream of data from all parts of the body. To preserve homeostasis, the CNS requires a constant supply of oxygen, **glucose**, and other nutrients. Should the data stream or the body's internal equilibrium be disrupted, the brain will quickly lose its ability to respond appropriately, resulting in a condition known as altered mental status (**Figure 11-1**).

Altered mental status is an abnormal change in a person's level of awareness or responsiveness. Altered mental status is a potentially serious problem that indicates that something is wrong within the brain. There are many causes of altered mental status, some are life-threatening. Signs and symptoms of altered mental status affect many parts of the body, or they may be seen in only one part of the body. Symptoms may vary widely and be subtle. Altered mental status can challenge OEC technicians who, without the benefit of diagnostic equipment, must gather key information quickly, assess the patient and the surroundings for associated clues, and differentiate among the various causes, allowing them to implement appropriate lifesaving care. To accomplish this, OEC technicians must first understand how various factors affect the brain and responsiveness. Then, by using a systematic approach, you will ensure that none of the major causes of altered mental status are overlooked.

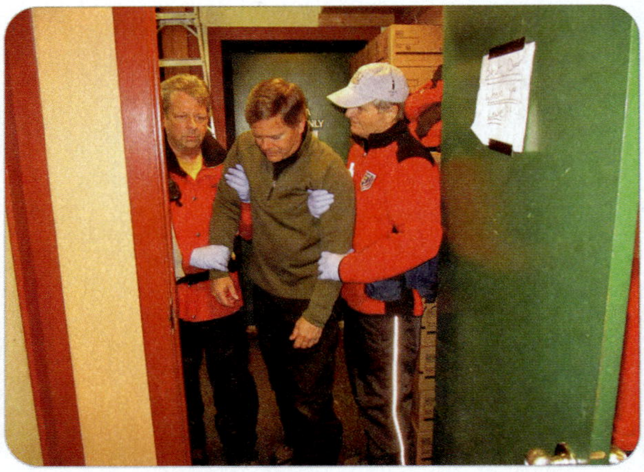

Figure 11-1 When the brain loses its ability to respond appropriately, this results in a condition known as altered mental status.

ANATOMY AND PHYSIOLOGY

Responsiveness is governed by a complex series of events that occur within the brain. One of the basic purposes of the nervous system is to sense the environment and to react to it. The nervous system helps us avoid extremes in temperature, seek oxygen or water, or find nutrients to sustain life. Humans have an extremely complicated nervous system capable of such highly evolved functions as speech, locomotion, and intellect. In biological terms, these functions are known as higher cortical functions. When these functions are compromised, the result is that the body's ability to sense and react is altered, resulting in the condition known as altered mental status.

The brain acts as a central processor that controls the rest of the body. The brain consists

CASE Presentation

In the bathroom at a ski resort, you find a woman on the floor. This middle-aged woman appears to be very confused and responds to verbal stimuli. Her radial pulse is fast and strong. Her skin is pale and cool to the touch, and she appears dyspneic (short of breath).

What should you do?

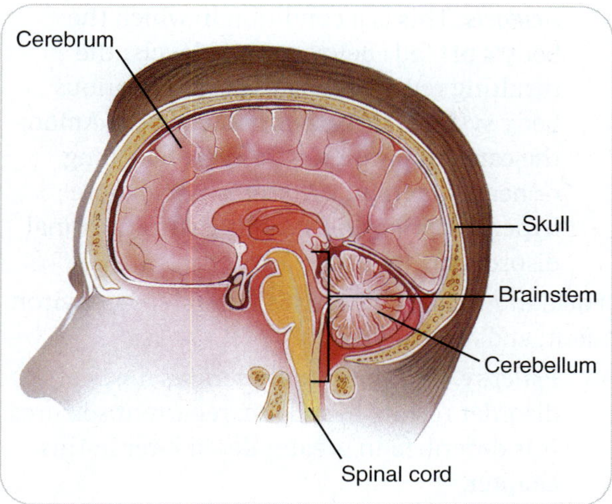

Figure 11-2 The different parts of the brain.

of three major parts: the brainstem, which controls functions necessary for life such as breathing, swallowing, responsiveness, heart function, and blood pressure; the cerebellum, which controls balance and coordination; and the cerebrum, which controls emotion, thought, speech, integration, and memory as well as sensation and motor function (**Figure 11-2**).

The lungs and vascular system provide oxygen to the brain. If this function is interrupted, altered mental status will occur.

The pancreas, an organ of the endocrine system, plays a unique role in human responsiveness due to its ability to regulate the supply of glucose, essential for proper brain and spinal cord function. The pancreas is an elongated organ located in the upper abdomen, posterior to the stomach (**Figure 11-3**). It secretes the hormones **insulin** and glucagon, which have a direct influence on circulating blood glucose (sugar) levels. Malfunction of the pancreas's hormonal system can cause blood sugar to be too high or too low, which in turn can affect mental status.

The pancreas constantly secretes insulin in low levels to maintain a constant level of sugar within the blood. After eating, blood sugar rises. In response, the pancreas secretes more insulin, which stimulates the muscle, liver, and fat cells to absorb glucose from the blood and lowers blood glucose back to normal levels. Excess glucose is converted to glycogen in the liver and muscle, or into fat and is stored for later use. Conversely, if

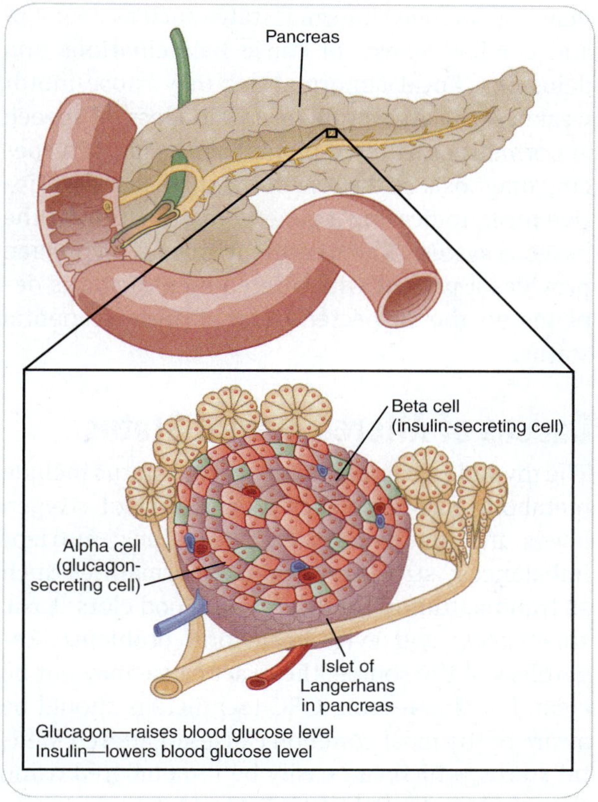

Figure 11-3 The pancreas makes glucose regulating hormones: insulin and glucagon.

the blood sugar level falls, as occurs during exercise or between meals, insulin secretion decreases, and the pancreas secretes glucagon. This hormone causes liver cells to release stored glycogen, which is then converted to glucose and released into the bloodstream. This ensures that the body has a constant supply of glucose even when food is not available. In diabetes, either enough insulin is not made by the pancreas, or insulin is not effective. If the regulation of blood sugar by these hormones becomes ineffective or altered, causing too high or too low a blood sugar, the result can affect the brain causing alterations in the level of sensory awareness or responsiveness.

ALTERED MENTAL STATUS

Malfunctions of the brain leading to altered mental status can affect all parts of the nervous system equally, or they can be localized, affecting only a portion of the body. Most changes typically present as decreased levels of responsiveness but may also include abnormal states such as **delirium** and combativeness, or cause hallucinations and delusions. Focal abnormalities may cause motor weakness, balance problems, vision loss, or speech abnormalities. Altered mental status is not a specific diagnosis or disease but is instead a descriptive term, indicating a general malfunction of the nervous system. The treatment an OEC technician provides a patient with altered mental status depends on the suspected cause of altered mental status.

Causes of Altered Mental Status

The myriad causes of altered mental status include metabolic disorders such as insufficient oxygen levels and low blood sugar; infections; nutrient imbalances; structural brain abnormalities such as trauma, tumors, and cerebral blood clots; toxic substances; and even behavioral problems. Regardless of the source, the exact cause may not be clear. For this reason, OEC technicians should be aware of the most common causes of altered mental status, which can easily be remembered using the acronym AEIOU-TIPS (**Table 11-1**):

The *A* in AEIOU-TIPS stands for alcohol and acidosis.

- *Alcohol.* It is the most widely abused drug in the United States and is among the leading causes of altered mental status in nearly every patient population group age 16 and older. This chemical depresses CNS function. A complete description of alcohol and its effects is presented in Chapter 12, *Substance Abuse and Poisoning*.

Table 11-1 Causes of Altered Mental Status: AEIOU-TIPS

A—Alcohol and acidosis
E—Epilepsy, environment, and electrolytes
I—Insulin
O—Oxygen (hypoxia) and overdose
U—Uremia (kidney failure)
T—Trauma, tumors, transient ischemic attack, and thirst
I—Infection (CNS, sepsis)
P—Poisoning and psychiatric conditions
S—Seizures, stroke, sleep, and syncope

- *Acidosis*. This is a condition in which the body's pH falls below normal levels; the resulting reduced effectiveness of various body systems threatens homeostasis. Among the causes of acidosis are decreased lung or heart function, kidney disease, severe hyperglycemia, and various gastrointestinal disorders.

The *E* in AEIOU-TIPS stands for epilepsy, environment, and electrolytes.

- *Epilepsy*. This potentially serious medical disorder results in sudden, recurrent seizures. It is described in greater detail later in this chapter.
- *Environment.* Changes in body temperature may also lead to altered mental status. The body must maintain a relatively constant internal temperature to function properly. Factors that cause core body temperature to rise above or fall below a tightly regulated temperature range can result in dramatic changes in a patient's level of responsiveness. Common conditions that can produce extreme temperature changes within the body are hypothermia (too cold) and hyperthermia (too hot), which are described in Chapter 25, *Cold-Related Emergencies*, and Chapter 26, *Heat-Related Emergencies*. Other environment-related causes of altered mental status include exposure to insect bites and stings.
- *Electrolytes*. These molecules within the body maintain energy gradients and help transmit electrical impulses within neurons. To maintain homeostasis, the body always requires that a careful balance of electrolytes be maintained. Any imbalance involving one or more electrolytes can affect cellular function, resulting in altered mental status. Electrolyte levels are affected by various conditions, including diet, exercise, medication use, and overall health. Factors such as excessive sweating, vomiting, or diarrhea can rapidly deplete electrolytes such as sodium, chloride, or potassium, resulting in an imbalance and altered mental status.

The first *I* in AEIOU-TIPS stands for insulin.

- *Insulin.* Any condition that adversely affects the production and use of insulin or the regulation of blood glucose levels can produce altered mental status.

The *O* in AEIOU-TIPS stands for oxygen and overdose.

- *Oxygen.* The brain requires an uninterrupted supply of oxygen to operate properly. Even minor decreases or short interruptions in oxygen levels result in an immediate decrease in CNS functioning and overall responsiveness. *Hypoxia is the most common cause of altered mental status.*
- *Overdose.* Overuse of drugs, whether prescription or illicit, is a cause of altered mental status that is frequently encountered by OEC technicians. Overdoses involving opiates and depressant agents are especially problematic because both depress CNS function and respiration, resulting in decreased oxygenation and altered levels of responsiveness. Heroin and fentanyl overdoses are common. Drug overdose is discussed in Chapter 12, *Substance Abuse and Poisoning*.

The *U* in AEIOU-TIPS stands for uremia.

- *Uremia.* This is a condition in which the kidneys are unable to effectively remove waste products from the body. Uremia causes lethargy, **coma**, and ultimately death unless the toxins are removed from the blood.

The *T* in AEIOU-TIPS stands for trauma, tumors, transient ischemic attack, and thirst.

- *Trauma.* Injury to the brain is an especially common cause of altered mental status (**Figure 11-4**). The resulting structural damage to the brain can cause focal altered mental status changes or more generalized alterations in the level of responsiveness. Bleeding from trauma or swelling of the brain from head injury reduces the amount of oxygen that reaches the brain's vital control centers. Brain injury is presented in more detail in Chapter 21, *Spine, Brain, and Nervous System Injuries*.
- *Tumors.* A tumor is an abnormal growth of cells that can be cancerous or malignant, or noncancerous or benign. Tumors within the brain or skull can impair normal brain function, causing both global and focal changes.
- *Transient ischemic attack (TIA).* A TIA is a reversible neurologic deficit that is caused by a *temporary* interruption of blood flow to an area of the brain. No permanent brain injury results, and the signs and symptoms resolve completely within 24 hours. TIAs are typically caused by a small embolus that only temporarily blocks a small artery within the brain. Signs and symptoms of a TIA appear when an embolus becomes temporarily lodged in and blocks one of the cerebral arteries.

  However, once the embolus dissolves, or no longer blocks the artery, the signs and symptoms quickly disappear. Although the symptoms often resolve spontaneously, a TIA serves as an early warning that a more serious stroke is likely to occur soon. About one in three patients that experience a TIA will eventually have a stroke. It is for this reason that patients who exhibit signs or symptoms of a TIA should seek immediate treatment at a hospital.
- *Thirst.* Dehydration, when significant, can also cause altered mental status.

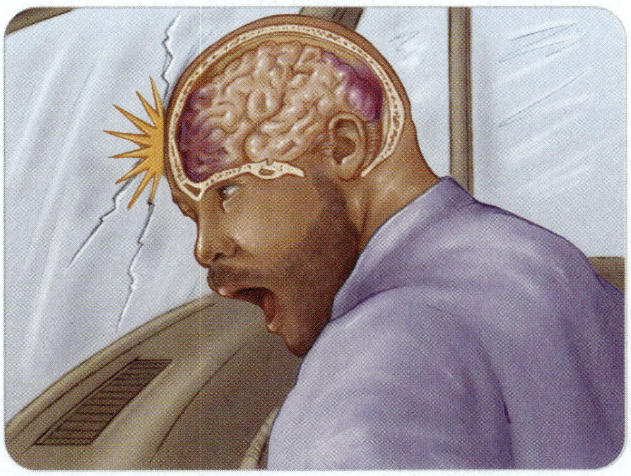

Figure 11-4 Different types of injury or trauma may cause altered mental status.

The second *I* in AEIOU-TIPS stands for infection.

- *Infection.* An infection anywhere in the body can spread through the bloodstream, a condition known as sepsis. Septic shock can affect mental status. Infections involving the brain and/or spinal cord (e.g., meningitis) also affect mental status.

The *P* in AEIOU-TIPS stands for poisonings and psychiatric conditions.

- *Poisoning.* A poison can cause altered mental status and injury or death. Described in Chapter 12, *Substance Abuse and Poisoning*, poisoning can be caused by innumerable substances and may occur accidentally or intentionally.

- *Psychiatric conditions.* A small percentage of patients with altered mental status may have a behavioral or underlying psychiatric disorder such as schizophrenia or manic-depressive disorder. Other common behavior-related disorders that can cause altered mental status are depression, Alzheimer disease, or **dementia**. Common psychiatric disorders are presented in Chapter 33, *Behavioral Emergencies and Crisis Response*.

The *S* in AEIOU-TIPS stands for seizure, stroke, syncope, and sleep.

- *Seizure.* A seizure is an electrical disturbance within the brain that causes alterations in awareness, attentiveness, responsiveness, behavior, or body movement.
- *Stroke.* This is a neurologic brain impairment resulting from low blood flow or a lack of blood flow to areas of the brain. Depending on what part of the brain is affected, different neurologic findings are present. OEC technicians should be familiar with two types of stroke and their signs and symptoms: ischemic (lack of circulating blood) and hemorrhagic (bleeding). The causes, signs, and symptoms of the two types of stroke are presented later in this chapter.
- *Syncope* (fainting). This temporary loss of responsiveness is due to a disruption in blood flow to the brain. Make sure the syncopal episode is not a function of a cardiac abnormality by asking appropriate questions and assessing vitals. Consider transport to a hospital.
- *Sleep.* Patients who suffer from even minor sleep deprivation may have altered mental status, decreased reaction times, poor memory, and irritability.

Conditions Associated with Altered Mental Status

Epilepsy

Epilepsy is a chronic medical condition that causes recurrent seizures in an otherwise healthy individual. According to the Epilepsy Foundation, approximately 3.4 million Americans have some form of epilepsy, and 150,000 new cases of epilepsy are diagnosed each year. Although the cause of this disorder is still relatively unknown, research has revealed several factors, including head injury and brain trauma, brain tumors, genetic conditions, and chemical imbalances.

With early diagnosis and proper treatment, patients with epilepsy can participate in a wide range of physically demanding activities. Therapeutic management of epilepsy is generally preventive in nature and involves the use of medications known as anticonvulsants, which help control seizure activity.

Seizures

A **seizure** is an electrical disturbance within the brain that causes alterations in awareness, attentiveness, responsiveness, behavior, and body movement. The signs and symptoms of seizures

CASE Update

An acquaintance states that she is unaware of the individual's past medical history. They were partying last night and drinking too much. The woman skipped breakfast. Her friend says that recently the woman has been drinking a lot of water and frequently goes to the bathroom. The friend says she has not fallen or been injured. At first you suspect she has hypoglycemia and you ask her to swallow. She can swallow, so you give her three packs of sugar dissolved in water. Her condition does not improve.

What should you do now?

can be mild or severe depending on the part of the brain affected. In its most dramatic form, a seizure results in violent, spasmodic movement of one or more opposing muscle groups and can cause a temporary loss of responsiveness. Seizures can last anywhere from seconds to hours, although most last 1 to 3 minutes. They usually end on their own and generally do not cause any long-term problems. Among the factors that may precipitate a seizure in susceptible individuals are pulsating lights or strobe lights and withdrawal from certain medications or alcohol. OEC technicians should be familiar with two types of seizures: focal (partial) seizures and generalized seizures.

Focal (Partial) Seizures

A focal or partial seizure can be simple (responsiveness is not altered) or complex (responsiveness is altered) and may involve sensory changes, involuntary skeletal muscle activity, or any combination of the two. A simple focal seizure originates in one side of the brain but under certain conditions can quickly spread to the other side. Thus, a simple focal motor seizure may present as an involuntary jerking motion of a specific muscle group such as those in the hand, or it can spread to involve the entire arm. Other signs associated with a simple focal motor seizure are grunting or incomprehensible vocalizations, tensing of the torso muscles, and facial twitching, usually on one side only.

A patient experiencing a simple focal sensory seizure may complain of blurred vision, seeing spots or flashing lights, abnormal smells, buzzing noises, hot or cold sensations, tingling, numbness, or abnormal metallic tastes. These types of seizures generally do not result in a loss of responsiveness. By comparison, a complex partial seizure starts in one area of the brain and results in a loss of responsiveness. Sometimes, individuals undergoing a complex focal seizure display repetitive actions, known as automatisms. Examples of these actions include lip smacking, tugging at their clothes, head twisting, or body turning.

Generalized Seizures

A seizure that typically affects both sides of the body equally and results in a decreased level of responsiveness is considered a **generalized seizure**. The mildest form, affecting mostly children and young adults, is called an **absence seizure**. This type of seizure, also called a petit mal seizure, is characterized by a vacant stare (i.e., "staring spells"), upward rolling of the eyes, or eyelid fluttering. An episode usually lasts less than 15 seconds and may not be noticed by others. The patient exhibits normal behavior immediately after and between episodes.

The most common type of generalized seizure, called a grand mal seizure, may occur without warning and is characterized by muscle tensing and contraction, better known as tonic-clonic activity. During **tonic activity**, the muscles of the body tightly contract, causing the patient to forcefully stiffen. During **clonic activity**, the muscle groups spasm violently. The two types of muscle activity can occur independently or simultaneously. A generalized seizure can occur at any time and has three distinct phases: the pre-ictal, ictal, and post-ictal phases.

- The *pre-ictal phase* occurs before the seizure and is sometimes preceded by a premonition of the impending seizure called an **aura**, a distinctive feeling or sensation that signals the patient a seizure is about to occur (**Figure 11-5**). Auras vary greatly among patients and are usually sensory in origin. They may present as a cognitive state such as déjà vu, a unique taste or smell, an auditory sensation or visual hallucinations. An aura usually lasts for only a few seconds but can last several minutes.
- The *ictal phase* usually begins with tonic (rigid, stiff) muscle activity during which

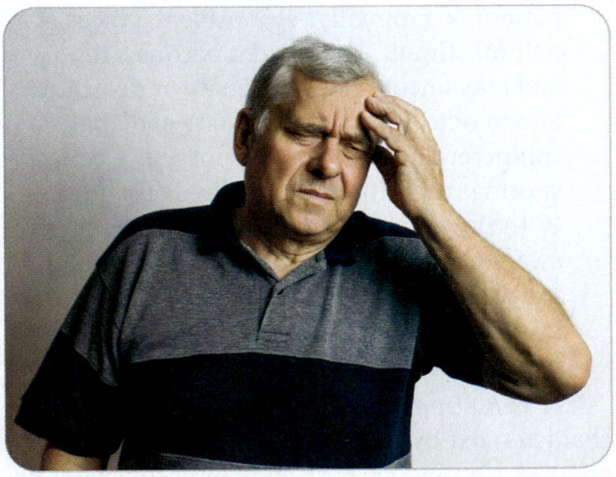

Figure 11-5 In the first, or pre-ictal phase an aura may be experienced.

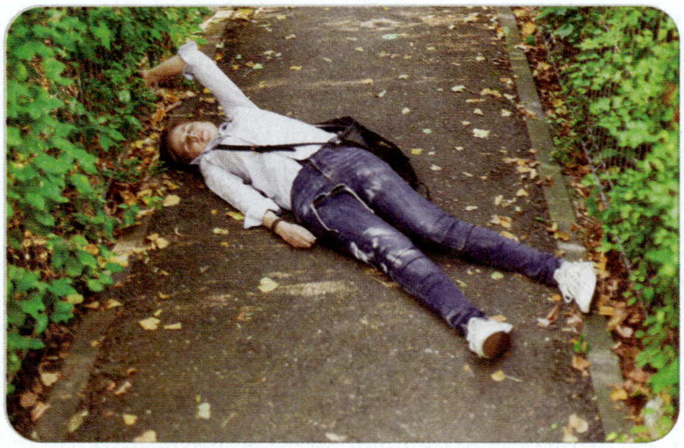

Figure 11-6 In the second, or ictal, phase of a grand mal seizure, the patient may first experience tonic movements followed by clonic muscle activity.

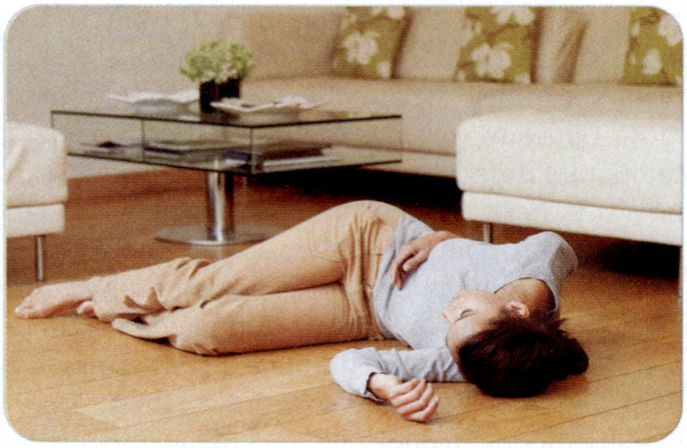

Figure 11-7 In the third, or post-ictal, phase of a grand mal seizure, the patient becomes flaccid and is minimally responsive.

the patient may cry out and or fall stiffly to the ground (**Figure 11-6**). Clonic (jerking) activity soon follows and may last for several minutes. During this phase the patient is unresponsive and may make grunting or gasping sounds. The jaw is usually clenched tightly, which can affect the patient's ability to breathe. In extreme cases, the patient may become slightly cyanotic, especially around the lips. The ictal phase typically lasts a very short time, usually 1 to 3 minutes. If the seizure lasts longer than 3 minutes, the cyanosis may become more pronounced.

- The *post-ictal phase* begins once tonic-clonic muscle activity stops. During this phase, the patient is minimally responsive to voices or painful stimuli. The patient becomes limp and may unconsciously urinate or defecate due to relaxation of the urinary and anal sphincter muscles. The patient may exhibit snoring respirations or appear disoriented. With time, the patient becomes increasingly aware of the surroundings while becoming fully responsive and completely oriented. It is common for OEC technicians to reach patients during this phase (**Figure 11-7**).

A condition known as status epilepticus is characterized by a seizure lasting longer than 10 minutes, a prolonged post-ictal unresponsive state, or three or more seizures without regaining consciousness or becoming responsive. This is a medical emergency that can cause permanent brain injury, because the tremendous amount of energy expended during a prolonged seizure quickly depletes the brain of important energy substrates, thereby destroying delicate brain neurons.

> **KEY POINT**
>
> **Seizure or Something Else?**
>
> Even though many people report having observed a seizure, often they saw some other medical condition that is unrelated to the brain. It is best to err on the side of caution: evaluate each report of seizure with the awareness that what you are seeing may be due to another medical condition and not a seizure.

Diabetes Mellitus

The body is very effective in maintaining a constant and appropriate supply of glucose in the blood (**Figure 11-8**). Normal blood sugar levels are between 80 and 140 mg/dL but may vary slightly depending on the individual's physiology and whether the person has recently eaten. When the body is no longer able to regulate the blood sugar level effectively and too much glucose is present in the blood, the patient is said to have diabetes mellitus, or simply "diabetes" (**Figure 11-9**).

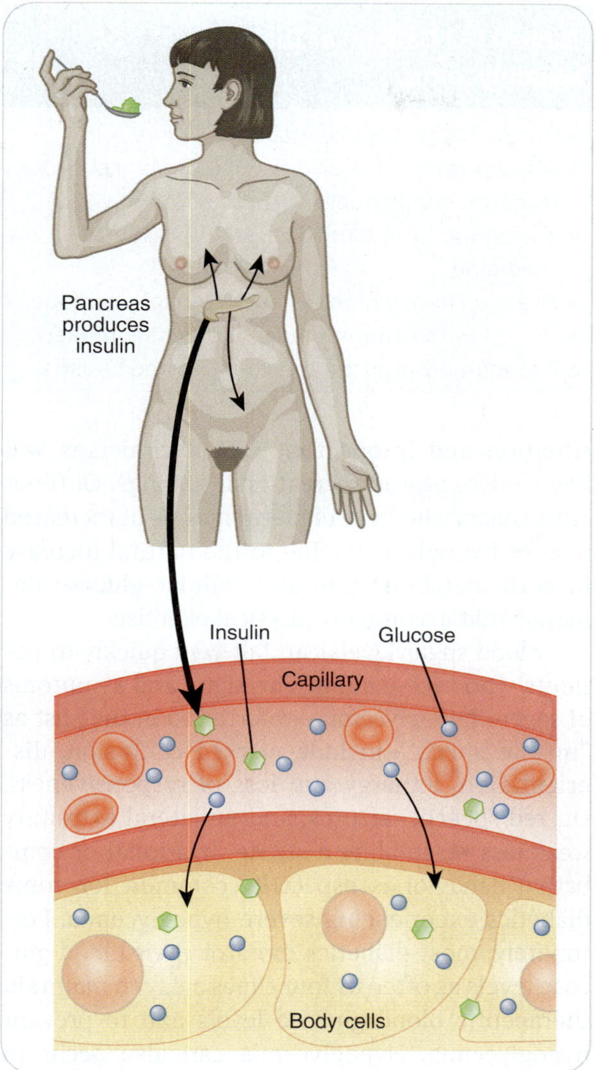

Figure 11-8 In a person without diabetes, the person eats, blood glucose levels rise, the pancreas secretes insulin into the blood, glucose enters the body's cells and is used for energy (glucose is also stored for glycogen in the liver and skeletal muscles for use later), blood glucose levels return to normal, and insulin stops being secreted.

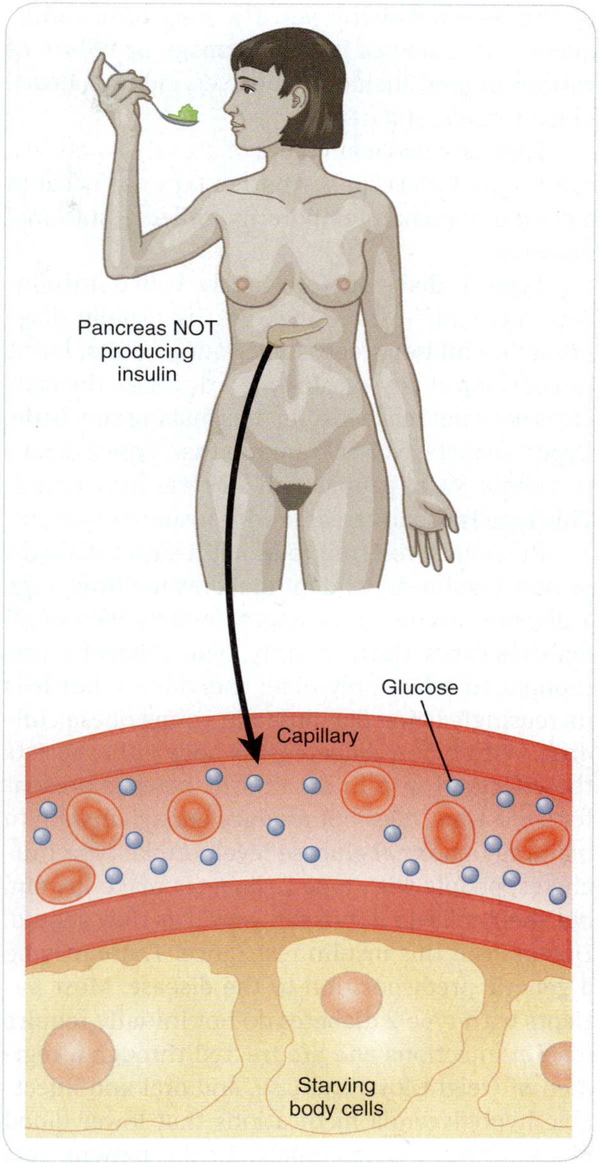

Figure 11-9 Glucose metabolism in a person with diabetes. Without insulin, cells starve because insulin is needed to allow glucose to enter and nourish the cells.

Diabetes is a chronic disease in which either the pancreas cannot produce enough insulin to meet metabolic needs, or the body's cells do not respond appropriately to insulin, or both. Normally, when a person eats a meal, glucose is absorbed from the small intestine into the bloodstream. The pancreas secretes insulin that allows glucose to move out of the bloodstream and into the cells for energy. Excess glucose is stored in the liver, muscles or fat. If not enough insulin is present, glucose cannot enter cells or be stored, so it accumulates in the bloodstream and raises circulating blood sugar levels. In 2018, 27 million people in the United States had diabetes. Another 86 million have prediabetes, meaning, their blood glucose is not normal but is not high enough to be considered diabetes yet. The long-term consequences of diabetes include damage or failure of various organs, including the eyes, kidneys, heart, blood vessels, and nerves.

There are two main types of **diabetes mellitus**, called type 1 and type 2. Another type can occur in a pregnant woman temporarily, called gestational diabetes.

Type 1 diabetes (previously called insulin-dependent or juvenile diabetes) is usually diagnosed in children, teens, and young adults, but it can develop at any age. In type 1 diabetes, the pancreas does not make insulin or is making very little. Type 1 diabetes is less common than type 2 diabetes; about 5% of people with diabetes have type 1. This type is usually treated with insulin injections.

Previously referred to as adult-onset diabetes or non-insulin-dependent diabetes mellitus, type 2 diabetes accounts for approximately 95% of all diabetes cases. Until recently, type 2 diabetes was thought to affect only older individuals, but it is increasingly being diagnosed in young obese children. With type 2 diabetes, the body either resists the effects of insulin or, after diabetes is present for some time, does not produce enough insulin to maintain a normal glucose level. Unlike type 1 diabetes, people with type 2 diabetes make insulin, but their cells do not use it as well as they should. Doctors call this insulin resistance. There may be a genetic predisposition to the disease. Most patients with type 2 diabetes do not initially require insulin injections and are treated through a regimen of weight loss, exercise, and oral and injectable hypoglycemia medications that lower blood glucose levels. Occasionally, as the patient gets older, low doses of insulin may be needed to regulate blood glucose levels.

Diabetic emergencies come to the attention of OEC technicians when the patient's circulating blood sugar level is either too low or too high. These conditions are known as hypoglycemia and hyperglycemia, respectively.

Hypoglycemia

When a blood sugar gets too low, **hypoglycemia** results. This condition most commonly occurs in a diabetic when the patient takes too much insulin or too much of an oral hypoglycemic medication. It may also occur if a person with diabetes takes a medication properly but fails to eat enough food or vomits a lot (**Table 11-2**). This is a common situation and is one that OEC technicians will likely encounter in recreational settings. Outdoor enthusiasts who have diabetes may be at increased risk for hypoglycemia due to the natural increase in both metabolic rate and cellular glucose demands that accompany physical exercise.

Table 11-2 Causes of Diabetic Hypoglycemia

- An excessive dose of insulin
- An excessive dose or overdose of an oral hypoglycemic medication
- Eating too little food after taking diabetes medicine
- Overexertion, which exhausts glucose supplies
- Illness with vomiting (loss of glucose intake)
- Combinations of the previously listed causes

Blood sugar levels can fall very quickly in patients who take insulin. The signs and symptoms of severe hypoglycemia—referred to in the past as "insulin shock"—include marked confusion, disorientation, lethargy and loss of responsiveness, slurred speech, seizures, and unilateral extremity weakness resembling a stroke. Irrational or combative behavior is especially common for some diabetics experiencing severe hypoglycemia. Fortunately, most diabetics monitor their blood glucose levels as often as four times a day to maintain therapeutic blood glucose levels and to prevent hypoglycemia. Hypoglycemia can also occur in people who do not have diabetes if they do not eat.

Hyperglycemia

High blood sugar, or **hyperglycemia**, is defined as an elevated circulating blood sugar level. In patients with known diabetes, the primary cause of hyperglycemia is failure to take diabetes medications, leading to a very high blood sugar level and **polyuria** (urinating a lot), **polydipsia** (thirsty all the time), dry mouth, and fatigue (**Table 11-3**).

Escalating blood glucose levels build up acids (ketones) within the blood. These patients have associated nausea, vomiting, abdominal pain, and varying degrees of altered mental status. Unless treated, the combination of high blood sugar and acidosis can result in coma, brain damage, or death. Fortunately, this condition occurs much less than hypoglycemia and typically comes on slowly over days to months.

Table 11-3 Comparison of Findings in Hypoglycemia and Hyperglycemia

Hypoglycemia
• Tremor • Anxiety • Headache • Diaphoresis • Dizziness • Confusion, disorientation • Slurred speech • Lethargy • Seizures • Weakness of one of more extremities • Irrational, combative behavior • Loss of responsiveness
Hyperglycemia
• Polyuria • Polydipsia • Dehydration • Warm, dry skin • Rapid weak pulse • Normal or low blood pressure • Sweet or fruity breath • Rapid, deep respirations • Less than A (alert) on AVPU scale

Many children and adults who are undiagnosed diabetics commonly present with signs and symptoms of hyperglycemia. When someone who denies having diabetes presents with altered mental status not from trauma, consider that they may have undiagnosed diabetes with hyperglycemia.

Stroke

Stroke is a general term that describes neurologic brain impairment resulting from low blood flow or a lack of blood flow to areas of the brain. OEC technicians should be familiar with the two basic types of stroke and their signs and symptoms.

Eighty percent of strokes are ischemic, caused by a disruption of blood flow to a portion of the brain (**Figure 11-10**). The primary cause of an ischemic stroke is foreign material (an embolus) that travels through the bloodstream until it lodges in an artery in the brain. Most emboli originate outside the brain. Examples of emboli that cause an ischemic stroke include blood clots, fat from bone marrow after a recent long-bone fracture, and cholesterol plaques that break loose from the heart chambers or carotid arteries. Once an embolus becomes lodged in an artery of the brain, blood flow to part of the brain may be reduced or completely stopped. Depending on the area affected, portions of the brain may cease to function properly, resulting in a variety of signs and symptoms. This type of stroke is also known as a "dry stroke" or "white stroke" because the brain's blood vessels, although blocked, remain intact and do not bleed.

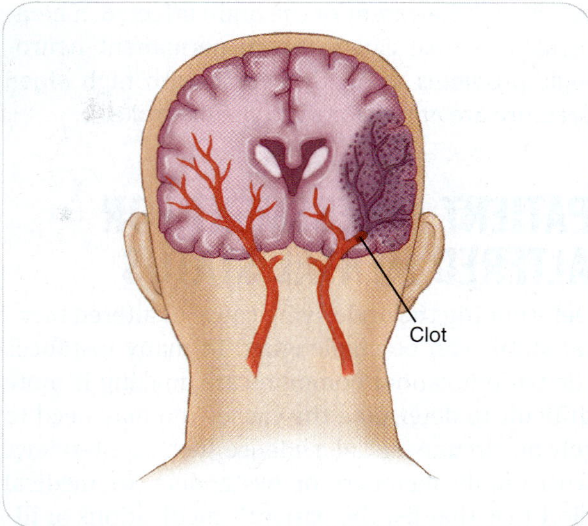

Figure 11-10 Ischemic stroke is caused by a disruption of blood flow to a portion of the brain.

The second type of stroke is a hemorrhagic stroke. This form, also known as an intracerebral hemorrhage, "wet stroke," or "red stroke," occurs when a blood vessel within the brain suddenly ruptures, releasing blood into the surrounding brain tissue. This not only reduces the amount of oxygen and nutrients available to the brain, but the resulting hematoma also places direct pressure on the delicate brain tissue confined within the skull. The most common cause of a hemorrhagic stroke is a structural weakness within the wall of a blood vessel within the brain. The constant force of blood pressing against the wall of the vessel can cause it to burst. A bulge, or aneurysm, present in an artery can burst open. The small, fragile "end arteries" located at the base of the brain are especially vulnerable to developing a weakness and rupturing. Depending on the size of the ruptured vessel and the extent of the brain affected, a hemorrhagic stroke can result in permanent neurologic problems or death. People with high blood pressure are at risk for this type of stroke.

PATIENT ASSESSMENT FOR ALTERED MENTAL STATUS

Determining the underlying cause of altered mental status can be challenging. In many instances the patient cannot communicate, making it more difficult to determine the cause. You may need to rely on circumstantial evidence such as interviews with family members or bystanders, or medical alert tags that list the patient's medications or illnesses. Altered mental status in younger individuals is more likely to be caused by a toxic overdose or trauma, whereas the cause in older individuals is more likely to be more complicated such as a heart problem or stroke. Diabetic, trauma-related, and epilepsy-related altered mental status can occur in any age group.

Some patients with psychiatric or behavioral illness may present a complicated picture of altered mental status. These patients should be considered to have a metabolic or structural lesion until proven otherwise at a definitive-care facility. Regardless of the underlying cause, altered mental status is considered an emergency until the cause can be determined and treated.

Begin the patient assessment process with a scene size-up, during which potential hazards are identified and removed. Then attempt to determine if the cause of altered mental status is traumatic or medical in origin, remembering that the two can occur together. If trauma is suspected, give careful consideration of spinal motion restriction when opening and maintaining the airway.

Once the scene size-up is complete, perform a primary patient assessment, control excessive bleeding, and carefully assess the ABCDs to ensure that they are intact. Evaluate the patient's level of responsiveness using the AVPU scale to determine the extent and severity of the altered mental status. Make sure the airway is open. If the patient is unresponsive, open the airway and simultaneously check for breathing and a carotid pulse. If no pulse, begin CPR. Activate advanced life support when needed for effective management of some of the more complex causes of altered mental status.

Perform a secondary patient assessment by first obtaining a complete SAMPLE history (if possible) and vital signs. A relative who is present may help you with the history if the patient is unresponsive. Look for a medical identification tag on a bracelet or necklace or for a medical identification card in the patient's pocket, wallet, or purse that may tell you of a medical condition, allergy, or medications the patient is taking. Some cell phones now have the patient's medical information in them. Ask responsive patients if they have taken their medications as prescribed. Remember to use AEIOU-TIPS when assessing for altered mental status.

Attempt to determine the exact time when the symptoms began or were first noticed, noting whether the symptoms came on suddenly or more slowly. Noting the onset time is very important for a stroke. If the patient had a seizure, investigate whether the seizure began in one part of the body and how long the convulsions lasted. Note whether the patient's speech appears impaired, such as the slurring of words, the misuse of words, or incomprehensible speech, which may result from alcohol or drug intoxication, hypoglycemia, stroke, or a behavioral condition. Also note if the patient repeatedly asks the same question or says the same phrase over and over. If, for example, the patient repeatedly asks, "What happened?" or keeps saying, "I need to find my poles," this disoriented behavior may be a clue to an underlying brain injury or a diabetes-related problem.

Perform a thorough physical exam. Look closely at the pupils and inside the patient's mouth. Note pupil size and response. Pinpoint pupils are often associated with a narcotics overdose, whereas unequal pupils are an ominous sign that generally indicates a buildup of pressure within the brain, often due to trauma or stroke. Examine the mouth for cuts on the tongue or inside the cheeks, which commonly result from inadvertent biting that occurs during a seizure or following a seizure. Then check the patient's skin, noting its temperature and overall condition. Pale, moist skin may be due to shock or hypoglycemia; hot, dry skin may result from hyperglycemia or hyperthermia. Skin that is hot and moist may also be caused by an infection. Also check to see if the patient is incontinent of urine or feces, which may indicate that the patient had a seizure.

Table 11-4 General Signs and Symptoms of Stroke

- Decreased responsiveness
- Severe headache
- Drooping eyelid and mouth on one side of the face
- Paralysis or weakness on one or both sides of the body
- Arm drift
- Loss of bowel or bladder control
- Change in personality
- Pupils unequal in size
- Loss of vision, dimness, or double vision
- Difficulty speaking or slurred speech
- Inability to speak
- Nausea or vomiting
- Sudden weakness or paralysis of the face, arm, or leg
- Possible seizures

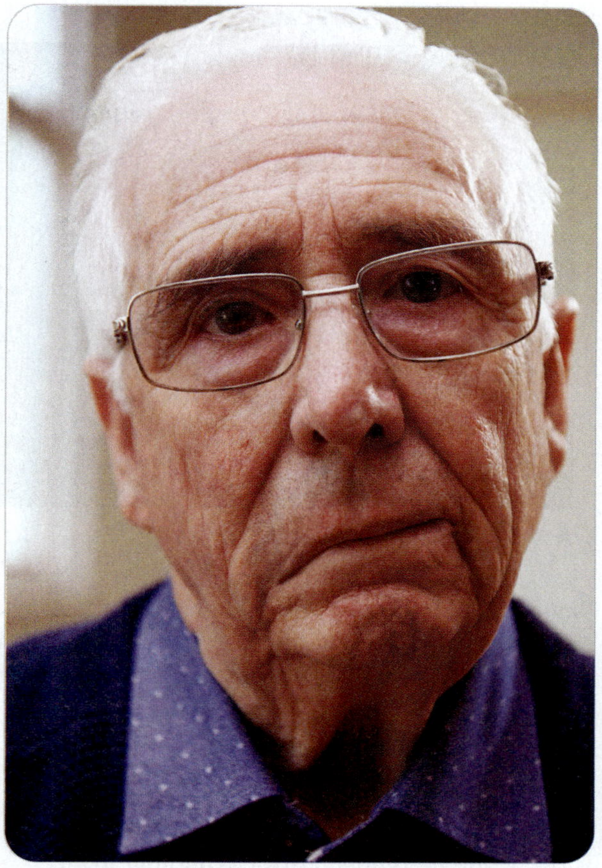

Figure 11-11 Facial feature showing effects of stroke.

Higher cortical function is checked by having the patient perform a task consisting of multiple steps. For instance, ask the patient to hold up two fingers on the right hand. This requires the brain to accurately process the request and to send the proper signal to the hand. The brain of a patient who is unable to perform the task accurately and quickly is not functioning properly, indicating an abnormality within the part of the brain that controls the higher cortical functions. The vocal-speech portion of the exam is assessed by having the patient repeat a phrase such as "Bananas are yellow, apples are red." A patient whose brain is not functioning properly cannot accurately repeat the phrase without such problems such as slurring the words.

OEC technicians must recognize the signs and symptoms of a stroke and recommend immediate evaluation at a clinic or hospital (**Table 11-4**). Signs and symptoms of a stroke include numbness and weakness or paralysis on one side of the body. A stroke may involve only the leg, the arm, or the face, or all of these. Speech and language may be affected as well. Sudden disorientation or inability to perform tasks such as buttoning a shirt, putting on a hat, or zipping a coat may be a sign of stroke.

Visual problems, such as blurry vision or loss of vision for part of the visual field, may be a symptom. As a result, patients may walk into objects they might otherwise see. Patients may exhibit a sudden inability to walk, dizziness, or clumsiness. Any of these signs and symptoms and the complaint of a sudden and unusually severe headache should alert OEC technicians to the possibility of a stroke. The patient may have experienced a TIA in which the signs and symptoms have resolved, or the signs and symptoms may be subtle.

Among the several stroke scales that have been developed to aid in the assessment of a stroke patient is the Field Assessment Stroke Triage for Emergency Destination (FAST-ED) scale.

F Face drooping (**Figure 11-11**): Look for paralysis of one side of the face, with drooping of the corner of the mouth when they smile or sagging of facial skin.

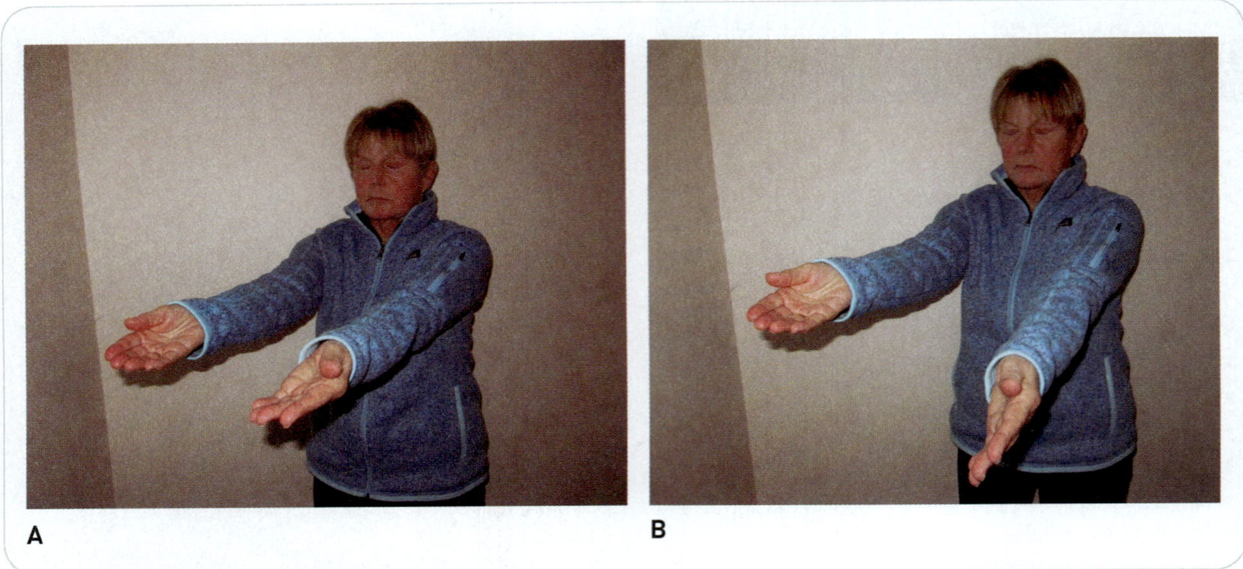

Figure 11-12 **A.** To perform the arm droop test, ask a potential stroke patient to extend the arms straight out in front with the palms facing up and the eyes closed. **B.** Patients who have had a stroke are often unable to hold both arms extended in front; one arm may drift downward or the palm may rotate downward.

- **A** Arm weakness: Have the patient raise both extended arms to shoulder level in front of them with eyes closed to see if one drifts down. The arm droop test is easy to perform in the field (**Figure 11-12**). Check to see if grip strength is equal in each hand.
- **S** Speech difficulty: See if their words are garbled or they cannot express themselves appropriately when you ask them to repeat a simple phrase.
- **T** Time to call: If you see any of these signs, call 9-1-1 immediately. If available, record the last known time the patient responded normally.
- **E** Eye deviation: Check extraocular eye motion. See if the eyes move appropriately in all directions. See Chapter 7, *Patient Assessment*, for more detail.
- **D** Denial/neglect: After you determine an arm is weak, ask the patient if they are weak anywhere. Touch the patient's arm and ask, whose arm is this? A positive finding is when the patient is in denial of the problem.

Both the public and prehospital responders are now using FAST-ED to identify a stroke victim. Although a complicated system assigning numbers to each category may be used to determine if someone is having a stroke, more important is for the patroller to understand and recognize each category listed.

Stroke Warning Signs and Symptoms

It is important that OEC technicians determine as near as possible the exact time of the onset of symptoms. Because the onset of symptoms may be painless and therefore silent, time of onset may be difficult to identify. Estimating the time of onset as accurately as possible is needed to establish a window for treatment, because treatment may be ineffective if therapy with medications (discussed later) is started outside the treatment window. If the time of onset of symptoms cannot be determined, the time of onset is the last time the patient was known to be normal.

In the early stages of a neurologic event such as a stroke, it is difficult to predict whether the symptoms will be reversible. Some conditions, such as a TIA, signal the potential for further episodes that may result in permanent injury. Thus, any patient presenting with altered mental status, including those with improving signs, should still be evaluated at a clinic or hospital. Early detection and rapid transport to an emergency care facility are the keys for improving the patient's survival after a stroke.

MANAGEMENT OF ALTERED MENTAL STATUS

The overall treatment of patients with an altered mental status is straightforward and centers on correcting any problems affecting the ABCDs, providing oxygen, giving sugar to an awake diabetic, and rapidly transporting the patient to a definitive-care facility. As basic as this sounds, strict attention to these management priorities will significantly improve the patient's outcome. Once the patient's ABCDs have been appropriately managed, OEC technicians may provide specific care depending on the possible cause, and then adopt a "load and go" principle for life-threatening conditions.

Be sure to protect patients against further injury. Monitor and pad any areas that may come into contact with pressure points, sharp objects, or temperature extremes, especially when prolonged transport is involved. Continue to reassess the neurologic findings for further deterioration or improvement. Document all findings and changes, including the time those findings were observed.

Check the patient's airway frequently, using suction as needed to ensure that it remains patent. Use the recovery position in patients who do not have the possibility of a spinal injury. Place a nasal or oral airway in the unresponsive patient to keep the airway patent. Spinal precautions should be taken for all unresponsive patients when the cause is unknown, because trauma may have produced a spine or other neurologic injury. The process for properly restricting spinal motion is presented in Chapter 21, *Spine, Brain, and Nervous System Injuries*. All other treatment is symptom based and is provided using the AEIOU-TIPS mnemonic as a guide.

A

- *Alcohol.* Altered mental status due to alcohol intoxication can be a true emergency, especially if CNS function is impaired. Patients who are unconscious and unresponsive and have diminished respirations must be immediately transported to a hospital for evaluation by a physician. During transport, place the patient in the left lateral recumbent position to avoid the aspiration of vomit. This position may be particularly important for longer backcountry extrications. If respirations become shallow, it may be necessary to support the patient's ventilation efforts using either a nasopharyngeal airway or an oropharyngeal airway and a bag-valve mask.
- *Acidosis.* Acidosis is a serious medical disorder that is best managed in a hospital by a physician. Hospital treatment of acidosis centers on identifying the underlying source of the acidosis and normalizing the body's pH, a process that can take several hours or days. It is difficult for an OEC technician to determine this cause.

E

- *Epilepsy.* Treatment of epilepsy is supportive. Any patient who is seizing must be protected from further traumatic injury. Treatment of seizures is described shortly. Careful suctioning may be needed to remove blood or mucus. Remove any broken teeth from the mouth to prevent their aspiration and to preserve any that may be salvageable. Be aware that the patient may accidentally bite down on your fingers.
- *Environment.* Regarding environment, both hypothermia and hyperthermia are treated by correcting the core body temperature, whether by warming or cooling the patient. For information concerning how to manage temperature-related problems, see Chapter 25, *Cold-Related Emergencies*, and Chapter 26, *Heat-Related Emergencies*.
- *Electrolytes.* Altered mental status associated with an electrolyte imbalance is a serious condition that warrants immediate referral to a hospital for electrolyte replacement therapy. Complex sports drinks may provide some short-term benefit, especially when the symptoms are minor.

I

- *Insulin.* A diabetic with altered mental status, whether on insulin or not, who can swallow should receive oral sugar. OEC technicians should always assume that the patient is hypoglycemic because hypoglycemia can quickly cause irreparable brain damage. If the patient was hyperglycemic, you will not cause further harm because the small amount of sugar that is administered will not make the patient worse.

Before administering oral glucose, be sure the patient can swallow. Never place oral glucose into the mouth of an unresponsive patient because this can result in aspiration and serious pulmonary problems. An unresponsive diabetic patient requires IV glucose or subcutaneous glucagon, which can be provided only by an advanced care provider. If an advanced provider is not immediately available, call for ALS. Check to see whether any family member present might be carrying an emergency glucagon kit and be trained in its use.

Give the patient oral glucose using either prepackaged chewable sucrose tablets, sugar packs, or prepackaged tubes of cake frosting. The sugar can be dissolved in water, or the person can drink water after eating the sugar. Orange juice has been found to be less effective than any of these forms for raising blood sugar levels. If symptoms resolve (usually within 15 minutes of treatment), the patient should consume a small meal to prevent recurrent hypoglycemia. If symptoms do not resolve, there may be another cause for the patient's altered mental status.

Patients often refuse further treatment or transport to a hospital once their level of responsiveness improves. This is especially common among patients who have had diabetes for a long time. OEC technicians should strongly recommend that such patients be evaluated further by a physician and document if the person refuses. Obviously if the patient has a hypoglycemic episode, their blood sugar is not well controlled.

KEY POINT

Administering Oral Glucose

Adult: Administer a commercially available 15-gram tube of glucose gel (**Figure 11-13**) or chewable tablets. An alternative is three or four commercial packets of sugar dissolved in a liquid for patient to drink.

Pediatric: For patients younger than 10 years of age, administer half the adult dose (e.g., two or three commercially available glucose tablets, two sugar packets).

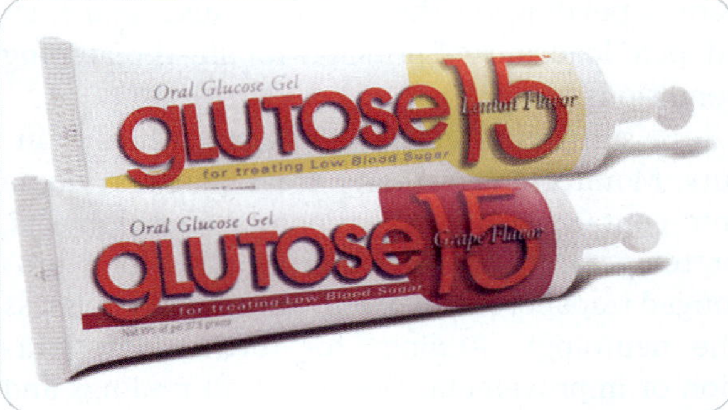

Figure 11-13 Glucose can come in a variety of forms that are easy to administer to a responsive patient.

O

- *Oxygen.* High-flow oxygen is recommended for all patients with hypoxia or shortness of breath. Hypoxia is the most common cause of altered mental status and is the easiest problem to correct.
- *Overdose.* The mainstay of overdose management is to maintain the ABCDs and prevent aspiration of gastric contents using the recovery position. This is especially important with overdoses involving opiates or other sympathetic nervous system depressants, which can depress respiratory effort. Rapid transport to the hospital is warranted because some overdoses can be reversed by administering a specialized class of medications known as antagonists. Some first responders may give naloxone (Narcan) to reverse narcotic overdoses. This is discussed in Chapter 12, *Substance Abuse and Poisoning.*

U

- *Uremia.* When OEC technicians encounter a patient in kidney failure resulting in uremia, they should try to make the patient comfortable and maintain the ABCDs. The patient needs to be transported immediately to a health care facility. This is rarely seen by OEC technicians.

T

- *Trauma.* The treatment of trauma-related altered mental status is covered in Chapter 21, *Spine, Brian, and Nervous System Injuries*. In general, the management of severe trauma, especially brain injuries, focuses on diligent maintenance of the ABCDs and rapid transport to a trauma center. Treat for shock, if present, as described in Chapter 10, *Shock*, and ensure that the patient is well oxygenated.
- *Tumors.* There is no specific prehospital treatment for a suspected tumor other than supportive care and rapid transport.
- *TIA.* If you encounter a patient with a possible TIA/stroke, the treatment provided is the same as for a stroke. Provide oxygen, note time of onset, and immediately transport to a hospital.

I

- *Infections.* Suspected infections, whether local or systemic, should be evaluated by a physician. Serious conditions such as sepsis, meningitis, or other infections involving the brain can be life threatening. In a remote setting in which the transport time is measured in hours to days, infected wounds should be cleaned as directed in Chapter 19, *Soft-Tissue Injuries and Burns*. Fevers, if present, may be initially treated with cool compresses and self-administration of acetaminophen, if your local, regional, and state protocol allows. Treat septic shock as discussed in Chapter 10, *Shock*.

P

- *Poisoning.* The treatment of poisoning is varied and depends on the type, potency, and quantity of the toxin. In most instances, treatment is supportive in nature, with emphasis on preserving the ABCDs. If the cause is carbon monoxide, treat with high-flow oxygen, keeping the SpO_2 between 94 and 99%. For other causes, refer to Chapter 12, *Substance Abuse and Poisoning*, or call the local poison center for specific treatment recommendations.
- *Psychiatric conditions.* The field treatment of psychiatric conditions is also supportive in nature but is focused on preventing patients from harming themselves. Specific treatment recommendations may be found in Chapter 33, *Behavioral Emergencies and Crisis Response*.

S

- *Seizure.* Seizures are generally self-limiting and usually end without intervention by an OEC technician. The primary goal is to protect the patient from further injury while letting the seizure run its course. OEC technicians often arrive during the post-ictal phase, during which care is generally supportive and emphasizes opening and maintaining the airway. Suction blood, mucus, and other secretions as necessary. Use an oropharyngeal airway or a nasopharyngeal airway and give oxygen if there is evidence of prolonged unresponsiveness or airway compromise. The preferred device in a seizure patient is a nasopharyngeal airway.

  If the patient is actively seizing upon your arrival or begins to seize in your presence, protect the patient from injury. Move hard or sharp objects away from the patient. Use padding to protect the patient's head from hitting the floor or from striking objects that cannot be moved. Do not place anything in the mouth or between the teeth of a seizing patient, especially your fingers, as this action may result in a dental injury, mouth lacerations, laryngospasm, or the loss of a finger (yours!).

  If the patient is seizing call ALS for treatment and transport. Intravenous medications are needed to stop the seizure. During transport, place seizing patients onto their side to allow blood and secretions to drain from the mouth. All first-time seizure patients also require further evaluation at a hospital. A patient with a history of seizures may have Diastat gel, which is a prescription medication given rectally, normally by family members, for seizures.
- *Stroke.* The definitive treatment for a patient who has had a stroke must be provided in

a hospital setting. OEC technicians can, however, greatly improve the patient's chances of survival by providing high-flow oxygen, protecting the airway, and rapidly transporting the person to a definitive-care facility, preferably a stroke center. Stroke is a time-sensitive condition because new therapies may reverse the effects if administered soon after symptoms develop. New "clot-busting" medications may reverse an ischemic stroke if given within several hours of onset. Do not delay transport unless spine trauma is highly suspected, in which case, apply spinal motion restriction and rapid transport to a hospital that cares for strokes. If possible, notify the receiving clinic or hospital that a potential stroke patient is coming to their location. Document the TLKW (time last known well), as this helps the doctor know if clot-dissolving medication can be given.

- *Syncope.* The treatment for syncope consists placing the patient on their back and keeping the patient warm. Because the underlying cause of syncope is often a problem originating within the cardiovascular system, any syncopal patient should be transported for evaluation by a physician.

VIOLENT BEHAVIOR AND ALTERED MENTAL STATUS

Any patient with altered mental status may exhibit violent, combative, or bizarre behavior. These patients can test your patience, as they are generally uncooperative and can endanger you and other rescuers if their behavior is not controlled. These patients are usually completely unaware of what they are doing and that their behavior is inappropriate. Many times, you will not be able to reason with these patients. The most difficult situation arises when trauma dictates that the spine must be protected using a cervical collar and long spine board. In these instances, try to remain calm, and reassure patients to keep them calm. Whenever possible, avoid the use of force, because using force may be more harmful than trying to get patients to cooperate or to lie still.

CASE Outcome

You realize the woman probably is not hypoglycemic, and you are unsure why she has altered mental status. You immediately call for ALS and transport. Several other patrollers arrive. Vital signs are stable. Following a secondary patient assessment, which reveals nothing, you get her to the waiting ambulance. Later you learn that she was admitted to the intensive care unit with hyperglycemia. She did not know she was a diabetic and had a blood sugar of 570 mg/dL on admission. Following the regulation of her blood sugar and starting insulin, she returns several weeks later to thank you.

CHAPTER REVIEW

In Summary

- Altered mental status describes an abnormal change in a person's level of awareness or responsiveness.
- The causes of altered mental status are numerous and may result in global or focal changes.
- The mnemonic AEIOU-TIPS can help determine the underlying cause of altered mental status.

  A—Alcohol and acidosis
  E—Epilepsy, environment, and electrolytes
  I—Insulin
  O—Oxygen (hypoxia) and overdose
  U—Uremia (kidney failure)
  T—Trauma and tumors, TIA, thirst
  I—Infection (CNS, sepsis)
  P—Poisoning and psychiatric conditions
  S—Seizures, stroke, sleep and syncope
- There are conditions associated with altered mental status.
  - Epilepsy
  - Seizures (focal and generalized)
  - Diabetes mellitus (hypoglycemia, hyperglycemia)
  - Stroke
- The Field Assessment Stroke Triage for Emergency Destination (FAST-ED) scale was developed to aid in the assessment of a stroke patient.
- Patients with altered mental status are considered "load and go" patients. Make the patient comfortable and maintain the ABCDs.
- High-flow oxygen is recommended for all patients with hypoxia or shortness of breath. The SpO_2 should be kept between 94 and 99%. Hypoxia is the most common cause of altered mental status and is the easiest problem to correct.
- Diabetics with altered mental status need sugar, but only if they can swallow.
- Any patient with unwitnessed altered mental status should be treated for spinal injury until proven otherwise.
- The definitive treatment for a patient who has had a stroke must be provided in a hospital setting.
- Seizures are usually self-limiting. Treatment focuses on protecting the patient from further harm.

Key Terms

Absence seizure A sudden, temporary loss of mental awareness and physical activity lasting a few seconds to several minutes; also known as a petit mal seizure.

Altered mental status A condition in which a person's level of awareness or responsiveness has changed.

Aura A subjective sensation that precedes a seizure.

Clonic activity The spasmodic jerking of muscles during a seizure.

Coma An abnormal loss of responsiveness during which the patient cannot be aroused by external stimuli.

Delirium A state of mental confusion and/or excitement characterized by disorientation with respect to time and place; may be associated with delusions and hallucinations.

Dementia A broad impairment of intellectual function (cognition) that usually is progressive and that interferes with normal social and occupational activities.

Diabetes mellitus A disease in which the body's ability to produce or respond to the hormone insulin is impaired, resulting in abnormal metabolism of carbohydrates (sugars) causing elevated levels of glucose in the blood and urine.

Epilepsy A disorder in which abnormal electrical discharges occur in the brain, causing seizure and possible loss of responsiveness.

Generalized seizure A seizure consisting of the sudden onset of unresponsiveness, tonic contraction of muscles, loss of postural control, and a cry caused by contraction of respiratory muscles that forces an exhalation; clonic contractions of muscles occur, followed by a period of somnolence.

Glucose A simple sugar that is the product of carbohydrate digestion in the body and the chief source of energy for most cells, especially neurons.

Hyperglycemia An excess of glucose in the blood; when severe, may be associated with confusion or changes in mental status.

Hypoglycemia An insufficient amount of glucose in the blood; may be associated with a myriad of signs and symptoms such as tremor, diaphoresis, drowsiness, headache, confusion, and lack of responsiveness.

Insulin A hormone produced in the pancreas that regulates blood sugar levels.

Polydipsia Excessive thirst and fluid intake.

Polyuria Frequent urination.

Seizure A neurologic episode caused by a surge of electrical activity in the brain; can be a convulsion characterized by generalized, uncoordinated muscular activity, and can be associated with loss of responsiveness.

Stroke An interruption of blood flow to the brain that results in the loss of brain function; also called a cerebrovascular accident (CVA).

Tonic activity A general stiffening of the muscles.

Chapter Questions

1. Altered mental status is defined as an abnormal change in a person's level of:
   a. awareness or responsiveness.
   b. oxygen in the brain.
   c. ability to do complex math.
   d. glucose in the brain.
2. You are called to a restaurant at your resort for an elderly woman who has altered mental status. You notice her slumped to one side of her chair. When you ask her name, she looks at you but does not respond. You decide to perform a stroke assessment and remember the acronym FAST-ED. You ask the woman to smile so that you can check for:
   a. hearing loss.
   b. speech difficulty.
   c. facial drooping.
   d. eye deviation.
3. Emergency care for a patient suffering from a stroke should focus on the ABCDs and:
   a. using padding to protect the patient's head.
   b. allowing the patient to rest during the post-ictal stage.
   c. providing the patient with oral glucose.
   d. arranging for immediate transport to a definitive-care facility.
4. Your patient is in the ictal phase of a grand mal seizure. Your emergency care should focus on:
   a. placing a tongue blade in the patient's mouth to prevent the patient from choking.
   b. protecting the patient from injury.
   c. restraining the patient.
   d. stopping the seizure.
5. A condition in which there is a temporary interruption of blood flow to an area of the brain resulting in no permanent brain injury is called a:
   a. generalized seizure.
   b. hemorrhagic stroke.
   c. partial seizure.
   d. transient ischemic attack.
6. Which type of stroke is characterized by a blood clot traveling through the bloodstream and lodging in an artery of the brain?
   a. Generalized
   b. Ischemic
   c. Hemorrhagic
   d. Partial

7. A Nordic skier is sitting on the side of a trail. He appears to be confused but can answer questions. He has been skiing for 3 hours without a break. The SAMPLE history reveals that the patient is a diabetic and his last oral intake was about 8 hours ago. You suspect that he is suffering from:
   a. hyperglycemia.
   b. hypoglycemia.
   c. epilepsy.
   d. uremia.
8. What is the first step you should take in caring for a patient with suspected hypoglycemia?
   a. Providing oral glucose
   b. Using the FAST-ED scale
   c. Placing the patient in the recovery position
   d. Arranging for immediate transport to a definitive-care facility
9. Your patient presents with an altered mental status. He has a weak, rapid pulse; warm, dry skin; deep, rapid respirations; and a fruity odor to his breath. He has a medical alert bracelet indicating that he is diabetic. His friend tells you that the patient has not been feeling well for about a week. These finding lead you to believe that the patient is suffering from:
   a. hyperglycemia.
   b. hypoglycemia.
   c. epilepsy.
   d. uremia.

Answers: 1. a, Objective 11-1, p. 240; 2. c, Objective 11-6, p. 251; 3. d, Objective 11-7, p. 253; 4. b, Objective 11-5, p. 255; 5. d, Objective 11-3, p. 243; 6. b, Objective 11-7, p. 249; 7. b, Objective 11-4, p. 248; 8. a, Objective 11-4, p. 254; 9. a, Objective 11-4, p. 248

CHAPTER 12

SUBSTANCE ABUSE AND POISONING

OBJECTIVES

Upon completion of this chapter, the OEC technician will be able to:

12-1 List and describe the four ways a drug enters and moves through the body.

12-2 List the four routes of absorption.

12-3 List and describe several commonly abused substances.

12-4 List the signs and symptoms associated with commonly abused substances and with common poisonings.

12-5 Describe and demonstrate the proper care of a patient who has abused a substance or been poisoned.

12-6 List and describe two emergency sources for poison-related or chemical-related information.

12-7 Define SLUDGEM and DUMBELS in the context of poisoning.

KEY TERMS

Absorption, p. 262
Dermal poisons, p. 265
Designer drugs, p. 266
Ingested poisons, p. 265
Inhaled poisons, p. 265
Injected poisons, p. 265
Opioids, p. 266
Poison, p. 265
Substance abuse, p. 265
Toxicological event, p. 270
Toxin, p. 265
Withdrawal, p. 265

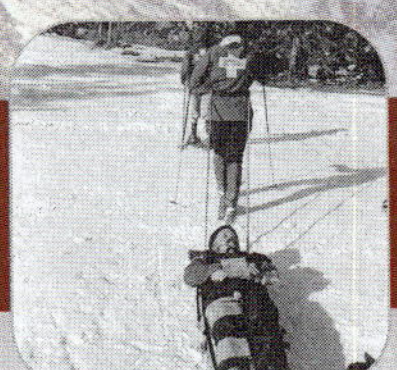

HISTORICAL TIMELINE **1968.** First Nordic ski patroller course conducted.

CHAPTER OVERVIEW

As an OEC technician, you will encounter patients who are experiencing problems resulting from an exposure to a substance. Depending on the substance involved, an exposure may be accidental or intentional. The effects of substances on the human body can vary greatly and can range from being medically therapeutic, to producing minor distortions in perception and coordination, to becoming immediately life threatening.

The use and misuse of a variety of substances in Western society, including the United States, are common. Any exposure, whether intentional or accidental, may pose direct risks to rescuers that must not be overlooked or ignored. OEC technicians must be alert when responding to a suspected case of substance abuse or poisoning to reduce the chances of becoming harmed through accidental exposure. This can be challenging because the effects of some poisons, including carbon monoxide or organic pesticides, may not be immediately apparent but can still pose a severe threat to everyone in the immediate vicinity.

One of the chief dangers posed by patients who have misused a substance is their false sense of reality and disturbed behavior and judgment. Sometimes the effects of the substance can mask or mimic other medical and psychological conditions.

This chapter provides an overview of substance abuse and poisoning. It includes the signs and symptoms that indicate that a toxicological exposure has occurred, a review of commonly abused substances and common poisons, and general guidelines for managing substance abuse and poisoning emergencies.

ANATOMY AND PHYSIOLOGY

Substances can exert many different effects on the body. Some, such as alcohol, act on multiple body systems; others, such as nerve agents, affect a specific body system, the nervous system. In the broadest context, a substance is anything that has mass and occupies space. In the context of this chapter, a substance is any matter that can harm the body. It can be a solid (e.g., a pill, a plant part), a liquid (e.g., alcohol, a drain cleaner), or a gas (e.g., smoke, carbon monoxide).

Physiological Actions

Substances enter, affect, and exit the body through four physiological actions: absorption, distribution, metabolism, and elimination.

Absorption

Absorption is the way in which a substance or poison enters the body. The four routes of absorption are ingestion, inhalation, transdermal absorption, and injection (**Figure 12-1**).

- *Ingestion* involves the intake of a substance through the mouth and its absorption through the gastrointestinal tract. Some substances are easily absorbed across the mucous membranes of the mouth. Substances that are not immediately absorbed travel down the esophagus to the stomach. Depending on the nature and strength of the substance, the delicate mucosa lining the mouth, esophagus, and stomach may be damaged by contact with the substance. Once in the stomach, the substance mixes with the stomach contents, which may slow the rate of absorption. If

CASE Presentation

You are called to the resort's cafeteria, where a male in his twenties is passed out on the floor. His friends, who are gathered around him, appear to be intoxicated and say he just passed out. They were drinking heavily on the bus that brought them to the ski area. They made one run and came in to have a few beers. Upon arousal, the patient moans incoherently.

What should you do?

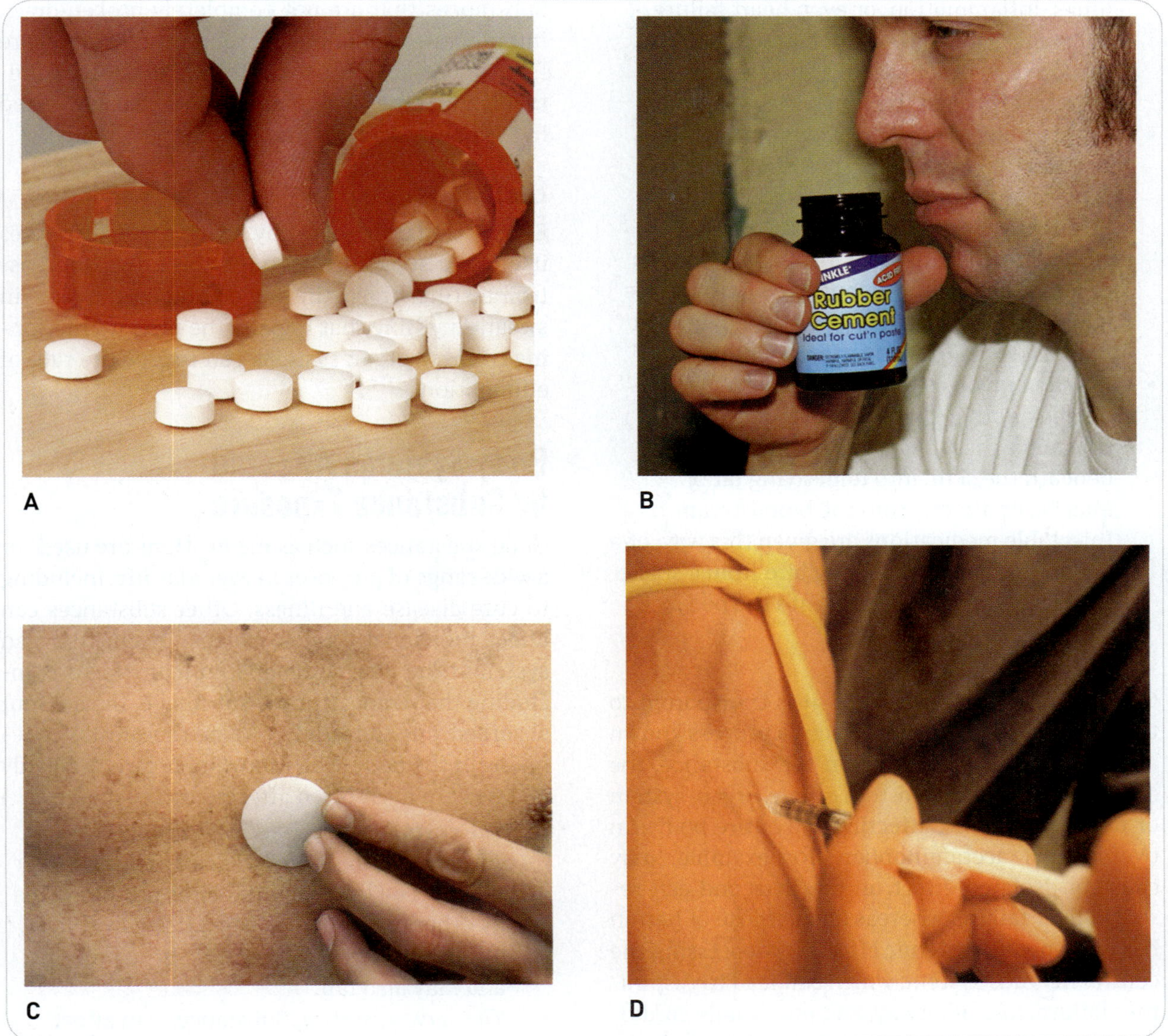

Figure 12-1 Substances can be absorbed into the body through four routes: ingestion (**A**), inhalation (**B**), transdermal absorption (**C**), and injection (**D**).

A: © Duplass/Shutterstock; **B:** © Jones & Bartlett Learning. Photographed by Kimberly Potvin; **C:** © Van D. Bucher/Science Source; **D:** © Oscar Knott/FogStock/Alamy Stock Photo.

the stomach is empty, the substance rapidly enters the intestines, which can quicken the rate of absorption. Little (if any) absorption occurs in the stomach; most absorption occurs within the small and sometimes the large intestines. Substances that are not absorbed are excreted from the body. Pills and liquids are commonly absorbed following ingestion. Some medications are extended release, which means they remain in the intestines for an extended period and then break down and release over a prolonged period.

- *Inhalation* is absorption through the lungs. Because the lungs have a rich vascular network, they are especially capable of absorbing many substances, including nicotine, carbon monoxide, and other gases. Some substances, however, are highly corrosive and when inhaled can damage the delicate lung tissue, causing swelling and bleeding. Other inhaled substances can travel through the bloodstream and affect other organs or body systems, such as the heart, and can cause excess fluid buildup in the lungs, inflammation, or even heart failure. Substances in smoke from marijuana and tobacco and other gaseous substances are absorbed through the lungs.

- *Transdermal absorption* occurs through the skin. As the largest body system, the skin is highly vascular and can absorb a variety of substances. Prescription medications administered transdermally may be worn as patches that contain scopolamine (to reduce nausea), nitroglycerin (to relieve angina), or opioids (to relieve pain), for example.
- *Injection* involves the use of a hypodermic needle or other sharp object to place a substance into the body's tissues, including beneath the skin, into underlying fat or muscle, or directly into the bloodstream. Injectable medications are given this way, or a stinger from a bee or a fang bite from a snake could inject toxic material into the body.

Distribution

Once a substance is absorbed, it is transported to the site where it exerts its effects, a process known as distribution. Depending on the substance, the effects may be isolated to a single organ system or may be systemic, affecting the entire body. An overdose of acetaminophen, for example, may cause an isolated effect on the liver and can result in liver failure, whereas an overdose of heroin has widespread, systemic effects by depressing the central nervous system, which can lead to respiratory failure, loss of airway, and potentially cardiovascular collapse.

Distribution is affected by several factors. Whether injected into muscle or fat, inhaled, ingested, or absorbed through the skin, once the substance is in the bloodstream, it will enter the entire circulatory system quite rapidly. Certain body systems have barriers that either limit or prevent distribution to them. The most commonly discussed is the blood–brain barrier, which limits the types and amounts of substances in the blood that can cross into the brain.

Metabolism

Metabolism is the process by which the body breaks down a substance. The primary site of metabolism is the liver. If the liver is diseased or injured, the time required for metabolism may be prolonged. Substances that are not completely broken down initially are recirculated through the liver, where further breakdown occurs through repeated metabolism. Some benign substances are converted in the body into ones that can harm the body.

Elimination

Elimination is a process by which the body purges itself of a substance through the urine, the gastrointestinal tract, the lungs, and/or the skin in sweat. Anything that impairs the proper functioning of these organ systems can reduce the rate of elimination.

Body Systems Affected by Substance Exposure

Good substances such as medications are used for a wide range of purposes in everyday life, including to cure disease and illness. Other substances can affect individual tissues, organs, or entire organ systems. The effects depend on many factors, including the strength of the substance, the amount absorbed, and the length of time the substance remains in the body. The following organs and body systems are most often affected by substances:

- *The gastrointestinal system.* Certain substances can harm liver cells, causing liver failure. The liver manufactures proteins used by other organs in the body. If the liver fails, other organs will not receive these proteins and may also fail.
- *The nervous system.* Substances can affect the central nervous system (i.e., brain and spinal cord), the peripheral nervous system (i.e., nerves), or both. Consequences depend on which part(s) of the nervous system are affected and may be localized or general.
- *The heart.* Substances can affect the heart muscle, either increasing or decreasing its contractility. They also can affect heart rate or the conduction system of the heart, causing dysfunction and disturbances in cardiac rhythm. In severe cases, they can cause total cessation of heart activity.
- *The eyes.* Substances can affect pupillary dilation or constriction, which can affect vision, and some substances affect the muscles responsible for coordinated eye movements.

- *The blood.* Substances can affect the blood's ability to clot or carry oxygen, or they can affect the bone marrow, the site of red blood cell formation. Some substances can directly destroy blood cells; the effects of this type of exposure may take a long time to become apparent.

COMMONLY ABUSED SUBSTANCES AND POISON-RELATED EMERGENCIES

Substance abuse is the intentional misuse of a substance that results in impairment or physical harm. Although teenagers and young adults may be particularly at risk for substance abuse, addictive dependence on substances can occur in individuals in any age group. Exposure at parties and social events often leads to the binge abuse of a substance. Addiction to a substance, a true medical/psychiatric illness, results when an individual's body craves the substance and when the absence of the substance results in some type of physical impairment due to **withdrawal**.

Drugs that are approved by the US Food and Drug Administration have legitimate medical uses when taken as directed. These same drugs, however, can have toxic effects if misused or abused. An overdose may occur when a person takes a larger dose of a drug than is safe. Often, the line between therapeutic benefit and toxic effect is a narrow one. Poisoning is a significant toxicological event that results in an injury, illness, or death following exposure to a harmful substance. A **poison** is a substance that causes harmful effects when introduced into the body. A **toxin** is a poison that comes from a living organism. Overdoses and poisonings can be accidental or intentional. In addition, any substance can have an unexpected and harmful effect unique to a specific person, referred to as an idiosyncratic reaction.

Poisons may be absorbed into the body through the same routes as any other substance. A substance does not become harmful (poisonous) until it enters the body, so it is important that you understand the specific mode of entry for a commonly encountered substance. For example, spray paint becomes harmful when an excessive amount of it is inhaled. It is unlikely to enter the body through other routes and poses no inhalation hazard unless a person deliberately inhales it to excess or fails to wear proper protective equipment while working in an environment saturated by its fumes. Understanding how a substance becomes poisonous will help you protect yourself and others from harmful exposures and will help you understand the physiological processes that a poisoned patient is experiencing. In your work, you may encounter **ingested poisons**, **inhaled poisons**, **injected poisons**, and **dermal poisons** (poisons that are absorbed transdermally, through the skin).

The following list presents the chief categories of poisons and substances of abuse.

- *Acids and bases* are substances that are commonly used in the household for a variety of purposes, such as in cleaning solutions. Acids (e.g., sulfuric, muriatic, hydrochloric) and bases (e.g., sodium hydroxide, potassium hydroxide) can cause direct tissue damage, especially to the respiratory tract and the delicate mucosa of the mouth and gastrointestinal tract.
- *Antianxiety drugs* are drugs that help relieve patients of anxious feelings. They are commonly prescribed for people with excessive emotions, panic disorders, or social disorders. Examples of these drugs include diazepam (Valium), alprazolam (Xanax), and lorazepam (Ativan).
- *Antidepressants* are medicines used to treat depression. Some newer antidepressants also are used to treat anxiety and panic. Older antidepressants, known as tricyclics, are particularly toxic to the heart. An example of a commonly prescribed tricyclic antidepressant is amitriptyline (Elavil). Although newer drugs may be safer, overdose can lead to heart arrhythmias, problems with perfusion, alterations in mental status, and seizures. Examples of newer antidepressants include sertraline (Zoloft) and fluoxetine (Prozac).
- *Antipsychotics (tranquilizers)* are used to treat psychoses (i.e., thought disorders). Overdose can cause low blood pressure or a disruption in the heart's conduction system, causing an irregular heartbeat. Both overdoses and normal doses can cause dystonic reactions

(abnormal muscle tone, especially in the neck, and facial movements). Examples of these drugs include haloperidol (Haldol) and chlorpromazine (Thorazine).

- *Depressants* are a class of drugs that decrease central nervous system activity. Common depressants include alcohol, tranquilizers, opioids, antipsychotics, and antianxiety drugs. When used in combination, these drugs have increased toxicity and can cause excessive sedation, respiratory depression, and death.
- *Designer drugs (club drugs)* are often used by teenagers and young adults. **Designer drugs** may impair brain function, causing seizures and coma. When combined with alcohol, some designer drugs can cause profound sedation and amnesia. Overdose can cause nausea and vomiting, respiratory difficulties, seizures, coma, and death. Some of these substances are made illegally, whereas others are prescription medications. Examples of these drugs include Ecstasy (MDMA), GHB, flunitrazepam (Rohypnol; a date rape drug), and "bath salts."
- *Hallucinogens* are drugs that distort sensory perceptions and impair emotion, judgment, and memory. Their chief danger lies in the loss of judgment by users and uncontrolled agitation and paranoia. Examples of these drugs include LSD, PCP, prescription ketamine (Special K), and peyote, a plant toxin.
- *Inhalants* are the chemical vapors from common household products such as cleaning solvents, aerosols, spray paints, commercial adhesives, model glue, and Freon. Inhaled substances can produce mind-altering effects like those of alcohol intoxication. Overdose can lead to the loss of sensation, unresponsiveness, shock, respiratory distress, and even death. Long-term effects can include permanent brain, lung, or heart damage.
- *Nerve agents* constitute a special class of chemicals used in warfare and acts of terrorism. These substances interrupt nerve impulses in the body, which can lead to profound shock, seizures, respiratory distress, and death. Poisoning typically occurs through inhalation or transdermal absorption. Examples of these agents include sarin, soman, tabun, and VX.
- *Opioids* are drugs derived from opium or opium-like compounds. Sometimes referred to as narcotics, **opioids** are medically used to relieve pain; however, they can affect mood and emotion. Technically, the term *opioids* refers to synthetically designed drugs such as fentanyl, and *opiates* refers to drugs derived naturally from the opium poppy plant such as morphine. In EMS, most medications administered by providers, and increasingly more drugs misused by patients, are opioids. We will use the term *opioids* in this chapter in a general sense, inclusive of true opiate drugs.

  Opioids affect the central nervous system, causing a surge of euphoria, then alternating wakefulness and drowsiness with impairment of mental functioning. Overdose can cause significant respiratory depression and death. Examples of common prescription opioids are morphine, oxycodone (OxyContin, Percocet), acetaminophen and hydrocodone (Vicodin), hydromorphone (Dilaudid), fentanyl, and meperidine (Demerol). Heroin is an illegal opiate.
- *Organophosphates* are chemicals used in insecticides, pesticides, and herbicides and are commonly found in household and commercial settings. Because of their broad application by agricultural spraying devices, the potential for many individuals to be simultaneously exposed is great. Poisoning most often occurs through inhalation, transdermal absorption, and ingestion (especially in children). The effects of organophosphate poisoning are like those caused by nerve agents.
- *Over-the-counter medications* are not considered dangerous by many people because they are not prescribed by a physician. Overdose or improper use, however, may have harmful side effects. Because of the easy access to these substances, several have become common drugs of abuse by some adolescents. Cough medicines have been identified as most commonly abused by adolescents. The ingredient used for nasal congestion and cough suppression, when taken in overdose, can cause hallucinations, which may be the

desired effect. But it can also cause seizures, arrhythmias, hyperpyrexia, and central nervous system depression.

- *Prescription drugs* are those drugs ordered by a licensed physician and are becoming increasingly misused by individuals of all age groups. Almost all prescription medications have potentially harmful effects if they are misused or not taken as directed. Many have toxic side effects if taken in excess. For some medications, the therapeutic dose (prescribed) is very close to the lethal dose. As examples, dosages for heart and blood pressure medications and those used to control seizures must be followed or toxic effects can occur. Overdose is often accidental and can occur when a person shares a medication with a spouse or other family members. Prescription drug overdose is especially common among elderly patients.
- *Sedatives* are drugs that help people relax. Examples are phenobarbital, zolpidem (Ambien), eszopiclone (Lunesta), and other sleep medications. Overdose and poisoning depress the central nervous system, leading to decreased levels of responsiveness and depressed respirations.
- *Stimulants* are substances that increase central nervous system activity. Overdose with a stimulant speeds up vital body functions (heart rate, blood pressure, metabolic rate) and commonly causes excitement and agitation that can lead to erratic and dangerous behavior and even seizures, hypertension, and stroke. Examples of stimulants include methamphetamine, cocaine, and crack.

Commonly Encountered Substances

OEC technicians are often required to respond to events involving the following substances:

- *Acetaminophen (Tylenol).* This over-the-counter drug is used to treat pain and help reduce fever. Acetaminophen is widely used and is a common ingredient in numerous combination medications, such as over-the-counter cold medications. One may take plain Tylenol in addition to the combination medication, and thus ingest too much acetaminophen. Overdose of acetaminophen is among the most common poisonings worldwide and can be life threatening. In toxic amounts, acetaminophen can cause irreversible liver damage.

KEY POINT

Polypharmacy

A term known as polypharmacy, in which substances are taken in combination, can be dangerous because the effects of the combination cannot always be accurately predicted. The effects of drugs taken in combination may be compounded, or one of the drugs may offset the effects of others. When the additive effects of polypharmacy produce a dangerous effect, the event is known as a multisubstance or polypharmacological overdose. Drug combinations with the potential for polypharmacological overdose include taking multiple prescription drugs, taking a prescription drug and an illegal drug together, using PCP and marijuana together (two illegal drugs), and consuming alcohol with any other substance (**Figure 12-2**). Polypharmacy is common among older patients and may become dangerous if they take multiple medications prescribed by different health care providers.

KEY POINT

Toxic Alcohols

Rubbing alcohol (isopropyl alcohol) and methanol can cause vomiting, confusion, slow breathing, seizures, low body temperature, pale or bluish skin, decreased level of responsiveness, and death. Homemade distilled liquor, or moonshine, can contain methanol.

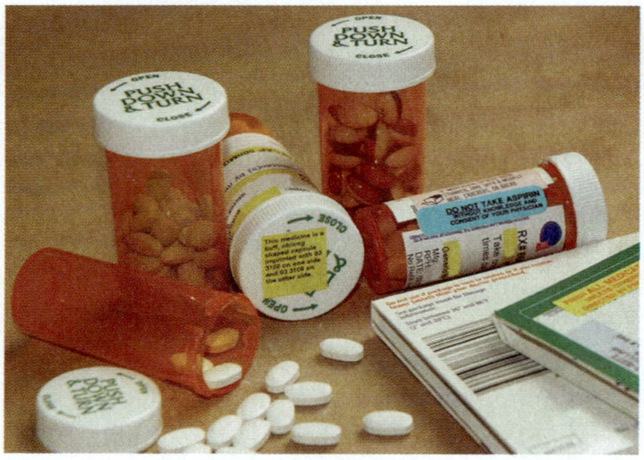

A

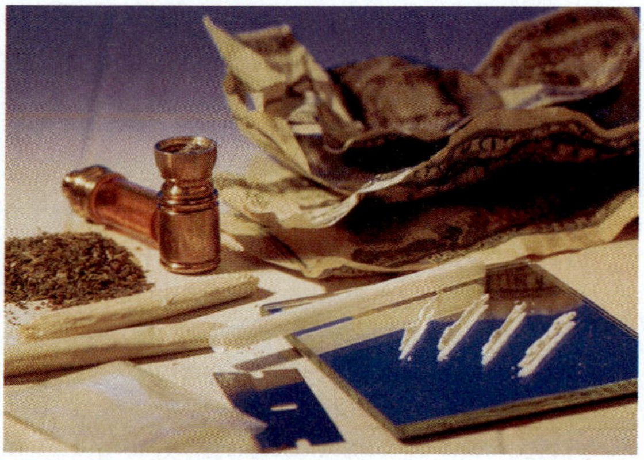

B

Figure 12-2 Patients who have ingested multiple drugs—whether legal, such as prescription medications (**A**), illegal, such as cocaine or THC (**B**), or a combination—can quickly overdose.

A: © Anne Kitzman/Shutterstock; B: © Comstock Images/Getty Images.

- *Alcohol.* Ethanol, the form of alcohol found in beverages, is the most commonly abused drug in the world. A disproportionate number of motor vehicle, aircraft, and recreational injuries are caused by the abuse of this mood-altering, central nervous system depressant. Alcohol-related emergencies are relatively common and can be serious, even life threatening.

  Alcohol has a wide range of effects and affects nearly every body system. Alcohol primarily inhibits central nervous system activity by slowing brain function, sensory input, and motor coordination. It also lowers one's inhibitions, which can lead to behavioral changes. Alcohol can depress the respiratory system, slowing both the rate and the depth of respirations. It is also a diuretic (increases urine output), possibly causing dehydration. In susceptible individuals, alcohol can lower blood sugar levels and enhance the effects of certain medications such as insulin and oral diabetes medications.

  One of the most common alcohol-related emergencies that OEC technicians may encounter is alcohol poisoning, a condition in which a person consumes too much alcohol and becomes severely impaired or even unresponsive. In severe cases, the person loses the gag reflex, aspirates oral secretions or vomit, and stops breathing. Patients also can develop seizures or hypothermia because of alcohol poisoning.

  Another condition that may be encountered is alcohol withdrawal. Most commonly, this is seen in people who have been drinking large amounts of alcohol over many years and then abruptly stop. Such sudden cessation can cause a variety of adverse effects, including muscle tremors, hallucinations, seizures, and even death.
- *Aspirin (acetylsalicylic acid).* Used to relieve pain and swelling and to reduce fever, aspirin is a common ingredient in many combination drugs. Before the widespread use of childproof caps, accidental aspirin overdose was relatively common and resulted in numerous deaths. Overdose is less common today but is still a very dangerous emergency. It can cause respiratory depression (although at first the patient breathes very fast, known as tachypnea), profound systemic acidosis (chemical imbalance in the blood), and death.
- *Carbon monoxide.* An odorless, colorless, and tasteless gas, carbon monoxide is a by-product of combustion (**Figure 12-3**). It impairs oxygenation of tissues by displacing oxygen molecules on red blood cells, thereby reducing the amount of oxygen in the blood. Effects of carbon monoxide poisoning range from mild to life threatening. Carbon monoxide poisoning is an extremely common cause of accidental death, especially in outdoor recreational settings involving stoves, vehicles, generators, and fires. It can occur in poorly ventilated tents, cabins, campers, and sheds. At high altitudes, where

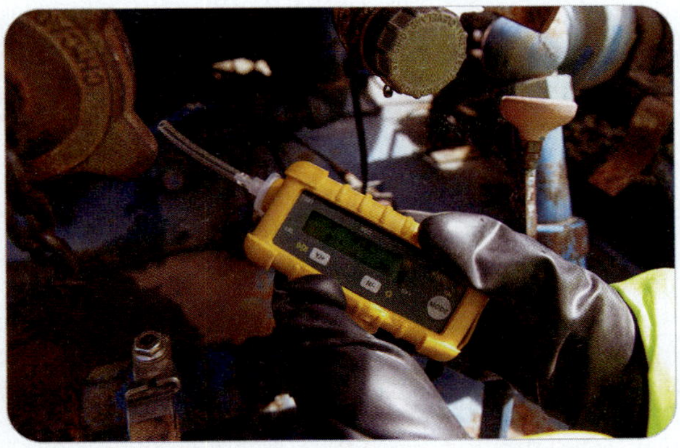

Figure 12-3 Carbon monoxide is hard to detect, and a monitor is required to identify it. If you have any concerns regarding carbon monoxide exposure, wait for fire services to check the area.

oxygen is less concentrated, the risks are even greater.

- *Cocaine (commonly referred to as coke, crack, snow, rock, or nose candy).* A powerfully addictive drug that affects the nervous and cardiovascular systems, cocaine makes the user feel euphoric and energetic and may be inhaled, ingested, injected, or absorbed through the skin or mucosa. Cocaine constricts peripheral blood vessels and stimulates the central nervous system, increasing the heart rate, blood pressure, and body temperature. These changes can cause heart attack, seizure, stroke, and respiratory failure. Because of cocaine's toxic effects on the heart, sudden death can occur at any time during its use, even upon an individual's first exposure to it.
- *Ethylene glycol.* Ingestion of this substance, which is a component of a variety of household and automotive products (including antifreeze), can cause organ damage, shock, and death.
- *LSD (lysergic acid diethylamide; commonly referred to as acid).* The effects of this powerful mood-changing drug are unpredictable and vary among individuals. Physical effects include elevated body temperature, heart rate, and blood pressure; sleeplessness; and loss of appetite. Large doses can cause delusions and visual hallucinations.
- *Marijuana (commonly referred to as pot, weed, cannabis, ganja, grass, or Mary Jane).* Marijuana has become legalized in a growing number of US states and is commonly used by individuals both medicinally and recreationally. It is smoked or ingested. The active ingredient in marijuana is tetrahydrocannabinol (THC). Marijuana distorts perceptions and affects thinking, memory, and learning. Marijuana may be used alongside other drugs, such as alcohol, or mixed directly with other drugs, such as PCP. Hashish is a form of marijuana that contains a higher concentration of THC. Commercial "vape" devices contain concentrated THC. Some vaping products have been found to be harmful to the lungs and may result in death.
- *Methamphetamine (commonly referred to as speed or meth).* The popularity of this drug, a powerful stimulant with a high potential for abuse and addiction, has grown significantly over the past decade. Methamphetamine produces a heightened state of arousal and physical activity and decreases appetite. Chronic use can lead to psychotic behavior, hallucinations, and stroke.
- *Methane.* This highly flammable gas displaces oxygen if present in an enclosed space. In high concentrations, methane can cause profound hypoxia in the body. Although rare, death can occur.
- *Opioids.* Addiction to opioids is a national crisis in the United States. Many who become addicted will eventually die. Fewer than 10% of people following inpatient treatment who are addicted to opioids succeed in recovery. Some researchers think there is no cure, only treatment with substitution using other medications. Opioids include heroin, fentanyl, morphine, codeine, oxycodone, and methadone. Naloxone (Narcan) when administered in a timely manner will reverse the effects of the overdose. However, effects may be transient, and additional doses may be needed. Some people overdose and are resuscitated, only to overdose again.
- *PCP (phencyclidine; commonly referred to as angel dust).* This veterinary tranquilizer was initially developed for use as an anesthetic in humans. PCP blocks the perception of pain and is commonly added to other drugs such as marijuana. Overdose can cause exceptionally violent or suicidal behavior and increases the user's risk of serious traumatic injury.

KEY POINT

Ethanol Percentages

The percentage of ethanol (i.e., grain alcohol) in a drink is expressed by a somewhat obsolete measure called "proof," which is defined as twice the proportion of a drink (by volume) that is ethanol. For instance, a liquor that is 40% grain alcohol is said to be 80 proof. The maximum proof is 200 (i.e., 100% pure, scientific-grade grain alcohol). By contrast, blood alcohol content is a measure of the mass of alcohol per volume of blood. For instance, if an individual's blood alcohol content is 0.10%, there is 1 gram of alcohol per 1,000 milliliters of blood.

KEY POINT

Toxic Plants

The ingestion of toxic plants represents 5% of all exposures to toxins. Exposure to plant toxins is the least toxic of all accidental ingestion-related poisonings. The most common victims of this type of poisoning are curious children, foragers (i.e., hobbyists who look for natural foods), herbalists, pleasure seekers, and people attempting suicide. See Chapter 27, *Plant and Animal Emergencies*, for more information about the ingestion of toxic plants.

PATIENT ASSESSMENT FOR SUBSTANCE ABUSE AND POISONING

As for any incident, the first action is to assess the scene. Pay careful attention to any potential hazards. Do not enter the scene if you suspect a hazardous chemical. Instead, request the assistance of a hazardous materials (hazmat) team. If illegal drugs are suspected, request law enforcement assistance. Requesting fire/Hazmat assistance is especially important if the incident is a **toxicological event** that could involve public safety or require special handling of toxic chemicals or gases or designer poisons such as those used in terrorism situations. Hazmat teams are specially trained and certified to handle these risks. Typical toxicological events include an overturned chemical tanker truck or a spill from a chemical storage site. If available, local police often provide crowd control and/or traffic control.

When responding to a toxicological event, OEC technicians should take the following actions:

1. Ensure scene safety.
2. Practice standard precautions.
3. Begin the primary assessment and correct any threats to life.

CASE Update

Immediately, you place the patient in the rescue position, on his side, in case he vomits. Going through the ABCDs, you make sure his airway is open and he has a pulse. You note gurgling sounds in his breathing, and he responds to pain, so is *P* on the AVPU scale. Next you call for help and crowd control. His friends have no information about him medically and keep saying, "He's just really drunk."

What should you do now?

4. Determine that the incident involves poisoning or substance abuse.
5. Search the scene for evidence of a substance or poison (e.g., pill bottles, spray cans).
6. Examine the patient for evidence of exposure to a toxic substance.
7. Manage and transport the patient.

Assess the ABCDs carefully and perform frequent reassessments to identify any changes. Chemical burns involving commercial cleaning agents can damage the oropharynx and can create enough swelling to cause airway obstruction. Inhalation exposures can cause swelling and inflammation of the respiratory system, resulting in difficulty breathing and hypoxia. Gases such as carbon monoxide can cause profound hypoxia. Opioids and depressants can decrease respiratory drive, leading to hypoventilation. Many poisons have toxic cardiovascular effects that can significantly alter heart rate, heart rhythm, and blood pressure. Also common are neurologic abnormalities that result in confusion, seizures, and coma.

Carefully assess the patient's level of responsiveness using the AVPU (alert, verbal, pain, unresponsive) scale. Depending on the substance involved, the patient's condition can change quickly.

Next, perform a secondary assessment. Obtain a complete SAMPLE history (signs and symptoms, allergies, medications, past medical history, last oral intake, events leading up to the problem), paying close attention to any mention of the use or misuse of any substances or exposure to a poison. Occasionally, the patient will volunteer this information. Bystanders should be questioned for this information. At the same time, carefully assess the scene for signs that suggest exposure to a harmful substance. Look for pill bottles, drug paraphernalia, suspicious containers or baggies, alcoholic beverage containers, or cans of spray paint or solvent. Be alert to peculiar odors such as gasoline, glue, or other chemicals. Collect all items, including pill bottles and commercial containers, because they can provide valuable information about the substance(s) involved. Remember not to touch hazardous materials. Send these items to the emergency department with the patient. Do not contaminate yourself or others with a suspected toxic substance. Try to determine the dosage of exposure and how long ago it happened. Determine whether the patient has other conditions (or injuries) that could complicate the situation. It is important for OEC technicians to recognize that a poisoning or substance abuse situation has occurred.

Perform a physical examination using the DCAP-BTLS mnemonic (deformity, contusions, abrasions/avulsions, punctures/penetrations, burns/bleeding/bruises, tenderness, lacerations, swelling), looking for any signs that indicate the patient may have been exposed to a poisonous substance. Many poisons depress the central nervous system, which can include blocking sensations of pain, so patients may be unaware that they have sustained any injuries. Nausea and vomiting are common with exposure to poisons. Obtain a complete set of vital signs. The signs and symptoms of toxic substances are presented in **Table 12-1**.

The mnemonic SLUDGEM or DUMBELS can help identify specific signs and symptoms associated with organophosphate poisoning or exposure to nerve agents (**Table 12-2**).

Table 12-1 Signs and Symptoms of Toxic Substances

Substance	Signs and Symptoms
Acetaminophen	Nausea, vomiting
Aspirin	Nausea, vomiting, ringing in the ears
Acids and bases	Pain, tissue damage
Alcohol/depressants/ sedatives	Altered mental status, confusion, poor coordination, abnormal gait, slurred speech, nausea, vomiting

(continues)

Table 12-1 Signs and Symptoms (*continued*)

Substance	Signs and Symptoms
Antipsychotics/ antidepressants	Abnormal heart rate, abnormal heart rhythm, confusion
Carbon monoxide	Decreased level of responsiveness, lightheadedness, nausea, confusion, depressed mental status, reddened skin (late sign)
Cocaine	Agitation, chest pain, elevated heart rate and blood pressure; psychosis may also be observed
Ethylene glycol	Nausea, vomiting, altered level of responsiveness, elevated heart rate and blood pressure, seizure, coma
Hallucinogens (LSD)	Agitation; restlessness; psychosis; hallucinations; elevated heart rate, blood pressure, and skin temperature
Inhalants	Respiratory distress, confusion, hypoxia, respiratory failure, decreased level of responsiveness, shock, coma
Marijuana	Decreased level of responsiveness, confusion, drowsiness
Methane	Decreased level of responsiveness, confusion, drowsiness, nausea, vomiting
Opioids (narcotics)	Euphoria, decreased level of responsiveness, respiratory depression
Organophosphates/ nerve agents	Excess salivation, tearing, coughing up mucus, respiratory depression, cardio-vascular arrest due to respiratory failure, arrhythmias, headache, depressed mental status, coma
PCP	Agitation, psychosis
Stimulants/ methamphetamine	Agitation, psychosis, chest pain, elevated heart rate

Table 12-2 SLUDGEM and DUMBELS

SLUDGEM	DUMBELS
S—Salivation	**D**—Defecation
L—Lacrimation (tearing)	**U**—Urination
U—Urination	**M**—Miosis (constriction of the pupils)/muscle weakness
D—Defecation	**B**—Bronchorrhea (discharge of mucus from the airways)
G—Gastrointestinal irritation (vomiting)	**E**—Emesis (vomiting)
E—Eye (pupillary) constriction	**L**—Lacrimation (tearing)
M—Miosis/muscle twitching	**S**—Salivation

MANAGEMENT OF SUBSTANCE ABUSE AND POISONING

Personal safety is of paramount importance. The first step, then, is to secure the scene. You must ensure that your safety is protected first and that further injury to the patient will not occur. This concern for personal safety is especially relevant at scenes involving gaseous poisons (e.g., carbon monoxide, chlorine) and other chemicals (e.g., insecticides, nerve agents). Do not enter the scene until it has been deemed safe by a hazmat team, fire officials, or both.

Treatment of a patient affected by a toxicological event is generally supportive in nature. It requires diligent attention to the patient's overall appearance, ABCDs, and vital signs. Perform the primary assessment and address any threats to life. Call early for transport and advanced life support (ALS) if needed. The patient's respiratory status should be continually monitored for changes. Manage airway and breathing problems as necessary.

Help Is Only a Phone Call Away

Many times, deciding on the best way to care for a patient is not easy, especially in outdoor environments, where transport times may be prolonged and treatment options are limited. Provided you have a radio or cell phone nearby, you may obtain immediate advice from a physician or medical toxicologist by first contacting medical direction per your local protocols. You also may contact the American Association of Poison Control Centers, which coordinates a network of every poison control center in the United States. It can be reached 24 hours a day, 7 days a week using the phone number 1-800-222-1222 (**Figure 12-4**). The poison control center can give you up-to-date information about a poison and its treatment and give you recommendations concerning the necessity for additional medical care.

If you happen upon an accident scene involving the transportation of a toxic chemical, your first call should go to the Chemical Transportation Emergency Center (CHEMTREC). CHEMTREC is a service of the American Chemistry Council. Registration of a chemical allows CHEMTREC to perform its emergency response function, which is to provide information concerning any of a registrant's products that may be involved in a transportation accident. A CHEMTREC-registered chemical is tagged with emergency information, including an emergency phone number, 1-800-262-8200, by which important information about the product can be obtained.

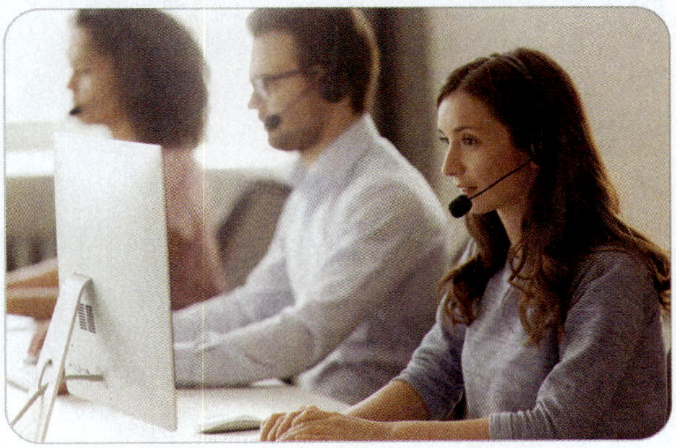

Figure 12-4 Poison control operators are standing by 24/7 to answer calls and provide help.

Relatively few toxicological emergencies can be effectively managed in the field. Beyond emergency interventions and normal supportive care, most toxicological emergencies require treatment in a definitive-care setting. High-flow oxygen, keeping the oxygen saturation level between 94% and 99%, is beneficial to toxic exposures that involve the respiratory system and is the primary treatment for events such as carbon monoxide poisoning and methane poisoning. Oxygen is also essential for patients exposed to any poisons that either stimulate or depress the central nervous system.

Beyond the initial assessment and stabilization of the patient, care for a victim of poisoning follows these steps: reduce further exposure, reduce absorption, and rapidly transport to a definitive-care facility.

Reduce Further Exposure

For ingested poisons, dilute the poison by having the patient drink water, but *only* if instructed by your medical director or the local poison center and if there are no contraindications (**Figure 12-5**).

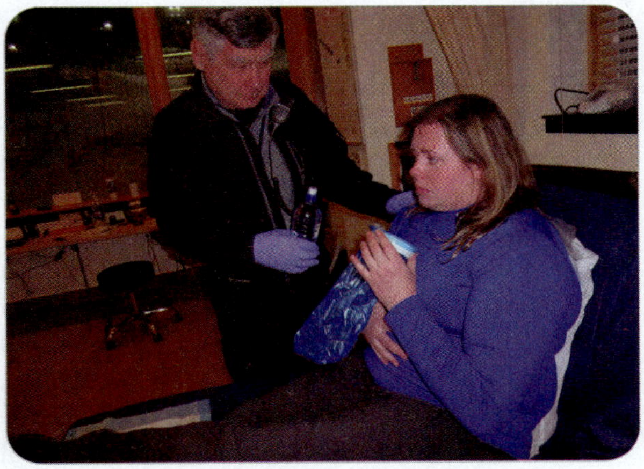

Figure 12-5 For ingested poisons, dilute the poison by having the patient drink water, if instructed to do so by your medical director or poison center, and if there are no contraindications.

General contraindications for giving a poisoning patient water by mouth include nausea/vomiting, depressed level of responsiveness, or having ingested a substance that has the potential to depress level of responsiveness. Although the administration of an emetic (an agent that induces vomiting) was once recommended for cases involving certain ingested substances, subsequent studies have shown that inducing vomiting can be dangerous and does not significantly reduce absorption. Therefore, OEC technicians should *never* induce vomiting in a poisoned patient.

For dry topical poisons absorbed through the skin, brush off the particles using and wearing appropriate personal protective equipment and rinse away any residue with water. First ensure that the poison does not react with water. For wet poisons, thoroughly rinse the affected area with water. If ocular exposure occurred, immediately irrigate the eyes with copious amounts of sterile water. Remember to always protect yourself from becoming contaminated.

For inhaled poisons, immediately remove the patient from the source of poisoning. Maintain the airway, administer high-flow oxygen via a nonrebreather mask, and consider transport with ALS if you observe a notable disturbance in coordination or balance, difficulty breathing, or altered mental status. If the inhaled poison is still present, do not attempt rescue until a hazmat team has removed the source, so you do not become a victim.

Reduce Absorption

Activated charcoal absorbs and binds many poisons. It is a relatively safe medication that has been shown to be most effective in decreasing absorption if given within 60 minutes following ingestion of a poison. Charcoal may also be beneficial after 60 minutes in patients who have ingested extended-release medications or have delayed emptying of the gastrointestinal tract. Therefore, activated charcoal may be administered *only* if authorized by a medical advisor or poison control center. Because activated charcoal is very difficult to remove from the respiratory system, it should *not* be given to any patient with a decreased level of responsiveness.

Specific Interventions

The following list provides guidance for responding to specific types of poisoning you may encounter in the field.

- *Opioid poisoning.* If you think the person has taken an opioid either by mouth or injection, using personal protective equipment, give naloxone if trained to use it and management has approved giving it (**Figure 12-6**). Continue to watch the patient if they respond to the medication. Call for an ALS ambulance. When you give naloxone, remember that the patient may wake up and react violently to the drug, potentially trying to hurt you.
- *Carbon monoxide poisoning.* Once the patient has been removed from the source of the carbon monoxide gas, administer 100% oxygen via nonrebreather, if available. Sometimes hyperbaric oxygen (i.e., oxygen at high pressure) is necessary for severely poisoned patients.
- *Inhalation poisoning.* Inhaled poisons, such as dust, fumes, and aerosols, may become deposited in the upper airways and cause damage, depending on the size of the particles. Inhaled poisons include natural gas and cyanide. Once again, 100% oxygen is the initial treatment of choice.
- *Organophosphate poisoning.* If you, a fellow rescuer, or a patient has been exposed to an organophosphate (e.g., insecticides) or

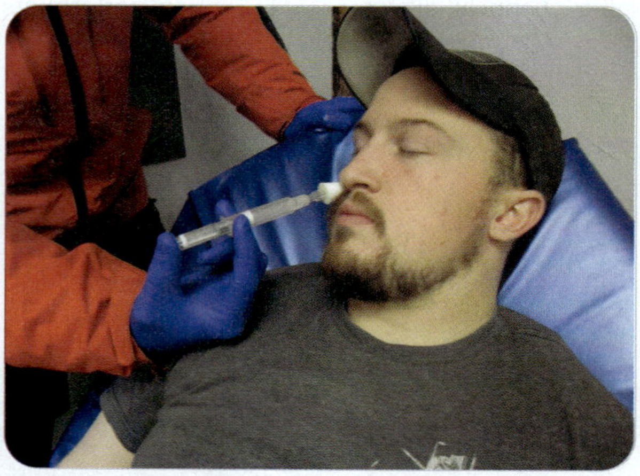

Figure 12-6 Naloxone can save a life when administered correctly and in time.

a chemical nerve agent, administering the Mark I or DuoDote antidote kit (discussed in Chapter 34, *Special Operations and Ambulance Operations*) can be lifesaving.

The approach to the ingestion of toxic plant material is like the approach used for other toxicological events. For more information about the treatment of toxic plant ingestions, see Chapter 27, *Plant and Animal Emergencies*. Specific treatments for other poisonings and toxic exposures are beyond the scope of training for OEC technicians. When in doubt, support the patient's ABCDs and transport the patient to an acute-care facility.

CASE Outcome

Suspecting acute alcohol intoxication, and possibly other issues from drugs, you call for transport and ALS. Further secondary examination does not reveal any other problems. Security arrives and provides crowd control. You continue to monitor the airway and provide oxygen, because his respirations are diminished. You watch for vomiting and have suction ready to prevent aspiration.

EMS arrives and takes the patient to the hospital. Later you find out he had a blood alcohol level of 0.35% which is very high. He recovers in an intensive care unit and was lucky he did not die.

CHAPTER REVIEW

In Summary

- Personal safety is always the first priority.
- Alcohol is the most commonly abused drug in the world.
- Carbon monoxide poisoning is a silent killer.
- Always try to identify the poison involved in an incident.
- Remember to use the mnemonics SLUDGEM and DUMBELS for organophosphate and nerve agent poisonings.
- In the United States, poison-related information is available 24 hours a day, 7 days a week, by calling the American Association of Poison Control Centers at 1-800-222-1222.
- If you encounter an accident scene involving the transportation of a toxic chemical, call CHEMTREC (1-800-262-8200) for information about the product.

Key Terms

Absorption The way in which a substance or poison enters the body. The four routes of absorption are ingestion, inhalation, transdermal absorption, and injection.

Dermal poisons Harmful substances that are absorbed through the skin.

Designer drugs Drugs that are constructed by a chemist to produce unique and specific effects.

Ingested poisons Harmful substances that enter the body through the mouth.

Inhaled poisons Harmful substances that are absorbed through the lungs.

Injected poisons Harmful substances that are injected into a vein or another tissue.

Opioids Drugs that are derived from opium or opium-like compounds; sometimes referred to as narcotics.

Poison Any substance that is injurious to health or dangerous to life.

Substance abuse The intentional misuse of a substance that results in impairment or physical harm.

Toxicological event An event in which a patient has been exposed to a harmful substance *or* an incident in which the intentional or unintentional use of a substance or poison endangers public safety and/or results in a medical emergency.

Toxin A noxious or poisonous substance that is produced by an organism.

Withdrawal The physical and mental readjustment that accompanies the discontinued use of an addictive substance.

Chapter Questions

1. The process by which the body breaks down a substance is called:
   a. absorption.
   b. distribution.
   c. metabolism.
   d. elimination.

2. Your patient encountered poison ivy on a trail at your resort 2 days ago. He is complaining of itching and burning sensations. This patient has absorbed a poison through which of the following means?
   a. Ingestion
   b. Injection
   c. Transdermal absorption
   d. Inhalation

3. A customer at your ski resort has intentionally misused opioids, resulting in an impaired ability to ski. This guest demonstrates:
   a. substance abuse.
   b. withdrawal.
   c. poison abuse.
   d. toxin abuse.

4. A class of drugs that includes heroin, fentanyl, morphine, codeine, and oxycodone is called:
   a. depressants.
   b. opioids.
   c. designer drugs.
   d. hallucinogens.

5. You are called to the maintenance shop where two mechanics have been working on snow grooming equipment. The outside temperature is below zero and the garage doors to the maintenance shop have been closed. The mechanics are complaining of headache, dizziness, nausea, and breathing difficulty. You recognize these symptoms to be associated with:
   a. food poisoning.
   b. carbon monoxide poisoning.
   c. alcohol abuse.
   d. PCP use.

6. The emergency care for patients who are suffering from substance abuse or poisoning should include:
   a. reducing further exposure and absorption.
   b. providing rapid transport to a definitive-care facility.
   c. contacting the poison control center.
   d. All of the above

7. You are called to the parking lot at your resort. Chemicals are spilling out of a truck. Important information about the chemicals can be obtained by calling:
   a. the American Association of Poison Control Centers.
   b. CHEMTREC.
   c. 9-1-1.
   d. your area manager.

8. The mnemonics SLUDGEM and DUMBELS can help identify specific signs and symptoms associated with poisoning. The "L" in these mnemonics stands for lacrimation, which means what?
   a. Drooling
   b. Vomiting
   c. Tearing
   d. Pupil constriction

Answers: 1. c, Objective 12-1, p. 264; 2. c, Objective 12-2, p. 264; 3. a, Objective 12-3, p. 265; 4. b, Objective 12-3, p. 266; 5. b, Objective 12-4, p. 268; 6. d, Objective 12-5, p. 273; 7. b, Objective 12-6, p. 273; 8. c, Objective 12-7, p. 272

CHAPTER 13

RESPIRATORY EMERGENCIES

OBJECTIVES

Upon completion of this chapter, the OEC technician will be able to:

13-1 Describe the physiology of breathing.

13-2 Identify the primary muscle of ventilation.

13-3 List the normal respiratory rate for individuals in the following age groups:
- Infant
- Child
- Adult

13-4 Identify the most common cause of airway obstruction.

13-5 List the signs and symptoms of the following respiratory emergencies:
- Asthma
- Chronic obstructive pulmonary disease (COPD)
- Hyperventilation syndrome
- Pulmonary embolism
- Pneumothorax

13-6 Describe and demonstrate how to assess a patient who is having difficulty breathing.

13-7 List the signs and symptoms of acute respiratory distress.

13-8 Describe characteristics of abnormal breathing.

13-9 Demonstrate how to assess lung sounds.

13-10 Describe and demonstrate the appropriate management of a patient in respiratory distress.

13-11 Demonstrate how to assist the patient with an inhaler.

KEY TERMS

Anoxia, p. 284
Bradypnea, p. 286
Bronchospasm, p. 283
Chronic obstructive pulmonary disease (COPD), p. 283
Crepitus, p. 287
Dyspnea, p. 280
Hyperventilation syndrome, p. 284
Hypoxia, p. 283
Inhaler, p. 292
Pleura, p. 282
Pleural space, p. 282
Pneumothorax, p. 284
Ventilation, p. 280
Wheezing, p. 286

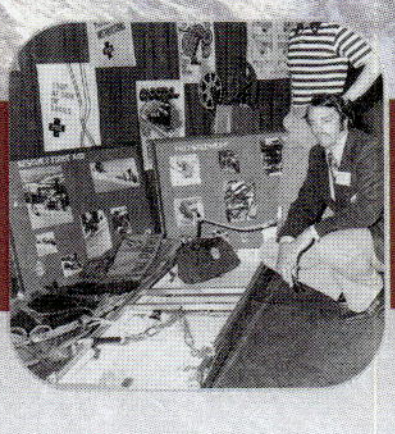

HISTORICAL TIMELINE **1970.** Patrol recruitment event during a period of expansive growth for the NSP.

CHAPTER OVERVIEW

OEC technicians may encounter patients with abnormal breathing. Problems can range from exercise-induced asthma, airway obstruction by a foreign body, to severe respiratory distress from pulmonary embolism. In addition, many patients can experience shortness of breath due to such medical conditions as heart attack, excessive blood loss, or conditions that have caused shock. A common patient complaint that OEC technicians encounter is **dyspnea**, which is difficult or labored breathing accompanied by feeling short of breath.

The oxygen supply to our brain cannot be interrupted for more than 4 minutes without severe and possibly even irreversible consequences. Caring for patients with respiratory problems requires OEC technicians to have a good understanding of the anatomy of the respiratory system.

The mechanical and physiological mechanisms by which the lungs take in oxygen from the air and expel carbon dioxide is called **ventilation**. Many other important terms associated with respiration will be introduced and explained so you will be able to communicate with peers and other medical personnel. By learning the normal ranges of respiratory rates for children and adults and learning how to assess the quality of breathing you will have the knowledge needed to assist patients with respiratory emergencies. The skills to provide ventilations or oxygen will be discussed. OEC technicians do not *diagnose* breathing problems, but they can perform a rapid, thorough respiratory assessment, identify potential threats to life, and initiate life-stabilizing therapy that includes oxygen delivery and transport to a higher level of care.

Many conditions and diseases causing breathing problems are discussed in this chapter. In 2015 almost 15% of adults in the United States had underlying pulmonary disease such as asthma, emphysema, or chronic bronchitis. Smoking is still a leading cause of lung disease.

This chapter begins by reviewing the major anatomical structures of the lower airway and the mechanics of breathing. It then discusses the most common types of respiratory emergencies that you will likely encounter, the signs and symptoms associated with each emergency, and their treatments.

ANATOMY AND PHYSIOLOGY

The anatomical structures that make up the respiratory system are described in detail in Chapter 6, *Anatomy and Physiology*. The airway begins at the mouth and nose and terminates in the lung tissue. Traditionally, the airway is divided at the epiglottis into two parts, the upper airway and the lower airway. The diaphragm and chest wall muscles mechanically expand the chest cavity, sucking outside air through the airway branches into the lung's many alveoli (**Figure 13-1**).

Air consists of 78% nitrogen, 21% oxygen, and 1% other gases. The relatively high oxygen concentration in air and the very low concentration of carbon dioxide drive the process of gas

CASE Presentation

A middle-aged man walks into the patrol medical room, saying "I can't breathe." You immediately have the man sit and begin your assessment. During your questioning, you find he is a smoker and 3 weeks ago had "minor knee surgery on his right leg." He said this is his first time out skiing since surgery. He is breathing at 28 breaths per minute and appears in distress. He has mild chest pain and cannot talk in complete sentences. His right calf is swollen and tender.

What should you do?

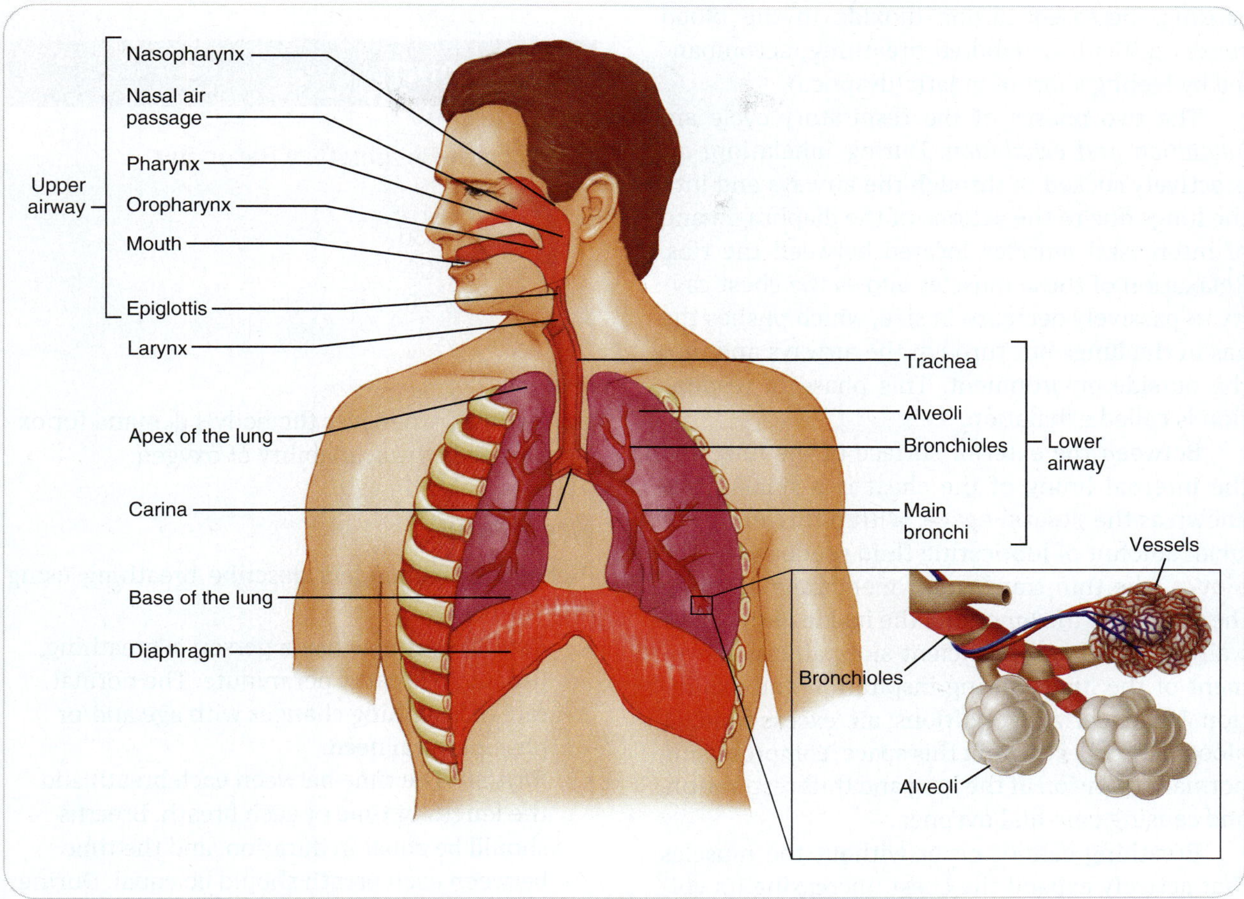

Figure 13-1 The respiratory system consists of all structures of the body that contribute to the process of breathing.

exchange at the alveolar level by a process called diffusion. The tiny air sacs called alveoli are organized into grape-like clusters and are the functional units of the pulmonary system. Each of the approximately 700 million alveoli serve as the sites of gas exchange. It is here that a thin membrane separates each alveolus from individual red blood cells traveling through microscopic capillaries. Oxygen moves by diffusion into the blood, in the capillaries of the alveoli, while carbon dioxide diffuses out of the blood in the capillaries of the alveoli, into the air that is exhaled. Once oxygen reaches the blood in the lung capillaries, it binds to hemoglobin in red blood cells and is carried throughout the body in the bloodstream. Carbonic acid, which is dissolved in the blood, is released from the capillaries as carbon dioxide, which is exhaled.

Respiratory rate and depth are controlled by the amount of acidity in the blood. More acid in the blood causes a lower "pH." A waste product from all our cells, carbon dioxide, combines with water in the blood to make carbonic acid, which lowers the pH of the blood. If there is excessive carbon dioxide in the blood making more carbonic acid, sensors located in the carotid arteries in the neck and in the aorta detect the lower pH and signal the brain to automatically increase the rate and depth of breathing. The increased respiratory rate blows off (exhales) excess carbon dioxide, raising the pH. Although this is a complex process, the important thing for OEC technicians to remember is that it is the amount of *carbon dioxide* dissolved in the blood that controls breathing, not the amount of oxygen in the blood. Any mechanical, structural, chemical, or neurologic disruption causing increased carbon dioxide in the blood causes difficult or labored breathing, accompanied by feeling short of breath (dyspnea).

The two phases of the respiratory cycle are *inhalation* and *exhalation*. During inhalation, air is actively sucked in through the airways and into the lungs due to the actions of the diaphragm and of intercostal muscles located between the ribs. Relaxation of these muscles allows the chest cavity to passively decrease in size, which pushes the gas in the lungs out through the airways and into the outside environment. This phase of respiration is called exhalation.

Between the exterior surface of the lung and the internal lining of the chest is a small space known as the **pleural space**. Within this space is a small amount of lubricating fluid produced by the **pleura** (the thin transparent membrane covering the outside of the lungs and the inside of the chest wall) that allows for efficient and painless movement of the lungs during inspiration and expiration. Under certain conditions, air, excess fluid, or blood may collect within this space, compromising normal expansion of the lung and thus respiration, and causing pain and dyspnea.

Breathing cannot occur without the muscles that actively expand the chest, increasing its volume and thus decreasing its internal pressure. The most important or primary muscle in this process is the diaphragm. This dome-shaped muscular sheet, which separates the thoracic and abdominal cavities, is the primary muscle of respiration. Upon inhalation, the diaphragm tightly contracts and flattens, which expands the volume of the chest, significantly lowering the pressure within the chest and sucking air into the lungs. During exhalation, the diaphragm relaxes and passively returns to its original position, reducing chest volume and increasing the pressure within the chest, which moves the air out of the body. Based on the blood's pH, the automatic part of the brain sends signals to nerves that come out of the cervical spine called the right and left phrenic nerves. These nerves go through the chest, inserting into the diaphragm and controlling this muscle's contractions.

Other muscles, including those of the chest, shoulder, neck, and abdomen, help to bring air into the lungs but have a less important role than the diaphragm. Those muscles, collectively referred to as the accessory muscles of respiration, are recruited whenever the body's demand for oxygen exceeds the availability of oxygen.

> **KEY POINT**
>
> **Normal Respiratory Rates per Minute**
>
> Infant: 20–60
> Child: 15–30
> Adult: 12–20

Breathing

Prehospital responders describe breathing using four terms:

- *Rate.* This is how fast a person is breathing, usually in breaths per minute. The normal rate of breathing changes with age and/or physiological need.
- *Rhythm.* The time between each breath and the length of time of each breath. Breaths should be equal in duration, and the time between each breath should be equal. During exercise, the rhythm remains the same, but the rate goes up.
- *Quality.* All breaths should produce very little external sound and should be inconspicuous except during exercise.
- *Depth.* The volume of air taken in for each breath. When more oxygen is needed, the chest will expand more on inhalation.

COMMON RESPIRATORY EMERGENCIES

The causes of respiratory emergencies are many and varied. The following sections describe the most common respiratory emergencies that you will encounter as an OEC technician.

Obstruction/Choking

For effective gas exchange to occur, airway patency must always be maintained. Any potential airway obstruction, from a foreign body (e.g., food, vomit, debris) or soft-tissue swelling (trauma or allergy/anaphylaxis), limits gas exchange and decreases

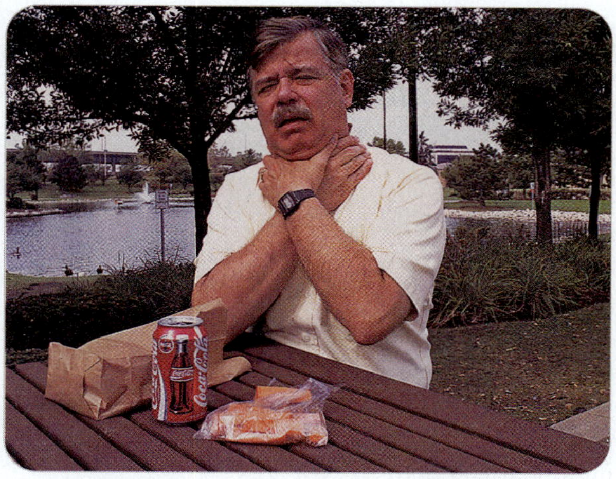

Figure 13-2 The universal sign of choking is a person who grasps his or her throat and has difficulty breathing.

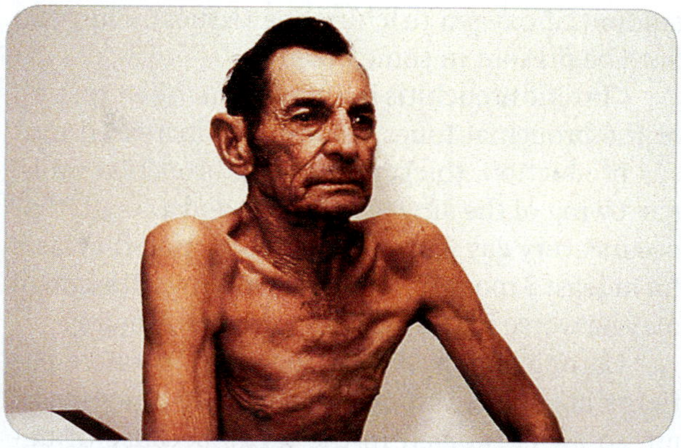

Figure 13-3 This person is suffering from severe COPD.

oxygen levels (**Figure 13-2**). *The tongue is the most common cause of airway obstruction.* In a patient who is lying down, the relaxed tongue can fall across the posterior pharynx and block the upper airway. In addition, foreign bodies that get past the epiglottis may become lodged in the trachea, a bronchus, or one of the lower airways, resulting in a foreign body obstruction. OEC technicians can remove obstructions from the airway by using the finger sweep, suction, gravity and positioning, or abdominal thrusts.

Asthma

Asthma is a respiratory disease characterized by sudden, recurrent lower airway constriction (bronchioles) and increased mucus production. Unlike chronic bronchitis or emphysema, an acute asthma attack can be reversed by treatment. In 2017, over 25 million children and adults in the United States had asthma. It can be life threatening and accounts for nearly 2 million visits to the emergency department each year. If left chronically untreated, permanent lung damage can occur.

Although the exact cause of asthma is not known, researchers believe that genetics and environmental triggers such as pollen, mold, allergens, or cold air can stimulate an intense reaction within the lower airways, resulting in acute **bronchospasm**, inflammation, and mucus accumulation. Strenuous physical activity also has been implicated as the cause of another, atypical variety of asthma, resulting in a condition known as exercise-induced asthma.

The condition called status asthmaticus involves a severe asthmatic attack that does not respond to inhaled medications. This condition requires the immediate dispatch of advanced life support and transport to the nearest hospital.

Chronic Obstructive Pulmonary Disease

Chronic obstructive pulmonary disease (COPD) is a chronic inflammatory lung disease that causes obstructed airflow by constricting the bronchi (the tubes) that carry air into and out of the lungs. Symptoms include breathing difficulty, cough, mucus (sputum) production and wheezing (**Figure 13-3**). COPD is most often caused by long-term cigarette smoking, but it also may be caused by certain diseases or by prolonged exposure to dust, chemicals, pollution, and other environmental irritants. According to a 2014 study by the Centers for Disease Control and Prevention, COPD is the third leading cause of death in the United States, with more than 15.7 million people diagnosed with COPD and many more undiagnosed.

People with COPD are at increased risk of developing heart disease, lung cancer, and a variety of other conditions. COPD cannot be cured but can be treated by improving oxygenation. OEC technicians should be familiar with two forms of COPD: chronic bronchitis and chronic emphysema. Both forms of COPD develop gradually and result in permanent lung damage and **hypoxia** (decreased amount of oxygen reaching the tissues). They can both be present in some people.

Chronic bronchitis is a persistent inflammation of the bronchial tubes resulting in increased mucus production, thickening of the bronchial walls, narrowing of the airway passages, and a cough that occurs every day with sputum production that lasts for at least 3 months, for 2 years in a row. The cough may be worse in the morning when awakening.

Chronic emphysema is a condition where patients are unable to exhale adequate amounts of air, so air is trapped in the lungs because of destruction of the tiny alveolar sacs where oxygen is absorbed. This results in the blood not being able to receive oxygen as well.

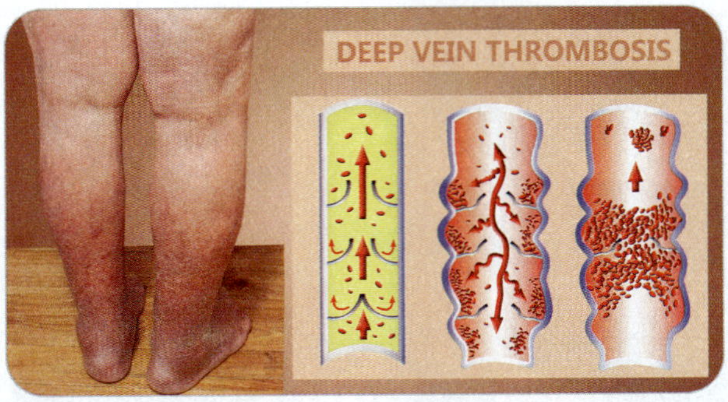

Figure 13-4 This swollen calf (right) could be caused by a deep vein thrombosis which is a blood clot. If the clot travels to the lung, it will form a pulmonary embolus.

Hyperventilation Syndrome

Hyperventilation syndrome (HVS) is a relatively common disorder that results in abnormally low levels of carbon dioxide in the blood. Excessive deep breathing, or hyperventilation, may be the body's response to some physiological insult such as uncontrolled diabetes, or it may be caused by psychological factors. HVS is often preceded by anxiety or a panic attack. Although the condition is usually benign, it can mimic other forms of deep breathing that have a more serious origin, such as heart attack, a diabetic emergency, or a head injury. In its most severe form, HVS can cause peripheral tingling, spasms in the hands and feet, chest tightness, tachycardia, and a temporary loss of responsiveness. It has also been known to cause seizures in patients who have seizure disorders.

Pulmonary Embolism

A pulmonary embolism is a condition where a blood clot becomes stuck in and blocks a pulmonary artery (**Figure 13-4**). The pulmonary artery is an artery that goes from the heart to the lung, where oxygen enters the blood. A blood clot, called a thrombus, travels from a distant location, usually a vein in the legs or pelvis. When the clot breaks loose, it can travel as an embolus through the right side of the heart, and lodge in the pulmonary artery. The resulting blockage disrupts the flow of blood through the lungs and back to the heart and prevents gas exchange in the lungs. Pulmonary embolism is rapidly fatal if it occurs in a large pulmonary artery and is not treated immediately.

Blood clots that often arise in the deep veins of either the lower legs or pelvis can break off and travel through the venous system through the right side of the heart and into the pulmonary circulation. In the legs the condition is characterized by a swollen tender calf caused by clots in the leg. This is called deep vein thrombosis (DVT). The causes of DVT are numerous and include prolonged sitting or immobilization, fracture of a long bone, recent surgery, heart disease, pregnancy, and certain inherited predispositions. A person who has had DVT previously is at an increased risk of a recurrence, especially if not taking medication to prevent reoccurrence.

Most cases of pulmonary edema (PE) affect only small portions of the lung; however, large blockages can obstruct blood flow to the entire lung, causing severe hypoxia or even **anoxia** (a condition characterized by the lack of an oxygen supply), with shock, and even death. The most lethal type of PE is a "saddle embolus," which occludes the lung's arterial circulation at the junction between the right and left pulmonary arteries, stopping blood flow into both of the lungs. Death from this form of PE can occur within minutes from acute right-sided heart strain, shock, and cardiac arrest.

Pneumothorax

A **pneumothorax** is an accumulation of air between the lung and inner chest wall (pleural space) (**Figure 13-5**). The most common cause of this condition is traumatic injury to the chest wall, ribs, or lung itself. However, chronic emphysema or severe acute asthma can cause alveoli to rupture spontaneously, causing air to escape from the lung into the pleural space. Depending on the size of the hole in the lung lining and subsequent air leakage, the problem may resolve spontaneously or cause profound hypoxia or shock requiring emergent hospital care. If there is blood instead of air in the pleural space it is called a hemothorax.

Other Respiratory System-Related Conditions

Among the variety of other medical conditions that can result in a respiratory emergency are trauma, altitude illness, pneumonia, and carbon monoxide poisoning. Trauma and altitude illness are covered in Chapter 18, *Principles of Trauma*, and Chapter 28, *Altitude-Related Emergencies*. It is important to remember that altitude illness can cause severe breathing problems and fluid in the lungs. This is called high-altitude pulmonary edema. Death can result if not treated rapidly.

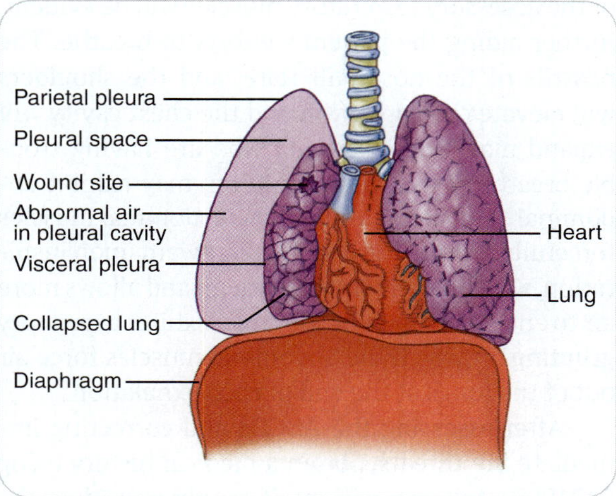

Figure 13-5 A pneumothorax is air inside the pleural cavity. This may collapse the entire lung.

Pneumonia, or inflammation of the lungs, can be caused by microorganisms, medications, and some medical diseases. The most common type, infectious pneumonia is caused by a bacterial, viral, parasitic, or fungal infection of the lung tissue. These pathogens cause the alveoli to become filled with fluid or pus, which reduces gas exchange, resulting in hypoxia. It is usually accompanied by fever. Pneumonia is a common disease, affecting more than 3 million people in the U.S. each year.

Carbon monoxide, an odorless, colorless gas that is a by-product of incomplete combustion, binds to red blood cells more easily than oxygen. As a result, not enough oxygen is absorbed by red blood cells, causing anoxia and eventually death.

Coronavirus: COVID-19

In 2020, COVID-19 was a global pandemic caused by a novel coronavirus. This virus was highly contagious, spread by airborne transmission. In many cases, symptoms included fever, cough, and shortness of breath. The elderly and people with compromised immune systems or serious medical problems were affected the most severely. At the time of the pandemic, there was no known vaccine or treatment. Social distancing, self-quarantining, PPE, and good handwashing was instituted but the virus continued to spread globally. This shows that an infectious disease can rapidly devastate mankind. OEC technicians should be ever-vigilant, using proper precautions when interacting with someone who has an infectious, airborne disease.

CASE Update

You place a pulse oximeter on his finger, which shows a pulse of 120 beats per minute and oxygen saturation of 85%. He becomes more anxious, and his respiratory rate is now 28 breaths per minute. Since he has chest pain and a low oxygen saturation with obvious respiratory distress, you place him on high-flow oxygen with a nonrebreather mask and have another patroller call for ALS transport. Your SAMPLE history only reveals recent knee surgery. While waiting for transport, you consider the possibilities of myocardial infarction, pulmonary embolism from blood clot (DVT) that came from the swollen calf, or other causes of acute breathing problems with chest pain. No matter what the medical problem is, transport is urgently needed.

How do you give a report to the prehospital ambulance personnel when they arrive?

PATIENT ASSESSMENT FOR RESPIRATORY EMERGENCIES

First do a scene size-up and ensure that the area is safe. As you approach the patient, note whether any signs of acute respiratory distress are apparent, or whether the patient's breathing is absent or noisy. Control severe bleeding. Conduct a primary patient assessment of the ABCDs, correcting any life-threatening conditions you identify, including opening and clearing the airway using any of the adjuncts identified in Chapter 9, *Airway Management*. If the patient has severe respiratory compromise, immediately call for ALS assistance. Assess the patient's circulation and level of responsiveness using AVPU.

Note the patient's overall appearance and any revealing signs. Does the patient appear ill at ease, restless, agitated, or confused? Does the patient seem thin or obese? Chronic bronchitis patients are generally overweight, have a productive cough, appear slightly cyanotic, and use their accessory muscles to breathe. Chronic emphysema patients are usually quite thin, have a barrel-shaped chest due to the trapping of air, and breathe through pursed lips; they seldom have a productive cough. Asthma patients generally appear very anxious, have rapid shallow breathing, and may have audible **wheezing**. Patients with pulmonary embolism may be cyanotic, may be panicked due to hunger for air, and have rapid, deep respirations. They may even be unresponsive, depending on the severity of the embolism and any resulting shock. Patients who are hyperventilating also may appear panicked and exhibit rapid, deep respirations, but their color is usually normal.

The hallmark of any respiratory-related emergency is dyspnea. Because "difficulty breathing" is a subjective term, it is essential that OEC technicians learn to recognize the signs and symptoms of acute respiratory distress, which provide valuable clues about the severity of the patient's condition and underlying hypoxia. These signs, which often precede complete respiratory failure, include the following:

- Choking or gagging
- Inability to speak
- Open-mouthed breathing
- Panting, gasping
- Breathing through pursed lips
- Tachypnea (greater than 30 breaths per minute in adults)
- **Bradypnea** (fewer than 10 breaths per minute in adults)
- Cyanosis
- Nasal flaring
- Sitting in an upright or tripod position
- Changes in level of responsiveness

In addition, patients who are having problems breathing will often assume a "tripod" position in which they sit upright while leaning forward with their hands near or gripping their thighs or knees (**Figure 13-6**). The elbows may be out from the body. This position lets gravity pull the chest wall outward and downward, which allows the lungs to expand more fully. In severe cases, involuntary use of the accessory respiratory muscles will be evident, further aiding the patient's efforts to breathe. The nostrils of the nose will flare, and the shoulders will elevate on inspiration and the chest cavity will expand maximally. Patients who are having trouble breathing, especially children, may exhibit abdominal breathing, in which the abdominal muscles forcefully expand the abdomen outward upon inspiration, which lowers the diaphragm and allows more air to enter the lungs, or they may exhibit expiratory grunting, in which the abdominal muscles force air out of the lungs at the end of each exhalation.

After assessing the ABCDs and correcting immediate life threats, obtain a medical history using SAMPLE. Ask the patient if anything makes the

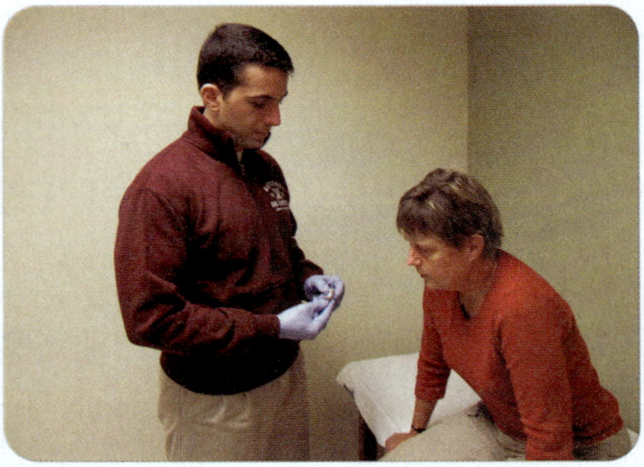

Figure 13-6 Finding a patient in the tripod position is a clue that the patient is having trouble breathing.

symptoms better or worse and be sure to query the patient about any medications the patient may be using, including over-the-counter drugs, herbs, and supplements. If you do not know what the medication is for, ask the patient. Find out if the patient uses an inhaler, and if so whether it is available. As part of the history, attempt to identify any associated symptoms such as a productive cough, fever, chest pain, or swelling of the lower extremities. Also ask about past medical problems such as blood clots or any underlying lung disease (e.g., COPD, asthma).

If the patient's history includes a respiratory ailment, ask how the current problem compares to previous episodes. Ask the patient if he or she could walk a short distance without becoming short of breath. This is important because the ability to ambulate to walk suggests that the underlying condition may be relatively minor, whereas shortness of breath while at rest or when walking only a short distance indicates a potentially serious condition.

Perform a secondary patient assessment, which includes a physical assessment and a check of the vital signs. Although it is evident the chief complaint is difficulty breathing, ask the patient if something else is wrong. Ask if there is chest pain. If the patient's dyspnea is relatively mild, the patient will provide this information with minimal effort and may even offer other unsolicited information, such as history of the problem, the duration of symptoms, and previous attempts at treatment. As you interview the patient, note whether the person can speak in complete sentences, or whether responses are broken into short groups of words. Severe dyspnea often limits the patient to one- or two-word answers. Frame your questions so that they may be answered with just a few words, or as short yes-or-no questions. Do not ask open-ended questions because the patient may not be able to answer due to a hunger for air.

Observe skin color for pallor or cyanosis, looking closely at the inside of the patient's eyelids, around the lips and at the fingernail beds (**Figure 13-7**).

Complete the rest of the physical examination in the usual fashion. For the chest exam, carefully palpate the skin of the patient's chest for the presence of any "crackling" or "Rice Krispies feeling" beneath the skin. This sign, known as subcutaneous emphysema or **crepitus**, is often due to a pneumothorax and indicates that air or gas is present beneath the skin. Other potential causes of subcutaneous crepitus include penetrating trauma and severe skin and tissue infections.

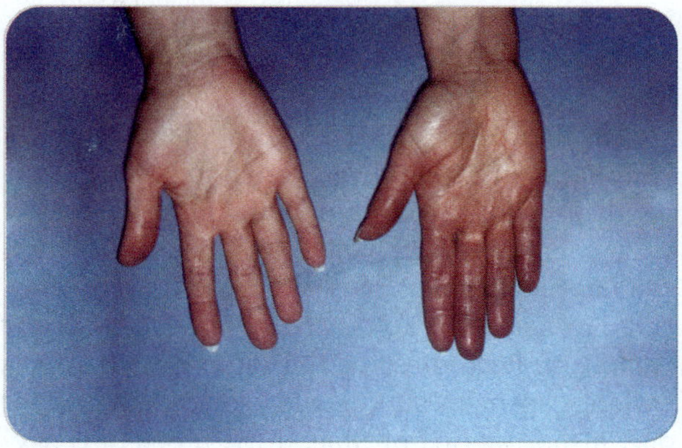

Figure 13-7 You can see the color difference between the cyanotic patient next to a patient with "normal" coloring.

> **KEY POINT**
>
> **Common Medications for Respiratory Conditions**
>
> - Albuterol (Proventil, Ventolin)
> - Albuterol/ipratropium (Combivent, Duoneb)
> - Aminophylline
> - Budesonide/formoterol (Symbicort)
> - Epinephrine (EpiPen)
> - Fluticasone (Flovent)
> - Fluticasone/salmeterol (Advair)
> - Ipratropium (Atrovent)
> - Prednisone
> - Terbutaline (Brethine)
> - Umeclidinium/vilanterol (Anoro Ellipta)

Obtain a complete set of vital signs, including the rate, rhythm, depth, and quality of respirations. Do not guess the respiratory rate; count the breaths for 30 seconds and multiply the count by 2 to determine the number of breaths per minute. Because vital signs change over time, repeat the vital signs frequently (every 5 minutes) in patients exhibiting signs of acute respiratory distress. *Vital signs are dynamic and change over time.* It is for this reason that several sets of vital signs usually provide more information than a single, isolated measurement and can serve as a marker for change, both favorable as well as unfavorable.

Respiratory rates less than 8 per minute or greater than 30 per minute in an adult are ominous and signify impending respiratory failure (remember that a normal respiratory rate for an adult is 12 to 20 per minute). Tachypnea and hyperventilation can have a variety of causes ranging from psychogenic in nature to a potentially lethal pulmonary embolism. Regardless of the underlying cause, a patient can maintain a rapid respiratory rate for only a short period of time. If the problem is psychogenic (e.g., hyperventilation), it will eventually resolve. If the problem is more serious, compensatory mechanisms will eventually be lost, and sudden respiratory failure will then result, especially in children.

Patients who are hyperventilating may complain of tingling or a "pins and needles" sensation around the lips, hands, or feet, a condition known as paresthesia. Patients also may complain of not being able to open their hands due to excessive muscle cramping. Upon observation, the hands and fingers may appear contorted. Although alarming to the patient, these findings are benign and will disappear once the patient's respiratory rate slows. Such psychogenic hyperventilation is typically seen in very anxious patients.

Breath Sounds

By listening to the patient's lungs using a stethoscope you can obtain valuable clues about the overall effectiveness of breathing efforts. Normal breath sounds are regular, relatively quiet (like a sigh), and equal for the two lungs. Abnormal breath sounds are diminished or absent, noisy (wheezes, crackles, gurgles), or unequal between the two lungs. It is beyond the scope of knowledge for OEC technicians to fully learn breath sounds. However, OEC technicians need to assess whether air is moving in and out of the lungs and to determine whether the patient is sufficiently oxygenated. This can be determined by assessing the patient's level of responsiveness, respiration quality and quantity, capillary refill, and skin color.

If you listen with a stethoscope, always tell the patient that you are going to listen to the lungs. When listening to breath sounds, place the patient in an upright position, preferably seated. The exception to this is when spinal injury is suspected, in which case the patient should remain in a neutral, supine position.

To avoid startling the patient with a cold stethoscope, warm it before use by vigorously rubbing it in a circular pattern on the palm of your hand. Also, place the stethoscope firmly against the patient's bare skin, not against clothing, as breath sounds may be subtle. Instruct the patient to breathe normally. If you are unable to hear the patient breathe, ask the patient to breathe through an open mouth or to breathe deeply. Using the large diaphragm of the stethoscope, listen at each location for approximately 15 seconds. As you listen, avoid unnecessary movement or talking, and do not allow the stethoscope tubing to rub against the patient's clothing or to bump into anything, because the resulting noise can make your assessment more difficult. Listen with a stethoscope over the eight locations seen in (**Figure 13-8**).

To assess lung sounds, follow the steps in **OEC Skill 13-1**.

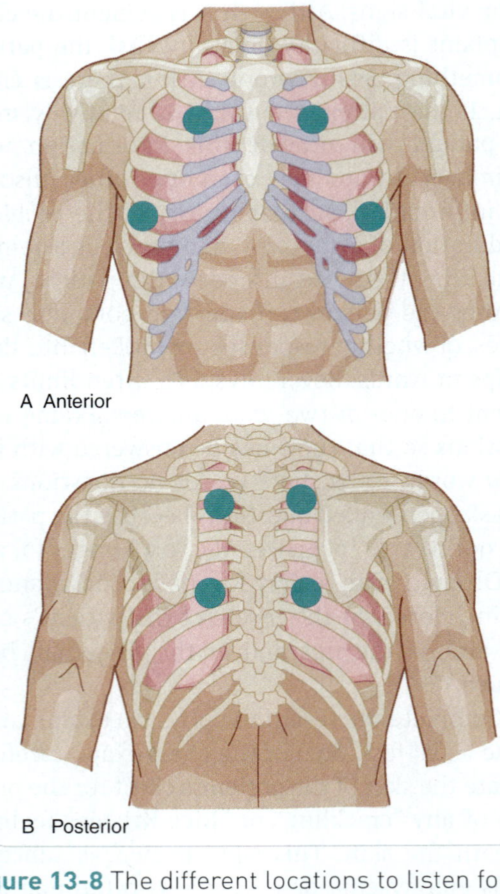

Figure 13-8 The different locations to listen for lung sounds.

OEC SKILL 13-1 Auscultation of Lung Sounds (8 Locations)

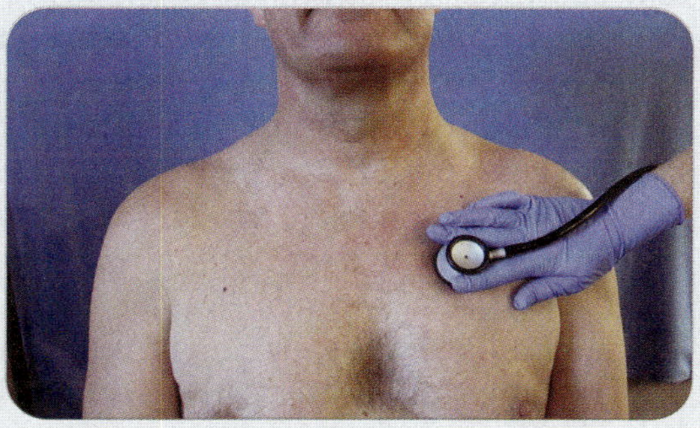

1 To listen to the **left upper lung lobes anterior**: place your stethoscope on the left side of the anterior chest 1.5 inches below the middle of the clavicle (midclavicular) (shown in Photo 1).

To listen to the **right upper lung lobes anterior**: place your stethoscope on the right side of the anterior chest 1.5 inches below the middle of the clavicle (midclavicular). Compare the results (Position 1 and 2).

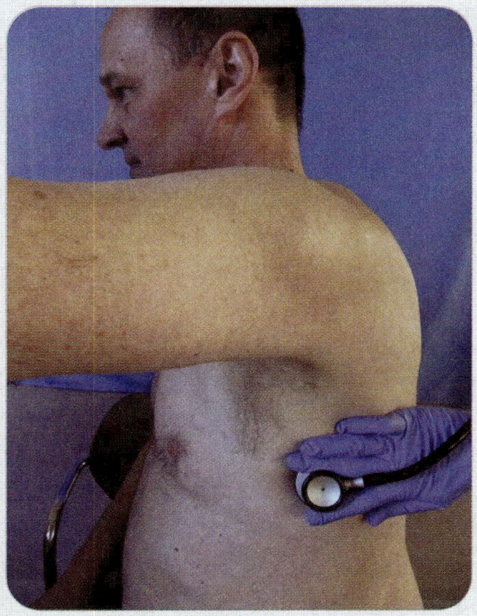

2 To listen to the **left lower lung lobe anterior**: place your stethoscope on the left midaxillary line between the 6th and 7th rib and under the armpit (shown in Photo 2).

To listen to the **right lower lung lobe anterior**: place your stethoscope on the right midaxillary line between the 6th and 7th rib and under the armpit. Compare the results (Position 3 and 4).

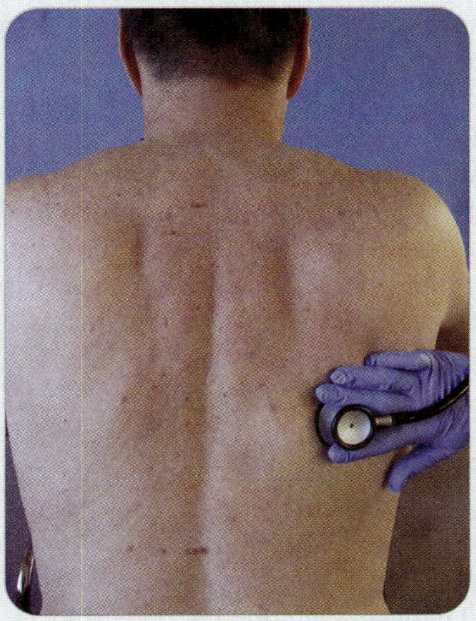

3 To listen to the **left upper lung lobe posterior**: place your stethoscope on the patient's left upper back between the top of the scapula and the spine, approximately 2 inches below the neck.

To listen to the **right upper lung lobe posterior**: place your stethoscope on the patient's right upper back between the top of the scapula and the spine, approximately 2 inches below the neck. Compare the results (Position 5 & 6).

To listen to the **left lower lung lobe posterior**: place your stethoscope on the patient's left lower back below the scapula and between the scapula and spine.

To listen to the **right lower lung lobe posterior**: place your stethoscope on the patient's right lower back below the scapula and between the scapula and spine (shown in Photo 3). Compare the results (Position 7 & 8).

KEY POINT

Wheezing

One of the most common abnormal breath sounds that OEC technicians will likely encounter is wheezing, which indicates constriction or narrowing of the lower airway passages. Wheezing is typically caused by asthma and is defined as a high-pitched respiratory sound that may be heard on inhalation, exhalation, or both. In most severe cases, wheezing can be heard without a stethoscope.

If you have a pulse oximeter and local protocol allows its use, assess the patient's blood oxygen concentration. Ideally, the patient's oxygen saturation should be between 94 and 99%. At high altitude the oxygen saturation may normally be slightly less than 94%. Any patient with a value below this should be given oxygen. Pulse oximetry is a useful tool for assessing oxygenation trends over time. Since the degree of dyspnea perceived by the patient may not correlate with the pulse oximeter readings, the instrument provides valuable information for deciding when to increase oxygen therapy or when to expedite the patient's transfer to a higher level of medical care.

If a patient with a pulse oximetry reading of 94% is cyanotic, breathing fast, and looks ill, trust your own observations and provide oxygen. Treat according to what the patient shows you, and not according to the number the pulse oximeter gives you. The pulse oximeter may not be giving a true reading.

MANAGEMENT OF RESPIRATORY EMERGENCIES

The treatment of a respiratory emergency by OEC technicians is straightforward and centers on improving the patient's overall oxygenation. Because breathing is essential to life, treatment begins by ensuring that the airway is open and clear, which is typically accomplished using one or more of the techniques or adjuncts described in Chapter 9, *Airway Management*. In addition, assess and monitor the pulse and treat for shock if found.

If the patient is choking, determine whether the patient can speak. If the person can speak, allow the patient to clear the airway on his or her own. If the patient is not able to speak, you must intervene quickly, or the patient will soon die. To clear the airway of a patient who is choking, whether responsive or unresponsive, follow the current American Heart Association guidelines or American Red Cross guidelines for performing abdominal thrusts. Refer to Chapter 9, *Airway Management*, for more information on clearing the airway.

If the patient is responsive and there is no indication of head or spine injury, allow the patient to assume a position of comfort that maximizes respiratory function. For most respiratory patients, this will be upright or a "tripod" position, which helps keep the abdominal contents from pushing upward on the diaphragm and maximizes the actions of the accessory muscles of respiration. OEC technicians should not place the patient in a supine position—unless signs of shock are present—because doing so will compromise the patient's breathing efforts and may even precipitate respiratory failure.

When having trouble breathing and shock is not present, load a patient into a ski toboggan with the patient's head uphill, elevating the chest and head slightly using an aid or equipment bag or a blanket. A patient on a backboard may need the head of the board to be raised slightly. Always administer supplemental oxygen for patients with a respiratory illness. As for whether to use a face mask or a nasal cannula, the simple answer is any patient with obvious respiratory distress should be placed on a nonrebreather mask initially at 15 liters per minute (LPM) (**Figure 13-9**). Lower the flow until the reservoir bag remains half full for every breath. High-flow oxygen administration through a properly fitting face mask can dramatically improve oxygen delivery to the tissues. If the patient has very mild shortness of breath and can speak in complete sentences, and the rate, rhythm, depth, and quality of respirations are normal, then a nasal cannula at 2 to 6 LPM may be used.

Most of the time if oxygen is given in the field, high-flow oxygen by nonrebreather mask is given (**Figure 13-10**). When in the aid room if pulse oximetry is used, after starting with high flow, adjust oxygen delivery to achieve an oxygen saturation level between 94 and 99%. As a rule, start oxygen delivery high and gradually reduce it as necessary

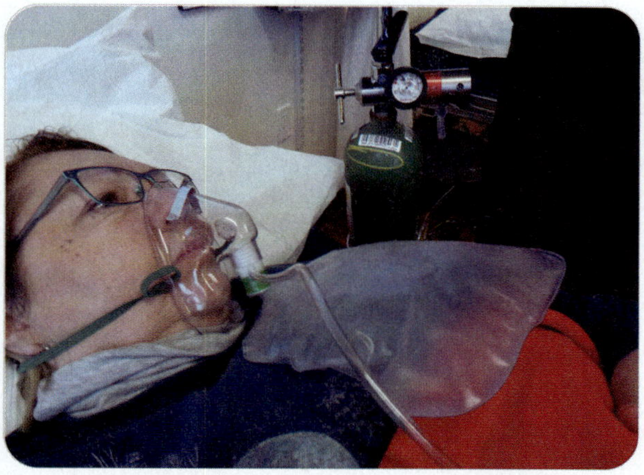

Figure 13-9 This patient is receiving high-flow oxygen via a rebreathing mask. The regulator is showing the flow rate (liters per minute, or LPM).

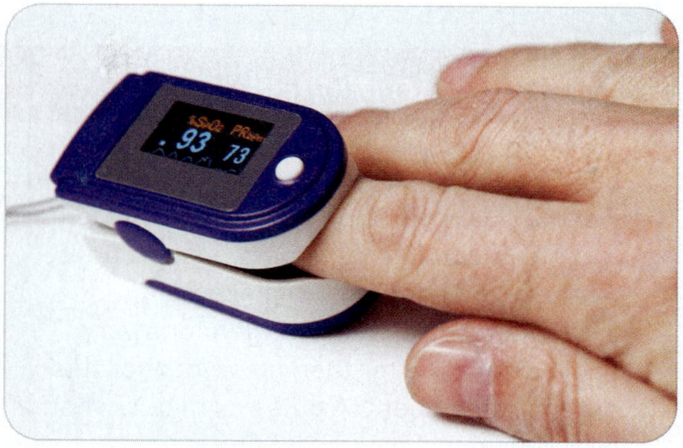

Figure 13-10 Pulse oximeter showing the oxygen saturation level in this patient.

("start high and titrate low"). If needed, assist the patient's ventilations using a bag-valve mask connected to oxygen.

Occasionally you will encounter a patient, especially a child, who refuses to wear a face mask, possibly from claustrophobia. Always encourage such patients to keep the face mask on, but if they refuse, hold the face mask as close to the face as possible, or use a nasal cannula at 6 LPM. This is better than not providing oxygen.

Altitude illness is treated by rapid descent to a lower altitude and using oxygen therapy. By descending several thousand feet, this condition usually improves. A full discussion of altitude illness is in Chapter 28, *Altitude-Related Emergencies*.

KEY POINT

Use of Oxygen: Adjust Appropriately with a Pulse Oximeter

Oxygen needs to be given appropriately. Recent medical evidence shows giving too much oxygen for certain medical conditions can expose tissues to an excess of oxygen, a condition called hyperoxia, which is not good for the patient. For example, too much oxygen, even for a short time, when given to COPD patients or some patients with stroke, cardiac conditions, or traumatic brain injury may be harmful. An excess of oxygen produces changes in the chemistry of the blood and in the response of the neurologic system and brain. These changes can alter breathing inappropriately and cause other adverse consequences in the tissues, making the patient worse. You should no longer "just give oxygen." For example, putting an oxygen mask on a *healthy* 20-year-old male with an isolated wrist fracture is not necessary.

Although no definitive threshold for a normal value exists, an oxygen saturation between 94 and 99% is accepted as healthy. Readings on pulse oximeters below 85% are less accurate but certainly indicate profound hypoxemia (not enough oxygen) and the need for oxygen therapy. When considering oxygen administration, the following recommendations will help you make the right decision.

In the field in cold weather when a person appears cyanotic or has an elevated breathing rate and/or heart rate and clinically needs oxygen, place a nonrebreather mask on the patient and turn up oxygen to 15 liters per minute. Adjust the flow to keep the reservoir

(continues)

KEY POINT (*continued*)

bag half full when the patient inhales. In cold weather, using a pulse oximeter in the field is difficult due to cold fingers, inappropriate readings, and difficulty in placement (removing glove). Using oxygen for a very short term is better than no oxygen for the appropriate patient. A pulse oximeter, when available, may be used outside in warm weather or in a warm building.

Once the patient is in an aid room and warm, take a reading using a pulse oximeter if available. If oxygen saturation is 100%, adjust the flow down continuously, watching the pulse oximeter to ensure the oxygen saturation reading is between 94 and 99%. If it goes below 94%, immediately adjust the flow upward, and then keep the pulse oximeter reading between 94 and 99%. After adjustment, it may take up to 1 minute to get an accurate reading on the pulse oximeter. Effectively maintaining the patient's oxygen saturation level is especially important if there could be a long wait for the appropriate transport.

If the oxygen saturation remains between 94 and 99% with the flow adjusted way down, take the mask off. If you find the oxygen saturation on room air with the mask off is between 94 and 99%, leave the mask off. Otherwise adjust the flow to keep the oxygen saturation between 94 and 99%.

For patients who you think are hyperventilating, use the pulse oximeter to obtain a reading. If the device reads 100%, reassure the patient and encourage the patient to breathe more slowly. A paper bag is no longer used. Oxygen is not needed, unless the oxygen saturation reading is less than 94%.

Always look at the patient clinically. If the patient is having difficulty breathing or appears cyanotic, use your clinical skills. Rarely, a pulse oximeter can give a false reading. For example, if the patient is wearing fingernail polish, has cold fingers, or has recently been exposed to carbon monoxide (such as by smoking a cigarette), the pulse oximeter may give false or no readings.

Remember, a sick patient's condition may change, and oxygen may be necessary later during your care, so watch the pulse oximeter for changes, just as you continually assess blood pressure, heart rate, and respirations. Recheck every 5 minutes for critical patients and every 15 minutes for stable patients.

Understand that not enough oxygen (hypoxemia) is much worse than too much oxygen (oxygen toxicity) in a patient with breathing problems. When in doubt, or unable to measure oxygen saturation reliably, give supplemental oxygen.

Using an Inhaler

Patients with a chronic respiratory illness such as asthma often carry a metered-dose **inhaler**, or "puffer," with them. A metered-dose inhaler, or MDI, is a small pressurized canister containing a powerful medication that dilates the bronchioles, opens the airways, and allows the patient to breathe more easily. A typical MDI consists of a medication canister, a plastic housing/mouthpiece, and a spacer.

If your local protocol allows it, you may *assist* patients having an asthma attack to use *their own* inhalers. Do not use someone else's inhaler, and make sure the inhaler's expiration date has not passed. To assist patients with the self-administration of their own MDI, perform the procedure shown in **OEC Skill 13-2**.

OEC SKILL 13-2 Assisting a Patient with a Metered-Dose Inhaler

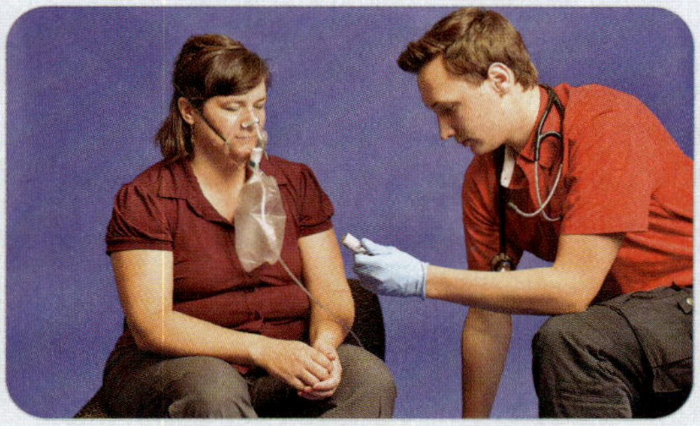

1 Check to make sure you have the correct medication for the correct patient. Check the expiration date. Ensure inhaler is at room temperature or warmer.

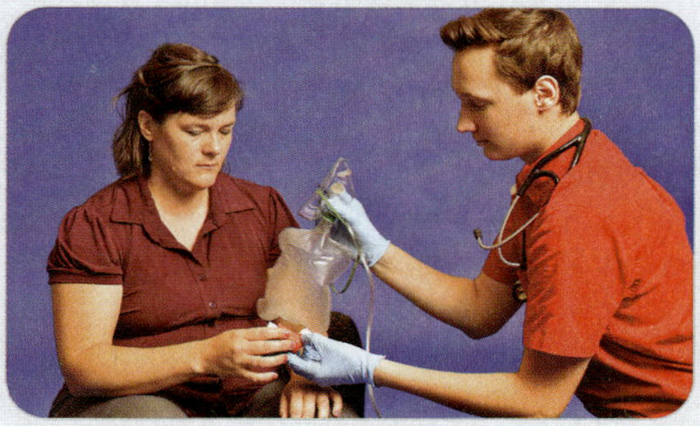

2 Remove the oxygen mask. Hand the inhaler to patient. Instruct the patient to hold the MDI upright and place their lips around the MDI tube, maintaining a good lip seal.

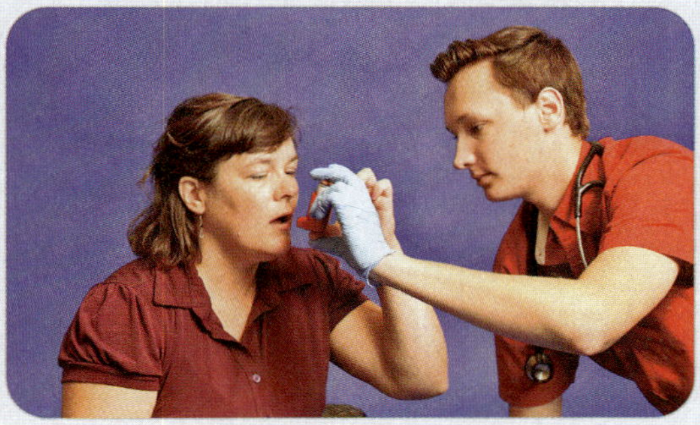

3 Instruct the patient to press the inhaler (assist if necessary) and inhale one puff. Instruct the patient to hold their breath for at least 10 seconds.

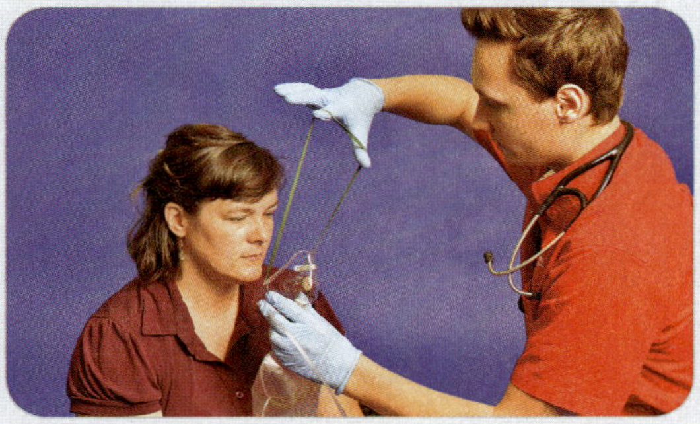

4 Reapply oxygen. After a 1 to 2 minutes, have the patient repeat the dose, if order or protocol allows.

CASE Outcome

Using a pulse oximeter, the patient's oxygen saturation is titrated and kept between 94 and 99%. You continue to take vital signs every 5 minutes, allowing the patient to continue to sit up. Ambulance personnel arrive. You explain the patient has had significant dyspnea and chest pain. He has been on oxygen with an oxygen saturation at 94%. You show the vital signs log, indicating elevated respirations and tachycardia. You explain the man had a knee arthroscopy 2 weeks ago.

Showing the swollen, painful calf to the paramedic, you both consider the possibility of a pulmonary embolism. Following rapid transport to a local hospital, further tests are completed, showing a blood clot in the man's lung. He is given medication to dissolve the clot, recovers, and comes back 3 weeks later to thank you.

CHAPTER REVIEW

In Summary

- Any mechanical, structural, chemical, or neurologic disruption causing increased carbon dioxide in the blood causes difficult or labored breathing, accompanied by feeling short of breath (dyspnea).
- The amount of carbon dioxide dissolved in the blood controls breathing.
- Breathing cannot occur without the muscles that actively expand the chest, increasing its volume and thus decreasing its internal pressure. The most important or primary muscle in this process is the diaphragm.
- The accessory muscles of respiration are used whenever the body's demand for oxygen exceeds the availability of oxygen.
- Prehospital responders describe breathing using four terms: rate, rhythm, quality, and depth.
- For effective gas exchange to occur, airway patency must always be maintained. OEC technicians can remove obstructions from the airway by using the finger sweep, suction, gravity and positioning, or abdominal thrusts.
- The causes of respiratory emergencies include obstruction/choking, asthma, chronic obstructive pulmonary disease, hyperventilation syndrome, pulmonary embolism, and pneumothorax. Other medical conditions that can result in a respiratory emergency are trauma, altitude illness, pneumonia, and carbon monoxide poisoning.
- It is essential that OEC technicians learn to recognize the signs and symptoms of acute respiratory distress.
- The use of accessory muscles of respiration is a sign of acute respiratory failure.
- By listening to the patient's lungs using a stethoscope you can obtain valuable clues about the overall effectiveness of breathing efforts.
- Always administer supplemental oxygen for patients with a respiratory illness. High-flow oxygen administration through a properly fitting face mask can dramatically improve oxygen delivery to the tissues.
- If the patient has very mild shortness of breath and can speak in complete sentences, and the rate, rhythm, depth, and quality of respirations are normal, then a nasal cannula at 2 to 6 LPM may be used.
- Start oxygen therapy high and titrate low. If a pulse oximeter is available titrate oxygen keeping the oxygen saturation between 94 and 99%.
- Check your local, state, or provincial protocols to determine whether you may assist a patient in the self-administration of a metered-dose inhaler.
- Consult with your local medical advisor and mountain management and follow local, state, or provincial laws in establishing a protocol for providing oxygen to patients.
- Respiratory emergencies are among the most common emergencies that OEC technicians will face.

Key Terms

Anoxia A condition characterized by the lack of an oxygen supply.

Bradypnea A decreased respiratory rate; in adults, less than 10 breaths per minute.

Bronchospasm The involuntary contraction of the bronchioles.

Chronic obstructive pulmonary disease (COPD) A chronic inflammatory lung disease that causes obstructed airflow by causing constriction of bronchi that carry air into and out of the lungs.

Crepitus A "crackling" feel of the skin of the chest that is detected by palpation; is caused by the presence of air trapped beneath the skin.

Dyspnea Difficult or labored breathing accompanied by feeling short of breath.

Hyperventilation syndrome (HVS) Abnormally low levels of carbon dioxide in the blood.

Hypoxia A decreased amount of oxygen reaching the tissues.

Inhaler A device that contains respiratory medicine and is used to improve breathing.

Pleura The thin transparent membrane covering the outside of the lungs and the inside of the chest wall.

Pleural space The potential space that lies within the pleura covering the outside of the lungs and the inside of the chest wall.

Pneumothorax An abnormal collection of air within the pleural space.

Ventilation The process by which air moves into and out of the lungs, so that oxygen can be exchanged for carbon dioxide in the alveoli.

Wheezing A high-pitched respiratory sound caused by a narrowing of the tubular airways.

Chapter Questions

1. The primary muscle of respiration is the:
   a. alveolus.
   b. diaphragm.
   c. lung.
   d. pleural space.
2. The site at which oxygen and carbon dioxide are exchanged between inhaled air and the bloodstream is called the:
   a. bronchi.
   b. bronchiole.
   c. trachea.
   d. alveoli.
3. When assessing a patient for normal breathing, consider:
   a. skin color.
   b. chest expansion.
   c. level of distress.
   d. Any of the above
4. You are assessing the respiratory rate of a 7-year-old boy. Your assessment finds that the boy is breathing 24 times per minute. You would describe this rate as:
   a. too slow.
   b. too fast.
   c. within normal limits.
   d. inconsistent.
5. The most common cause of airway obstruction is:
   a. the tongue.
   b. food.
   c. vomit.
   d. soft-tissue swelling.
6. You are asked to assist with a patient who is in acute respiratory distress. You might find this patient to be:
   a. gasping.
   b. having difficulty speaking.
   c. breathing through pursed lips.
   d. All of the above
7. An accumulation of air between the lung and the pleural space is called:
   a. pulmonary edema.
   b. COPD.
   c. a pulmonary embolism.
   d. a pneumothorax.

8. A blockage in the artery that carries blood from the right side of the heart to the lungs is called:
   a. pulmonary edema.
   b. COPD.
   c. a pulmonary embolism.
   d. a pneumothorax.

9. You are completing a report on a patient who was found to be breathing 8 times per minute. Which term best describes this rate?
   a. Tachypnea
   b. Bradypnea
   c. Cyanosis
   d. Crepitus

Answers: 1. b, Objective 13-2, p. 282; 2. d, Objective 13-1, p. 281; 3. d, Objective 13-8, p. 286; 4. c, Objective 13-3, p. 282; 5. a, Objective 13-4, p. 283; 6. d, Objective 13-7, p. 286; 7. d, Objective 13-5, p. 284; 8. c, Objective 13-5, p. 284; 9. b, Objective 13-3, p. 286

CHAPTER 14

ALLERGIES AND ANAPHYLAXIS

OBJECTIVES

Upon completion of this chapter, the OEC technician will be able to:

14-1 List four routes by which an allergen may enter the body.

14-2 List four potential allergy causes.

14-3 List the signs and symptoms of an allergic reaction.

14-4 Demonstrate the steps for properly using portable epinephrine auto-injectors.

KEY TERMS

Allergen, p. 301
Allergic reaction, p. 300
Anaphylaxis, p. 301
Angioedema, p. 302
Antibody, p. 301
Histamine, p. 301
Hypersensitivity, p. 301
Pruritus, p. 302
Urticaria, p. 302

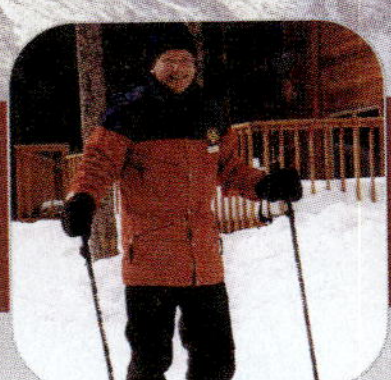

HISTORICAL TIMELINE 1970. Warren Bowman becomes NSP National Medical Advisor.

CHAPTER OVERVIEW

Many people have medical problems caused by allergies. There are many different substances that can cause an allergic reaction in people. Substances causing allergies are everywhere. These substances can be in the air such as pollen or be from common foods such as peanuts or shellfish. Many people are allergic to medications.

Allergies can be more than a simple nuisance; in their most severe form they can be deadly. Allergies affect 30% of the adults and 40% of children in the United States, with 4% of adults and 5% of children having food allergies. Interestingly, people who live in developed nations are far more likely to have allergies than those who live in undeveloped nations. The reasons for this are unclear, although some think it is due to exposure to possible allergens at an earlier age in undeveloped countries. What is clear, is that the prevalence of allergies is rising at an alarming rate. OEC technicians are increasingly likely to encounter patients who are experiencing an **allergic reaction**. Allergy-related signs and symptoms can vary widely, from a simple runny nose, to hives, to shortness of breath, to life-threatening shock (**Figure 14-1**).

As an OEC technician, you need to have a basic understanding of the causes of allergies and their effects on the body. You must be able to recognize the signs and symptoms of an allergic reaction and be ready to help at a moment's notice. This is especially true for severe allergic reactions, in which death can occur from anaphylaxis within minutes if the problem is not quickly treated. OEC technicians are in a unique position to assist allergy patients because they are typically the first to arrive at the patient's side. The correct and timely responses to the situation may lessen the overall effects of an allergic reaction. You may even save the patient's life by assisting them with their emergency allergy medications in the event of a severe allergic reaction.

ANATOMY AND PHYSIOLOGY

The immune system is a complex collection of the body's cells, proteins, and organs that protect the body from foreign substances, including viruses, bacteria, and other microorganisms. Chief among the immune system's primary components are white blood cells, hormones, lymph nodes, bone

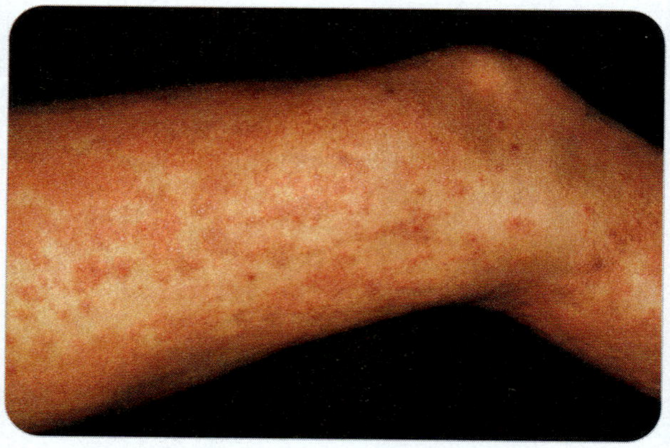

Figure 14-1 Allergic reactions can result in skin reactions such as a rash or hives.

CASE Presentation

You arrive on scene to assist a 16-year-old girl who is complaining of shortness of breath in the resort's picnic area. In very short phrases, she states, "I have . . . a hard time . . . breathing." She appears to be very anxious and says, "My tongue feels fat." She denies any preexisting medical problems but states, "I am deathly . . . allergic to peanuts." Her mother says she had a reaction to peanuts twice before. The last time required hospitalization. She appears to be very afraid. Just then you notice only a few feet away a small girl eating a peanut butter and jelly sandwich.

What should you do?

marrow, the thymus, and the spleen. Without the immune system, your body would be constantly invaded by pathogens that could easily harm or even kill you. The immune system is highly specialized and can distinguish between the body's normal cells and millions of foreign substances, known as antigens. When antigens get into the body, this stimulates the production of an antibody. These foreign substances could be allergens, toxins, bacteria, foreign blood cells, or the cells of transplanted organs.

Under normal conditions, when an antigen is first introduced into the body, the immune system quickly responds by identifying it and then developing antibodies against it. An **antibody** is a protein that helps destroy specific antigens. When mobilized, antibodies target the offending antigen. This triggers a chain of events, known as antigen–antibody reaction, which results in the immune system attacking and destroying the antigen without harming normal body cells.

The antibodies produced from an initial exposure to the antigen are specific to that antigen, and those antibodies continue to be present in the body. So the next time that antigen enters the body, the immune system is ready. This explains why a person who contracts a disease such as measles enjoys life-long protection if exposed to the disease again.

Occasionally, and for reasons unknown, the immune system overreacts to a substance that is otherwise harmless to humans (e.g., pollen) and develops a **hypersensitivity** to it. When this occurs, subsequent exposures cause the immune system to exaggerate its response by producing excessive amounts of antibodies. We know this hypersensitivity as an allergy, and the exaggerated response is better known as an allergic reaction. A severe allergic reaction, known as **anaphylaxis**, can result in life-threatening shock (anaphylactic shock) (**Figure 14-2**). Allergies can affect anyone and at any time, regardless of age.

Any antigen that triggers an allergic response is known as an allergen. An **allergen** can enter the body via four routes. They can be inhaled, ingested, injected, or touch the skin (topical). Once a person develops an allergy to a specific allergen, repeated exposure will again produce an allergic reaction. How the body responds to an allergen and how long the effects last depend on the body's sensitivity to the substance. A mild reaction typically causes skin-related effects, such as a rash or itching, whereas a severe antigen–antibody reaction stimulates a massive inflammatory response due to the release of a chemical called **histamine** into the bloodstream, an event that can result in cardiovascular collapse and death.

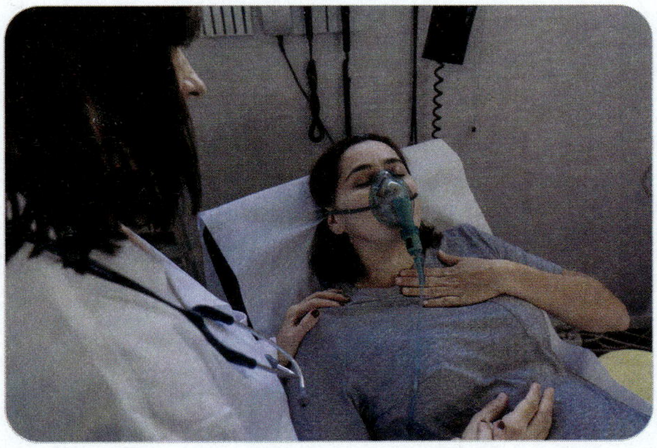

Figure 14-2 This patient is having a severe allergic reaction, which requires assistance with oxygen.

Histamine is a protein produced by specialized cells in the immune system called mast cells. Histamine causes local and peripheral edema (swelling), bronchoconstriction (contraction of smooth muscles in the bronchi), vasodilation (blood vessels dilate), hives, itching, and pain. It is the primary culprit in the production of an allergic reaction. Most allergic reactions occur within minutes to hours following the *subsequent* exposure to the allergen. However, some allergic reactions occur much later, after repeated exposure to an allergen and once the body develops a hypersensitivity to the substance.

COMMON CAUSES OF ALLERGIES

Allergies can occur throughout the year (chronic allergies) or they can be seasonal, affecting an individual only during certain times of the year. Allergies have a variety of causes, including the following (**Figure 14-3**):

- Foods (e.g., peanuts, sesame seeds, shellfish, nuts, soy, milk, eggs, chocolate)
- Insect bites and stings
- Environmental irritants (e.g., smoke, airborne particles)
- Pollen and plant parts (e.g., weeds, grasses, trees)

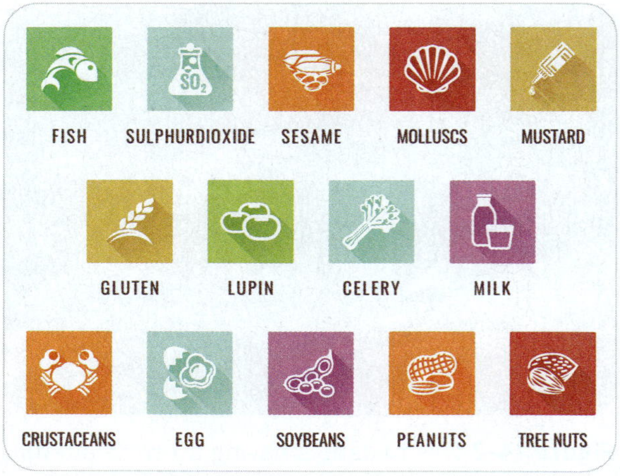

Figure 14-3 Some of the many things that can cause an allergic reaction.

- Molds (e.g., mildew, spores)
- Animal dander (e.g., skin flakes, fur)
- Medications (e.g., antibiotics, pain medications)
- Chemicals (e.g., latex)
- Other causes (e.g., blood transfusions, organ transplants, radiographic dyes)

Peanuts are the number one cause of allergic reactions to food in the world. The exact reason for this is unknown. In the United States in 2019, approximately 3 million people were allergic to peanuts. Studies indicate that children are more prone to peanut allergies than are adults. Dust mites, which are commonly found in household dust, are another leading allergen.

Chemicals such as natural rubber and latex are known to induce allergic reactions. Medical personnel, including OEC technicians, are strongly encouraged to use latex-free medical supplies and equipment. Even severe stress can evoke an allergic reaction in susceptible individuals. Allergies may also have a genetic component.

Categories of Allergic Reactions

Allergic reactions are categorized according to their effects as mild, moderate, or severe. Unfortunately, most people do not realize they are allergic to a substance until they have a reaction.

Mild Allergic Reactions

Mild allergic reactions typically result in skin reactions such as a rash or hives, known as **urticaria**. The rash may appear anywhere on the body. Flushed and/or itchy skin, known as **pruritus**; tingling in or around the mouth; swelling of the nasal mucosa, a runny nose, and nasal congestion; sneezing; watery reddened eyes; and a general feeling of being tired or "run down" can also be seen in a mild reaction (**Table 14-1**). Depending on the person's sensitivity to the allergen, signs and symptoms may take minutes, hours, or even days to develop. The effects usually disappear over time or with treatment.

Table 14-1 Mild Allergic Reaction

- Itching/scratching
- Flushed skin
- Rash or hives
- Watery, reddened eyes
- Nasal congestion
- Increased heart rate (over normal resting rate)
- Tingling in/around the mouth
- Fatigue

Moderate Allergic Reactions

The effects of moderate allergic reactions include all those that occur in mild reactions, but they are more pronounced (**Table 14-2**). Hives can appear on the chest and arms, and itching is worse. Additionally, the skin can become flushed or pale. **Angioedema**, the swelling or "puffiness" of the tissues beneath the skin, is common around the eyes, mouth, and hands (**Figure 14-4**).

Table 14-2 Moderate Allergic Reaction

- Anxiety, confusion
- Tightness in the throat
- Difficulty swallowing
- Difficulty breathing
- Wheezing
- Rash or hives on the face, neck, chest, or arms
- Persistent itching/scratching
- Angioedema of the face or hands (patients often complain that rings feel tighter)
- Abdominal pain or cramping
- Nausea and/or vomiting
- Elevated vital signs

Moderate allergic reactions also affect the respiratory system. Breathing may become mildly compromised as the bronchioles constrict and secretions within them thicken. Wheezing (high pitched whistling sound) is often present and may be pronounced. Swelling can become more pronounced in and around the face and lips. The tongue may also

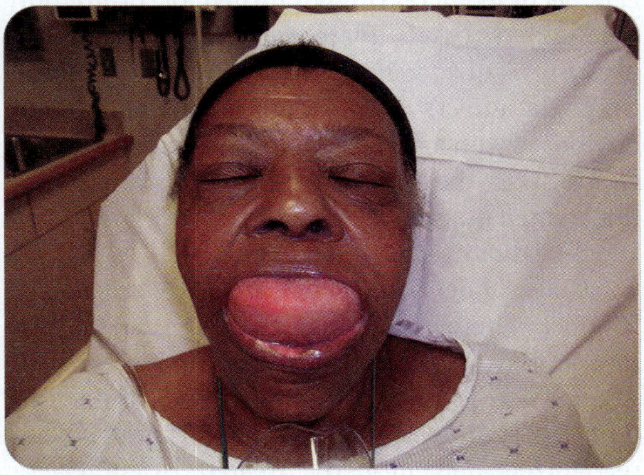

Figure 14-4 This patient is having a reaction with angioedema being present. Note the swollen tongue.

begin to swell, which can further hinder breathing. As breathing becomes compromised, the amount of oxygen reaching the brain may be reduced.

Gastrointestinal distress is common in moderate allergic reactions. This includes release of hydrochloric acid by the stomach's lining, creating heartburn, and contraction of intestinal wall smooth muscle, causing diarrhea. Also seen are intestinal cramping, nausea, and vomiting.

As with mild reactions, all these effects may appear within a few minutes after exposure to an allergen, or they may take several hours to become apparent. Depending on the person's individual physiological makeup, including the effectiveness of the immunologic response, these effects may dissipate on their own or increase in severity to a life-threatening problem.

Severe Allergic Reactions

Anaphylaxis is the most severe type of allergic reaction and results in collapse of the respiratory and circulatory systems (**Figure 14-5**). Severe allergic

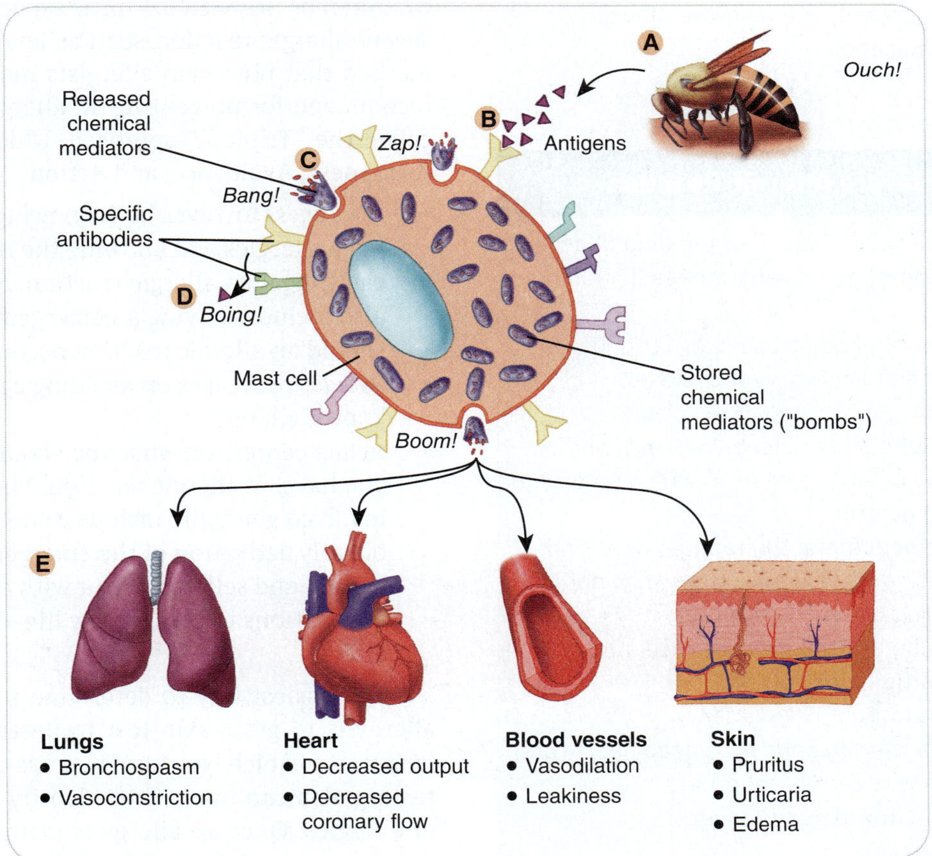

Figure 14-5 The sequence of events in anaphylaxis.

reactions cause major changes within the respiratory, integumentary, circulatory, and gastrointestinal systems due to the release of massive amounts of histamine (**Figure 14-6 and Table 14-3**). Within the respiratory system, the smooth muscles of the bronchioles tightly constrict, making wheezing severe and frequently audible. Ventilations, if any, may be minimal and often result in virtually no gas exchange within the alveoli because the airways become occluded due to the combination of tight bronchoconstriction and edema.

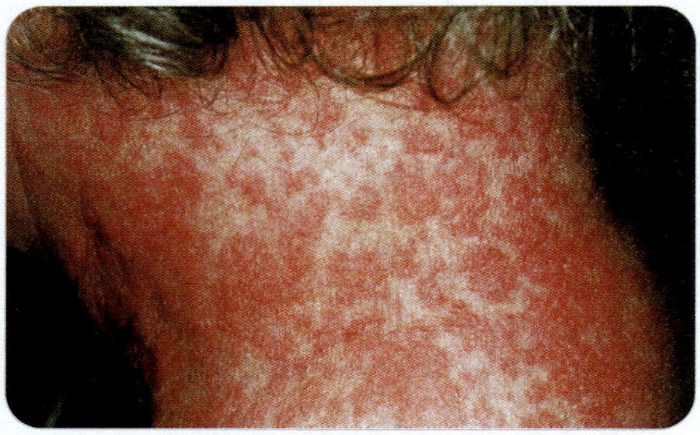

Figure 14-6 A patient with a severe allergic reaction to medication.

Table 14-3 Severe Allergic Reaction
• Severe anxiety, feelings of impending doom • Decreased level of responsiveness (including coma) • Severe respiratory distress (e.g., "tripod" position, use of accessory muscles of respiration) • Abnormal lung sounds (can vary from audible wheezing to a "silent chest" in which no breath sounds are heard) • Severe angioedema of the tongue, face, and hands (eyes can swell shut, rings may not be able to be removed) • Hives (may be located over the face, neck, chest, abdomen, and arms) • Inability to swallow • Tachycardia (significantly increased heart rate) • Weak or absent peripheral pulses • Hypotension (low blood pressure) • Pallor (pale skin) • Cyanosis around the lips and face

Additionally, the tongue and lips may become so swollen that they completely block the upper airway. Angioedema may progress to the point that the eyes and upper airway swell completely shut. Hives may cover the entire upper body. The skin can become increasingly flushed or profoundly pale. Blood vessels dilate, causing a fall in blood pressure. Unlike mild or moderate allergic reactions, the effects of a severe reaction are usually obvious within a few seconds to minutes following exposure to the eliciting antigen. If patients are not treated quickly, the result can be anaphylactic shock and/or death.

Unless quickly corrected, anaphylaxis can lead to shock, where blood pressure falls to dangerously low levels and tissue hypoxia becomes critical. Anaphylactic shock is a serious medical disorder that almost always leads to death if it is not quickly recognized and properly treated. Anaphylactic shock is covered in detail in Chapter 10, *Shock*.

Prevention

As with many medical disorders, allergic reactions can often be prevented. This is especially true of a severe allergic reaction such as anaphylaxis. The method that physician allergists most commonly recommend for preventing an allergic reaction is called the "Triple A" approach, which centers on *A*wareness, *A*voidance, and *A*ction.

- *Awareness* involves both knowing that you have allergies and knowing the things that can trigger an allergic reaction. Awareness also includes having an emergency plan should an allergic reaction occur.
- *Avoidance* focuses on avoiding contact with known allergens.
- *Action* centers on what you should do if you have an allergic reaction. The actions involved generally include a combination of early activation of the emergency care system and self-treatment with one or more medications to combat any life-threatening effects.

The easiest way to determine if you have an allergy is to get a skin test to determine the allergens to which you are hypersensitive. Blood testing also can be used to identify the presence of allergies. Once an allergy is identified, the patient may be advised to undergo "allergy shots" administered on a regular schedule. Although the

CASE Update

You move the patient to a safe area and begin to assess her condition. She looks pale and appears to be in moderate respiratory distress, and she has a wheeze. Once you determine that the ABCDs are intact, you notify dispatch to send additional personnel with oxygen and an airway kit. You also request that an ALS provider respond. Secondary patient assessment reveals no extremity, spinal, or abdominal problems. Respirations are 38 breaths per minute and labored. The patient's face appears swollen. You then ask her if she has an epinephrine auto-injector. The mother says she has the girl's EpiPen in the car. You reassure the mother that you will watch the girl while she goes to get the injector.

What should you do now?

shots do not cure the person's allergies, they usually provide significant relief from the effects of allergic reactions.

PATIENT ASSESSMENT FOR ALLERGIC REACTIONS

Assessment of a patient with a suspected allergic reaction starts with scene safety considerations. This is particularly important if rescuers will be exposed to the suspected allergen, especially if those rescuers also have the same allergy as the patient. For instance, if a beehive has been disturbed and a swarm is present, it may be necessary to move the patient to another location before the assessment process can be initiated. Any rescuer who has the same allergy as the patient should not risk exposure.

The primary patient assessment using ABCD is performed in the usual manner. Treat any immediate threats to life. Depending on the severity of the patient's distress and available resources, OEC technicians may need to care for life threats and not perform a secondary patient assessment until additional rescuers arrive. However, if no immediate threats to life are apparent, proceed with obtaining a medical history and performing the secondary patient assessment. If an allergic reaction is suspected, continue to monitor the patient's ABCDs carefully.

Remember that the signs and symptoms of an allergic reaction are often evolving; they may not be immediately apparent and can change over time. As a rule, signs and symptoms associated with respiratory impairment (e.g., increasing dyspnea, difficulty swallowing, tongue swelling) are especially ominous and indicate a potentially serious reaction.

Obtain a SAMPLE history, paying close attention to any known allergies, including medications, and details of previous allergic reactions. For patients with known allergies, specifically ask if they have ever had a severe allergic reaction or an anaphylactic reaction. Be sure to ask patients whether they have taken any medications to self-treat this current allergic reaction (**Table 14-4**).

Table 14-4 Common Oral Allergy Medications

Brand Name	Generic Name
Allegra	fexofenadine
Astelin	azelastine hydrochloride
Benadryl	diphenhydramine
Clarinex	desloratadine
Claritin	loratadine
Chlor-Trimeton	chlorpheniramine
Dimetane	brompheniramine
Zyrtec	cetirizine
Tavist	clemastine

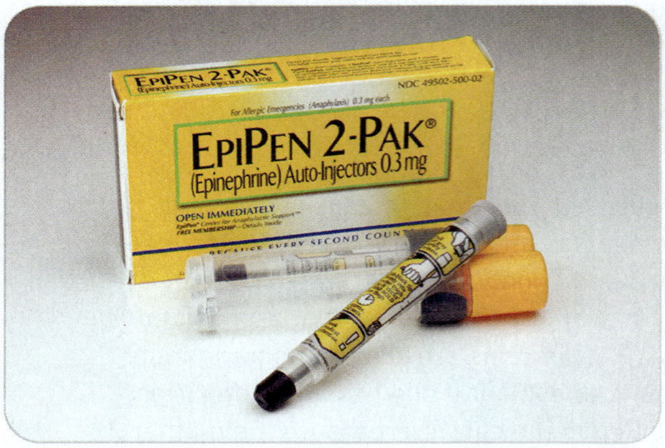

Figure 14-7 Patients who experience allergic reactions often carry their own prescription epinephrine.

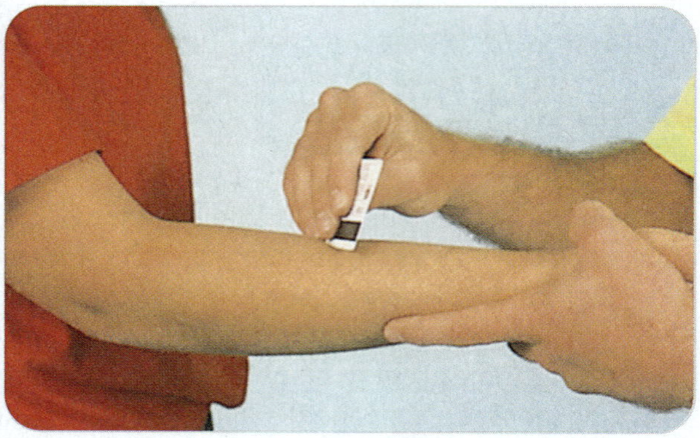

Figure 14-8 Scraping the skin with the edge of a stiff object such as a credit card is one technique for removing a stinger, which prevents further injection of venom.

The patient may have their own epinephrine auto-injector (EpiPen) (**Figure 14-7**). Patients who are highly allergic often are prescribed an epinephrine auto-injector in the event they experience a severe allergic reaction and are unable to reach a medical facility within a few minutes. In this situation, an auto-injector can be truly lifesaving.

Anaphylactic Shock

Anaphylactic shock is identified by the simultaneous presence of the signs of a severe allergic reaction and shock (nonhemorrhagic hypovolemic shock), which include the following:

- Systolic blood pressure below 90 mm Hg
- Respirations greater than 20 breaths per minute
- Heart rate greater than 110 beats per minute; in some cases, the patient may have a pulse rate less than 60 beats per minute
- Level of responsiveness decreased; AVPU scale less than *A* (alert)
- Pulse oxygen saturation levels less than 90%; may be less than 80%

MANAGEMENT OF ALLERGIC REACTIONS

The initial management of an allergic reaction is taking care of the ABCDs. Try to identify the allergen, as this knowledge might change the care you provide. If possible, remove the patient from the source of the allergen. If during the primary patient assessment you find that the airway is open, breathing and circulation are normal, and there are no neurologic problems, then the patient needs to be treated symptomatically. Any injuries or other medical problems should be treated if the patient is stable. You need to decide if the patient's allergic reaction is truly life-threatening (anaphylactic shock). If so, a broken arm may be of secondary concern and immediate transport may be needed. Monitor the patient frequently, as the person may have only a mild rash at first and then over time develop into a full-blown anaphylactic reaction. Take vital signs frequently watching for changes that indicate a worsening condition. If the patient *appears* to be developing anaphylaxis, you should immediately treat the ABCDs, call for ALS support, and transport.

If the source of an allergic reaction is a bee, hornet, or wasp sting, locate and remove the stinger. Use the flat edge of a credit card, fingernail, plastic knife, or similar object to scrape along the surface of the skin to dislodge the stinger (**Figure 14-8**). If you decide to pull the stinger out using your thumb and index finger, pinch the skin *around* the site to raise the stinger above the level of the skin before grasping the stinger as close to the skin as possible. If all else fails, remove the stinger using tweezers. Once the stinger is removed apply ice to the site to minimize the pain.

Moderate and Severe Allergic Reactions

Moderate and severe allergic reactions and anaphylaxis constitute a true emergency that must be treated immediately to prevent life-threatening shock. Begin treatment by correcting any ABCD-related problems. Open the airway. If the patient has an EpiPen assist the patient as soon as possible by delivering the shot of epinephrine. Oxygen should be given using a nonrebreather mask at 15 liters per minute (LPM). If necessary, assist the patient's ventilations with a bag-valve mask. Arrange transport and notify advanced life support immediately. Severe anaphylaxis may require CPR.

Remove any tight-fitting necklaces, scarves, or bandanas from around the neck. Additionally, remove tight-fitting watches, rings, and bracelets, all of which can restrict or occlude blood flow through swollen distal structures. Place the patient into a position of comfort. In most instances, this will be a seated and slightly forward position. If the patient exhibits signs of shock or a decreased level of responsiveness, place the patient in a supine position.

If an allergic reaction is suspected, determine whether the patient has an epinephrine auto-injector. Do not use anyone else's epinephrine auto-injector.

Epinephrine Auto-Injector

An epinephrine injector contains epinephrine, the drug of choice for managing severe allergic reactions. It promotes bronchodilation and vasoconstriction, thereby relieving dyspnea and hypotension. These auto-injectors come prepackaged as a single-dose or dual-dose portable auto-injector sold under brand names such as Epi E-Z Pen, EpiPen, and Auvi-Q (**Figure 14-9**). A portable auto-injector administers the proper dose of epinephrine using an automatic needle-injection system. Most auto-injectors look like a fountain pen with a cap on it. The injectors come in adult and pediatric doses.

To use or help a patient use an auto-injector, follow the steps in **OEC Skill 14-1**.

Epinephrine is a fast-acting drug. In most cases, a single dose will relieve the patient's symptoms within a few minutes. In severe cases, however, the patient may require additional doses of epinephrine; this is especially true for prolonged transport situations. A second dose of epinephrine is indicated if the patient's symptoms have not resolved within 10 minutes, or if they reoccur. Several epinephrine auto-injectors now have two doses of epinephrine in them, and thus can be used twice. Monitor the patient's breathing, lung sounds, and vital signs every 5 minutes, noting any

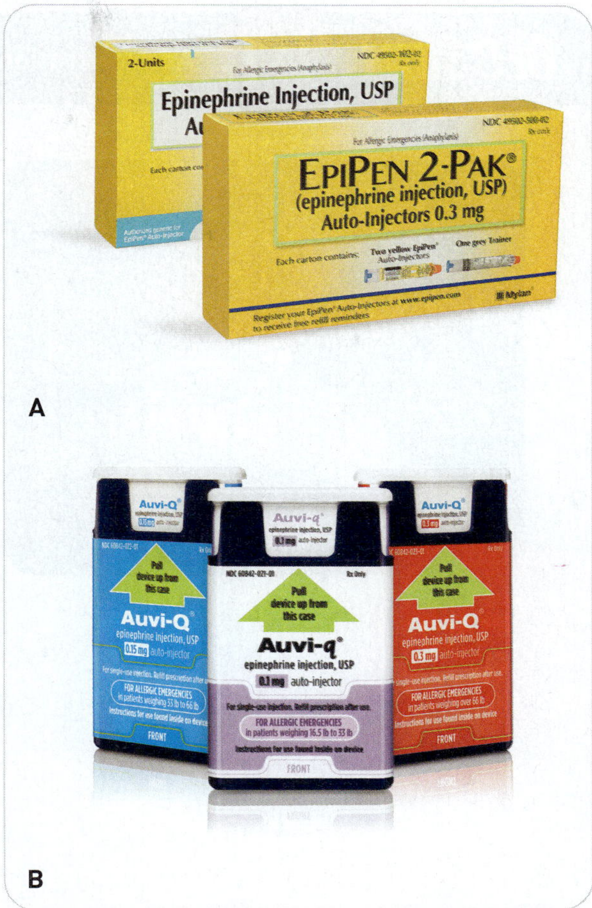

Figure 14-9 Different types of auto-injectors that an OEC technician might come in contact with include the EpiPen (**A**) and Auvi-Q (**B**).

A: Courtesy of Mylan Specialty L.P.; **B:** Courtesy of kaleo, Inc.

changes. Ideally, the patient's condition should rapidly improve following the administration of epinephrine. Improvement includes the patient being able to breathe more easily and normal vital signs. Signs of shock also should quickly diminish.

Administration of a person's auto-injector is a lifesaving measure. After usage, adverse reactions may occur. These side effects are usually benign. Anxiety, restlessness, tremor, weakness, dizziness, sweating, palpitations, pallor, nausea, vomiting, headache, and rarely heart rhythm irregularities can occur.

When you have any patient who experiences a moderate to severe allergic reaction, you should always call for ALS and transport early. They need to go to the hospital even if their condition improved using the auto-injector. Anyone who accidentally injects epinephrine into a thumb or finger also should be transported to the hospital for a follow-up evaluation.

OEC SKILL 14-1 Administration with an Auto-Injector (EpiPen)

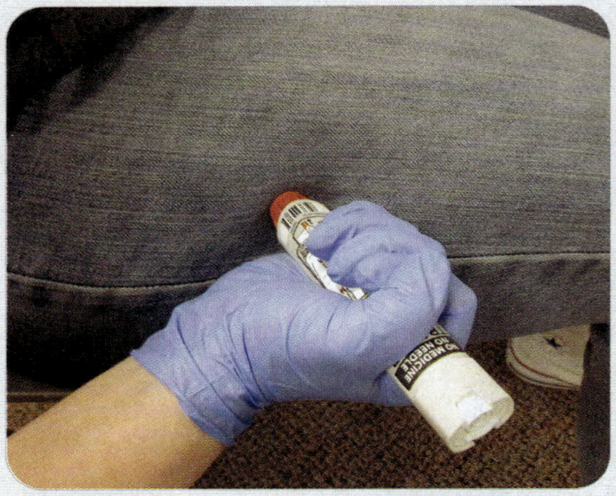

1 Ensure that the medication is prescribed for the patient by checking the name on the medication. Remove the medication from its protective package. Do not use if expired or discolored. Remove the safety cap from the auto-injector. Use your dominant hand to grasp the auto-injector firmly.

2 Do not place your thumb over either end of the auto-injector, because doing so could result in the accidental injection of the medication into *your thumb*. Place the tip of the auto-injector against the patient's outer thigh muscle (halfway between the hip and knee). If possible, wipe the skin with an alcohol wipe first. In an extreme emergency, the auto-injector may be administered through clothing. Firmly push the tip against the thigh until the needle deploys. (You should hear an audible "click" as the medication is being injected into the thigh muscle.) Maintain firm pressure for 10 seconds so that needle does not come out of skin. Remove the auto-injector, and dispose of it in a suitable container. Massage the injection site for 10 to 20 seconds. Note the time and dose at which the drug was administered, and document.

CASE Outcome

Another OEC technician arrives with oxygen. You place the patient on a nonrebreather mask at 15 LPM. Her mother arrives with the girl's EpiPen and you assist her in administering the medication in the lateral side of her thigh. Within a few minutes, she is breathing more easily, and her facial swelling begins to diminish. Shortly thereafter, an ALS provider arrives on scene. Together, you transport the girl to the parking lot, where an ambulance takes her to a nearby hospital. She makes a full recovery, thanks to your quick action.

CHAPTER REVIEW

In Summary

- An allergy is the body's overreaction to a foreign substance.
- Allergies are caused by antigens called allergens. Allergens can be inhaled, ingested, injected, or topical.
- Foods, insect bites and stings, environmental irritants, pollen and plants, molds, animal dander, medication, and chemicals are common causes of allergies.
- Many people do not know they have an allergy until they suffer an allergic reaction.
- Peanuts are the number one food allergy in the world.
- Allergic reactions are categorized according to their effects as mild, moderate, or severe.
  - A mild reaction typically causes skin-related effects, such as a rash, hives, or itching.
  - The effects of moderate allergic reactions include all those that occur in mild reactions, but they are more pronounced, and they also affect the respiratory system and gastrointestinal system.
  - Anaphylaxis is the most severe type of allergic reaction and results in collapse of the respiratory and circulatory systems. Anaphylaxis can lead to shock, where blood pressure falls to dangerously low levels and tissue hypoxia becomes critical. Anaphylaxis can be fatal unless rapidly treated.
- Allergic reactions may be prevented using the Triple A approach: *A*wareness, *A*voidance, and *A*ction.
- Don't hesitate to assist the patient by administering an EpiPen to a patient who is experiencing a severe reaction.
- Usually, severe allergic reactions show signs and symptoms early, while mild to moderate reactions evolve more slowly.
- When you have a patient who experiences a moderate to severe allergic reaction, you should always call for ALS and transport early.

Key Terms

Allergen A foreign substance (antigen) whose presence in the body stimulates an allergic reaction.

Allergic reaction A series of signs and symptoms that occur in response to exposure to an allergen.

Anaphylaxis A severe allergic reaction that can result in serious cardiac or respiratory compromise.

Angioedema Swelling that occurs beneath the skin or mucosa because of an allergic reaction.

Antibody A protein that is produced by the body to neutralize or destroy specific antigens.

Histamine A chemical that is released in the body because of an allergic reaction.

Hypersensitivity An exaggerated immune response to an allergen, drug, or other foreign substance.

Pruritus Severe itching; frequently occurs in the skin during mild and moderate allergic reactions.

Urticaria Hives or rashes that accompany an allergic reaction.

Chapter Questions

1. Allergens enter the body through several routes, including:
   a. inhalation.
   b. ingestion.
   c. injection.
   d. All the above

2. Topical exposure of an allergen directly affects which part of the body?
   a. Heart
   b. Sinuses
   c. Skin
   d. Connective tissues
3. You are called to the cafeteria where a guest is displaying symptoms of tingling around the mouth, mild rash, itching, and flushed skin. As you collect information, the patient tells you she is allergic to peanut butter. What is your determination?
   a. The guest is reacting to a peanut product.
   b. The guest is anxious about her allergy to peanuts.
   c. The guest is suffering from the flu.
   d. The guest is tired and does not want to ski.
4. Common causes of allergies would include, but not be limited to, which of the following?
   a. Mold
   b. Medications
   c. Chemicals
   d. All the above
5. Which of the following signs would indicate anaphylactic shock?
   a. Slow respirations
   b. Systolic blood pressure above 110 mm Hg
   c. Respirations greater than 20 breaths per minute
   d. Pulse oxygen saturation greater than 94%
6. A mountain biker fell off his bike, fracturing his forearm, and landed in a bee's nest. He received multiple stings, resulting in an anaphylactic reaction. You have secured the scene. Your next step is to:
   a. splint the fractured forearm.
   b. supply the patient with water so he does not become dehydrated.
   c. transport the patient.
   d. move the patient away from the nest (scene safety), assess the ABCDs, monitor vital signs, and call for ALS transport.
7. A medication used for a patient having an anaphylactic reaction is:
   a. aspirin.
   b. epinephrine.
   c. Benadryl.
   d. Tylenol.
8. You are called to the scene of a hiker who is experiencing an allergic reaction. The hiker has an epinephrine auto-injector in her possession. You have determined that administration of the epinephrine is appropriate. Your next step is to:
   a. remove the medication from its protective package.
   b. check the name on the mediation to ensure it belongs to the patient.
   c. remove the safety cap from the auto-injector.
   d. shake the auto-injector to evenly distribute the medication inside the pen.

Answers: 1. d, Objective 14-1, p. 301; 2. c, Objective 14.1, p. 301; 3. a, Objective 14-2, p. 302; 4. d, Objective 14-2, p. 302; 5. c, Objective 14-3, p. 306; 6. d, Objective 14-3, p. 305; 7. b, Objective 14-4, p. 307; 8. b, Objective 14.4, p. 308

CHAPTER 15

CARDIOVASCULAR EMERGENCIES

OBJECTIVES

Upon completion of this chapter, the OEC technician will be able to:

15-1 List the arrhythmias associated with sudden cardiac death.

15-2 Demonstrate how to assess and treat a patient with a cardiovascular emergency.

15-3 Describe what you should ask a patient who takes a heart medication.

15-4 Explain what an anticoagulant ("blood thinner") is.

15-5 List the signs and symptoms for each of the following cardiovascular disorders:
- Acute myocardial infarction
- Congestive heart failure
- Aortic aneurysm
- Pericardial tamponade

15-6 Give the indications and contraindications of aspirin and nitroglycerin therapy.

15-7 Describe and demonstrate assisting a patient in taking nitroglycerin and/or aspirin.

KEY TERMS

Acute myocardial infarction (AMI), p. 318
Angina pectoris, p. 318
Aorta, p. 313
Aortic aneurysm, p. 320
Arrhythmia, p. 319
Asystole, p. 319
Atherosclerosis, p. 317
Automated external defibrillator (AED), p. 327
Automatic implantable cardioverter defibrillator (AICD), p. 328
Cardiopulmonary resuscitation (CPR), p. 320
Congestive heart failure (CHF), p. 317
Coronary arteries, p. 313
Coronary artery disease, p. 317
Defibrillation, p. 327
Hypertension, p. 317
Hypotension, p. 324
Ischemia, p. 318
Myocardium, p. 312
Pericarditis, p. 320
Pulmonary edema, p. 317
Sudden cardiac arrest (SCA), p. 319
Ventricular assist device (VAD), p. 328
Ventricular fibrillation (VF), p. 319
Ventricular tachycardia (VT), p. 319

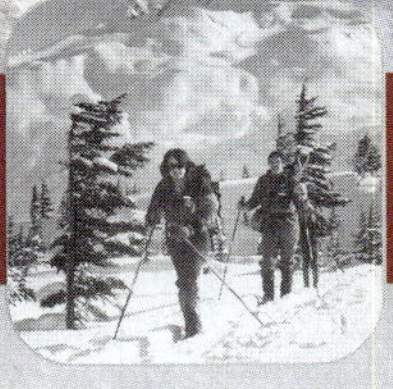

HISTORICAL TIMELINE **1975.** NSP Board votes to modify the NSP emergency care course to better address the needs of patrollers.

CHAPTER OVERVIEW

Cardiovascular disease is the leading cause of death in the United States. It includes pathologic conditions of both the heart and blood vessels. This chapter discusses problems that occur with the heart and major blood vessels. Deep vein thrombosis and pulmonary embolism, where a blood clot in a vein travels to the lung, is discussed in more detail in Chapter 13, *Respiratory Emergencies*. Stroke, an occlusion or rupture of an artery or vein in the brain, is discussed in Chapter 11, *Altered Mental Status*.

Many cardiac emergencies occur outside the hospital setting so you as an OEC technician will very likely have to care for a patient suffering a cardiac emergency. Because many cardiovascular disorders can be immediately life threatening, it is important for OEC technicians to identify the signs and symptoms of these emergencies quickly, render appropriate care quickly, and transport with advanced life support (ALS) assistance.

ANATOMY AND PHYSIOLOGY

The cardiovascular system consists of three major components: the heart, blood vessels, and blood. The cardiovascular system is responsible for providing oxygen and nutrients and carrying waste products in the blood. It takes carbon dioxide to the lungs and other waste products to the kidneys, so these waste products can be excreted. Blood is pumped by the left-side of the heart through the arteries starting with the largest artery, the aorta, to all parts of the body.

Arteries continue to divide into progressively smaller arteries and arterioles and then the capillaries, which serve as the bridge between arterioles and venules. The walls of the capillaries are only one cell thick and are permeable, allowing nutrients and oxygen in the blood to diffuse into the tissues, and waste products to diffuse out of the tissues into the bloodstream and to the kidneys for excretion.

The Heart

The heart is a thick muscular organ located behind and just to the left of the sternum and is approximately the size of a closed fist. It is enclosed within a tough, fibrous pericardial sac, which contains a small amount of pericardial fluid that allows friction-free movement of the heart within the sac.

The heart has four compartments or "chambers" (**Figure 15-1**). It is divided into right and left sides, with two chambers on each side. The right side accepts deoxygenated blood from the body and pumps it to the lungs to remove carbon dioxide and to receive fresh oxygen. The oxygenated blood then moves from the lungs to the left heart which pumps the oxygenated blood to the brain, muscles, and other organs. Each side has an upper chamber called the atrium which serves as a primer pump for the lower, larger, and more powerful ventricle.

Cardiac muscle is called **myocardium**. The heart's pumping function is coordinated through the cardiac conduction system, an electrical pathway that has a pacemaker function located in the atrium that initiates an automatic electrical impulse (**Figure 15-2**). This impulse goes through

CASE Presentation

You are called to assist a 65-year-old man who is complaining of chest pain. Upon arrival, you find the patient sitting on a log. He appears to be in considerable distress. The patient tells you that he was hiking on snowshoes when he suddenly experienced a "crushing pain" in his chest that radiated down his left arm. He has a history of "heart problems" but has never experienced pain this bad before. He also complains of feeling weak and slightly nauseated. He is pale and is sweating profusely.

What should be your first step in providing care?

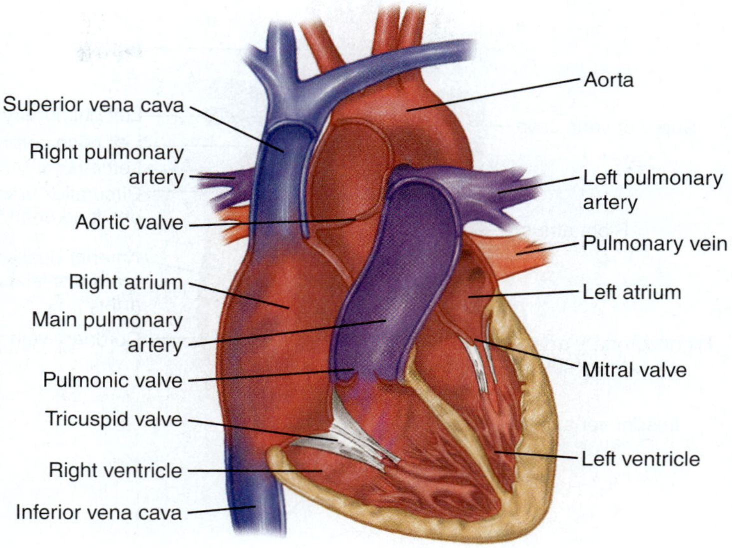

Figure 15-1 The heart is a four-chambered muscle that pumps blood to all parts of the body.

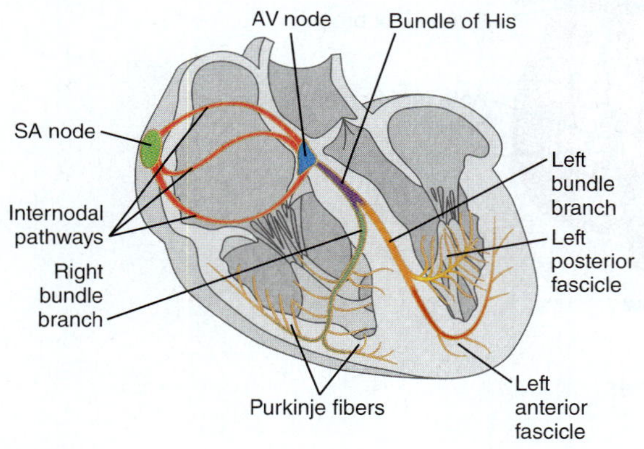

Figure 15-2 The electrical conduction system within the myocardium.

the heart stimulating the myocardium to contract in an organized and efficient manner. This electrical system creates the regular "beat" of the heart. The efficiency of the pump depends on four valves situated between each of the chambers and the major blood vessels, the opening and closing of which allows for only forward flow of the blood. The heart has arteries that come off the first part of the aorta and provide oxygen and nourishment to the heart muscle (**Figure 15-3**).

Blood Vessels

There are different types of blood vessels that serve different purposes. They are the arteries, arterioles, capillaries, veins, and venules. Arteries and arterioles carry blood away from the heart. Veins and venules bring blood back to the heart. Capillaries connect the arteries to the veins.

It is important to know where the major arteries are located (**Figure 15-4**). The largest artery in the body, the **aorta**, carries blood out of the left side of the heart to smaller arteries that travel through the entire body. The **coronary arteries**, which carry oxygen-rich blood to the heart muscle, leave the aorta just above the heart. Next are the carotid arteries in the neck, which supply blood to the brain. The subclavian arteries under the clavicles supply the arms through the brachial, radial, and ulnar branches. In the torso, the aorta supplies blood to the internal organs, then the pelvis and legs through the iliac and femoral arteries. In the legs, the femoral arteries divide into the tibial and peroneal arteries. On top of the foot is the dorsalis pedis artery. Several of these arteries

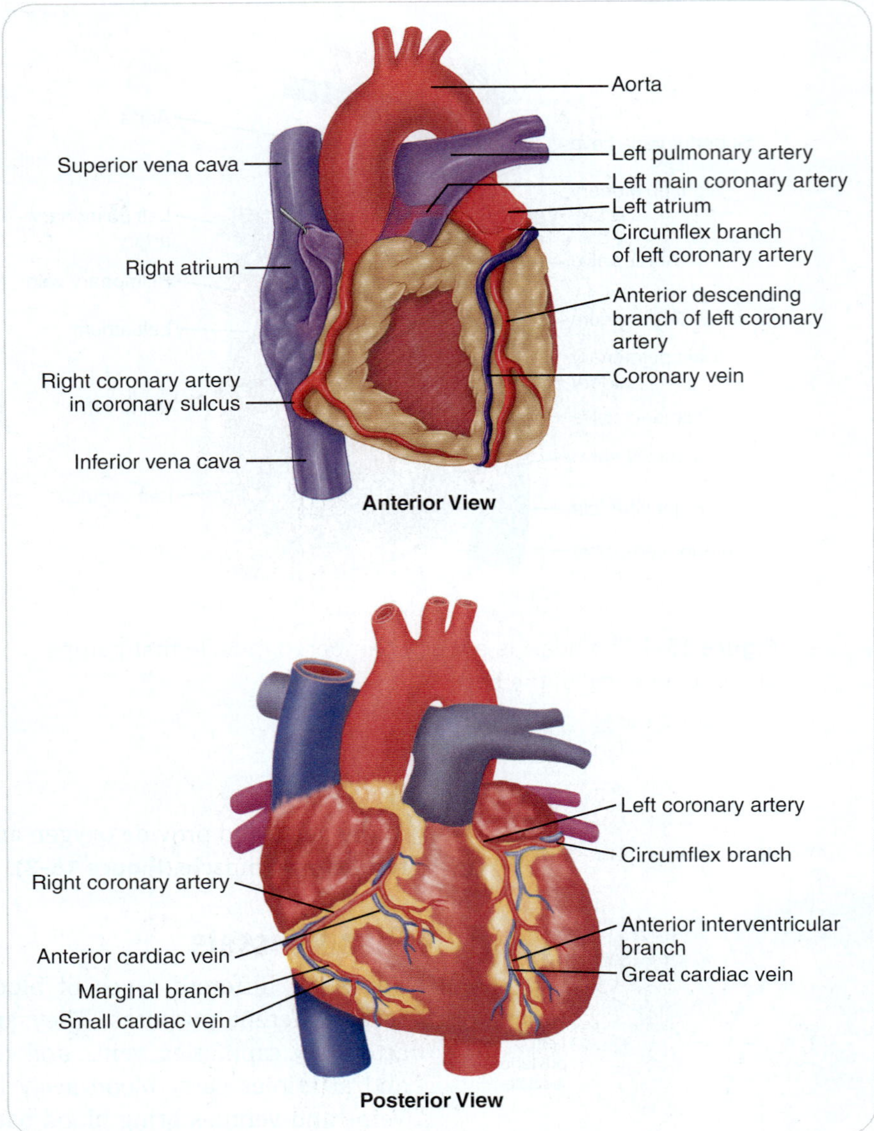

Figure 15-3 The heart and coronary arteries.

are just under the skin, where you can take a pulse (**Figure 15-5**).

Veins transport oxygen-depleted blood back to the right side of the heart. Venules are the smallest component of the venous circulation. They drain into progressively larger venules and veins, then through two major veins: the superior and inferior venae cavae which drain into the right side of the heart. Venous blood from the head, arms, and chest drains into the superior vena cava, whereas blood from the legs and abdomen drains into the inferior vena cava. The blood then goes through the right side of the heart to the lungs where carbon dioxide is excreted, and oxygen is taken in. This blood goes back to the left side of the heart, and the cycle is repeated.

The Blood

There are four main components of blood: red blood cells, white blood cells, platelets, and the straw-colored liquid in which they are suspended, called plasma. The function of the red blood cells is to carry oxygen to the body's cells and assist in removing carbon dioxide from them.

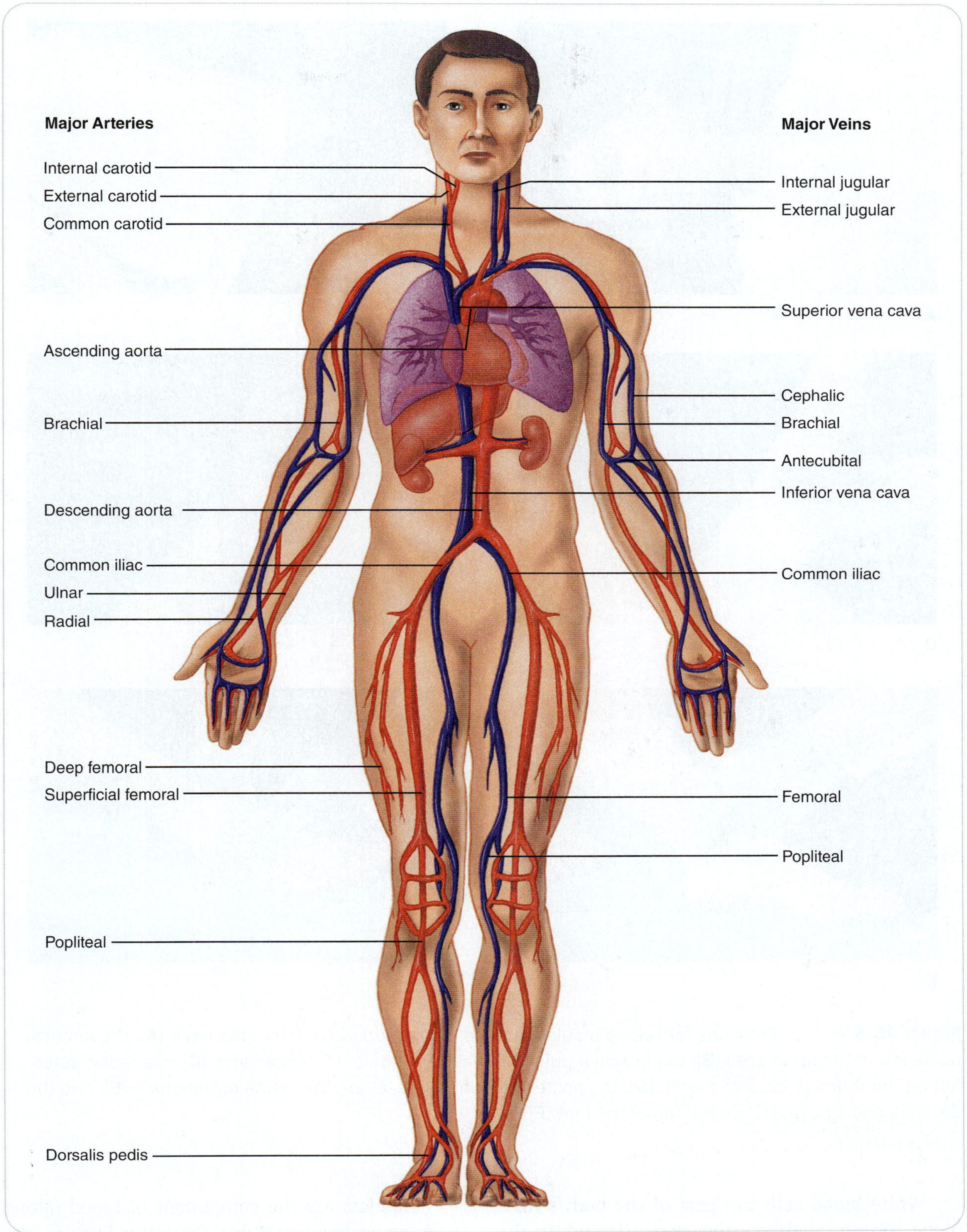

Figure 15-4 The major arteries in the human body.

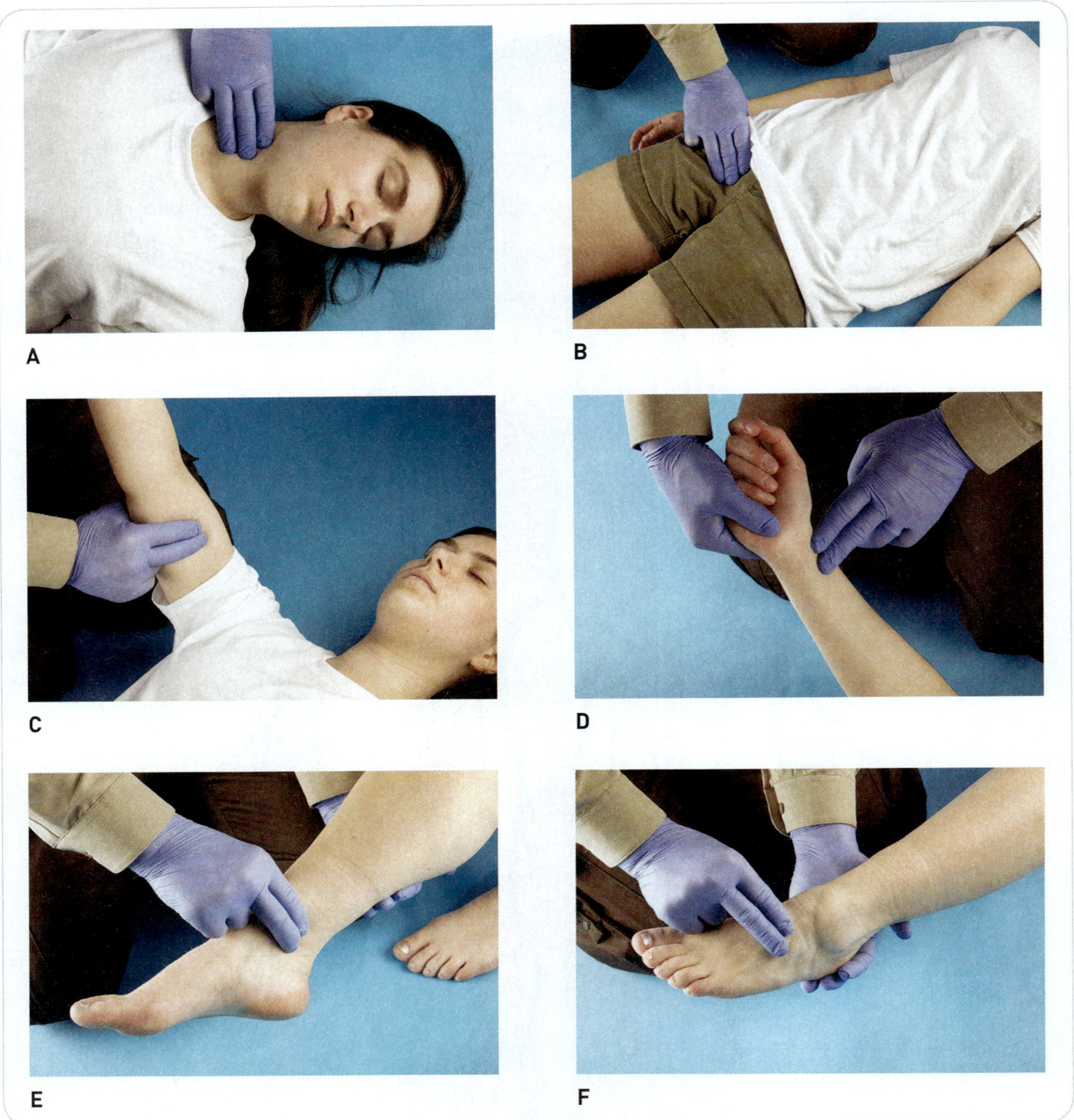

Figure 15-5 Various locations for taking a pulse include the carotid pulse felt in the neck (**A**), the femoral pulse felt in the groin area (**B**), the brachial pulse felt on the inside of the upper arm (**C**), the radial pulse felt on the thumb side of the wrist (**D**), the posterior tibial pulse felt on the inside of the ankle (**E**), and the dorsalis pedis pulse felt on the top of the foot (**F**).

White blood cells are part of the body's immune system, helping the body defend itself against infection. There are several types of white blood cells, each providing defense against different microorganisms.

Platelets are the component of blood (along with specialized proteins from the liver in the plasma) that forms blood clots to stop bleeding.

Plasma carries the blood cells and nutrients to the tissues, carries waste products away from the organs, and transports other important chemicals such as hormones.

CARDIOVASCULAR EMERGENCIES

Most causes of cardiovascular system failure can be traced to cardiovascular disease, a generic term that describes several diseases that affect the heart and blood vessels. Cardiovascular disease can cause a host of problems, including high blood pressure, congestive heart failure, acute myocardial infarction, and stroke. A "heart attack," or acute myocardial infarction, is more common in individuals 40 to 70 years of age but can occur as early as one's twenties and remains a significant problem in the elderly. Although the underlying causes of cardiovascular disease are many, most are attributed to **coronary artery disease**, or **atherosclerosis** of the arteries of the heart. A feared complication of a heart attack is triggering a lethal arrhythmia (ventricular fibrillation or pulseless ventricular tachycardia) leading to sudden cardiac arrest because the heart cannot pump blood.

Atherosclerosis

Atherosclerosis, or "hardening of the arteries," is a disease in which plaques form along the inner lining of arteries. These plaques consist of cholesterol, lipids, calcium, and proteins, and are deposited throughout a lifetime. During their initial formation, plaque deposits typically remain undetected. However, as they grow, they can decrease the internal diameter of an artery decreasing blood flow to tissues. When this happens in the femoral arteries, pain may occur in the affected leg with exercise and then is relieved with rest. In the coronary arteries this may cause chest pain with exertion when the demand for blood flow to the myocardium increases but cannot be met. This is called angina pectoris or "angina." A plaque in the vessel can "rupture," usually causing a complete blockage of a critical coronary artery. This is the most common cause of an acute myocardial infarction (AMI) or heart attack.

Hypertension

Hypertension, or abnormally high blood pressure, is a common cardiovascular disorder. According to the American Heart Association, hypertension affects nearly one billion people worldwide. In 2018 in the United States more than 75 million people had hypertension. Only about 50% of people in the US who have high blood pressure are treated. Many do not know they have it.

Blood pressure within the arteries is abnormally elevated with hypertension. Clinical hypertension is defined as a systolic pressure greater than 130 or a diastolic pressure greater than 80. Hypertension occurs when the internal diameters of small arteries and arterioles narrow due to atherosclerosis or from other causes that restrict blood flow through the arterial system. To get the same amount of blood flowing through the narrowed space in the arteries, pressure must build up. The increased pressure damages small arteries in many of the body's organs. Hypertension can lead to other serious health problems, including stroke and kidney failure. In addition to atherosclerosis, high salt intake, chronic kidney disease, genetic predisposition, and other medical problems can cause hypertension.

Untreated, hypertension predisposes a person to heart disease because of the damage it causes to the heart's arteries over time. Fortunately, the condition can be treated through medications and by eliminating controllable risk factors such as smoking, excessive salt intake, and obesity.

Congestive Heart Failure

When the heart cannot adequately pump blood to body tissues, blood backs up into the major blood vessels that lead to the heart and certain organs. This condition is called **congestive heart failure (CHF)**. One or both sides of the heart can fail. Right-sided CHF results in the backup of blood in the venous system (the body's blood return circuit), causing leakage of the fluid part of the blood into the extremities, commonly the legs, ankles and feet (**Figure 15-6**). The swelling caused by this is referred to as pedal edema. Left-sided CHF causes blood to backup in the lungs, resulting in shortness of breath and fluid in the lungs. This condition is called pulmonary edema, and causes difficulty breathing.

Pulmonary Edema

Pulmonary edema is an accumulation of fluid in the lungs. The cause may either be due to the

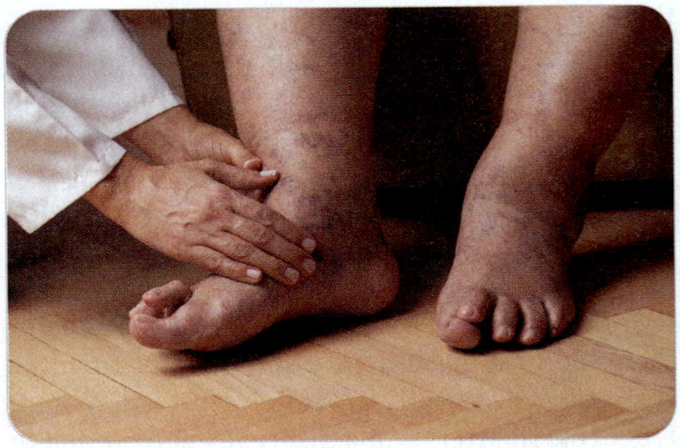

Figure 15-6 Pedal edema.

heart failing or due to other non-heart-related causes. It is from the inability of the left ventricle to pump blood effectively to the body. A common cause is related to heart damage from an AMI, but many other conditions can lead to this including untreated hypertension, heart valve disease, direct trauma to the lung tissue, and certain drugs (heroin). When the left ventricle is no longer able to pump blood effectively, blood backs up into the lungs. This causes an increase in fluid pressure within the pulmonary capillaries. As a result, fluid seeps into the alveoli and prevents proper exchange of oxygen and carbon dioxide. This can lead to moderate-to-severe hypoxemia (low oxygen in the blood) with associated respiratory distress. To compensate for poor tissue perfusion, the respiratory centers within the brain signal the body to breathe faster.

As the lungs become more damaged, red blood cells leak into the alveoli, causing frothy, blood-tinged fluid to be coughed up. Eventually the patient develops cardiogenic shock from profound hypoxia. Another cause of pulmonary edema is altitude illness, which is discussed in a later chapter.

Angina Pectoris

Angina pectoris, or simply angina, is chest pain or discomfort caused by **ischemia** (lack of oxygen) of the myocardium (heart muscle). The heart muscle is not getting enough oxygen. Angina pectoris is a common occurrence among patients with significant coronary artery disease.

The most common cause is a narrowing of the internal diameter of the coronary arteries due to atherosclerotic plaque. The coronary arteries provide oxygenated blood to the heart. During routine daily activities, a heart with a normal coronary arterial supply receives enough oxygen and nutrients. However, stressors such as physical activity, cold weather, and certain drugs place increased oxygen demands on the heart. If blood flow through the coronary arteries is reduced by plaque, the increased demand and insufficient blood supply overtaxes the heart, leading to ischemia of the myocardium. This is typically manifested as chest discomfort. When the stressor is eliminated, the pain usually subsides.

Another cause of angina is vasoconstriction or spasm of a coronary artery. If a heart's artery is suddenly narrowed due to constriction, the amount of blood flowing through the vessel will not be adequate to meet the heart's nutrient and oxygen needs. Coronary artery vasospasm may occur in response to certain drugs (e.g., methamphetamine, cocaine) or for other reasons.

Myocardial Infarction

A myocardial infarction or an **acute myocardial infarction (AMI)** is a blockage in one or more of the coronary arteries that results in ischemic death of heart muscle that is supplied by the blocked artery(s) (**Figure 15-7**). A blood clot is the most common source of the blockage, representing approximately 90% of all myocardial infarction cases. After a small atherosclerotic plaque in the coronary artery has ruptured or dislodged, a blood

> **KEY POINT**
>
> **"The Widow Maker"—Left Main Coronary Artery**
>
> The left main coronary artery supplies most of the oxygenated blood to the muscle of the left ventricle, which pumps blood to the body. When a blood clot forms in this artery, a dangerous, often deadly heart attack occurs because a large amount of the heart muscle becomes ischemic.

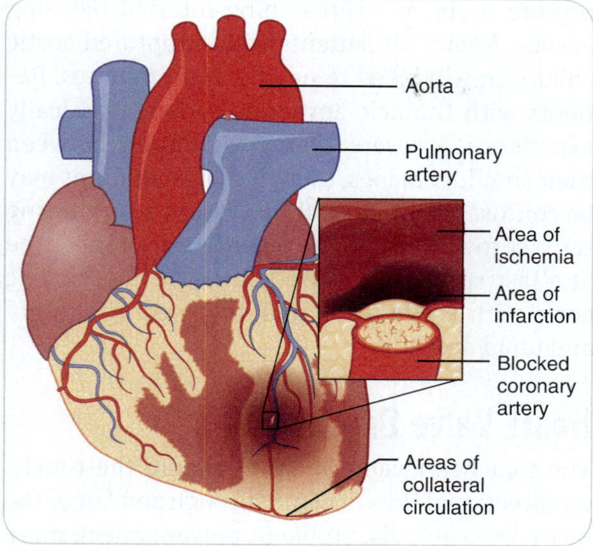

Figure 15-7 Myocardial infarction.

clot forms to repair the rupture, and the coronary artery can become completely blocked, preventing blood flow past the blockage. Another cause of myocardial infarction is the gradual growth of plaques in coronary vessels until they completely prevent blood flow through the vessels.

When the heart tissue supplied by an obstructed coronary artery becomes oxygen starved, the tissue begins to die. This area of dead heart muscle is referred to as an infarct. If enough heart muscle is damaged, the heart cannot pump effectively, which can lead to a host of other life-threatening problems, including cardiac arrhythmias, CHF, cardiogenic shock, and death.

Cardiac Arrhythmias

Built into the heart is a pathway with a coordinated electrical signal that makes the heart beat in a normal rhythm. Any abnormality in this process can lead to an irregular heart beat or heart rhythm, known as an **arrhythmia**, which can compromise normal heart function. A blockage of the electrical pathway through the heart muscle, or an abnormal electrical signal somewhere in the heart muscle can cause an arrhythmia.

Sudden life-threatening arrhythmias may be caused by ischemia (lack of oxygen) of the heart muscle. Although the identification of cardiac arrhythmias is beyond the scope of this text, their effects are straightforward: they either slow the heart rate to below 60 beats per minute (bradycardia), speed it up to above 100 beats per minute (tachycardia), alter the regularity of the rhythm, or stop the heart. Many arrhythmias affect the ability of the heart to pump blood causing a severe drop in blood pressure, leading to cardiogenic shock.

Not all arrhythmias cause immediate life-threatening problems. Some chronic arrhythmias are relatively benign, although they indicate a problem with the heart's electrical system. Chronic cardiac arrhythmias can cause blood to stagnate and clot within the heart. Such clots can break free and travel to the brain or elsewhere in the body, where they may block blood flow. A blood clot that ends up in the brain is likely to cause a stroke. People who have certain chronic arrhythmias are put on medications that prevent the blood from clotting.

Cardiogenic Shock

If enough of the heart muscle is suddenly and severely damaged, the heart may no longer pump effectively. This diminished pumping ability can cause blood pressure to fall resulting in cardiogenic shock. Cardiogenic shock is a condition in which the heart cannot adequately pump blood, resulting in poor cardiac output. The most common cause of cardiogenic shock is myocardial infarction. Many patients with cardiogenic shock will die, regardless of treatment. If the amount of heart muscle damaged is not too severe, emergent care by a cardiologist in a definitive-care facility can potentially save these patients.

Sudden Cardiac Arrest

Sudden cardiac arrest (SCA) is the abrupt cessation of *effective* pumping of blood from the heart into the coronary arteries, the brain, and other vital organs. This condition is caused by an arrhythmia. These include **ventricular fibrillation (VF)** (chaotic and ineffective contraction of the ventricles that leads to cardiac arrest), **ventricular tachycardia (VT)** (rapid regular contraction of the ventricles that can lead to ineffective blood flow to the body tissues and eventually cardiac arrest), or **asystole** (an abrupt cessation of all cardiac electrical activity). These conditions occur without warning. A patient that is affected by SCA (also known as sudden cardiac death or simply, cardiac arrest) will not have a pulse. According to the American Heart Association, SCA is a leading cause of death in the United States, resulting in more than 475,000 deaths each year, with 350,000 of these deaths occurring outside a hospital. Without **cardiopulmonary resuscitation (CPR)** and use of an automated external defibrillator (AED), nearly all with SCA will die. Prompt treatment of pulseless VT or VF with CPR and an AED may result in restoration of an effective heartbeat. Asystole is usually fatal, unless an underlying reversible cause or source is rapidly found and corrected.

Pericarditis and Pericardial Tamponade

Pericarditis is an inflammation of the pericardial sac that surrounds the heart. Among the numerous causes of pericarditis are myocardial infarction, bacterial and viral infections, and trauma. The inflammation can cause the pericardium to rub against the heart, resulting in severe pain, especially upon deep inhalation or coughing. In some cases, excess fluid may build up within pericardial sac, applying external pressure to the heart preventing adequate filling of the heart with blood, a condition known as pericardial tamponade, which restricts the heart's ability to pump effectively. Pericarditis develops slowly, whereas pericardial tamponade from trauma usually occurs suddenly, rapidly leading to death without treatment at a hospital.

Aortic Aneurysm/Aortic Dissection

An aneurysm is a localized dilation in a blood vessel that is either congenital (born with the condition) or results from the degenerative weakening of the vessel wall over time. It is like a "bubble" that forms on an overinflated bicycle inner tube. If not congenital, common causes of an aneurysm are atherosclerosis, hypertension, and smoking.

An **aortic aneurysm** is an aneurysm that occurs anywhere along the length of the aorta. Potentially deadly aneurysms occur in the abdomen (known as an abdominal aortic aneurysm, or AAA) or in the chest (known as a thoracic aortic aneurysm). Aneurysms also may occur in blood vessels within the brain.

Aortic dissection is a condition in which the lining of this large artery's inner wall tears away from the outer wall. Due to the high pressure within the aorta, the tear grows and can penetrate the other layers of the vessel, weakening the vessel wall and making it susceptible to rupture. Should rupture occur, life-threatening internal bleeding ensues. Nearly all patients with a ruptured aortic aneurysm will bleed to death within minutes. Patients with thoracic aortic dissections classically experience a severe tearing sensation between their shoulder blades, though their symptoms may be confused with an AMI. An abrupt stop causing trauma to the chest, like when a skier hits a tree at a fast speed, can cause tearing of the thoracic aorta with aortic dissection, followed by rupture and rapid death.

Heart Valve Disorders

The four heart valves help to ensure the timely, unidirectional flow of blood through and out of the heart. Occasionally, problems prevent one or more of these valves from functioning properly. When this happens, the heart may have to work harder, blood may leak backward, or blood may pool and/or clot within the heart. Most heart valve problems are congenital (the valve formed improperly before birth). Valve-related problems also are caused by heart disease, myocardial infarction, infection of the valve, and trauma.

PATIENT ASSESSMENT OF CARDIOVASCULAR EMERGENCIES

Begin your assessment as you would for any patient—by ensuring that the scene is safe. Next, perform a primary patient assessment in which any problems related to the ABCDs are addressed. Patients in cardiac arrest will be unresponsive, apneic, and pulseless, so immediately begin CPR, call for an AED and ALS. Do not delay transport, except to use an AED.

If the ABCDs are stable, obtain a SAMPLE history as you begin a secondary patient assessment, paying close attention to any complaints of chest pain and any cardiac medications that the patient may be taking such as nitroglycerin or aspirin. If the patient just took nitroglycerin, ask if the symptoms went away, diminished, or stayed the same.

Patients experiencing a cardiovascular emergency may have difficulty communicating, so you may have to gather historical information from a relative or friend at the same time you are performing an intervention to stabilize a patient. If a patient tells you they take a medication, especially

KEY POINT

Agonal Respirations

Patients early in cardiac arrest may have reflexive gasping called "agonal respirations." Agonal respirations are occasional gasping breaths that occur when the heart has stopped. They are associated with increased likelihood of successful resuscitation. Do not let agonal respirations confuse you: start CPR!

KEY POINT

What Is Nitroglycerin?

Nitroglycerin is a medication that causes first veins and then arteries to dilate. Nitroglycerin is commonly prescribed to patients who have a history of angina. Smaller doses cause dilation of the peripheral blood vessels reducing the amount of blood that enters the heart, decreasing the heart's overall workload. A larger dose causes dilation of the coronary arteries during myocardial ischemia improving blood flow to the myocardium. It comes in several forms, including a paste or patch that is applied directly to the skin, a pill that is placed under the tongue, and a metered spray that is applied beneath the tongue.

Table 15-1 Common Cardiac Medications

Drug Name (Generic Name)	Mechanism of Action
Plavix (clopidogrel), aspirin	Prevents clumping of platelets, thereby preventing the formation of clots
Nitroglycerin	Causes dilation of both arteries and veins
Tenormin (atenolol), Toprol/Lopressor (metoprolol)	Lowers blood pressure, slows the heartbeat
Prinivil/Zestril (lisinopril)	Lowers blood pressure, treats CHF
Lipitor (atorvastatin), statins	Lowers harmful cholesterol levels
Repatha	Improves lipid chemistry
Lasix (furosemide), HCTZ (hydrochlorothiazide)	Removes excess fluid from the body
Cordarone (amiodarone)	Used to treat certain arrhythmias, makes heartbeat more regular
Coumadin/Jantoven (warfarin)	Oral anticoagulant, used to treat blood clots, and certain arrhythmias
Eliquis (apixaban)	Oral anticoagulant
Pradaxa (dabigatran)	Oral anticoagulant
Savaysa (edoxaban)	Oral anticoagulant
Aspirin	Oral anticoagulant
Xarelto (rivaroxaban)	Oral anticoagulant

a "heart" medication, ask what is, and why they take it. Usually the patient or a family member knows what the medication is for (**Table 15-1**).

If the patient complains of chest discomfort or pain, assess its nature and characteristics using the OPQRST mnemonic. Cardiac chest pain is usually described as either "heavy," "crushing," or "tight." Less commonly, patients with a cardiovascular emergency may describe the pain as "sharp," may indicate that the pain increases during inspiration, or may locate the pain in the chest wall or over the stomach (**Figure 15-8**). Be sure to ask patients if the pain is only in the chest or radiates into the jaw, abdomen, back, or down the arm. Such referred pain can indicate a myocardial infarction. Patients with a pulmonary embolism can have significant chest pain. As an OEC technician, you will not be able to determine if a patient is having an AMI or a pulmonary embolism; both are emergencies.

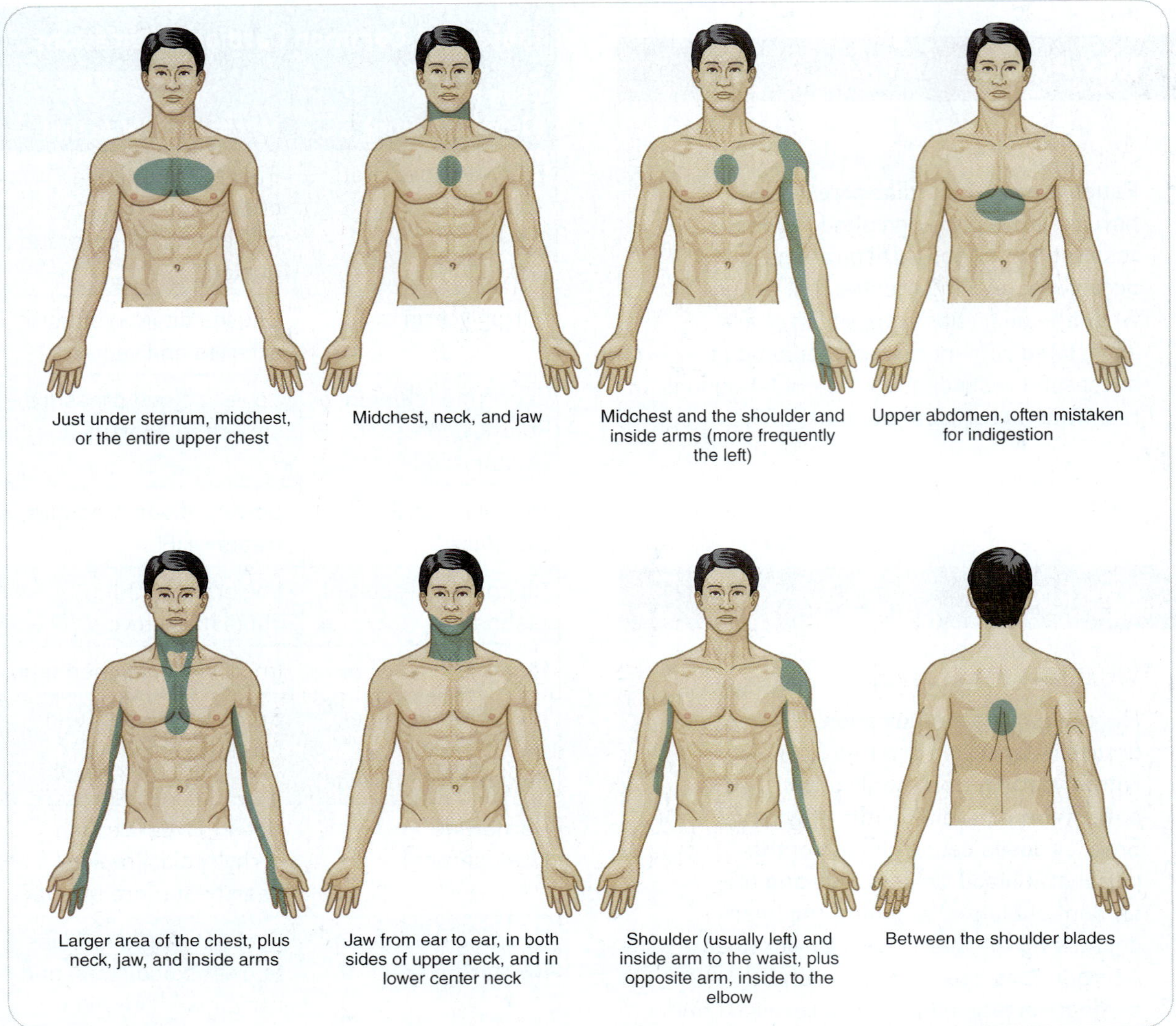

Figure 15-8 Typical sites of chest discomfort and referred pain associated with cardiac emergencies.

Patients with an aortic dissection often describe the pain as "tearing." Depending on the site of the dissection, the pain can be abdominal or acute severe back pain.

Ask patients whether the pain or other symptoms improve with rest or remain constant. Also ask about a patient's medical history, including potential risk factors for cardiovascular disease (**Table 15-2**). Do not be afraid to ask about the use of street drugs—specifically, cocaine and methamphetamine, because use of these increases the risk for AMI.

Next, perform a physical exam and assess vital signs while you are waiting for transport. Patients with cardiac emergencies are usually short of

Table 15-2 Risk Factors for Cardiovascular Disease

1. Uncontrolled high blood pressure
2. Smoking
3. Diabetes
4. Lack of exercise
5. Obesity
6. Elevated lipids (cholesterol and triglycerides)
7. Poor diet
8. Depression
9. Family history
10. Excessive alcohol intake, or cocaine or methamphetamine use

CASE Update

After ensuring that the scene is safe, you call for transport with ALS assistance and begin your assessment. You note a pulse of 128 beats per minute, respirations of 28 breaths per minute and shallow, and blood pressure of 164/94 mm Hg. The physical exam reveals an overweight man who is short of breath and appears to be very anxious. He is pale and diaphoretic. He describes the chest pain as a "9" on a scale of 0 to 10. Upon further questioning, you discover that he has a history of angina pectoris, but according to him, "This is the worst it's ever felt." He also says, "I feel like I'm going to die!"

What should you do?

breath. Carefully assess cardiac output by checking pulses, capillary refill, and level of responsiveness, each of which provides evidence as to whether tissue perfusion is effective. Assess the skin for color, temperature, and profuse sweating or diaphoresis, which is caused by ischemia during an AMI. When outside the aid room, take a radial pulse; if present the systolic blood pressure is at least 80 mm Hg. In the aid room, take a blood pressure with the equipment available.

Reassess the patient and the vital signs at regular intervals, every 5 minutes if the patient is unstable, or every 15 minutes if the patient is stable. Record the vital signs and compare the results to previous findings. Vital signs that are deteriorating indicate that a patient has a serious medical problem.

You should never delay transport for a patient you think is having a cardiovascular emergency. Call for transport early, and as soon as transport arrives, interrupt your assessment and ship the patient unless you have a specific treatment that will benefit the patient on scene, such as using an AED. Going through a full history and physical on the side of a mountain will not help the patient when ALS care and transport to a hospital are needed.

Hypertension

The effects of hypertension generally do not become apparent or produce detectable signs and symptoms until blood pressure reaches high levels. The actual pressure at which symptoms become evident varies from person to person. When present, signs and symptoms of hypertension include headache, vision disturbances, seizures, nausea and/or vomiting, facial flushing, and a bounding pulse. Patients with dangerous levels of hypertension typically complain of chest pain, shortness of breath, and/or confusion. When any medical condition causes blood pressure to elevate to a very high level *rapidly*, transport with ALS is indicated.

Angina and Myocardial Infarction

Because patients with either angina pectoris or myocardial infarction lack enough delivery of oxygen to the heart muscle, both types of patients may present with the same signs and symptoms. Although the chest pain is often described as "crushing" or "heavy," patients may describe the pain in a vague way, such as severe "heartburn." The pain may be only in the chest or it may radiate into the jaw, arm, or back. Other signs and symptoms may include anxiety, dizziness, nausea, diaphoresis, and feelings of impending doom or death. Women have chest pain as a presenting complaint commonly but may also have an atypical presentation, such as a painless myocardial infarction, more than men.

Heart Attack Without Chest Pain

A "silent myocardial infarction" refers to a condition in which a patient is having an AMI without chest pain. Up to a third of all patients presenting with an AMI will have no chest pain, per the National Registry of Myocardial Infarction II. Although silent MIs are more common in women, diabetics, and the elderly, they can occur in any population. Patients having an AMI will always have some symptoms. The two most common complaints in patients having an AMI without chest pain are shortness of breath and fatigue. Other complaints include upper back pain, abdominal pain, and nausea. Some people do not seek care for a silent AMI, but the fact that they had one will show up on an EKG done later in life.

Cardiogenic Shock

Patients who are in cardiogenic shock appear deathly ill and exhibit signs of shock, including pale skin, diaphoresis, anxiety, and respiratory distress. If the cause of the shock is AMI, the patient will likely be tachycardic and hypotensive. If the cause of the shock is an abnormal heart rhythm, the patient may be bradycardic or tachycardic and hypotensive. Any patient with suspected AMI should be evaluated for decreased perfusion and shock.

Congestive Heart Failure

Patients with CHF can display a wide range of signs and symptoms, depending on which side of the heart is affected. Right-sided CHF causes edema in the lower extremities, manifested by swollen ankles that may or may not be painful to the touch. With time, the swelling can become severe and may progress up the leg. Pressing the swollen area gently with a finger may leave an indentation. This sign, known as "pitting edema," is a common finding. The more pronounced the swelling, the more severe are the effects of heart failure. Because left-sided CHF causes blood to back up into the lungs, patients may have shortness of breath that may be mild or a profound dyspnea with audible "bubbling" sounds or gasping breaths due to fluid in the lungs. Patients can have both right-sided and left-sided CHF at the same time.

Pericardial Tamponade

As with cardiogenic shock, patients with pericardial tamponade appear gravely ill. Most are short of breath, appear anxious or restless, and have pale, cool, diaphoretic skin. Chest pain and tachycardia are common with **hypotension** due to decreased cardiac output. The hallmark signs of pericardial tamponade are hypotension and distended neck veins. Additionally, the pulse pressure narrows meaning the systolic and diastolic blood pressure numbers get closer. The systolic pressure is lower because the left ventricle cannot force as much blood out when the heart contracts, because the fluid in the pericardium limits the filling capacity of the left ventricle. The diastolic pressure gets higher due to the external pressure on the heart when it relaxes. However, patients with gradual onset pericardial tamponade may initially present with fatigue and tachycardia only.

Aortic Aneurysm/Dissection

A patient with a thoracic aortic dissection commonly complains of severe chest pain and occasionally back pain described as tearing, ripping, or stabbing. The pain frequently radiates to the back between the shoulders. Unless the dissection has ruptured, the patient may be hypertensive. Rupture of the thoracic aorta can occur when a person hits a fixed object with his or her chest when moving rapidly.

Abdominal aortic aneurysms often present in an older age group with abdominal pain radiating to the groin or back pain. If you suspect that the patient has an abdominal aortic aneurysm, abdominal exam should not be performed. There will be decreased pulses in the groin or legs. If the aneurysm ruptures, the patient goes into profound shock with hypotension and diaphoresis and is at great risk for dying. Be sure to assess vital signs and note any abnormalities.

Pulmonary Embolism (Thromboembolism)

The hallmarks of pulmonary embolism are a sudden onset of chest pain, shortness of breath, rapid breathing, and tachycardia. The pain is often described as "sharp" and increases with deep breaths. The patient also may be cyanotic. If you have a pulse oximeter, you may find the patient to be hypoxic if they do not compensate by breathing fast.

For patients you suspect have pulmonary embolism, look for the presence of deep vein thrombosis (DVT). The signs and symptoms of DVT typically affect only one leg and include severe pain, tenderness to touch, and swelling, usually in the calf. The most dangerous DVTs form in the larger pelvic veins and are often asymptomatic (without symptoms) until they break loose from within the vessel causing a pulmonary embolism. While finding a DVT will not affect your acute management, it can help support the diagnosis. For more information about pulmonary embolism, refer to Chapter 10, *Shock*.

MANAGEMENT OF CARDIOVASCULAR EMERGENCIES

Time is of the essence when caring for a patient with a suspected life-threatening cardiovascular problem. If the patient is having an AMI, the more time that passes without medical intervention, the greater the extent of the myocardial infarction, the greater the heart damage, and the more likely this situation will proceed to SCA. Studies also show that SCA occurs most often within the first hour of AMI. Accordingly, transport with ALS assistance should be requested immediately. Also call for oxygen and an AED as soon as possible. If the patient becomes hypoxic or cyanotic, use oxygen. Initial care is directed toward correcting any problems related to the ABCDs. If the patient is having severe difficulty breathing, make sure the airway is open, assist the patient's breathing efforts, and provide high-flow oxygen with a nonrebreather mask. When inside the aid room, regulate the use of oxygen with a pulse oximeter to keep the oxygen saturation between 94 and 99%. If the patient is diaphoretic and cyanotic, use oxygen immediately.

Care for Patients in Cardiac Arrest

Most cardiovascular emergencies need rapid primary patient assessment, correction of threats to life that may include CPR and the use of an AED, and rapid transport using ALS. If rapidly available, oxygen can be provided.

During assessment, always evaluate the ABCDs and treat problems as they are found. However, for that small percentage of patients who are unresponsive, pulseless, and apneic, recognize the primary problem is lack of circulation and immediately begin CPR. Any *unresponsive* patient should be assessed following a CAB approach.

KEY POINT

CPR and AED

CPR is the first and most important intervention for someone in cardiac arrest. It must be done as quickly as SCA is recognized and should be performed at right rate, right depth, and with full recoil with minimal interruption. Use of an AED should be done as quickly as can be accomplished. CPR pauses associated with AED application should be avoided. Survival following defibrillation after extended periods of CPR is well documented.

Using CAB assesses circulation first. In an unresponsive patient, immediately check for a pulse. If no pulse, begin chest compressions. You will need to open the airway and simultaneously check for breathing. If a patient is in cardiopulmonary arrest as indicated by absent pulse and breathing, begin basic life support (BLS) measures immediately.

The five links in the adult out-of-hospital chain of survival are as follows (**Figure 15-9**):

1. Recognition of early warning signs and immediate activation of the emergency medical services
2. Immediate CPR with an emphasis on high-quality chest compressions
3. Rapid defibrillation
4. Basic and advanced emergency medical services
5. Advanced life support and post-arrest care

Recognition of Early Warning Signs and Immediate Activation of the Emergency Medical Services

Immediate recognition of cardiac arrest and activation of the emergency response system is the first link in the chain of survival and focuses on recognizing the signs and symptoms of SCA. Trained ALS medical personnel with specialized equipment and medications are needed rapidly. Delays in seeking assistance or providing CPR significantly decrease the patient's chances of survival.

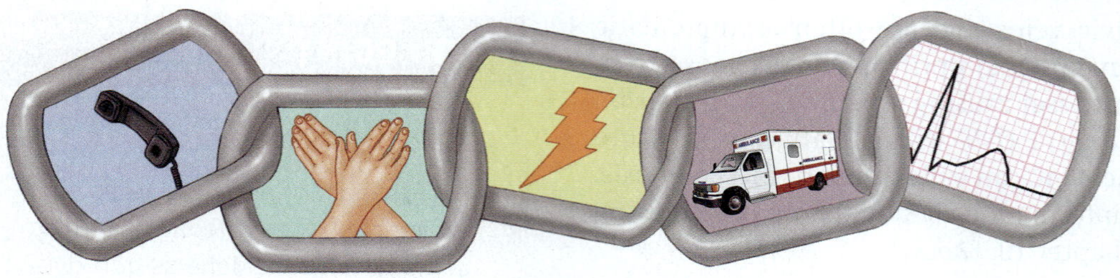

Figure 15-9 The links in the chain of survival.

KEY POINT

CPR Technique

All OEC technicians need to know the most current CPR skills for all ages, as recommended by authoritative sources such as the American Heart Association or American Red Cross. All OEC technicians must maintain a current CPR/AED certification.

Annual demonstration of these skills is required by the National Ski Patrol.

KEY POINT

Cause of Cardiac Arrest in Children

The most common cause of cardiac arrest in children and infants is respiratory failure.

This text does not teach CPR techniques. There are many approved programs that teach CPR following the lead of the American Heart Association Emergency Cardiac Care standards. It is mandatory for all OEC technicians to maintain current certification in CPR and AED methods. In addition, they must demonstrate CPR skills annually to a CPR instructor.

Immediate CPR with Emphasis on High-Quality Chest Compressions

Survival rates fall drastically when CPR is delayed. Because of this, CPR must be initiated as quickly as possible to anyone needing it. The goal of effective CPR is to pump remaining oxygenated blood from the heart to other vital organs. The most critical step in the performance of CPR is the effective use of chest compressions, minimizing any interruption of compressions. The current philosophy in CPR care is "Push hard, push fast" (at least 100 times a minute) while allowing time for full recoil of the chest to occur.

Once begun, CPR should not be stopped unless:

- The patient improves [Return of Spontaneous Circulation (ROSC)].
- An AED has been attached to the patient and is ready to be used. The emphasis in the current approach is to not stop compressions until the AED is attached, powered on, and ready to analyze.
- Rescuers are too tired to continue.
- Care has been transferred to another health care provider of equal or higher competency.
- The patient is declared dead.

Rapid Defibrillation

The third link in the chain of survival is to correct life-threatening arrhythmias such as VF and VT as soon as possible. While CPR is important to maintain circulation to vital organs, the key is to reestablish cardiac circulation. This is done by **defibrillation**, using a defibrillator. The device used in the field for defibrillation by BLS providers is called an **automated external defibrillator (AED)** (**Figure 15-10**). It delivers an electric shock (defibrillation) to convert VT or VF to an effective heartbeat. When an AED delivers a shock, it temporarily stops the heart's electrical activity, thereby allowing the heart's internal pacemaker cells to reset and if the heart is capable, resume directing the heartbeat in an organized fashion. Since both trained and lay rescuers can now effectively use an AED, patient survival from SCA has recently doubled in some communities. In the US, when an AED is used during out-of-hospital care, survival is greatly improved. This percentage varies by location in the US.

An AED must be applied quickly, as its effectiveness decreases very rapidly over several minutes. After 10 minutes of pulseless cardiac arrest due to VT or VF without CPR, the heart is nearly completely nonresponsive to electrical stimulation. CPR can expand the window of time for which defibrillation may be effective. When two trained rescuers are on scene with a patient who has SCA, one-person CPR should be performed while the second rescuer seeks an AED.

If CPR is in progress and an AED is available, continue CPR while the pads are applied, and the AED is turned on. Stop CPR only when the machine is ready to analyze and directs everyone to stand back and not touch the patient. Although originally designed for use on adults only, recent studies indicate that an AED may be safely used on cardiac arrest patients of any age.

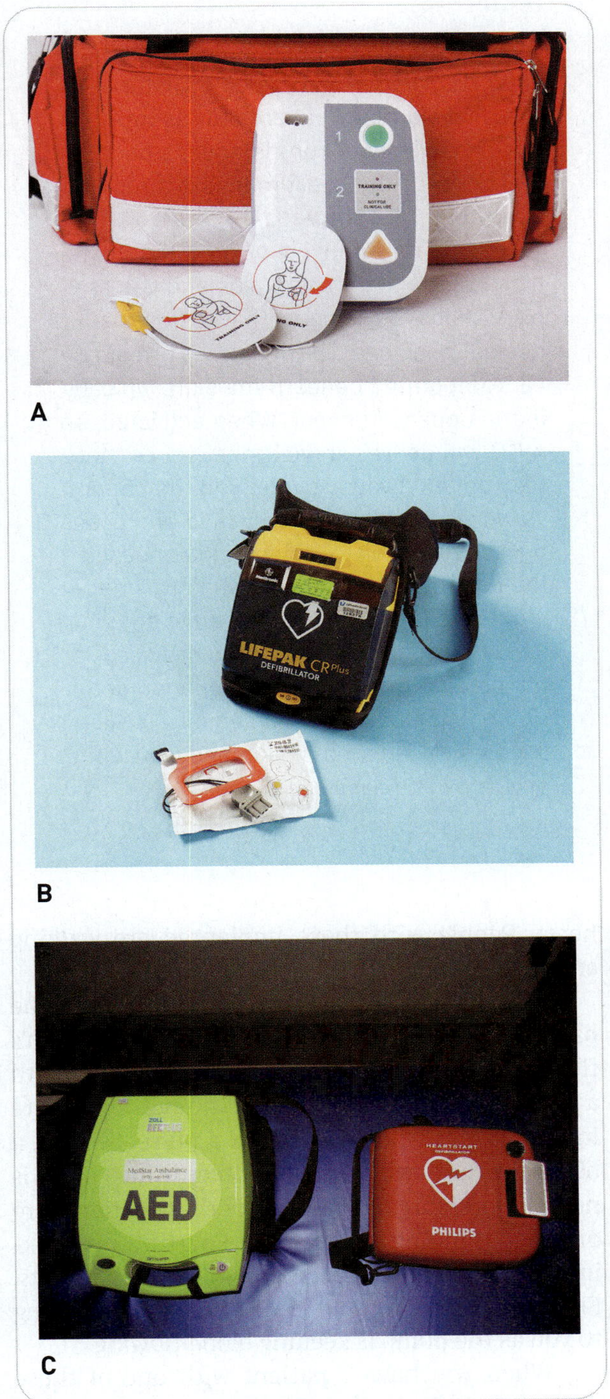

Figure 15-10 Various types of AEDs.

A: © Photographee.eu/Shutterstock; B: © Jones & Bartlett Learning.

KEY POINT

Automated External Defibrillators (AEDs)

What is an AED? An AED is a portable device that identifies lethal arrhythmias (e.g., VF, VT) and tells you to press a button to deliver an electrical shock to stop the lethal arrhythmia to restore an effective heartbeat. AEDs are increasingly available in public areas, and most provide step-by-step voice instructions. They are now used by people who have no formal medical training.

Basic and Advanced Emergency Medical Services

The fourth link is basic and advanced emergency medical services. These providers can provide valuable interventions and lifesaving medications for cardiac arrest patients. Calling for ALS early is important, so advanced interventions can be given to the patient.

Advanced Life Support and Post-Arrest Care

The final link provides advanced life support and transport and care at a critical care facility.

Definitive care at a hospital is part of the last link in the chain of survival. Because of technological advancements, the survival rate from an AMI is better, provided the chain of survival is maintained. Once at the hospital, the following therapies and interventions may be used to restore effective circulation to the heart:

- *Thrombolytic therapy*. In this approach, medications commonly referred to as "clot busters" are injected into the patient to dissolve any blood clots or thrombi that may be occluding the coronary arteries.
- *Angioplasty.* In this surgical technique, a small balloon is inserted into a blocked coronary artery. Once positioned next to the site of the occlusion, the balloon is inflated, thereby restoring effective circulation.
- *Cardiac stent*. This device, a small wire-mesh tube, is surgically inserted into a formerly blocked coronary artery to keep the vessel open and to prevent its reocclusion. Stents are commonly inserted during a heart catherization.
- *Coronary artery bypass grafting*. This procedure involves taking a vein from the patient's leg, arm, or chest and inserting it in such a way that it bypasses a blocked coronary artery.

> **KEY POINT**
>
> **Automatic Implantable Cardioverter Defibrillator**
>
> Technology has enabled many cardiovascular disorders to be corrected, which has allowed many patients to resume an active lifestyle. For instance, a pacemaker helps the heart maintain a regular heartbeat. An **automatic implantable cardioverter defibrillator (AICD)** detects life-threatening arrhythmias and can apply a shock to the heart that restores a normal heartbeat. Both devices are surgically implanted beneath the skin, typically in the upper left chest. When activated, an AICD will deliver an electrical shock that may be felt if you are touching the patient. However, the shock is very mild and poses no risk to rescuers. Upon being shocked the patient will feel pain, usually grimacing. An AED can be used on a patient who has either of these implanted devices. Do not place the pads over the location of the implantable device, which usually is visible as a raised area of skin and where the device can be easily palpated.

Ventricular Assist Device

The **ventricular assist device (VAD)** is implanted in the chest, with a battery pack outside the chest. It is a pump that helps the failing heart with poor muscle. If connected to the left ventricle (LVAD) it assists pumping blood into the aorta or if connected to the right ventricle (RVAD) it assists pumping blood into the pulmonary arteries. It is not an artificial heart but assists the patient's heart. People with these implanted are walking around in public.

Patients with a VAD need special care. First, the patient will not have a pulse, as the artificial pump's flow is continuous and not intermittent like with a normal heart, so there will be no pulse pressure in the arteries where you check a pulse. Second, a blood pressure will be hard to obtain since there is no pulse pressure. Third, most of these patients are on blood thinning medications. Fourth, a pulse oximeter does not read accurately in these patients. Fifth, the patient may be in VT or VF and be talking to you as the pump is keeping blood flowing.

When you have a patient with one of these devices, help is needed. The patient's family will usually know quite a bit about the device. There is usually an emergency number to call for immediate help that the patient or the loved ones may have. If not, call 9-1-1 immediately if a patient with one of these devices implanted has a problem. Routine CPR with defibrillation can be done, but whether chest compressions can be done without damaging the device is controversial.

Cardiovascular Patients Who Are Not in Cardiac Arrest

Responsive patients with a suspected cardiovascular emergency may go into cardiac arrest at any time. Call immediately for assistance, oxygen, AED, and transport with ALS. Attempt to keep patients calm because doing so will help reduce both anxiety and stress on the heart. Place the patient into a position of comfort. For patients with chest pain, this is usually sitting up. Place *hypotensive* patients into a supine position and keep them warm. If CHF or pulmonary edema is suspected, the patient will likely prefer to be seated upright because this helps breathing. If possible, allow a CHF patient's legs to be in a dependent position (i.e., below the level of the heart as in sitting in a chair), which allows excess fluid to pool in the lower extremities. This can also permit the patient to breathe more easily.

Oxygen Therapy

Because respiratory distress and myocardial ischemia are commonly associated with cardiovascular-system disorders, it is important to maintain *normal* blood oxygen levels. In the outside prehospital environment, it is difficult to measure blood oxygen levels, so when *clinically indicated with hypoxemia or cyanosis*, oxygen therapy should be initiated as soon as possible. Administer high-flow oxygen at 15 LPM via a nonrebreather mask (**Figure 15-11**). However, after getting the patient inside, if a pulse oximeter is available, titrate the oxygen flow, maintaining an oxygen saturation between 94 and 99%. Oxygen may not be needed if the patient can maintain oxygen saturation between 94 and 99% without increased respirations.

For patients with cardiovascular disease who are claustrophobic when an oxygen mask is used, continue to calm the patient as you render care, to avoid worsening their anxiety and increasing oxygen demands on the heart. You may have to weigh the relative risks and benefits of using a mask compared to a nasal cannula. If an agitated patient continues to remove the mask, administering

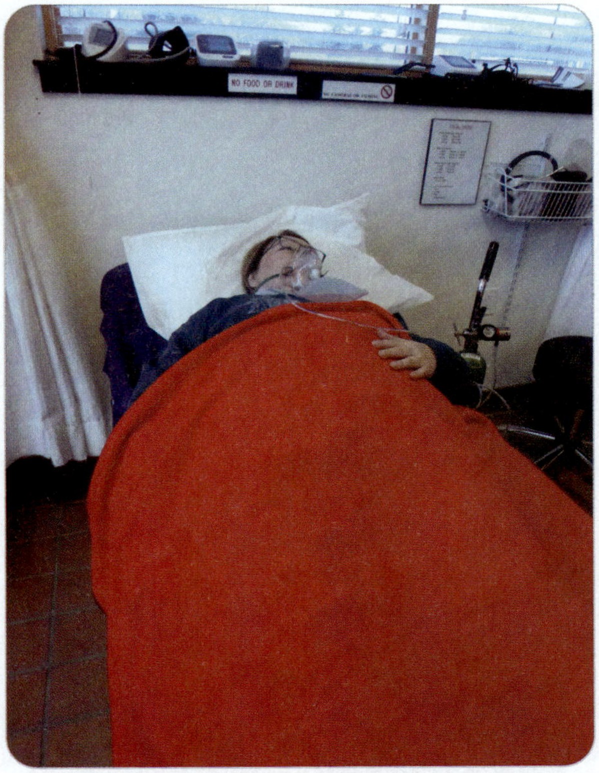

Figure 15-11 This patient is receiving oxygen therapy in the aid room while awaiting EMS transport.

oxygen at 4 to 6 LPM by nasal cannula is better than no oxygen, but the use of a mask is preferred.

Nitroglycerin

Some patients with angina pectoris may carry their own nitroglycerin, a medication used to relieve chest pain (**Figure 15-12**). As with all prescribed medications, this drug may be used only by the patient for whom it has been prescribed. If the *patient's own* nitroglycerin is available, you may need to assist the patient in taking this medicine. Check your area, state, or provincial protocols to determine if you are permitted to assist a patient in taking nitroglycerin. OEC technicians should call for transport and ALS even though a patient takes nitroglycerin.

Nitroglycerin should be given only to a patient with chest pain who is awake and responsive. It should NOT be given to patients if any of the following contraindications pertain:

- The nitroglycerin is expired.
- The nitroglycerin is not prescribed for that patient.

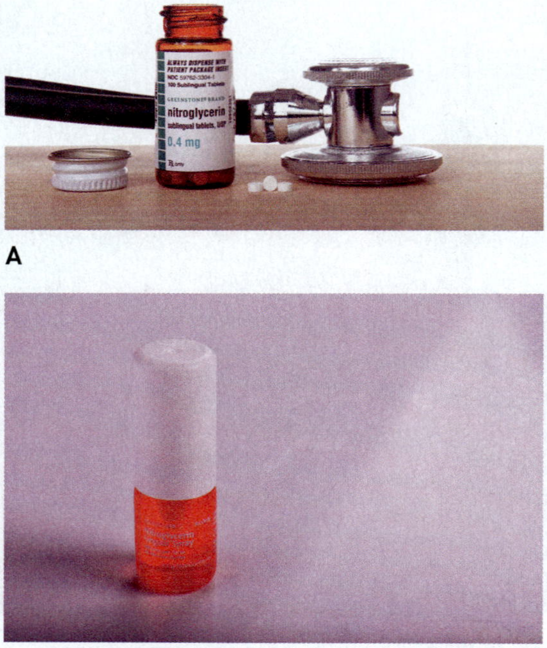

A

B

Figure 15-12 Nitroglycerin can come as sublingual tablets (**A**) or a spray (**B**) and is used for angina pectoris.

A: © Sheila Fitzgerald/Shutterstock; **B:** © Tony Savino/Shutterstock.

- Systolic blood pressure is less than 100 mm Hg.
- The patient has taken three doses of nitroglycerin for this episode of chest pain.
- The patient has used a medication for erectile dysfunction or altitude illness prevention (e.g., Viagra, Levitra, Cialis) within the past 24 hours.
- Chest pain is due to trauma (is not cardiac in origin).

To assist patients in taking their own nitroglycerin tablets, follow these steps:

1. Check systolic blood pressure to ensure it is over 100 mm Hg.
2. Check to make sure the medication is prescribed for this patient and that it has not expired.
3. Put on your disposable gloves, and then remove one tablet from the bottle and place the tablet in the patient's hand.
4. Instruct the patient to place the medication under the tongue and to allow it to dissolve completely. Tell the patient not to chew or swallow the tablet. If necessary, assist the patient by putting the medication in place once the patient has lifted the tongue.

To assist patients in taking their own nitroglycerin sublingual spray, follow the steps in **OEC Skill 15-1**.

If the patient is still experiencing chest pain, you may assist the patient in taking two more doses of nitroglycerin, for a total of three doses, at 5-minute intervals. This total of three doses includes any nitroglycerin the patient may have taken immediately before your arrival on scene. Recheck the patient's blood pressure after each dose. If systolic blood pressure is less than 100 mm Hg, do not give more nitroglycerin.

After taking nitroglycerin, the patient will likely experience a burning sensation beneath the tongue and may get a headache. Both symptoms are normal and indicate that the medication is working properly. Reassure the patient that these are commonly occurring symptoms with this type of medication. Document in your notes the date, time, and dosage (if known) at which the drug was administered. Reassess the patient frequently for signs of improvement (e.g., decreased severity of pain) and recheck the vital signs at regular intervals.

Aspirin

Evidence-based medicine now recommends that a layperson assist a person who is having a myocardial infarction (heart attack) chew and swallow an adult (325 mg) or four pediatric (81 mg) aspirin tablets as soon as symptoms appear. Most myocardial infarctions are caused by a blood clot in a coronary artery. This blood clot consists of platelets in the blood sticking together. Aspirin is a medication that helps prevent platelets from sticking together. If you suspect a patient is having AMI and you are authorized by your local medical advisor to assist the administration of aspirin, do so. Do not give aspirin to anyone who is either allergic to or sensitive to aspirin or wintergreen. Give aspirin only to patients who are fully responsive and can swallow.

To assist a patient in taking aspirin, follow these steps:

1. Confirm that the patient is not allergic to aspirin.

OEC SKILL 15-1 Administering Nitroglycerin

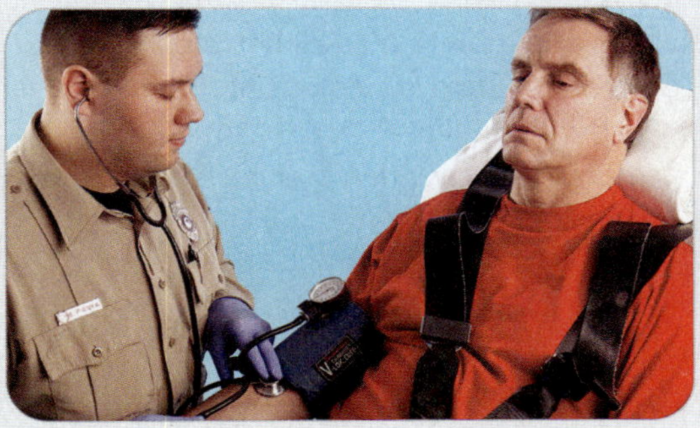

1. Check systolic blood pressure to ensure it is over 100 mm Hg.
2. Check the medication to ensure it is prescribed for the patient and that it has not expired. Do NOT shake the metered-dose spray.
3. Instruct the patient to lift the tongue.
4. Apply one spray beneath the patient's tongue.

2. Confirm there is no obvious GI bleeding (no vomiting of blood or blood in stool).
3. Select the proper dosage of aspirin. Use either one adult buffered aspirin (325 mg per tablet) *or* four chewable baby aspirins (81 mg per tablet for total of 324 mg). The baby aspirin are preferred and easier for a patient to chew and swallow.
4. Check the expiration date of the aspirin; do not use the medication if it has expired.
5. Put on your disposable gloves and place the aspirin in the patients hand. Instruct the patient to chew the aspirin before swallowing it.
6. A sip of water may help get the aspirin into the stomach.

Document the date, time, and dosage administered. Reassess the patient frequently, including the vital signs.

Whenever possible, minimize the patient's physical exertion because exertion increases the oxygen demand on the heart. This may be difficult, however, in backcountry settings, especially if resource availability requires the patient to self-evacuate under his or her own power. If available, use one of the transportation methods described in Chapter 5, *Moving, Lifting, and Transporting Patients*.

Conditions such as aortic aneurysm, aortic dissection, pulmonary embolism, and pericardial tamponade all have high mortality rates if lifesaving interventions are not rendered quickly. Unfortunately, the field care for these threats to life is limited to treating the patient for shock, providing oxygen if readily available, and providing rapid transport with ALS to a definitive-care facility.

KEY POINT

What Does Aspirin Do?

Aspirin blocks the clumping of platelets, components of blood that clump together and stimulate the formation of a clot that repairs a ruptured blood vessel. During AMI, platelets tend to clump together to repair a ruptured plaque within a coronary artery. However, in this case the repair of the ruptured plaque is harmful, because it leads to the formation of a thrombus that can occlude the artery, causing the cardiac muscle distal to the artery to become ischemic and die. Therefore, by blocking the clumping of platelets, aspirin also blocks thrombus formation, thereby preventing the development of a myocardial infarction and if an AMI has occurred, decreasing its level of severity.

CASE Outcome

You administer oxygen by nonrebreather mask at 15 LPM and maintain SpO2 between 94-99%. The man is more comfortable sitting. Soon after ALS personnel arrive, you assist them in transporting the patient to an ambulance waiting at the trailhead. Later, you learn that the patient had a myocardial infarction. He underwent a cardiac catherization placing a stent into the blocked coronary artery and is expected to make a complete recovery.

CHAPTER REVIEW

In Summary

- Cardiovascular disease is the leading cause of death worldwide.
- Cardiovascular disease can cause a host of problems, including high blood pressure, congestive heart failure, acute myocardial infarction, and stroke.
- Most cardiovascular emergencies need rapid primary patient assessment, correction of threats to life that may include CPR and the use of an AED, and rapid transport using ALS. If rapidly available, oxygen can be provided.
- Time is of the essence when caring for a patient with a suspected life-threatening cardiovascular problem.
- Responsive patients with a suspected cardiovascular emergency may go into cardiac arrest at any time.
- Always evaluate the ABCDs. For unresponsive, pulseless, and apneic patients, recognize the primary problem is lack of circulation and immediately begin CPR.
- The five links in the adult out-of-hospital chain of survival include recognition of early warning signs and immediate activation of EMS, immediate CPR with an emphasis on high-quality chest compressions, rapid defibrillation, basic and advanced emergency medical services, and advanced life support and post-arrest care.
- Evidence-based medicine now recommends aspirin for a patient who is having a myocardial infarction (heart attack).

Key Terms

Acute myocardial infarction (AMI) The interruption of blood supply to part of the heart from a blocked artery, causing death of heart muscle. Also known as a heart attack.

Angina pectoris Sudden chest pain due to an inadequate supply of oxygen to the heart muscle; also called angina.

Aorta The largest artery in the body, carries blood out of the left side of the heart to smaller arteries that travel through the entire body.

Aortic aneurysm An aneurysm that occurs anywhere along the length of the aorta.

Arrhythmia Abnormal heart rhythm.

Asystole A complete absence of a heartbeat due to a lack of electrical activity within the heart.

Atherosclerosis A form of arteriosclerosis in which cholesterol and lipid plaques form within the walls of arteries.

Automated external defibrillator (AED) A medical device used to deliver an electrical shock to a patient to restore an effective heart rhythm.

Automatic implantable cardioverter defibrillator (AICD) A defibrillator that recognizes common lethal heart rhythms and then delivers an electrical shock to the heart to restore an effective heart rhythm.

Cardiopulmonary resuscitation (CPR) A procedure to revive a patient who is pulseless and not breathing.

Congestive heart failure (CHF) Failure of the heart to efficiently pump blood to body tissues.

Coronary arteries Two arteries that come off the first part of the aorta, that provide oxygenated, nutrient rich blood to the heart muscle.

Coronary artery disease Narrowing of the coronary arteries, which supply blood and oxygen to the heart muscle.

Defibrillation The restoration of a normal rhythm of the heart by electrical shock.

Hypertension Abnormally high blood pressure.

Hypotension Abnormally low blood pressure.

Ischemia A deficiency in blood supply (and thus a deficiency of oxygen and nutrients) to a tissue; if prolonged, may result in death of tissue.

Myocardium Heart muscle tissue.
Pericarditis Inflammation of the pericardium or sac surrounding the heart, causing chest pain.
Pulmonary edema An accumulation of fluid in the lungs.
Sudden cardiac arrest (SCA) The abrupt cessation of an effective heartbeat.
Ventricular assist device (VAD) A device implanted into the chest that assists the heart's ventricle circulate blood to the body.
Ventricular fibrillation (VF) Chaotic and ineffective contraction of the ventricles that leads to cardiac arrest.
Ventricular tachycardia (VT) Rapid regular contraction of the ventricles that can lead to ineffective blood flow to body tissues and eventually cardiac arrest.

Chapter Questions

1. A visitor is in the lodge watching a skiing event and he is complaining of left arm pain, is sweating, and has mild shortness of breath. He may be experiencing which of the following?
   a. Indigestion from eating lunch
   b. A common cold
   c. An acute myocardial infarction
   d. The flu
2. A patient who has fallen on his chest while skiing and presents with chest pain and a blood pressure of 110/102 mm Hg may have which of the following?
   a. Acute pericardial tamponade
   b. Muscle strain from the fall
   c. Anxiety from the fall
   d. Respiratory insufficiency
3. The most common arrhythmias associated with SCA are:
   a. normal sinus rhythm and premature ventricular contractions.
   b. atrial fibrillation and premature ventricular contractions.
   c. ventricular fibrillation, ventricular tachycardia, and asystole.
   d. couplets, premature atrial contractions, and asystole.
4. The first steps to care for patients in SCA are:
   a. assess the pulse, perform chest massage, and use an AED.
   b. connect the AED, assess the airway, and call for help.
   c. call for help and wait for them to arrive.
   d. perform rapid primary assessment, perform CPR and AED if needed, and provide rapid transport.
5. You are asked to assess a 55-year-old patient in the aid room who is complaining of chest pain after skiing several times down the mountain. The patient states he took one dose of his nitroglycerin tablet about 30 minutes ago. His blood pressure is 150/99 mm Hg, and his pulse is 98 beats per minute. Following your assessment, the best care consists of:
   a. assessing vital signs and encouraging the patient to repeat his nitroglycerin.
   b. calling EMS, assessing vital signs, and consulting another patroller.
   c. assessing vital signs, calling EMS, and laying the patient down.
   d. calling EMS, administering oxygen, assessing vital signs, encouraging the patient to repeat his nitroglycerin if he still has chest pain and if his systolic blood pressure is at least 100 mm Hg.
6. True/False: It is standard procedure to give an oral dose of aspirin and nitroglycerin to an unresponsive patient who just had a myocardial infarction.
7. A man who has been skiing and has a known history of angina pectoris just took his nitroglycerin and comes to the patrol room for assistance. How can you assist him?
   a. Assist the patient with taking another dose of nitroglycerin and call EMS.
   b. Assess the patient, call EMS, administer oxygen, and assist the patient with taking up to two more doses of nitroglycerin provided his blood pressure is above 100 mm Hg.

c. Assess the patient's blood pressure, call EMS if his blood pressure is below 100 mm Hg, administer oxygen, and ask the patient not to take any more medication.

d. Assess the patient; if his blood pressure is above 100 mm Hg, contact EMS and assist the patient with as much nitroglycerin as he wants.

8. A patient needs to take another nitroglycerin pill for chest pain and is having some trouble getting the bottle open. He seems rather weak. How would you help the patient?
   a. Watch the patient struggle to take the pill.
   b. Check the blood pressure. If over 100 mm Hg, put on some gloves, remove a pill, and place it in the patient's hand with the instruction that the patient is to place it under the tongue. Tell the patient not to chew the pill.
   c. Check the pulse, if the pulse is over 100 beats per minute, put on some gloves and ask a relative to take the pill out and give it to the patient.
   d. Check the pulse, if the pulse is under 100 beats per minute, put on some gloves and give it to the patient to chew.

9. A female patient tells you that she takes several heart medications. You should:
   a. have the patient spell the medicines.
   b. ask the patient what the medications are and why she takes each of them.
   c. ask a friend if these are necessary medications.
   d. ask a relative to go home to get the medications.

10. True/False: Blood thinners (anticoagulants) reduce the amount of red blood cells circulating in a patient's body.

Answers: 1. c, Objective 15-5, p. 318; 2. a, Objective 15-5, p. 320; 3. c, Objective 15-1, p. 319; 4. d, Objective 15-2, p. 320; 5. d, Objective 15-6, p. 330; 6. False, Objective 15-6, p. 330; 7. b, Objective 15-6, p. 330; 8. b, Objective 15-6, p. 330; 9. b, Objective 15-3, p. 320; 10. False, Objective 15-4, p. 321

CHAPTER 16

GASTROINTESTINAL, GENITOURINARY, AND REPRODUCTIVE SYSTEM EMERGENCIES

OBJECTIVES

Upon completion of this chapter, the OEC technician will be able to:

16-1 List the possible causes of emergencies involving the gastrointestinal, genitourinary, and reproductive systems.

16-2 List the signs and symptoms of emergencies involving the genitourinary system.

16-3 List the signs and symptoms of emergencies involving the gastrointestinal system.

16-4 List the signs and symptoms of emergencies related to the reproductive system.

16-5 Describe and demonstrate how to assess the abdomen.

16-6 Describe and demonstrate the management of a patient with a gastrointestinal, genitourinary, or reproductive emergency.

KEY TERMS

Acute abdomen, p. 347
Bladder infection, p. 345
Ectopic pregnancy, p. 347
Guarding, p. 344
Hematemesis, p. 346
Jaundice, p. 344
Melena, p. 346
Ovarian cyst, p. 347
Pancreatitis, p. 343
Pelvic inflammatory disease, p. 347
Peritoneum, p. 348
Peritonitis, p. 348
Referred pain, p. 339

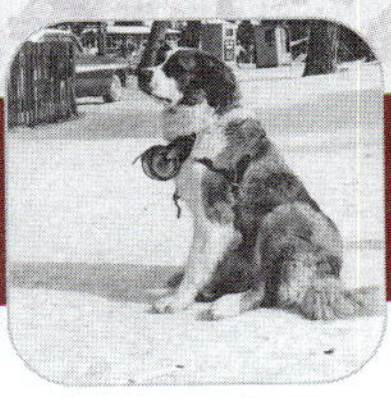

HISTORICAL TIMELINE **1977.** NSP adopts "Rusty," a St. Bernard wearing a first-aid belt, as a mascot.

CHAPTER OVERVIEW

The functions of the gastrointestinal (GI), genitourinary (GU), and reproductive organs include digestion of food, regulation of water balance, elimination of wastes, and reproduction. Some of these organs make important hormones that regulate our body functions. Understanding the location and basic function of the major organs within the abdominal and pelvic cavities will greatly assist OEC technicians in identifying common disorders of these systems. Patients with acute abdominal or pelvic pain can present unique challenges to OEC technicians: a patient's symptoms may be vague or misleading, patients often do not seek care until their symptoms are unbearable, and severe pain or embarrassment may make a thorough exam difficult (**Figure 16-1**).

Men have reproductive organs (testes) outside the pelvis, presenting problems different from those of women. Conditions relating to the female reproductive organs can mimic GI or GU pathology, since these organs are inside the pelvic cavity. Although rarely seen in the outdoor environment, childbirth can occur outside the hospital. As an OEC technician, you should know the basics of this process and how you can assist the pregnant patient. More information about this topic is provided in Chapter 17, *Childbirth, Obstetric Emergencies, and Sexual Assault*.

With a basic understanding of the anatomy and physiology of abdominal and pelvic structures and of the types of medical conditions that could be encountered, OEC technicians can effectively manage initial care of most GI, GU, and gynecologic problems. The goal is not to diagnose the *exact* cause of the problem but to rapidly identify

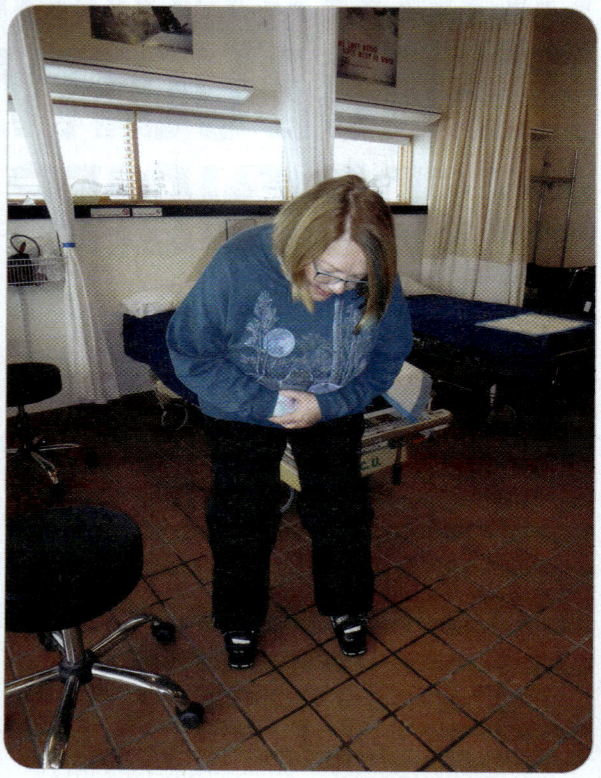

Figure 16-1 OEC technicians must be prepared to care for patients experiencing abdominal pain.

CASE Presentation

You are working first-aid duty in the patrol room when a 25-year-old woman slowly walks in holding her abdomen and complaining of severe abdominal pain. You steer the patient to the nearest exam table and begin to assess her condition. Moments later, she vomits. The vomit is clear and does not appear to contain blood. The patient apologizes and states that she started feeling ill this morning but decided to come skiing anyway to be with her family. She has not suffered any recent trauma and is not currently taking any medications. There is nothing pertinent in the patient's past medical history. She says that she has never experienced anything like this before and describes her abdominal pain as "intense."

What should you do?

any potentially serious emergency, render emergency care, and move the patient quickly toward definitive care.

ANATOMY AND PHYSIOLOGY

It is important for an OEC technician to know where all organs are in the abdomen and pelvis. The abdomen is divided into four quadrants: the right upper, left upper, right lower, and left lower (**Figures 16-2**). It is important to know what organs are in each quadrant because when examining the abdomen, each quadrant is examined separately.

The abdominal organs digest food, eliminate waste, make hormones, and assist with other body functions. These organs can be solid or hollow. The stomach, gallbladder, small and large intestines, appendix, ureters, and urinary bladder are hollow. These organs contain food, bile, feces, and urine. Inside the intestines are bacteria that help digest food. Because hollow organs contain possible irritants and contaminants, injury can lead to spillage into the otherwise sterile abdominal and pelvic cavities.

The solid organs within the abdomen are the liver, pancreas, spleen, and ovaries. The liver is a chemical powerhouse that makes proteins, synthesizes blood-clotting chemicals, and produces bile to aid in the digestion of fat. The pancreas produces digestive enzymes and hormones to regulate blood sugar. The spleen stores blood cells and helps to make antibodies for fighting infections. The ovaries in a woman make hormones and eggs for reproduction. Because the solid organs are highly vascular, damage to them can result in profuse internal bleeding that can lead to hemorrhagic shock.

The kidneys and ureters, which are just outside the abdominal cavity in the flanks, filter and excrete liquid waste and transport it into the bladder in the pelvis. Because they are not inside the abdomen, they are in the retroperitoneal space (the area behind the peritoneum or abdomen). The peritoneum is the lining of the inside of the abdomen (**Figure 16-3**).

Large blood vessels are also found within the abdominal cavity (**Figure 16-4**). The two largest are the abdominal aorta and inferior vena cava, which like the kidneys have a retroperitoneal position just in front of the spine. The pelvic cavity contains numerous vascular structures that are generally well protected by the pelvic bones but can be injured during pelvic trauma. Disorders affecting any of these large blood vessels within the abdominal, pelvic, or retroperitoneal cavities can quickly lead to life-threatening blood loss, shock, and even death.

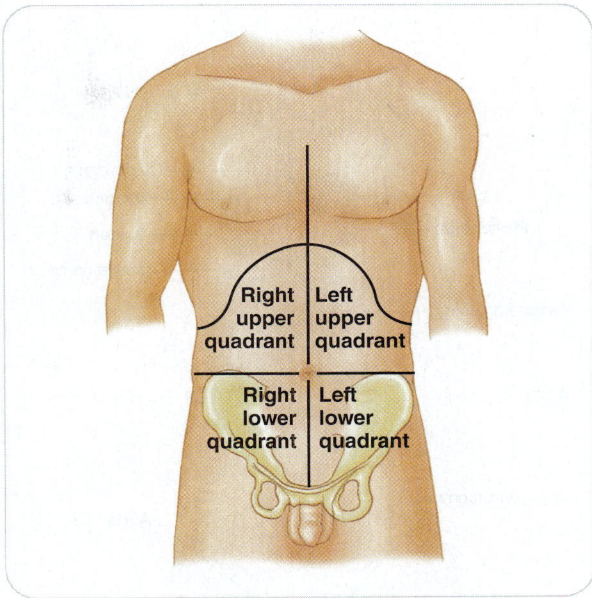

Figure 16-2 The four quadrants of the abdomen.

Abdominal pain may be felt in a specific organ, in a general area of the body, or in a part of the body distant from the source of the pain. Sensory nerves, which enable a person to perceive touch, pressure, heat, cold, and pain, are in the skin of the abdominal wall and within the peritoneum. When sensory nerves become irritated, the location of the pain can be precisely pinpointed; that is, the patient *can* point to the exact location of the pain. This condition is known as parietal pain. In contrast, visceral pain is caused by irritation of visceral nerves and is described as diffuse or spread over a large area. With visceral pain, the patient *cannot* point to the exact location of the pain. Additionally, distention or contraction of the peritoneum stimulates various visceral stretch receptors that can cause pain to be perceived at a distant location, such as the back or shoulder; this condition is known as **referred pain** (**Figure 16-5**).

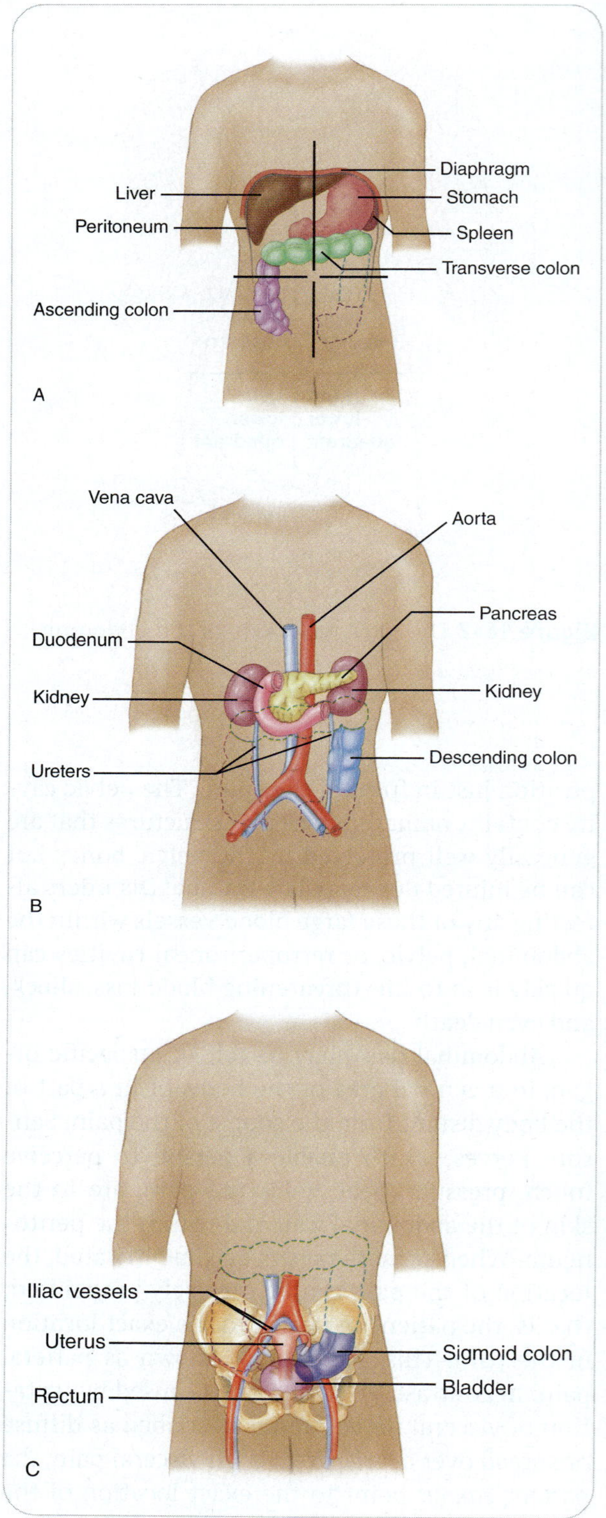

Figure 16-3 Location of organs within the peritoneum (**A**), the retroperitoneal space (**B**), and the pelvis (**C**).

The female reproductive organs are in the abdominal and pelvic cavities (**Figure 16-6**). The ovaries are located in the abdomen. They produce eggs, which are essential for reproduction. The fallopian tubes connect the ovaries to the uterus in the pelvis, allowing for the movement of the eggs into the uterus. The cervix and vagina are in the pelvis. The external parts of the female anatomy include the clitoris and labia. Urine exits the body through the urethra, a tube that connects the bladder to an outside opening just below the clitoris.

The male reproductive system is inside and below the pelvic cavity (**Figure 16-7**). It includes the testes, which are located inside the sac, or scrotum, that hangs below the penis. Sperm, made in the testes, is collected in the epididymis and travels through a tube called the vas deferens to the urethra. The sperm exits the urethra through the penis during intercourse. The prostate and vas deferens make the liquid part of the ejaculate, which is added to the sperm inside the urethra before ejaculation.

MEDICAL PROBLEMS OCCURRING IN THE GI, GU, AND REPRODUCTIVE SYSTEMS

Gastroenteritis

An inflammatory condition involving the stomach lining and/or intestines called gastroenteritis is one of the most common GI problems that OEC technicians will encounter. It is typically caused by a bacterial, viral, or parasitic infection. Patients with gastroenteritis present with cramping abdominal pain, bloating, nausea, vomiting, and diarrhea. Fever may or may not be present, depending on the cause of the inflammation. Pain may be localized to the upper quadrants or may be diffuse. Generally, gastroenteritis is not life threatening, and the symptoms resolve quickly. If vomiting and diarrhea symptoms persist for over 24 hours, the patient could become dehydrated. If blood appears in vomit or stool, the condition may be due to undiagnosed GI bleeding. Regardless of the cause, the patient should be encouraged to seek follow-up care at a medical facility.

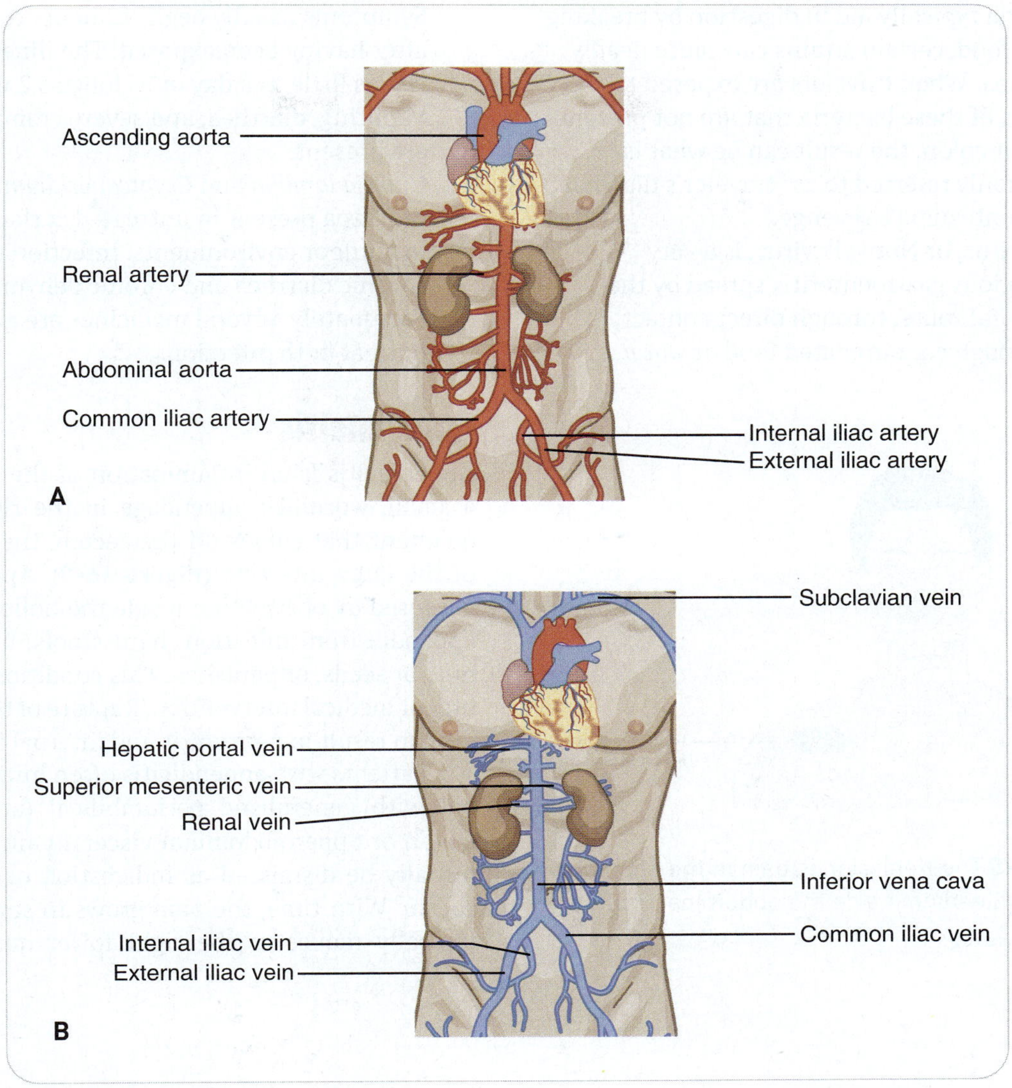

Figure 16-4 The arteries (**A**) and veins (**B**) of the abdomen.

Bacteria, Viruses, and Protozoa

Several bacteria, viruses, and protozoa warrant mention because they can also cause pain and diarrhea. Depending on the causative microorganism, some illnesses are self-limiting, lasting generally less than 24 hours, whereas others can be deadly, especially in the young, elderly, or infirm. Prominent among the bacterial, viral, and protozoan, agents of GI ailments are the following organisms:

- *Staphylococcus* bacteria grow everywhere in the environment. Unrefrigerated mayonnaise may be contaminated with certain strains of *Staphylococcus* (commonly referred to simply as "staph"). Acute diarrhea and vomiting occur for 1 to 2 days.
- *Salmonella* bacteria in undercooked poultry can cause the same problems as *Staphylococcus* food poisoning. Although salmonellosis is usually self-limiting, the illness lasts longer than food poisoning with *Staphylococcus*, lasting up to 3 or 4 days.
- *Escherichia coli* (*E. coli*) bacteria are normal residents in all human colons. Although these

bacteria typically aid in digestion by breaking down food, certain strains can cause deadly diarrhea. When travelers are exposed to strains of these bacteria that are not present in their colon, the result can be what is commonly referred to as "traveler's diarrhea" or "Montezuma's revenge."

- Norovirus, or Norwalk virus, is a very contagious gastroenteritis spread by the fecal/oral route, through direct contact, or through contaminated food or water. Symptoms usually begin 12 hours to 4 days after having been exposed. The illness may last as little as a day or as long as 2 weeks. Vomiting, diarrhea, and severe cramping are present.
- *Giardia lamblia* and *Cryptosporidium* are protozoa present in untreated surface water in outdoor environments. Infection causes chronic diarrhea and chronic dehydration. Fortunately, several medicines are available to treat both infections.

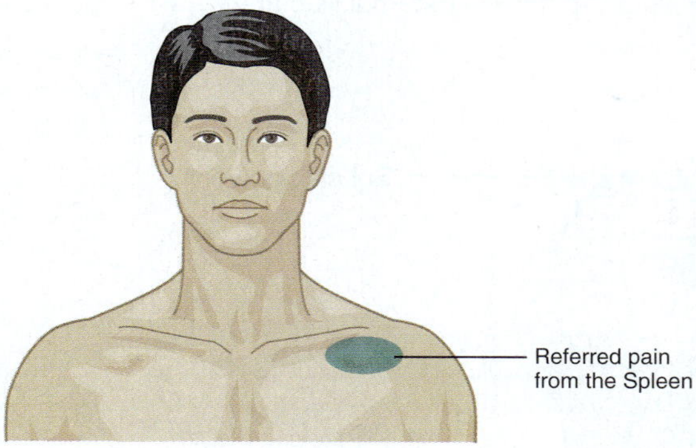

Figure 16-5 The Kehr sign is pain in the shoulder caused by bleeding inside the abdominal cavity.

Appendicitis

Appendicitis is an inflammation of the appendix, a small, wormlike appendage in the right lower quadrant that comes off the cecum, the first part of the large intestine (**Figure 16-8**). Appendicitis is caused by obstruction inside the hollow tubular appendix from infection, hard stools, undigested nuts or seeds, or parasites. This condition requires urgent medical intervention. Rupture of the appendix can result in peritonitis and internal bleeding.

Patients with appendicitis often initially present with generalized periumbilical (around the navel) or upper abdominal visceral pain that may initially be dismissed as indigestion or a muscle spasm. With time, the pain grows in severity and typically moves to the right lower quadrant as

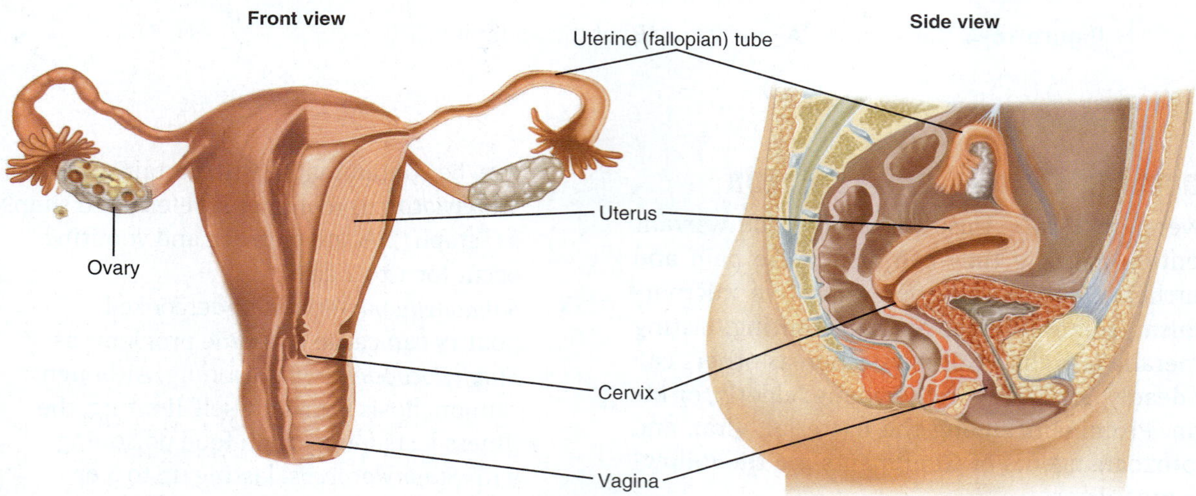

Figure 16-6 The female reproductive system.

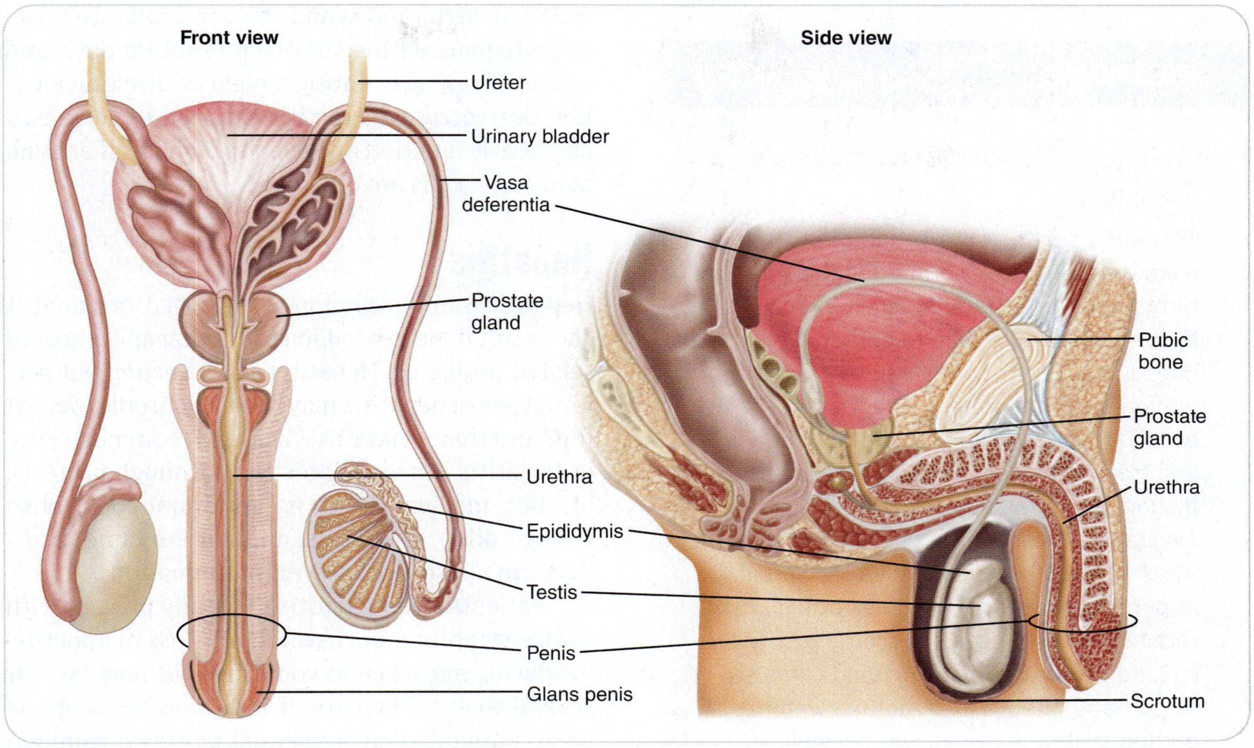

Figure 16-7 The male reproductive system.

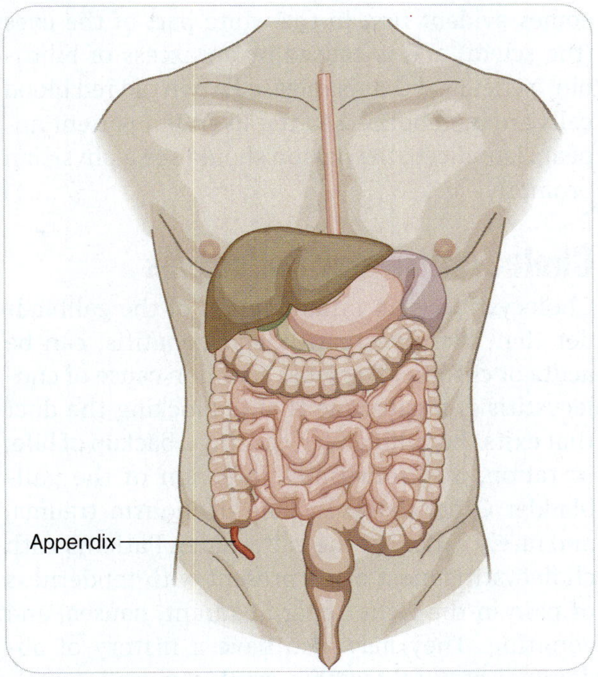

Figure 16-8 This is the location of the appendix in the abdominal cavity.

parietal pain. The pain is often accompanied by abdominal guarding, nausea, vomiting, and fever, but rarely diarrhea.

In 2018, several medical articles suggested a link between the appendix and Parkinson disease. People who had an appendectomy early in life had a lower risk of Parkinson disease.

Pancreatitis

Pancreatitis is a very painful condition in which the pancreas becomes inflamed. Pancreatic damage happens when the digestive enzymes are activated before they are released into the small intestine and begin attacking the pancreas (resulting in autodigestion, meaning the pancreas tries to break itself down). Pancreatitis can be mild or life threatening and can occur suddenly or become chronic, recurring throughout one's life. The number one cause of pancreatitis is excessive long-term alcohol consumption, followed by gallstones (which block the pancreatic duct), medications, trauma, viral infections (e.g., hepatitis), and pancreatic tumors or cancer.

KEY POINT

Traveler's Diarrhea (Montezuma's Revenge)

Traveler's diarrhea is a condition resulting from ingesting water or food that is contaminated by bacteria. It can be prevented by meticulous attention to personal cleanliness. Wash your hands before preparing and eating food, protect food from spoilage or flies that carry bacterial contamination, and treat drinking water either by filtering, boiling, or chemically decontaminating it. Avoidance of eating raw or undercooked meat and seafood, vegetables, or fruit is imperative. Peeling vegetables or fruit can reduce one's chances of becoming sick. Ice and water used to wash food can also be contaminated, so use bottled water or bottled beverages whenever possible.

Montezuma II was an Aztec ruler 500 years ago. Today travelers to Mexico who get diarrhea humorously name this condition after him.

Acute pancreatitis is a serious emergency that can result in death if not treated quickly. Patients present with a sudden onset of moderate-to-severe parietal pain in both upper quadrants, often with referred pain to the back or left shoulder. The pain is usually constant and worsens with movement, coughing, or deep inspiration, or if the patient is placed in a supine position. The abdomen is usually distended and is very tender to palpation. **Guarding** (spasm of abdominal wall muscles when palpated) is present. Nausea and vomiting are common and may be accompanied by a low-grade fever. The vital signs may be elevated. In severe cases, the patient may present with shock-like signs (e.g., rapid pulse and breathing, low blood pressure, sweating) from multiple-organ failure; this is considered a life-threatening situation.

Chronic pancreatitis is an ongoing condition that causes scar tissue to form within the pancreas, which results in decreased pancreatic function. Signs and symptoms are similar to those of acute pancreatitis, may be present for days, and often worsen after eating a meal or drinking alcohol. Untreated, pancreatitis can lead to decreased pancreatic function and even to diabetes if enough pancreatic cells are destroyed.

Hepatitis

Hepatitis is inflammation of the liver. Untreated, it can result in decreased liver function and a host of related problems. Hepatitis can be acute, but certain types of hepatitis may become chronic (persist for more than 6 months). The most common cause of hepatitis is a viral infection, although bacteria, alcohol, medications (e.g., acetaminophen, birth control pills), chemicals, and autoimmune disorders can also result in liver inflammation.

Patients with hepatitis generally present with flulike symptoms such as fatigue, loss of appetite, headache, nausea, and vomiting that may last for several weeks. The patient may have a low-grade fever. Parietal-type abdominal pain is a common finding and is typically located in the right upper quadrant and/or in the epigastrium, which is the area just below the sternum. The hallmark sign of hepatitis is **jaundice**, a dull yellowing of the skin and mucous membranes. Jaundice usually becomes evident first in the white part of the eyes (the sclera) and is caused by an excess of bilirubin, a chemical that is released when old red blood cells are metabolized by the liver. If a patient appears jaundiced, the person should see a physician promptly.

Cholecystitis and Gallstones

Cholecystitis is an inflammation of the gallbladder that, like pancreatitis and hepatitis, can be acute or chronic. The most common cause of cholecystitis is a gallstone that is blocking the duct that exits the gallbladder, causing a backup of bile, irritation, and sometimes infection of the gallbladder. Other causes include alcoholism, trauma, and rarely cancer of the gallbladder. Patients with cholecystitis most often present with tenderness or pain in the right upper quadrant, nausea, and vomiting. They may also have a history of abdominal pain following a meal, especially meals involving fatty or greasy foods. Patients may or may not have a fever and may occasionally exhibit jaundice.

Bladder Infections and Pyelonephritis

The urine in the bladder is sterile. When bacteria get into the bladder, cystitis or a **bladder infection** occurs. This infection results in painful urination, blood in the urine, fever, and sometimes severe abdominal/pelvic pain. Untreated, the bacteria can travel up the ureters and infect the entire urinary system.

Pyelonephritis is a bacterial infection involving one or both kidneys and the ureters, the tubes leading to the urinary bladder. The condition can occur acutely or be chronic. Over time, repeated infections can cause decreased kidney function, septic shock, and even death in rare cases. The young, elderly, and people with poor health are very susceptible to kidney infections.

Pyelonephritis is caused by a bacterial infection that typically begins in the urinary bladder. Bacteria enter the urinary tract through the urethra and travel up to the urinary bladder. Left untreated, the bacteria continue to grow and travel up the ureters to the kidneys. Due to the short length of the female urethra, women are more prone to urinary tract infections than are men. Complications of pyelonephritis can include infection throughout the body, known as sepsis, kidney stones, and kidney failure.

Patients with a kidney infection appear ill and present with a variety of signs and symptoms, including severe abdominal, flank, or back pain; fever; warm or hot skin; chills and shivering; nausea and vomiting; pain or increased frequency of urination; or abnormal urine (discolored urine, blood in the urine, foul-smelling urine).

Nephrolithiasis is the presence of kidney stones, which are formed when mineralized salts within the kidneys crystallize into small, hardened deposits that grow over time. Stones may travel out of the kidney and become trapped within one or both ureters. When this occurs, urine flow may become blocked, causing pressure, spasm, and intense pain within the affected ureter. Causes of kidney stones include increased levels of stone-forming chemicals within the kidney, dehydration, and congenital kidney defects. Certain medical conditions such as obesity and gout increase the risk of kidney stones.

Patients with a kidney stone that has become lodged within a ureter are usually in severe distress and are generally in excruciating pain. The pain may be localized in the abdomen or (more commonly) the flank, and it may radiate into the groin area. The pain is often described as "tearing" or "stabbing," and often the patient is unable to sit still due to the intensity of the pain. Other signs and symptoms include pain upon urination, blood in the urine, nausea, and vomiting.

Bowel Obstruction

Bowel obstruction is a serious medical emergency in which a segment of either the small intestine or the large intestine gets partially or completely blocked inside, so food is unable to be pushed along the intestinal path, causing a partial or complete blockage (**Table 16-1**). As a result, solids and/or liquids cannot move normally through the digestive tract.

Patients with bowel obstruction commonly present with a history of constipation, abdominal pain, guarding, profound nausea, and vomiting. Fever may or may not be present. The patient's abdomen may be bloated or grossly distended. Vital signs may initially be elevated, indicating severe distress, but can quickly fall, leading to shock and even death if the condition is not recognized and treated rapidly.

Perforated Bowel

A perforated bowel is a true emergency where a hole or tear develops in the intestinal wall,

Table 16-1 Causes of Bowel Obstruction
Previous abdominal surgery resulting in the development of scar tissue
Structural intestine problems such as twisting, herniation, and the presence of foreign bodies or impacted feces
Diet-related problems such as a low-fiber diet, failure to adequately chew solid foods, and insufficient water intake (dehydration)
Medications that may cause constipation such as oxycodone (a narcotic pain medication) and loperamide (an antidiarrhea medication)
Chronic medical conditions such as Crohn's disease or diverticulitis
Tumors that obstruct the lumen of the intestines

resulting in the contents leaking into the abdominal cavity. This condition can rapidly lead to peritonitis, sepsis, and death if not rapidly corrected by surgery. The causes of perforated bowel include bowel obstruction, excess stomach acid, ulcerative disease, trauma, cancer of the bowel, a ruptured appendix, and chronic weakness of the intestinal wall. Patients with a perforated bowel present with intense, visceral abdominal pain that worsens with movement or deep inspiration and is accompanied by guarding, high fever, severe nausea, and intense vomiting.

Inflammatory Conditions of the Stomach, Esophagus, and Upper Small Intestine

Gastritis, or inflammation of the stomach, can occur due to many reasons, including alcohol use, chronic vomiting, use of certain medications, and infections. It causes "heartburn"-type symptoms. The stomach makes hydrochloric acid to help digest food. When too much acid is made, the wall of the stomach becomes inflamed, a condition commonly referred to as indigestion.

Esophagitis is caused by gastro-esophageal reflux disease (GERD), a condition in which stomach contents mixed with hydrochloric acid flow back into the esophagus. A hiatal hernia is usually the cause. This hernia allows the sphincter or valve at the bottom of the esophagus to malfunction. Normally this valve allows food into the stomach, but not back up into the esophagus. Food and acid reflux into the bottom of the esophagus, damaging this tube that empties into the stomach.

Peptic ulcer disease is a condition in which excess stomach acid creates a defect of the lining of the esophagus, stomach, or duodenum (the first section of the small intestine) (**Figure 16-9**). The most common causes of peptic ulcers are infection with the bacterium *Helicobacter pylori* and long-term use of aspirin and nonsteroidal anti-inflammatory drugs (NSAIDs; e.g., Advil, Aleve). Factors that can cause excessive acid production in the stomach include smoking and consumption of fatty foods, caffeine, and alcohol. Although stress and spicy foods do not cause peptic ulcers, they can make symptoms worse.

Patients with inflammation of the upper GI tract may present with chest pain, upper abdominal pain, nausea, or a complaint of a sour taste in the mouth. The heartburn pain is often described as "gnawing." At times, it may be difficult to differentiate pain from these conditions from pain resulting from acute heart disease. OEC technicians should assume that the pain is of a serious nature until proven otherwise.

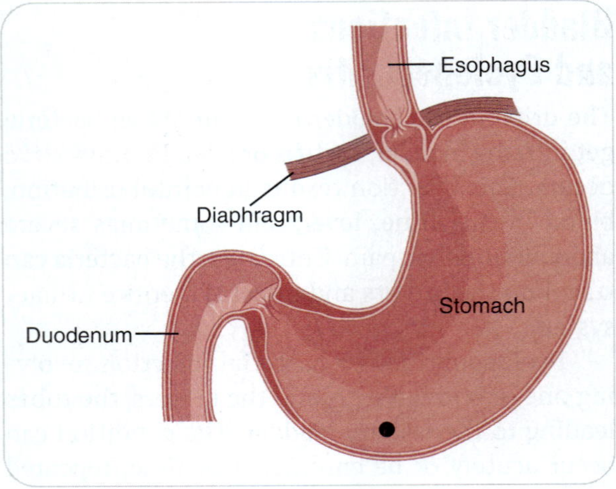

Figure 16-9 Peptic ulcer disease occurs when excess stomach acid penetrates the wall of the stomach, duodenum, or esophagus. Note the ulcer in the stomach, represented by the black dot.

In severe cases of inflammation of the upper GI tract, erosions (damage to the inside wall of the GI tract) can penetrate a blood vessel within the upper GI tract, causing a life-threatening hemorrhage known as a GI bleed. GI bleeding, which can occur in any part of the GI tract, can be caused by use of certain medications (e.g., aspirin), alcohol consumption, tears within the esophagus or intestines, ulcers, or ruptured blood vessels.

Upper GI bleeding can present as blood-tinged vomit, known as **hematemesis**. Acute bleeding is bright red, whereas older blood has a "coffee grounds" appearance. OEC technicians should recommend EMS transfer to hospital care for any patient who presents with blood or "coffee grounds" in the vomit, or significant bright red blood in stools or black stools, called **melena**.

Abdominal Aortic Aneurysm

Over time, the abdominal aorta's wall can become weakened and develop a bulge or ballooning, known as an aneurysm. Chronic, uncontrolled high blood pressure, arteriosclerosis, and genetic factors are usual causes. Rupture of an aneurysm is usually fatal due to massive blood loss. If the aneurysm is leaking slowly, it may be possible to save the patient.

Patients with an abdominal aortic aneurysm typically present in shock and may complain of flank, lower back, or abdominal pain, weakness, and/or dizziness. The medical history often includes recent fainting spells, smoking, and alcoholism. Patients with abdominal aortic aneurysm often have unequal femoral pulses.

Conditions of the Reproductive System

Female Reproductive Organ Conditions

The abdominal and pelvic cavities contain the structures of the female reproductive system, which, when affected by disease, can cause signs and symptoms similar to those of acute abdomen (discussed in the next section). Common conditions related to obstetrics and gynecology are ectopic pregnancy, ovarian cysts, bladder infections, and pelvic inflammatory disease.

Following fertilization of an egg, which normally occurs in the fallopian tube, the egg travels down the tube and implants into the uterine wall. If the egg implants in the fallopian tube or somewhere outside the uterus, an **ectopic pregnancy** occurs. The fetus (developing baby) cannot grow in the small fallopian tube. As the fetus grows in this tube, severe pain occurs as the tube dilates. Bleeding usually occurs and can be massive.

An **ovarian cyst** is fluid-filled sac or pocket in an ovary or on its surface. Eggs (ova), which develop and mature in the ovaries, are released in monthly cycles during the childbearing years. Many women have ovarian cysts at some time. Most ovarian cysts present little or no discomfort and are harmless, but some may cause problems such as rupture, bleeding, or pain. The majority disappear without treatment within a few months. However, some ovarian cysts, especially those that have ruptured, can cause serious symptoms, similar to those of an acute abdomen. Pelvic pain, fullness in the abdomen, and bloating are common symptoms. If fever, vomiting, or severe pain occur, rapid medical follow-up is needed. When internal bleeding occurs from an ovarian cyst, shock can occur. Moreover, surgery may be required in certain situations to remove the cyst(s).

Pelvic inflammatory disease is an infection of the organs of a woman's reproductive system. The infection can occur in the uterus, ovaries, fallopian tubes, and cervix. It is usually caused by a sexually transmitted infection, such as chlamydia or gonorrhea, and is treated with antibiotics. Other infections that are not sexually transmitted can also cause pelvic inflammatory disease. A woman can present with severe abdominal pain, but usually this condition is painless. When severe, pelvic inflammatory disease might cause fever, chills, severe lower abdominal or pelvic pain, and bowel discomfort (**Table 16-2**).

Male Reproductive Organ Conditions

Trauma to the testicles is very painful and can cause severe problems with swelling, bleeding into the scrotum, rupture of the testicle, and later infection inside the scrotum. Severe trauma usually requires follow-up with a physician, especially if swelling occurs.

Testicular torsion is a condition in which a testicle rotates, twisting the spermatic cord and artery that brings blood to the testicle. The reduced blood flow causes sudden and often severe pain and swelling. Testicular torsion is most common between the ages of 12 and 18 years but can occur at any age. It usually requires emergency surgery. If treated quickly, the testicle can usually be saved. When blood flow has been cut off for too long, a testicle may be so damaged that it may have to be removed.

The Acute Abdomen

Sudden, severe pain in the abdomen is referred to as an **acute abdomen** and encompasses many

Table 16-2 Signs and Symptoms of Pelvic Inflammatory Disease

- Pain in a woman's lower abdomen and pelvis
- Heavy vaginal discharge with an unpleasant odor
- Abnormal uterine bleeding, especially during or after intercourse, or between menstrual cycles
- Pain or bleeding during intercourse
- Fever, sometimes with chills
- Painful or difficult urination

different medical problems that occur in the abdominal or pelvic cavities (**Table 16-3**). Rapid recognition of this condition is important because advanced medical care is urgently needed. Although many intra-abdominal conditions can result in an acute abdomen, correctly identifying the source of the problem is often difficult. Without advanced testing, physicians accurately diagnose the exact cause of acute abdomen only 50% of the time. It is more important for OEC technicians to recognize that a patient is very ill and needs to go to the hospital than to pinpoint the source of the problem.

The hallmark of acute abdomen is severe pain from inflammation of the peritoneum, known as **peritonitis**. The **peritoneum** is a thin membrane that lines the abdominal cavity. When contacted by blood or contaminants (e.g., gastric contents, urine, feces), nerve endings become irritated, resulting in pain. Patients with an acute abdomen often have guarding, making the abdominal wall rigid and hard.

Table 16-3 Causes of Acute Abdominal Pain

- Abdominal aortic aneurysm
- Appendicitis
- Bleeding or perforated ulcer
- Bowel obstruction
- Ectopic pregnancy
- Gastritis and GI bleeding
- Gastroenteritis
- Ovarian cyst rupture
- Pancreatitis

KEY POINT

Myocardial Infarction Versus Acute Abdomen

A myocardial infarction can present as acute abdominal pain.

KEY POINT

Peritonitis

When an abdominal hollow organ leaks anything, especially bacteria, due to either a rupture or a laceration during trauma, the result is peritonitis, or inflammation of the lining of the abdominal cavity (the peritoneum). Peritonitis can cause intense abdominal pain, nausea, vomiting, fever, and shock.

CASE Update

On examination of the patient, you notice that she is pale, is sweating, and feels warm to the touch. She relates that her pain was originally near her navel but has now "moved down and to the right." Her last menstrual period was 2 months ago. Examination of the abdomen reveals severe tenderness in the right lower quadrant. She tells you that every bump in the road on the way to the ski hill felt like she was "being stabbed in my gut." The patient's heart rate is 116 beats per minute, blood pressure is 132/88 mm Hg, and respirations are 20 breaths per minute and shallow.

What do you think is wrong with the patient?

PATIENT ASSESSMENT FOR GI, GU, AND REPRODUCTIVE SYSTEM EMERGENCIES

After ensuring that the scene is safe, begin the assessment process by looking for excessive bleeding, and examining the patient's ABCDs (airway, breathing, circulation, and disability) and vital signs. Obtain a thorough medical history and perform a physical exam. OEC technicians should ask patients about their medical history and pain symptoms using the mnemonics SAMPLE (signs and symptoms, allergies, medications, past medical history, last oral intake, events leading up to the problem) and OPQRST (onset, provocation, quality, radiation, severity, and time).

Attempt to determine if pain is constant or intermittent, how long the pain has been present, and whether the pain has moved since its initial onset. Ask the patient about any factors that aggravate or relieve the condition, such as motion, coughing, breathing, belching, or urination. Finally, determine whether any associated signs and symptoms, such as nausea, vomiting, diarrhea, bloody stool, fever, or loss of appetite, are present (**Table 16-4**).

Due to the number and complexity of GI, GU, and reproductive organs, there are many possible causes of acute abdominal and pelvic problems beyond those described in this chapter. As previously indicated, this wide range of possibilities can make assessment of the abdomen and the pelvic region extremely difficult.

Your understanding of the various abdominal problems and use of available information, including vital signs, presentation of the medical problem, and findings such as blood in the vomit or stool, will help you determine the status of the problem. If there is a serious concern, such as the patient going into shock, immediate transport with ALS is needed.

Because emergent conditions involving the GI, GU, and reproductive systems rarely present without pain, it is important to examine patients to identify the nature and extent of their pain. Again, the role of OEC technicians is not to diagnose the underlying cause but to recognize the signs and symptoms associated with an emergent condition and initiate lifesaving care if needed.

Table 16-4 Signs and Symptoms of Abdominal Problems

Signs and Symptoms	Description
Pain and tenderness	Pain that is sharp, dull, localized, generalized, or rigid, and pain referred to another location
Nausea and vomiting	Stomach upset with regurgitation
Anorexia	Lack of desire to eat
Fever	Increased core body temperature
Jaundice	Yellow skin and mucous membranes
Tachycardia	Rapid heart rate
Hypotension	Low blood pressure
Hematemesis	Blood in the vomit; may be red or black and resemble coffee grounds
Hematochezia	Bright red stools indicating recent bleeding in the lower GI tract
Melena	Black, tarry stools indicating bleeding in the upper GI tract
Hematuria	Blood in the urine

Nausea and Vomiting

When the muscles in the wall of the stomach violently contract, stomach contents (partially digested food and digestive acid) are sent up the esophagus and out the mouth. Vomiting is usually preceded by a feeling of impending vomiting, more commonly referred to as nausea. Common causes of nausea and vomiting include motion sickness, altitude, food poisoning, viral or bacterial infections, irritating drugs or chemicals (e.g., aspirin, alcohol), ulcers, tumors, kidney stones, bowel obstruction, and abdominal trauma.

Vomiting that is excessive or occurs over time without fluid replacement can cause a host of other problems, most notably dehydration. Vomiting that occurs in an unresponsive patient is especially serious if the vomit is aspirated into the trachea and lungs. Aspiration, where foreign material gets into the lungs, can lead to a lung infection, a potentially life-threatening condition. Therefore, quickly clean or suction vomit out of the upper airway of an unresponsive patient to prevent aspiration pneumonia. Place unresponsive patients in the recovery position.

Colic

Colic is intermittent, severe abdominal pain caused by the obstruction and distention of a hollow organ. It is caused when strong muscular contractions within the wall of a hollow organ such as the gallbladder, bowel, or ureter are unsuccessful in forcing the organ's contents past the obstruction. Gallstones, tumors, a twisted bowel, trapped gas or a mass of hard stool within the bowel, and kidney stones are all common sources of colic. Colicky bowel pain is generally first experienced around the navel but can be located anywhere within the abdominal and pelvic cavities and can move over time. When a ureter is blocked by a kidney stone, colicky pain occurs in the flank and radiates to the groin.

Diarrhea and Bloody Stool

Diarrhea is defined as the passage of frequent, liquid stools. It is caused by viruses, bacteria, protozoa, chemicals, and other gastric irritants, and by medical conditions such as bowel disease, intestinal tumors, and food allergies. Untreated, some of these conditions can become chronic. Like vomiting, excessive or prolonged diarrhea can lead to profound dehydration.

In outdoor environments, most cases of acute diarrhea are caused by contaminated water or food. In urban settings, modern sanitation has largely eliminated most causes of diarrhea. However, bowel infections with certain viruses such as adenovirus, norovirus, and rotavirus commonly cause diarrhea in urban population centers and on cruise ships.

GI bleeding can also present as hematochezia, which are bright red stools. Stool that contains bright red blood typically indicates that recent bleeding is occurring within the *lower* GI tract, most commonly from a hemorrhoid or from the colon. Hematochezia could also result from a serious upper GI bleed with rapid evacuation of the stool. Tarry, black, foul-smelling stools, or melena, indicate bleeding that originates within the *upper* GI tract. Slow bleeding from the upper GI tract takes time to pass into the colon. As a result the digested blood becomes black. People who take chronic oral iron supplements can have stools that resemble melena.

Constipation

Constipation is the inability to excrete feces, a condition that nearly everyone suffers occasionally. Manifested by unusually large, hard, and dry stools that are passed infrequently, constipation can occur due to physical inactivity, dehydration, lack of dietary fiber, or a more urgent condition such as a tumor blocking the intestinal canal. Outdoor enthusiasts who do not eat enough fiber or drink enough water over several days are especially vulnerable to constipation. Obstipation, or chronic constipation, can sometimes cause a bowel obstruction.

PHYSICAL EXAM OF THE ABDOMEN

Begin your physical examination of patients with acute abdominal or pelvic pain by calming the patients to ease their anxiety. Ask permission to examine the abdomen and explain what you are going to do before starting any examination. Place the patient into a position of comfort: a supine position with the knees slightly flexed allows the abdominal and pelvic muscles to relax. If possible, move the patient to a warm location, as this will make the exam much easier. Make sure your hands are warm when conducting this exam.

Examination of the abdomen and pelvic region in indoor settings is typically a two-step process involving inspection and palpation. During the inspection step, the area is exposed and observed for clinical signs such as trauma, distention, bulging, or discoloration. Note whether the patient is motionless or is unable to sit still, as well as how the abdominal wall moves with the patient's respirations. If pain is present, ask the patient to use one finger to point to the site at which the pain is most intense (**Figure 16-10**). If the pain is diffuse, ask the patient to use a finger to draw a circle indicating the boundaries of the pain.

The second step, palpation of the abdomen, is a systematic process that involves physically compressing each of the four quadrants to determine the presence or absence of pain, masses, tensing, guarding, or rigidity (**Figure 16-11**). OEC technicians should not be afraid to palpate the abdomen. Before palpating the abdomen, OEC technicians should ensure that their hands are warm, because placing cold hands on the abdomen of unsuspecting patients can cause the patients to tense their abdominal muscles, which can complicate the exam process.

Begin palpating the abdomen in the quadrant farthest away from the site of the pain; examine the painful quadrant last. Place one hand atop the other and gently place them on the patient's abdomen. Rest your hands in this position for a moment to allow the patient to become comfortable. Then, moving slowly, apply firm but gentle downward pressure; note the patient's response and whether the abdominal muscles suddenly tense in response. Slowly release the pressure, gently gliding your hands from one quadrant to the next, and then repeat the process for each quadrant. Note any evidence of tenderness upon examination. Palpate gently just above the pubic bone in the midline, where the bladder is located. Also inspect and palpate the right and left flank areas individually, noting any discoloration or tenderness.

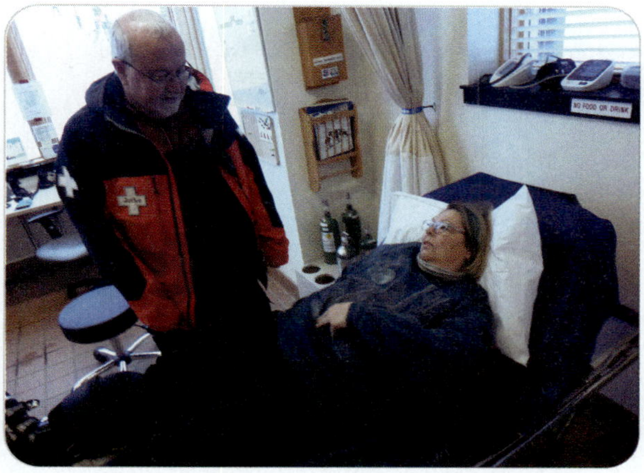

Figure 16-10 Ask the patient to point to the area of pain, which helps the OEC technician pinpoint the area of concern.

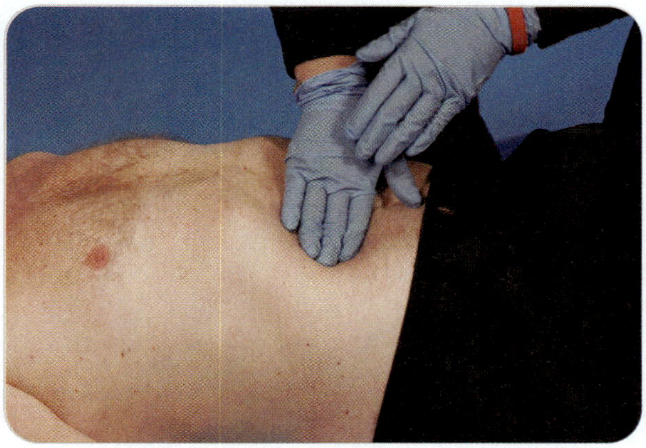

Figure 16-11 OEC technician palpating the abdomen.

MANAGEMENT OF GI, GU, AND REPRODUCTIVE SYSTEM EMERGENCIES

The treatment of patients with an abdominal problem in outdoor settings generally involves supportive care. Many serious conditions require an in-depth evaluation by a physician, and surgical correction and/or long-term care are often required. Still, OEC technicians can do many things to improve a patient's overall comfort and the subsequent outcome. The OEC technician needs to determine if the problem is serious and requires further care, not what the specific abdominal problem is.

Initial treatment includes assessing and correcting any problems involving excessive bleeding and the ABCDs. If possible, move the patient to a location that has a comfortable temperature. If outdoors, keep patients warm by using jackets or blankets as needed. During the physical exam of the abdomen, place the person in a position of comfort. For most patients, this is either a supine

KEY POINT

Shock

If shock exists, lifesaving care should be initiated while simultaneously referring the patient to a higher level of care with ALS.

position with the knees slightly flexed or a seated position with the head raised 45 to 60 degrees. Place a patient who is vomiting repeatedly in the recovery position. Patients may be restless, so be empathetic to their discomfort and help them remain calm.

Provide supplemental oxygen as needed for serious problems such as shock, typically using a nonrebreather mask and pulse oximeter. Anticipate vomiting and be ready to clear the airway by removing the oxygen mask and turning the patient onto his or her side. If the patient continues to vomit, consider placing the patient on a nasal cannula. Suction the airway as needed to prevent aspiration. Despite their requests, do not give patients anything to eat or drink because some abdominal and pelvic conditions require surgical intervention. The presence of food or liquids in the stomach can worsen some problems, can cause the patient to vomit, and can make surgery, when needed, more dangerous.

Continue to monitor the patient's vital signs, because they can change rapidly. Anticipate shock and treat accordingly if the patient exhibits the characteristic clinical signs (e.g., fast pulse, rapid breathing, low blood pressure). With few exceptions, patients with significant abdominal or pelvic pain require further evaluation. Transfer these patients to a higher level of care or encourage them to seek physician evaluation and definitive treatment. When the problem is severe, transfer by ambulance using ALS if available.

CASE Outcome

As you examine the patient and listen to her story, you become concerned that the patient may have an acute abdomen, possibly appendicitis, ectopic pregnancy, or ruptured ovarian cyst. You place the patient on oxygen, keep her comfortable, and have her transported to the hospital. A week later, the patient's sister comes to the patrol room to thank you and the other patrollers for taking such great care of her sister. She reports that she had surgery for acute appendicitis and is now doing well. It was important that you recognized she had a serious problem, not what the exact problem was.

CHAPTER REVIEW

In Summary

- The abdominal and pelvic cavities contain solid and hollow organs, reproductive organs, major blood vessels, and nerves.
- The abdomen can be divided into four quadrants: the right upper, left upper, right lower, and left lower.
- Patients with abdominal or pelvic pain may not present until their signs and symptoms are unbearable.
- Abdominal pain may be the first indication of a life-threatening emergency.
- Abdominal assessment includes an inspection and examination of all four abdominal quadrants. All patients with abdominal pain should be taken seriously and either referred to a physician or transported to a hospital.
- An understanding of the various abdominal problems and use of available assessment information will enable the OEC technician to determine the seriousness of the patient's problem and the need for immediate transport with ALS.
- Do not give a patient complaining of abdominal pain anything by mouth.
- A heart attack can present as abdominal pain.
- Acute abdominal pain may be a symptom of intra-abdominal trauma, such as a ruptured spleen or a kidney injury.
- Conditions relating to the female reproductive organs can mimic GI or GU pathology, since these organs are inside the pelvic cavity. Common conditions related to obstetrics and gynecology are ectopic pregnancy, ovarian cysts, bladder infections, and pelvic inflammatory disease.

Key Terms

Acute abdomen A condition of sudden onset of pain within the abdomen, usually indicating peritonitis; immediate medical or surgical treatment is necessary.

Bladder infection A condition in which bacteria enter the bladder, potentially causing a serious infection with fever and chills.

Ectopic pregnancy A condition in which the fertilized egg attaches outside of the uterus.

Guarding An involuntary action in which the abdomen becomes rigid upon examination.

Hematemesis Vomit that contains blood in it.

Jaundice A dull, yellow color of the skin, whites of the eyes, and mucous membranes caused by an excess of bilirubin; usually indicates liver disease.

Melana Stools that appear black and tarry due to digested blood in the bowel.

Ovarian cyst A fluid-filled sac or pocket in an ovary or on its surface.

Pancreatitis A painful condition in which the pancreas becomes inflamed.

Pelvic inflammatory disease An infection of the organs of a women's reproductive system.

Peritoneum A membrane that covers the organs of the abdomen and also lines the inner wall of the abdominal cavity.

Peritonitis Inflammation of the peritoneum of the abdominal cavity, typically caused by leakage of hollow organ contents; it is usually worse if caused by bacteria from inside the intestines.

Referred pain Pain that originates in one part of the body but is felt in another part of the body.

Chapter Questions

1. Your patient is a 25-year-old female with severe abdominal and pelvic pain. The most likely cause of the pain is:
   a. abdominal aortic aneurysm.
   b. ovarian cysts.
   c. kidney stones.
   d. pancreatitis.

2. A common GI problem is gastroenteritis, which involves inflammation of the stomach lining and intestines. This condition is typically caused by:
   a. a bacterial, viral, or parasitic infection.
   b. the crystallization of mineralized salts in the kidney.
   c. a fertilized egg implanting in the fallopian tube.
   d. bowel obstruction.
3. Your patient complains of blood in his stool. This is a sign of bleeding that is occurring in the:
   a. GI system.
   b. GU system.
   c. reproductive system.
   d. endocrine system.
4. When assessing the vital signs of a patient suffering from an abdominal problem who has tarry stools, you might expect to note:
   a. tachycardia and hypotension.
   b. bradycardia and hypertension.
   c. tachycardia and hypertension.
   d. bradycardia and hypotension.
5. When assessing a patient with abdominal pain in the right upper quadrant, you should begin palpating the abdomen in the:
   a. right upper quadrant.
   b. left upper quadrant.
   c. right lower quadrant.
   d. left lower quadrant.
6. When preparing to conduct a physical exam of a patient with an acute abdomen, it is helpful to:
   a. explain what you will be doing before you start.
   b. warm your hands.
   c. place the patient in a position of comfort.
   d. All of the above
7. Your patient is complaining of severe abdominal pain and has vomited several times. Your assessment does not reveal any conditions other than an acute abdomen. The best way to position this patient is:
   a. supine.
   b. prone.
   c. in the recovery position.
   d. seated.
8. Management of a patient with an acute abdomen includes:
   a. transferring the patient to definitive care.
   b. providing water for the patient to drink.
   c. providing an energy bar to the patient.
   d. All the above
9. For a woman with severe abdominal pain, vomiting of blood, tachycardia, and hypotension, you should:
   a. make every attempt to determine the cause of the problem.
   b. watch the patient in the aid room for a short time to see if she gets better.
   c. arrange rapid transfer with ALS.
   d. take her temperature to see if she has a fever.

Answers: 1. b, Objective 16-1, p. 347; 2. a, Objective 16-1, p. 340; 3. a, Objective 16-3, p. 346; 4. a, Objective 16-5, p. 349; 5. d, Objective 16-5, p. 351; 6. d, Objective 16-5, p. 350; 7. c, Objective 16-6, p. 348; 8. a, Objective 16-6, p. 352; 9. c, Objective 16-4, p. 352

CHAPTER 17

CHILDBIRTH, OBSTETRIC EMERGENCIES, AND SEXUAL ASSAULT

OBJECTIVES

Upon completion of this chapter, the OEC technician will be able to:

17-1 Explain the normal reproductive cycle of a woman.

17-2 List the normal changes in vital signs a woman experiences during pregnancy.

17-3 Explain how to take a blood pressure in a pregnant woman.

17-4 Describe what happens to the mother and fetus during shock.

17-5 Describe the three trimesters of a normal pregnancy.

17-6 Describe possible complications of pregnancy.

17-7 Demonstrate how to examine a female patient with abdominal or pelvic pain.

17-8 Describe the special considerations that are needed when using spinal motion restriction for a pregnant woman.

17-9 Describe the management of a pregnant patient with abdominal trauma.

17-10 Describe and demonstrate the process of assisting a woman during a delivery.

17-11 Explain what to do when there is a possible sexual assault of a woman.

17-12 Describe the basic care for a newborn.

KEY TERMS

Abruptio placentae, p. 361
Eclampsia, p. 362
Ectopic pregnancy, p. 360
Gestational period, p. 358
Meconium, p. 366
Menstruation, p. 358
Miscarriage, p. 361
Placenta previa, p. 361
Preeclampsia, p. 362
Reproductive age, p. 358

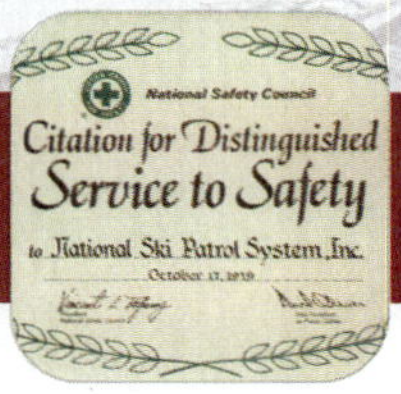

HISTORICAL TIMELINE **1979.** NSP is awarded the National Safety Council's Distinguished Service to Safety Award.

CHAPTER OVERVIEW

A woman's anatomy enables reproduction and the continuation of humanity. Fertilization of an egg inside a woman results in pregnancy. Following fertilization, a fetus grows inside a woman's uterus for approximately 9 months, when delivery of a newborn baby occurs. During pregnancy, many changes happen to a woman's body that a ski or bike patroller must understand when caring for the pregnant woman.

Many athletic women continue to exercise and enjoy outdoor activities during the first several months of pregnancy. Some women participating in sports may not even know they are pregnant. Pregnant women nearing childbirth may stay in the lodge while their family is out skiing or biking (**Figure 17-1**). As an OEC technician, you may be called upon to care for a pregnant woman in a wide range of scenarios, from a medical or traumatic emergency to delivery of a baby.

For thousands of years, women have been delivering babies without the assistance of medical personnel. Women who have a normal, uncomplicated childbirth need very little help. However, even in an uncomplicated childbirth, the right assistance can enhance safety and comfort for the mother and child. Helping the mother when complications arise can prove lifesaving for the woman, the newborn, or both. Thus, it is important for OEC technicians to understand key concepts relating to pregnancy, labor, and delivery.

Some women have medical conditions while pregnant such as high blood pressure or diabetes (which during pregnancy is called gestational diabetes). Trauma can potentially result in the injury or death of two patients—the mother and the fetus. The goals for management of obstetric emergencies and pregnancy complications are the rapid identification of a potentially serious or life-threatening condition followed by immediate prehospital care and evacuation to a medical center.

ANATOMY AND PHYSIOLOGY

The woman's reproductive system is located within the abdominal and pelvic cavities. In pregnancy, the woman's uterus expands upwards and is no longer protected by the pelvic bone. The major internal structures of the female reproductive system are the ovaries, fallopian tubes, uterus, and vagina (**Figure 17-2**).

Ovaries

An ovary is one of two solid reproductive organs located in the right and left lower quadrants. The ovaries contain the eggs, called ova, and produce the female hormones progesterone and estrogen.

Fallopian Tubes

The fallopian tubes are two hollow structures that begin in the right and left lower quadrants, near

CASE Presentation

Late one afternoon, you are called to assist a woman who is having medical problems in a second-floor condo just off a ski slope. Upon arrival, you knock on the door and a frantic woman's voice inside says come in. In the bathroom you find a 29-year-old woman who is standing in front of the sink, half-dressed, and a lot of blood on the floor. She is screaming, complaining of severe abdominal pain, and saying she has never bled this much in her life. She is alone and says her husband and two children went skiing while she stayed behind to fix dinner. The toilet bowel is full of blood clots. As you assess the patient, you notice her radial pulse is quite weak and seems faster than normal.

What should you do?

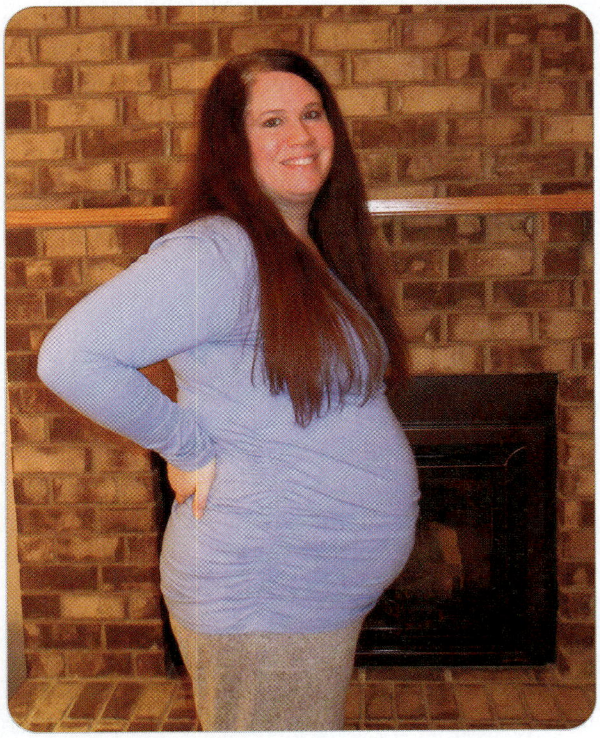

Figure 17-1 Remember that when caring for a pregnant woman, you are taking care of two patients.

the ovaries, extend downward into the pelvic cavity, and connect onto either side of the uterus. An ovum is typically fertilized inside a fallopian tube, which connects the ovary to the uterus.

Uterus

The fertilized egg develops into a fetus inside this hollow muscular organ. The uterus is about 3 inches in length in a nonpregnant female and is supported in the pelvic cavity (behind the urinary bladder and in front of the rectum) by various ligaments. The large, upper, rounded end of the pear-shaped uterus is known as the fundus; the elongated lower portion, or cervix, ends in an opening known as the os. The uterus is normally palpable only during pregnancy. At full term during pregnancy, the uterus enlarges to the size of a watermelon.

Vagina

The vagina is a hollow, muscular tube extending from the uterus to an exterior opening, the vulva. It serves as a passageway for menstrual flow and is a part of the birth canal. This part of the woman's anatomy facilitates intercourse.

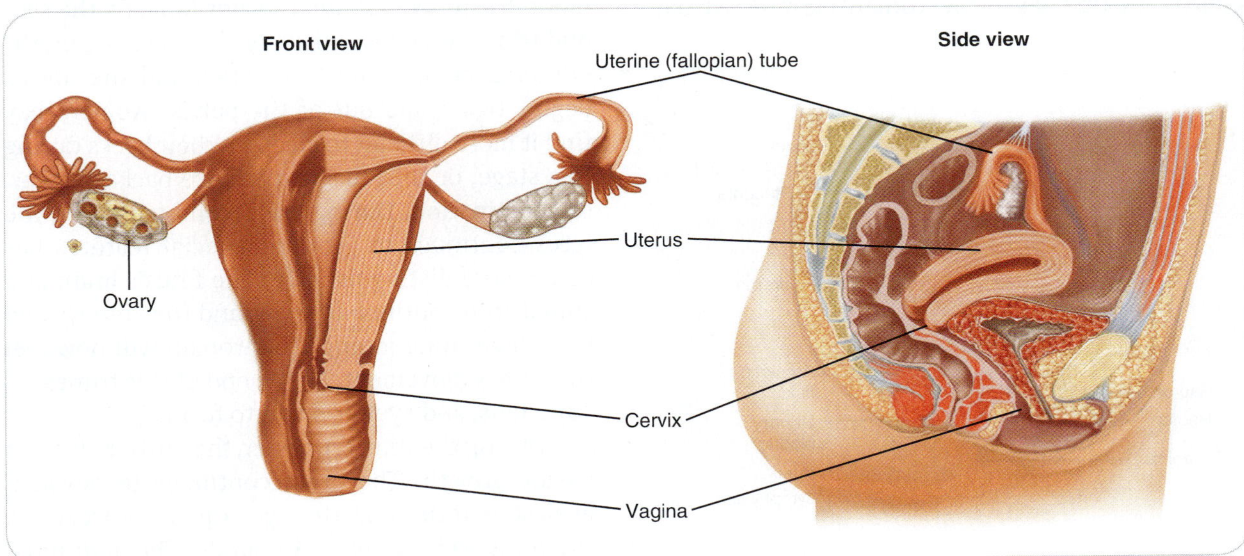

Figure 17-2 The female reproductive system.

Perineum

The perineum is the outer soft tissue in a female extending from the vaginal opening to the anus. The perineal area may be torn during childbirth.

The Reproductive Cycle

This cycle occurs about once every 28 days during a woman's reproductive years. The female reproductive cycle begins with ovulation, when an ovum or egg is released from an ovary. The ovum travels through a fallopian tube to the uterus. For pregnancy to occur, the ovum must be fertilized by a sperm while in the fallopian tube. The fertilized ovum then continues into the uterus, which has become thicker and richer in blood vessels because of hormones (**Figure 17-3**). The fertilized egg implants and grows in the lining of the uterus. If not fertilized, the ovum dies, and the lining of the uterus breaks down and is expelled through the vagina in the form of **menstruation**, or a menstrual period, which normally lasts for 5 to 7 days. **Reproductive age** is approximately ages 12 to 49 years.

Following fertilization of an ovum by a sperm, an embryo is formed. The embryo becomes a fetus from the beginning of the 9th week of pregnancy until delivery. In humans, birth normally occurs between 37 to 42 weeks of pregnancy.

The average **gestational period** in humans is 280 days, or 40 weeks. The gestational period begins on the first day of the woman's last menstrual period. The gestational period is divided into three trimesters of 12 weeks each. Delivery before 37 weeks is considered "preterm" or premature and can result in a wide spectrum of problems for the infant, most of which result from immature lungs that cannot absorb oxygen. In general, an infant born before the third trimester of pregnancy has a very low chance of survival.

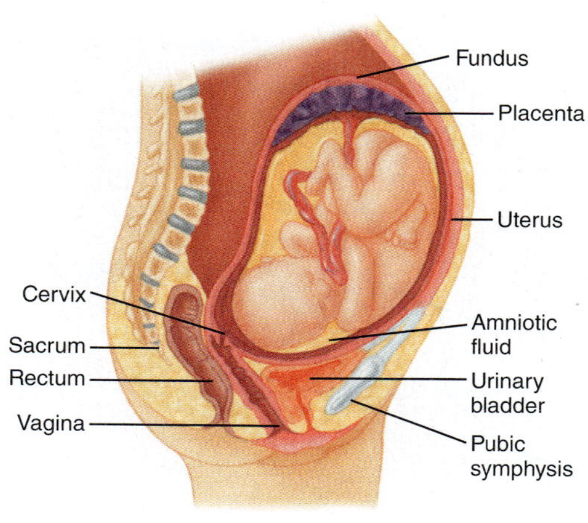

Figure 17-3 The structures within a woman during a full-term pregnancy.

Changes to the Mother and Development of the Fetus in the Uterus

As the fetus develops, a woman's body changes during pregnancy. During the first trimester, a pregnant woman may notice swelling of her breasts, fatigue, nausea, and the need to urinate frequently. Vomiting is common, especially in the morning, and when severe or protracted it may prompt the woman to seek medical attention.

The fetus develops within the mother's uterus inside a bag-like amniotic sac filled with up to a liter of clear amniotic fluid. This fluid helps to insulate, cushion, and protect the developing baby. Nourishment is provided from the mother from a vascular placenta, which adheres to the uterine wall and is connected to the baby by the umbilical cord.

By the end of the 12th week, the baby's vital organs have developed, its bones start developing, and the limbs become more pronounced. At this point, the fetus is about 4 inches long. By the second trimester, nausea usually resolves. The mother's breasts continue to enlarge, and the uterus begins to expand out of the pelvis. Women may find it more difficult to sleep on their backs during this stage, or they may experience backache, gas, or constipation. During the second trimester, the fetus continues to grow, and facial features become more distinguishable. The fetus's brain and spinal cord continue to grow, and the kidneys and liver begin functioning. The woman will now feel the baby's movement. By the end of this trimester, hair, nails, and eyelids begin to form.

During the third trimester, the fetus maintains steady growth. The brain continues to develop, eyelashes form, and the eyes open. By week 30, the fetus weighs about 3 pounds. The additional weight gain can make a pregnant woman feel off balance, creating a risk for falls, especially during outdoor recreational activities. Some swelling of the feet and hands is common, as are indigestion, fatigue, difficulty sleeping, and difficulty breathing (due to the growing uterus expanding high into the abdomen). By the end of the third trimester, the fetus usually rotates within the uterus to a head-down position in preparation for delivery (**Figure 17-4**).

Early in pregnancy, the uterus and developing fetus are protected by the pelvic bones and are not palpable. After 12 to 13 weeks, however, the uterus emerges from this protective bony enclosure, making it vulnerable to direct trauma. By 20 weeks, the uterus rises to the level of the umbilicus. Toward the end of pregnancy, the uterus can extend as high as the diaphragm. Thus, the uterus may be found in all four quadrants of the abdomen as well as the pelvis at the end of a full-term pregnancy.

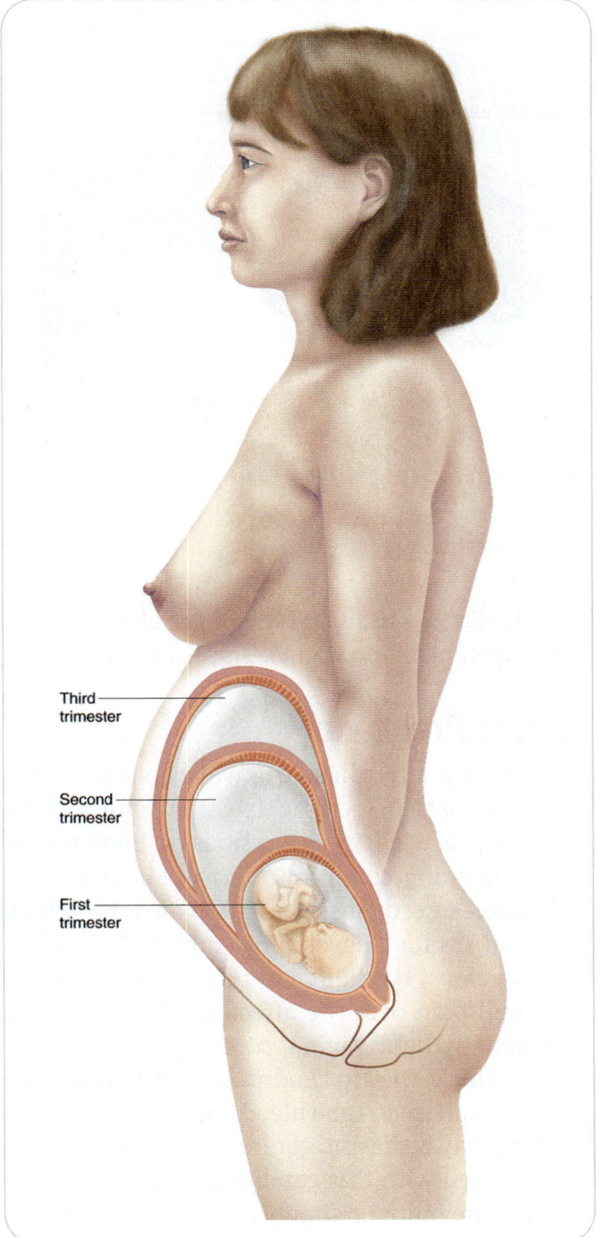

Figure 17-4 The three trimesters of pregnancy.

A woman has changes to her vital signs that are normal during pregnancy. The maternal heart rate increases by 15 to 20 beats per minute (beats/min) by the third trimester. The respiratory system is also subject to changes during pregnancy. As the uterus expands, the diaphragm is pushed upward into the thorax, and the ribs compensate by flaring out. The mother's need for oxygen increases as the fetus and uterus grow and as blood volume increases. The respiratory system adapts to this need through a variety of mechanisms that result in a slight increase in respiratory rate. The pregnant woman's normal blood pressure also changes. Systolic and diastolic blood pressures decrease by 4 to 6 mm Hg and 8 to 15 mm Hg, respectively, reaching their lowest point in midpregnancy before returning to normal levels by full term.

Significance to an OEC Technician

What do these insights into the anatomy and physiology of pregnancy mean for OEC technicians who are assessing a pregnant woman? First, blood pressure, pulse rate, or respiratory rate may not change during the first trimester. However, from the midsecond trimester on, a healthy woman with a typical uncomplicated pregnancy may have a *normal* blood pressure of 96/60 mm Hg and a pulse of 100 beats/min—values that would potentially be considered indicative of shock in a nonpregnant female. Accurate blood pressure measurements are obtained with the patient lying on her left side (take pressure from the right arm), a position that prevents the pregnant uterus from placing pressure on the inferior vena cava that returns blood to the heart.

Any vaginal bleeding during pregnancy is abnormal, until time of delivery. After 28 weeks of gestation, maternal blood volume (both red blood cell and plasma components) rises. Because of this, a woman may lose 30% to 35% of her blood volume to *any* hemorrhage before showing any signs of shock. However, even though a woman's vital signs may appear stable, her fetus will be in shock due to the combination of decreased blood flow from the uterus to the placenta and the shunting of blood away from the fetus. The mother is kept alive with the fetus suffering the consequences of shock first. OEC technicians should always anticipate the development of shock in a pregnant trauma patient and in her fetus.

COMMON OBSTETRIC EMERGENCIES

Vaginal Bleeding and Hemorrhage

Vaginal bleeding is normal during a menstrual period. In a nonpregnant female, the most common cause of vaginal bleeding is menstruation, the cyclical discharge of about 25 to 65 mL of blood and tissue beginning approximately 2 weeks after ovulation if fertilization does not occur. Bleeding usually lasts for 5 to 7 days and gradually decreases in flow. The amount of bleeding varies from female to female and is usually quantified by the number of pads or tampons used per day (or per hour for heavier bleeding).

For most women, the amount of bleeding is relatively consistent from one menstrual period to the next. On occasion, however, an increase in flow—possibly related to hormonal fluctuations or stress—causes a woman to seek medical attention. In addition, some women will develop midcycle bleeding that simulates a period. These episodes, referred to as "abnormal vaginal bleeding," may have benign causes (such as stress) or may result from more serious diseases (such as uterine or cervical cancer). Fortunately, most abnormal vaginal bleeding does not cause significant hypovolemia, even when it occurs over several days. Abnormal vaginal bleeding always requires further evaluation by a physician, especially if accompanied by signs or symptoms of shock, such as dizziness, shortness of breath, fainting, pale skin, tachycardia, or hypotension, or if the bleeding is heavy enough to require a new pad or tampon every 15 minutes or is associated with the passage of large clots. If any of these findings are noted, immediately call for an ambulance to transport the patient to an emergency department. Several causes of vaginal bleeding are related to problems during pregnancy, and these women need to be seen by an obstetric practitioner (**Table 17-1**).

A "bloody show" occurs at full-term pregnancy when the woman is about to go into labor. The cervix starts to dilate, and a *small* amount of blood appears at the opening of the vagina. This is normal.

Table 17-1 Causes of Vaginal Bleeding During Pregnancy

- Ectopic pregnancy
- Miscarriage (or threatened miscarriage)
- Placenta previa
- Postpartum hemorrhage
- Trauma
  - Uterine rupture
  - Abruptio placentae
  - Amniotic sac rupture

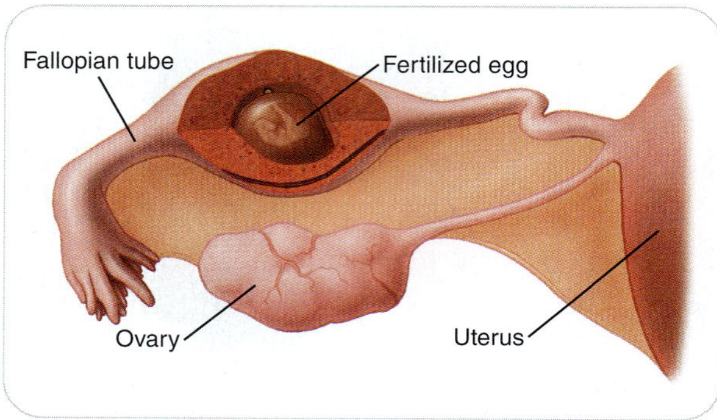

Figure 17-5 An ectopic pregnancy occurs when the fertilized egg implants in one of the fallopian tubes.

Ectopic Pregnancy

Occasionally, a fertilized egg will implant outside the uterus, or at an "ectopic" location (**Figure 17-5**). An **ectopic pregnancy** is a serious and potentially life-threatening condition. Up to 95% of ectopic pregnancies occur inside a fallopian tube, which is too narrow for a developing embryo. As the embryo develops, the fallopian tube stretches, causing a dull pain over the affected lower quadrant. Occasionally light vaginal bleeding or "spotting" occurs during the first months of pregnancy because the fallopian tube bleeds as it stretches. The spotting may be misinterpreted as a menstrual period. Women with this condition may be unaware they are pregnant or simply deny being pregnant. With time the tube ruptures, resulting in major internal bleeding, severe pain, and hemorrhagic shock or even death. Blood within the abdomen may cause referred pain in the left shoulder. Up to 50% of women with ectopic pregnancies have a history of prior pelvic inflammatory disease.

Miscarriage

A **miscarriage**, or spontaneous abortion, is the loss of a pregnancy prior to 20 weeks of gestation, before the fetus can survive outside the uterus. Any fetus at less than 24 weeks will have little chance of survival, and even at 24 weeks, the chances of survival are slim. Spotting or bleeding is the primary sign, and it may be accompanied by lower abdominal cramping. About a fourth of all pregnant women will have a miscarriage. This percentage increases as the age of the pregnant woman increases. In many miscarriages, there is a birth defect, stopping the pregnancy. At times, only a portion of the tissues are expelled, resulting in an incomplete abortion and heavy, continuous vaginal bleeding accompanied by cramping and the passage of clots.

Placenta Previa

After the first trimester, bleeding may result from a placenta that is implanted abnormally low, *covering* the opening of the cervix, a condition known as **placenta previa** (Figure 17-6). This abnormality initially presents with painless, dark-red vaginal bleeding. Since the placenta is above the os (opening) of the cervix, blood leaks out of the cervix and can result in termination of the pregnancy, and severe maternal bleeding.

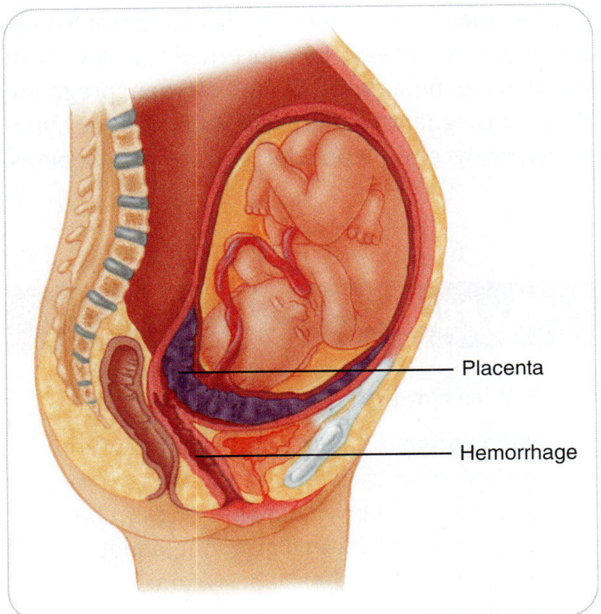

Figure 17-6 Placenta previa.

Postpartum Hemorrhage and Uterine Atony

Following delivery of a newborn, hormones are released that cause the uterine muscle to contract, making the uterus smaller; the hormones also cause blood vessels in the wall to contract, slowing bleeding. Occasionally this process does not occur, resulting in atony (no muscular tone). Also, a piece of the placenta can remain in the uterus. Both conditions can result in excessive continued bleeding (500 mL or more), and maternal shock can follow rapidly.

Trauma During Pregnancy

As an OEC technician, you are more likely to provide emergency care to a pregnant woman who is injured while participating in a sport such as skiing than you are to deliver a baby. Women who are fit or athletic may continue to ski through the second trimester. Occasionally they ski or bike during the third trimester, although most obstetricians do not recommend this. The two main risks for pregnant women who participate in sports are falling and collisions. An indirect blow to the abdomen can be just as dangerous as a direct blow and could harm the developing fetus or the woman's enlarged uterus.

Three potentially dangerous consequences from trauma are uterine rupture, abruptio placentae, and the rupture of membranes (amniotic sac). Uterine penetration by a foreign body is also possible but is exceedingly rare.

Uterine Rupture

Trauma to the abdomen during pregnancy can result in rupture of the uterus. When this occurs, the muscular wall of the uterus tears, massive bleeding results, the fetus usually dies, and the mother's life is in jeopardy. This is a true emergency, with shock to both mother and fetus occurring rapidly.

Abruptio Placentae

After the death of the mother during pregnancy, the most common cause of fetal death is **abruptio placentae**. This condition is typically the result of a shearing force produced when the body stops

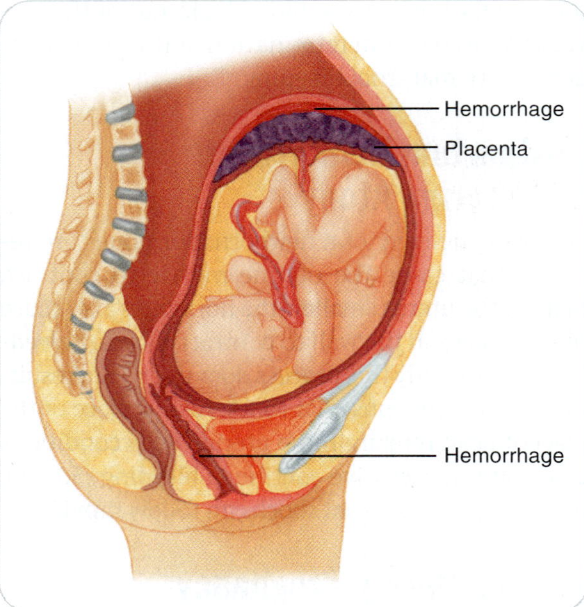

Figure 17-7 Abruptio placentae.

moving before the internal organs (uterus) stop (**Figure 17-7**). The amount of shearing force and the extent of the resultant indirect injury are determined by the rate of deceleration, and not necessarily by how fast the body was moving. When shearing forces cause the placenta to separate from the uterus, all blood flow and nutrient transfer to the fetus is interrupted, resulting in fetal death. Classic signs and symptoms include vaginal bleeding, abdominal pain, constant uterine contractions, and expanding uterine height from bleeding inside the uterus.

Rupture of the Amniotic Sac (Ruptured Membrane)

Premature rupture of the amniotic sac before full term often causes leakage of clear or blood-tinged fluid from the vagina. This condition can occur spontaneously but usually occurs following trauma. Early labor usually occurs once the sac is torn. Fluid, sometimes blood-tinged, will leak out of the vagina. Normally the sac ruptures spontaneously just before birth at full term.

Other Complications of Pregnancy

Pregnancy-Induced Hypertension

Pregnancy-induced hypertension, or "toxemia," is a form of high blood pressure that develops during pregnancy. Also known as **preeclampsia**, pregnancy-induced hypertension develops after the 20th week of gestation and is more common in a first-time pregnancy, twin pregnancies, and women with preexisting diabetes. OEC technicians may observe the following two characteristics of this condition:

1. Blood pressure greater than 140/90 mm Hg (or a significant rise in one or both pressures)
2. Edema of the face and/or hands

Pregnancy-induced hypertension may be complicated by seizures, a condition known as **eclampsia**. This severe form of pregnancy-induced hypertension usually develops late in pregnancy, close to the time of delivery.

Supine Hypotensive Syndrome

After 20 weeks of gestation, the enlarged uterus can compress the inferior vena cava when a pregnant woman is in a supine position. Such compression decreases blood return to the heart and subsequently decreases cardiac output by 30% to 40%, resulting in profound maternal hypotension. In general, place a pregnant woman on her *left* side to take the pressure off the vena cava.

Diabetes of Pregnancy

As pregnancy progresses, some women may develop gestational diabetes. Following delivery, most women's blood sugar levels will return to normal. However, always be concerned that a woman could have new-onset diabetes when pregnant. When a pregnant woman shows findings of hypo- or hyperglycemia, consider gestational diabetes.

KEY POINT

One Victim but Two Patients

When caring for a pregnant trauma victim, you are really caring for two patients. The expectant mother will understandably be very concerned, even distraught, about potential injury to her baby. A calm, reassuring manner will help ease her anxiety.

CASE Update

Realizing the woman has severe vaginal bleeding, you ask for permission to help her. Somewhat embarrassed, she says, "Please help me." You rapidly place her supine, putting several blankets on her to keep her warm. Soon two other patrollers arrive, one a woman. Vital signs are obtained, with a carotid pulse of 112 beats/min and respirations of 20 breaths/min. Her radial pulse is absent. You instruct the female patroller to help you, since hypovolemic shock is present. You instruct the other patroller to tell dispatch to send the ambulance directly to the condo parking lot. The female patroller calms the patient. The patient's history reveals she is healthy with no medical problems, but she missed her last two periods and could be pregnant. She takes no medications. Oxygen is placed on the woman by mask with rebreather.

What should you do next?

First responder care is the same for anyone with diabetes, but the patient needs referral to a qualified medical professional for definitive care.

PATIENT ASSESSMENT FOR OBSTETRIC EMERGENCIES

The assessment of a woman with an obstetric or abdominal complaint is unique because the history must include information concerning her reproductive cycle. Obstetric emergencies can threaten the life of both the woman and the fetus. In addition, because a woman may not be aware she is pregnant, always consider the possibility any female patient of reproductive age is pregnant.

Begin the assessment, as always, with an evaluation of the ABCDs (airway, breathing, circulation, and disability) and vital signs (Figure 17-8). Use the SAMPLE acronym (signs and symptoms, allergies, medications, past medical history, last oral intake, events leading up to the problem) and the OPQRST mnemonic (onset, provocation, quality, radiation, severity, and time) to guide you in obtaining both a general medical history and a history of the current illness or injury.

If you suspect the woman to be pregnant, ask these questions:

1. When was your last (normal) menstrual period, and when is the next period expected?

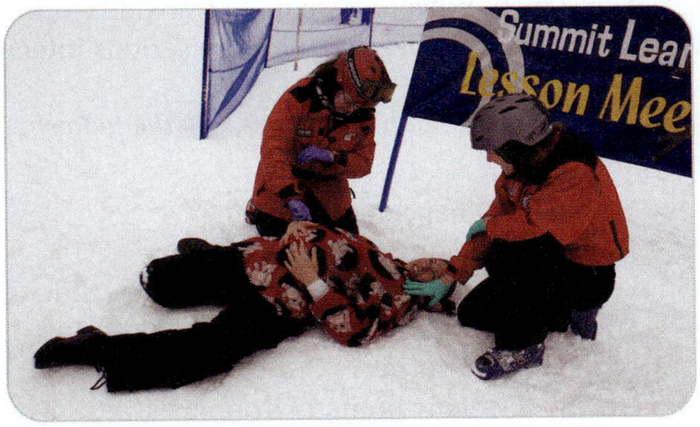

Figure 17-8 Begin your assessment of a pregnant woman as you would any other assessment—with an evaluation of the ABCDs and her vital signs.

2. If you are late for an expected menstrual period, could you be pregnant?
3. Have you had a recent pregnancy test?

The woman's responses to these questions will tell you if she is, or could be pregnant, allowing you to care for the woman appropriately.

If her complaint is related to vaginal bleeding, ask the following questions:

1. How many pads or tampons have you used in the past 24 hours?
2. Have you passed any clots?
3. Have you noted any dizziness upon standing?
4. Have you received any trauma to your genital area?

If many pads or tampons were used, suspect significant bleeding. Clots could mean heavy bleeding or possible miscarriage. Dizziness could indicate hypovolemia from blood loss. Trauma could be from an accident or from sexual abuse.

If her complaint is related to abdominal pain, ask these questions:

1. Have you experienced this type of pain before (with menstruation, or between menses)?
2. Have you noted any recent vaginal bleeding or spotting?
3. Do you have any abnormal vaginal discharge, burning during urination, fever, or back pain?

Some women have heavier bleeding with menstruation normally. Generally, women have the same amount of bleeding during each cycle. Unusual bleeding or spotting may indicate an early miscarriage, or other significant problems with the woman's reproductive system. Abnormal discharge may indicate a sexually transmitted infection, a bladder infection, or more serious infection of the kidneys.

If she is known to be pregnant, ask the following questions:

1. When is the expected due date?
2. Have you had any prenatal care?
3. Have you been pregnant before? If yes, did you have any deliveries, and were there any problems delivering?
4. Do you have any prenatal or preexisting medical conditions such as gestational diabetes, or a history of high blood pressure or twins?
5. Has your water broken (membranes ruptured)?
6. Have you noted any vaginal bleeding since the injury?
7. Have you felt the baby move since the injury?

Knowing the due date will help you determine if delivery is imminent. A woman who has not had prenatal care is more likely to have untreated problems of pregnancy. Women who have had several previous vaginal deliveries usually have a more rapid subsequent delivery. If the woman has had trouble with a previous delivery, there may be problems with other deliveries. Gestational diabetes can be recurrent, as can high blood pressure during pregnancy. Women who have had fraternal twins are more likely to have them again.

When the amniotic fluid discharges, delivery is imminent. When trauma has occurred in a pregnant woman, you must consider a ruptured uterus, with harm to the baby, mother, or both. If the mother says she has recently felt the baby move inside her, that is a good sign.

EXAM OF A PREGNANT WOMAN

Always be mindful of a woman's need for privacy. Although a gynecologic or obstetric history is crucial, try to ask the necessary questions in a way and in a place where others cannot overhear your conversation. In general, undressing a woman in an outdoor environment to perform an examination is not necessary; wait until she has reached a patrol facility or other first-aid facility where a female assistant can help with the inspection of the affected areas in privacy. If evacuation will take a long time and the woman is in labor, you need to inspect for crowning, which is the appearance of the infant's head at the vaginal opening. Improvise some screening using clothing, sheets, towels, or sleeping bags.

Always ask for permission to examine a woman. When examining a nonpregnant woman who has abdominal pain or vaginal bleeding, place her in a position of comfort—usually, supine with her knees flexed to allow the abdominal and pelvic muscles to relax. Look at the abdomen, noting any distention or discoloration. Have the patient use one finger to point to where her pain is most intense. Also, if abdominal pain is present in a pregnant woman, determine the quality, location, and timing, and whether any back pain is present. Remember, conditions other than pregnancy may be the cause of the pain. Next, gently palpate the four quadrants of the abdomen and

KEY POINT

Fetal Movement

Fetal movement can be detected by a pregnant woman after about 20 weeks of gestation and is a good sign of fetal well-being.

the suprapubic region, as described in Chapter 16, *Gastrointestinal, Genitourinary, and Reproductive System Emergencies*. Note whether the woman reveals tenderness or shows guarding. OEC technicians should not examine a nonpregnant woman's genital region unless she has a history of trauma and ongoing hemorrhage. If the responder is male, and a female responder is immediately available, consider having the woman conduct the exam. Patrollers should only visually inspect the female genitalia. Internal palpation is done only by a qualified medical professional.

For a woman with a known pregnancy, note whether the uterus feels tight, as during a uterine contraction, or if there is tenderness upon palpation. If the uterus is easily palpable, attempt to detect any fetal movement. Also look for a bloody show or amniotic fluid leaking from ruptured membranes.

MANAGEMENT OF OBSTETRIC EMERGENCIES

The general management of a pregnant woman who is bleeding or has serious trauma is like that of any other trauma victim, but with a few additional considerations. Vaginal bleeding *cannot* be stopped using dressings or bandages or by packing the vagina. You can use an external pad to absorb the blood, but this will not control it. Pregnant women may lose 30% to 35% of their blood volume before showing signs of shock. While the woman's vital signs may appear stable, the fetus will be in shock due to decreased blood flow from the uterus to the placenta and the shunting of blood. Thus, OEC technicians should always anticipate the development of shock in a pregnant trauma patient and her fetus, even when vital signs are normal. Provide oxygen when needed to keep the oxygen saturation between 94 and 99%, rapid evacuation, and immediate transport using an ALS provider to a definitive-care facility.

Postpartum (following childbirth) hemorrhage is bleeding in excess of 500 mL following a vaginal delivery. Firm, downward massage of the woman's lower abdomen after delivery stimulates the uterus to contract and can promptly resolve this form of bleeding.

If possible, position the woman on her left side. If her injuries prevent this, elevate her right hip, displacing the uterus to avoid possible supine hypotension from pressure on the vena cava. When using spinal motion restriction for a pregnant woman on a backboard, avoid placing any straps directly over her abdomen (**Figure 17-9**). After securing her to the backboard, tilt the backboard approximately 4 to 6 inches to the patient's left by placing a patrol pack or a folded blanket under the right side of the backboard. Abdominal pain may be associated with nausea or vomiting, so anticipate this. Suction as needed to clear the patient's airway.

Transport rapidly but gently, reassessing the patient regularly. In late stages of pregnancy, the

KEY POINT

First Steps in Treating a Pregnant Trauma Patient

Early critical intervention for a pregnant woman with trauma includes placing her on high-flow oxygen if her oxygen saturation is less than 94% and positioning her on her left side (perhaps by tilting the patient to the left). Treat her for shock even in the presence of normal vital signs.

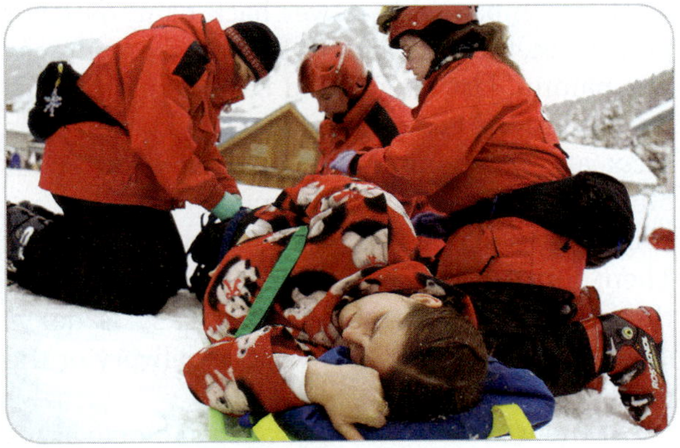

Figure 17-9 If possible, place the woman on her left side, or elevate her right hip or manually displace the uterus. Avoid placing straps over her abdomen.

uterus pushes up toward the diaphragm and makes it more difficult to take a deep breath. Transport a woman in her third trimester with her head uphill in a toboggan. In the case of shock or suspected fetal shock for which transport in a head-downhill position is needed, an object such as a fanny pack can be placed under the head of the board to bring the board to a more neutral position, thus lessening respiratory difficulties while simultaneously treating shock.

CHILDBIRTH

Few emergencies cause more anxiety for an OEC technician than an emergency delivery; however only a century ago, almost all childbirth took place outside of a hospital, usually at home. As an OEC technician, the most likely scenarios encountered are a miscarriage, spontaneous abortion, or an obese female who denies being pregnant but complains of regular intermittent abdominal pain and has physical findings consistent with pregnancy (for example, an enlarged uterus, a lack of menstrual periods, stretch marks, and fetal movement). Today, delivery outside of a hospital is more common in women with little or no prenatal care and in women who have had multiple pregnancies. Babies of these women have a higher incidence of fetal mortality than babies delivered in the hospital.

Childbirth begins with labor, which can be gradual or abrupt in onset and is divided into three stages. The first stage begins with irregular lower abdominal uterine contractions and is often accompanied by lower back pain. As labor progresses, the contractions become more intense and painful, last longer, and become more regular. Toward the end of the first stage, contractions recur at 3- to 4-minute intervals and last about 50 to 60 seconds. The cervix gradually dilates, becoming large enough for the baby to be delivered. Then, during the second stage, the fetus descends through the birth canal and the baby is delivered. The third stage involves the delivery of the placenta.

If the woman is in early labor and delivery is not imminent, place the patient on her left side while arranging transport to a hospital with ALS. If delivery is imminent, the following signs may be present.

1. Bloody show (passage of the mucus plug that seals the cervix throughout pregnancy)
2. Rupture of the amniotic sac (the "ruptured membrane"), with fluid coming out of the vagina
3. The urge to push or defecate

Leaked fluid is usually clear but may also appear tea-stained or be pea-colored from fetal stool, known as **meconium**. The urge to have a bowel movement is a normal sensation indicating delivery is about to occur. Do not allow the patient to go to a bathroom, and reassure her this is a normal sensation that means she is about to deliver the baby. If she feels the urge to push or to have a bowel movement, inspect the vagina for bulging or for crowning.

Ideally, have a second OEC technician (a woman if immediately available) present for this examination and/or to assist with the delivery. At the same time, look for a prolapsed umbilical cord, in which case the umbilical cord extends out of the vagina (**Figure 17-10**). If the umbilical cord or any part of the baby besides its head (a foot, for example) is visible at the vaginal opening, instruct the woman to stop pushing, and assist her into a knees-to-chest position. Place the mother on

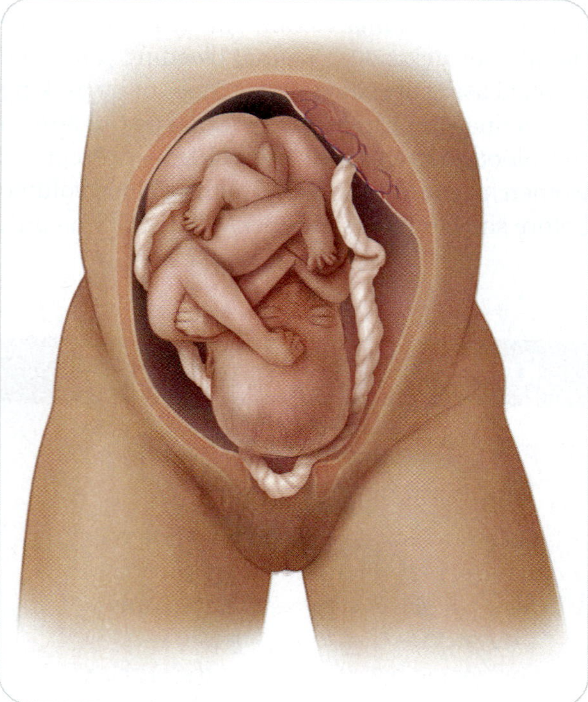

Figure 17-10 Prolapsed umbilical cord, where the umbilical cord extends out of the vagina, requires emergent transfer to advanced medical care.

KEY POINT

Always be Prepared for an Emergency Delivery

When assisting with an emergency delivery, always use standard precautions, and wear a face mask with an eye shield or safety glasses. Consider having a commercial obstetric delivery kit available in the aid room for emergencies.

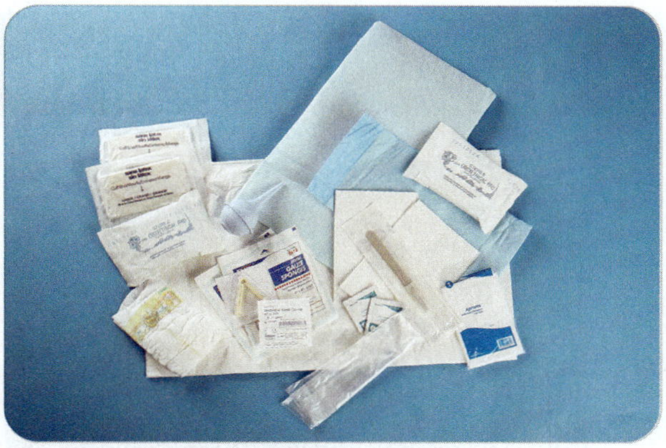

Figure 17-11 A sterile obstetric kit.

supplemental oxygen if the oxygen saturation is less than 94%. Arrange emergent transfer to advanced medical care.

Transport a woman in labor to a higher level of care under the following circumstances:

- Transport time is less than 20 minutes.
- The umbilical cord is visible before the baby is born in the vagina (a prolapsed cord).
- Any part of the baby other than the top of the head is visible in the vagina.
- The woman states that her doctor says she will need a cesarean section.
- This delivery is the woman's first, and the amount of the baby's head that is visible is smaller than 1 inch across.

Preparing for Delivery

Use a sterile disposable obstetric delivery kit (OB kit), if available (**Figure 17-11**). If one is not available, improvise by obtaining clean towels and sheets, a blanket for the baby, 4-inch by 4-inch gauze sponges, scissors, a soft rubber bulb syringe, white cloth tape, and two clean cotton shoelaces, all of which should be sterilized with boiling water if there is time to do so. Always use standard precautions, including a face mask with an eye shield or glasses. A gown may prevent splashing of body fluids on you during the delivery. Following delivery, place all supplies soiled with body fluids in a biohazard bag and dispose of them properly.

Remove the woman's clothes from the waist down, placing her in a semi-Fowler position (patient sitting with back at a 45-degree angle and knees bent) on a firm, sturdy padded table if available (a bed may be too low or too soft). If such a table is not available, use any firm, elevated flat surface. Use a folded blanket or large towel to elevate her buttocks 2 to 4 inches in relation to the middle of her back. Bend her hips and flex and spread her knees apart, always protecting her modesty with a sheet. Place one end of a clean sheet or large towel under her buttocks and allow the other end to unfold to the floor, creating a clean delivery "field." Sit or stand in front of the women so that you can see between the woman's legs, and place other sheets or towels in front of you to soak up blood or amniotic fluid during the delivery. Put your OB kit or other sterile supplies on a firm level surface beside you. Station another OEC technician at the woman's head to provide reassurance.

The Delivery

Any signs of imminent delivery require OEC technicians to be prepared to assist with immediate delivery. Time the woman's contractions from the start of one contraction to the start of the next. Then, while feeling the abdomen, note the duration of a single contraction by recording the time between the onset of a contraction and its completion. Encourage the woman to rest (and pant) between contractions.

If the baby is crowning (top of the infant's skull is showing), perform the following steps of **OEC Skill 17-1** to assist the woman with an emergency delivery.

After birth, put a sanitary pad over the mother's vagina and have her lie on her back with her legs straight. Vaginal bleeding slows after the

OEC SKILL 17-1 Assisting with Childbirth

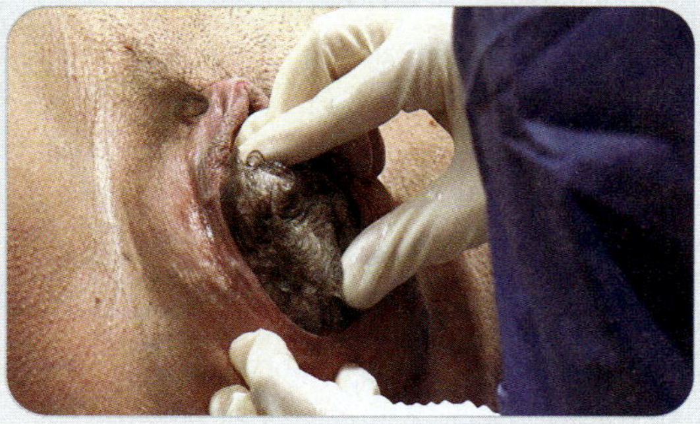

1 Once the baby is crowning, allow the woman to push the baby's head out; support its head with your gloved hand as it emerges. Applying gentle pressure to the top of the baby's head with your hand will allow the head to come out in a controlled fashion and help prevent the baby's head and body from suddenly popping out. Applying this gentle pressure can markedly reduce the severity of tearing to the woman's perineal tissues. The head usually emerges facedown. Once the head has emerged, it will rotate slightly, allowing easier access to the baby's face and airway. Do not twist the baby's neck. Next, feel for the umbilical cord around the baby's neck. If present, gently lift the cord over the baby's head. If unable to lift the cord over the baby's head, immediately place two clamps or umbilical ties around the cord 2 to 4 inches apart and at least 6 inches from the child, then cut the cord between the clamps.

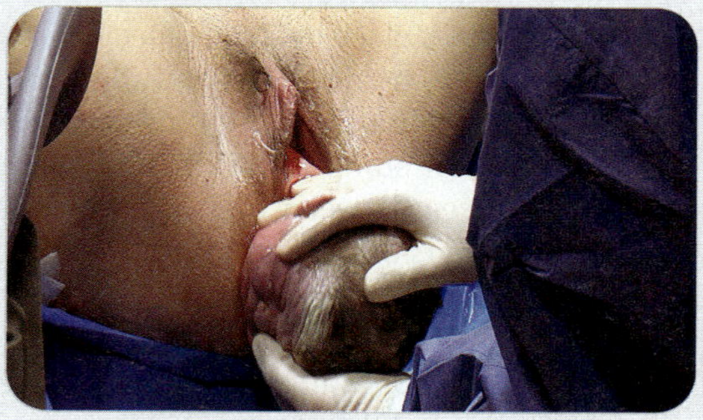

2 After delivering the head, you should see the baby's upper shoulder. With one hand on either side of the baby's head, gently guide the head down slightly to help deliver the upper shoulder as the woman pushes. After the upper shoulder is delivered, you may need to guide the head up slightly to deliver the lower shoulder. Support the baby's head with one hand and its upper body with your other hand as the shoulders are delivered. Never pull the baby from the birth canal.

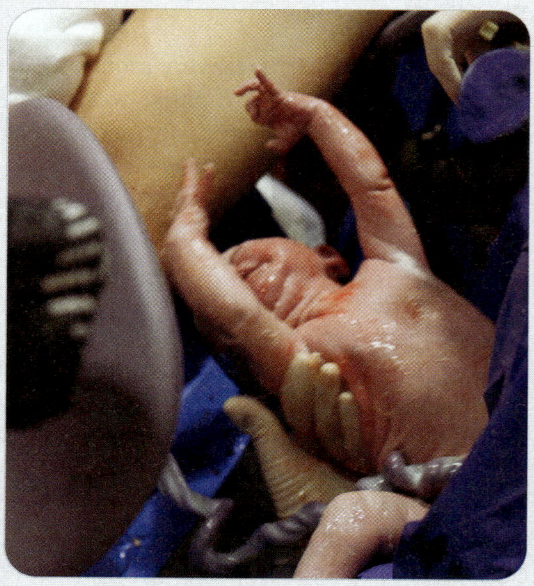

3 Once the head and shoulders are delivered, the rest of the baby slips out quickly because its body is covered with a white, cheesy substance (vernix caseosa). Be prepared to catch the baby! Once the baby emerges, rotate it 180 degrees so the supine newborn is against your body, with one hand holding the head and neck, and the torso resting on the same hand's forearm. Hold the newborn with the head slightly lower than the body to facilitate drainage of secretions. Always hold the baby's head and neck in a neutral position to maintain an open airway. Have an assistant record the time and location of the birth for later entry on a birth certificate.

OEC SKILL 17-1 Assisting with Childbirth (*continued*)

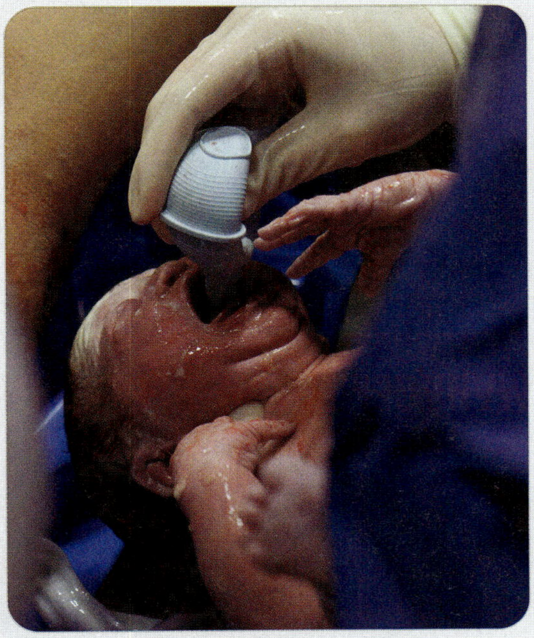

4 If there is *obvious obstruction* to the baby's spontaneous breathing, immediately suction the baby's mouth and then the nostrils, using a soft rubber bulb syringe. Squeeze the bulb *before* inserting it into the baby's mouth and let the bulb suck once in the mouth. Suctioning the nostrils before the mouth may stimulate the baby to gasp and thereby aspirate any fluid in the nose or pharynx. Note if the fluid in the baby's mouth and nose does not appear clear, a sign of meconium (stool) in the amniotic fluid. This condition is called meconium aspiration and causes inflammation in the baby's lungs after birth. If you believe that you have seen this condition, make sure you tell the EMS personnel.

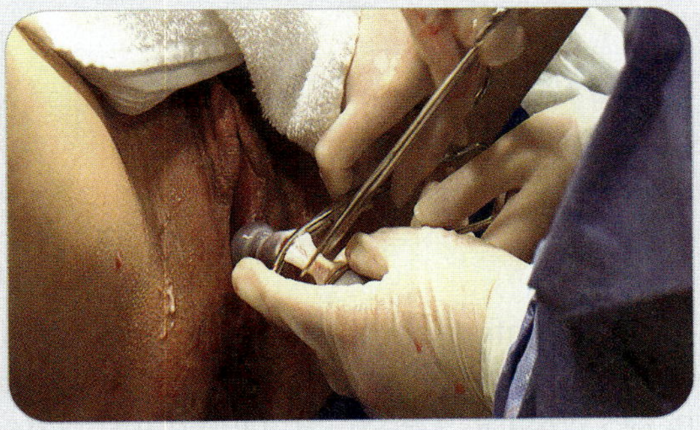

5 You will need to cut the umbilical cord. Place two clamps or tie two cloth shoelaces about 6 inches from the baby and about 2 to 4 inches apart, then cut the cord between the clamps or laces.

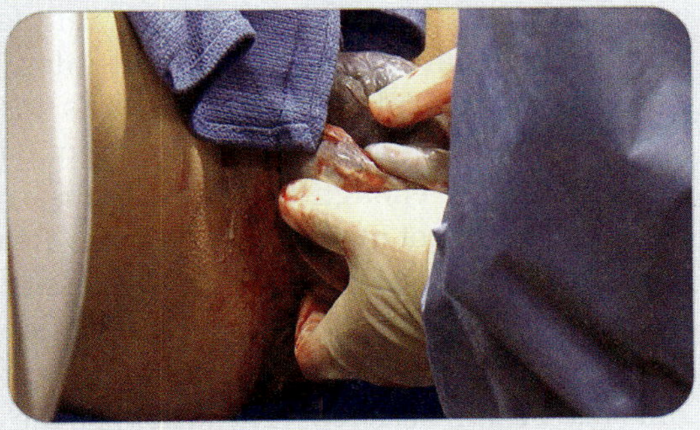

6 The delivery of the placenta is the third stage of labor. Allow the placenta to come out of the vagina by itself. Pulling on the umbilical cord that is still attached to the placenta can be harmful. The placenta should separate from the inside wall of the uterus about 20 to 30 minutes after the baby is delivered. If transport is available once the baby is born, do not wait on the delivery of the placenta. However, if the placenta does come out of the vagina, put it in a plastic bag and send it to the hospital with the mother and her baby. It will need to be inspected by the receiving physician.

KEY POINT

Caution in Suctioning the Baby's Airway

ONLY if there is obvious obstruction to the baby's spontaneous breathing will you immediately suction the baby's mouth and then the nostrils, using a soft rubber bulb syringe.

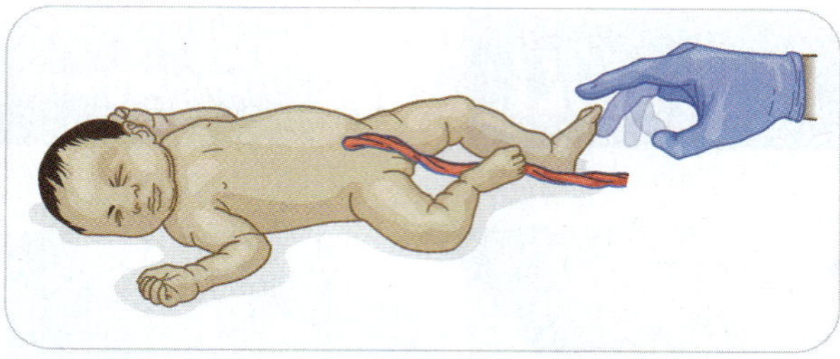

Figure 17-12 To stimulate a newborn to breathe, flick the soles of the feet or rub the back.

placenta is out and the uterus starts to shrink. Massage the mother's lower abdomen in a circular motion where the uterus is located to help her uterus shrink and to aid in the production of oxytocin, a hormone that makes the uterine muscles contract.

Always have the mother, baby, and placenta transported to the hospital. If there is excessive bleeding, keep the mother in the supine position, provide supplemental oxygen, and monitor her vital signs. Apply sanitary napkins to the perineum, as needed, an especially helpful practice when bleeding is the result of lacerations of the birth canal or perineum. Do not place a tampon or any dressings inside the vagina.

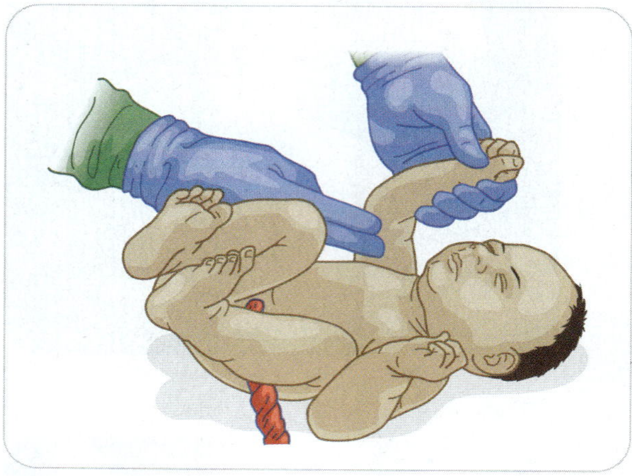

Figure 17-13 Always use the brachial pulse when checking the heart rate of a newborn/infant.

BASIC CARE OF NEWBORNS

Once an infant is delivered, vigorously dry it off and wrap it in a blanket or towel, covering the entire baby except for its face. Begin your evaluation of a newborn with the ABCDs. The airway may be suctioned after the head is delivered and again after the baby is delivered, but *only* if there is obvious obstruction to spontaneous breathing. When using a bulb syringe, always blow the air out before suctioning the airway (do not blow air into the airway). Usually an infant begins crying vigorously within 15 to 20 seconds after delivery, often while being dried. If not, use your fingers to either flick the soles of the infant's feet or rub the infant's back (**Figure 17-12**). Do not spank the baby. If the infant does not begin to breathe after 10 to 15 seconds, begin resuscitation.

If the infant appears to be breathing well, determine its pulse rate by palpating the brachial pulse (**Figure 17-13**). A newborn's pulse rate should be between 90 and 180 beats/min. If it is less, begin gentle positive-pressure ventilations with supplemental oxygen using an infant bag-valve mask (BVM) placed over the baby's nose and mouth at a rate of 40 to 60 breaths/min. Bag the baby using just enough pressure to observe the chest rising. Do not overinflate the lungs. Reassess the pulse rate after 90 seconds, and if less than 60 beats/min, give oxygen at low concentrations, increasing it as needed until the heart rate is at least 100 beats/min. Assisted ventilation is the most effective action in neonatal resuscitation and usually brings the heart rate up to 100 beats/min. Once the pulse rate reaches 100, gradually reduce the rate and pressure of the BVM ventilations until it is apparent the infant is breathing well on its own and is maintaining good color.

An infant's skin color is another indicator of its well-being. A lack of oxygen in the infant's bloodstream causes cyanosis of the face and trunk, normally for up to several minutes after delivery as the hemoglobin becomes saturated with oxygen. Full oxygen saturation takes up to 10 minutes. Therefore, newer evidence has shown clinical assessment of skin color is a very poor indicator of the newborn's oxygen saturation of hemoglobin during the period immediately after birth. For infants with strong, regular respirations *and cyanosis*, administer high-flow oxygen using "blow-by oxygen," in which the end of the tubing is placed close to the infant's nostrils (**Figure 17-14**). If the newborn is not breathing, begin ventilation with room air first and increase the oxygen percentage in the ventilations slowly. There is growing evidence that brief hypoxia of the newborn can result in an adverse outcome.

Infants with a pulse rate lower than 60 beats/min, or a pulse rate remaining between 60 and 100 beats/min despite adequate ventilation with supplementary oxygen for 30 seconds, should be given chest compressions (CPR) (**Figure 17-15**). In this situation, even though a pulse may be palpable, the heart rate and cardiac output are inadequate for supporting the infant's life. Perform the chest compression technique and compression rates specified by current standards for health professionals as published by approved NSP CPR certification program providers. CPR should be continued until the infant responds with adequate respirations and a heart rate greater than 60 beats/min, or until pronounced dead by a physician. Although it can be distressing to perform CPR on an infant, remember that infants are quite resilient and can survive prolonged effective CPR without brain damage.

If the baby is doing well, place the baby in an improvised crib so you don't drop it. This crib could be a basket or a cardboard box padded with blankets. Keep the baby warm, as a baby's body temperature can drop very quickly. Neonatal hypothermia is reported in about half of all prehospital deliveries.

While drying and stimulating the baby, assess its Apgar score, a scoring system used to evaluate a newborn's health status. (Although *Apgar* is used as an acronym, the term is actually named after its creator, Virginia Apgar, and therefore is not written in all capital letters.) In determining an Apgar score, either 0, 1, or 2 points are assigned at 1, 5, and 10 minutes after birth for each of the following five categories (**Table 17-2**):

Appearance
Pulse
Grimace or irritability
Activity or muscle tone
Respirations

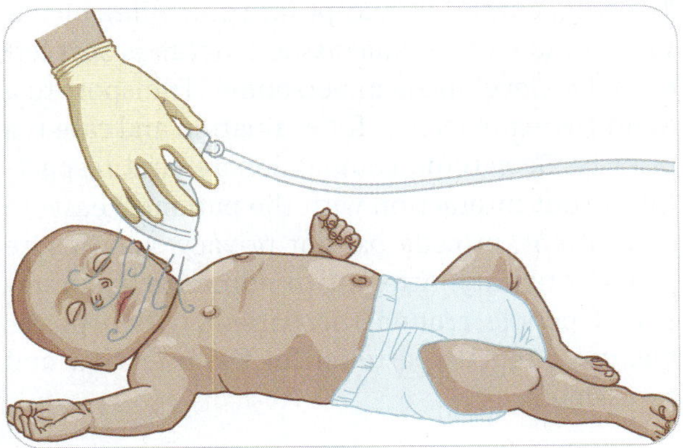

Figure 17-14 Provide blow-by oxygen by placing the oxygen tubing, or a mask or paper cup connected to the end of the tubing, near the infant's nostrils.

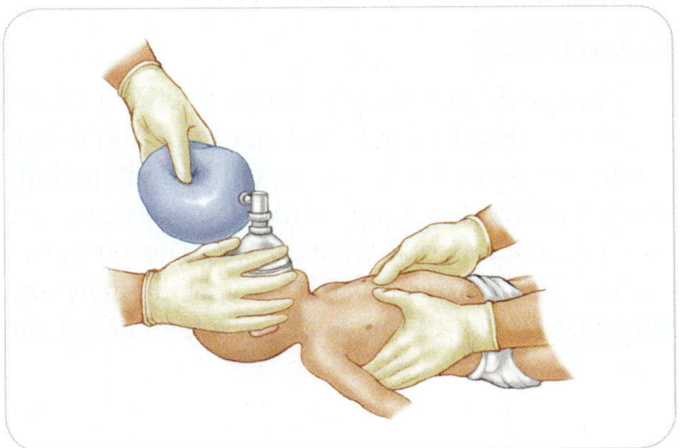

Figure 17-15 Infants with an inadequate pulse rate require chest compressions.

Table 17-2 Apgar Scoring System

Category	Points		
	2	1	0
Appearance	Body completely pink	Body pink, limbs blue	Body completely blue or pale
Pulse (beats/min)	Greater than 100	Less than 100	Absent
Grimace or irritability	Crying	Feeble cry when stimulated	Does not cry or react to stimuli
Activity or muscle tone	Active	Some weak motion	Body limp, no tone
Respirations	Strong cry	Weak cry	None

The Apgar score is helpful in determining if the baby is doing well outside the uterus or if it needs resuscitation. If the infant needs resuscitation before the 1-minute score, do not wait; begin resuscitation efforts. Should the 5-minute score be less than 7, continue obtaining scores every 5 minutes up to 20 minutes.

GYNECOLOGIC SEXUAL ASSAULT

Sexual assault is a form of trauma defined as any physical contact of a sexual nature without voluntary consent. Forms of sexual assault include inappropriate touching, child molestation, and vaginal, anal, or oral penetration. The perpetrator may be of either sex but is typically male and someone known to the victim or a member of the victim's family, rather than a total stranger. Many victims are adolescent females and children.

In a survey conducted in the United States in 2016, one woman in six reported being the victim of an attempted or completed rape in her lifetime. The rate of sexual assault and rape has fallen 63% since 1993, from a rate of 4.3 assaults per 1,000 people in 1993, to 1.2 per 1,000 in 2016. From 2009 to 2013, an average of 63,000 children were victims of sexual abuse each year. In 2013, 89,000 women reported they were raped in the United States. There are estimates that only 30% of sexual assaults are reported, although this percentage seems to have increased with the 2018 "Me Too" movement, as more women are now reporting abuse.

Sexual assault may occur with enough force to cause physical trauma, both internal and external. Other health problems resulting from rape include sexually transmitted infections, chronic abdominal pain, and headaches. The psychological trauma is often more severe than the physical trauma and is potentially long lasting. Victims of sexual assault often suffer from anxiety, fearfulness, eating disorders, and chronic depression that may even lead to suicide. In most states, OEC technicians are mandated by law to report suspected sexual assault to law enforcement officials.

Sexual assault is a serious problem. Reassure the patient and contact the proper authorities, usually law enforcement, immediately. If there is bleeding, control it. Except for controlling bleeding, an exam of a sexual assault victim is best left to higher-level medical personnel. Transport to a definitive-care facility for evaluation and care is a priority. Be careful, compassionate, and respectful in your interaction with the patient. Reassure the patient, provide patient privacy, and ensure confidentialiuty. Attempt to minimize the number of people around the patient. When possible, use a female patroller for the interview and assessment.

CASE Outcome

The patient continues to complain of severe abdominal pain, and reassessment shows more vaginal bleeding with clots. A paramedic arrives with the ambulance crew. You explain what you have done to the crew. An IV line is started on scene, and transport is rapidly carried out. Just before transport, the woman's husband and children arrive. The female patroller takes the children to the side and comforts them, while the husband accompanies his wife to the hospital. You tell the husband his children will be taken to and cared for in the patrol family room until another relative can pick them up. Later that day, a sister of the patient retrieves the children. Two days later the husband returns and says his wife was nearly 3 months pregnant and had a miscarriage. She was in shock when arriving at the hospital and received three units of blood. She is improving and should be OK. He tearfully notes that without your prompt care he could have lost his wife.

CHAPTER REVIEW

In Summary

- Gynecologic emergencies are related to a woman's reproductive organs.
- Always consider the possibility of pregnancy in a female of reproductive age.
- The goals for managing obstetric and gynecologic emergencies are rapid identification of a potentially serious or life-threatening condition, immediate care, and evacuation to definitive care.
- A pregnant woman may lose 30% to 35% of her blood volume from hemorrhage before showing signs of shock.
- Maternal hemorrhage places the fetus at high risk for shock.
- All pregnant trauma patients need to be evaluated for *possible* shock.
- Prevent maternal hypotension by placing the patient on her left side.
- Always respect a woman's privacy.
- Women with an obstetric problem will require further evaluation by a physician at a medical facility.
- Be prepared to deliver a baby, if a pregnant woman is having contractions.
- If a woman is in labor, immediately contact EMS, while you prepare for delivery of the baby.
- Be prepared to resuscitate a newborn if the Apgar scores are poor.
- Always contact the proper authorities when you suspect sexual assault.

Key Terms

Abruptio placentae The premature separation of a normally situated but improperly implanted placenta; usually occurs late in pregnancy but may occur during labor.

Eclampsia A potentially life-threatening disorder in pregnant women characterized by hypertension, generalized edema, and proteinuria (protein in the urine); involves the seizures of the convulsive stage of preeclampsia-eclampsia syndrome, which are not attributable to another cerebral condition such as epilepsy.

Ectopic pregnancy A pregnancy occurring in a site other than within the uterus.

Gestational period The time from the first day of a woman's last normal menstrual period before fertilization, which is about 2 weeks before fertilization, until birth.

Meconium Fecal stool found in amniotic fluid.

Menstruation The processs in a woman of discharging blood and other materials from the lining of the uterus at intervals of about 1 month; occurs from puberty until menopause.

Miscarriage A common term for a spontaneous abortion; the spontaneous termination of a pregnancy before about 20 weeks of gestation, at which time the fetus is not yet sufficiently developed to survive.

Placenta previa Low implantation of the placenta where it partially or completely covers the internal opening of the uterus. Upon the onset of any contractions and cervical dilation, or when the cervix begins to dilate at the onset of labor, the placenta is stretched and pulled from the uterine wall, producing painless bleeding that may be life threatening to both mother and fetus.

Preeclampsia A toxemia during pregnancy characterized by high blood pressure and edema of the hands or face; also called pregnancy-induced hypertension.

Reproductive age The years when a woman can become pregnant, approximately age 12 to 49 years.

Chapter Questions

1. The female reproductive cycle begins with ovulation when an ovum or egg is released from the:
   a. fallopian tube.
   b. uterus.
   c. vagina.
   d. ovary.
2. During pregnancy, which of the following changes in vital signs would be considered normal?
   a. Decrease in heart rate
   b. Decrease in respiratory rate
   c. Decrease in blood pressure
   d. All of the above
3. A pregnant woman may lose 30% to 35% of her blood volume before showing signs of shock. If this occurs:
   a. allow the mother to drink and replenish fluids.
   b. be aware that the fetus will be in shock due to decreased blood flow.
   c. position the mother on her right side.
   d. monitor the mother closely and if further blood loss occurs, transport to the hospital.
4. Swelling of the feet and hands, indigestion, fatigue, and difficulty breathing are signs symptoms commonly experienced by women in which trimester of pregnancy?
   a. First
   b. Second
   c. Third
   d. Fourth
5. Swelling of the breasts, fatigue, nausea and vomiting, and the need to urinate frequently are signs and symptoms commonly experienced by women in which trimester of pregnancy?
   a. First
   b. Second
   c. Third
   d. Fourth
6. Initial movement of the fetus is commonly experienced by women in which trimester of pregnancy?
   a. First
   b. Second
   c. Third
   d. Fourth
7. A life-threatening condition that occurs when a fertilized egg implants outside the uterus, is called:
   a. placenta previa.
   b. ectopic pregnancy.
   c. preeclampsia.
   d. abruptio placentae.
8. You are assisting a woman who has gone into labor. After a successful delivery of the baby, you should now prepare to:
   a. allow for the delivery of the placenta.
   b. pull on the umbilical cord to ensure placenta delivery.
   c. transport the mother and baby prior to placenta delivery.
   d. All of the above

9. The emergency care management of a pregnant woman who has experienced trauma should include:
   a. anticipating and treating for shock even in the absence of signs and symptoms.
   b. positioning the patient on her left side when possible.
   c. providing rapid transport to definitive care.
   d. All of the above

10. Your patient is a woman who has experienced a possible sexual assault. Your emergency care should include:
    a. reassuring the patient.
    b. transporting to a definitive-care facility.
    c. reporting the incident to the proper authorities.
    d. All of the above

Answers: 1. d, Objective 17-1, p. 358; 2. c, Objective 17-2, p. 359; 3. b, Objective 17-4, p. 359; 4. c, Objective 17-5, p. 358; 5. a, Objective 17-5, p. 358; 6. b, Objective 17-5, p. 358; 7. b, Objective 17-6, p. 360; 8. a, Objective 17-10, p. 369; 9. d, Objective 17-9, p. 365; 10. d, Objective 17-11, p. 372

CHAPTER 18

PRINCIPLES OF TRAUMA

OBJECTIVES

Upon completion of this chapter, the OEC technician will be able to:

18-1 Define mechanism of injury.
18-2 Describe the five mechanisms of injury.
18-3 Describe why specific patients should be sent to a trauma center versus a community hospital.
18-4 Describe and demonstrate the management of a trauma patient.

KEY TERMS

Golden hour, p. 386
Injury pattern, p. 378
Kinetic energy, p. 378
Trauma, p. 378
Trauma center, p. 382

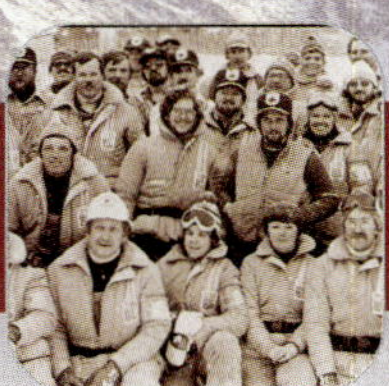

HISTORICAL TIMELINE

1980. NSP patrollers provide coverage of 1980 Winter Olympic Games in Lake Placid, New York (the first volunteer Nordic patrol at a major international event).

CHAPTER OVERVIEW

Trauma is the leading cause of death in the United States for individuals up to the age of 45 years. Trauma is also the fourth leading cause of death overall for all ages, sixth leading cause of death worldwide (resulting in 5 million deaths annually, which is 10% of all deaths), and the fifth leading cause of significant disability worldwide.[1] Because trauma is the most common emergency that OEC technicians will encounter, it is essential that OEC technicians have a firm understanding of the causes and basic management of **trauma**, or physical injury caused by an external source. Injuries in an urban setting that are considered survivable after rapid transport to a trauma center are more difficult to manage in remote locations, especially when weather is a factor.

KINETIC ENERGY AND INJURY PATTERN

Kinetic energy is an important concept in trauma. Kinetic energy is the energy of a moving object. For example, when a skier or cyclist is traveling fast and comes to an abrupt stop, a large amount of energy is absorbed, resulting in a more severe injury. When traveling slowly, less energy is absorbed, with less trauma to the body. *The speed of the individual is the important factor, not the person's size or weight.*

An **injury pattern** is a set of problems associated with a specific source of trauma. For example, someone who falls from a height, landing on their feet will more likely have injuries to their feet, ankles, and lower back. If they fall forward, they are likely to injure their wrists. Someone who dives into shallow water headfirst will likely injure their head and neck. A cyclist who stops quickly may have pelvic, genital, and abdominal injuries from hitting the handlebars. By knowing what happened to the patient, you can better assess what the mechanism of injury (MOI) could be. The MOI is the type of force that acts on the body to cause injury or the method of trauma causing an injury.

Another concept relevant to injury patterns is "stopping distance," or the amount of space necessary for kinetic energy to dissipate during an impact. Imagine if instead of hitting a tree, a snowboarder struck a pliable net that could stretch to absorb the impact (**Figure 18-1**). Once completely stopped, the amount of kinetic energy transferred

KEY POINT

Calculating Kinetic Energy

Physicists use the following equation to calculate kinetic energy:

$$\text{kinetic energy (KE)} = \frac{\text{mass} \times \text{velocity}^2}{2}$$

The patient's velocity is *squared*, making speed of the patient a more important factor than mass (size and weight) of the patient in high-energy trauma.

CASE Presentation

A bicyclist is racing on a course at a ski area in the summer. At a high rate of speed, he loses control and hits a tree. Upon your arrival on scene, you find the patient lying up against the tree which has some bark missing. He is complaining of pain in his groin and chest. Bystanders state the fall was "nasty" and that the crash "was very bad." The patient is short of breath, and says, "I think I'll be all right." The handlebars are bent.

What should you do?

would be the same, but the distribution and severity of injury would be vastly different because the flexibility of the object the person struck spread the transfer of the energy over distance and time. So, both speed and stopping distance are key factors that dramatically affect both injury potential and the severity of injuries that occur.

Just as the type of material the body strikes can influence injury severity, so does the type of body tissue that takes the impact. Different body parts have different densities; they absorb kinetic energy differently. Hollow organs such as the lungs and intestines are filled with air, whereas solid organs such as the kidneys and muscles are filled with fluid, which is much denser than air. Still other body parts, such as bone and cartilage, are more rigid and have even greater density. Because each of these structures absorbs and transmits energy differently based on their densities, they have different "thresholds of injury."

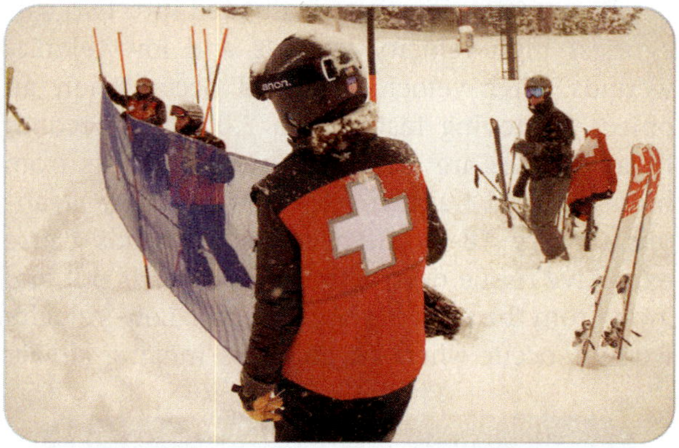

Figure 18-1 A soft-pliable barrier will allow the energy to be dissipated, possibly reducing the injury to the patient.

Bone is well suited to protecting underlying structures because it is more resistant to blunt force and punctures than is skin. When a bone breaks, it absorbs kinetic energy and reduces the amount of trauma to less-dense structures that lie beneath. Organs within the chest cavity are protected by the ribs, sternum, and spine.

Hollow ("air-dense") organs are less likely to rupture than are solid ("water-dense") organs (**Figure 18-2**). The urinary bladder is considered an air-dense organ when empty. When the bladder is full, it is a solid organ and more likely to rupture. The spleen and liver are dense; thus, they rupture with blunt force trauma. The intestines are hollow, so they are harder to rupture.

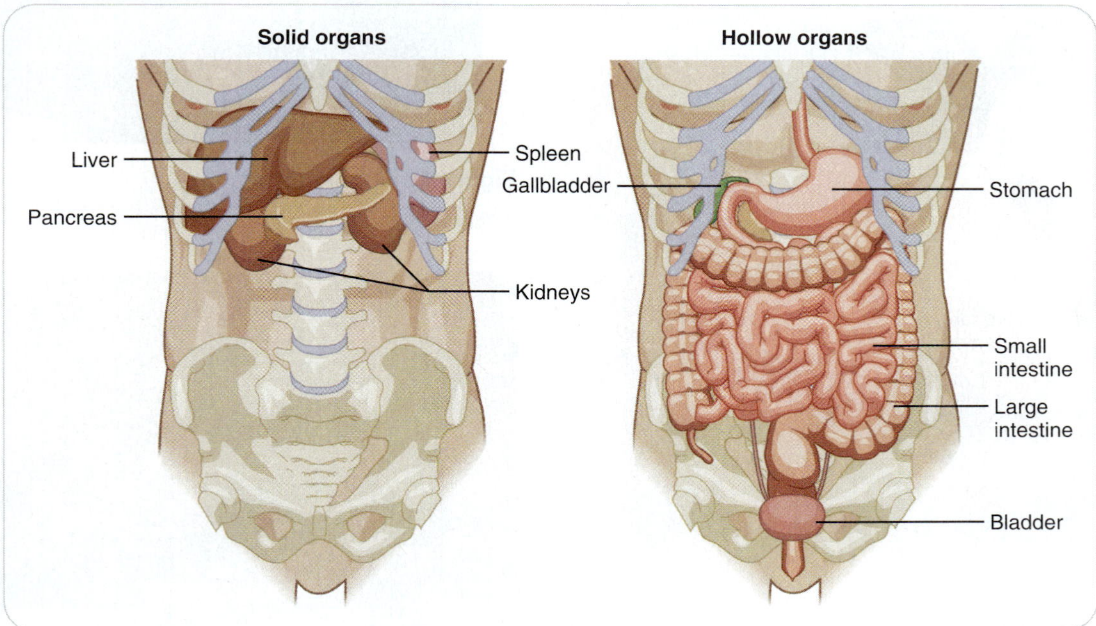

Figure 18-2 Solid organs are denser than hollow organs and thus are more likely to rupture upon impact.

MECHANISMS OF INJURY

Different types of MOIs will produce many types of injuries. OEC technicians should be familiar with the following five major MOIs:

1. Impact/blunt injury
2. Penetrating injury
3. Rotational injury
4. Crush injury
5. Blast injury

Impact/Blunt Injury

The severity of bodily injury from blunt trauma is directly related to three factors: the amount of kinetic energy absorbed, the direction the energy travels through the body, and the density of the body structures impacted (**Figure 18-3**). An impact/blunt, or "closed," injury is one in which kinetic energy is transmitted through, but does not break, the skin. Instead, it is transmitted to underlying structures, resulting in injuries such as bruised tissues, internal bleeding, broken bones, and organ damage. Impact/blunt injuries are commonly seen in falls, ski slope collisions, snowmobile accidents, and as a result of physical assault.

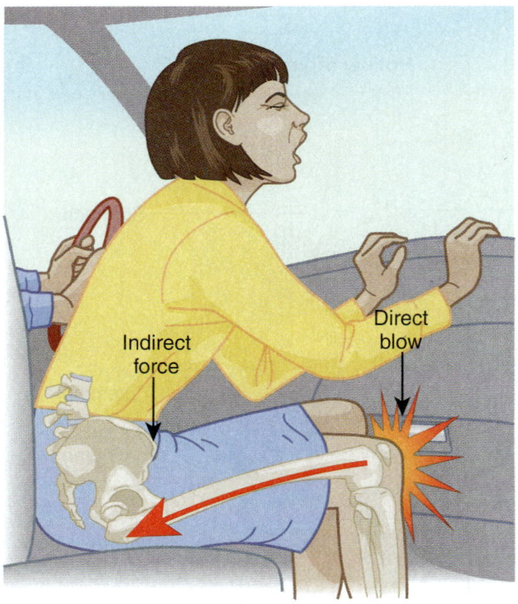

Figure 18-3 With blunt force injuries, the kinetic energy is transmitted through the skin to the underlying bones/organs.

Penetrating Injury

A penetrating, or "open" injury, is one that breaks the skin and damages underlying structures (**Figure 18-4**). A smaller surface of the skin is affected when an object in motion, such as an ice tool, a knife, or a bullet, strikes the body with enough kinetic energy to pierce the skin. It can also occur when the body is moving with enough kinetic energy to impale itself upon an object such as a tree branch, a ski pole, or an ice axe.

Penetrating injuries are divided into two categories: high-velocity wounds and low-velocity wounds. High-velocity wounds occur when an object is moving faster than 2,000 feet/second; these injuries are usually caused by bullets from high-powered hunting rifles and military weapons (**Figure 18-5**). High-velocity wounds cause extensive tissue destruction that spreads out and away from the path of the projectile. Low-velocity wounds occur when an object is moving slower

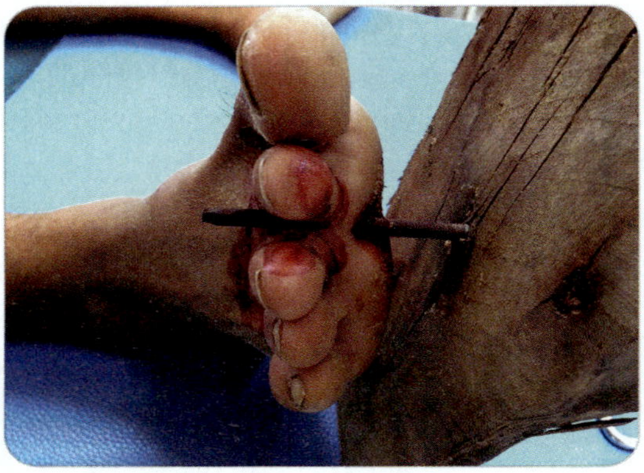

Figure 18-4 A penetrating injury.

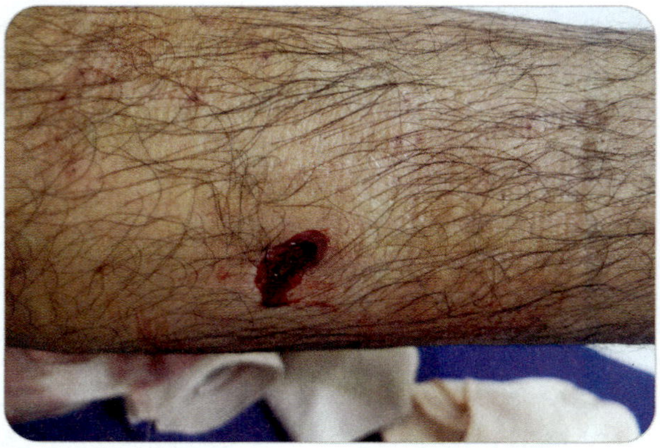

Figure 18-5 A high-velocity entrance wound.

than 2,000 feet/second. Gunshot wounds from handguns and stab wounds are examples of low-velocity wounds. Tissue destruction is limited to the actual path of the moving object.

Rotational Injury

Rotational injuries occur when energy is transmitted to the body in a twisting direction (Figure 18-6). This can happen to a joint when it is twisted through an abnormal range of motion. Examples include turning an ankle while hiking, dislocating a shoulder after catching a ski pole on a tree branch, or twisting the lower leg and causing a spiral tibia fracture. The primary factor in a rotational injury is the direction the energy is traveling through the body, as opposed to the amount of energy absorbed in the impact of an object that strikes the body. The energy travels through the body in a rotational or twisting direction.

Crush Injury

A crush or compression injury occurs when a body part is caught between two or more hard objects and is subjected to significant compressive force or pressure (Figure 18-7). This type of injury can produce devastating wounds that include penetrating trauma, blunt trauma, or both. Such injuries are common in river sports, backcountry skiing, and mountaineering. For example, when a person's arm is pinned between a large rock and a tree for an extended period of time, the tissue begins to die. Avalanche victims can also suffer from crush injuries from heavy packed snow.

Blast Injury

Blast injuries are caused by an explosive force and are divided into four categories: primary, secondary, tertiary, and miscellaneous (or quaternary) injuries (Figure 18-8).

Primary blast injuries are due to a massive pressure wave that strikes the body following the rapid release and expansion of gases. Solid and water-dense tissues (such as the liver or urinary bladder) are minimally affected, whereas air-dense tissues (such as the lungs, ears, or intestines) can be contused or ruptured. Secondary blast injuries are caused by airborne objects that strike the body. Tertiary blast injuries occur when the body is forcibly thrown and strikes other objects such as a wall or the ground.

Tertiary blast injuries are usually seen only in high-energy explosions. Miscellaneous, or quaternary, injuries are caused by other blast-related factors such as exposure to steam or burning materials, inhalation of toxins, or impact by debris from a collapsing building. When aggravated by a blast, illnesses including asthma, angina, hypertension, and anxiety are also considered quaternary injuries.

Blast injuries are more commonly associated with an industrial accident or a military/terrorist event, but they could be encountered in kitchens or backcountry environments. Examples include a camp stove explosion, a mountain lodge kitchen

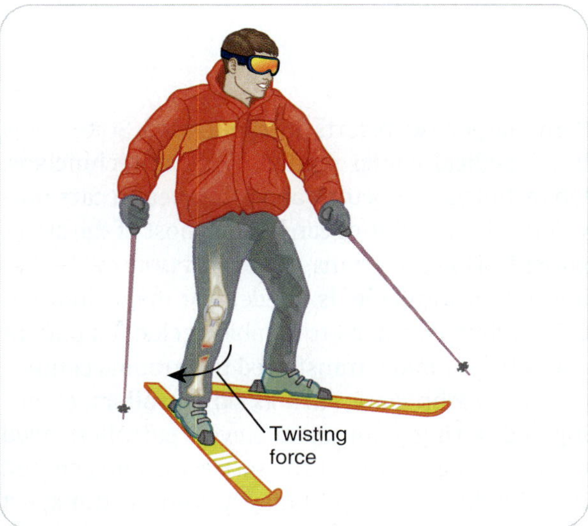

Figure 18-6 A rotational injury.

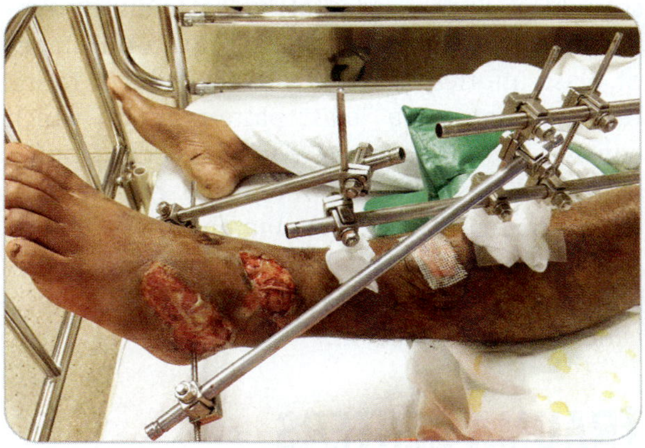

Figure 18-7 A crush injury.

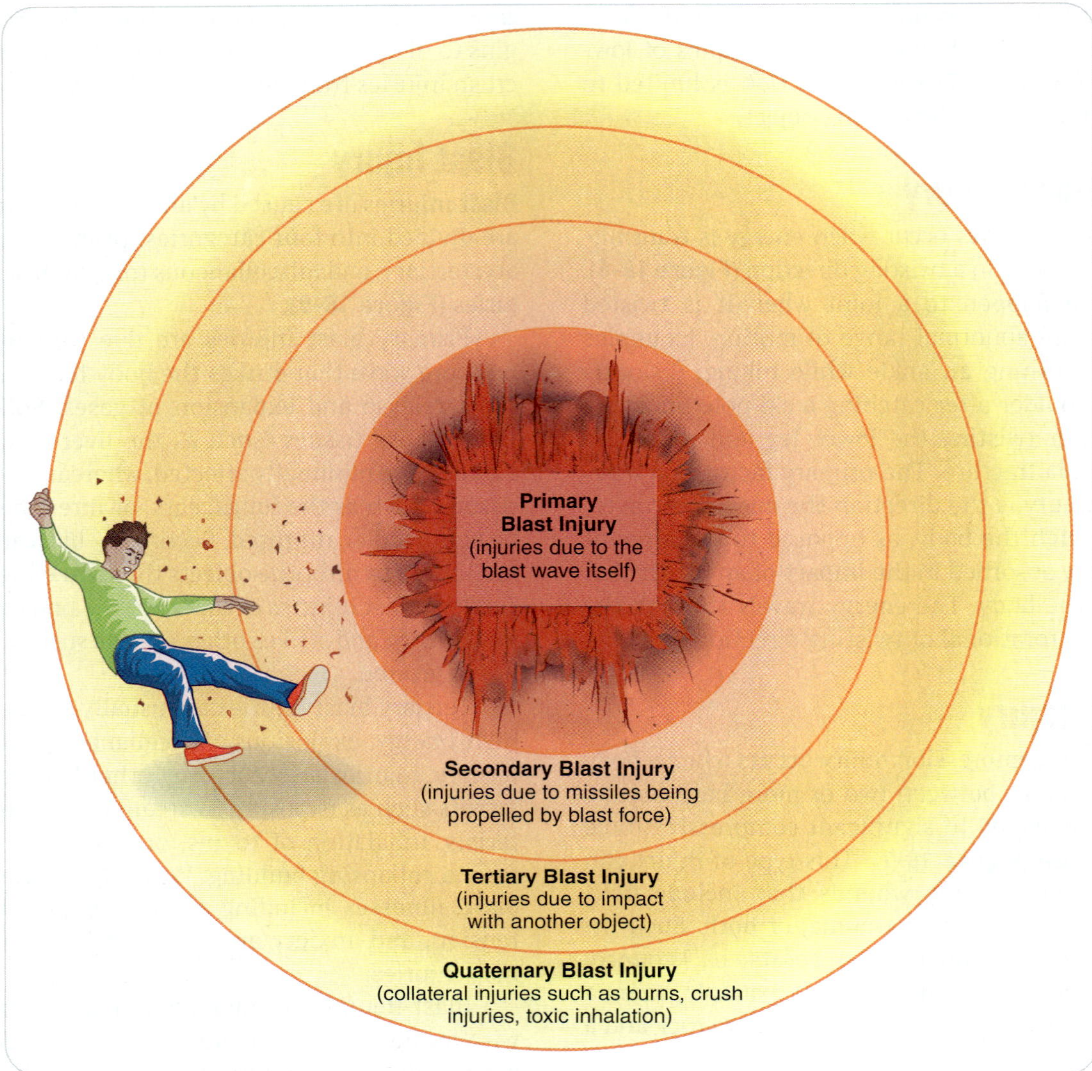

Figure 18-8 The mechanisms of blast injuries.

stove blast, or an accidental explosion during avalanche control measures. During the initial stages of blast injuries, patients often exhibit a reflex response, termed a "blast pattern triad," which consists of initial apnea ("wind knocked out"), bradycardia (slow heart rate), and hypotension (low blood pressure). Fortunately, these abnormal vital signs usually return to pre-blast values within a relatively short time unless other significant injuries are present.

TRAUMA CENTERS

Most minor injuries you will encounter can be seen in local or community outpatient hospital setting. Some larger ski resorts in the United States now have medical clinics staffed by x-ray technicians, lab technicians, doctors, and other health care providers. These facilities can handle most of the area's patients. However, transport to a **trauma center** using ALS, if available, is needed for major injuries. OEC technicians need to be able decide if a patient needs to be rapidly transferred to a trauma center.

OEC technicians such as ski patrollers, climbing and rafting guides, and bicycle patrollers need to know the location of the nearest trauma center. If available, air transport may hasten the transport time to these specialized centers (**Figure 18-9**). With the help of the local EMS system, develop a local protocol regarding air transport.

A national system of designated accredited trauma centers has been established in the United States to provide specialized care to multisystem trauma patients. Trauma centers are equipped to provide care to trauma patients at any time and are specifically designed to manage patients whose injuries involve two or more body systems, a condition known as multisystem trauma. Examples of patients with multisystem trauma are a patient with a possible fractured femur and internal abdominal injuries. Definitive care at these centers is coordinated by a trauma surgeon, who is a physician with specialized training in the treatment of severely injured patients. This doctor usually takes the lead, calling on specialists when needed.

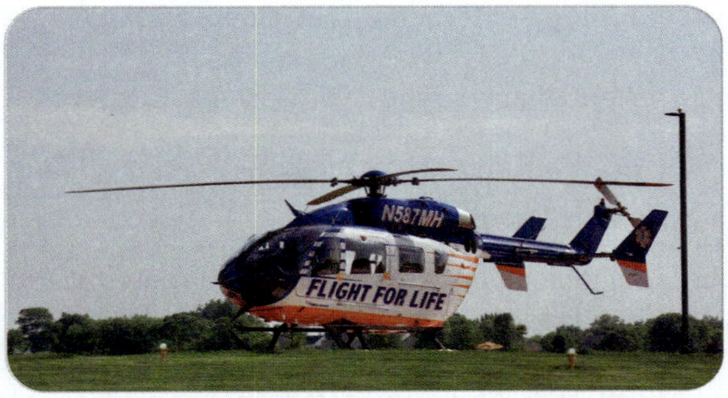

Figure 18-9 The severity of the patient's injuries might require air transport to get to a trauma center as quickly as possible.

Destination Selection

The American College of Surgeons (ACS) designates each trauma center at one of five levels based on the specialization, complexity, and availability of care that the facility can accommodate (**Table 18-1**). Also, some trauma centers are now designated as pediatric trauma centers, specializing in children's trauma care. Burn centers, handling severely burned patients are also available. An OEC technician should work with the local EMS system's providers to determine the level of care needed for serious patients. It is important to understand that some states or territories do not follow ACS guidelines or designations.

PATIENT ASSESSMENT FOR TRAUMA

Assessment begins with a scene size-up where potential hazards are identified and addressed (**Figure 18-10**). Because traumatic injuries often include the presence of body fluids such as blood, urine, and cerebrospinal fluid, OEC technicians must follow standard precautions using appropriate protective gear.

The scene size-up includes determining the MOI. If the MOI has produced severe injuries, assess the need for spinal motion restriction. If indicated, manually restrict the motion of the neck. Determine whether the incident involves multiple patients, or whether the injuries incurred require

CASE Update

You are concerned that the patient's MOI—slamming into the handlebars and then a tree at a high rate of speed—may have caused internal injuries. After making the scene safe, you check for life-threatening bleeding and assess the ABCDs. The patient talks to you in short sentences. You complete your primary patient assessment and radio for extra help and equipment.

The patient's initial pulse was 92 beats per minute and respirations were 18 breaths per minute; they are now 140 beats per minute and 26 breaths per minute. You suspect that the deterioration in condition is due to internal injuries caused by blunt trauma. You notify the dispatcher to activate EMS and request air transport. The pain in the patient's anterior pelvic area and chest is significant.

What should you do now?

Table 18-1 Key Elements for Trauma Centers

Trauma Center Level	Elements of the Trauma Level
I	• 24-hour in-house coverage by general surgeons, and prompt availability of care in specialties such as orthopedic surgery, neurosurgery, anesthesiology, emergency medicine, radiology, internal medicine, plastic surgery, oral and maxillofacial, pediatric, and critical care. • Referral resource for communities in nearby regions. • Provides leadership in prevention, public education to surrounding communities. • Provides continuing education of the trauma team members. • Incorporates a comprehensive quality assessment program. • Operates an organized teaching and research effort to help direct new innovations in trauma care. • Provides program for substance abuse screening and patient intervention. • Meets minimum requirement for annual volume of severely injured patients.
II	• 24-hour in-house coverage by general surgeons, as well as coverage by the specialties of orthopedic surgery, neurosurgery, anesthesiology, emergency medicine, radiology, and critical care. • Tertiary care needs such as cardiac surgery, hemodialysis, and microvascular surgery may be referred to a Level I trauma center. • Provides trauma prevention and continuing education programs for staff. • Incorporates a comprehensive quality assessment program.
III	• 24-hour immediate coverage by emergency medicine physicians and the prompt availability of general surgeons and anesthesiologists. • Incorporates a comprehensive quality assessment program. • Has developed transfer agreements for patients requiring more comprehensive care at a Level I or Level II trauma center. • Provides backup care for rural and community hospitals. • Offers continuing education of the nursing and allied health personnel or the trauma team. • Involved with prevention efforts and must have an active outreach program for its referring communities.
IV	• Basic emergency department facilities to implement Advanced Trauma Life Support (ATLS) protocols and 24-hour laboratory coverage. Available trauma nurse(s) and physicians available upon patient arrival. • May provide surgery and critical-care services if available. • Has developed transfer agreements for patients requiring more comprehensive care at a Level I or Level II trauma center. • Incorporates a comprehensive quality assessment program • Involved with prevention efforts and must have an active outreach program for its referring communities.
V	• Basic emergency department facilities to implement ATLS protocols • Available trauma nurse(s) and physicians available upon patient arrival. • After-hours activation protocols if facility is not open 24 hours a day. • May provide surgery and critical-care services if available. • Has developed transfer agreements for patients requiring more comprehensive care at a Level I though III trauma centers.

Reproduced from Trauma Center Levels Explained, Designation Vs. Verification. American Trauma Society. Retrieved from https://www.amtrauma.org/page/TraumaLevels. Accessed December 4, 2019.

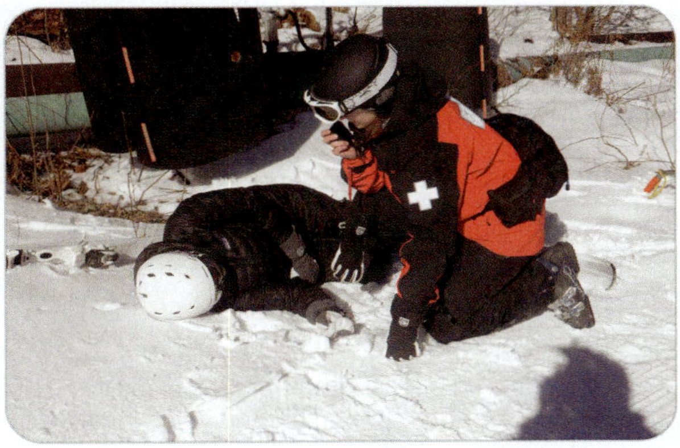

Figure 18-10 Scene size-up, addressing life threats, and assessing the patient's ABCDs are the first steps of the patient assessment process.

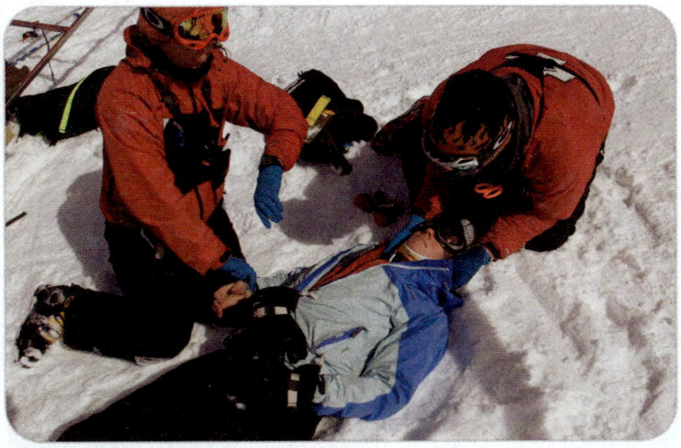

Figure 18-11 Obtaining a baseline set of vital signs is an important part of the secondary patient assessment.

immediate EMS intervention and/or rapid evacuation to a trauma center.

A trauma assessment should include a quick evaluation of the patient's level of responsiveness followed by a primary assessment of the ABCDs, with initial emphasis on identifying the need for lifesaving interventions such as controlling life-threatening bleeding. This should take no more than 30 seconds to complete. Once immediate threats to life have been corrected, obtain a medical history. Obtaining a complete medical history is a critical part of the patient assessment process. As part of the history taking process, use OPQRST to assess pain. If the patient is unresponsive and there were no witnesses to the incident, a good history may not be attainable. You must then base your assessment of what happened on what the scene tells you. For example, if you find an unresponsive patient with a deformed thigh lying beneath a cliff, the person most likely fell off the cliff. Also, check patients for a medic alert tag. In addition to a standard SAMPLE history, obtain trauma-specific information. Look at the forces involved. In unwitnessed trauma patients, assessment of many suspected trauma injuries may be based only on a good understanding of how the trauma occurred. Based on the MOI, a thorough evaluation of a body part suspected to be injured is important.

Next, perform a full hands-on head-to-toe secondary physical assessment examining the head, neck, chest, abdomen, pelvis, legs, back, and arms for other injuries. When there is multiple trauma, this exam may find additional injuries that were overshadowed by another more painful injury. Do this in unresponsive patients also, as a hands-on exam of a long bone may reveal a possible fracture. The DCAP-BTLS method is a very helpful tool that can facilitate this process, with the head-to-toe exam taking 2 minutes or less. Obtain a set of vital signs during the secondary patient assessment (**Figure 18-11**). Take the pulse and respirations; blood pressure may be approximated by finding a carotid, femoral, or radial pulse, as described in Chapter 7, *Patient Assessment*.

Well-meaning bystanders often attempt to render aid to an injured person. Unfortunately, their actions may have unintended consequences or even cause additional injury. Examples include moving a patient with a spinal injury, blocking the airway by placing a jacket under the patient's head, pulling out an impaled object, or applying an inappropriate tourniquet.

The information obtained through the patient assessment should enable you to formulate a treatment plan and help you decide if the patient's injuries require immediate transport (**Figure 18-12**). When making a transport decision, consider whether evacuation is necessary because this may warrant the mobilization of a helicopter, an extrication vehicle, or a specialized wilderness search-and-rescue team. Other factors such as current weather conditions, expected weather changes, terrain, temperature, time of day, and altitude must also be considered.

Monitor and reassess the patient frequently by taking vital signs every 5 minutes for critical

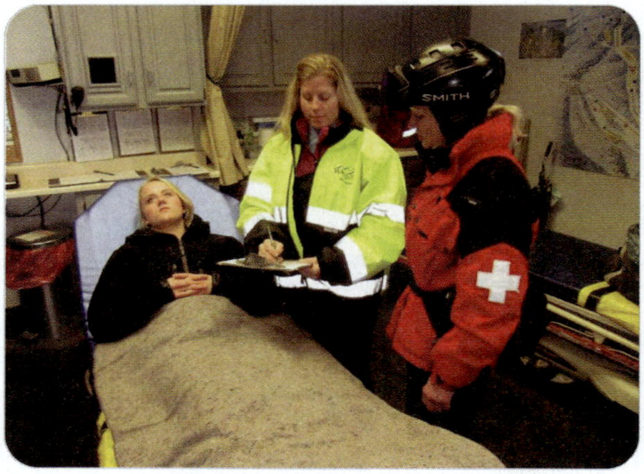

Figure 18-12 With the information from the patient assessment, you will be able to determine the best method of transportation for your patient.

> **KEY POINT**
>
> **Golden Hour**
>
> The first hour following a life-threatening injury is a crucial period during which survival rates may be improved if critical injuries are identified and properly managed. This period is referred to as the **golden hour**. In backcountry settings, caring for these life threats can be difficult, and thus immediate evacuation to a specialized definitive-care facility, known as a trauma center, becomes important.

patients, and every 15 minutes for noncritical patients. Reassess the area of injury frequently to ensure that, for example, bleeding that had been controlled has not started again.

MANAGEMENT OF TRAUMA

Management of trauma patients varies greatly and depends on the MOI, injury severity, available resources, and distance to a medical facility.

As for any patient, the first step in managing a person who has been injured is to mitigate any hazards that may be present. Next, correct any immediate threats to life (ABCD). Control excessive bleeding. If the patient is unresponsive, it is important to open the airway, simultaneously assess breathing, and make sure there is a carotid pulse (feel for 10 seconds). If the patient is not breathing and there is no pulse, immediately begin CPR. If indicated, stabilize the patient's spine by applying manual stabilization to the head and neck. This must be maintained until replaced with mechanical stabilization.

Critical multisystem trauma patients may need a "load-and-go" approach. Manage the ABCDs, control bleeding, stabilize the spine if needed, load the patient into the toboggan or onto the litter, and transport with as little delay as possible.

Once all life threats have been managed in severely injured patients, if oxygen is immediately available, administer oxygen at 12 to 15 liters per minute by nonrebreather mask. Titrate oxygen with a pulse oximeter, if available, keeping the oxygen saturation between 94 and 99%. If a patient needs rapid transport for life threats you cannot correct, do not wait for oxygen to arrive on scene; transport and provide oxygen when available (**Figure 18-13**).

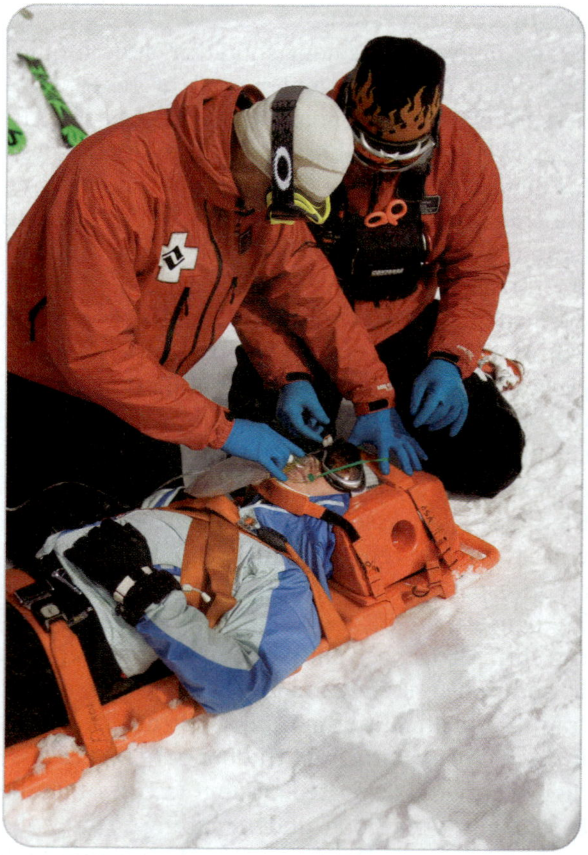

Figure 18-13 Transport the patient as soon as possible for critical trauma patients.

Monitor patients for shock and treat accordingly, being careful to keep them warm because hypothermia can hasten the effects of shock.

For patients who are stable and do not require load-and-go transport, turn your attention to any less critical injuries or problems that may exist, such as stabilizing long-bone fractures by applying splints. Then, prepare patients for transport to a medical care facility or, when appropriate, to a trauma center. The mode of transportation largely depends on your findings during the assessment. In general, protect trauma patients who need spinal motion restriction from the elements and secure them either to a long backboard or in a basket-style litter. Base your additional treatment decisions on reassessment findings. Finally, document your assessment findings and the treatments you provided on a patient care report, and if local protocol allows, send a copy with the patient to the hospital.

CASE Outcome

As other patrollers arrive with oxygen and equipment, you inform them that you believe the patient is suffering from blunt trauma and has a high potential for serious internal injury. Given the MOI, the patient's deteriorating state, and your assessment findings, you suspect a fractured pelvis with internal bleeding, and an internal chest injury.

Recognizing that this is a load-and-go situation, you place the patient on high-flow oxygen by nonrebreather mask and prepare to evacuate him from the slopes as expeditiously as possible. The patrollers use a pelvic binder to stabilize the pelvis and use spinal motion restriction with a long backboard. By radio, you notify the base clinic of your impending arrival. After delivering the patient, an ALS provider starts an IV. Soon after, a helicopter crew arrives and begins administering blood to the patient. They transport him past the local community hospital, which is only a few miles away, in favor of a Level II trauma center just a few air miles farther.

Later that day, the clinic physician joins you during a break in the patroller hut. He tells you that he received a call from a trauma surgeon congratulating him and his staff on the rapid and comprehensive field care of the patient, who broke his pelvis in four places and had a collapsed lung. The patient is now stable and expected to make a full recovery.

CHAPTER REVIEW

In Summary

- The more energy or force the body receives during trauma, the greater the possibility of serious injury.
- The MOI will give important clues to help assess the injuries sustained.
- The speed of a person who strikes a fixed object is a more important factor for determining seriousness of trauma than is the size of the person.
- Hollow organs are less likely to rupture than are solid organs.
- The five mechanisms of trauma are impact/blunt, penetrating injury, rotational injury, crush injury, and blast injury.
- A trauma center is a specialized medical facility geared toward addressing the specific needs of trauma patients.
- Whenever possible, multisystem trauma patients should be taken to a trauma center.
- When indicated by the MOI and patient findings, spinal motion restriction is essential.
- The three goals of serious trauma management are early recognition, correction of threats to life, and rapid transport to a trauma center.

Key Terms

Golden hour The first 60 minutes following a serious traumatic event, during which prompt medical treatment may prevent death.

Injury pattern A combination of injuries commonly seen in a patient based on the mechanism of injury.

Kinetic energy The energy generated by a body in motion.

Trauma Physical injury caused by an external force.

Trauma center A specialized hospital providing 24-hour trauma care, including stabilization, critical care, subspecialty care, and nursing care.

Chapter Questions

1. Mechanism of injury results from:
   a. the amount of kinetic energy absorbed.
   b. the direction the energy travels through the body.
   c. the density of the body structures impacted.
   d. All of the above
2. Which of the following is one of the five types of injuries that can be considered a mechanism of injury in trauma?
   a. Penetrating injury
   b. Rotational injury
   c. Crush injury
   d. All of the above
3. Rotational injuries occur when:
   a. energy is transmitted to the body in a twisting direction.
   b. energy is transmitted through, but does not break, the skin.
   c. a body part is caught between two or more heavy objects
   d. a body part is subjected to a blast.
4. Crush injuries occur when:
   a. energy is transmitted to the body in a twisting direction.
   b. kinetic energy is transmitted through, but does not break, the skin.
   c. a body part is subjected to minimal pressure.
   d. a body part is subjected to significant compressive force or pressure.
5. What is the term for the first hour following a life-threatening injury, during which survival rates may be improved if critical injuries are identified and properly managed?
   a. The golden hour
   b. The 11th hour
   c. The news hour
   d. The last hour

6. Assessment and management of the trauma patient should include:
   a. reassessing the patient every 30 minutes.
   b. transporting trauma patients without a scene size up.
   c. initiating CPR on all patients with chest trauma.
   d. determining the mechanism of injury.

Reference

[1] American Association for the Surgery of Trauma. n.d. Trauma facts. http://www.aast.org/trauma-facts. Accessed December 4, 2019.

Answers: 1. d, Objective 18-1, p. 380; 2. d, Objective 18-3, p. 380; 3. a, Objective 18-2, p. 381; 4. d, Objective 18-2, p. 381; 5. a, Objective 18-3, p. 386; 6. d, Objective 18-4, p. 383

CHAPTER 19

SOFT-TISSUE INJURIES AND BURNS

OBJECTIVES

Upon completion of this chapter, the OEC technician will be able to:

19-1 List the four functions of the skin.
19-2 List the layers of the skin.
19-3 Explain the difference between arterial and venous bleeding.
19-4 Explain how to assess a soft-tissue injury.
19-5 Describe and demonstrate care for the following closed soft-tissue injuries:

- Contusion
- Hematoma
- Crush injury
- Compartment syndrome

19-6 Describe and demonstrate care for the following open soft-tissue injuries:

- Abrasion
- Amputation
- Avulsion
- High-pressure injection injury
- Incision
- Laceration
- Mechanical tattooing
- Open crush injury
- Puncture, including impaled object

19-7 Explain the difference between thermal, chemical, electrical, lightning, and radiation burns, and the treatment for each.
19-8 Explain how to assess and care for sunburn, and what SPF means for sun creams.
19-9 Explain how to assess and care for a burn.
19-10 Explain and describe how to classify burns by depth of injury.
19-11 Explain and demonstrate the different methods to control bleeding, including application of a tourniquet.
19-12 Explain the difference between a bandage and a dressing.
19-13 Describe and demonstrate how to apply a dressing and bandage, including occlusive and stabilizing dressings.
19-14 Explain which burn patients need to be transferred to a "burn center."
19-15 Explain how to assess and treat an individual struck by lightning.

KEY TERMS

Amputation, p. 398
Avulsion, p. 398
Bandage, p. 413
Burn, p. 399
Compartment syndrome, p. 397
Compression (pressure) dressing, p. 409
Crush injury, p. 396
Dressing, p. 413
Ecchymosis, p. 395
Exsanguination, p. 411
Hematoma, p. 395
Hemorrhage, p. 408
Hemostatic dressing, p. 410
Impaled object, p. 421

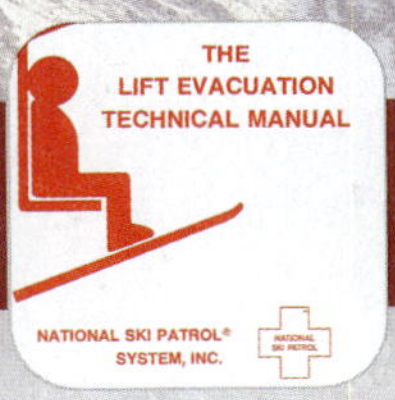

HISTORICAL TIMELINE **1982.** NSP co-publishes "Lift Evacuation Technical Manual" with the National Ski Areas Association (NSAA).

Incision, p. 397
Laceration, p. 397
Mucous membranes, p. 395
Occlusive dressing, p. 414
Puncture, p. 398
RISE, p. 419
Scald, p. 400
Subungual hematoma, p. 396
Tourniquet, p. 408
Universal dressing, p. 413

CHAPTER OVERVIEW

Soft-tissue injuries are common occurrences in outdoor recreation and are an inherent risk of nearly every outdoor sport and activity. These injuries are among the most common emergencies that OEC technicians will encounter. Identifying various soft-tissue wounds, controlling external bleeding, and caring for these injuries are essential skills.

Soft-tissue injuries encompass wounds of the skin and all soft tissues, down to and including muscle. They include everything from abrasions, simple lacerations, and bruises to life-threatening bleeding and major amputations. Burns can be devastating injuries, especially if much of the surface of the body is involved.

The skin has several functions, the most important of which is to serve as a protective barrier to external contaminants. In addition to its protective functions, the skin contains millions of tiny nerves that continually send sensory information to the brain. Although it is flexible and resilient, the skin is not impervious to injury and is easily damaged when exposed to abrasive or sharp objects or to heat, cold, or caustic substances. When penetrated, the skin's underlying structures and organs may be exposed to a variety of bacteria that can establish infections.

ANATOMY AND PHYSIOLOGY

The skin is the body's largest organ and covers its entire external surface. It serves many purposes, including acting as a protective barrier, regulating body temperature, maintaining water balance, and synthesizing vitamin D.

CASE Presentation

As a member of your area bike patrol, you are called to assist a participant in a summer bicycle race who apparently lost control on the curve of a steep gravel road. As you approach the patient, you can see that his wrist and leg are covered with blood. He is responsive and alert but in obvious pain. After the scene is safe, you introduce yourself and ask him what happened. He says, "I lost it in the gravel." The patient is wearing a helmet and denies striking his head. He denies any neck or back pain. You note a deep, actively bleeding laceration over the cyclist's left wrist and "road rash" on his left leg. Immediately you put on protective medical gloves and notify dispatch that you will need EMS for significant bleeding.

What should you do?

Skin Anatomy

As described in Chapter 6, *Anatomy and Physiology*, the skin consists of two layers: the epidermis, which lies on the surface and is several layers thick, and the dermis, which lies beneath the epidermis and contains several unique structures (**Figure 19-1**). Beneath the dermis are the subcutaneous tissue, muscles, bones, and other underlying structures.

The epidermis continuously produces new skin cells that steadily migrate toward the surface. As these cells become more superficial, they are bonded securely together by an oily material to form a watertight, protective layer that helps the body retain water and prevents bacteria and other organisms from entering the body. The outermost epidermal cells are continually being rubbed away by normal daily activities and bathing and are replaced by new cells from below. The epidermis is very thick on the soles of the feet, the palms of the hands, the back, and the scalp, but it is very thin in other areas of the body, such as the back of the hand. Pigment granules in the epidermis along with small blood vessels in the dermis combine to produce skin color.

The dermis is the layer of the skin deep to the epidermis, and it contains several important structures, including hair follicles, sebaceous (oil) glands, sweat glands, blood vessels, and specialized nerve endings.

Hair follicles are the structures that produce hairs. Adjacent to each follicle are both a sebaceous gland and a very small muscle. Sebaceous glands secrete an oily substance, known as sebum, onto the skin surface. In addition to its waterproofing function, sebum helps keep the skin supple and prevents it from cracking. The adjacent muscle fibers cause the hair to stand on end when a person becomes cold or frightened.

Sweat glands secrete a liquid that helps cool the body. Sweat is released from the dermis onto the surface of the skin through small pores, or ducts, that pass through the epidermis. Blood vessels that provide nutrients and oxygen to the skin are found in the dermis and send small branches up to the bottom layer of the epidermis.

Specialized nerve endings found within the dermis detect and then transmit to the brain data concerning heat, cold, body position, external pressure, and painful and pleasurable stimuli.

The subcutaneous tissue lies beneath the dermis and is composed almost entirely of fat, which insulates the body and stores energy. The amount, thickness, and composition of subcutaneous tissue vary greatly from one area of the

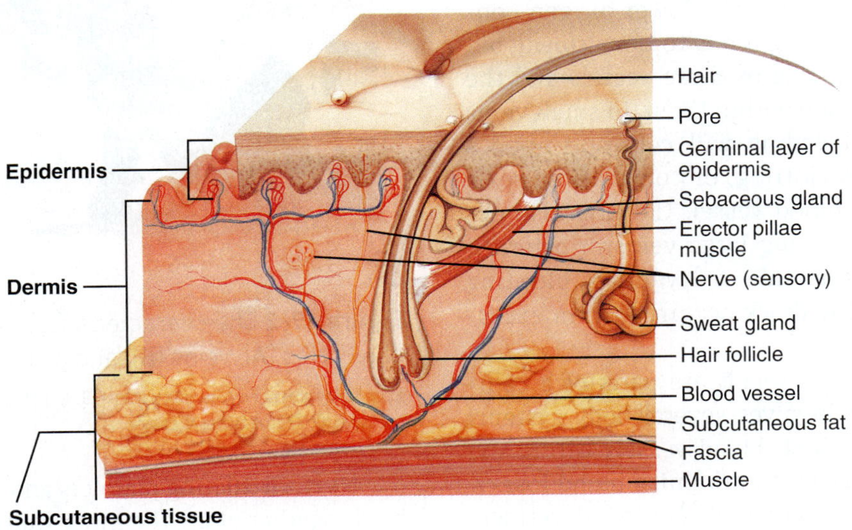

Figure 19-1 The layers of the skin and underlying structures.

body to another and from one individual to another. The body's musculature and the bony skeleton are found directly beneath the subcutaneous tissue and are discussed in more detail in other chapters.

In addition to its function as a protective barrier, the skin participates in the regulation of body temperature. In a cold environment, hair follicles become erect to trap warm air near the skin's surface. At the same time, when you are cold, blood vessels within the dermis and subcutaneous tissue constrict to shunt blood away from these areas, which helps to slow heat loss. In a hot environment, dermal blood vessels dilate, causing the skin to become warm and flushed, which allows heat to radiate away from the body and into the environment. Additionally, sweat glands secrete sweat onto the surface of the skin, where it evaporates and thus cools the skin (and body temperature) through the process of evaporation.

Physiology of Bleeding and Clotting

Bleeding results from a leak or breakage in an artery, a vein, and/or tissue capillaries (**Figure 19-2**). If an artery is damaged, the high arterial pressure within produces pulsating spurts of blood that is bright red because of its higher oxygen content. Conversely, blood from a lacerated vein flows freely and evenly under less pressure and is slightly darker red due to its lower oxygen content. Capillary bleeding tends to ooze slowly because of the small size of these vessels and the low pressure of blood within them. In small veins and capillaries, bleeding will continue until a process known as clotting, or coagulation, seals off the damaged blood vessel. Clotting also occurs in bleeds involving large veins or arteries; however, without outside intervention, bleeding may continue, with shock occurring from excessive blood loss.

Clotting and skin repair are parts of a complex process that involves several body systems working together. First, blood vessels within the affected area constrict to minimize blood loss. A blood vessel that is completely cut in half retracts into the soft tissue around it, slowing down the flow. A vessel that is cut on only one side will not retract and bleeds more.

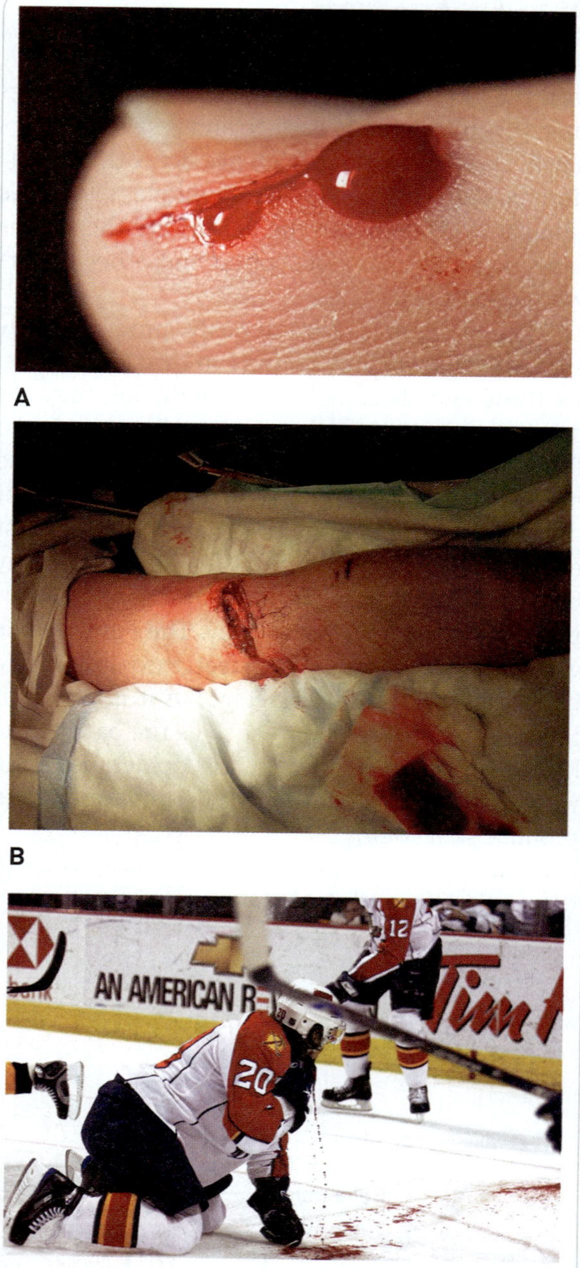

Figure 19-2 The characteristics of bleeding from capillaries (**A**), veins (**B**), and arteries (**C**).

A: © Sasha Radosavljevic/iStock/Getty Images; **B:** © E.M. Singletary, M.D. Used with permission; **C:** © Brian Slichta/AP Images.

Next, circulating platelets and plasma proteins bind together along the inner wall of the damaged vessel to form a temporary "plug," thereby sealing the hole in the vessel. At the same time, an inflammatory response causes swelling in the area, pushing the sides of the wound closer together. Additional platelets and plasma proteins bind at the periphery of the wound, forming a scab, which acts as a temporary barrier that keeps out bacteria and other contaminants. White blood cells migrate to the wound to fight infection. Within a few days, the scab is replaced underneath by epidermal cells that have quickly multiplied. These cells form "new" skin as a scar. Depending on the size and depth of the wound, complete tissue replacement may take several days to weeks. When a scab forms, it is best to not remove it, as it acts as a human Band-Aid.

Some patients take prescribed "blood thinning" medications. These medications, called anticoagulants, do not really thin the blood; instead, they therapeutically slow the normal clotting process for patients with certain medical conditions, such as a heart arrhythmia or a history of a blood clot in the leg, lungs, heart, or brain. Bleeding is more difficult to control in these patients. Ask patients if they take a "blood thinner" such as aspirin, warfarin (Coumadin), dabigatran (Pradaxa), or clopidogrel (Plavix). There are many other anticoagulants.

TYPES OF SOFT-TISSUE INJURIES

The soft tissues are commonly injured because they are in the more superficial layers of the body. OEC technicians should be familiar with three types of soft-tissue injuries:

- Closed injuries
- Open injuries
- Burns

Closed Injuries

Closed soft-tissue injuries result in damage to structures beneath the skin or **mucous membranes** while the overlying skin surface remains intact. These injuries run the gamut from mild to severe, depending on the mechanism of injury.

OEC technicians most commonly encounter the following four types of closed soft-tissue injuries:

- Contusions
- Hematomas
- Crush injuries
- Compartment syndrome

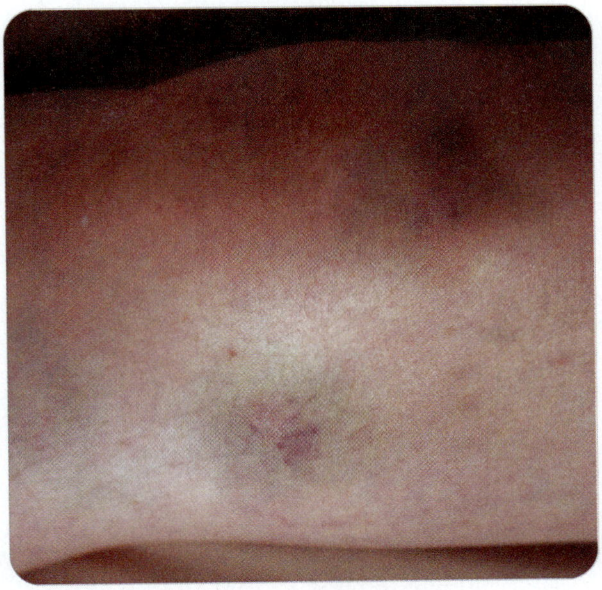

Figure 19-3 An example of a contusion.

Contusions

In contusions, the epidermis, or outer layer of skin, is not disrupted, but cells within the dermis are injured and the smallest blood vessels are torn. Contusions are typically produced when a blunt force strikes the body or when the body strikes an immovable surface. The extent and severity of the injury depend on the amount of energy absorbed by the soft tissue. Cellular fluid and blood leak into the injured area, causing tenderness, pain, and localized swelling. The breakdown of blood cells that leak out of capillaries beneath the dermis eventually produces a characteristic blue or black skin discoloration known as a bruise, or **ecchymosis**. As the injury heals, the bruise will change in color from black or purple to yellow or green (**Figure 19-3**). Eventually, a bruise will disappear as the leaked blood is reabsorbed by the body.

Hematomas

A **hematoma** is a collection of blood that has leaked from a blood vessel and is confined to a localized area inside the body, usually as the result of a blunt soft-tissue injury (**Figure 19-4**). It is a collection (mass) of blood between the tissues. Hematomas are produced when an injured blood vessel bleeds, bone marrow leaks out of a broken

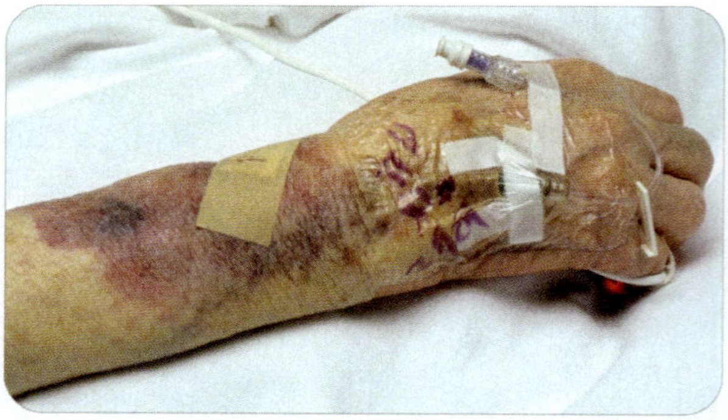

Figure 19-4 A hematoma, or collection of blood under the skin.

Courtesy of Rhonda Hunt.

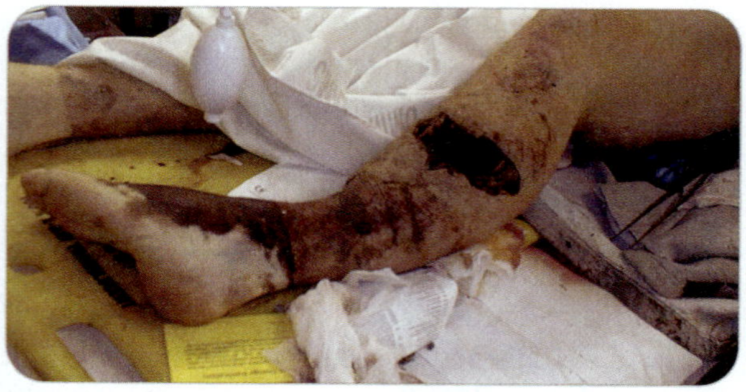

Figure 19-6 An example of a crush injury. Note the extreme swelling resulting from compression of the soft tissues.

© Andrew Pollak, MD. Used with permission.

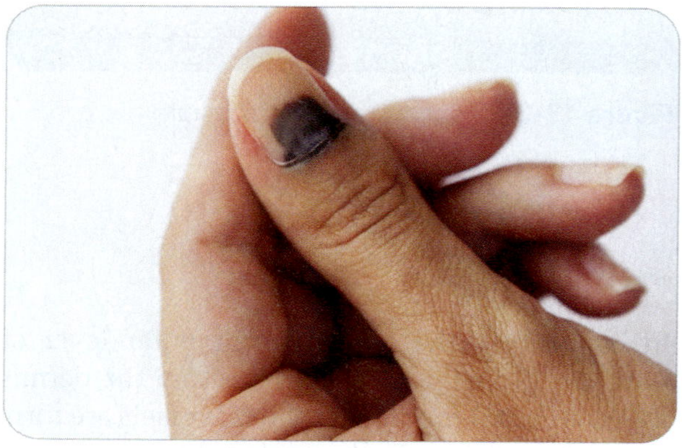

Figure 19-5 Subungual hematoma.

© Maxim Ahner/Shutterstock.

bone, or a highly vascularized solid organ is damaged. In severe cases, a large hematoma can contain enough blood to cause hemorrhagic shock.

A **subungual hematoma** is a special type of hematoma that occurs beneath a nail bed (**Figure 19-5**). This type of hematoma, which also is caused by blunt trauma, can be very painful due to the buildup of pressure within the affected area.

Crush Injuries

A **crush injury** is produced when an excessive force strikes the body suddenly or when a force is continuously applied to the body over an extended period. The resulting degree of tissue damage depends on several factors: the amount of force involved, the severity of the crushing, and the duration of the force applied. In addition to causing immediate direct soft-tissue injury, sustained compression eventually interrupts circulation within the tissues, thereby producing further cell damage and/or tissue death (**Figure 19-6**). If, for example, a tree trunk has fallen on and trapped a patient's legs, the sustained damage to leg tissues due to crushing (compression) will continue until the weight of the tree is removed.

KEY POINT

Relieving the Pressure of a Subungual Hematoma

In the rare instance when emergency care is many hours away, it may become necessary to relieve the pressure of a subungual hematoma. To decompress this type of painful injury, follow these steps:

1. Gently wash the fingertip. Heat a paper clip or the blunted end of a needle or pin with a lighter, a match, or an open flame until the metal is red hot.
2. Touch the hot tip of the paper clip in the center of the darkened nail bed and gently push down to allow the paper clip to burn through the nail *only*. The trapped blood will suddenly escape as the pressure is released, providing immediate relief from severe pain.
3. Immediately remove the paper clip to prevent it from penetrating the nail bed.
4. Dress and bandage the wound.

Compartment Syndrome

Another injury resulting from significant trauma to the tissues of an extremity, usually from compression, is called **compartment syndrome**. In this type of injury, damaged cell walls begin to leak fluid into the potential space that lies between them. If this resultant swelling, or edema, continues to expand within a large muscle's connective tissue covering, the pressure within the tissues may increase to dangerous levels. It is important to note that the connective tissue forms a compartment around the muscle that will not allow the edematous muscle to expand. Eventually blood vessels in the edematous area become compressed, thereby diminishing or even interrupting blood flow to the injured soft tissue, resulting in tissue death. Compartment syndrome is a true emergency that requires rapid transport to a trauma center to prevent the loss of the limb.

Open Injuries

Open soft-tissue injuries involve disruption of the skin and possibly damage to the soft tissue underneath. These injuries can result in extensive external bleeding. Because the integrity of the epidermal layer is compromised, the wound may be exposed to microorganisms or become contaminated by foreign bodies such as dirt, rocks, or other debris.

There are nine types of open soft-tissue wounds:

- Abrasion
- Incision
- Laceration
- Avulsion
- Amputation
- Puncture
- Open crush injury
- High-pressure injection
- Mechanical tattooing

Abrasion

An abrasion involves the outermost layer of skin (**Figure 19-7**). It is caused when a body part scuffs or grates across a rough, abrasive surface such as a gravel road, a rocky protrusion, corn snow, or some other rough surface. Usually an abrasion does not extend through the dermis, although blood may seep outward from injured capillaries in the dermis. These injuries, called a variety of slang names such as a strawberry, road rash, and road burn, may be extremely painful.

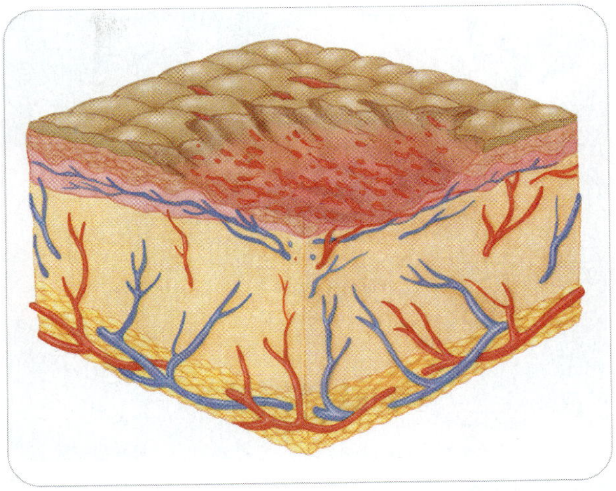

Figure 19-7 In an abrasion, or "road rash," the top layer of skin is injured and does not bleed a lot.

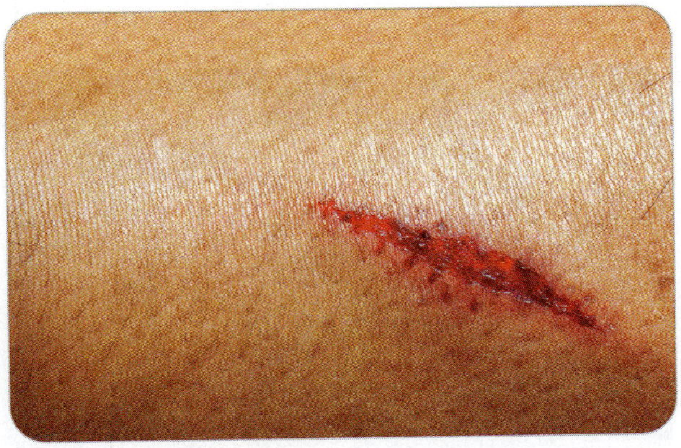

Figure 19-8 An incision is a smooth-edged cut.

Incision

An **incision** is a cut caused by a sharp object and has clean, *smooth* edges (**Figure 19-8**). This type of injury can be superficial, extending only through the skin and subcutaneous tissue, or it can be deep, involving underlying muscle and adjacent nerves and blood vessels. A knife or other sharp object causes incisions.

Laceration

A **laceration** is a cut caused by forces that tear or crush the skin and tends to have *jagged* edges

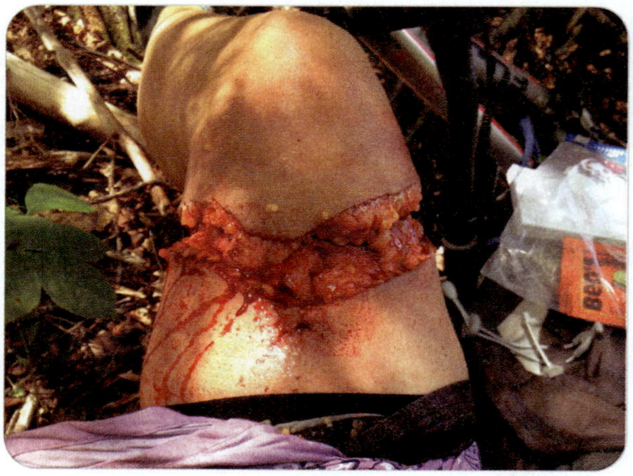

Figure 19-9 Lacerations tend to have jagged edges and can differ in depth. The amount of bleeding will depend on the location and depth of the cut.

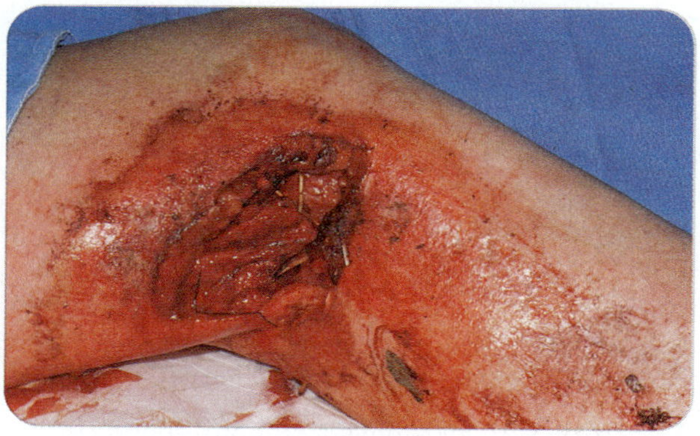

Figure 19-10 An avulsion may result in tissue hanging as a flap.

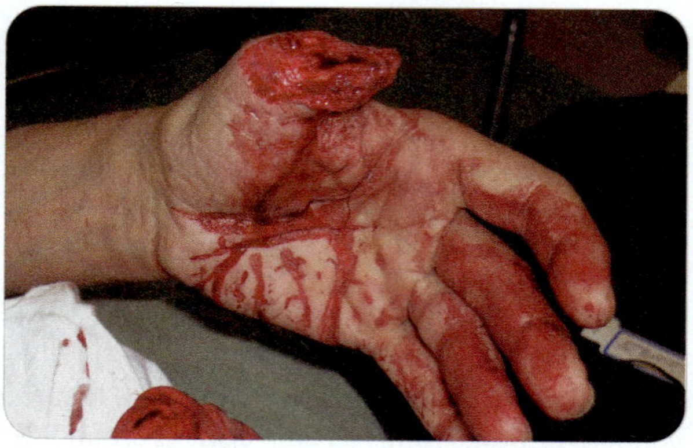

Figure 19-11 An amputation occurs when the limb or digit is completely or nearly completely separated from the body.

(**Figure 19-9**). Like an incision, a laceration can be superficial or deep. A laceration that is irregular is called stellate. Lacerations that sever arteries typically result in severe bleeding.

Avulsion

An **avulsion** is the incomplete or complete separation of the soft-tissue layers (most often between the subcutaneous layer and the underlying fascia) where the injured tissue is left dangling as a flap (**Figure 19-10**). The flap also may no longer be connected to the body. Because the soft tissue is torn, the resultant skin edges are irregular. Significant bleeding usually accompanies this type of injury. If the avulsed tissue is hanging by only a small bridge of skin, circulation in the avulsed segment may be lost.

Amputation

An **amputation** is the complete or nearly complete separation of a body part or limb (**Figure 19-11**). Amputations are serious injuries that may involve an entire extremity (e.g., arm, leg), an appendage (e.g., hand, foot, finger, toe), or some other anatomic part (e.g., ear, nose, lips). Bleeding from this type of wound can be severe, even life threatening.

Puncture

A **puncture** is an injury involving the penetration of skin. Pointed objects, such as sticks, nails, tree limbs, ski poles, tent stakes, or ice tools, are common causes of this type of injury. Bullets or knives may also cause puncture wounds. An accidental stick from a hypodermic needle causes a puncture. Even though the entrance wound may be small, serious damage to underlying structures can occur. If the puncture penetrates the chest, abdomen, or a major artery, it can cause severe, potentially fatal bleeding.

Open Crush Injury

Open crush injuries, as with closed crush injuries, may damage underlying internal organs, fracture adjacent bones, and/or generate widespread soft-tissue damage (**Figure 19-12**). Even if the external bleeding caused by such an injury appears negligible, internal bleeding may be extensive and can produce life-threatening hypovolemic shock. If the patient survives a massive crush injury, the

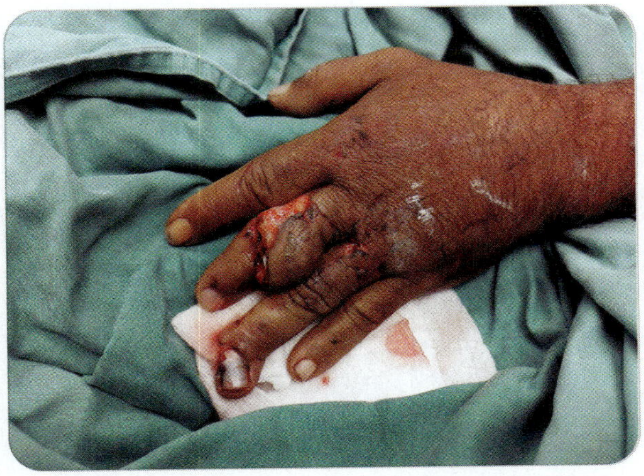

Figure 19-12 Crush injuries can damage the underlying organs or cause extensive soft-tissue damage.

result is often a permanently painful and deformed area of the body.

High-Pressure Injection

A high-pressure injection injury involves the introduction of a liquid or gas into the body from a pressurized source. In many instances, the presenting wound is very small and may initially be thought of as minor. High-pressure injection injuries can cause severe damage to underlying tissues, blood vessels, and nerves. Because the substance is injected into the tissues with great force, high-pressure injection injuries must be considered serious until proven otherwise. These injuries may result in surgical amputation of the affected part. Common sources of high-pressure injection injuries include high-pressure water sprayers, grease guns, paint sprayers, and pneumatic tools. Most injuries involve the hands, arms, or legs.

Mechanical Tattooing

Mechanical tattooing is a form of open soft-tissue injury that occurs when foreign debris such as dirt, rocks, or tar is ground into a wound or the adjacent skin (**Figure 19-13**). Such injuries can leave indelible marks on the skin. Powder residue from a gunshot wound suffered at close range also can result in mechanical tattooing. In the case of cosmetic tattooing, the person deliberately etches ink into the skin.

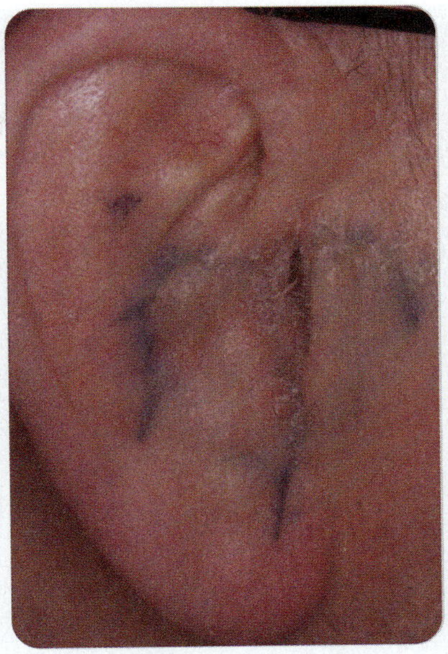

Figure 19-13 This ear had previous injury, with dirt ground into tissue from mechanical trauma.

Burns

A **burn** is a unique type of soft-tissue injury that is caused by exposure to excessive ultraviolet light (sunburn), thermal heat, heat resulting from friction, chemicals, electricity, lightning, or nuclear radiation. Each year, burns account for approximately 700,000 emergency department visits, nearly 45,000 hospitalizations, and more than 3,000 fatalities.

Sunburn

Sunburn is a superficial burn of the skin caused by medium-wavelength ultraviolet (UV) light in sunlight (**Figure 19-14**). While also a type of radiation burn, discussed in a following section, sunburn is a unique consideration for the OEC technician. Repeated excessive sun exposure over many years may lead to chronic degenerative skin changes, such as excessive wrinkling, darkening, and thickening. Localized benign growths are common. Repeated sunburns are associated with an increased incidence of cancerous lesions. All these changes can be delayed by avoiding excessive sun exposure and using proper skin protection.

Environments in which sunlight is more intense, such as at high altitude, or where sun is reflected, such as on snow or water, increase the risk of sunburn. At higher altitudes, sunburn occurs upon shorter exposure to sunlight because the less-dense atmosphere at greater elevations provides less protection against UV rays. Even on cloudy days, significant sunburn can occur to the skin or eyes in these environments. In general, individuals with fair skin, light-colored hair, or a

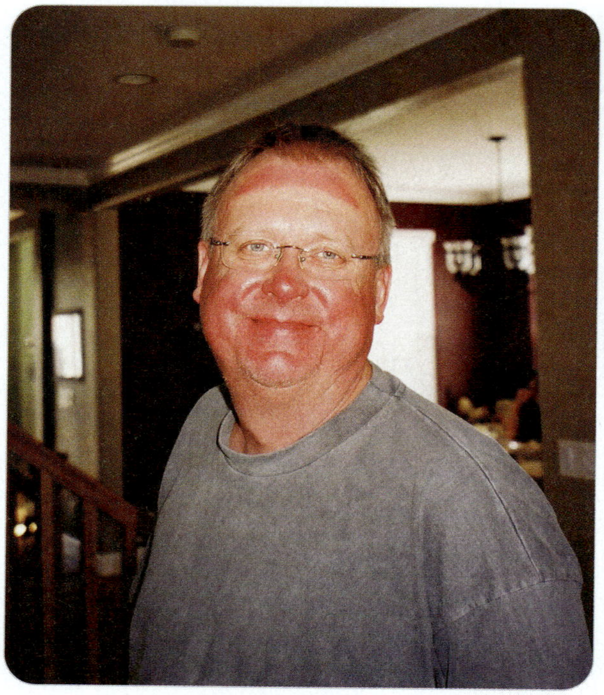

Figure 19-14 A sunburn is a superficial burn.

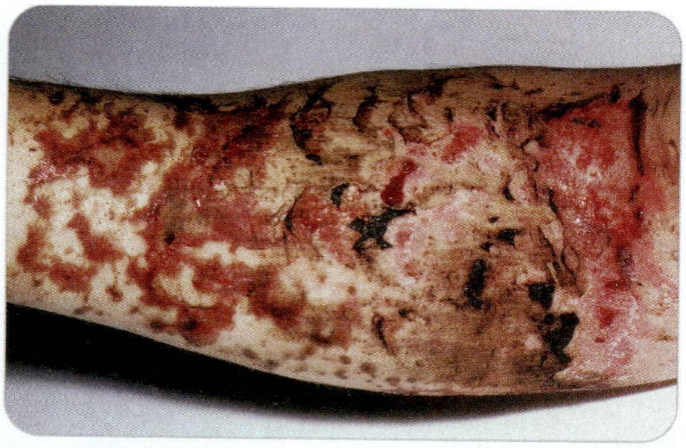

Figure 19-15 Thermal burns can come from a variety of hot surfaces or steam and can occur both internally and externally.

prior history of sun burning easily should be more careful when at high altitude, on snow, or on water.

Sunscreen can protect the skin by providing a mechanical or chemical barrier to sunlight. Zinc oxide and titanium dioxide are examples of mechanical (or physical) barriers that reflect the UV light in sunlight when applied to the lips and nose. Chemical components of sunscreen absorb, rather than reflect, harmful UV rays.

Most manufacturers of sunscreen creams, lotions, and lip salves specify the sun protection factor (SPF) on the label. This number, which usually ranges from 4 to 100, refers to how long the skin is protected before becoming red from exposure to the sun. "SPF 15" means that 1⁄15 of the burning radiation reaches the skin through the recommended thickness of sunscreen.

Sunscreen with an SPF of 50 or greater should be used in outdoor environments, especially at high altitude and on snow. There is probably no additional benefit to sunscreens with an SPF that is higher than 50. The key is to apply a thick coat of sunscreen on the skin before exposure to sunlight, and then to reapply it every few hours. Most individuals do not apply enough sunscreen and do not apply it frequently enough, particularly when it is lost through sweating or water immersion.

Thermal Burn

The most common type of burn suffered is a thermal burn, caused when heat comes directly into contact with the skin (**Figure 19-15**). Temperatures greater than 46°C (115°F) are enough to inflict a thermal burn. Common causes of thermal burns include open flames; hot water, hot steam, or superheated air, which cause a **scald**; and physical contact with a hot object such as an iron, a stove, molten tar, or a lightbulb. While most thermal burns occur on the skin surface, they can also occur inside the body under certain circumstances. For example, patients who breathe heated air or hot steam into their lungs may receive an inhalation burn that causes extensive damage to delicate lung tissue.

Chemical Burn

Chemical burns result from exposure to acids or bases, depending on the substance's potential of hydrogen (pH)—the concentration of hydrogen ions in solution. The pH scale ranges from 1 (strong acid) to 14 (strong base); a pH of 7 is considered neutral because it is neither acidic nor basic.

The extent of injury resulting from exposure to caustic substances varies with the concentration of the chemical, the amount of chemical involved, and the duration of contact. Alkaline (or basic) chemicals tend to cause more extensive chemical burns than acids because they penetrate

Table 19-1 Common Acids and Bases

Acids (pH <7)	Bases (pH >7)
• Sulfuric acid • Hydrochloric acid • Hydrofluoric acid • Muriatic acid • Carbolic acid (phenol) • Phosphoric acid • Nitric acid • Acetic acid	• Sodium hydroxide (caustic soda) • Potassium hydroxide (caustic potash) • Lye • Lime • Calcium chloride • Chlorine bleach

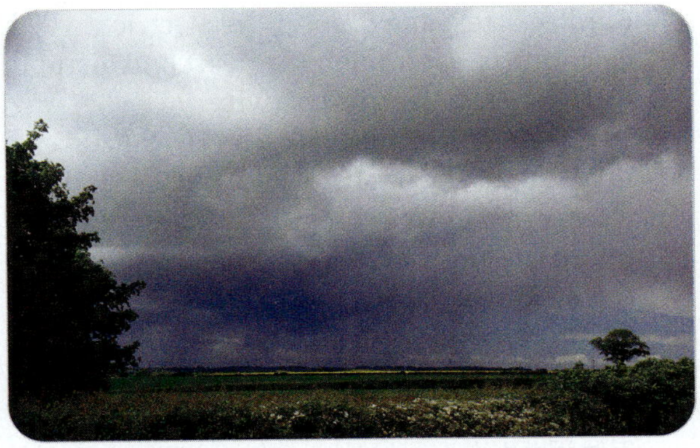

Figure 19-16 These cumulonimbus clouds ("thunderheads") could well generate lightning.

the skin more deeply. Mucous membranes, especially in the mouth, can be burned if the patient has ingested a caustic chemical.

Acidic and alkaline solutions are commonly found in commercial settings such as a mountain resort or backcountry lodge, often in cleaning solutions (**Table 19-1**). Unlike most household equivalents, commercial cleaners are typically in concentrated forms that require dilution before use. In addition to acids and bases, chemical burns can be caused by substances such as mustard gas, a powerful vesicant (blister-producing agent). These substances are used as chemical weapons.

Electrical Burns

When the body encounters an electrical current, an electrical burn can occur. Many factors determine the severity of an electrical burn, including the amount and type of electricity contacted, where the electricity enters and exits the body, and the duration of contact. Under normal conditions, electricity flows from some electrical source to an electrical ground following the "path of least resistance," or the pathway that has the highest conductivity and the least resistance. The importance of this knowledge to OEC technicians is that skin is a relatively poor conductor with high resistance. When skin becomes wet or oily, its conductivity increases, and its resistance markedly decreases, so electricity travels through the skin easier. Internal structures such as blood vessels and nerves are highly conductive and have low resistance, which is why electrical injuries traveling through the body produce severe internal injuries.

OEC technicians should always consider internal injuries whenever a patient has been exposed to a significant electrical current, which can pass into and burn (essentially cook) any organ in the body. The heart can be significantly damaged or can stop altogether when significant electrical current travels through it.

Lightning Injuries

Technically a type of electrical burn, lightning injuries present unique considerations for the OEC technician. Lightning is an atmospheric discharge of electricity that can generate 300,000 amps and 2 billion volts (**Figure 19-16**). Although it depends on the resistance of the human body, which varies greatly among individuals, under the right conditions, it takes only 500 milliamps of direct current to kill someone.

According to the National Weather Service, the odds of being struck by lightning during a lifetime of 80 years are 1 in 15,300. The average number of lightning deaths from 1989 to 2018 was 43 per year. The number is trending downward, with only 27 lightning fatalities per year from 2009 to 2018. (This figure may be deceptively low due to underreporting.)

Facts About Lightning-Caused Injuries

- Lightning injury is caused by direct electrical current at high voltage that lasts only 0.1 to 0.001 seconds.
- Respiratory arrest can result from injury to the respiratory control center of the brainstem.

- Cardiac arrest can occur if the electrical current passes through the heart and disrupts its organized electrical activity.
- Severe tissue damage by an electrical current may lead to the breakdown of muscle and the release into the circulation of chemicals that injure the kidney.
- Lightning can cause unpredictable neurologic effects such as pain, paralysis, blindness, numbness, weakness, loss of hearing or speech, and unresponsiveness.
- Significant internal tissue damage may not be obvious from the external burns at the sites at which electricity entered or exited the body.
- Electrical current from lightning can cause muscular contractions that throw the patient off balance and cause injurious falls.
- The fatality rate from a direct lightning strike is 30%; cardiac arrest is the most common cause of death.
- The characteristic lightning-induced skin injury is known as "feathering" or "ferning" (**Figure 19-17**).

Reducing the Risk of Lightning Strikes

Although lightning is unpredictable, several commonly accepted techniques can reduce the risk of injury or death associated with lightning strikes. When lightning is in the area, or during a storm, do the following:

- Seek shelter away from high points, exposed ridges, solitary trees, and trees taller than surrounding trees.
- Seek shelter in a forested area among trees or bushes, or in an area containing rocks of uniform size.
- Avoid open areas where you are one of the tallest objects.
- Avoid extremes of high ground or low ground.
- Do not stand in or near bodies of water.
- Avoid contact with metal objects.
- Put your feet together, squat low, tuck your head, and cover your ears. If possible, place your feet on a nonconductive material. Soil, nonmetallic substances, and plastics may be used. Avoid being close to others; stay about 15 feet apart.
- Seek shelter deep in a dry cave, and stay away from the sides and the ceiling. Avoid small caves in which you must remain close to the walls or ceiling, because ground currents may flow through your body instead of taking a longer path through the cave wall.
- If you are boating, attempt to get to shore, waves and distance to the shoreline permitting.
- If you are on a chairlift or other elevated structure, get off as soon as possible.
- If available, large buildings and enclosed vehicles are usually safe.

The National Weather Service supports the use of the 30/30 rule: If you see lightning, count the time until you hear thunder. If this time is 30 seconds or less, immediately seek safe shelter, and wait 30 minutes or more after hearing the last clap of thunder before leaving your shelter. Even if you cannot see lightning, hearing thunder indicates that lightning is likely within striking range. The 30/30 rule cannot protect against the first lightning strike, so it is important to know the local weather forecast and to seek appropriate shelter at the first sign of an impending storm.

If lightning overtakes you, the first precaution should be to descend as far as possible off exposed ridges or move out of clearings to lower, more-sheltered areas. Keep away from metal

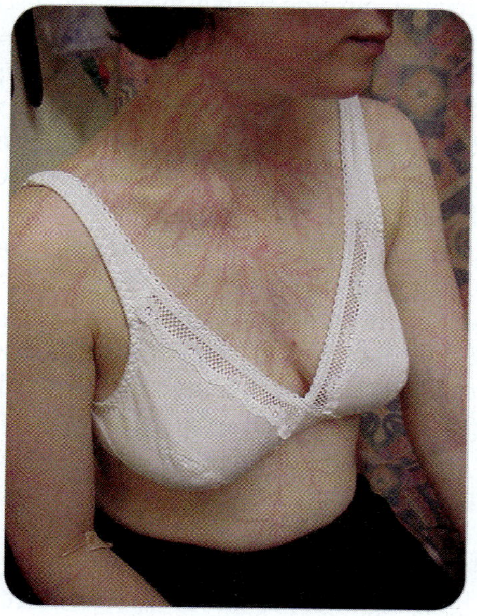

Figure 19-17 A "feathering" or "ferning" pattern of a burn caused by a lightning strike.

objects; remove your crampons, and place ski poles and ice axes a distance from your location. If there is no possibility of descending out of open areas to lower terrain, then you and all the members of your group should spread out and squat down, preferably while standing on insulated material, if possible. Stay away from exposed rock overhangs, where a ground current may pass through individuals seeking shelter. Within a ski area, clear all lifts of people when the danger of a lightning strike exists.

Radiation Burns

Following exposure to an object, substance, or element that emits radiation, a radiation burn may occur. Depending on the source, exposure may be brief or prolonged. Radiation is transmitted in the form of rays or particles and may be transmitted by a variety of sources, including tanning beds, plant and grow lights, heat lamps, black lights, radioactive materials, medical X-ray machines, welding equipment, and other industrial or military equipment. The sun is another source of radiation; as discussed, it transmits UV light, which can burn the skin. Sunburn or burns associated with welding equipment are the radiation burns most likely to be encountered by OEC technicians.

PATIENT ASSESSMENT OF SOFT-TISSUE INJURIES

Soft-tissue injuries may look very impressive, especially when they are associated with significant external bleeding. The assessment of soft-tissue injuries must be approached like any other medical or traumatic emergency: It begins with a scene size-up. Start by donning appropriate personal protective equipment (PPE) and ensuring that the scene is safe to enter.

Once the scene is secured, control serious external bleeding first then perform a primary assessment of the patient's ABCDs (airway, breathing, circulation, disability) to identify potential threats to life, correcting any that may be present. Assess the patient's level of responsiveness using the AVPU scale (alert, verbal, pain, unresponsive). If spinal injury is suspected, ensure manual stabilization of the cervical spine.

Upon completion of the primary assessment, perform a secondary assessment using DCAP-BTLS (deformity, contusions, abrasions/avulsions, punctures/penetrations, burns/bleeding/bruises, tenderness, lacerations, swelling), and obtain a thorough medical history. Collect a SAMPLE history (signs and symptoms, allergies,

CASE Update

You instruct a race official to close the site to ensure that no other cyclists crash into the scene. The patient can speak to you normally, so he has an airway and is breathing, and his heart is pumping blood. Using standard precautions, you apply direct pressure to the "spurting" wrist laceration using a sterile dressing. The deep laceration over the patient's wrist continues to bleed. A large bruise over the superior-lateral aspect of the patient's left shoulder is tender to the touch, and multiple abrasions are apparent over the lateral aspect of the patient's lower leg. Many of the abrasions contain dirt and small stones that appear to be ground into the skin and are slowly oozing blood. The cyclist also has large abrasions on the palms of both hands. He can rotate his left arm in all directions without an increase in pain. SAMPLE is noncontributory. All extremities have normal motor and sensory function. The patient's pulse is 100 beats per minute, and his respirations are 16 breaths per minute.

What should you do now?

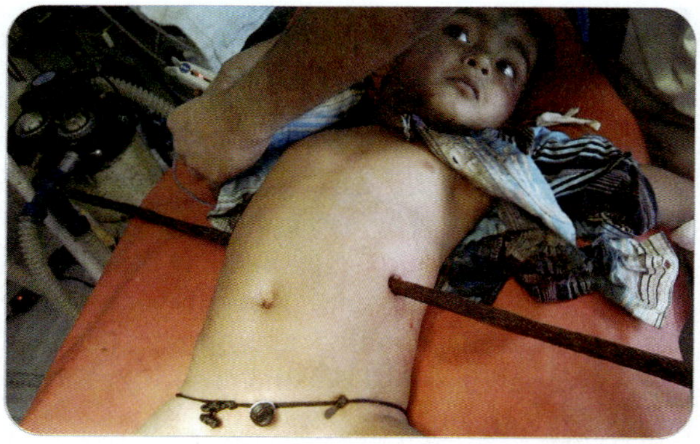

Figure 19-18 A patient with an obvious injury may have more serious, less-apparent injuries.

medications, past medical history, last oral intake, events leading up to the problem). Consider asking if the patient is taking an anticoagulant, especially if there is bleeding that is difficult to control.

As you assess the patient, remember that the forces that produce closed soft-tissue injuries also can damage underlying structures, bones, and internal organs. Maintain a high index of suspicion and presume that any patient who has an obvious soft-tissue injury, regardless of whether it is closed or open, has other more serious hidden injuries (**Figure 19-18**). For example, a patient who has an obvious puncture wound in the chest may have internal bleeding and a lung injury.

Carefully assess the patient for signs of shock. Be sure to check distal circulation, movement, and sensation (CMS) in all extremities, even with seemingly minor soft-tissue injuries. Obtain a complete set of vital signs.

Thoroughly document the circumstances surrounding the injury, the patient's general condition, and your assessment findings on a patient care report. Many shooting- or stabbing-related incidents end up in court. The initial caregiver could be required to testify in court later. Ensure that your written report accurately reflects all the assessment performed and treatment rendered.

PATIENT ASSESSMENT OF BURNS

The priority when assessing a burn patient is to ensure that the scene is safe to enter. Put out any fires, turn off the electricity, and have any chemicals removed. Call a fire department and request a hazardous materials (hazmat) team respond if the scene contains any chemicals or radiation that could harm you or others. Touching a patient who is still in contact with a live electric wire can be dangerous, perhaps even fatal. Only after all potential dangers have been abated may you begin the assessment process. If the source of the burns is not obvious, attempt to identify it as part of the scene size-up because this information may be useful both in performing the assessment and in making treatment decisions.

As soon as you are aware that a toxic substance or bodily fluids may be present, use standard precautions. At a minimum, use eye, face, and hand protection. For chemical burns, consider using chemical-resistant gloves and a protective gown or overgarment. Do not overlook this critical step; some chemicals may not be readily apparent, and failure to adequately protect yourself increases your risk of injury. Some chemicals give off toxic gases that can cause damage to the eyes and lungs, and burns can expose structures beneath the skin to potential contaminants and pathogens.

The next step is to control serious bleeding and assess the ABCDs, beginning with evaluating the patency of the airway. Patients who are exposed to thermal sources or caustic chemicals, especially those involving inhaled substances such as smoke, heat, or chemical vapors, are at high risk for serious airway injuries. Burn injuries to the upper airway may require prompt ALS airway evaluation for potential emergent intubation. The lower airway, although better protected by the larynx from direct heat, can still suffer inhalation injuries. These injuries may not be immediately apparent but can cause sudden respiratory compromise.

KEY POINT

Protect Yourself

Caution! When treating a burn patient, ensure your own safety by protecting yourself from sources of heat, chemicals, and electricity. Wearing protective gear is required.

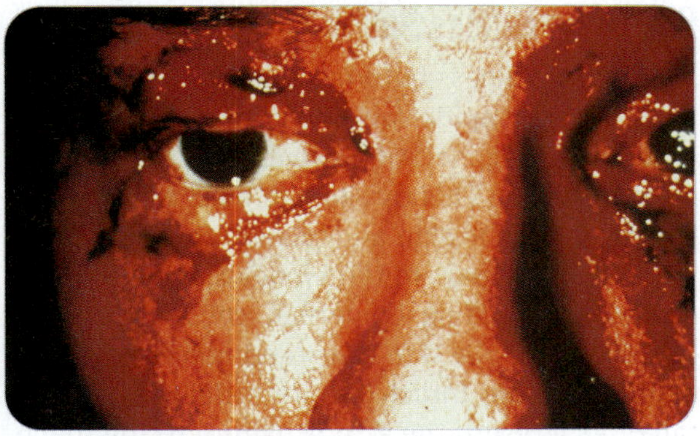

Figure 19-19 Burns to the face suggest respiratory tract involvement or injuries to the eyes.

Signs and symptoms associated with an inhalation injury include the following:

- Obvious burns involving the head, face, or neck (**Figure 19-19**)
- Singed hair, including the eyebrows, nose hairs, and facial hair
- Soot and other by-products of combustion on the face, in the mouth, or around the nostrils
- Hoarseness or voice changes
- Airway swelling
- Difficulty swallowing
- Darkened oral or nasal discharge, known as carbonaceous sputum

Finish the primary assessment by determining the patient's level of responsiveness and distal neurologic function.

Perform a thorough secondary assessment and take vital signs. Use the SAMPLE acronym to obtain a medical history, which can reveal valuable clues regarding the mechanism of injury and may help to identify other possible injuries and preexisting medical conditions such as diabetes, prior myocardial infarction, or pulmonary disease, which can be exacerbated by the stress of burn injuries. Obtain information regarding the patient's medications and tetanus immunization status.

If the source of the burn involves flames that occurred in an enclosed area, assume that the patient may have carbon monoxide poisoning. Symptoms of elevated carbon monoxide levels include headache, nausea, and altered mental status. Even though cherry-red skin is often described as a feature of carbon monoxide poisoning, it is rarely observed in prehospital environments and occurs only after significant exposure. In this situation, skin redness is probably the result of burns. If exposure to carbon monoxide is expected, after all flames are extinguished, give the patient high-flow, high-concentration oxygen through a nonrebreather mask. Note: Pulse oximetry (SpO_2) is not effective when a patient has carbon monoxide poisoning.

If the source of the burn is a hot liquid, attempt to determine how long the liquid was in contact with the skin. Find out if the burn was irrigated with water or if a cream or lotion was applied to the burn before your arrival.

If you suspect the burn results from exposure to a chemical, attempt to identify the chemicals involved by examining the container, paying attention to the identities and concentrations of the active ingredients. Do not expose yourself or others to the chemical.

If the burn source is electricity, attempt to determine which body part was in direct contact with the electrical source and for how long. Attempt to identify the source of the electricity (e.g., an electrical outlet in the lodge, the power supply to the lift motor). In injuries involving electricity, the patient's burns are usually more extensive than is first apparent, because the greatest injuries are often internal and involve deep tissues or organs. Moreover, the patient is at greater risk for cardiac-related injury or arrest when electricity is involved. Determining the path of the electrical current through the patient's body (as indicated by the sites of entrance and exit burns) and applying your knowledge of human anatomy can help you identify which internal structures may have been affected.

Once the initial threats to life have been mitigated, the history obtained, and the secondary assessment completed, the next step is to evaluate the severity of the burns by classifying them using either the degree-based or the thickness-based method.

The Classification of Burns

Burns are classified according to the depth of skin damage using two methods: the thickness-based method, which classifies burns as superficial burns, partial-thickness burns, or full-thickness burns, and the degree-based approach, which classifies burns as first-degree burns, second-degree burns, third-degree burns, and fourth-degree burns. Both methods are commonly used in emergency and burn medicine, often in conjunction with one another (**Table 19-2**).

Accurately classifying burn injuries is an important skill for OEC technicians to learn because this information is used to determine initial treatment, subsequent therapy, and whether hospitalization should occur in a specialized burn center. In the sections that follow, we consider the classification of burns.

Superficial Burns

A superficial burn (first-degree burn) is the mildest form of burn and affects the epidermis only (**Figure 19-20**). It is characterized by skin that is hot, dry, and reddened. Although the epidermis remains intact, mild swelling may occur. Pain and tenderness are mild to moderate due to intact but irritated nerve endings. Healing is usually spontaneous, occurs within a few days, and may be accompanied by superficial sloughing of the epidermal layer ("peeling"). Too much exposure to the sun and remaining too long in a tanning bed are the most common sources of superficial burns. Depending on the amount of UV radiation exposure, sunburns are usually first-degree burns, but can blister and result in second-degree burns.

Partial-Thickness Burns

A partial thickness burn (second-degree burn) affects both the epidermis and dermis but does not exceed the regenerative capabilities of the skin (**Figure 19-21**). This category of burn is characterized by reddened skin and blisters that form from plasma (liquid part of the blood) leaking into the spaces surrounding epidermal cells. Unless the blisters break, the skin is dry and reddened. Nerve endings remain intact but are inflamed and irritated. As a result, the skin is painful to the touch, with the pain described as moderate to severe. OEC technicians should consider calling for ALS to provide intravenous pain medication for patients with extensive partial-thickness burns.

Full-Thickness Burns

A full-thickness burn is a devastating injury. In those classified as third-degree burns, all layers of the skin and possibly the underlying structures are destroyed (**Figure 19-22**). Those classified as fourth-degree burns are even more extensive, affecting muscle and bone. When full-thickness burns cover a large surface area of the body, the mortality rate is high.

In a full-thickness burn, the skin takes on a white or charred "leathery" appearance and is usually dry. Pain is usually absent in that specific area due to complete destruction of nerve endings; however,

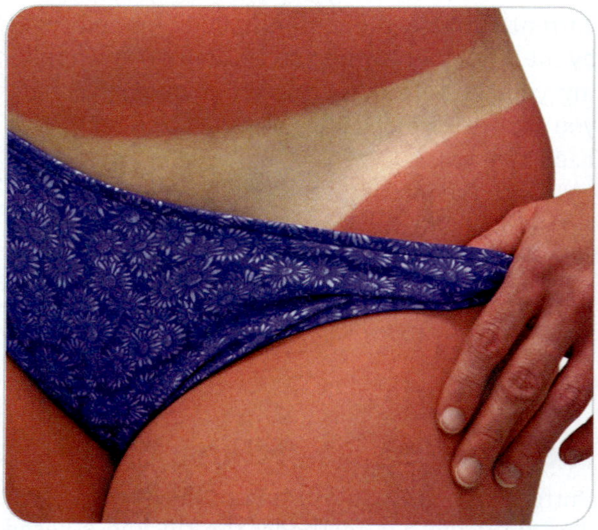

Figure 19-20 Superficial, or first-degree burns affect only the epidermis.

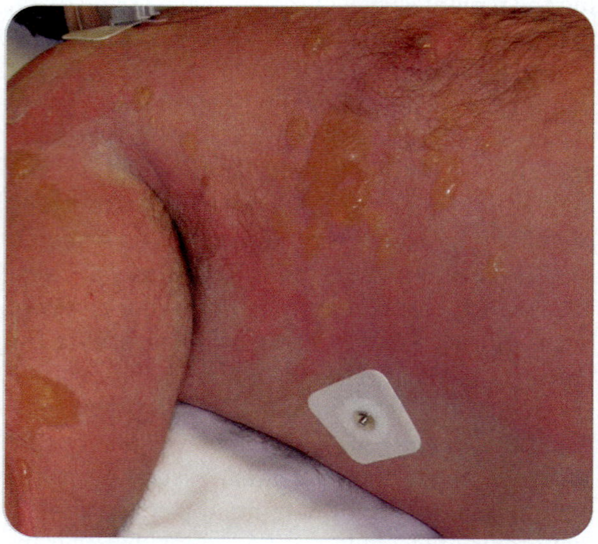

Figure 19-21 A partial-thickness burn. Note the redness and blisters.

the site may be surrounded by partial-thickness and superficial burns that are painful. Skin does not grow back, because the growing layer of skin has been destroyed. Skin grafts are needed.

Thermal burns, such as boiling water, scalds, or direct contact with an open flame, are the most common sources of full-thickness burns. Such serious burns also are more prone to infection than are superficial or partial-thickness burns.

Calculation of Burn Area

Next, calculate the total area of skin that has partial-thickness or full-thickness burns; superficial burns should be described and noted but are not included in this calculation. This calculation is accomplished using the Rule of Nines. In this method, the surface of the body is divided into the 11 sections shown in **Figure 19-23**, each of which represents approximately 9% of total body surface area (TBSA).

> **KEY POINT**
>
> **Potential Airway Injury**
>
> A hoarse voice can be a sign of injury to the airway. Always assess patients with hoarseness for potential respiratory compromise.

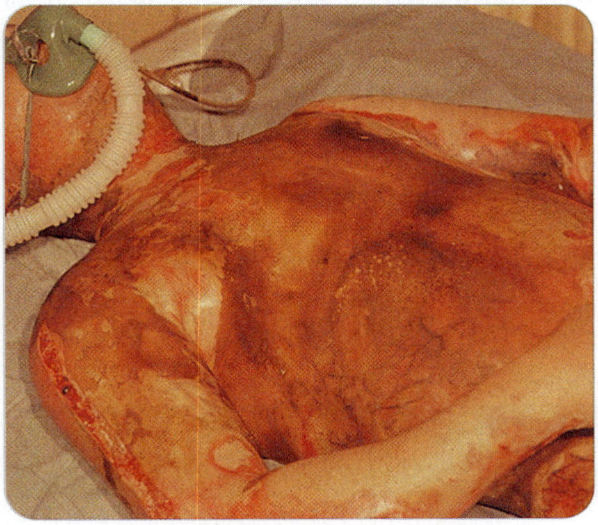

Figure 19-22 Full-thickness burns destroy all layers of the skin.

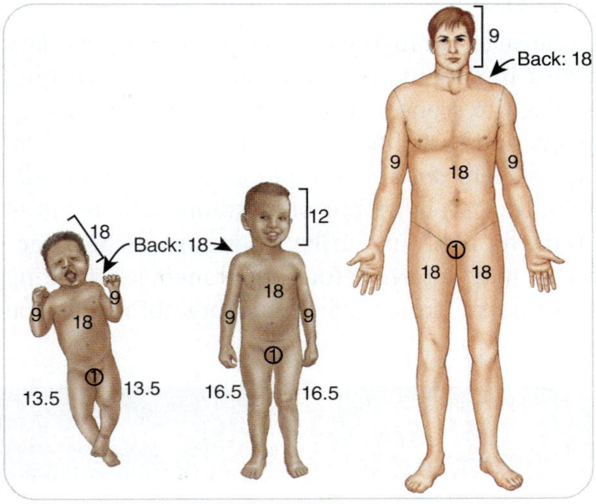

Figure 19-23 The Rule of Nines for estimating the proportion of the body surface affected by burns.

Table 19-2 Burn Classification

Burn	Appearance of Skin	Skin Layers Affected	Pain
Superficial (first-degree burn)	Red, no blisters	Epidermis	Significant
Partial thickness (second-degree burn)	Blisters, wet appearance	Epidermis and dermis	Intense
Full thickness (third-degree burn)	Charred or white, dry	Epidermis, dermis, and underlying soft tissues	None
Full thickness (fourth-degree burn)	Black	Muscle and bone	None

KEY POINT

Pediatric Considerations

When treating pediatric burn patients, always consider the possibility that the injuries were not accidental. Given the high index of suspicion for child abuse, determine whether the injuries you observe are consistent with the circumstances of the incident as reported to you.

Patient Assessment of Lightning Strikes

Because of the high incidence of cardiopulmonary arrest in patients who have sustained a lightning strike, the scene size-up, primary patient assessment, and basic life-support measures are critical. Assessment should be rapid and include the ABCDs. Look for burns and other trauma that resulted from the lightning strike. Spontaneous heart activity may return before spontaneous breathing returns, so prolonged rescue breathing may be necessary. Unlike patients who are still in contact with the source of an electrical shock, patients struck by lightning are not electrically charged and pose no threat to rescuers.

MANAGEMENT OF BLEEDING

Controlling Bleeding

Management of bleeding is a fundamental OEC skill. As part of your primary patient assessment, when managing the ABCDs, control any severe bleeding first. The OEC technician needs to determine *immediately* if the bleeding is a life-threatening problem. The treatment for minor bleeding and major bleeding is different. Bleeding from a minor cut can be treated with a small dressing or Band-Aid. In most situations, more extensive external bleeding, whether arterial, venous, or capillary, can usually be controlled by applying direct pressure. Then, if needed, apply additional dressings, or use a compression dressing. When bleeding is life threatening with larger or deeper wounds, or when bleeding is more intense, other measures such as packing the wound, using hemostatic dressings, or using a **tourniquet** are needed. More severe bleeding is called **hemorrhage**.

To control bleeding, follow the steps in **OEC Skill 19-1**.

OEC SKILL 19-1 Controlling Bleeding

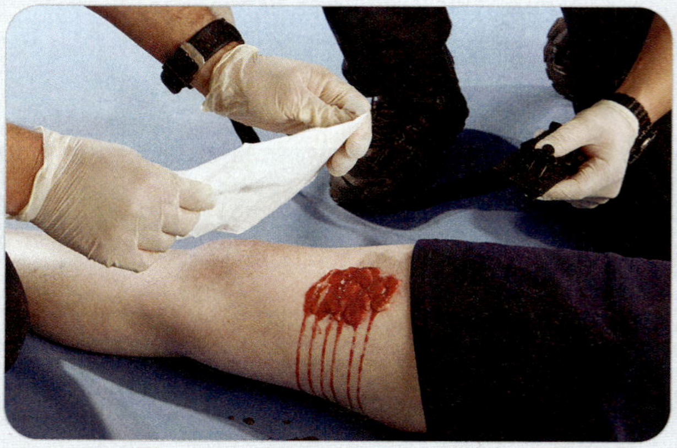

1. Expose the area to see the wound. Open, cut, or remove clothing. Place a sterile dressing over the wound and apply direct pressure. If you find life-threatening bleeding, control this immediately.

2. If the bleeding does not stop, add other sterile dressings over the first dressing and again apply direct pressure. When applying direct pressure to a wound, always observe standard precautions by wearing appropriate PPE.

3. Bandage extremity.

KEY POINT

Stop the Bleed

The OEC technician must immediately decide whether bleeding is minor or life threatening. According to the Stop the Bleed campaign by the American College of Surgeons, life-threatening bleeding is indicated by any of the following:

- Blood that is spurting out of the wound
- Blood that won't stop coming out of the wound
- Blood that is pooling on the ground
- Clothing that is soaked with blood
- Bandages that are soaked with blood
- Loss of all or part of an arm or leg
- Serious bleeding in a patient who is now confused or unconscious

Direct Pressure

Direct pressure, the primary method used to control *any* external bleeding, is performed by applying firm direct pressure with a gloved hand, or both hands if bleeding is severe (**Figure 19-24**). Direct pressure can even stop major arterial bleeding. If a sterile dressing (e.g., 4×4, 4×8) is available, place this on the wound and then apply and maintain continuous firm pressure. This technique occludes underlying blood vessels until normal clotting mechanisms can seal them.

If the situation is urgent and a sterile dressing is not available, use any clean soft material or even the palms of your gloved hands to apply direct pressure. People who are on anticoagulants ("blood thinners") will need to have pressure applied for a much longer time, sometimes 30 minutes. If for some reason you do not have medical gloves, leave your ski gloves on. It is better to protect yourself and have your ski gloves cleaned later.

Application of Additional Dressings

For non-life-threatening bleeding not controlled by the initial application of a dressing, add additional sterile dressings over the initial dressing. Once applied, do not remove the original dressing. Instead, add to the base layer, because removing the primary dressing will disrupt any clotting that has occurred and cause additional bleeding. Continue to place pressure on the wound with both hands. If bleeding continues, additional measures are needed.

Compression Dressing

A **compression (pressure) dressing** maintains direct pressure on a bleeding wound. It consists of several sterile dressings secured in place by a firmly applied roller bandage. When two OEC technicians are available, one should hold direct pressure with both hands over the wound while the second OEC technician applies the pressure dressing, removing the first person's hand as it is positioned.

To apply a pressure dressing, begin distal to the injury and wrap the roller bandage over the dressing, all the time moving proximally and tying

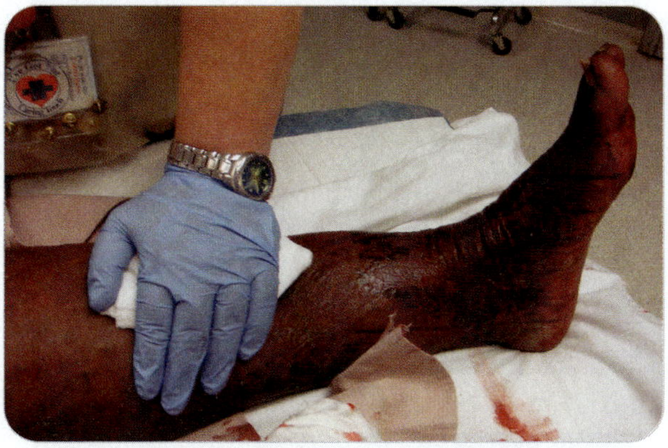

Figure 19-24 Direct pressure is always the first thing to try when attempting to control bleeding.

Courtesy of Rhonda Hunt.

KEY POINT

Elevation of Bleeding Extremity—Not Recommended

In the past, some prehospital authorities recommended the elevation of bleeding extremities to assist in stopping the bleeding. This technique has *not been shown to help control bleeding* and will distract providers from the proven technique of direct pressure.

the knot directly over the wound. If needed, a cravat can then be applied to add more pressure. In the event you do not have access to a roller bandage, a cravat wrapped around the wound several times and then tied tightly over the wound will work. Check CMS distally before and after applying the pressure dressing (**Figure 19-25**).

Severe Life-Threatening Bleeding

Stop the Bleed is an educational program created for prehospital providers in 2015 by the American College of Surgeons. It uses a step-by-step approach for controlling life-threatening bleeding. The primary principles of the program include notifying the EMS system of a patient with severe bleeding, while at the same time finding the source of the bleed and applying pressure to stop the bleeding. Based on local protocol, an OEC technician should notify dispatch to call EMS. To stop severe bleeding, first cover the wound with a sterile dressing or clean cloth and apply pressure with both gloved hands. If this does not work, use a tourniquet, or pack (fill) the wound with gauze or a clean cloth and apply pressure with both hands. Hemostatic dressings (discussed later) may also be used in treating severe bleeding.

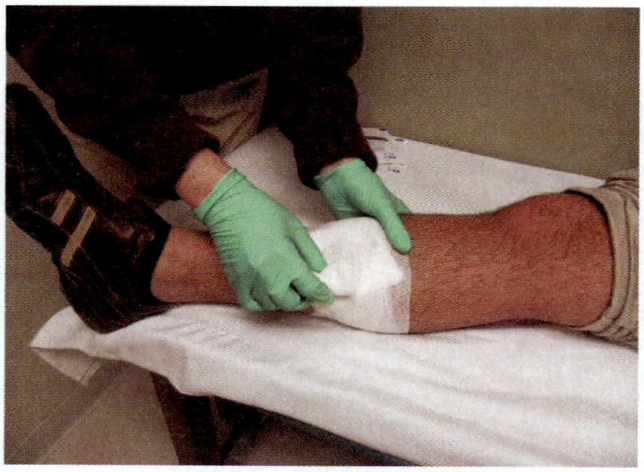

A

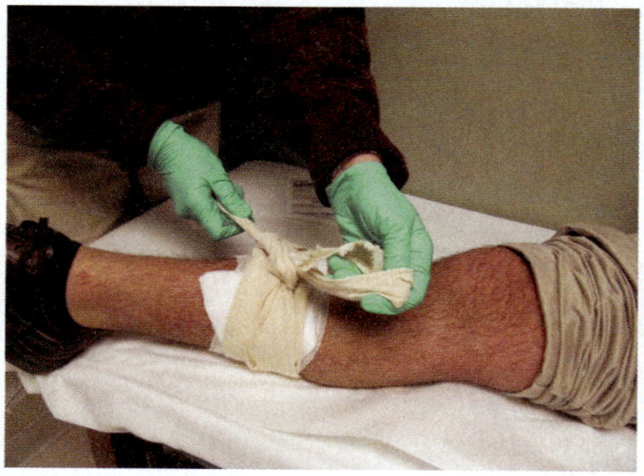

B

Figure 19-25 A. When applying a pressure dressing, wrap the roller bandage starting at the distal aspect of the injury and wrap in a proximal direction. **B.** If necessary to stop bleeding, secure the roller bandage in place with a cravat knotted over the wound to add pressure.

Packing the Wound

Although packing can also be used on large or deep extremity wounds with severe bleeding, it is better to use a tourniquet when available. Packing the wound is necessary for life-threatening bleeding from locations where a tourniquet cannot be used, namely the neck, shoulder, torso, abdomen, chest, or groin (**Figure 19-26**).

To pack a wound, fill the wound with gauze, hemostatic dressing, or a clean cloth and then apply pressure with both hands. A pressure dressing using a cravat can then replace your hands if the bleeding is controlled, except on the neck, where you must continue to maintain pressure with your hands.

Hemostatic Dressings

A **hemostatic dressing** contains a topical hemostatic agent that promotes clotting. Originally used by the military successfully, then by EMS, some ski patrols now have these dressings available. A variety of sizes are sold individually wrapped in a vapor barrier. They are latex-free. The cost of these dressings and shelf life need to be considered

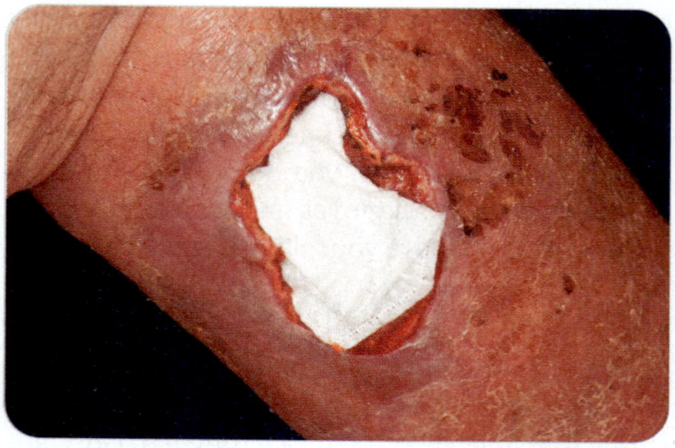

Figure 19-26 Packing the wound is the treatment of choice when you are unable to use a tourniquet.

when developing a local protocol for use of these products.

These dressings are not needed for small cuts and abrasions where bleeding can be controlled by simple means. A panel of experts in prehospital trauma from the American College of Surgeons in 2014 recommended the use of hemostatic gauze (which can be used for wound packing) where direct pressure alone is ineffective or not practical, and in cases where tourniquet application is not possible due to anatomic limitations.

Hemostatic dressings must be placed directly on the wound to be effective (**Figure 19-27**). If severe bleeding exists initially that cannot be controlled and the location of the wound makes the use of a tourniquet difficult, and if a hemostatic gauze dressing is available, this can be an effective way to control bleeding. Apply direct pressure first to the wound to stop the bleeding, then apply the hemostatic dressing as the first layer, and add more sterile gauze on top. Make this into a pressure dressing.

Tourniquets

The use of a tourniquet to control *severe* bleeding in an extremity is well accepted. Tourniquets should be used only on extremities. If the bleeding is severe and places the patient at great risk for bleeding to death, an event known as **exsanguination**, a tourniquet can be lifesaving and needs to be applied. A tourniquet is an effective method to completely stop blood flow distal to the area of application. These devices are applied only when hemorrhaging from an extremity cannot be controlled by other methods. Two situations that might warrant use of a tourniquet *immediately* are when a you are unable to control severe bleeding with direct pressure or when you have a patient with significant bleeding from an extremity and simultaneously other major problems—for example, airway issues. The use of the tourniquet will allow you to stop the bleeding from that extremity while you are dealing with other lifesaving issues. Always make the tourniquet tight. If you apply a tourniquet and it is completely tight and the bleeding does not stop, leave the first tourniquet on and apply a second tourniquet *above* (proximal to) the first one.

You can place a tourniquet directly over clothing. You must remove bulky items before placing a tourniquet. When applied, a tourniquet will hurt, *a lot*. Do *not* loosen it if the patient complains of pain. Never remove a tourniquet in the prehospital setting once it is applied.

Use of a tourniquet always is accompanied by the risk of the patient losing the limb. No amputations have been caused by leaving tourniquets in place for fewer than 2 hours. It is best to get the patient to a trauma center as soon as possible so that bleeding can be completely stopped and the tourniquet removed (**Figure 19-28**). Write the time at which the tourniquet was applied either directly on the patient's forehead or on a piece of tape applied to the patient's forehead.

To apply a tourniquet, follow the steps of **OEC Skill 19-2**.

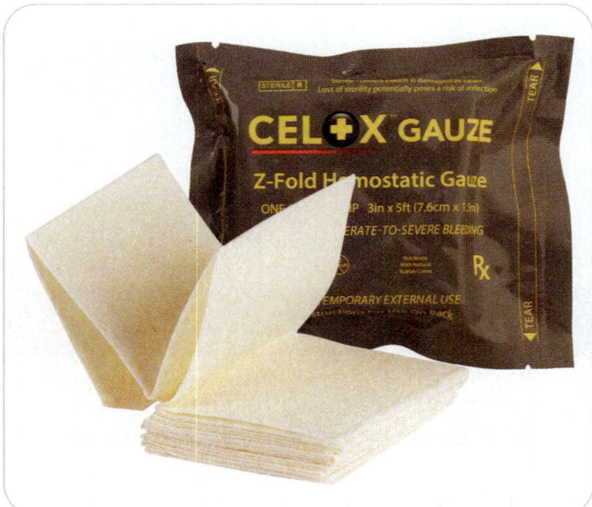

Figure 19-27 Hemostatic dressings must be placed directly on top of the wound to be effective.

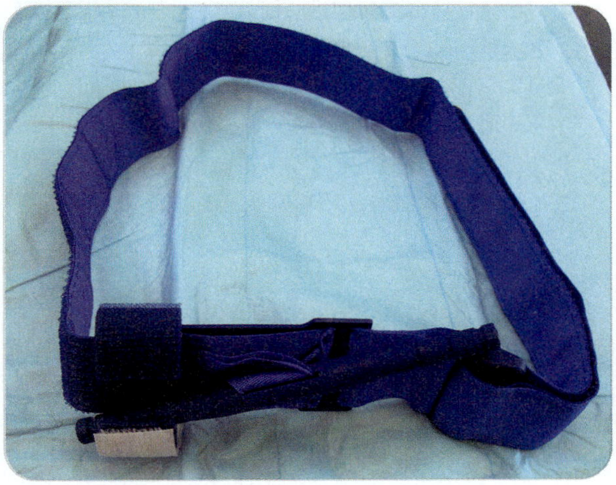

Figure 19-28 Tourniquets have improved and do not necessarily cause the loss of the limb distal to the tourniquet.

Courtesy of Peter T. Pons, MD, FACEP.

OEC SKILL 19-2 Applying a Tourniquet

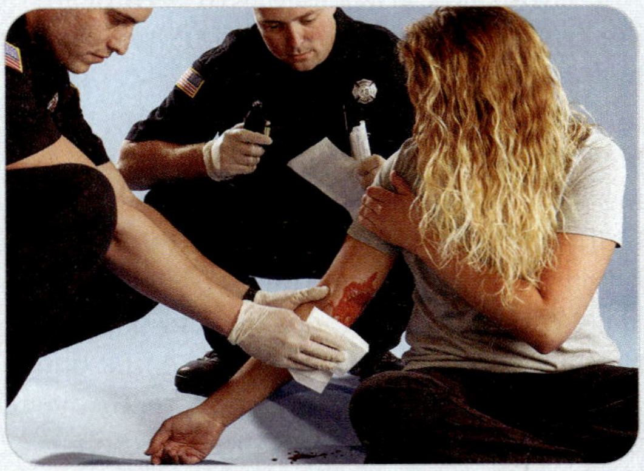

1 While preparing the tourniquet, apply direct pressure to a dressing placed over the wound.

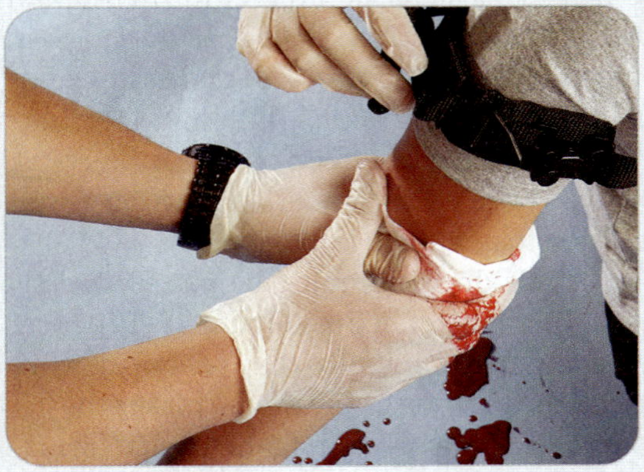

2 Place the tourniquet around the injured extremity several inches above (proximal to) the injury but not over a joint.

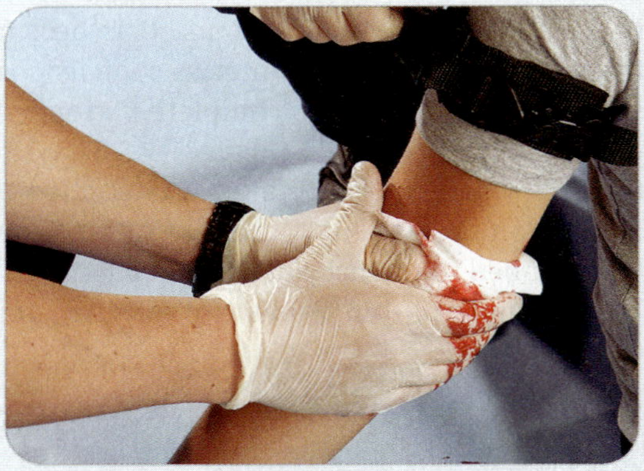

3 Pack large wounds with gauze. Twist the rod to tighten the tourniquet only to the extent needed to control the bleeding.

KEY POINT

Do Not Remove the Tourniquet

Never release a tourniquet! Doing so will result in more blood loss.

KEY POINT

Basic guidelines for tourniquets can be remembered by the principle of twos and threes. They should be at least 2 inches wide, at least 2 inches proximal from the wound, and at least 3 inches from a joint.

Dressings and Bandages

A **dressing** is a piece of material, usually cloth or a cloth-like fabric, that is placed directly on a wound. Ideally, the dressing should be sterile, come prepackaged, and be large enough to extend at least 1 inch beyond all wound edges.

Conventional sterile gauze pads, sized as 4 inches by 4 inches (4×4) or 4 inches by 8 inches (4×8), soft self-adherent roller dressings, and assorted small adhesive-type dressings (Curads, Band-Aids) work well to cover most wounds that you will encounter (Figure 19-29). The **universal dressing**, sometimes called the trauma dressing, which measures 9 inches by 36 inches and is made of a thick, absorbent cotton material, is well suited for covering large open wounds and works well to pad rigid splints. All these dressings are commercially available in compact, individually wrapped sterile packages. Occlusive dressings (e.g., Vaseline gauze, aluminum foil, plastic cling wrap) are used in special situations in which the wound requires an occlusive dressing.

A **bandage** is a piece of material that is used to hold a dressing or splint in place. The term *bandaging* usually refers to the process of applying both a dressing and a bandage. Most wounds require dressings and bandages to prevent further contamination and to absorb blood and wound secretions. Become familiar with the indications, functions, and proper application of each of the many types of bandages.

Self-adhering roller bandages (e.g., Kerlix), rolls of soft gauze (e.g., Kling), triangular bandages folded into 2- to 3-inch wide strips, or adhesive tape are used to secure dressings in place. Kerlix is a commercial self-adherent roller bandage that is available in multiple widths and is considered by many to be the most effective because its elasticity makes it easy to apply. Kling is a commercially available, tightly woven, light gauze wrap that also may be used to secure a dressing in place but is less elastic than Kerlix, which is a loosely woven gauze wrap (Figure 19-30). Triangular bandages can be used to secure dressings in place.

OEC Skill 19-3 explains how to use a self-adhering roller bandage.

Principles of Bandaging

Most bandages that are placed on an extremity are wrapped entirely around the body part, which

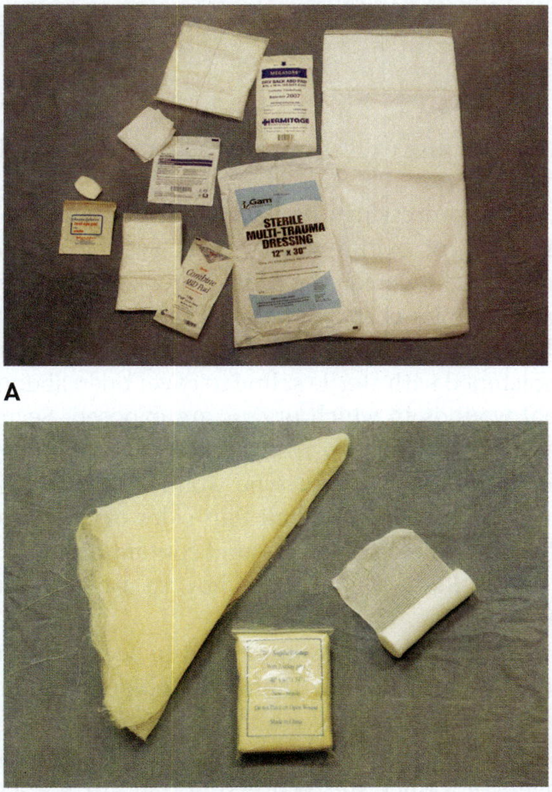

A

B

Figure 19-29 A. Many types of sterile dressings are used for covering open wounds, including universal dressings, gauze pads, adhesive dressings, and occlusive dressings. **B.** Bandages keep dressings in place and include soft roller bandages, triangular bandages, and adhesive tape. Splints may also be used to hold dressings in place.

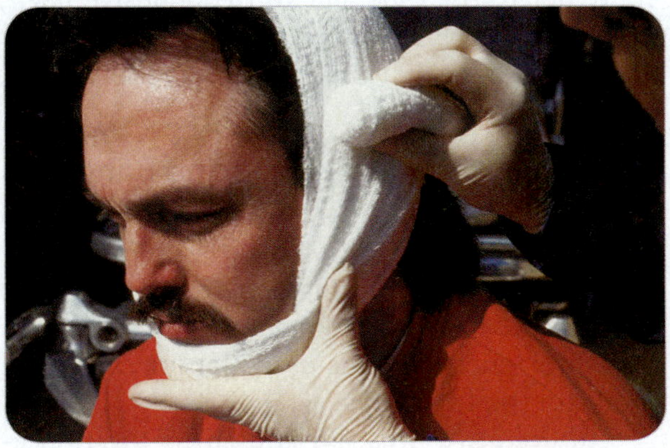

Figure 19-30 A roller gauze bandage can be used to secure a dressing in place.

OEC SKILL 19-3 Using a Self-Adhering Roller Bandage

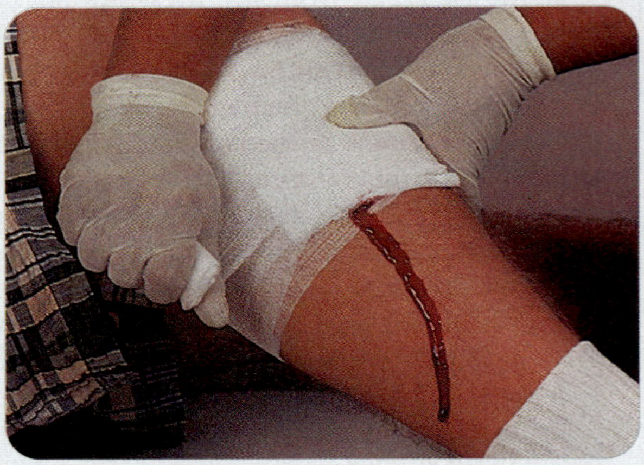

1. Use your hand to hold the dressing in place and secure the roller bandage with several wraps around the wound.
2. After the dressing and bandage are anchored, continue to wrap the bandage around the wound, overlapping it and keeping it snug.
3. After covering an area larger than the wound, tie the bandage in place or secure it with tape.

introduces the danger of restricting circulation if the bandage is too tight. For this reason, always leave fingers and toes exposed so that you can perform CMS checks distal to any bandage that has been applied. Obviously, a tourniquet for uncontrolled bleeding is not a bandage.

Do not use elastic bandages, because they tend to tighten on the injured part. In some instances, an Ace wrap may even function like a tourniquet and subsequently cause additional tissue damage or loss of limb.

Adhesive tape can be used to secure small dressings (4×4s) in place and is helpful in closing/securing larger dressings. Remember that allergies to adhesive tape are common. (The allergy is generally not to the tape, but to the adhesive itself, which contains latex.) If you discover during your SAMPLE history that the patient has this allergy, use latex-free tape.

Special Types of Dressings and Bandages

OEC technicians must be able to provide emergency care for all types of soft-tissue injuries. A necessary skill for treating soft-tissue injuries is the ability to tie a square knot (left over right, then right over left), which is essential for successful bandaging and splinting.

An **occlusive dressing** is used to cover sucking chest wounds and open neck wounds with an airtight layer of sterile Vaseline gauze, plastic cling wrap, or aluminum foil. Commercially available sterile occlusive dressings are packaged individually wrapped.

These dressings prevent air and liquids from entering (or exiting) the wound. Sealing all four edges might worsen the problem if used for a chest wound, so for chest wound, seal only three sides to allow air to escape. Use a sterile universal dressing moistened with sterile saline to cover open abdominal wounds in which organs are exposed. Secure with a dry universal dressing taped to the abdomen. For all other puncture-type wounds to the head, neck, or abdomen, seal all four sides of the occlusive dressing to prevent wound contamination.

OEC Skill 19-4 explains how to use an occlusive dressing.

A *stabilizing dressing* is used to secure an impaled object in place. Taking the object out could result in more damage to the tissues or cause significant bleeding. The dressing consists of several layers of a thick sterile dressing that are wrapped around the object and held in place by tape or a self-adhering roller bandage. Fully stabilizing the object may require wrapping several layers of folded cravats around the object to form a doughnut (**Figure 19-31**). If you do not have a stabilizing dressing, stabilize the object with several cravats and secure it with a square knot.

Bandaging Problem Areas

Moveable joints and irregularly shaped areas of the body require special bandaging techniques, as do

OEC SKILL 19-4 Using an Occlusive Dressing

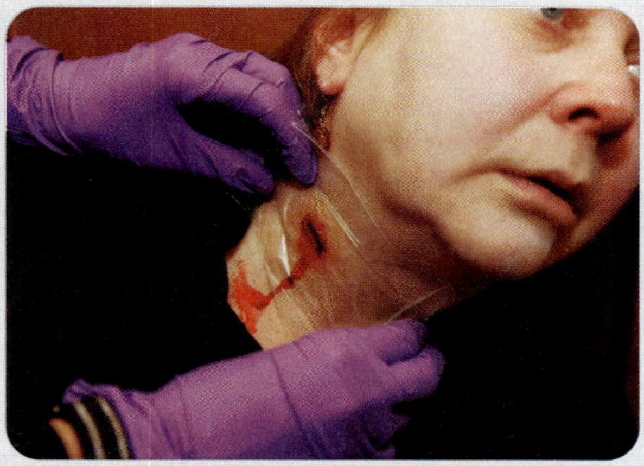

1 Cover neck wound with an airtight dressing and apply manual pressure. Do not compress both carotid arteries at the same time as this may impair circulation to the brain.

Note: In the case of an open chest wound seal only 3 sides of the occlusive dressing to allow air to escape on expiration.

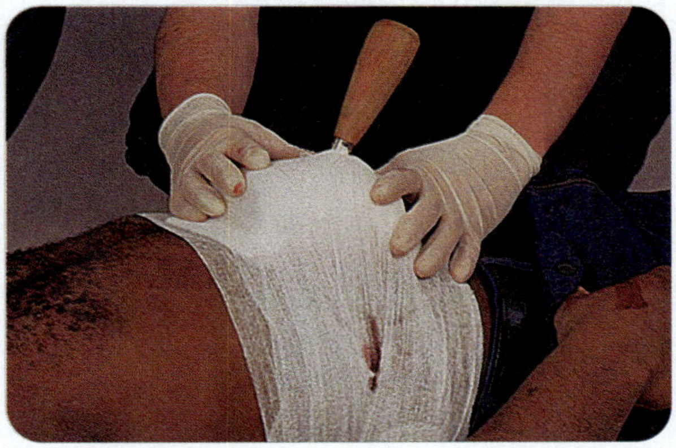

Figure 19-31 Stabilize an impaled object with a bulky dressing or several layers of cravats.

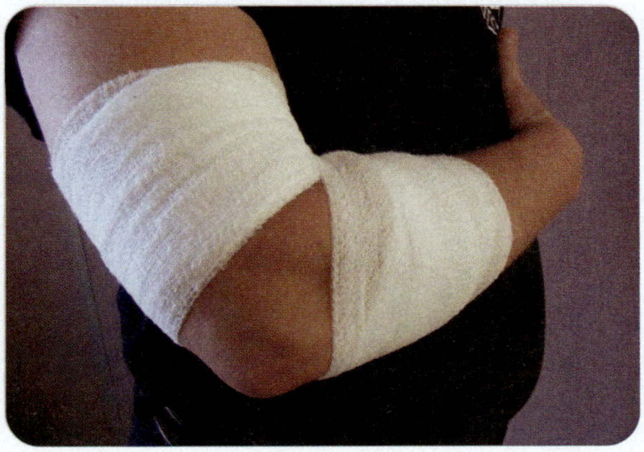

Figure 19-32 When dressing an elbow, secure it with a roller bandage in a figure-eight pattern.

spherical and conical anatomic regions. Because bandages tend to loosen when the joints beneath them move, choose a 3- to 6-inch self-adherent roller bandage to secure a sterile dressing applied to wounds near joints. Begin applying the bandage from below the joint and move diagonally in a figure-eight pattern to above the joint and then back down, overlapping the wrap as you go (**Figure 19-32**). Either tuck in the free end or secure it with adhesive tape. If roller bandage is not available, multiple 3- to 6-inch wide strips made from cravats may be used.

Conical regions such the arm, forearm, thigh, and leg are also best bandaged using a self-adherent roller bandage. Make several turns below the dressing, and then continue up, over, and above the dressing, overlapping the edges as you wrap. Anchor the loose end either under an edge of the bandage or with a strip of tape.

It is difficult to keep a dressing in place on the head (**Figure 19-33**). Either secure the dressing using a 2- to 3-inch self-adherent roller bandage as a compression band or create a bandana wrap using a triangular bandage, as explained in **OEC Skill 19-5**.

Because hands are always moving, even after being injured, bandages tend to work loose

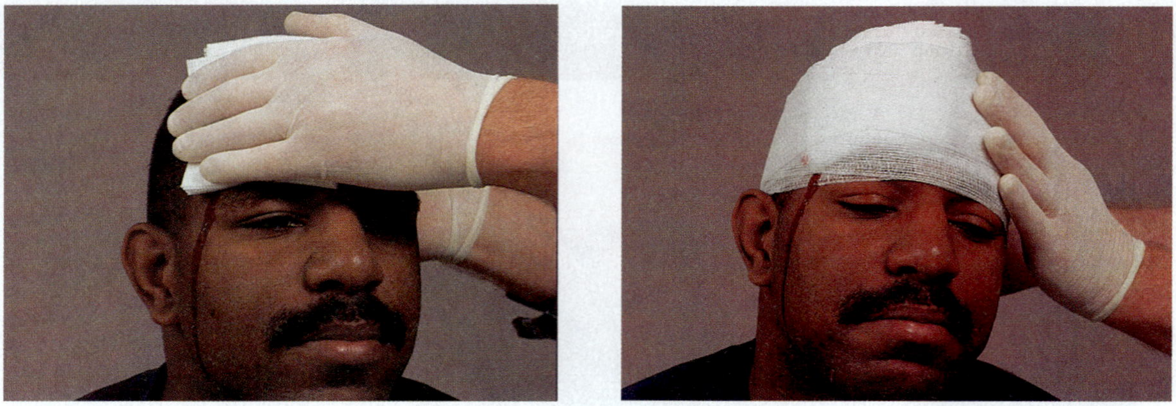

Figure 19-33 Head bandaging is difficult to keep in place.

OEC SKILL 19-5 Using a Triangular Bandage Bandana Wrap

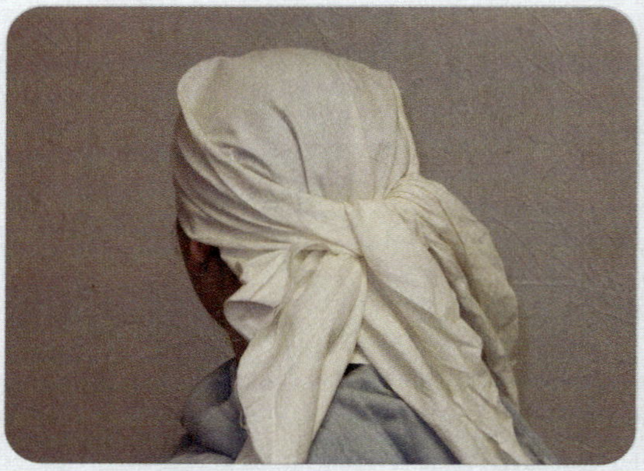

1. Fold a triangular bandage making a 3" hem. Position over the head with the point hanging down the back of the neck.

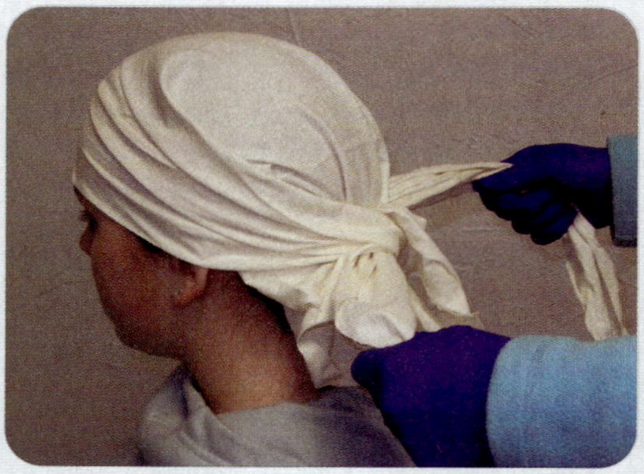

2. Draw the ends together and tie at the back of the head.

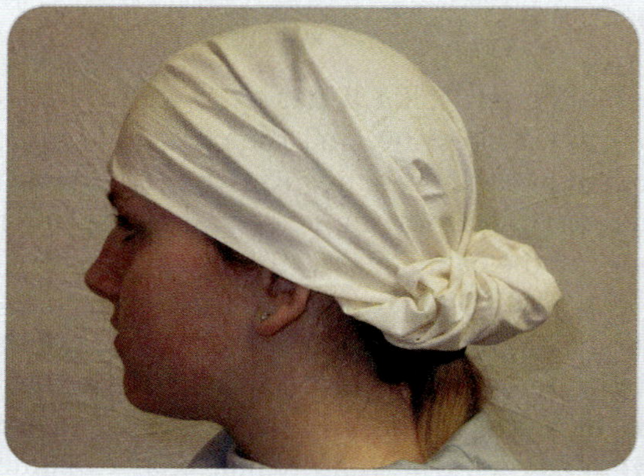

3. Lift the point of the triangular bandage, fold it over, and tuck it behind the knot. Smooth the bandage.

easily. An effective technique for bandaging wounds involving the palm or the back of the hand is to immobilize the entire hand. This is accomplished by placing small sterile pads (2×2) between the fingers and a roller gauze in the palm, putting the hand into the "position of function" (**Figure 19-34**). Next, wrap the hand with nonelastic bandage, elevate it above heart level, and sling and swathe it into place. When wrapping the gauze, try to leave the thumb and the fingertips exposed to facilitate CMS checks. When the patient's fingers must be left relatively free, so the hand can be used during rescue, use a suitable alternate bandaging technique for palm and dorsal hand wounds. Employ a modified figure-eight bandage or apply a short splint to the hand and distal forearm.

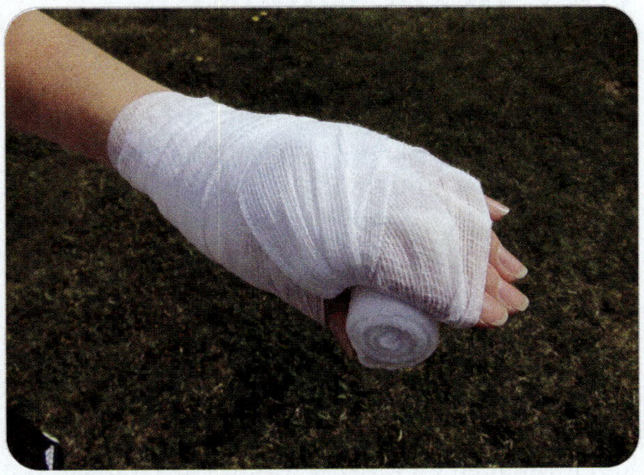

Figure 19-34 One method to splint two fingers together providing support to the injured digit.

A finger is a difficult structure to bandage because of its cylindrical shape and ability to move in multiple directions. If possible, use 1-inch roller gauze for smaller wounds, and a bulky hand bandage for large finger wounds. An alternative finger bandage is the modified figure-eight hand bandage, in which the finger is wrapped in an overlapping circular fashion with 1/2- or 1-inch roller gauze, which is then brought diagonally through the palm and around the wrist several turns. The free end is secured with adhesive tape. Do not wrap bandages around a finger too tightly, because doing so can compromise capillary refill.

OEC Skill 19-6 explains how to bandage a finger.

OEC SKILL 19-6 Bandaging a Finger

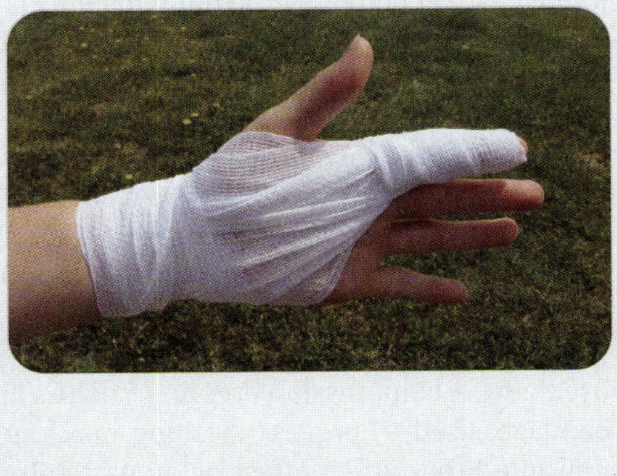

1. While supporting the injured finger, secure the dressing and begin to wrap the finger with a roller bandage.
2. Secure the bandage with adhesive tape.
3. If appropriate, apply a splint to the finger.
4. Secure the splint to the finger.
5. Use either a roller bandage or tape to secure the bandage to the hand.

KEY POINT

Geriatric Considerations

As members of our aging population spend more time outdoors, OEC technicians are increasingly likely to encounter patients who are taking warfarin, clopidogrel, aspirin, or other anticoagulants to reduce their risk of blood clot–related cardiovascular problems. Because these medications prolong bleeding time, they can result in life-threatening hemorrhage from seemingly innocuous internal and external wounds (**Figure 19-35**).

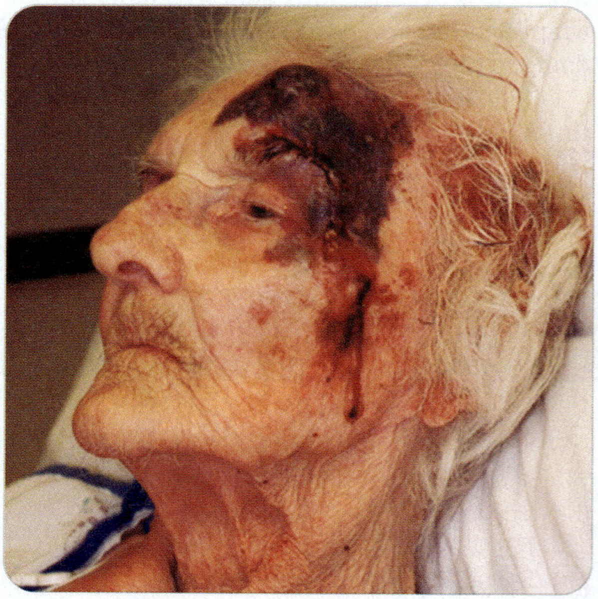

Figure 19-35 Be aware that a relatively minor injury in a geriatric patient on blood thinners could be life threatening.

Courtesy of Rhonda Hunt.

Splinting

Splinting also will help with bleeding. By immobilizing a fractured extremity, the bone ends are held still, allowing a solid internal hematoma to form at the fracture. Movement of a fractured and bleeding arm or leg allows internal bleeding to continue from both the damaged soft tissue and the fracture site. In severe pelvic fractures, the reason to use a pelvic sling is that it holds the bones still and together and slows bleeding.

MANAGEMENT OF SPECIFIC SOFT-TISSUE INJURIES

Contusions

For years, ski patrollers have been following the RICE protocol when caring for contusions, as recommended initially by Dr. G. Mirkin back in the 1970s. RICE stands for *r*est, *i*ce, *c*ompression, and *e*levation. Splinting was later added, creating RICES.

In 2019, Dr. Mirkin modified his opinion about ice. Ice or cooling works by decreasing the blood flow to an area, preventing the swelling and inflammation. In the 1970s we knew very little about the healing process. We did not understand that inflammation is actually a very important part of the healing process. Blood vessels in an injured area dilate, causing swelling and warmth. The increase in blood flow brings in very potent chemicals, proteins, and cells. Those chemicals and cells cause inflammation, initiating the healing process, and tissue repair begins. Recent medical literature shows that slowing or inhibiting the inflammation will delay the natural healing process.

However, applying ice initially makes an injured area feel better, by the numbing effect. Using ice immediately following an injury and for several hours is acceptable, but only for short "bursts" of time. Ice the injury for 5 minutes at a time and then leave it off for at least 30 minutes to allow the blood flow to return to the area. Always put cloth between the ice and the skin, so you do not freeze the tissue. After a few hours, the ice will no longer be effective in managing the pain and should be avoided.

Also, compressing an injured extremity is not used now. A compression dressing, such as an ACE bandage, used to prevent swelling may cause an unwanted tourniquet effect on an extremity. This can damage skin and soft tissue while decreasing blood flow that starts the healing process.

Initial splinting still is important, as decreasing initial movement helps to reduce pain and

OEC SKILL 19-7 Treating Closed Soft-Tissue Injuries

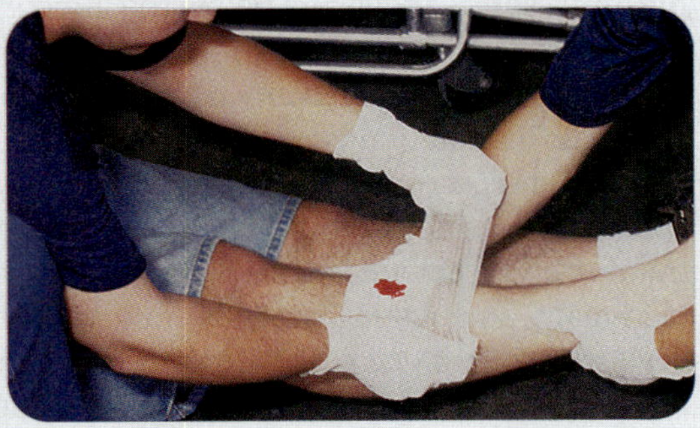

1 R—Rest: Cease activity or the use of the affected limb. Inactivity helps to reduce pain.

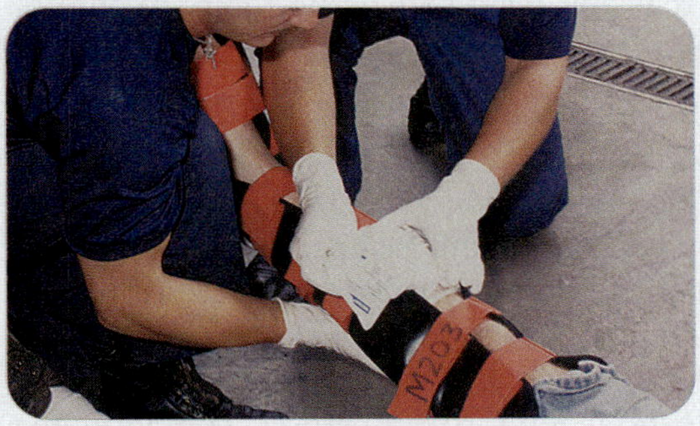

2 I—Ice: Apply cold packs or ice for pain control. Use only for short intervals.

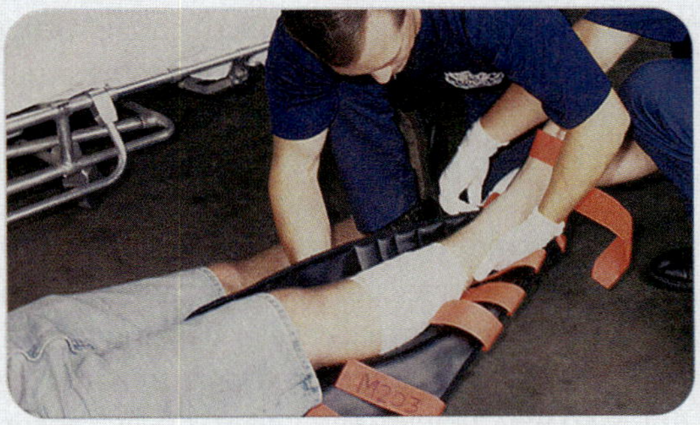

3 S—Splint: Immobilize the injured part using either a commercial splint or one fabricated from available materials. Splinting helps decrease pain.

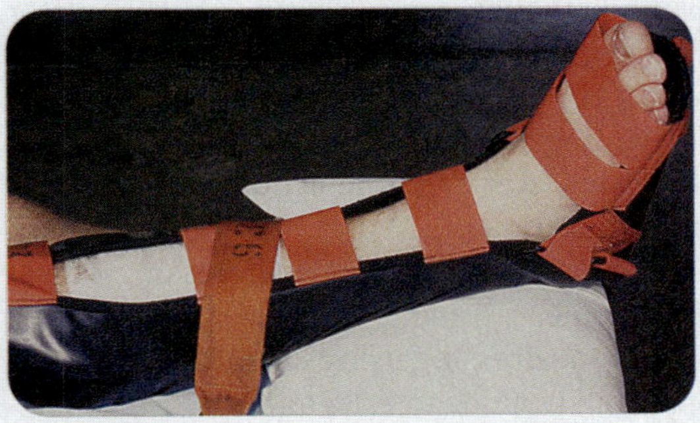

4 E—Elevate: Elevate the injured area above heart level to reduce pain.

slow bleeding in the case of fractures. Also, elevation will help initially with pain.

Therefore, the current recommendation is to use **RISE**, as explained in **OEC Skill 19-7**.

- **R—Rest:** Cease activity or the use of the affected limb. Inactivity helps to reduce pain.
- **I—Ice:** Apply cold packs or ice for pain control. Use only for short intervals.
- **S—Splint:** Immobilize the injured part using either a commercial splint or one fabricated from available materials. Splinting helps decrease pain.
- **E—Elevate:** Elevate the injured area above heart level to reduce pain.

Open Injuries

Open soft-tissue injuries require a different approach in order to reduce the risk of wound contamination and infection. In general, most open soft-tissue injuries that are minor—that is, abrasions, cuts that do not require suturing, and small lacerations—and that have not had significant bleeding or contamination can be treated in a definitive-care facility within several hours.

Treat any open soft-tissue injury in the following manner:

1. Control bleeding while observing standard precautions.
2. Once bleeding is controlled, provide wound care. If the wound is superficial, irrigate with sterile water (tap water if sterile water is not available) to clean the wound. If it is deep, leave the wound to be cleaned at the hospital. For dirty and grossly contaminated wounds when definitive medical care is more than 90 minutes away, carefully expose the wound and control initial active bleeding in the usual fashion. Then, carefully wash around all open wounds with soap and water, and *gently* irrigate all open wounds copiously with a 20- to 30-mL syringe if available containing sterile water or saline solution. If sterile water or saline is not available, use tap water.
3. Cover the wound with a clean dressing, sterile if available.
4. Secure the dressing using a bandage.
5. Splint all wounds in extremities and elevate the injured area above the level of the heart to reduce swelling.

Complex Soft-Tissue Injuries

Complex soft-tissue injuries such as avulsions, amputations, high-pressure injuries, and impaled objects require specialized treatment.

Avulsions

Control bleeding first. Cleanse the injury site as previously described to remove any debris. If the flap of skin is still attached, replace the flap in its original position and apply a sterile bandage to help reduce blood loss and contamination, and possibly to restore blood flow to the avulsed tissue.

Amputations

Control bleeding first. For any amputation with associated severe bleeding, directly apply several pressure bandages; if that is not effective, apply a tourniquet as previously described. Additional treatment will vary slightly depending on whether the amputation is incomplete or complete.

With an incomplete amputation, immobilize the injured part with a bulky compression dressing and a splint above and below the affected area to protect against further injury or further tissue separation. Never detach any partial amputation.

If the amputation is complete, preserve all amputated parts, no matter how damaged they may appear to be. Thanks to advances in microsurgical training and techniques, today's surgeons can reattach many amputated limbs, even those that have been without a blood supply for several hours. The key to success is appropriate care of the amputated part, both at the incident scene and en route to the hospital.

Check with local EMS regarding care for the amputated part (**Figure 19-36**). Some recommend wrapping the amputated part in a couple of layers of saline-moistened (not soaked) gauze. Others recommend wrapping a dry sterile dressing around the part. After this, put the part in a sealed plastic bag and place it in a container with ice. The amputated part should not be placed directly on the ice because doing so could result in a frostbite injury to the tissues. The objective is to keep the detached part cool without allowing it to freeze or develop frostbite. Do not submerge an amputated part in water because doing so will damage the tissue. Always ensure that the amputated part is transported with the patient. Replantation of an amputated part is ideally performed within 4 to 6 hours after injury, but success has been reported up to 24 hours after the injury if the amputated part has been kept cool.

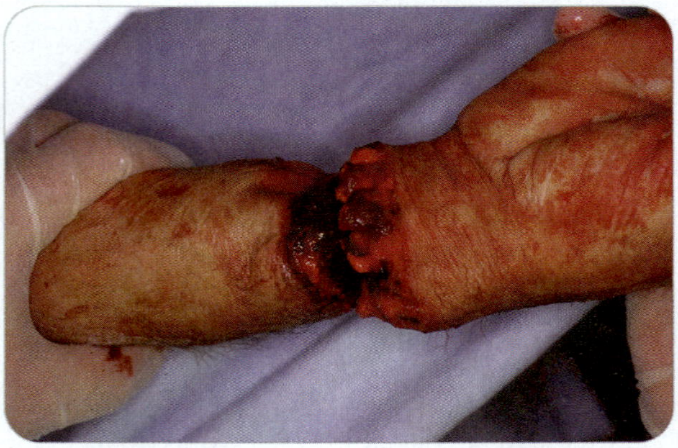

Figure 19-36 Amputated hand.

High-Pressure Injection Injuries

These injuries are very serious. Do not try to clean the injected material out of the tissue. Apply sterile dry bandages, splint the extremity, and transfer to a trauma center immediately.

Impaled Objects

An object that causes a puncture wound and remains embedded in the patient's body is known as an **impaled object**. Objects may be impaled in any part of the body and can occur accidentally or intentionally. Common impaled objects include knives, sticks, tree limbs, fence posts, rebar, glass shards, ski poles, fishhooks, arrows, and nails. As with any puncture wound, an impaled object can cause serious damage to underlying tissues. After controlling bleeding, the primary goal of treatment for a patient with an impaled object is to stabilize the object in the position you found it (**Figure 19-37**). The impaled object may effectively seal the wound, thereby preventing life-threatening bleeding. An impaled object should be removed by a physician in an operative setting (in an emergency department or in surgery).

In rare instances, impaled objects are removed in the field when they hinder rescue efforts or compromise the patient's airway. An impaled object that obstructs the airway (e.g., cheek, mouth, throat) should be removed to open the airway.

To stabilize an impaled object, follow the steps of **OEC Skill 19-8**.

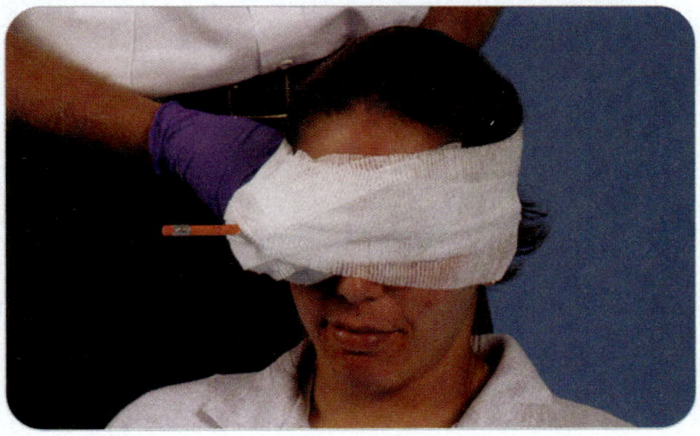

Figure 19-37 Unless the impaled object is obstructing the airway of the patient, it is best to leave the item in place, stabilize the object for transport, and transfer care to EMS as soon as possible.

OEC SKILL 19-8 Stabilizing an Impaled Object

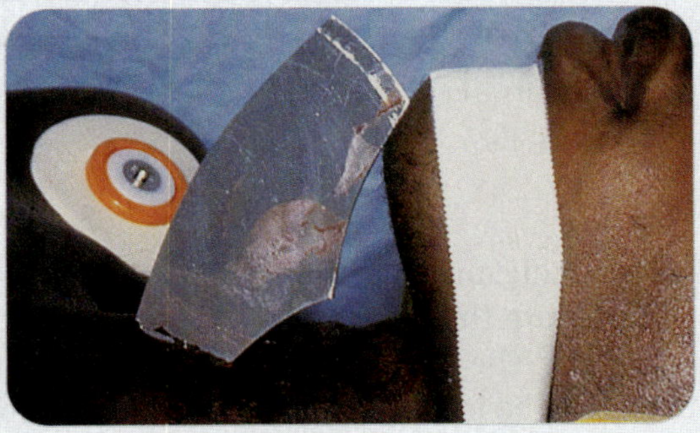

1 Manually stabilize the object so that it cannot move and damage surrounding and underlying tissues while you perform the next steps in this procedure.

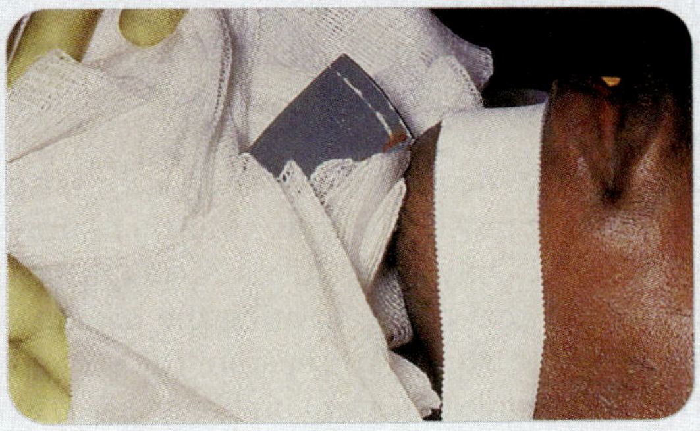

2 Remove or cut away all clothing surrounding the impaled object. Control bleeding by direct pressure. Apply a donut dressing around the impaled object. Stabilize the impaled object against the body.

(continues)

OEC SKILL 19-8 Stabilizing an Impaled Object (*continued*)

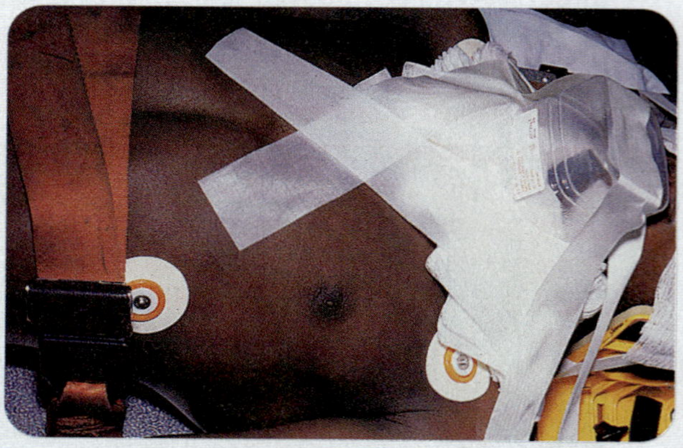

3 Apply a bulky dressing around the object. If the object is long or unwieldy, it may be necessary to shorten it by cutting off some of the exposed portion. Keep the object from being nudged or moved during transport by stabilizing it with tape or bandages. If available, consider securing a plastic cup, a bowl, or half of a plastic water bottle over the object after it has been stabilized.

MANAGEMENT OF BURNS

Continue to ensure your safety and that of other rescuers, which takes precedence over the treatment of patients. OEC technicians should wear special chemical-resistant gloves that provide protection from strong acids or bases when touching patients whose skin is still contaminated with such chemicals. Do not go near a patient who is contaminated by radioactivity; instead, wait for specially clothed and equipped personnel to arrive. Do not allow sloppy hazard mitigation or decontamination practices to decrease a patient's chances of survival because rescuers have become injured.

The primary focus of initial burn care is to stop the burning process to prevent further injury (**Figure 19-38**). Only after this is accomplished can the second goal begin: treating the patient's injuries. The first step is to separate the patient from the burn source. A patient on fire needs to be rolled on the ground or covered with a blanket or jacket to put out the fire. Obviously, such actions are performed during the scene size-up and before any assessment is begun.

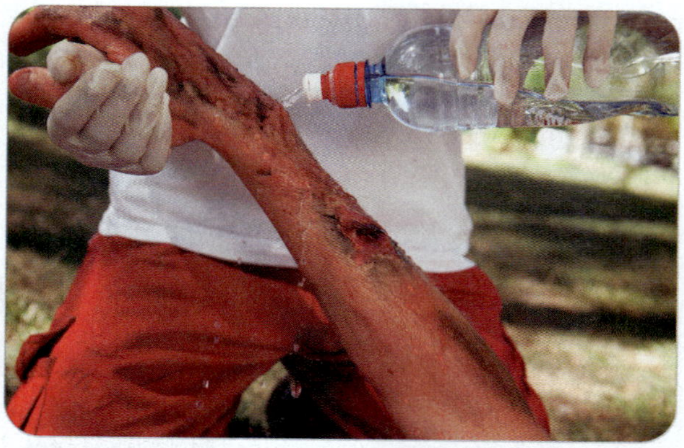

Figure 19-38 The first goal of initial burn care is to stop the burning process.

In general, treatment of burn patients, like that for any patients, starts with correcting any ABCD-related problems. The airway can be compromised in burn patients. Upon recognizing these signs and symptoms of an airway problem, OEC technicians must begin immediate treatment and activate the emergency care system for rapid transport. The window of time during which patients can be intubated by an ALS provider before airway swelling becomes too great is typically narrow.

Burns that affect the chest wall, especially full-thickness burns and burns that encircle the trunk, can compromise chest wall expansion, leading to restricted breathing. In such cases, assist the patient's respirations, as needed, using appropriate airway adjuncts and supplemental oxygen. Apply high-flow oxygen at 15 liters per minute via a nonrebreather mask to patients who can breathe on their own. Adjust the flow so that the oxygen saturation is equal to or higher than 94% by pulse oximeter. This will not only help reduce the likelihood of shock but also may provide some measure of pain relief. Remember that oxygen is highly flammable and its use near an open flame is extremely dangerous.

Electrical burns are associated with heart conduction problems, so initiate CPR if the patient is pulseless.

Patients with burns often have another mechanism of injury—for example, a blast injury, which can cause additional injuries such as fractures, head injuries, or internal bleeding. Care for these and any other injuries as needed. Use a cervical collar and protect the spine if indicated.

Remove charred clothing and any jewelry the patient may be wearing as soon as reasonably possible. If clothing is synthetic, it may have melted into the tissues and be difficult to remove; in that case, do not pull it off but instead cut off any pieces of cloth that are not imbedded in the wound. Cool and irrigate burned tissue with room-temperature tap water or (better yet) sterile saline solution. Complete immersion of the burned body part in water is advisable only for small, localized burns for which the patient still has sensation. Monitor the patient throughout this process because cooling with water in outdoor environments can result in hypothermia.

Once a larger burn has been sufficiently cooled, cover it with dry, sterile dressings (**Figure 19-39**). If no dressings are available, use a clean, cotton-based article of clothing, preferably one that is lint-free.

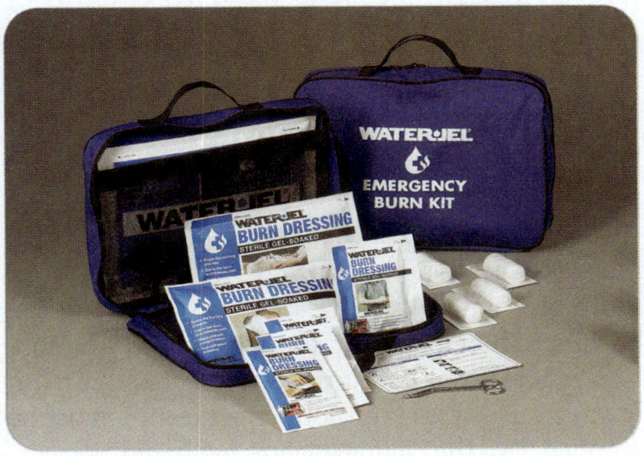

Figure 19-39 Emergency supplies needed to care for burns.

Courtesy of Water-Jel® Technologies.

Burns that are smaller than 5% of total body surface area (TBSA) may benefit from the application of a clean, wet, and cool dressing. Except for minor sunburn, do not apply antimicrobial ointments, creams, aloe vera burn cream, or other emollients because their use complicates future hospital care.

Keep patients warm by covering them with a clean sheet or blanket. Applying clean linens can also decrease pain severity by reducing air movement over burned tissue. Continuously monitor the patient and treat for shock, which can occur even with burns that are less than 5% of TBSA.

For significant upper body burns, elevate the patient's head and chest 20 to 30 degrees to minimize upper body edema. If the burn is accompanied by suspected spinal injury, secure the patient on a long spine board with full spinal immobilization and elevate the head end of the board. Be prepared to provide considerable emotional support to the patient.

Additional treatment for specific types of burns follows.

Sunburn

Treatment for sunburn includes cool compresses and skin lotions containing aloe vera. Until the sunburn has resolved, prevent reexposure to sunlight by wearing clothing that covers the affected areas.

Thermal Burns

The priority, as previously indicated, is to extinguish any burning or smoldering clothing using the National Fire Protection Association's time-honored practice of "Stop, Drop, and Roll." With this technique, a person on fire is instructed not to run, but to drop to the ground immediately and then roll back and forth or be rolled by rescuers until the flames are extinguished. At the same time, rescuers can cover the patient with a coat or

KEY POINT

Stop the Burn

1. Stop the burning process.
2. Remove clothing and jewelry near the affected area.

blanket to smother the flames if water or a carbon dioxide fire extinguisher is not immediately available. Do not use a chemical fire extinguisher. Do not swat at the flames with a blanket or jacket; doing so only fans the flames and makes them larger. Extinguish the flames and then remove any clothing that is burned, singed, or smoldering.

If thermal burns are due to a hot liquid, remove all wet items of clothing (especially diapers) because they can hold the hot liquid against the skin, increasing the duration and thus the severity of the burns. Additionally, some fabrics, especially those used in outdoor athletic apparel, melt when sufficiently heated and may leave a hot adherent residue on the patient's skin. Do not attempt to pull this material from the skin because doing so may cause additional damage.

Do not break any blisters that are present because this action increases the risk of infection. Do not apply cold compresses because their use may precipitate hypothermia.

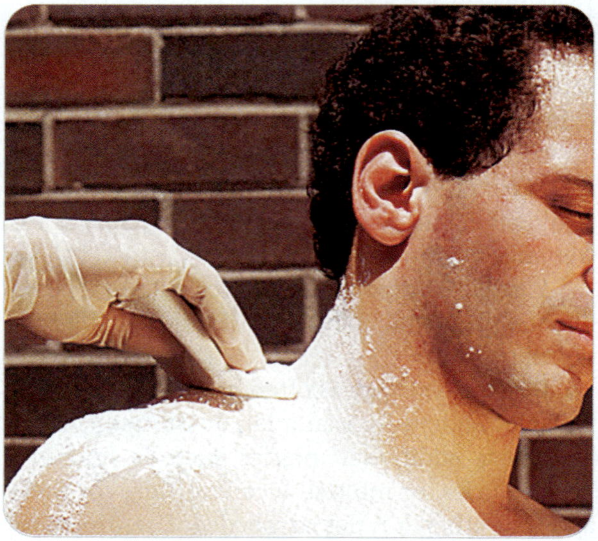

Figure 19-40 Brush off dry chemicals that remain on the patient after clothing has been removed.

Chemical Burns

For burns resulting from contact with a caustic substance, quickly remove all the patient's clothing (including undergarments and socks) and jewelry—regardless of whether they appear contaminated—to ensure full removal of the chemical and to minimize tissue damage. In the process, use PPE to protect yourself, especially your hands, from the caustic substance. If large amounts of the chemical are present, consider mobilizing a hazmat team for achieving full decontamination.

Because some dry chemicals become even more caustic when activated by water, brush off any dry chemical residues that may remain on the patient (**Figure 19-40**).

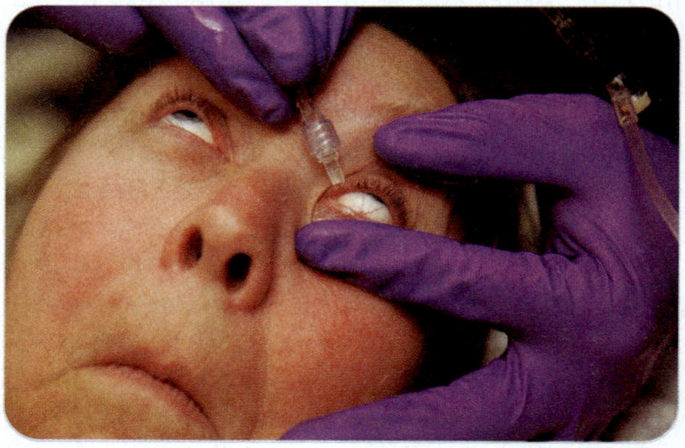

Figure 19-41 Flush the eyes with a copious amount of water and then bandage the eyes and transfer the patient to EMS.

Immediately irrigate the chemically burned areas with large amounts of tepid water for at least 15 minutes, or until the burning sensation ceases. This includes the eyes, which should be bandaged after irrigation is complete (**Figure 19-41**). Because alkali burns penetrate more deeply than acid burns, they may require longer irrigation times to completely clear the chemical. During irrigation, avoid extending burns to uninjured areas by turning the patient so that the irrigating water flows away from unaffected skin. Avoid causing further tissue injury by not forcefully directing water onto the injury. Do not rub the injured tissue because doing so will likely result in massive tissue sloughing.

If you are in an outdoor environment in which tap water is not available, remember that your first objective in treating any burn is to stop the burning. Therefore, even though the risk of infection is increased if you rinse a patient's burns in water from a stream or pond, the burning must be stopped. Use the cleanest water available.

Once irrigation is complete, cover all burned areas in the manner previously described. If at any time you are unsure about the specific chemical

KEY POINT

Chemical Burn Alert

Caution! When managing chemical burns, do not apply a neutralizing agent because this may cause a thermal reaction, worsening the injury. Dust off any dry chemicals and irrigate the area with room-temperature water. Note as well that the application of water to some chemicals also produces heat.

you are dealing with or have treatment-related questions, you can obtain emergency information 24 hours a day by calling CHEMTREC, the national emergency chemical information center, at 1-800-262-8200.

Electrical Burns

The first step in managing a patient with an electrical burn is to *make sure the power source is turned off*. This cannot be overstated; fatal injuries can occur if you or anyone else comes into contact with the electrical current or with a patient who is still in contact with the electrical current. If available, have specially trained personnel separate the patient from the power supply.

All patients who have been electrically shocked should be fully immobilized using spinal motion restriction (SMR). Move the patient to a safe area, protecting the spine by manually stabilizing the neck. Maintain the airway and give supplemental oxygen. Evaluate for shock and treat appropriately. Cardiac arrest resulting from electrical injury is common. If the patient goes into cardiopulmonary arrest, treat in the usual manner by beginning CPR and attaching an automated external defibrillator (AED), if available.

During the secondary assessment of a patient with electrical burns, look for the points of entry and exit, which can help you determine which underlying structures may have been affected by the current (**Figure 19-42**). Whereas entrance wounds are often small, exit wounds are usually extensive and deep. Cover all wounds in the usual manner.

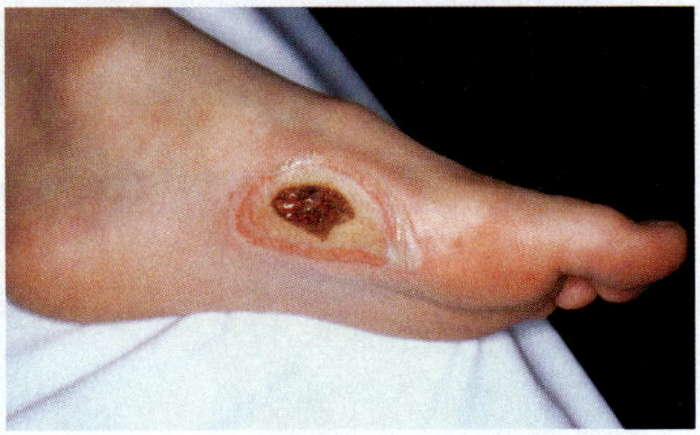

A

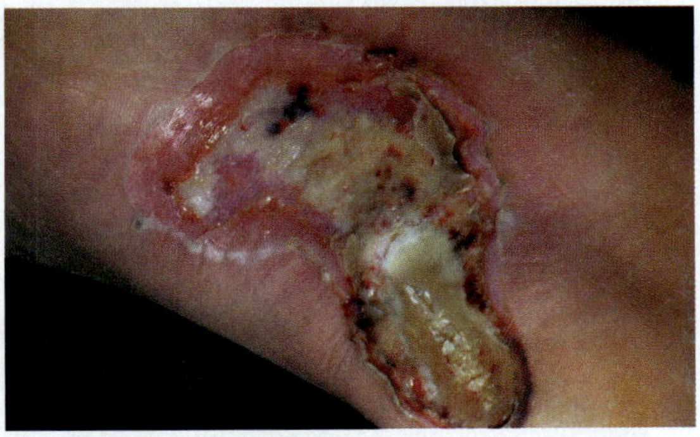

B

Figure 19-42 When treating an electrical burn patient, always look for the entry (**A**) and exit (**B**) burns.

OEC Skill 19-9 describes how to care for burns.

Lightning Strikes

Care for patients who have sustained a lightning-strike injury in the same way as you would for any unresponsive patient: Perform an appropriate primary assessment. You cannot be shocked by touching a patient who has been struck by lightning. Open the airway using the jaw-thrust maneuver and simultaneously check for breathing and a carotid pulse. Always protect the spinal column using spinal motion restriction (SMR) because the patient could have a spinal injury. If breathing and a pulse are not present, begin CPR. If there is no pulse, early defibrillation with an AED is best. Because damage to the circulatory and respiratory systems is usually temporary and patients may be capable of full recovery, continue CPR. If a pulse returns but the patient is not breathing, continue rescue breathing as long as possible. Use a bag-valve mask and high-flow oxygen, if available.

OEC SKILL 19-9 Caring for Burns

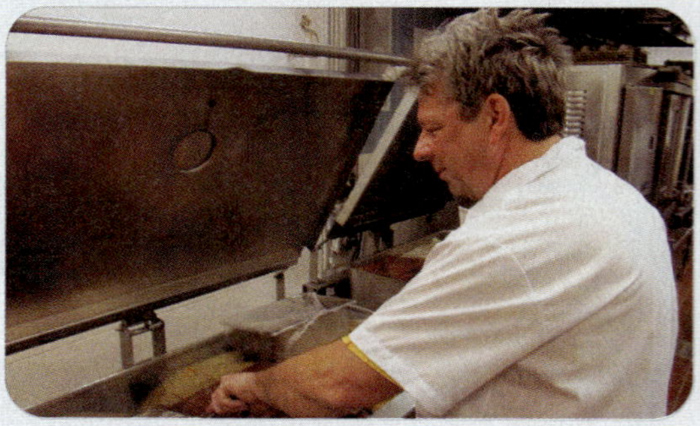

1 Burns can happen unexpectedly.

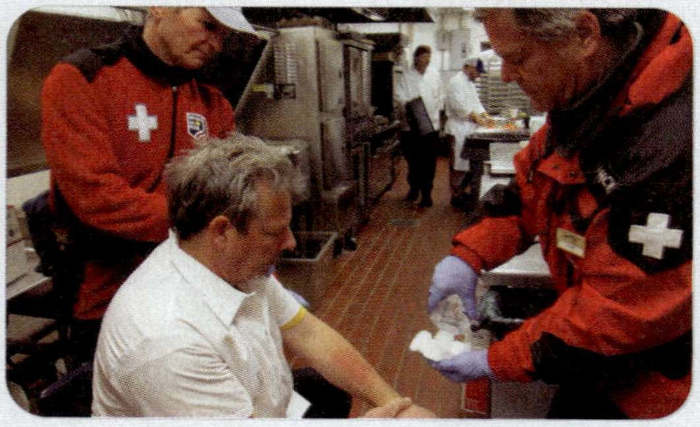

2 Remove any affected clothing, stop the burning process, and cool the burn.

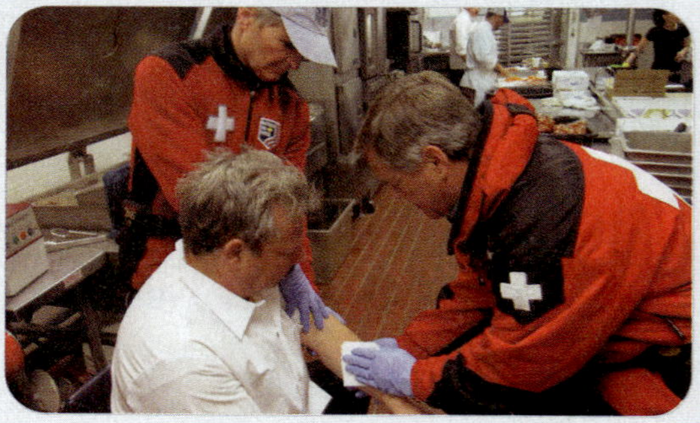

3 Apply a sterile gauze dressing to the wound. Wet the dressing only if the wound is less than 5 percent of TBSA.

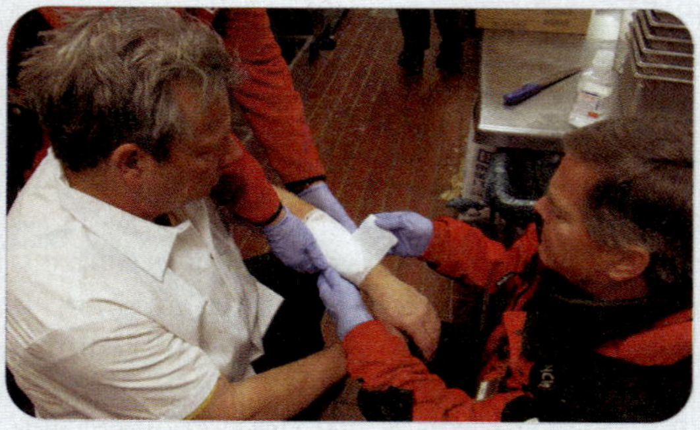

4 Bandage the wound to keep the dressing securely in place. Then prepare to assist the patient to find further medical treatment.

For lightning-strike incidents involving multiple victims, care first for those in cardiac or respiratory arrest. This approach, called "reverse triage," is based on the assumption that patients who show signs of life (pulse and respirations, and perhaps movement, moaning, or talking) are likely to survive and thus should be treated *after* CPR is attempted on patients who appear to be dead. Quick treatment is crucial for increasing the chances that lightning-strike victims who are in cardiac or respiratory arrest can be successfully resuscitated. Remember, lightning-strike victims do not carry any residual electrical charge and are safe to touch.

Radiation Burns

Radiation burns other than those resulting from exposure to UV light require specialized equipment and management techniques that are beyond the scope of this text. Patients can become contaminated by radioactive material with or without direct contact with the source. Patients who have been contaminated by radiation should be approached only by hazmat team members wearing special protective gear. If radiation injury resulted from an industrial accident or a terrorist attack, do not enter the area; instead, notify a team that specializes in such incidents. UV-related

> **KEY POINT**
>
> **Entrance and Exit Wounds**
>
> Remember that patients injured by electricity often appear to be much better off than they are because many of their burns are beneath the surface. Take vital signs frequently and be prepared for extensive resuscitation (CPR and AED).

> **KEY POINT**
>
> **Extensive Burns**
>
> Remember that with extensive burns, patients lose the ability to thermoregulate. Make sure they do not become hypothermic by wrapping them in warm, dry sheets.

burns are typically treated in the same manner as first-degree burns.

Further Care and Transport of Burn Patients

Although most burns are minor, severe burns can develop numerous complications, including shock, sepsis, respiratory distress, and cardiac arrest. Patients who have extensive burns must be transported to a definitive-care facility, preferably a designated burn center, because of the likelihood of extensive tissue damage, underlying injuries, and the need for long-term care. If a burn center is not available, transport the patient to the nearest trauma center.

The area of the body with partial-thickness and full-thickness burns (or second-degree and higher burns) is important in determining the care of a patient. The more severe the burns and the greater the amount of TBSA involved, the more difficult it is to manage the injuries, and the higher the mortality rates. OEC technicians must be able to quickly identify burn patients whose injuries are considered critical and require immediate treatment and rapid transport. According to the American Burn Association, patients who meet any of the following criteria are considered critical and should be taken to one of the nation's 125 designated burn centers:

- Burns to a child younger than 10 years or to an adult older than 65 years
- Burns involving more than one body part (e.g., torso and leg)
- Burns involving the head, neck, hands, feet, genitals, or major joints
- Inhalation injury or burns
- Burns associated with difficulty breathing or hoarseness
- Chemical or electrical burns (including lightning injury)
- Partial-thickness (second-degree) burn greater than 10% of TBSA
- Any full-thickness (third- or fourth-degree) burn
- Burns associated with trauma
- Burns with a serious underlying medical disorder (e.g., diabetes, heart disease)
- Burns in a patient who has special social, emotional, or physical needs
- Exposure to radioactive materials

If possible, summon advanced care providers to transport the patient, because they can administer pain medications and other advanced therapies that can make the patient significantly more comfortable and lessen the incidence of shock. However, do not delay transport if ALS is not readily available.

Transport burn patients on a clean, dry sheet to prevent the person from sticking to the backboard, toboggan, litter, or stretcher. Provide the transporting crew or hospital staff a complete oral handoff report that includes the source of the burn, any pertinent history, clinical findings and treatment administered, and the patient's responses to the treatment.

CASE Outcome

You apply more dressings over the wrist, and bleeding continues. Thinking the man cut his radial artery, you pull your tourniquet out of your pack and place it on his arm above the cut and below the elbow, tightening it appropriately. The bleeding stops. You mark the time the tourniquet was applied on the arm bandage. Realizing you have a major bleed, you call base, requesting immediate transport, saying you have applied a tourniquet. While waiting on transport, you wrap the lower leg abrasions with a roller bandage. Next, you bandage the patient's hands to prevent further contamination. You then recheck the distal circulation, motor function, and sensation to ensure that the bandages are not too tight. A sling is placed on the arm with the shoulder injury. An ambulance arrives shortly thereafter and transfers the patient to a trauma center that is 30 minutes away. The patient has surgery to repair the lacerated radial artery.

CHAPTER REVIEW

In Summary

- The skin is the largest organ in the body, and it serves four purposes: it provides a protective barrier, it functions in the control of body temperature, it acts as a sensory organ, and it helps synthesize vitamin D.
- The three types of soft-tissue injuries are closed injuries, open injuries, and burns.
- External bleeding is controlled using direct pressure, a pressure dressing, additional dressings, or, rarely, a tourniquet.
- When applying a dressing to control bleeding, do not remove it because doing so can disrupt clots and cause more bleeding. Instead, add additional dressings.
- Hemostatic bandages contain a substance that helps stop external bleeding.
- Do not use elastic bandages to secure dressings.
- Splinting a soft-tissue injury helps decrease bleeding and reduces pain.
- Applying an effective field dressing and bandage is an important skill for OEC technicians.
- Always make sure the scene is safe before caring for a burn patient, then stop the burning process.
- Patients with extensive burns need to go to a burn center.
- Patients struck by lightning are not electrically charged and (unlike victims of electrical injury) pose no threat to rescuers.
- In a triage situation, care first for lightning-strike victims who appear dead.

Key Terms

Amputation The complete or nearly complete separation of a body part or limb.

Avulsion The incomplete separation of the soft-tissue layers where the injured tissue is left dangling as a flap.

Bandage A strip or roll of gauze or other material used for wrapping or binding a body part.

Burn A lesion of the skin caused by thermal or frictional heat, chemicals, electricity, or nuclear radiation.

Compartment syndrome A condition in which the swelling of injured muscles within their connective tissue coverings causes pressure that can damage tissue and cut off blood flow.

Compression (pressure) dressing A dressing that closes bleeding blood vessels by compressing the wound.

Crush injury A compression injury in which a great amount of force is applied to the body.

Dressing Any material (preferably sterile) used for covering and protecting a wound.

Ecchymosis A bruise; discoloration of the skin associated with a closed wound; signifies bleeding within the skin.

Exsanguination Massive blood loss resulting in death; the process of bleeding to death.

Hematoma A localized collection of blood inside the body that has leaked from a blood vessel.

Hemorrhage The escape of blood from the vessels; bleeding.

Hemostatic dressing A surgical gauze/mesh impregnated with a material that stops arterial and venous bleeding in seconds.

Impaled object A foreign object that remains in the body in a puncture wound.

Incision A cut caused by a sharp object; has clean, smooth edges.

Laceration A cut caused by forces that tear or crush the skin; tends to have *jagged* edges.

Mucous membranes The linings of body cavities and passages that are in direct or indirect contact with the outside environment.

Occlusive dressing A dressing made of Vaseline gauze, aluminum foil, or plastic wrap that prevents air and liquids from entering or exiting a wound.
Puncture An injury that is caused by a pointed object that penetrates the skin.
RISE Rest, ice, splint, elevate, the sequence of actions that providers should take when caring for contusions.
Scald An injury caused by a hot liquid or a hot, moist vapor.
Subungual hematoma A painful collection of blood under a nail.
Tourniquet An instrument that when tightened around an arm or leg temporarily arrests the flow of blood through a large artery.
Universal dressing A sterile, soft, highly absorbent, individually wrapped dressing that provides superior padding and protection for major wounds; usually measures 9 inches by 36 inches; also called *trauma dressing*.

Chapter Questions

1. The functions of the skin include:
   a. acting as a protective barrier.
   b. regulating temperature.
   c. maintaining water balance.
   d. All of the above
2. Which layer of the skin contains hair follicles, sebaceous (oil) glands, sweat glands, blood vessels, and specialized nerve endings?
   a. Epidermis
   b. Dermis
   c. Subcutaneous tissue
   d. Arteries
3. If your patient presents with a laceration that has bright red blood spurting from it, the cause is most likely a cut in:
   a. an artery.
   b. a vein.
   c. a capillary.
   d. subcutaneous tissue.
4. When assessing a soft-tissue injury, it is important to:
   a. remember that forces causing the injury could damage underlying structures.
   b. approach it like any other medical traumatic emergency.
   c. ask the patient if he or she is taking an anticoagulant.
   d. All of the above
5. The objective for caring for a detached body part is:
   a. placing the detached body part directly on ice.
   b. submerging the detached body part in sterile water.
   c. covering the detached body part with an occlusive dressing.
   d. keeping the detached body part cool without freezing.
6. The cook at the ski area has spilled boiling water onto himself, burning his arm. This type of burn is called a:
   a. thermal burn.
   b. chemical burn.
   c. electrical burn.
   d. radiological burn.
7. Your patient has a partial-thickness burn. You would expect that the affected skin would be:
   a. charred and dry.
   b. black.
   c. blistered and reddened.
   d. waxy looking and dry.
8. An adult patient has burned her entire back and the posterior portion of both legs. What is the total body surface area that is burned?
   a. 36%
   b. 27%
   c. 18%
   d. 9%

9. The simplest way to control most bleeding is application of:
   a. a tourniquet.
   b. a hemostatic dressing.
   c. direct pressure with a dressing and an additional dressing if needed.
   d. an occlusive dressing.

10. You control bleeding by placing a 4-inch by 4-inch gauze pad over a small wound. This pad is called a(n):
    a. dressing.
    b. bandage.
    c. cravat.
    d. occlusive closure.

11. Your patient has been struck by lightning and is found lying unresponsive on the ground. During the assessment of this patient, it is important to be mindful of the high likelihood that the patient could be:
    a. electrically charged.
    b. in cardiac arrest.
    c. suffering from anaphylaxis.
    d. suffering from sepsis.

Reference

National Weather Service. n.d. How dangerous is lightning? https://www.weather.gov/safety/lightning-odds. Accessed December 13, 2019.

Answers: 1. d, Objective 19-1, p. 392; 2. b, Objective 19-2, p. 393; 3. a, Objective 19-3, p. 394; 4. d, Objective 19-4, p. 404; 5. d, Objective 19-6, p. 420; 6. a, Objective 19-7, p. 400; 7. c, Objective 19-9, p. 406; 8. a, Objective 19-9, p. 407; 9. c, Objective 19-11, p. 408; 10. a, Objective 19-12, p. 409; 11. b, Objective 19-15, p. 401

CHAPTER 20

MUSCULOSKELETAL INJURIES

SECTION 1: ANATOMY, PHYSIOLOGY, INJURIES, AND ASSESSMENT

OBJECTIVES

Upon completion of this section of this chapter, the OEC technician will be able to:

20-1.1 Identify and define the functions of the following structures:
- Bones
- Cartilage
- Joints
- Muscles
- Synovium
- Tendons
- Ligaments

20-1.2 Describe how musculoskeletal tissues heal.

20-1.3 Explain the difference between a sprain and strain.

20-1.4 Describe and demonstrate the general assessment of musculoskeletal injuries.

20-1.5 List the signs and symptoms of sprains, strains, ruptured tendons, dislocations, and fractures.

KEY TERMS

Acromioclavicular (A/C) joint, p. 448
Angulation, p. 450
Articular cartilage, p. 434
Articulation, p. 461
Bone crepitus, p. 445
Cartilage, p. 434
Cortex, p. 435
Dislocation, p. 441
Dorsal, p. 453
Dorsiflex, p. 456
False movement, p. 452
Fracture, p. 438
Guarding, p. 443
Immobilization, p. 438
Joints, p. 434
Joint capsule, p. 435
Ligaments, p. 434
Meniscus, p. 459
Musculoskeletal system, p. 434
Periosteum, p. 435
Plantarflex, p. 456
Popliteal fossa, p. 461
Skeletal muscle, p. 437
Sling and swathe, p. 468
Splint, p. 467
Sprain, p. 439
Strain, p. 439
Subluxation, p. 441
Synovium, p. 435
Tendons, p. 434
Traction, p. 472
Traction splint, p. 472
Zone of injury, p. 439

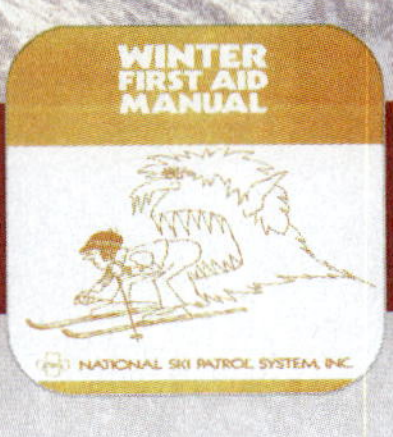

HISTORICAL TIMELINE **1986.** Field trials of the new Winter First Aid program begin.

CHAPTER OVERVIEW

This chapter has three sections. Section 1 includes general information about the musculoskeletal system, including anatomy, physiology, common injuries, and assessment of musculoskeletal injuries. It is important to understand these concepts before proceeding to Section 2, which discusses the various musculoskeletal injuries. Section 3 details how OEC technicians care for musculoskeletal injuries.

The body's **musculoskeletal system** allows the body to stand and walk upright and perform tasks. The system's primary components are the muscles and the bony skeleton, but the system also includes **joints**, the **cartilage** on the ends of bones at joints, synovial fluid that lubricates the joints, **ligaments**, **tendons**, and the interface between the nervous system and the muscles. Ligaments hold joints together, while tendons go from muscles to bones.

The bones and muscles protect vital organs within the body's cavities. This protection can occur directly, when the vertebrae of the spinal column protect the spinal cord, or indirectly, when one holds up a forearm to prevent an object from striking the body.

This chapter provides a review of the anatomy of the various components of the musculoskeletal system. It is important that you know the names of the major bones, muscles, and joints, as well as how ligaments, tendons, and joints work. The chapter also discusses the physiology of movement, and how the musculoskeletal system repairs itself. Common musculoskeletal injuries, including strains, sprains, dislocations, ruptures of tendons, and fractures are discussed with respect to both assessment and management.

ANATOMY AND PHYSIOLOGY

The various components of the skeleton are crucial to the makeup and function of the musculoskeletal system. OEC technicians need to have a good understanding of the parts of the musculoskeletal system, including the names of major bones, muscles, and joints.

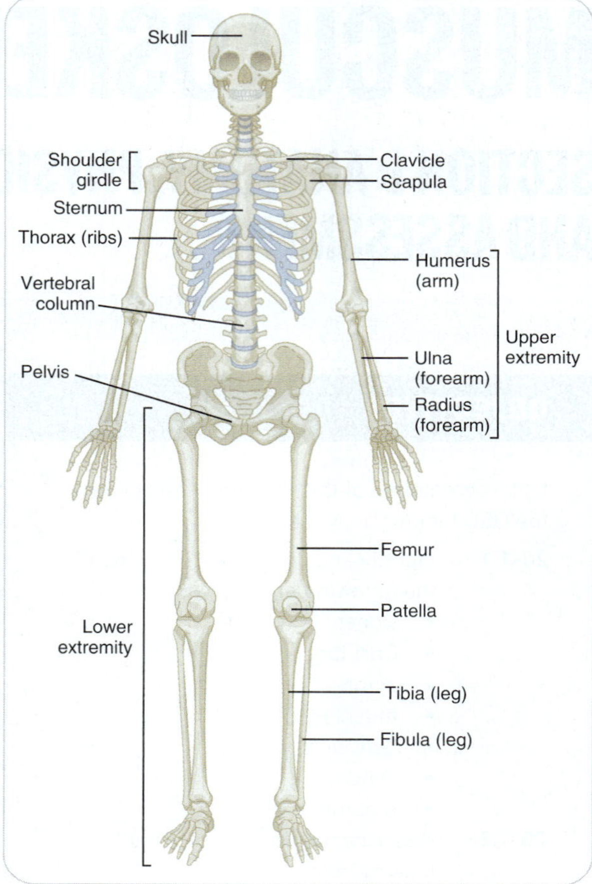

Figure 20-1 The human skeleton.

The Skeleton

The skeleton functions as a rigid framework to protect the internal organs, provides the body form we recognize as human, and produces blood cells. The skeleton consists of bones, connective tissue, and cartilage (**Figure 20-1**).

The skeleton has seven areas:

1. Head, skull, facial bones
2. Spine
3. Shoulder
4. Upper extremities (arms)
5. Rib cage (thorax)
6. Pelvis
7. Lower extremities (legs)

Bone ends are covered with **articular cartilage**, which provides a nearly friction-free

CASE Presentation

On a great day for spring skiing, a call comes over the radio for someone to respond to Fiddler's Elbow for a possible leg injury. Getting off the top of the lift, you find a helmeted teenager on twin-tipped skis, just below a rail sitting on the ground. He is in severe pain, complaining that his left knee hurts and "feels funny." You notice his left shoulder seems lower than the right one. One of his buddies standing nearby says, "Wow, that was awesome."

What should you do?

surface, allowing bone ends to move smoothly against one another. Children's bones grow longer near the ends, along the growth plate. Fractures occurring in the growth plate during childhood can damage the cells needed for bone growth, creating abnormal bone growth and deformity.

The dense vascular layer on the outside of a bone is the **periosteum** (**Figure 20-2**). Beneath the periosteum is the hard **cortex**. Within the cortex is the bone marrow, a less-dense region where blood cells are made. Bones are highly vascular and receive 10% to 20% of the blood pumped by the heart. When the cortex of a bone breaks, the highly vascular marrow may bleed severely.

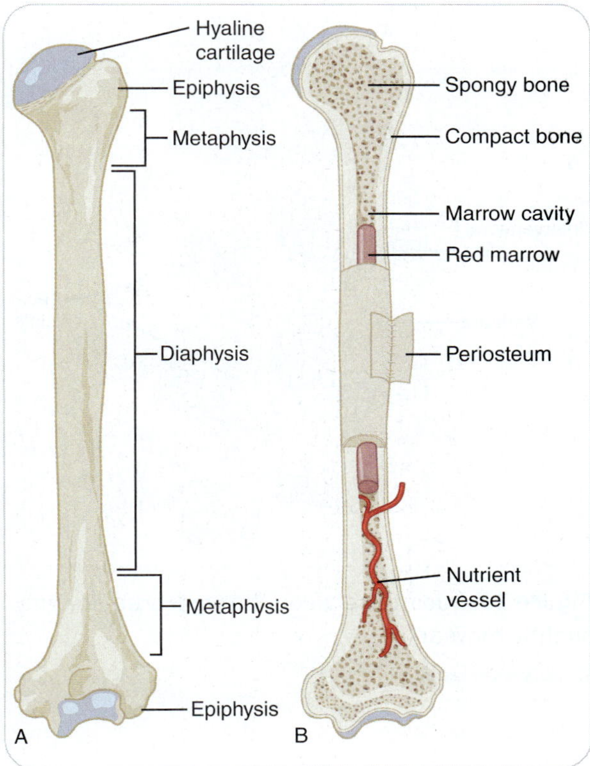

Figure 20-2 The components of a long bone. **A.** Humerus. **B.** Longitudinal section of the humerus.

Joints

The site at which two or more bones make contact is known as a joint. Joints enable all body movements, including bending and straightening. The connective tissue that surrounds, stabilizes, and supports the joint is called the **joint capsule**. This capsule contains a slippery lubricant, known as synovial fluid, made by the lining of the joint, which is called the **synovium**. This fluid, along with the bones' articular surfaces, allows the bones to move freely within the joint capsule.

Joints provide different degrees of movement. Many joints, such as the knee, hip, elbow, and shoulder joints, are essentially *freely movable* (**Figure 20-3**). A few joints, such as those between vertebrae, are *slightly movable* (**Figure 20-4**). Other joints, such as the acromioclavicular joint of the shoulder, permit

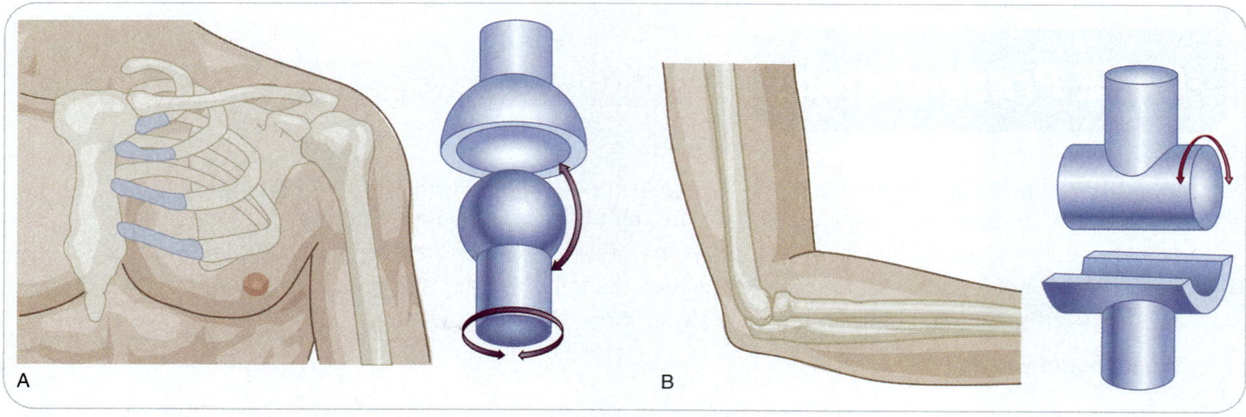

Figure 20-3 A. The shoulder is a ball-and-socket joint. **B.** The elbow is a hinge joint, which allows motion in only one plane.

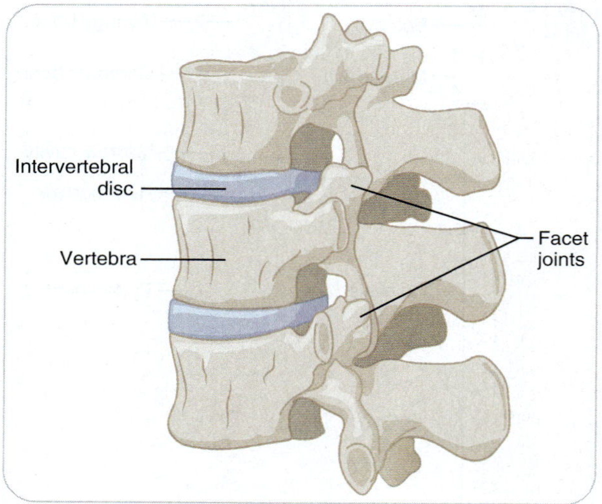

Figure 20-4 Joints between the vertebrae are only slightly moveable.

minimal movement because thickened fibrous ligaments firmly stabilize the bone ends.

Ligaments

Ligaments are thick bands of tissue that connect two bones together. Composed of strong connective tissue, ligaments resist stretching, restricting joint movement to the range of normal motion. By holding one bone to another bone, ligaments provide structure and stabilize the skeleton.

In the knee, ligaments located on each side connect the femur to the tibia medially, and the femur to the tibia and fibula laterally (**Figure 20-5**). The anterior and posterior cruciate ligaments are inside the knee, providing anterior/posterior stability. This forms a stable hinge joint, allowing motion only in the anterior/posterior plane. Conversely, the shoulder joint, with only a few restrictive ligaments, can move in almost any direction.

Joint movement is determined by the degree of tightness or laxity of the ligaments and capsule that hold the bone ends together, and by the orientation of the bone ends to each other. The amount and type of motion differ from joint to joint, with all joints restricting motion to some degree. When a joint is

KEY POINT

Ligament or Tendon?

Ligament: a tissue that connects one bone to another bone.

Tendon: a tissue that connects a muscle to a bone.

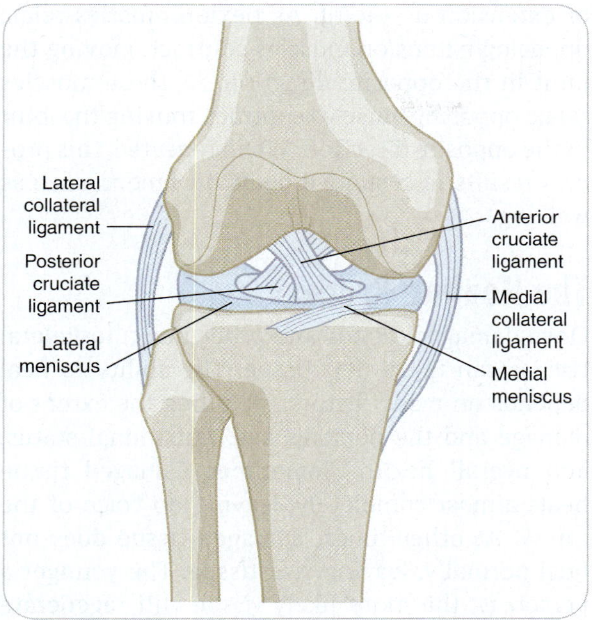

Figure 20-5 The anatomy of the knee. Ligaments connect bone to bone and are an essential part of the skeletal system.

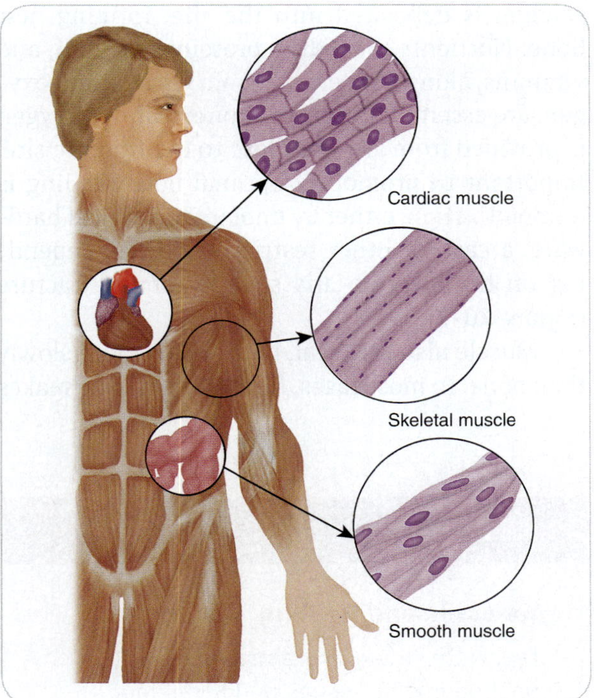

Figure 20-6 The three types of muscle.

pushed beyond this limit, damage occurs. The supporting ligaments can overstretch or tear, or the capsule can tear open. Regardless, the joint becomes unstable, which can limit function and cause pain.

Muscle

The body has three types of muscle, each of which has a unique function (**Figure 20-6**). These muscles are classified as skeletal, smooth, and cardiac. Smooth and cardiac muscle were discussed in the anatomy chapter. The musculoskeletal system has only **skeletal muscle**. Skeletal muscle makes up the major visible muscle mass in the body and is named for its close association with the skeleton.

Muscle is a unique type of tissue that, when stimulated, can contract. After a muscle has contracted, it passively returns to its original length during the relaxation phase. The combination of contraction and relaxation enables the body to move the extremities, walk, and perform normal daily activities. Muscles respond to chemical and electrical signals that travel from the brain through the spinal cord to peripheral nerves, causing the movement of a specific body part. If the signal from the nerve cannot reach the muscle because of disease or injury, the muscle can no longer contract, and muscle function is reduced or lost.

Most of the more than 600 muscles in the skeletal muscular system are divided into complementary pairings. For instance, in the upper arm the biceps and triceps are paired muscles: Contraction of the biceps muscles enables us to bend (flex) the elbow, whereas contraction of the triceps muscles enables us to straighten (extend) the elbow (**Figure 20-7**). These complementary pairings are essential for effective movement and for the manipulation of objects.

Tendons

Tendons are the strap-like continuations of a muscle that connect a muscle to a bone across a joint (**Figure 20-8**). This tissue is very strong and transmits the force of a contracting muscle to the bone. Like ligaments, tendons can be damaged through overstretching and tearing. When a tendon is damaged, the effectiveness of a muscle is significantly reduced or can become nonfunctional.

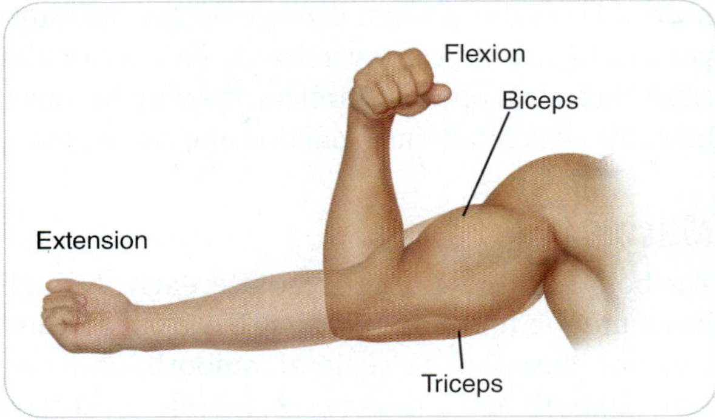

Figure 20-7 Flexion and extension are the two main movements of the elbow.

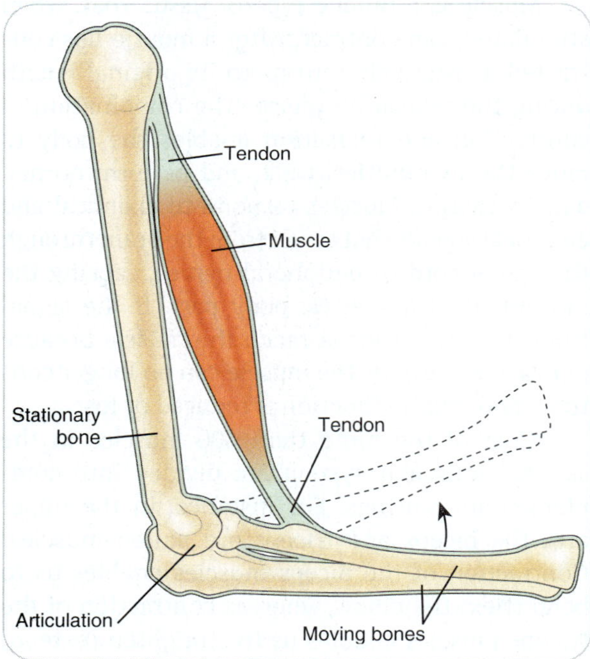

Figure 20-8 Tendons attach muscles to bone.

THE PHYSIOLOGY OF MOVEMENT

Body movement is a coordinated process in which skeletal muscles receive a signal from the brain to contract. This signal may produce voluntary movement, such as when you lift an object, or it may produce involuntary movement, such as when you quickly pull your hand away from an open flame. The contraction of muscles causes flexion or extension of a joint. As flexion muscles relax, opposing extension muscles contract, moving the joint in the opposite direction. As these muscles relax, opposing muscles contract, moving the joint in the opposite direction. When repeated, this process results in sustained body movement, such as walking.

The Healing Process

Once damaged, bones and other musculoskeletal tissues can make new tissue. The ability to heal depends on many factors, including the extent of damage and the person's age, nutritional status, and overall health. Sometimes damaged tissue heals almost completely, leaving no trace of the injury. At other times, damaged tissue does not heal normally, leaving scar tissue. The younger a person is, the more likely tissue will regenerate without excessive scar tissue formation.

Although bone tissue is strong, it can break. The site of a break in bone is called a **fracture**. The break causes the bone to bleed, and a hematoma forms around the fracture site. Over the next several weeks, this hematoma, or collection of blood, organizes into a substance called callus. Later, calcium is deposited into the site, forming new bone. Nutrients, including proteins, calcium, and vitamins, along with energy from glucose and oxygen, are essential for proper bone healing. Oxygen is provided from arteries close to the fracture site. Important to promoting optimal bone healing is **immobilization**, either by implanted surgical hardware, a cast, or other restrictive device, depending on the location and severity of the fracture (**Figure 20-9**).

Muscle also can heal, but it heals more slowly than bone. In most cases, fibrous scar tissue makes

> **KEY POINT**
>
> **Smoking and Healing**
>
> Cigarette smoking drastically slows healing in soft tissues and bone. In a person who smokes even one cigarette a day, a fractured bone may take much longer to heal or not heal at all.

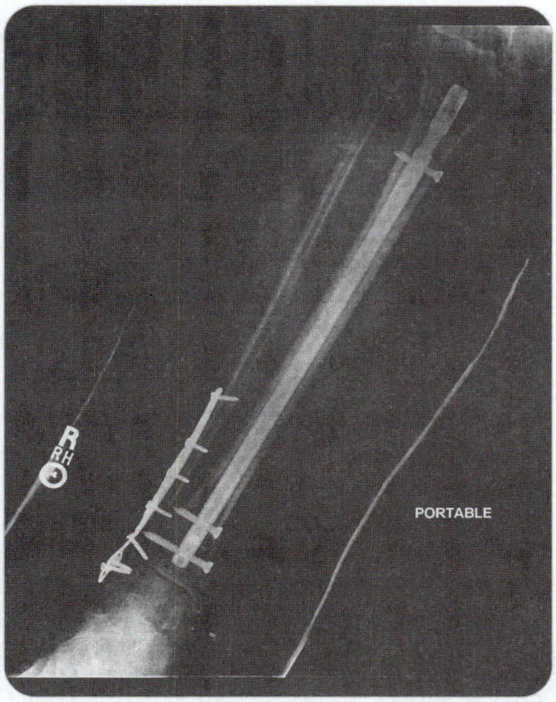

Figure 20-9 An X-ray image of a lower leg showing surgical hardware and a surrounding cast.

© Nancy Pitstick.

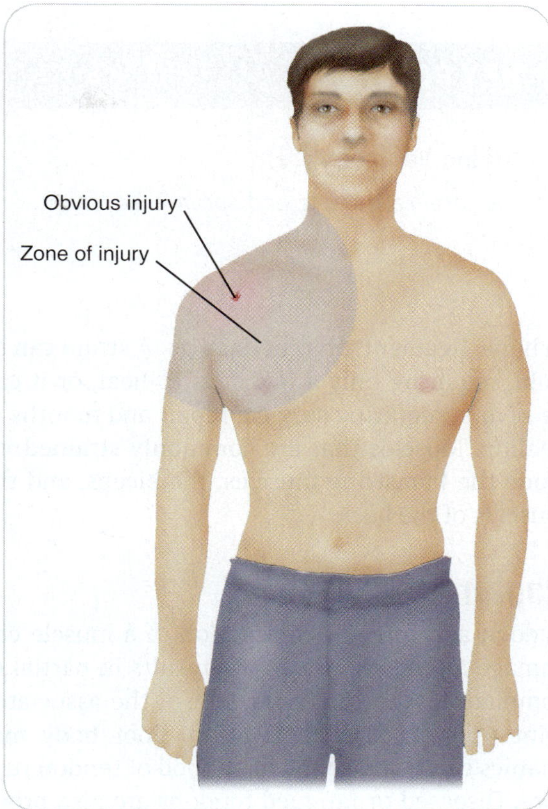

Figure 20-10 Zone of injury.

© Jones & Bartlett Learning.

up some of the new tissue. Ligaments also heal slowly and with some scar tissue. Like bones, the healing process for muscles and ligaments involves the formation of a hematoma that is later replaced by new fibrous tissue; however, calcium is not deposited. This healing process can take 6 weeks or longer. New ligament tissue can take up to a year to mature.

Tendons heal similarly but need to be protected for several months then be increasingly stressed so they can take the stress on them when a muscle pulls hard. Cartilage does not heal very well, because the blood supply to this tissue is poor. In general, traumatically torn cartilage is removed, although in some instances it can be surgically repaired, especially in children.

COMMON MUSCULOSKELETAL INJURIES

The area of damage to the surrounding soft tissues, nerves, and blood vessels around a bone or joint injury is known as the **zone of injury** (**Figure 20-10**). This zone can be large or small depending on the amount of force (kinetic energy) that caused the trauma.

Sprains

A **sprain** is an injury involving the stretching or tearing of a *ligament*. This type of injury occurs when a joint is forced beyond its normal range of motion. Sprains typically affect the ligaments on one side of a joint and may occur with other musculoskeletal injuries. Mild ligament sprains heal relatively quickly, usually in several weeks, whereas most completely torn ligaments need surgical repair. In outdoor sports, sprains most often involve the knee, shoulder, wrist, or ankle, but a sprain can affect any joint.

Strains

A **strain** is a stretched or torn *muscle*. Commonly referred to as a "pulled muscle," a strain is often caused by overexertion and poor body mechanics. Strains affect muscle tissue only and do not result

KEY POINT

Strain Versus Sprain

You *strain* a muscle and *sprain* a ligament.

in bone, ligament, or joint damage. A strain can be mild, requiring only a few days to heal, or it can be severe, requiring surgical repair and months of healing. Muscles that are commonly strained include the hamstring muscles, the biceps, and the muscles of the back.

Ruptured Tendons

Sudden and forceful contraction of a muscle can damage a tendon. This injury results in partial or complete loss in the movement of the associated joint upon muscle contraction. Poor body mechanics can increase the likelihood of tendon rupture. Diseased or fatigued tendons are also prone to rupture. Common tendons that rupture are the Achilles tendon in the ankle, the biceps tendon at the shoulder or elbow, the rotator cuff tendons in the shoulder, and the flexor tendons in the fingers (on the palm side of the hand). Other tendons that rupture less frequently include the tendons above and below the patella (kneecap).

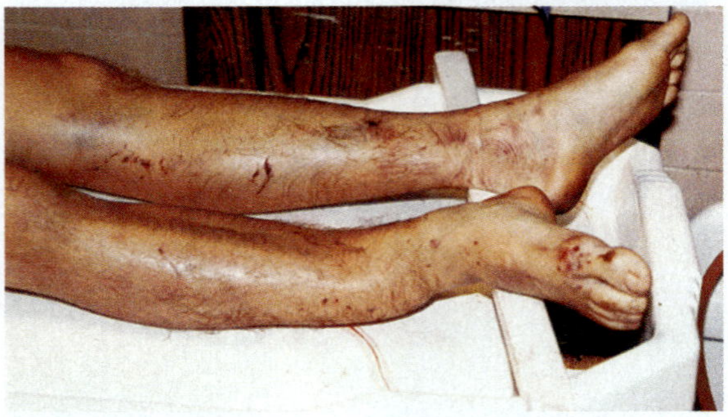

A

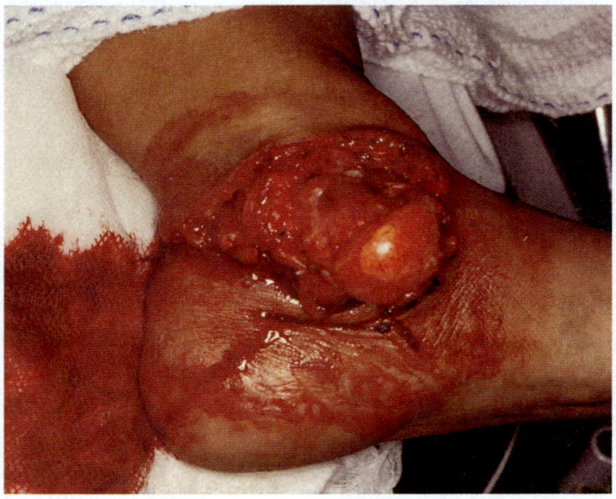

B

Figure 20-11 A. A closed fracture. **B.** An open fracture/dislocation.

Fractures

A fracture is a break in a bone. Although most fractures are caused by trauma, they may also result from bone disease. A fracture may occur anywhere along a bone and can affect any bone. OEC technicians must be familiar with different types of fractures; the most common categories are closed fractures and open fractures.

A closed fracture is one in which the overlying skin surface has not been disrupted (**Figure 20-11A**). An open fracture is one in which the overlying skin has been opened (**Figure 20-11B**). Also known as a compound fracture, this injury occurs when either an external force penetrates the skin and fractures the underlying bone, or more commonly the sharp ends of a broken bone come through the surface of the skin. Open fractures are a true emergency because the opening in the skin allows contaminants to enter the body. Bacteria entering the wound may cause infection of the bone and local tissues.

Fractures may be further classified according to whether the broken bone remains in normal anatomic alignment. In a *nondisplaced* fracture, the ends of a fractured bone remain in alignment. An extremity with a nondisplaced fracture might appear normal except for swelling at the fracture site. Nondisplaced fractures are often difficult to detect by exam, even for experienced physicians, so X-ray imaging is required to identify many of these injuries. A *displaced* fracture causes the affected extremity to appear bent, crooked, shortened, or rotated (**Figure 20-12**). This abnormal appearance is caused by the ends of a fractured bone being anatomically misaligned.

Some fractures are named according to either the specific mechanism of injury or the shape of the fracture line (**Figure 20-13**).

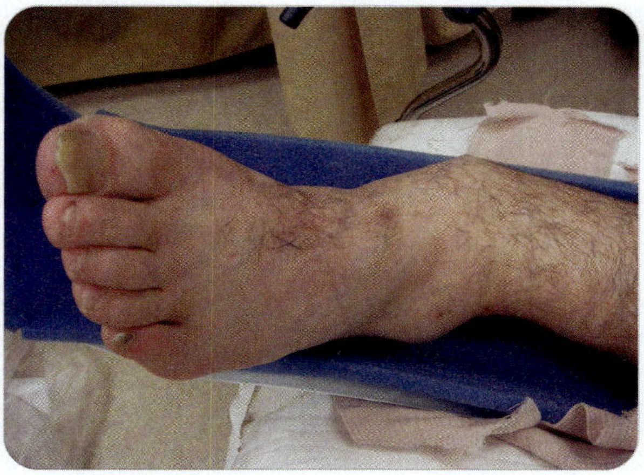

Figure 20-12 A displaced fracture.

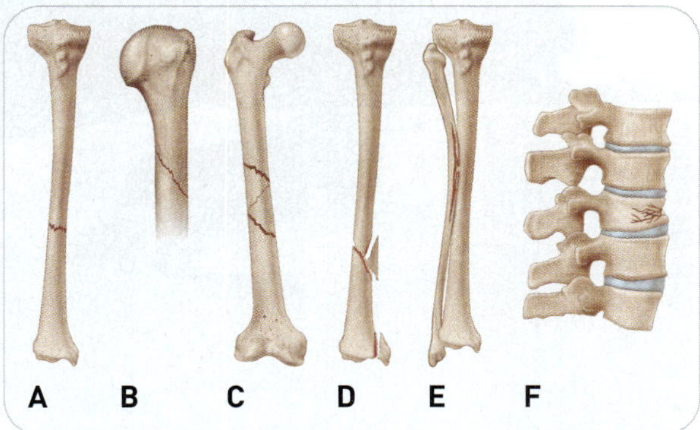

Figure 20-13 Types of fractures. **A.** Transverse fracture of the tibia. **B.** Oblique fracture of the humerus. **C.** Spiral fracture of the femur. **D.** Comminuted fracture of the tibia. **E.** Greenstick fracture of the fibula. **F.** Compression fracture of the vertebral body.

Due to the vascular nature of bones and surrounding tissues, certain fractures can result in significant internal and/or external blood loss. Closed fractures are associated with internal blood loss, which generally stops due to the limited space available for blood to accumulate (**Table 20-1**). If the space for blood to accumulate inside the body is large, as is the case for the thigh with a femur fracture or inside the pelvis when the pelvis is fractured, a significant amount of blood can be lost internally. Open fractures may result in a greater loss of blood because local soft tissues do not restrict the bleeding.

Table 20-1 Potential Blood Loss From Fracture Sites

Fracture Site	Potential Blood Loss (mL)
Pelvis	1,500–3,000
Femur	1,000–1,500
Humerus	250–500
Tibia or fibula	250–500
Ankle	250–500
Elbow	250–500
Radius or ulna	150–250

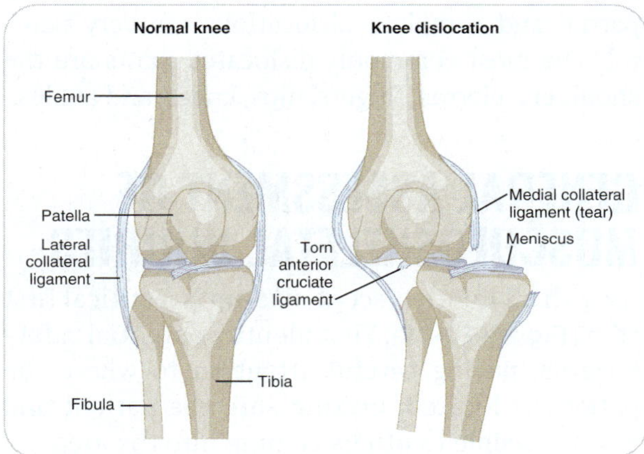

Figure 20-14 A dislocation of the knee.

Dislocations

A **dislocation** is a separation or displacement of the bones of a joint (**Figure 20-14**). This injury usually results from forceful trauma. In some people who have previously dislocated a joint, minimal force may be all that is necessary to dislocate that joint again.

When a joint dislocates, the joint capsule and surrounding ligaments can stretch or tear. Additionally, the soft tissues, blood vessels, and nerves surrounding the joint are often damaged. Some specific dislocations can be true orthopedic emergencies due to neurovascular compromise. A joint can partially dislocate and then return to its normal anatomic position, a condition known as **subluxation**, or it can be completely dislocated or "locked" out of normal anatomic position. When the bone ends remain out of position, joint movement can

CASE Update

After making sure the scene is safe, placing crossed skis above the site, and taking standard precautions, you perform a primary patient assessment, also looking for severe bleeding. The patient states that he caught "way too much air and crashed." Airway, breathing, and circulation are normal. There is no bleeding. Both his knee and shoulder do not look normal. You immediately call for assistance.

What should you do next?

be dramatically, often completely, restricted. Both partial and complete dislocations are very painful. The most commonly dislocated joints are the shoulders, elbows, fingers, hips, knees, and ankles.

GENERAL ASSESSMENT OF MUSCULOSKELETAL INJURIES

As with all injuries, scene size-up is a critical first step (**Figure 20-15**). First identify potential safety hazards, paying careful attention to where the patient is located, making sure the patient and you are visible to others coming into the area.

Following scene size-up and making the scene safe, go through all the steps in the primary patient assessment process before focusing on the musculoskeletal injury. Carefully examine the patient for external bleeding, which may not be apparent if the patient is wearing bulky clothing or multiple layers. Control any excessive bleeding. Assess the patient's ABCDs (airway, breathing, circulation, disability) and correct any threats to life. If the patient is unresponsive, immediately open the airway and simultaneously check for breathing and a pulse. If there is no pulse, start CPR. Assess responsiveness using the AVPU scale (alert, verbal, pain, unresponsive). Following the primary patient assessment, after other rescuers arrive, manually stabilize the head and spine if neurologic injury is suspected. Be sure to assess the mechanism of injury, which may provide helpful clues that can help you better understand the patient's *possible* injuries (**Figure 20-16**). As a rule, any patient who has a potential threat to life, or is unstable, unresponsive, or has suspected multiple fractures, is considered a high priority and should receive immediate care and rapid transport.

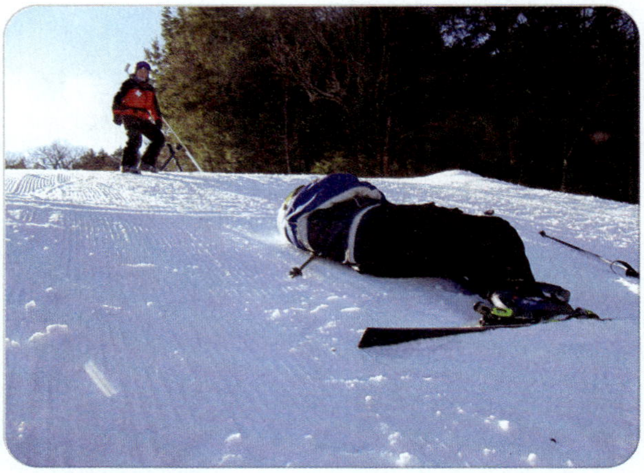

Figure 20-15 Scene size-up is an especially important part of a primary patient assessment when patients may be out of view of oncoming skiers.

Once the ABCDs have been managed, correcting life threats, perform a secondary patient assessment. Determine the patient's chief complaint. Next obtain a SAMPLE history (signs and symptoms, allergies, medications, past medical history, last oral intake, events leading up to the problem). The most common symptom of a musculoskeletal injury is pain. Ask the person to point with one finger to where it hurts. If the area of pain or tenderness is quite large, ask the patient to draw a circle around the site with a finger (**Figure 20-17**). Assess the nature and quality of the patient's pain on a scale of 0 to 10.

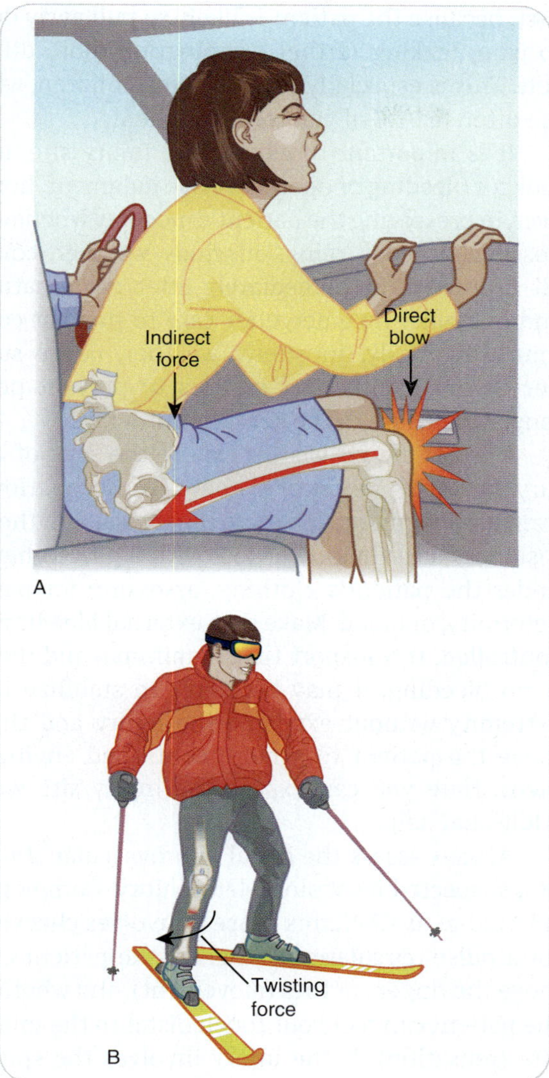

Figure 20-16 **A.** Multiple injuries may occur depending on the force and the mechanisms of injury. **B.** Knowing the mechanism of injury, such as that it resulted from a twisting force, may provide helpful clues about the patient's injury.

KEY POINT

Point Tenderness

Ask the patient to point with one finger to where it hurts. This gives you the best idea where the injury is located.

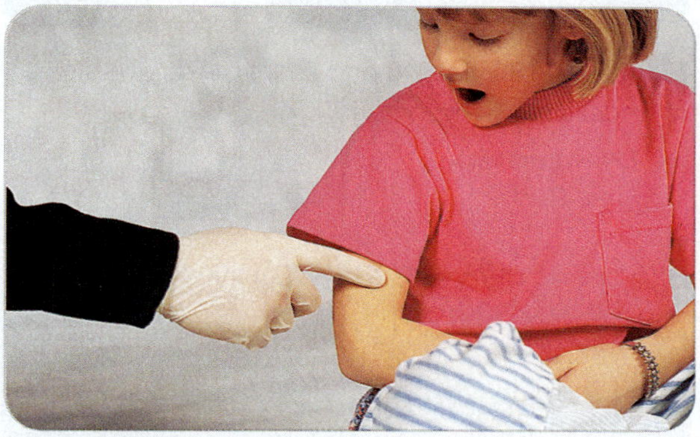

Figure 20-17 An important aspect of a secondary patient assessment is locating the point of tenderness. This is the location that the patient pointed to as being painful.

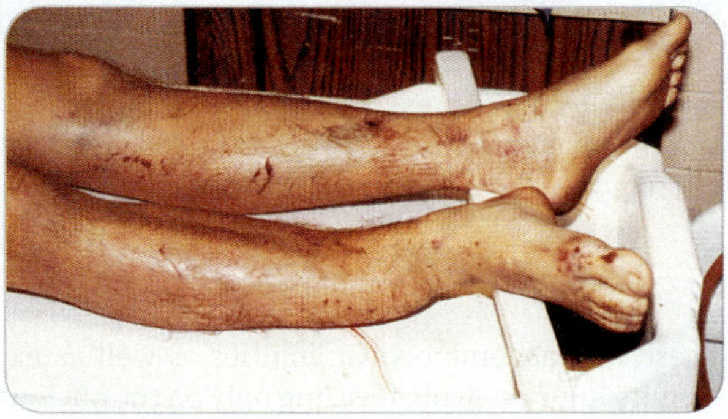

Figure 20-18 Deformity often indicates a musculoskeletal injury.

Deformity is a common finding that generally indicates musculoskeletal injury (**Figure 20-18**). Mild deformity is generally caused by swelling or internal bleeding but can be caused by a fracture (**Figure 20-19**). Gross deformity usually results from a fracture or a dislocation. For patients who suffer a musculoskeletal injury, try to protect the site from further injury. For instance, a person with a sprained wrist or a broken radius bone will typically hold the forearm close to the body and be reluctant to move it. This sign is known as **guarding** (**Figure 20-20**).

Perform a physical exam using DCAP-BTLS (deformity, contusions, abrasions/avulsions, punctures/penetrations, burns/bleeding/bruises, tenderness, lacerations, swelling). Make sure you perform a full-body assessment, looking for head,

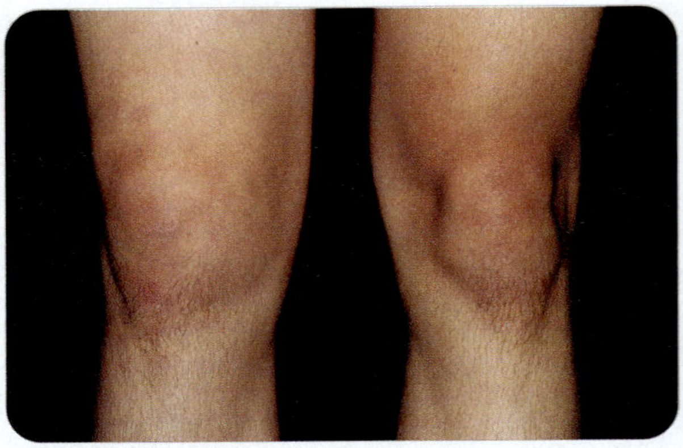

Figure 20-19 Swelling and ecchymosis are signs of underlying hemorrhage.

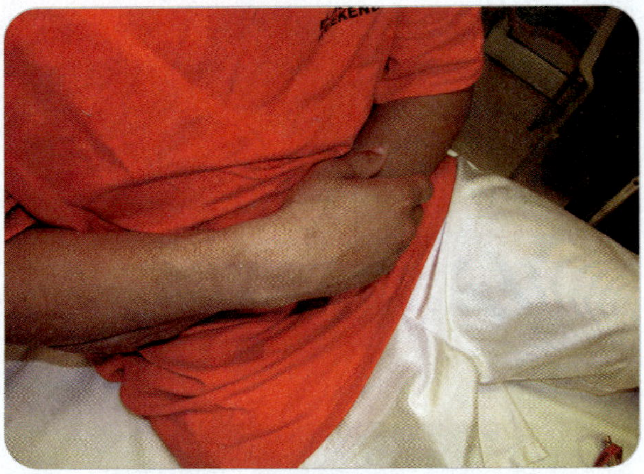

Figure 20-20 The presence of musculoskeletal trauma is often indicated by a sign called guarding.

chest, and abdominopelvic injuries as well as extremity injuries. Avoid focusing only on the obvious musculoskeletal injury. Focusing your attention on a leg that is bent at an unnatural angle may cause you to overlook a serious head or internal abdominal injury.

Once you have located the zone of injury, unless there is major bleeding that needs to be controlled immediately, examine the rest of the extremity first. Do not palpate the zone of injury first, because the patient is likely to pull away due to pain, making further examination more difficult. This is especially true in young children, who are often fearful of you touching them.

It is important to expose the injury site and look for bleeding or open skin. Use judgment, however, in preserving the patient's modesty whenever possible. In cold, rainy, or windy weather, cover all exposed skin immediately after examination and/or rendering emergency care to prevent cold injury. Similarly, in sunny weather, cover suspected musculoskeletal injuries to prevent prolonged exposure to the sun's harmful rays.

It is not always wise to expose the zone of injury by cutting jacket or ski pants on scene. However, use judgment, and do so if necessary. In these instances, briefly look or feel with a gloved hand under the patient's clothing, assessing for pain, deformity, or blood. Make sure external bleeding is controlled. If transport time is minimal and there is no bleeding, it may be better to stabilize the extremity without exposing the injury and then move the patient to a more controlled environment. Here you can expose the injury site with additional help.

Always assess the distal neurovascular status of a suspected musculoskeletal injury. Commonly referred to as CMS, this process involves checking for a pulse (*c*irculation), whether the patient can move the fingers or toes (*m*ovement), and whether the patient can feel your touch distal to the injury site (*s*ensation). If the injury involves the spine, assess distal CMS in all limbs. These findings should be documented.

During the assessment, begin formulating a plan concerning what you will do to manage the injured body part(s), which mode of transport to use, and any special considerations. Determine what equipment, including splints, may be needed, and request that these items be brought to the scene. If a toboggan, litter, ambulance, or other mode of transport will be needed, notify dispatch as soon as possible. Call for ALS if required and remember that ALS can be very beneficial for pain control.

Reassess the patient frequently, including the vital signs and distal CMS. Document any changes.

Signs and Symptoms of Common Musculoskeletal Injuries

1. Sprains:
   - Point tenderness over the injured ligament(s)
   - Swelling and bruising within the zone of injury
   - Joint instability, which is characterized by abnormal motion of the affected joint, but may be masked by major joint swelling, severe tenderness, and/or guarding
   - Decreased motion due to pain, swelling, and/or ligament instability
   - Difficulty bearing weight on the injured joint (in the lower extremities)
2. Strains:
   - Point tenderness over a muscle or a portion of a muscle
   - Pain when using the injured muscle to flex or extend an extremity
   - Bruising over a muscle
   - Swelling or hematoma over a muscle
3. Tendon injuries:
   - A noticeable "gap" under the skin where the tendon has ruptured (this is a hallmark sign for this type of injury)
   - After initial severe pain, minimal pain due to minimal nerve involvement.
   - Little bruising or swelling (tendons contain few blood vessels)
   - Lack of joint movement because the tendon no longer connects the muscle to the bone
4. Fractures:
   - Pain at the fracture site that worsens upon movement of the affected bone
   - Tenderness to palpation
   - Swelling due to internal bleeding from the fracture site
   - Ecchymosis (bruising)
   - Decreased motion due to pain, and lack of bone continuity
   - Deformity due to bone misalignment
   - Tenting on the skin
   - **Bone crepitus** (a noise or palpable feeling of crackling when fractured bone ends rub together)
5. Dislocations:
   - Pain
   - Swelling
   - Deformity
   - Reduced joint motion
   - Joint "locking" or "freezing" (a complete inability to move the joint)
   - Numbness or tingling distal to injury

Section 1 Questions

1. Factors that impact the healing of damaged bones and other musculoskeletal tissues include:
   a. age of person and extent of damage.
   b. sex of person and location of injury.
   c. equipment used and snow conditions.
   d. environmental temperature and muscle tone.
2. A patient is diagnosed with a strain to the lower right leg. Which of the following structures is the primary structure affected in that injury?
   a. A joint
   b. A ligament
   c. A muscle
   d. A bone
3. What is the term for is a tissue that connects a bone to another bone?
   a. Joint
   b. Muscle
   c. Tendon
   d. Ligament
4. What isolated musculoskeletal injury is marked by initial severe pain followed by minimal pain due to little nerve involvement?
   a. Fracture injury
   b. Tendon injury
   c. Strain injury
   d. Sprain injury
5. During your assessment of a young snowboarder who is complaining of significant pain in her elbow, you find diminished CMS of her fingers. CMS stands for:
   a. color, muscle tone, stability.
   b. color, movement, sensation.
   c. circulation, movement, stability.
   d. circulation, movement, sensation.
6. A skier is complaining of significant pain in his lower left leg. During your assessment, you find swelling and ecchymosis just above the top of his ski boot. With this information, you suspect a:
   a. significant sprain.
   b. ruptured tendon.
   c. fracture injury.
   d. strained hamstring.
7. You offer to help another OEC technician with a patient. She tells you that during her assessment she found that a fractured tibia bone has broken the skin. You identify this as a(n):
   a. nondisplaced fracture.
   b. open fracture.
   c. closed fracture.
   d. displaced fracture.
8. During the assessment, the patient has identified a zone of injury. To further identify the injury, next steps include:
   a. examining the rest of the extremity.
   b. exposing the injury.
   c. assessing the distal neurovascular status.
   d. All of the above

Answers: 1. a, Objective 20-1.2, p. 438; 2. c, Objective 20-1.3, p. 439; 3. d, Objective 20-1.1, p. 436; 4. b, Objective 20-1.5, p. 445; 5. d, Objective 20-1.4, p. 444; 6. c, Objective 20-1.5, p. 445; 7. b, Objective 20-1.5, p. 440; 8. d, Objective 20-1.4, p. 444

SECTION 2: ASSESSMENT OF SPECIFIC MUSCULOSKELETAL INJURIES

OBJECTIVES

Upon completion of this section of this chapter, the OEC technician will be able to:

20-2.1 Describe and demonstrate how to assess injuries in the following parts of the body:

- Shoulder and clavicle
- Humerus
- Elbow
- Forearm
- Wrist
- Hand and finger
- Pelvis
- Hip
- Femur
- Knee
- Tibia and fibula
- Ankle
- Foot and toe

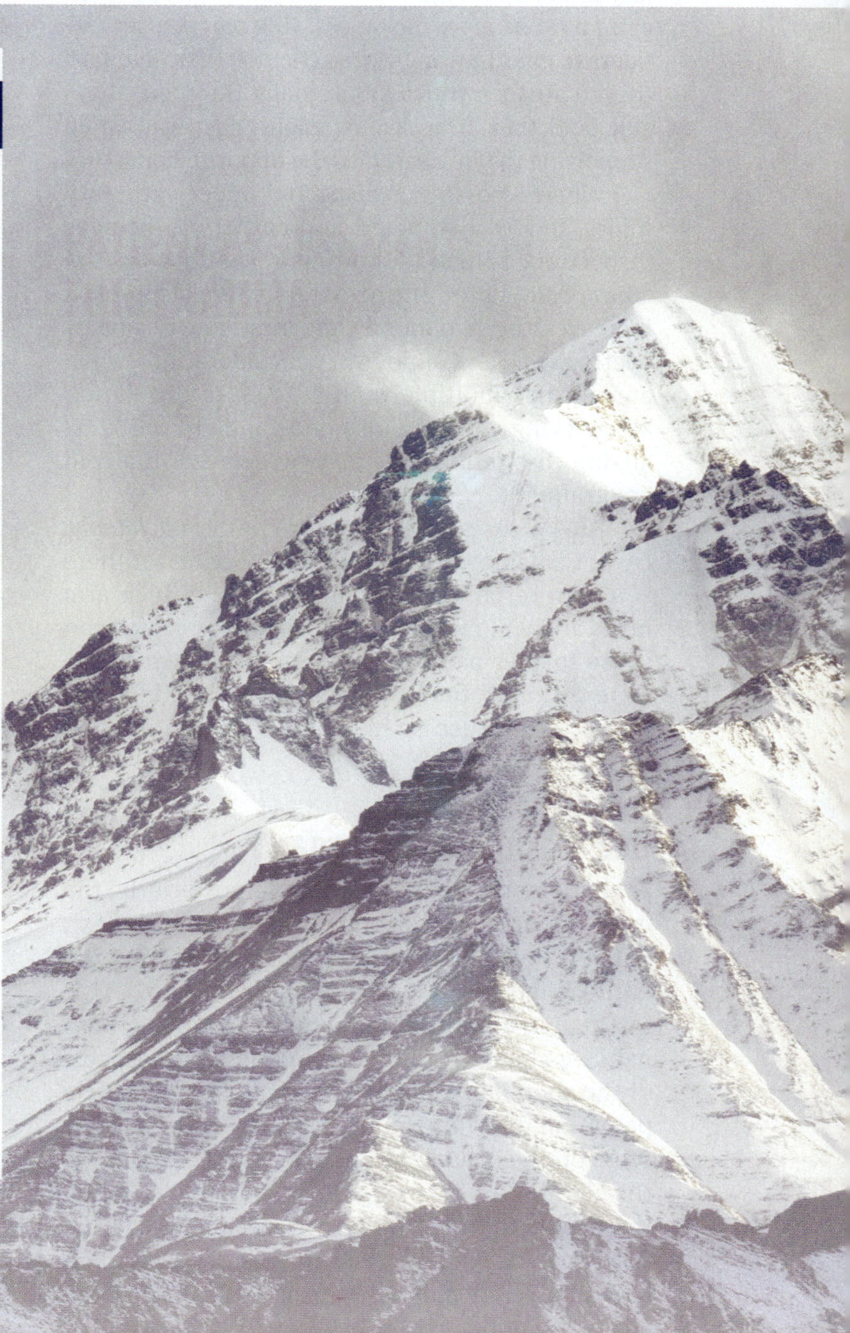

ASSESSMENT OF UPPER EXTREMITY INJURIES

Upper extremity injuries are commonly encountered in participants of outdoor activities. Most are caused by falling onto an outstretched hand, an elbow, or a shoulder.

The pain associated with an upper extremity injury is almost always increased by movement of the extremity. In many instances, this pain causes patients to guard the injury in a characteristic manner: they rotate their shoulder internally, flex their elbow, and hold their arm against their chest wall while supporting the forearm with the opposite hand.

When assessing a suspected upper extremity injury, follow a standard approach that includes inspection, palpation, and neurovascular assessment (CMS) of the entire extremity. This approach increases the likelihood that injuries will not be overlooked, an important consideration when an arm has multiple injuries. Assess circulation by checking a distal pulse and capillary refill, realizing that refill times may be delayed in a cold environment.

Always assess each upper extremity individually. Do not palpate both arms at once, because if there is a pain response, you will not know which arm hurts and will need to repeat the exam, which can cause further pain. Have the patient identify the zone of injury first and examine it last unless a threat to life such as bleeding is associated with the zone.

Use a Standard Approach

Examine and palpate the scapula posteriorly, the most proximal part of the upper extremity. Next, in the front, palpate the sternoclavicular joint, the entire length of the clavicle, the **acromioclavicular (A/C) joint**, and the acromion process. Using both hands, palpate the anterior and posterior aspects of the shoulder, and proceed with gentle but firm palpation down the humerus to the elbow. Gently press on the inside, the outside, and the "point" of the elbow. Continue palpating down the length of the radius and ulna to the wrist. Palpate each of the bones of the hand and fingers. Be sure to go back and *gently* palpate the zone of injury at the end of the upper extremity exam.

Evaluation of movement of an extremity should be attempted only if it does not cause pain, because excess movement can cause additional damage to surrounding tissues, bones, blood vessels, and nerves. If movement is assessed, proceed carefully, having the patient move the extremity. Stop at the first indication of increased pain. Touch the skin of the extremity to assess sensation.

The assessment of specific upper extremity injuries is described in the sections that follow.

Clavicle and Shoulder Injuries

The clavicle, or collarbone, is located on the upper portion of the anterior chest wall. This bone has a joint on either end and it is the only bone of the arm to articulate (form a joint) with the chest wall. The sternoclavicular joint attaches the clavicle to the sternum, whereas the A/C joint attaches the clavicle to the acromion of the scapula (**Figure 20-21**). The clavicle is the most frequently fractured bone in the body.

The clavicle commonly fractures in the middle or distal portions of the bone. As a result, the skin may "tent" over the fracture site due to a fractured end protruding up, resulting in deformity. This injury can be quite painful, and any movement of the arm hurts. Young children may say that the entire arm hurts. Patients will typically self-splint the arm to the chest wall as previously described. Swelling, tenting of the skin, bruising, and point tenderness are hallmarks of a clavicle fracture (**Figure 20-22**).

The distal end of the clavicle articulates with the acromion process or superior part of the

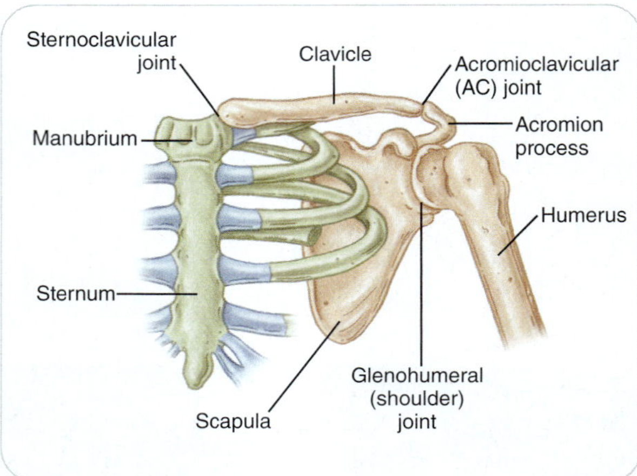

Figure 20-21 The shoulder girdle includes the clavicle and the scapula.

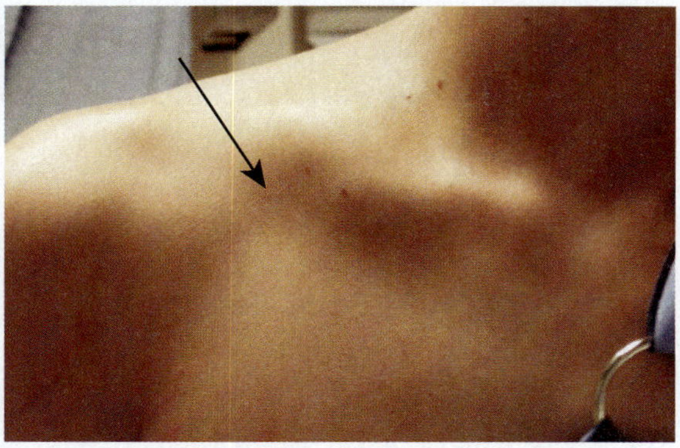

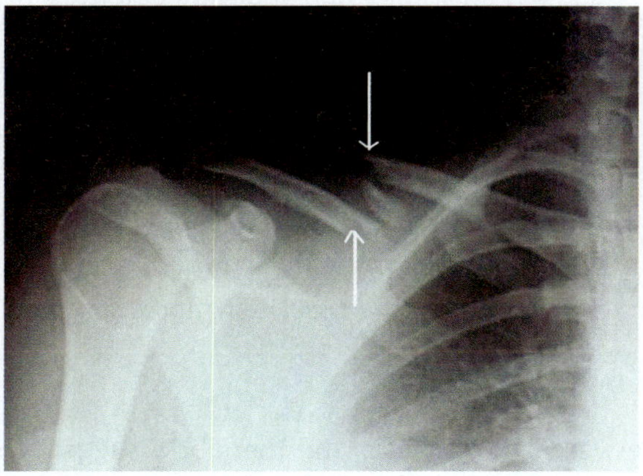

Figure 20-22 A. The "tenting" of the skin over a fractured clavicle. **B.** An X-ray image of a fractured clavicle.

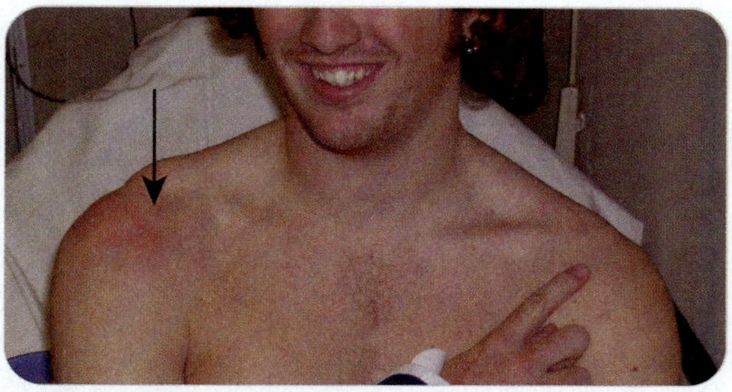

Figure 20-23 In an A/C separation, the end of the right clavicle sticks out.

scapula, forming the A/C joint. The A/C joint is frequently sprained or dislocated when a person falls on the "point" of the shoulder. This injury is referred to as an A/C separation, or sometimes a shoulder separation. Some may confuse this injury with a fracture of the distal clavicle (**Figure 20-23**).

An A/C separation is different from a true shoulder *dislocation* between the glenoid cavity (socket) and the humeral head (ball). Point tenderness is present over the A/C joint and just medial and inferior to the joint. A mild deformity to the distal end of the clavicle may be present. Rarely, the distal end of the clavicle will stick significantly upward. A skier who falls forward or a biker who goes over the handlebars may incur this injury by landing on the shoulder.

The shoulder's ball-and-socket joint, called the glenohumeral joint, has a very loose capsule, and the ligaments that hold the shoulder in position are not very strong. Because of this, the shoulder can easily dislocate, especially if forces are applied from certain directions. This type of injury can occur in violent falls during skiing or snowboarding and may be seen in accidents relating to kayaking and mountain biking. This joint is the most frequently dislocated large joint in the body. Over 95% of shoulder dislocations are anterior, where the humeral ball comes out in the front. If an OEC technician suspects a shoulder dislocation, the mechanism of injury may help identify the direction in which the humeral head is dislocated.

The mechanism for anterior dislocation is forceful abduction and external rotation of the arm at the shoulder or falling backwards on an outstretched arm that is away from the body. The arm usually "locks" in this position, making an OEC technician's job of packaging the patient somewhat difficult (**Figure 20-24**). Patients guard the dislocated shoulder aggressively, usually by sitting, holding the shoulder up and out with the other hand, and not allowing you to lower the arm. They may, however, hold their arm against their body with their hand on the abdomen. Exposing the shoulder will reveal a skin "dent" under the acromion, where the humeral head has dislocated down and anteriorly. Any dislocated shoulder is very painful, and occasionally the patient will complain of some numbness of the outside of the shoulder.

Posterior shoulder dislocations are rare and are most commonly seen in vehicle collisions in which a person reaches out and puts a hand on the car's dashboard just before impact, causing the humeral head to be forced directly posterior. These

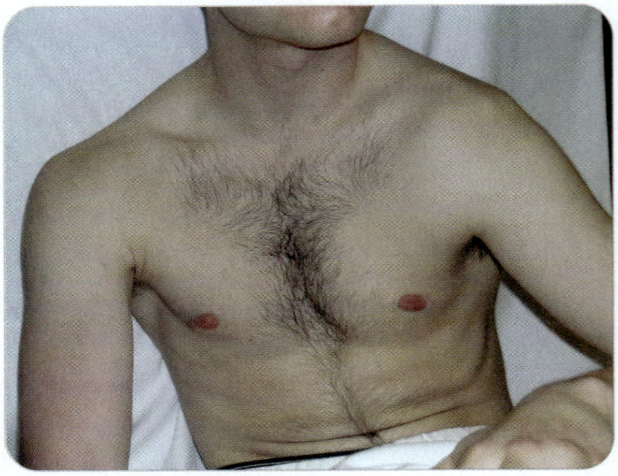

Figure 20-24 An anterior dislocation of the shoulder is the most common dislocation of the shoulder.

are also seen in patients who have had a seizure or an electric shock. The same mechanism of injury is seen when someone falling forward "breaks the fall" using an arm in which the elbow is locked, which pushes the humeral head out posteriorly.

Another injury of the shoulder, a fracture of the scapula on the posterior chest wall, is rare and usually indicates a severe mechanism of injury. Injuries to the chest wall (rib), internal chest, and spine are common when the scapula is fractured due to large forces. The socket part of the shoulder, or glenoid process, which is part of the scapula, can be fractured when significant force is applied to the outside of the shoulder, pushing the humeral head in and fracturing the underlying glenoid. Patients with a fractured scapula hold the arm very still and resist any movement of the limb.

Humerus Fractures

Starting at the top of the humerus, the ball can be broken, although the "neck" just below the ball is more frequently fractured, especially in children and older adults. More commonly the cause is a hard direct blow to the shoulder. The top of the humerus can break into several pieces. The patient complains of pain directly over the fracture site. Deformity is uncommon because the large muscles over the proximal humerus hide the fracture, even if it is angulated.

Fractures involving the shaft of the humerus are common. Signs such as point tenderness, swelling, and **angulation** (deviation from straight) between the shoulder and the elbow suggest the presence of a midshaft humerus fracture. Such fractures can be very unstable and often result in movement of the bone at the fracture site. Humerus fractures can be significantly angulated. The radial nerve spirals around the middle of the back of the humerus. Bone fragments can damage this nerve, resulting in a wrist drop (inability to raise the back of the hand up).

> **KEY POINT**
>
> **Hints for Determining Type of Shoulder Injury**
>
> Patients with A/C injuries, clavicle fractures, scapular fractures, and humeral head and neck fractures generally hold their arm against their abdomen; patients with posterior shoulder dislocations hold their arm against their abdomen and will not let you bring the arm away from the abdomen. By contrast, patients with anterior dislocated shoulders hold their arm out and up (occasionally patients with dislocated shoulders hold their arm the same as if they had an A/C injury). The position in which a patient holds the injured arm can help you identify the possible injury.

Elbow Injuries

The elbow joint is composed of the ends of three bones: the radius, the ulna, and the humerus (**Figure 20-25**). Elbow injuries are very painful, can present with gross deformity at the elbow, and can have significant neurologic and/or vascular complications. Because many elbow injuries, especially involving young children, can result in permanent damage if not managed in a timely manner, all elbow injuries should be examined by an advanced health care provider after prehospital care.

The soft tissue around the elbow contains many veins, large nerves, and the brachial artery, all of which can be injured. Adults, and more commonly children, fracture the distal humerus just above the elbow, because the bone is not very thick here. This fracture, called a supracondylar fracture of the

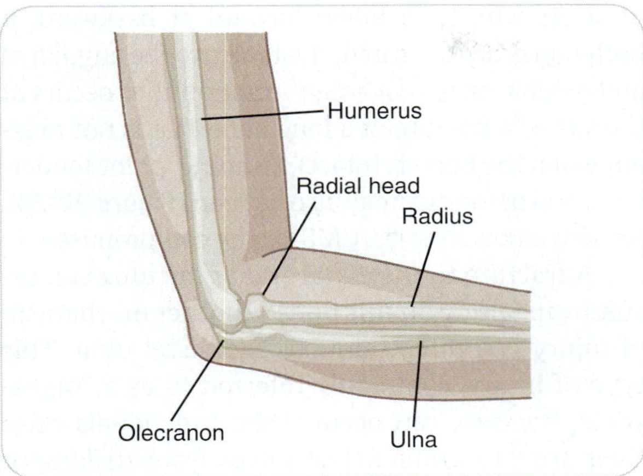

Figure 20-25 The bones that form the elbow.

elbow, can have disastrous early and late complications in children, including nerve damage, arterial interruption, crooked healing, or muscle damage in the forearm from loss of blood supply. This injury is most often caused by falling directly onto the elbow. Signs and symptoms can include gross deformity, severe pain, swelling, and possible CMS deficits.

Fractures can also occur to the olecranon process, or to the radial head. The olecranon, or "point," of the elbow can be fractured by falling directly on it. Signs include swelling over the tip of the elbow, and possibly a gap between the fractured bone ends. Additionally, the patient will not be able to extend the arm at the elbow.

A radial head fracture occurs when the radius is forced up into the distal end of the humerus. The most common source of this injury is falling on an outstretched hand. Pain will be present on the lateral side of the elbow. Movement, especially turning the palm down or up (pronation/supination), is very painful.

An elbow dislocation may occur if a patient falls on an outstretched hand with the elbow in partial flexion (**Figure 20-26**). As a result, the joint becomes locked, usually at about 40 to 50 degrees of flexion. Pain is severe and is aggravated by movement. Swelling develops rapidly, and CMS function can be compromised.

Nursemaid's elbow, an injury seen in toddlers younger than 5 or 6 years old, results when an adult, who is walking beside the child and holding the child's hand, impatiently jerks the child's hand, dislocating the head of the radius in the elbow joint. Nursemaid's elbow can also be caused by "swinging" a young child by the hands. Symptoms include self-splinting (holding the arm against the body), slight flexion of the arm, and pain. Often, the child will cry if you touch or move the arm.

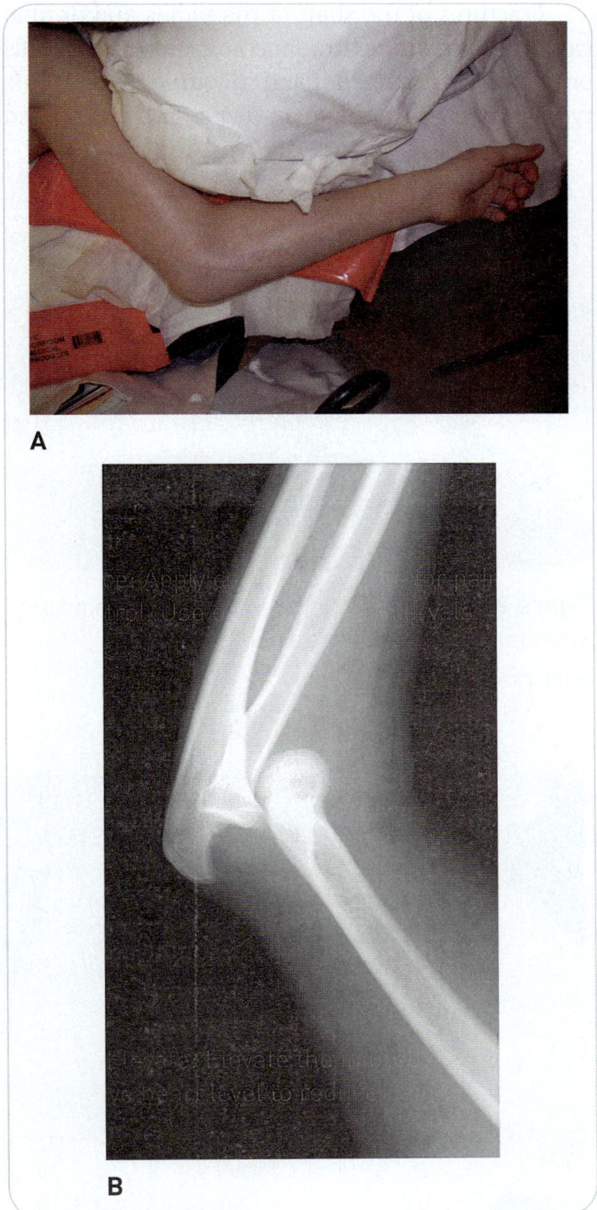

Figure 20-26 An elbow dislocation. **A.** The clinical appearance. **B.** An X-ray image.

Forearm Injuries

Direct or indirect trauma to the arm between the elbow and wrist can cause a variety of injuries, including fractures. Without X-ray imaging, it may be difficult to differentiate between a fracture and a soft-tissue injury such as a contusion.

Fractures of the shaft of the radius and/or ulna can occur from direct trauma or when a person falls onto an outstretched hand (**Figure 20-27**). This type of injury is common among snowboarders and bicyclers who have fallen forward or backward. If both bones are fractured, the limb may be angulated and exhibit **false movement** (motion that occurs at the site of a fracture of a long bone that is not present when the bone is intact). Swelling, point tenderness, and deformity may also be seen (**Figure 20-28**). As with elbow injuries, CMS can be compromised.

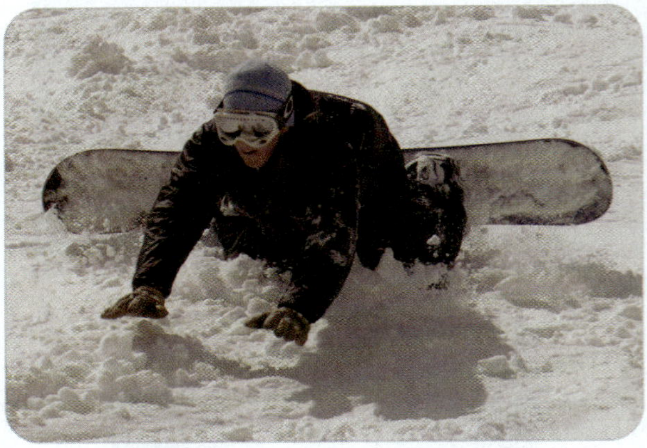

Figure 20-27 Injuries to the forearms often occur when falling onto outstretched hands.

A fracture to the distal end of the ulna can result from falling on this bone. Another mechanism of injury is a direct blow to the distal ulna. This type of injury, commonly referred to as a "nightstick" fracture, can occur when individuals raise their arms to protect themselves from striking or being struck by a solid object. A large tree branch, a hockey stick, or a snowboard rail is commonly involved in this type of injury.

Wrist Injuries

Falling forward on the palm of the hand can result in fractures to the distal radius and ulna. This

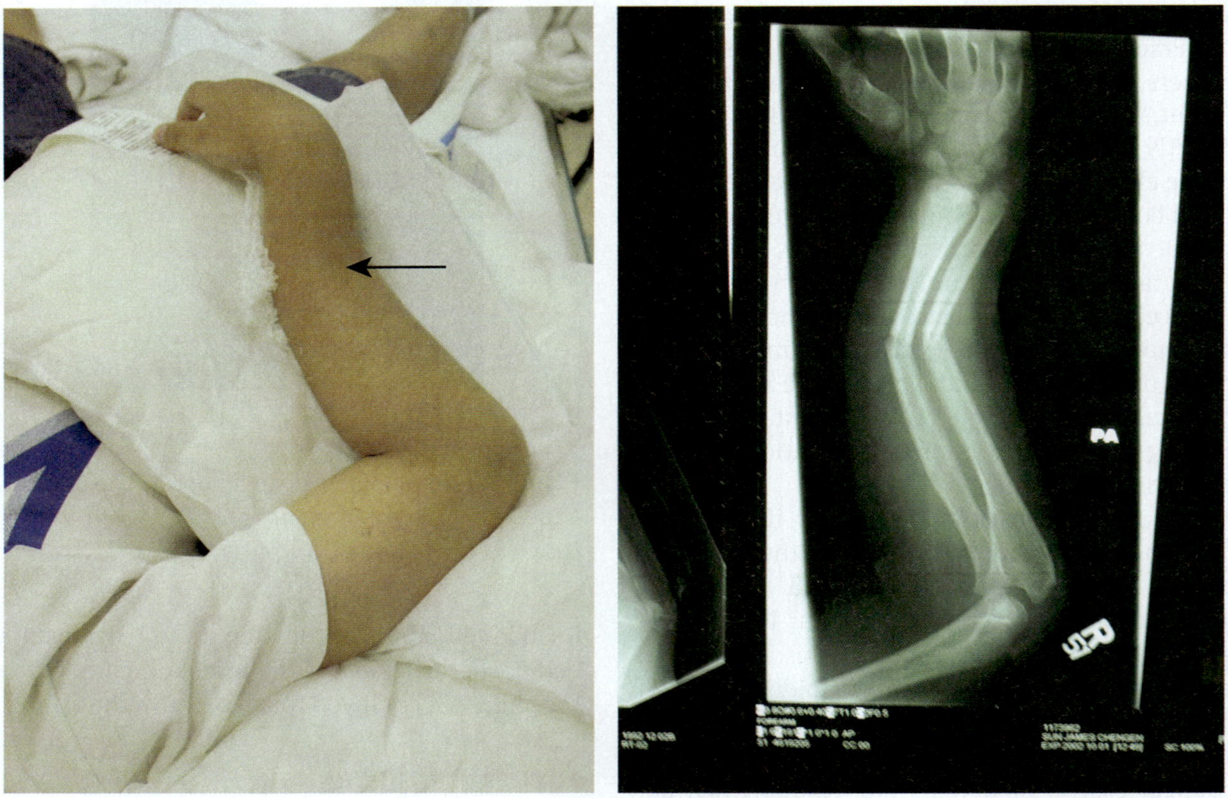

A B

Figure 20-28 **A.** A forearm injury. **B.** An X-ray image showing a fractured radius and ulna.

KEY POINT

Colles Fracture

Dr. Abraham Colles was an Irish surgeon who wrote a paper in 1814 titled "On the Fracture of the Carpal Extremity of the Radius." This paper, describing distal radial fractures, was far ahead of its time, being published decades before xray came into use. The type of wrist injury he described continues to be known as a Colles fracture.

injury, known as a Colles fracture or "silver fork" fracture, results in a characteristic injury pattern in which the displaced wrist bones resemble an overturned fork. The distal end of the fractured radius is pushed in the direction of the back of the hand. Deformity, pain, swelling, and false movement are common. A Colles fracture is a common snowboarding injury. Rarely, one can fall on the dorsum (back) of the hand, causing a reverse Colles, or Smith, fracture in which the fractured end of the radius is displaced toward the palm.

The most commonly fractured of the wrist's eight carpal bones is the scaphoid, also known as the navicular bone. Like other upper extremity injuries, this injury is caused by falling on an outstretched hand and is a rather common injury among snowboarders who fall forward on the toe side of their board, a fall known as a "mousetrap." It can also result from falling off a bicycle or horse, or while rock climbing. Among the symptoms are pain in the lateral side of the wrist joint in the "snuffbox," the area distal to the end of the radius and proximal to the base of the thumb's metacarpal (**Figures 20-29** and **20-30**). Other carpal bones may also fracture. Dislocation or fracture–dislocation of the carpal bones results in a deformed wrist, severe pain, swelling, and reduced motion. The patient is often found cradling the injured wrist in the opposite hand.

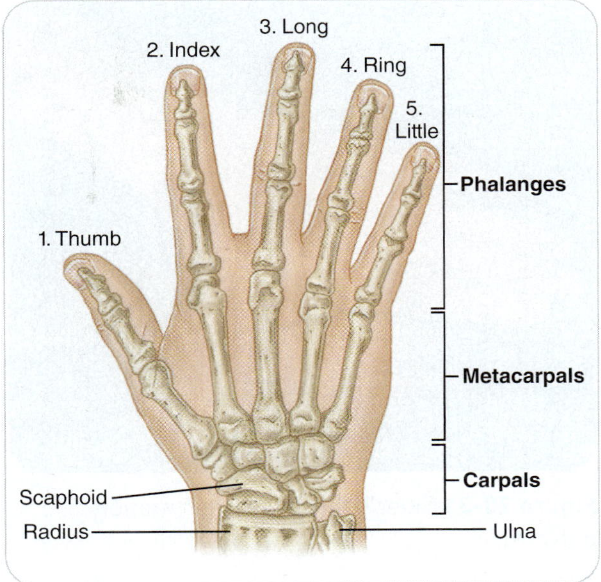

Figure 20-29 The anatomy of the hand and wrist.

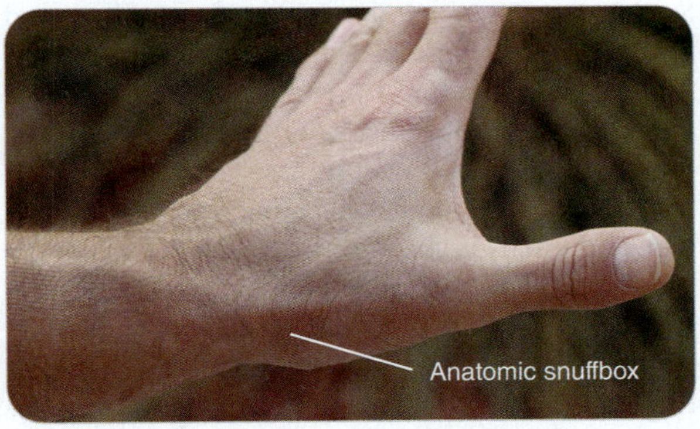

Figure 20-30 Pain is present in the snuffbox of the wrist when the scaphoid bone is broken.

Hand and Finger Injuries

A common skiing injury to the upper extremity is a sprain of the ulnar collateral ligament of the thumb. This injury, called skier's thumb, occurs when a ski pole catches on the snow and bends the thumb in a lateral and **dorsal** (backward) direction, disrupting the ligament at the base of the thumb next to the web between the thumb and index finger (**Figure 20-31**). This injury can also occur in hikers who fall while using walking poles.

Any of the bones of the hand may be fractured or dislocated. If the first metacarpal (the bone at the base of the thumb) is fractured, the thumb may appear dislocated where it attaches to the hand. One of the most common hand injuries is a "boxer's fracture," a fracture of the fifth metacarpal bone that is caused by punching a hard object or falling on the hand when it is clenched in a fist.

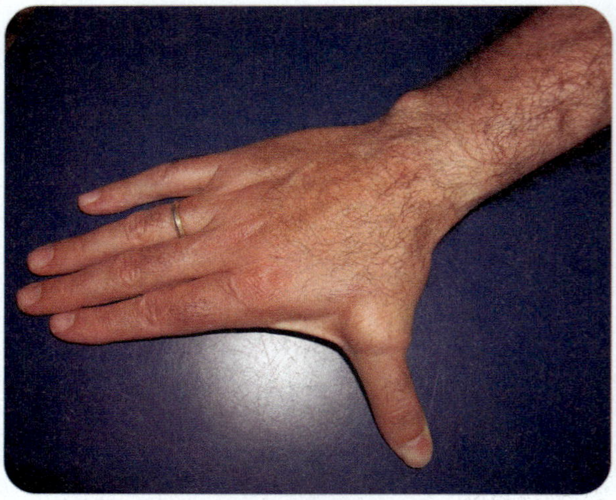

Figure 20-31 Skier's thumb: excess motion outward.

Other hand and finger injuries can involve damaged tendons, creating severe disability. Symptoms may include pain and swelling, and always loss of motion. Depending on the forces involved, the fractured fingers may be angulated, and deformity may result. For experienced OEC technicians, a good way to assess the neurologic function of the hand's three nerves (median, radial, and ulnar) is shown in **Table 20-2**.

Amputations involving the fingers may be partial, in which the finger is still attached to the hand by a tendon or skin, or complete, in which the finger is entirely separated from the hand. See Chapter 19, *Soft-Tissue Injuries and Burns*, for more information about caring for amputations.

One of the worst injuries to the hand can result from trying to remove a stuck object from a running snowblower. When an object gets stuck, the blades stop spinning, so the tendency is to reach into the blade area and pull the object out. If you have not turned off the machine, the blades will immediately start turning again once the object is

Table 20-2 Sensation and Motor Assessment of Three Nerves of the Hand

Nerve	Motor Action That Results	Location of Sensation
Median	Makes a fist or flexes the fingers	Palm side of thumb
Radial	Extends the fingers	Back of thumb
Ulnar	Spreads fingers apart	Palm side of fifth finger (pinkie)

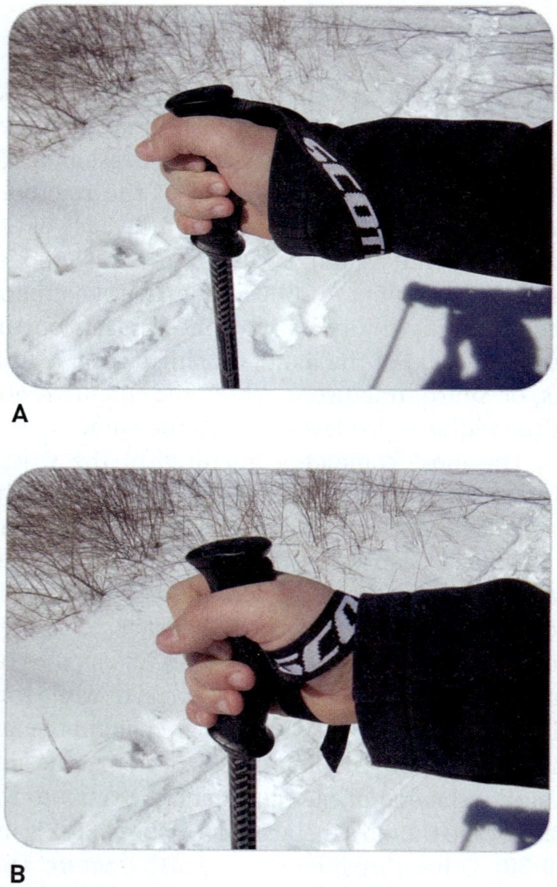

Figure 20-32 The incorrect way to hold a ski pole with straps. (**A**) and the correct way to hold a ski pole with straps (**B**).

KEY POINT

Pole and Strap Injury

It is important to learn and remember the proper way to hold a ski or walking pole with straps. If you hold it the wrong way, when you fall, the strap of the pole may torque the thumb, causing the injury known as skier's thumb (**Figure 20-32**).

free, potentially severely damaging the hand. *Always shut off the snowblower first and use a stick or pole to push out the stuck object.*

ASSESSMENT OF LOWER EXTREMITY INJURIES

The process for evaluating a leg is like that for an arm. As before, assess the mechanism of injury, check distal CMS, then inspect and palpate the entire extremity. Assess each leg separately and systematically. Avoid touching the zone of injury, unless exposure reveals bleeding, until after you have examined the entire leg. Always control bleeding first. Ask permission to examine the pelvic bones and upper legs and explain what you are doing.

Because patients with fractures or dislocations in one or both legs do not want to move the affected limb(s) and are very sensitive to any movement, try not to move the extremity unnecessarily as you examine it. If appropriate and conditions permit, expose the area being evaluated before palpating it.

Begin the field exam by palpating the pelvis. Although the pelvis is not really part of the leg, the ball of the femur fits into the acetabulum or socket of the pelvis. Although a more detailed description of a pelvic exam is described in Chapter 24, *Abdominal and Pelvic Trauma*, a brief explanation of a pelvic exam is presented here.

Assess the stability of the pelvic bones by gently pressing medially (inward) on the iliac crests at the same time (**Figure 20-33**). You can assess the front of the pelvis by placing the patient's uninjured hand on the bones in the front above the genitalia (**Figure 20-34**). Then push gently on the patient's hand looking for pain. This protects the person's modesty. Below the iliac crests where the top of the femur connects to the pelvis is the hip joint. Assess each hip by gently pushing medially (inward), feeling for tenderness and bone stability.

Next, examine each leg individually. Using two hands, one on the inside of the leg and one on the outside of the leg, start near the groin and gently but firmly palpate down the femur to the knee (**Figure 20-35**). Palpate the knee over the patella in the front, medially and laterally, and in the back. If pain is present, perform a more detailed knee exam in a controlled environment. Continue palpating down the lower leg (tibia and fibula) to the ankle. If the patient is wearing a ski boot or

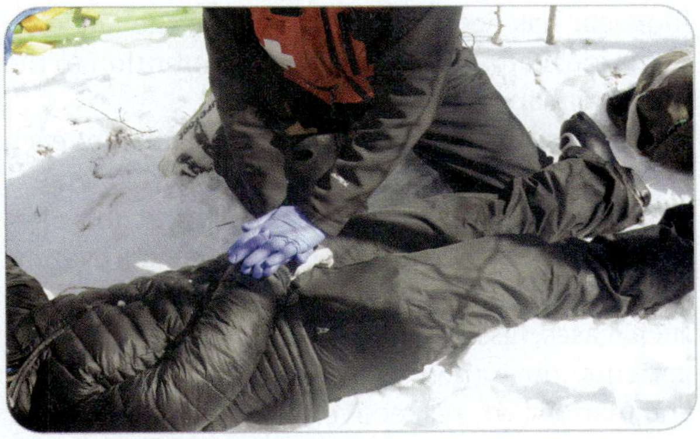

Figure 20-34 Assess the front of the pelvis by placing the patient's uninjured hand on the bones in the front above the genitalia.

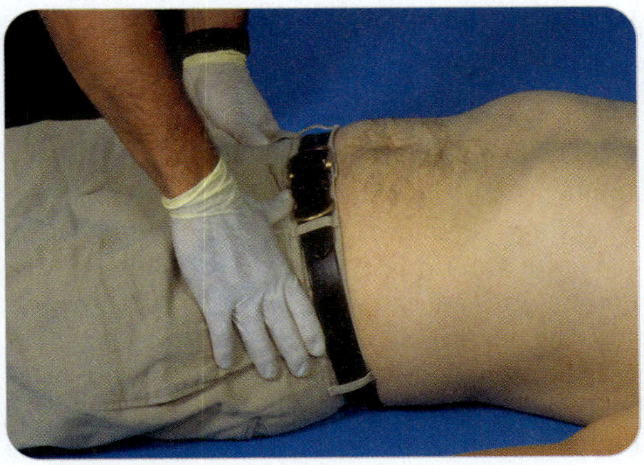

Figure 20-33 Assess the pelvic bones by pressing gently medially on the iliac crests.

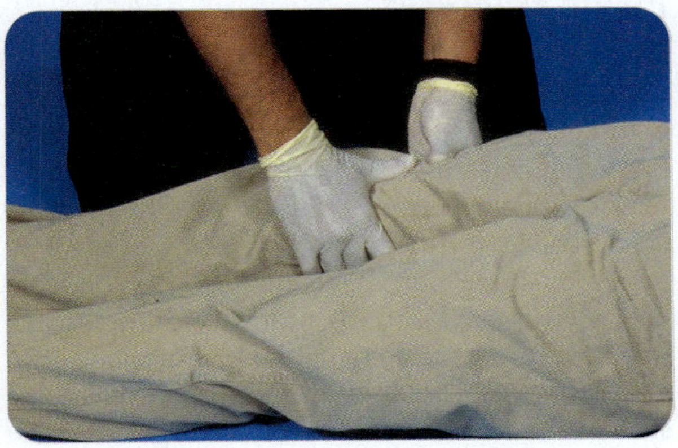

Figure 20-35 Assess the leg from the femur to the knee.

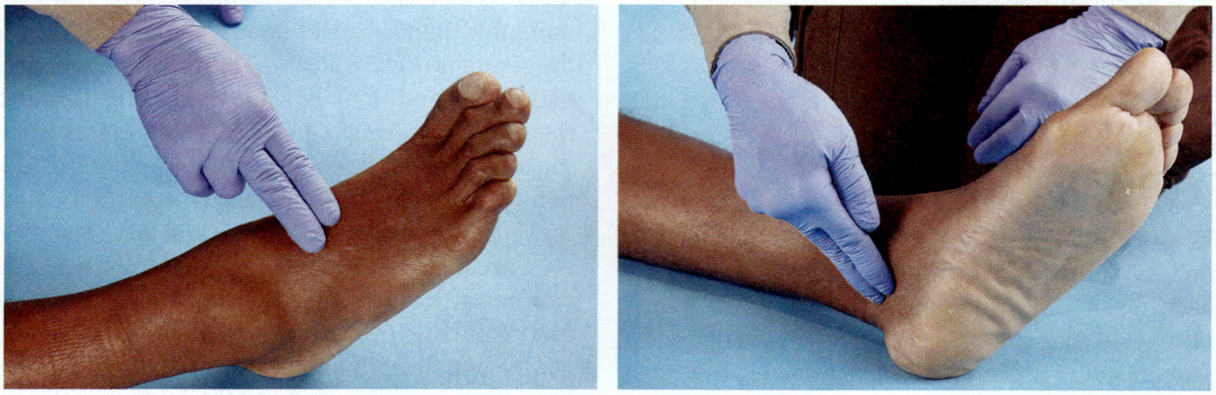

Figure 20-36 Check distal pulses in the foot—dorsalis pedis (**A**) and posterior tibialis (**B**).

other heavy footwear, consider leaving it on until the patient has been moved indoors. After the footwear has been removed, palpate the ankle on each side. Palpate the foot, paying attention to the heel, arch, and outside of the foot.

Assess the distal neurovascular status of each leg. In the event of serious leg injury, inclement weather, or heavy clothing/footwear, it may not be possible to perform a complete neurovascular exam until the patient is moved indoors. In such cases, assess movement by simply having patients move their toes up and down (**dorsiflex** and **plantarflex**, respectively). Determine whether patients can feel the toes wiggling inside the boot. Assess distal pulses (dorsalis pedis pulse) as soon as possible after the removal of the patient's footwear (**Figure 20-36**).

Pelvic Fractures

Fractures involving the pelvic bones usually require great force and should be suspected in high-speed collisions, falls from 20 feet or higher for adults and from 10 feet or higher for children, motor vehicle crashes, pedestrian-vehicle collisions, pelvic gunshot wounds, or any other type of direct blunt trauma (**Figure 20-37**). Because the pelvis is such a sturdy protector of the organs within it, forces great enough to fracture the pelvic bones may result in injuries to internal structures such as the urinary bladder and blood vessels. The most significant complication of a pelvic fracture is acute internal bleeding. Because the pelvis forms a ring, it is likely to fracture in more than one location.

Hip Fractures

The hip is a joint with a socket (acetabulum) and ball (top of the femur). Fractures involving the proximal femur are commonly referred to as "hip fractures." Older individuals, whose bones are more brittle, experience these fractures much more commonly, often from simple falls. Most patients with a *displaced* proximal femur fracture present with the affected leg shortened and externally rotated. The patient usually will not want to move the injured leg. Pain is extreme and is generally located in the groin or inner aspect of the thigh. Occasionally pain is referred to the knee, even though the knee is not injured. Movement makes the pain worse. The patient will complain of pain with gentle, *very* slight movement of the leg by rolling the knee medially and laterally. This finding will usually help you determine this injury. Always check CMS.

Hip Dislocations

The hip joint is a ball-and-socket joint with strong ligaments that hold the bones in position. Significant force is required to dislocate the hip, which can occur anteriorly or posteriorly (**Figure 20-38**). Both injuries are extremely painful and are aggravated by movement of the affected leg.

Signs of the less common anterior hip dislocation include abduction of the thigh and external rotation of the knee. Over 90% of hip dislocations are posterior dislocations. The mechanism of injury for a posterior hip dislocation is a significant force applied to the knee of a person who is sitting. In this position, the *flexed* hip is pushed out

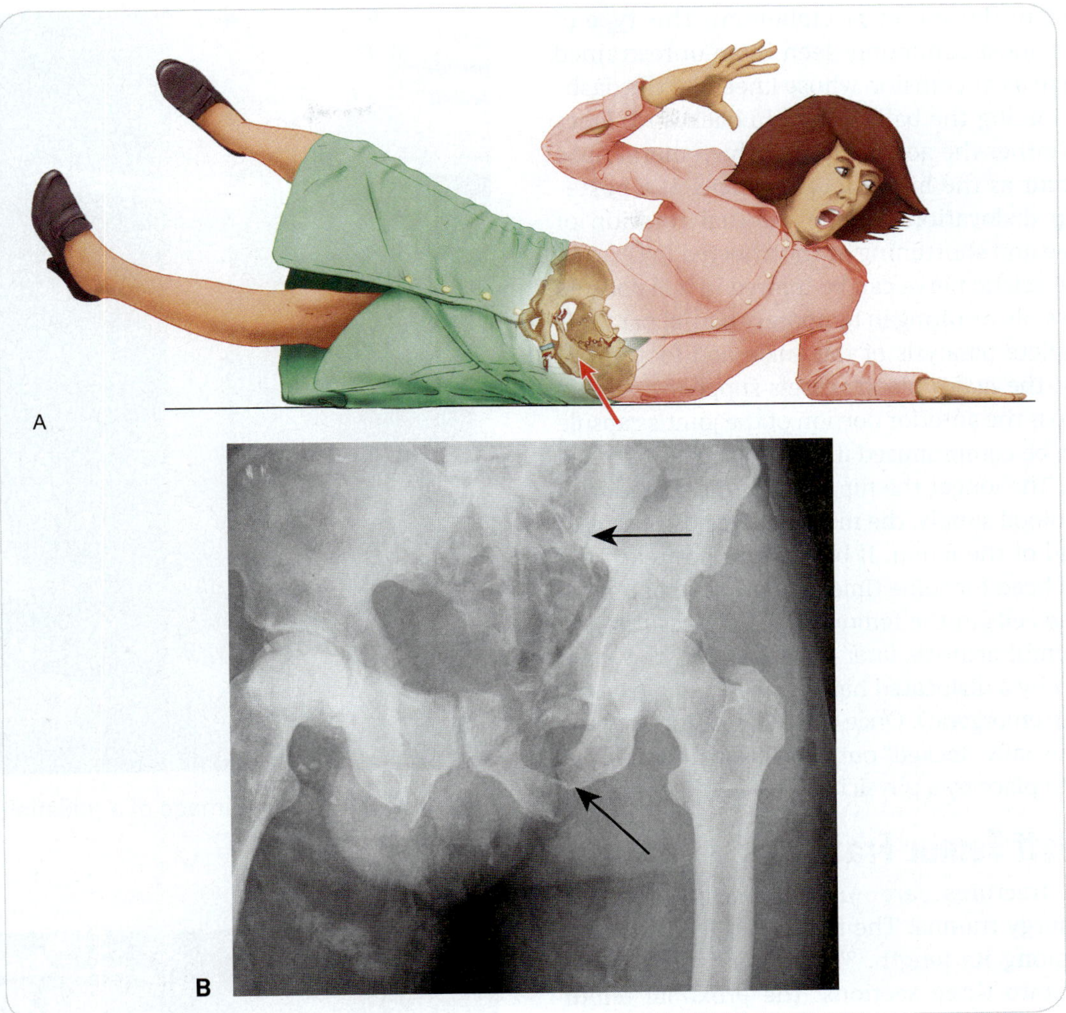

Figure 20-37 **A.** A lateral compression injury to the pelvis. **B.** An X-ray image of a lateral compression injury.

A: © Jones & Bartlett Learning; B: Courtesy of Andrew N. Pollak, MD, FAAOS.

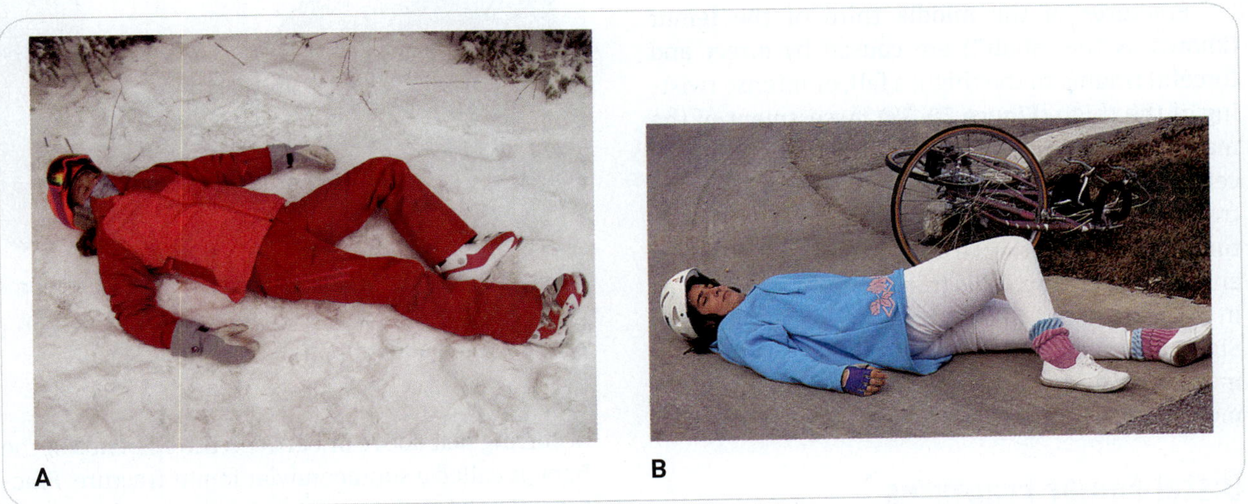

Figure 20-38 **A.** An anterior hip dislocation. **B.** A posterior hip dislocation.

A: Edward McNamara; B: © Jones & Bartlett Learning. Courtesy of MIEMSS.

the back of the socket (acetabulum). This type of injury is most commonly seen in an unrestrained person in a car collision whose knee hits the dashboard, forcing the ball of the hip backward. Fracture of either the acetabulum or the femoral head may occur as the hip dislocates. Signs of a posterior hip dislocation include internal rotation of the knee and shortening of the affected leg.

The sciatic nerve can be injured in a dislocated hip, possibly resulting in temporary partial paralysis or complete paralysis of the ankle and foot. Additionally, the major blood vessels supplying the hip joint cross the anterior portion of the joint's capsule and can be compromised if the capsule is stretched or torn. The longer the hip remains dislocated with lack of blood supply, the more damage can occur to the head of the femur. If blood does not reach the femoral head for some time (usually several hours), the bone cells in the femoral head die, resulting in very painful arthritis later in life. This is the main reason why a dislocated hip is considered a true orthopedic emergency. Once a hip has dislocated, the joint is usually "locked" out of position until it is put back into place by a physician.

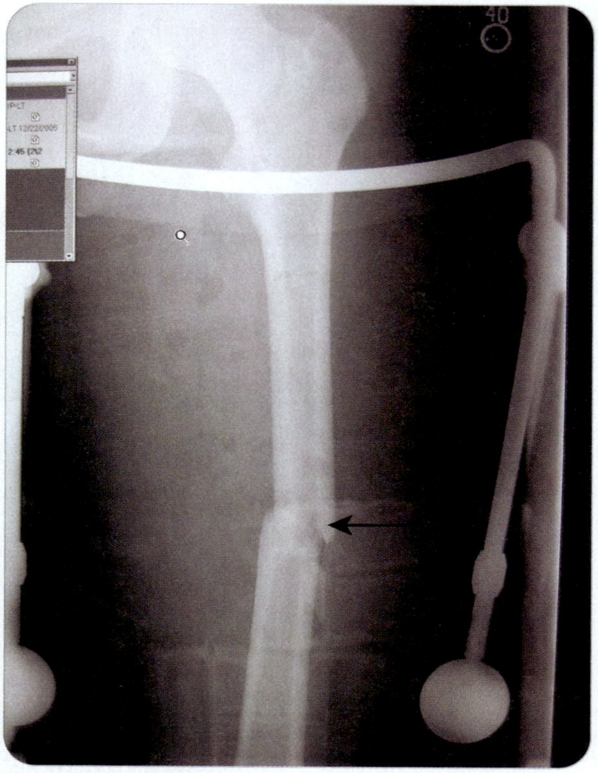

Figure 20-39 An X-ray image of a midshaft fracture of the femur.

Midshaft Femur Fractures

Femur fractures are usually seen only in high-energy trauma. The femur can fracture anywhere along its length. The femur is commonly divided into three sections: the proximal femur (hip), the shaft, and the distal femur. It is important for the OEC technician to be able to recognize where the femur is possibly injured, as prehospital immobilization is different for each section.

Fractures of the middle third of the femur (known as the "shaft") are caused by direct and forceful trauma to the thigh, a fall, or intense twisting of the thigh (**Figure 20-39**). Assessment of the mechanism of injury generally provides clues concerning the forces involved (**Figure 20-40**). Direct trauma results in a transverse (straight across) fracture, whereas twisting results in a spiral fracture or an oblique fracture. Falls from a height often result in a comminuted (more than two parts) fracture. Signs and symptoms of a femur fracture include intense pain, deformity, thigh swelling, and false movement. The bone may also be angulated.

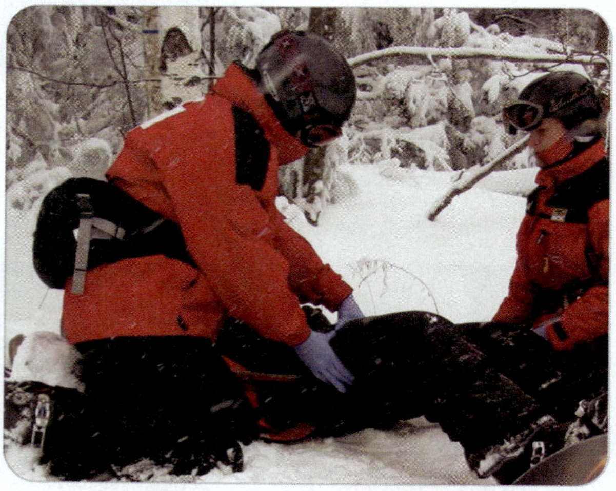

Figure 20-40 Information concerning the mechanism of injury and a thorough assessment of the patient provide clues about the nature of a thigh injury.

Distal Femur Fractures

The distal end of the femur has two large flared ends known as the medial and lateral condyles. A fracture occurring just above or between the two ends of the bone is called a supracondylar femur fracture. Fractures involving this area are characterized by severe pain and swelling just above the knee, deformity, inability to move the knee, and spasm of the thigh muscles. Just behind the distal end of the femur are the large popliteal artery and its branches, the popliteal veins, and the major nerves to the lower leg. These structures can be damaged by jagged bone ends of a distal femur fracture. If this occurs, distal CMS may be compromised, resulting in poor blood perfusion, decreased motor function, and decreased sensation in the lower leg.

Knee Injuries

Knee injuries are a common occurrence in many other outdoor activities, especially those involving twisting of the knee during running and jumping (**Figure 20-41**). Most knee injuries are sprains involving the four main ligaments that support the knee joint. The medial collateral and lateral collateral ligaments act as hinges on each side of the knee. Inside the joint are the anterior and posterior cruciate ligaments, which prevent forward and backward motion of the femur on the tibia. Depending on the mechanism of injury, one or more of these ligaments can be stretched or torn.

A common ski injury is a medial collateral ligament sprain. This injury occurs when the knee is stressed while in a valgus position (when the knee is forced medially into an extremely "knock-kneed" position). Symptoms of this injury include point tenderness above, below, or over the joint line on the inside of the knee. Much less frequent is an injury to the lateral collateral ligament, which can occur if the knee is stressed in the opposite or varus position, in which the knee is forced laterally (as if the limb were suddenly made bow-legged). With this injury, pain is localized to the lateral part of the knee.

The anterior cruciate ligament can be torn when a skier "sits back" and falls, or when someone is running and stops abruptly. Typically, the patient will report feeling or hearing a "pop" and has immediate pain in the knee. This common injury is a big problem for all outdoor recreationists and athletes, as it may require surgical reconstruction and lengthy rehabilitation.

Knee injuries involving the articular cartilage are also common. Articular cartilage is firm tissue that acts like a cushion attached on the end of a bone where it forms a joint. The cartilage on the ends of the femur and tibia where they come together to form the knee joint can be damaged when the knee is injured. Additionally, on the medial side of the knee is a C-shaped cartilage, known as the medial **meniscus**, whereas on the lateral side is a nearly O-shaped cartilage called the lateral meniscus (**Figure 20-42**). These menisci cushion the knee and help stabilize the joint by increasing the depth of the "dish" on each side of the knee where each round femoral condyle articulates with the tibia. The menisci can be damaged or torn when the knee joint is compressed or twisted. Injuries often cause the meniscus to become torn, causing pain, swelling or fluid in the knee joint, and reduced mobility. When a piece of meniscus gets "stuck" in the joint space, the knee can become locked.

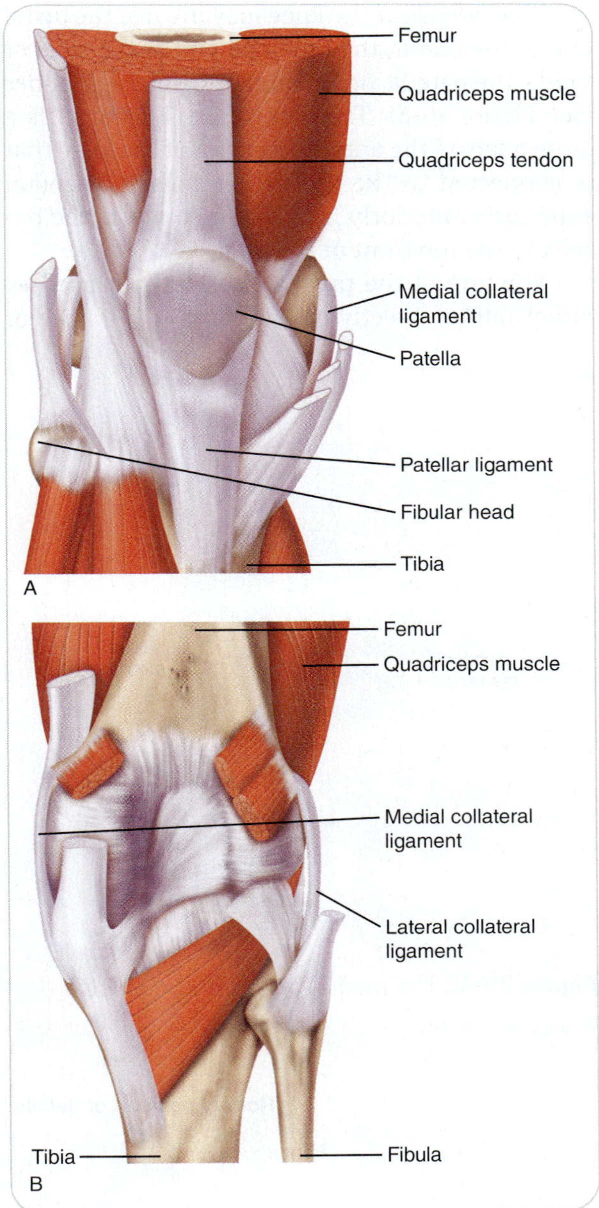

Figure 20-41 The knee. **A.** Anterior view. **B.** Posterior view.

Fractures near the knee may involve the distal end of the femur, the proximal end of the tibia or fibula, the patella, or a combination of these bones (see Figure 20-5). The patella, or "kneecap," is a large bone on the anterior portion of the knee that is connected to the quadriceps muscle's tendon superiorly. Inferiorly, a ligament connects the patella to the top front of the tibia.

Fracture of the patella is typically caused by either falling directly on the front of the knee or receiving a significant direct or blunt force on the anterior knee. The amount of force necessary to fracture the patella is great, as it is a dense bone. Patella fractures may be open, so expose the zone of injury to assess for bleeding.

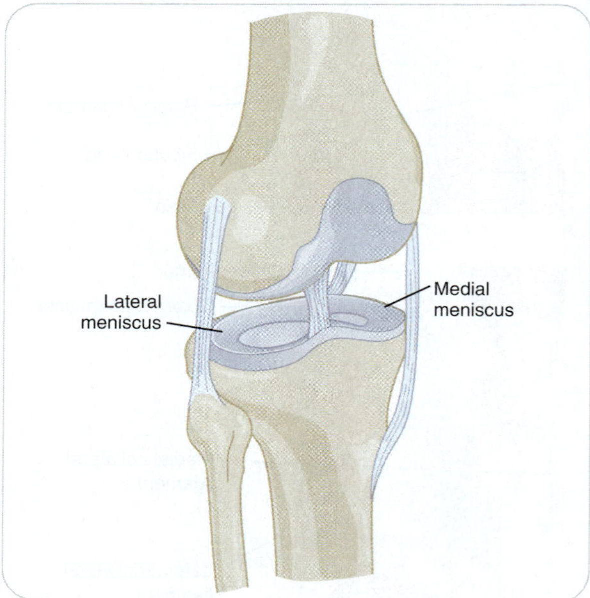

Figure 20-42 The medial and lateral menisci.

Dislocation of the patella is common, and most busy OEC technicians will see a patellar dislocation sometime during their career (**Figure 20-43**). This injury occurs more frequently in teens and in women because the knees are in a valgus position (knock-kneed). The common mechanism of injury involves twisting the knee in a slightly flexed position while forcefully contracting the quadriceps muscle. Excessive direct force to one side of the patella or the other can also dislocate it. Once a patella dislocates, the risk for future dislocations is great. Nearly all patella dislocations are *lateral* (to the outside) because the tissue holding the patella in place is disrupted on the medial side of the knee. This results in a knee that is flexed and has a large firm bulge (the patella) on the lateral side of the knee. The isolated deformity is significant and characteristic, but it is not limb threatening. Often, the patella will "pop" back into place spontaneously if the leg (knee) is straightened. If this occurs before an OEC technician has examined the knee, the medial aspect of the knee will be tender to the touch, and both ecchymosis and swelling may be present.

A patella dislocation should not be confused with a *dislocated knee*, which is a much more serious

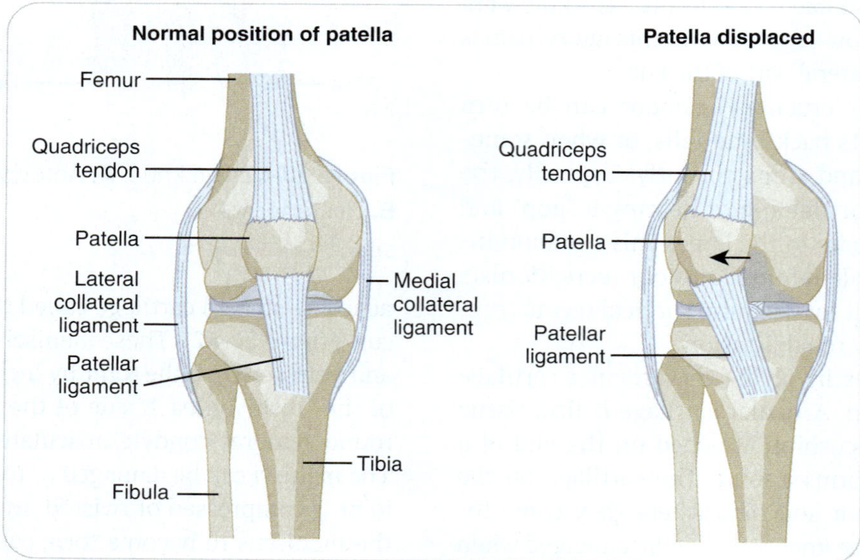

Figure 20-43 A dislocation of the patella.

CASE Update

You perform a secondary assessment. The patient's shoulder shows tenderness at the end of the clavicle where it attaches to the shoulder. Because of the extreme pain in the teen's knee, you cut the ski pants. You find a grossly deformed knee, with the tibia shifted laterally from under the femur. No other injuries or problems are seen. You call base and request EMS transport.

What do you do now?

problem. Refer to a patella that is out of place as a dislocated patella, not as a dislocated knee.

A knee dislocation is a true orthopedic emergency (see Figure 20-14). It occurs rarely. However, once an OEC technician has seen one, it will never be forgotten. The injury is associated with massive trauma in which at least three (if not all four) of the ligaments of the knee are completely torn. This allows the actual knee joint, not just the patella, to move into an abnormal anatomic position. There is gross deformity, in which the proximal tibia is in front of or behind the femur. Additionally, the leg may be severely angulated at the knee joint. Because there is no longer any true **articulation** in this portion of the leg, important neurovascular structures in the **popliteal fossa** are frequently damaged, resulting in severe neurovascular compromise. The most important of these structures is the popliteal artery, which can be lacerated or compressed, causing a pulseless, pale, and cold foot. The pain with this injury is severe. Since the mechanism of injury is severe, a complete patient assessment is needed to ensure that no potential threats to life are present.

Rupture of the quadriceps tendon or patellar ligament is another knee-related injury that OEC technicians may encounter. This injury may be caused by an excessively forceful contraction of the quadriceps muscle that rips the quadriceps tendon off the top of the patella. The same mechanism of injury can cause the patellar ligament to rip below or off the bottom of the patella. This injury is more common in weight lifters and in individuals with chronic disease such as diabetes. With either injury, the patient will likely report hearing a "pop." A palpable "gap" is present above or below the kneecap where the tendon or ligament ruptured, and the patient will be unable to straighten the affected leg at the knee. Swelling from internal bleeding occurs in the zone of injury.

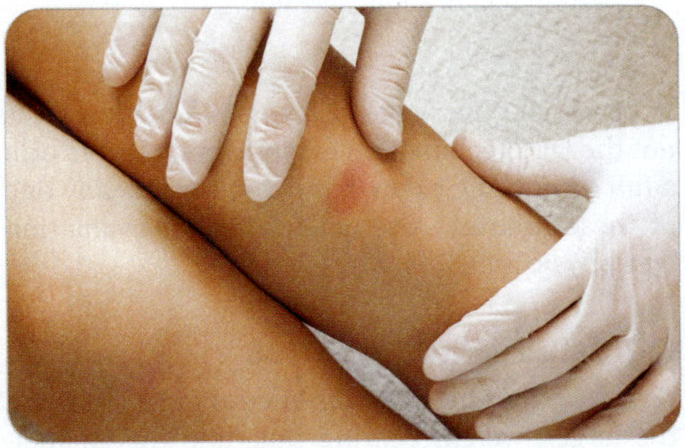

Figure 20-44 When assessing the knee, look for swelling, point tenderness, and bruising.

Assessment of a knee injury at the accident scene should be brief. It is not necessary to diagnose the injury in the field; instead, try to establish a mechanism of injury; attempt to isolate the part of the knee that is injured; assess injury severity, deformity, and CMS; and plan immobilization and transport.

Further assessment of the knee is best performed in a controlled environment such as a warm aid room. Expose the leg from midthigh to the toes. Look for swelling, point tenderness, bruising, or deformity (**Figure 20-44**). Ask the patient to point with one finger to where it hurts the most. Tenderness along the outside or the inside of the joint usually indicates a ligament or cartilage injury, whereas pain over the distal femur, patella,

KEY POINT

Knee Joint Trauma

Following trauma, the knee joint can fill up with blood, excess synovial (lubricating) fluid, or both. In all cases, a large, swollen knee joint usually means something is seriously wrong with the knee. *Rapid* swelling of the knee joint usually indicates a buildup of blood and a more serious injury. A buildup of excessive synovial fluid in the knee takes longer, usually hours, resulting in gradual swelling.

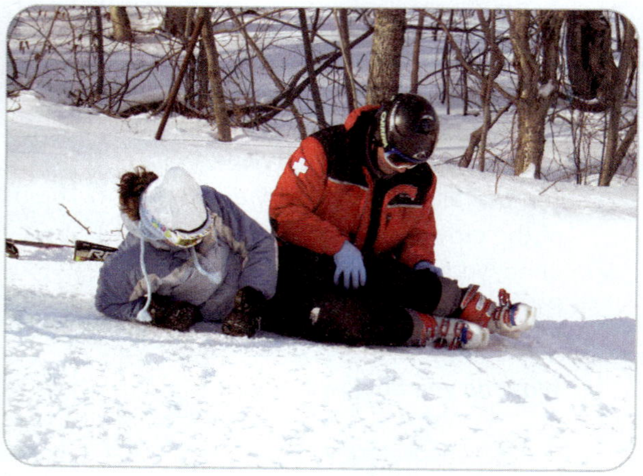

Figure 20-45 A compression fracture of the proximal tibia is a common injury among skiers.

or proximal tibia suggests a possible fracture. It is not the OEC technician's responsibility to perform a full orthopedic exam, but if you suspect any one of these injuries, recommend further evaluation by a physician.

Tibia and Fibula Injuries

The two bones between the knee and the ankle are the larger, weight-bearing tibia and the smaller, non-weight-bearing fibula. The two bones are connected to the femur and the ankle/foot by muscles and ligaments. Both the knee and ankle are hinge joints. The tibia and the femur come together to form the knee joint, whereas the ankle joint is a "mortise" joint formed where the talus bone fits into the space created by the tibia and fibula.

Proximal tibia fractures can be extremely painful and may occur when someone falls from a height or simply lands flat when performing a jump in a terrain park. In this injury, the bottom of the femur is forced into the top of the tibia, compressing the tibia and causing a compression fracture of the top of the bone just below the joint line (**Figure 20-45**). This injury is becoming increasingly frequent in older skiers.

Fractures to the shafts of these bones can occur anywhere along the bone. Tibia and fibula fractures are often seen in skiers, especially those using snowblades (very short skis slightly longer than a ski boot) that do not have release bindings. The incidence of this injury is lower in snowboarders. Frequently, both lower bone shafts in the same leg will break at the same time, a condition known as a "tib-fib" fracture. Less often, direct trauma or other infrequent mechanisms of injury can break the shaft of one bone only. Open fractures involving the tibia can easily occur because the entire anterior bone is just under the skin (**Figure 20-46**). Compartment syndrome can be seen with tibia and fibula fractures.

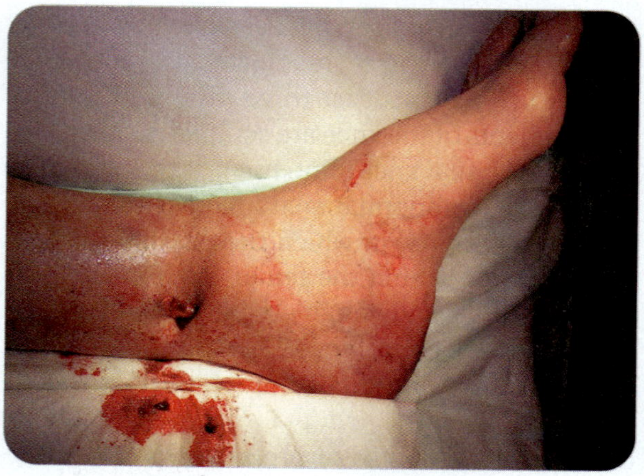

Figure 20-46 An open fracture of the tibia.

Compartment syndrome is a condition in which a muscle swells but is constricted by the connective tissue around it, which cuts off the blood supply to the muscle. It is a true emergency that can happen rapidly following an injury to an extremity and requires rapid transport.

Injuries that occur while skiing include a *boot top* fracture (**Figure 20-47**), in which the fibula or

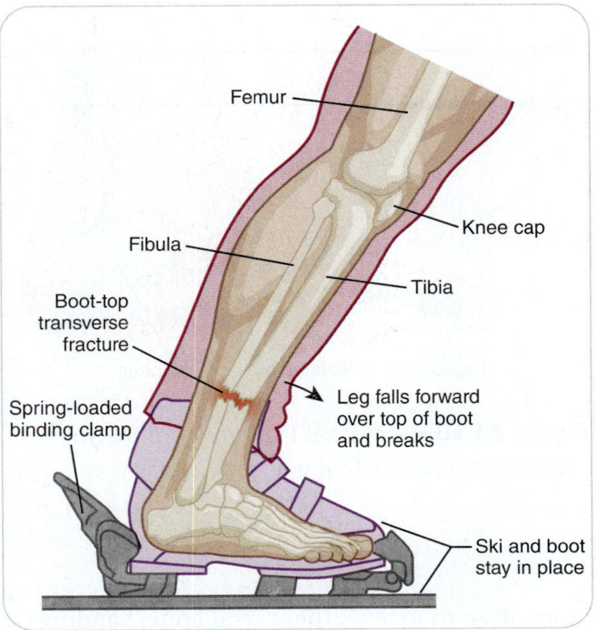

Figure 20-47 A boot top fracture can involve the tibia, the fibula, or both bones.

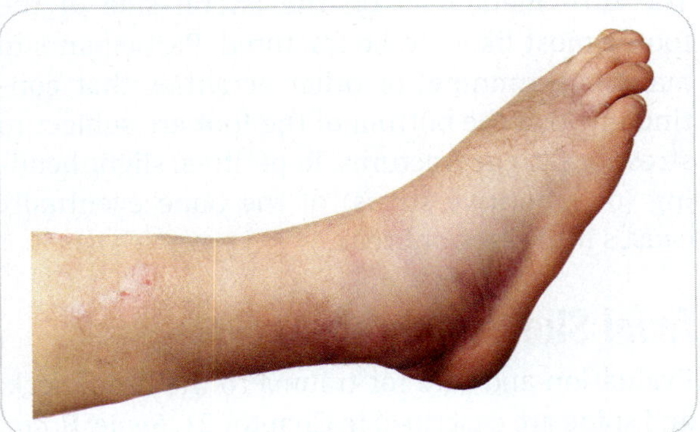

Figure 20-48 Ankle injuries commonly occur on rough or uneven terrain.

the tibia and fibula can undergo a transverse fracture; a *spiral* fracture, in which the tibia is broken in the middle and the fibular shaft is broken above or below the tibial fracture; and a *direct blow* fracture, in which either bone is broken crosswise.

Ankle Injuries

Ankle injuries are common among outdoor enthusiasts, especially those who walk in uneven terrain (**Figure 20-48**). OEC technicians see many types of ankle injuries, from a mild sprain to a deformed, open fracture–dislocation. Sneakers, soft snowboard boots, soft alpine boots, and low-top cross-country ski boots give little support to the ankle, allowing it to twist or bend sideways. When a foot slips off the pedal of a bicycle, the ankle can be injured. Most ankle injuries are due to "rolling" the joint, which typically occurs in one of two ways: either by stepping on the outside of the foot and turning the arch up (a condition known as *inversion*) or by coming down on the inside of the foot and flattening the arch (known as *eversion*). Of the two injury types, inversion is more common and results in a sprain or fracture to the outside of the ankle. High lace-up hiking boots and plastic-shelled alpine ski boots hold the ankle in a more rigid position, reducing both the incidence and the severity of ankle injuries. However, the likelihood of tibial shaft fractures and knee injuries increases with stiffer or higher boots.

Three ligaments on the lateral side of the ankle may be injured by inversion. One symptom of this injury is tenderness *below* the lateral ankle bone, known as the lateral malleolus of the fibula. If the bone is tender, a fracture is more likely than a sprain. By palpating the lateral (outside) ankle bone, you can determine if it is a possible ankle fracture. Pain over the bone usually means a fracture, but only X-ray imaging can determine if it is broken.

The medial malleolus is the large bulge located at the distal end of the tibia on the medial (inside) side of the ankle. One large wide ligament located there may be injured when the ankle everts (turns outward). Tenderness above this ligament suggests the presence of a medial malleolus fracture (**Figure 20-49**).

Snowboarders can have a unique ankle injury that appears to be a sprain but is a fracture that, left untreated, can result in serious disability. A bone in the middle of the ankle, the talus, is broken beneath the lateral ankle ligaments when the snowboarder jumps and lands on a "flat," severely dorsiflexing the ankle (shoving the foot up toward the shin). X-ray images may not show this injury, and a computed tomography (CT) scan is needed to detect it. Surgery may be needed to prevent future disability, so any injured snowboarder with lateral ankle pain should see an orthopedist.

Other mechanisms that cause ankle injury include axial compression due to a fall from a

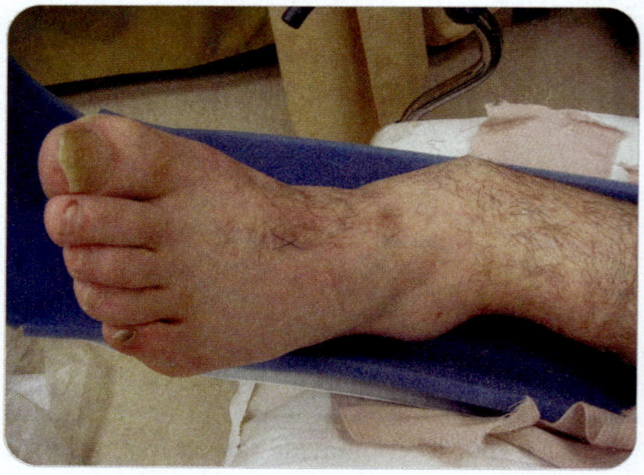

Figure 20-49 A fracture of the medial malleolus of the ankle and a fracture dislocation.

Courtesy of Rhonda Hunt.

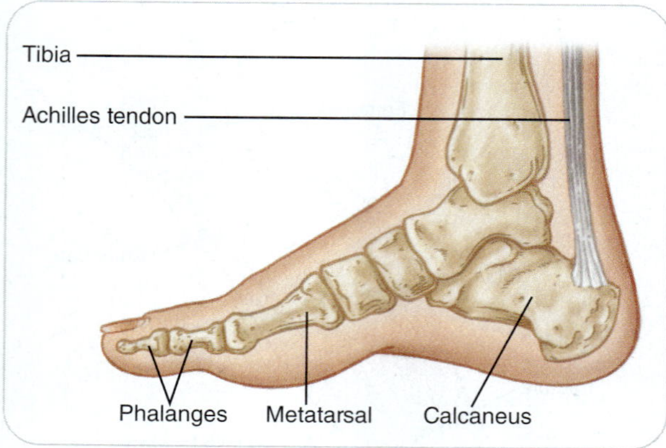

Figure 20-50 Metatarsal fractures are the most common traumatic foot injuries.

height, twisting, or shearing. When combinations of forces are involved, more severe injuries result.

Ankle injuries can range in severity from mild to severe. Additionally, one side of the ankle could be fractured, the other side sprained, or both sides could be broken. Determining whether an ankle injury is a sprain or a fracture requires X-ray imaging. Most ankle injuries present with point tenderness, swelling, ecchymosis, and reduced motion of the joint. Patients may or may not be able to bear weight on the joint. It is not true that individuals can walk on a sprained ankle but cannot walk on a fractured one.

Foot and Toe Injuries

In snow sports, the foot is usually held to a flat surface (e.g., ski, snowboard, snowshoe), and the type of boots worn generally holds the foot immobile. As a result, fractures involving the foot and toes are uncommon. However, they do occur in other winter sports (e.g., tubing, ice skating). Foot injuries occur more frequently in recreational activities and sports like cycling where the shoes worn are soft and the foot can twist. Toe and metatarsal fractures are common, as are sprains of the midfoot and great toe joint (**Figure 20-50**). Toe injuries most commonly occur when a person kicks a fixed object. The calcaneus (heel bone) is broken more often than any other tarsal bone. Landing on the heel during a jump or fall from height is the most common mechanism of injury for a calcaneal fracture. Metatarsal fractures occur frequently in jumping sports such as basketball or volleyball. The fifth metatarsal on the lateral side of the foot is most likely to be fractured. Participants in marching, running, or other activities that continually load the bottom of the foot are subject to stress or fatigue fractures. Repetitive, slight bending (or repetitive stress) of the bone eventually causes it to crack or break.

Axial Skeleton Injuries

Evaluation and care for trauma to the head, neck, and spine are described in Chapter 21, *Spine, Brain, and Nervous System Injuries*. Significant axial injuries generally take precedence over injuries to an extremity unless severe bleeding in a limb must be managed. A patient can have both spinal trauma and an extremity injury at the same time. As a result, OEC technicians must be able to rapidly evaluate and care for the extremity while simultaneously managing significant spinal trauma or other life-threatening problems. Injuries to the axial skeleton are associated with numerous outdoor activities, including skiing, snowboarding, snowmobiling, tubing, sledding, white-water rafting, mountain biking, and climbing.

Section 2 Questions

1. When you are assessing a suspected injury on an extremity, what standard approach should you follow?
   a. Ask the patient if it hurts and do not palpate.
   b. Palpate both sides of the body at the same time.
   c. Inspect and palpate the part of the body.
   d. Inspect, palpate, and perform a neurovascular assessment.
2. Which of the following statements about humerus fractures is most accurate?
   a. They are very uncommon.
   b. They happen only near the elbow.
   c. They are common and can cause nerve damage.
   d. They are never angulated.
3. A snowboarder in the terrain park has a deformed elbow. What might you find when assessing him?
   a. The elbow joint is locked at about 40 degrees.
   b. The pain is severe and aggravated by movement.
   c. CMS is compromised.
   d. All of the above
4. A mountain maintenance worker was snowblowing a walkway at a resort. The snow was wet and heavy, resulting in the center blade becoming jammed. The next step should be to:
   a. carefully use your hand to free up the heavy snow.
   b. shut off the snowblower before putting anything near the blade.
   c. try to rev the machine up to free the blade.
   d. run the snowblower at idle speed and use a stick or pole to push out the stuck object.
5. A boot top fracture could involve the:
   a. tibia only.
   b. fibula only.
   c. tibia, fibula, or both bones.
   d. kneecap and femur.
6. If your assessment indicates a pelvic fracture, you might also see:
   a. injuries to internal structures such as the bladder and blood vessels.
   b. injuries to the diaphragm and lungs.
   c. injuries to metatarsals.
   d. injuries to the stomach and pancreas.
7. You are on scene caring for a patient with a knee injury. As you gather information during your survey, you find out this patient has chronic knee pain from an old injury. Your next step is to:
   a. not splint since this problem has happened many times before.
   b. splint in the position of comfort and transport.
   c. use a traction splint to safely secure the leg.
   d. backboard and transport to the local hospital for X-ray imaging.
8. In skiing, snowboarding, and snowshoeing, the foot is supported and held in a flat position, resulting in the foot being immobile. As a result:
   a. foot and toe fractures are less common.
   b. foot and toe fractures are more common
   c. femur fractures are common.
   d. patella dislocations are more common.

Answers: 1. d, Objective 20-2.1, p. 448; 2. c, Objective 20-2.1, p. 450; 3. d, Objective 20-2.1, p. 450; 4. b, Objective 20-2.1, p. 454; 5. c, Objective 20-2.1, p. 463; 6. a, Objective 20-2.1, p. 456; 7. b, Objective 20-2.1, p. 459; 8. a, Objective 20-2.1, p. 464

SECTION 3: MANAGEMENT OF MUSCULOSKELETAL INJURIES

OBJECTIVES

Upon completion of this section of this chapter, the OEC technician will be able to:

20-3.1 Explain the general management of a patient with a musculoskeletal injury.

20-3.2 List and demonstrate the use of the following types of splints:
- Sling and swath
- Quick splint
- Soft splint
- Rigid splint (e.g., airplane, quick, wooden, SAM)
- Traction splint (the one you use at your resort/area; e.g., Kendrick, Hare, Slishman, Sager)

20-3.3 Explain the difference between traction and tension.

20-3.4 Discuss the general principles of splinting.

20-3.5 Demonstrate how to care for an injured extremity when there is neurovascular compromise.

20-3.6 Demonstrate how to care for the following injuries:
- Shoulder, clavicle, and scapula
- Humerus fracture
- Elbow
- Forearm
- Wrist
- Hand and finger
- Pelvis
- Hip
- Femur
- Knee
- Tibia and fibula
- Ankle
- Foot and toe

20-3.7 Define and demonstrate the proper care for an open (compound) fracture.

20-3.8 Demonstrate how to remove a ski boot, hiking boot, or snowboard boot when the patient has an injury to that leg.

OVERVIEW OF MUSCULOSKELETAL INJURY MANAGEMENT

The early management of musculoskeletal injuries is the same as that for other injuries. Begin with a scene size-up, eliminating any hazards that may be present. Next, manage any life-threatening problems and assess ABCDs in a primary patient assessment. Bleeding is common with musculoskeletal injuries and can be severe, especially with open fractures. Take standard precautions, and control external bleeding. Bandage wounds appropriately, using sterile dressings that completely cover the wound. Cover exposed bone ends to keep them from becoming contaminated. When appropriate, call for ALS personnel, especially for open fractures, and severely angulated extremities. Apply high-flow oxygen *as needed* based on breathing rate and clinical picture. Titrate with a pulse oximeter, keeping the oxygen saturation between 94 and 99%. Generally, patients with fractures that can bleed a lot—femoral, pelvic, and open fractures—may need high-flow oxygen. Rarely does a person need oxygen for an isolated broken ankle or wrist.

The methods described in this section, although commonly used by OEC technicians and other emergency medicine professionals around the world, may differ slightly from area to area due to local protocols or a medical director's guidance.

The ability to differentiate one musculoskeletal injury from another can be difficult in the field. The general care of sprains, dislocations, and fractures is essentially the same and involves the following actions:

1. Use standard precautions to avoid contaminating yourself or others.
2. Formulate a plan of action early, get the right equipment for the patient's injuries, and summon EMS transport if needed. Request ALS if there are threats to life or if pain medication may be needed.
3. Expose the zone of injury to look for bleeding, abrasions, lacerations, contusions, punctures, swelling, or deformity.
4. Bandage any wound appropriately, applying a pressure bandage if there is active bleeding. Use sterile dressings, and completely cover the wound. Make sure bleeding is controlled and check the wound frequently for additional bleeding. *When needed*, use a tourniquet.
5. Use the correct splint or other immobilization device for the injury. When a fracture is immobilized, there is usually less pain. Avoid letting an injured extremity move uncontrollably, as this may cause more tissue damage and pain.
6. Always immobilize the joint above and below the injury.
7. Check CMS before and after splinting. If normal CMS becomes compromised after the splint is applied, readjust the splint and/or bandage *once* to improve CMS. Rapid transport to advanced care is needed if CMS has been compromised, even if it returns.
8. Use some cooling method (e.g., ice or snow in a plastic bag) early to treat pain. Do not keep ice on for longer than 15 minutes. Cover the skin with a cloth or a bandage and place the ice on the cloth so that the skin is cooled but is not allowed to freeze.
9. Make sure the patient is comfortable during transport, especially if an extremity is immobilized in an unusual position.
10. Provide oxygen if appropriate, titrating to an oxygen saturation of equal to or greater than 94% with a pulse oximeter. The majority of musculoskeletal injuries do *not* require oxygen.
11. Transport as soon as is practical to a higher level of care.

SPLINTING

Splinting is a skill that all OEC technicians should practice and master. A **splint** is a piece of equipment—whether commercially made, homemade, or improvised on scene—that is used to safely immobilize an extremity or other body part. The steps for applying various splints are given in the OEC Skills throughout this chapter.

Reasons for Splinting

- To decrease the movement of the ends of broken bones and to allow a hematoma at the fracture site to clot, thus preventing further blood loss
- To decrease pain at the fracture site
- To reduce muscle spasms, by placing the limb in better anatomic alignment

- To prevent a sharp bone end from penetrating the skin and making a closed fracture an open fracture
- To prevent any further damage to soft tissues, including muscles, nerves, and blood vessels
- To allow easier transport because the body is in better anatomic alignment
- To prevent spinal cord damage using spinal motion restriction (using a backboard, large vacuum splint, or other appropriate motion restriction devices/equipment) when indicated for spine injuries (discussed in Chapter 21, *Spine, Brain, and Nervous System Injuries*)

Types of Splints

OEC technicians have various types of splints at their disposal. Many splints may be used for a variety of injuries, although some are designed for a specific type of injury. Knowing when and how to use each type of splint effectively is one of the hallmarks of a highly trained OEC technician. There are four main types of splints: soft, rigid or semi-rigid, traction, and improvised.

Soft Splints

Sling and Swathe Splints

A **sling and swathe**, made from two triangle-shaped cravats, is used to immobilize upper extremity injuries, including clavicle fractures, shoulder separations, humerus and elbow injuries, and wrist injuries (**Figure 20-51**). A sling and swathe provides a stable platform for the arm and can be used to either immobilize just the arm or the arm with an additional rigid splint in place. Properly applied, a sling and swathe holds the arm close to the body, thereby preventing further movement. It is the most commonly used splint by OEC technicians. There are two ways to apply a sling and swathe. Depending on the injury, one method may be better than the other.

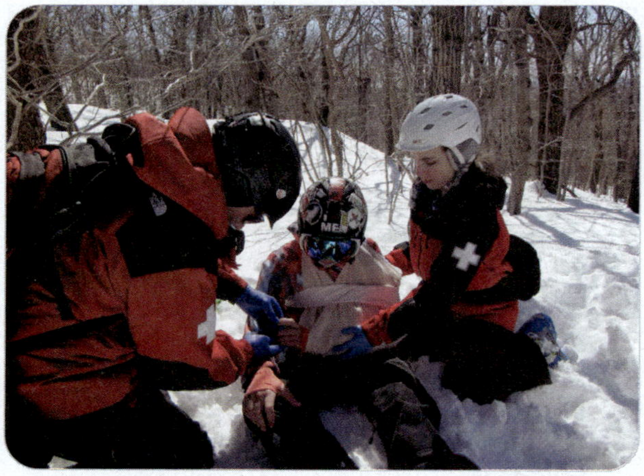

Figure 20-51 A sling and swathe is used primarily to immobilize injured upper extremities.

Air Splints

An air splint is a dual-walled, tube-shaped device used to temporarily immobilize a long bone. Constructed of clear, soft plastic, an air splint is applied around an extremity and secured in place, usually by a zipper. It is then inflated with air to form a rigid splint around the injured extremity. By applying constant external pressure to a wound, it also helps control bleeding. Air splints are most often used to immobilize injuries below the elbow or knee. Some air splints are shaped like an extremity, so they can be applied to an elbow or ankle; others can splint an entire leg or arm. Air splints are commonly used within emergency care systems, where they are simple to use, inexpensive, and easier to clean than other splints.

Despite these advantages, the use of air splints in outdoor settings is limited for several reasons. First, because they are made of plastic, they can be easily punctured by sharp or abrasive objects, rendering them unusable. Second, they are affected by temperature and altitude. In very cold weather, the plastic can become stiff or brittle, making the splint difficult to use. Additionally, changes in temperature and altitude cause the air inside the splint to contract or expand, which can cause the splint to become too loose or too tight. For these reasons, air splints are not commonly used by OEC technicians.

Vacuum Splints

A vacuum splint is a device that consists of a closed, airtight plastic bag that contains thousands of small plastic pellets (**Figure 20-52**). Following its application to the injured extremity, the air is sucked out of the splint with a special pump, forming a rigid enclosure around the body part. Vacuum splints are available in a variety of sizes, ranging from small ankle or forearm splints to full-body splints used to

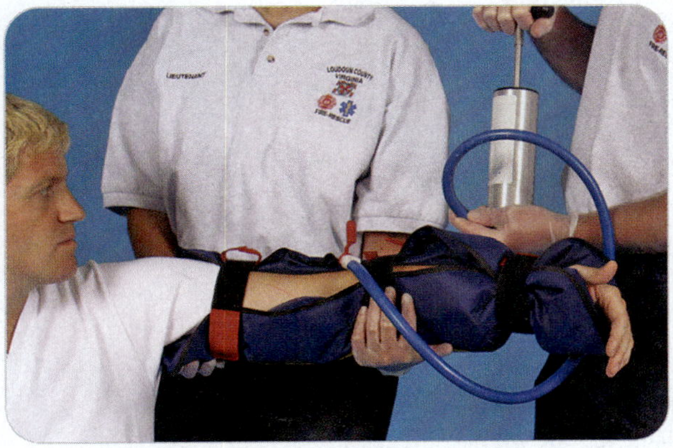

Figure 20-52 A vacuum splint can be used on an injured arm.

immobilize the spine. Vacuum splints provide excellent insulation in cold weather. However, they can cause heat retention in warm or hot weather, which may not be ideal. Also, it is not possible to apply an ice or other cold compress over the splint, because the cold cannot penetrate this splint. Like air splints, vacuum splints can be easily punctured. Despite this, vacuum splints are widely used by ski patrols in Europe and are becoming more widely used in North America, including use by ski patrols. Large, full-body vacuum splints are being used more for spinal motion restriction; however, because of their expense, long spine boards are still used by most ski areas in 2020.

Blanket Roll/Pillow Splint

A blanket can be fashioned into a splint to fit around or beside nearly any joint, whether large (e.g., shoulder, knee) or small (e.g., elbow, ankle). When fashioned into a tight roll, a blanket is especially effective for injuries in which patients will not allow their arm to be brought to their side, such as a shoulder dislocation (**Figure 20-53**).

For shoulder injuries that need to be held firmly with the elbow away from the body, fashion a blanket into a special splint known as a blanket roll splint. A blanket roll can also be used under a knee as a splint. Pillows and other soft materials can also be used effectively to splint various joint injuries, most notably elbow and ankle injuries, especially when these joints are severely dislocated (**Figure 20-54**).

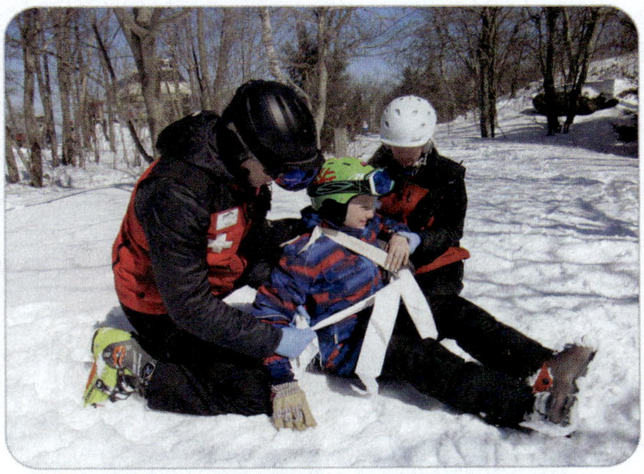

Figure 20-53 Blanket roll splints are a good option for splinting an upper extremity injury where the patient is unable to bring the injured arm to the body.

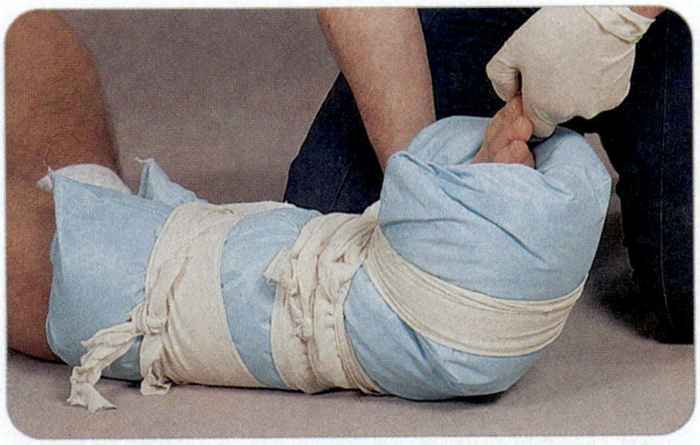

Figure 20-54 A pillow splint can be used when rigid splints are not available.

Pelvic Binders

Because fractures of the pelvis often cause life-threatening blood loss, they are among the most devastating musculoskeletal injuries. Pelvic fractures should be stabilized emergently in the field, if possible before the patient is transported. Two methods of pelvic binding are commonly used to manage these injuries: a sheet wrap and a commercial pelvic sling (**Figure 20-55**). Refer to Chapter 24, *Abdominal and Pelvic Trauma*, for details regarding how to apply a pelvic binder.

Rigid or Semi-rigid Splints

Cardboard, Wood, or Metal Splints

As the name implies, rigid splints are constructed of stiff materials such as heavy cardboard, wood,

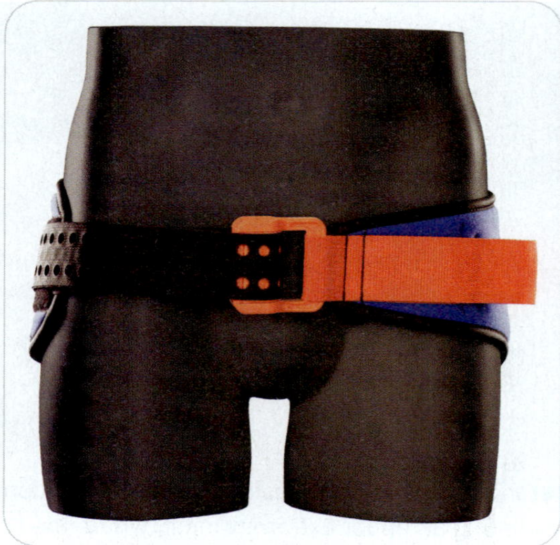

Figure 20-55 A SAM pelvic sling.

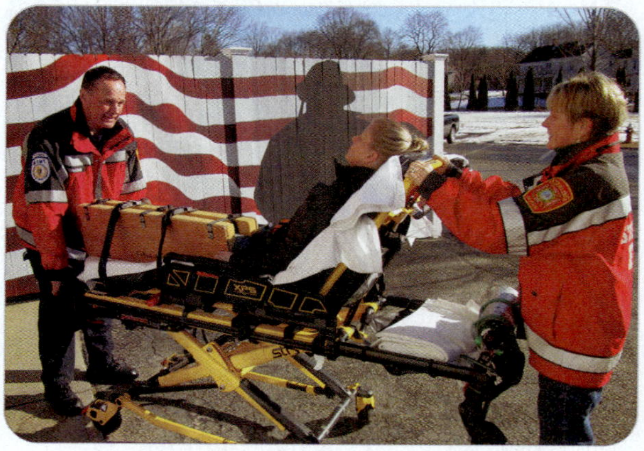

Figure 20-56 EMTs taking a patient with a rigid splint out of the patrol room to a hospital.

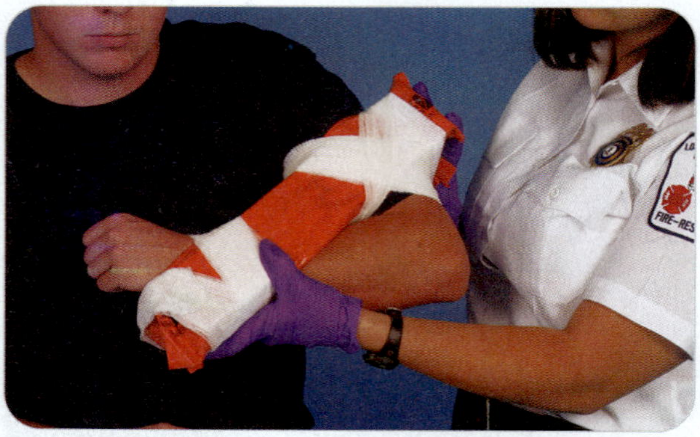

Figure 20-57 Rigid splints are held in place with roller gauze or cravats.

or metal. OEC technicians commonly use these splints because of their reliability, low cost, effectiveness in all weather and altitude conditions, and ease of use. Some are available commercially, whereas others may be fashioned from readily available materials and are just as effective (**Figure 20-56**). Rigid splints are applied to the sides, front, and/or back of an injured limb and are generally held in place by roller gauze (bandage) or cravats, not Ace bandages (**Figure 20-57**). The compression from an Ace bandage can cause circulation problems distally. Cardboard splints are used primarily to splint an arm or leg. Cardboard splints are best used in dry environments unless they are specially treated with a water-resistant coating. Cardboard is reasonably inexpensive, so when the patient leaves while wearing a cardboard splint, it does not need to be retrieved.

Although cardboard splints are commercially available, they are easy to make using corrugated cardboard. The most useful splint to hold a lower leg firmly is 15 inches by 42 inches, with folds and cuts placed in the correct places (**Figure 20-58**). For an elbow or a forearm, a double thickness of cardboard 3 inches by 12 to 15 inches is effective.

Wood splints are more rigid than cardboard and provide very effective immobilization. Like cardboard splints, wood splints are available commercially or can be homemade. Some commercial wood splints are padded and are enclosed in a water-resistant shell. Homemade splints should be sanded smooth on all sides and sealed to prevent splintering. Wood splints are available in a variety of sizes; they may be constructed of quarter-inch exterior-grade plywood, 3 inches wide and 12 to 36 inches long. Wood splints are commonly used to immobilize long bones (radius, ulna, humerus, tibia, and fibula) and joints (elbow, knee, and wrist).

Quick Splint

The Quick Splint has been used by ski patrols for many years (**Figure 20-59**). Made of lightweight plastic or plywood, they are the mainstay of care for lower leg injuries among ski patrollers. They are especially effective for knee, tibia, or fibula injuries. A Quick Splint is easy to use and may be applied rapidly by one or two people. Its compact design allows it to easily fit on a fully loaded toboggan.

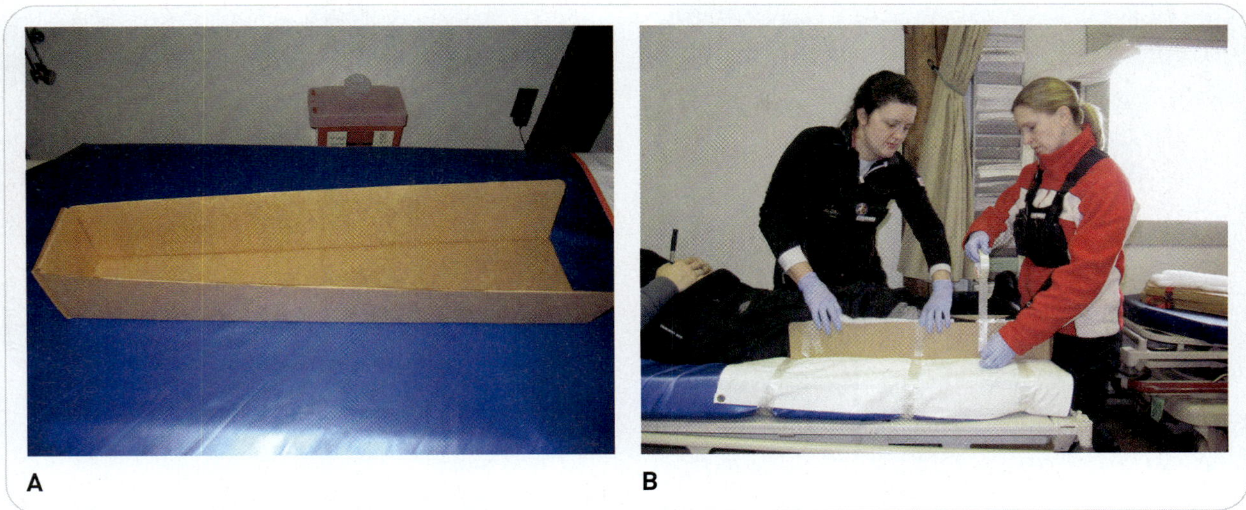

Figure 20-58 Cardboard splints are used in dry environments to splint an arm or leg. **A.** A cardboard splint used for the leg. **B.** The cardboard splint applied to a patient.

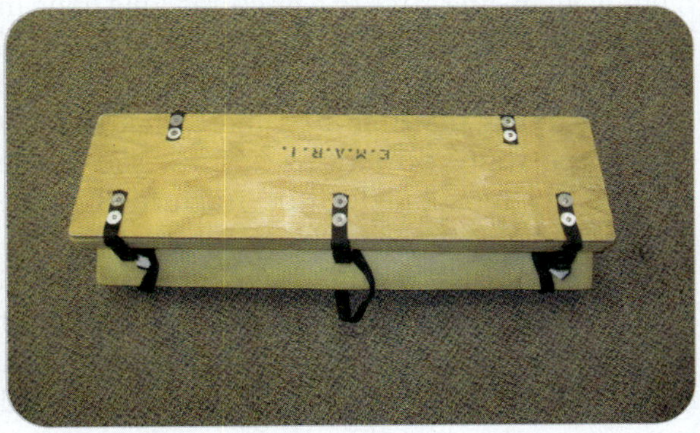

Figure 20-59 A Quick Splint.

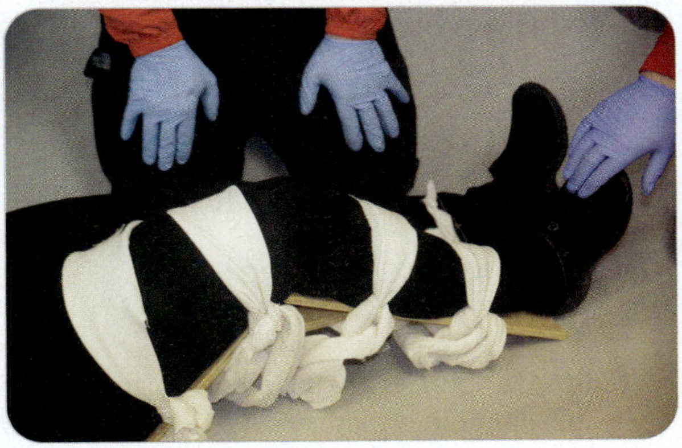

Figure 20-60 An airplane splint applied.

Airplane Splint

An airplane splint is a special-purpose rigid splint fabricated from two 4-inch by 12-inch wooden boards that are held together with a hinge that allows the device to be adjusted to different angles. The splint is secured into position with cravats. It may be used in conjunction with a Quick Splint to secure an injured knee in the bent position (**Figure 20-60**). It may also be used in place of a blanket roll to hold an arm up in a shoulder injury.

Malleable Metal Splints

These splints are made of lightweight aluminum or wire mesh. As their name implies, malleable splints can be molded to fit the injured extremity. Wire, ladder, and padded aluminum splints are commercially available. You can also fabricate a ladder or wire splint from wire mesh obtained from a hardware store. These splints can be shaped to fit precisely around an elbow or ankle joint in a *sugar tong* configuration (**Figure 20-61**). They can also immobilize a body part in either the position in which it was found or a position of function. Once applied, a roller bandage or several cravats hold the splint in place. Wire and ladder splints generally come in 3-inch by 30- or 36-inch sizes and can be folded to fit in a backpack. Metal splints should be padded for the patient's comfort.

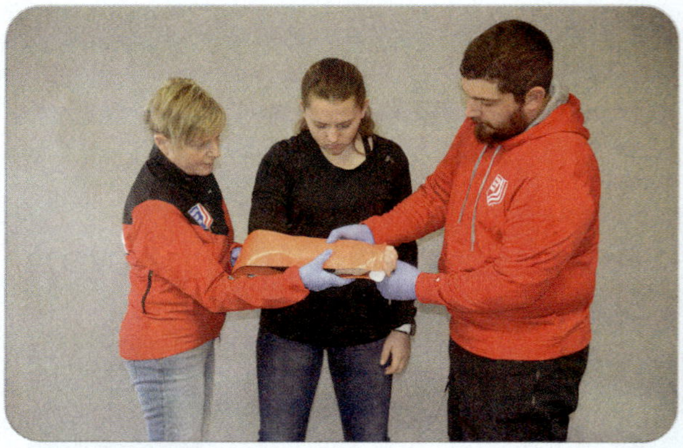

Figure 20-61 Sugar tong splint for forearm fractures.

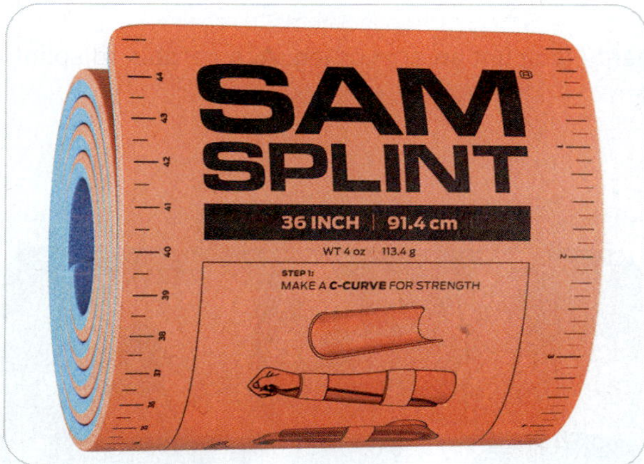

Figure 20-62 A SAM Splint.

The SAM Splint is a 4-inch by 36-inch piece of malleable aluminum that is covered on both sides by a thin layer of foam. Developed by orthopedic surgeon Sam Scheinberg upon his return from the Vietnam War, the SAM (Structural, Aluminum, Malleable) splint is used by the US military and is very popular among emergency and rescue professionals worldwide (**Figure 20-62**). It can be easily shaped to better conform to the patient's anatomy or position and comes packaged as a 3-inch cylinder for easy transportation. If one looks at the original scheme of how to apply a SAM Splint, it involves creasing the splint for its entire length in the middle, making a short "T" of the splint, with the bottom of the "T" doubled so it is rigid. Without the "T," when applied it takes the shape of a "U" and is less rigid. Applying a SAM Splint involves folding and molding the material into shapes that are rigid and firmly immobilize the injured extremity.

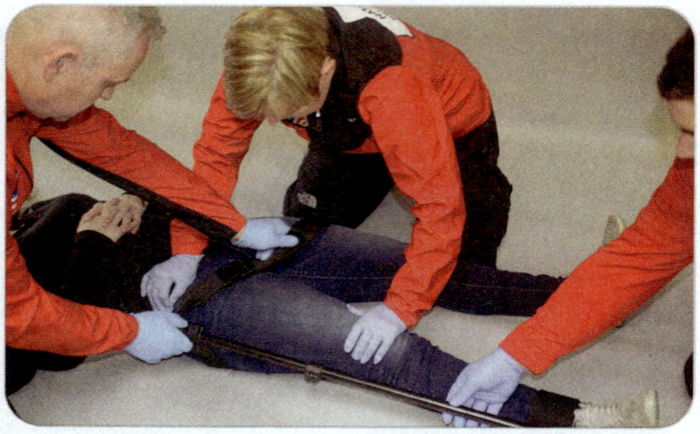

Figure 20-63 A Slishman traction splint.

Traction Splints

A **traction splint** is a device that applies longitudinal traction to a fractured femur. In emergency care, **traction** is defined as a safe mechanism for immobilizing a broken bone. Traction is the placement of an in-line force to a fractured long bone in the direction of its normal alignment for the purpose of regaining bone length and reducing pain. Traction aligns the limb in a more anatomically neutral position, preventing further soft-tissue damage. By immobilizing the fracture site, the splint also helps to reduce blood loss. Because excessive traction is harmful to an injured limb, OEC technicians should set and control the amount of traction being applied. A traction splint does not reduce a fracture, but it does align the fractured bone in a more anatomically favorable position. This type of splint can also make transportation easier.

Many different types of femoral traction splints are commercially available, including splints made by Sager, Slishman, and Kendrick (**Figure 20-63**). Although each has its own advantages and "ease of use," they work in a similar fashion by splinting the femur exerting mild traction.

Traction splints are used primarily for fractures involving the middle third of the femur. Some EMS programs and traction splint manufacturers (Sager) have advocated the use of these devices, *using tension*, for proximal femur fractures, including classical hip fractures. Generally, hip fractures can be immobilized well with the use of a backboard and straps used as a litter. Check with both your local medical advisor and the manufacturer of your traction device to determine if your equipment may be used in this manner. Traction splints are contraindicated in fractures of the distal third of the femur and on any upper extremity fracture.

The Hare splint has also been reported to have been used successfully with less tension applied for tibial shaft fractures (**Figure 20-64**). In this setting, the Velcro attachments applied below the knee and above the ankle (but not over the fracture site) help hold the tibia in position. If no other device is available, a traction splint could be used in this fashion. However, a Quick Splint is a better choice for a tibia fracture. A femoral traction splint with stabilizing rods on both sides can be used in a "floating knee" (a fracture of the femur and tibia in the same leg), as discussed later.

KEY POINT

Thomas Splint

The original lower extremity traction splint was developed by British surgeon Dr. Hugh Owen Thomas in 1875 and dubbed "The Knee Appliance" (**Figure 20-65**). It received great reviews for its use in helping wounded soldiers during World War I. When applied, this device prevented hypovolemic shock by allowing the hematoma around the femur fracture to stabilize.

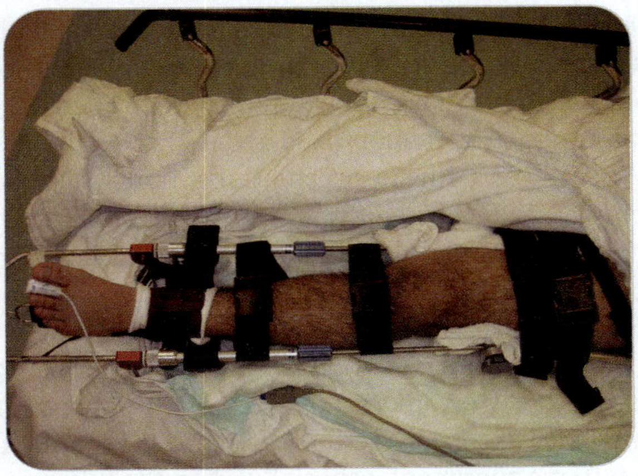

Figure 20-64 A Hare traction splint.

Improvised Splints

Occasionally, you may need a splint but find that one is not readily available. In these instances, an effective splint may be fashioned from available materials. For instance, a magazine can be made into a splint for a forearm, a foot, or an ankle. A plastic knife from the cafeteria or a Popsicle stick can be used to splint a finger when a tongue blade is not available (be sure to tape the serrated portion first so patient does not get cut). For Nordic skiers, off-road bicyclers, or rafters, larger splints can be made from ski poles, tree branches, oars, or any other long, stiff object (**Figure 20-66**). There are countless ways to splint an extremity. Imaginative OEC technicians who understand the principles of splinting, both for immobilization and traction, can treat nearly any extremity injury they

KEY POINT

Traction Versus Tension

When applying a traction splint for certain femur fractures, OEC technicians must apply *traction* to align the leg. Usually, this requires pulling on the foot with about 15 pounds of force. The force of traction should be no more than 10% of total body weight. When alignment is necessary for other long-bone fractures, *tension* is used. Tension involves pulling with less force, generally 7 to 8 pounds, or only enough force to align the bone. After the proper application of traction or tension, patients will generally tell you that the limb feels better.

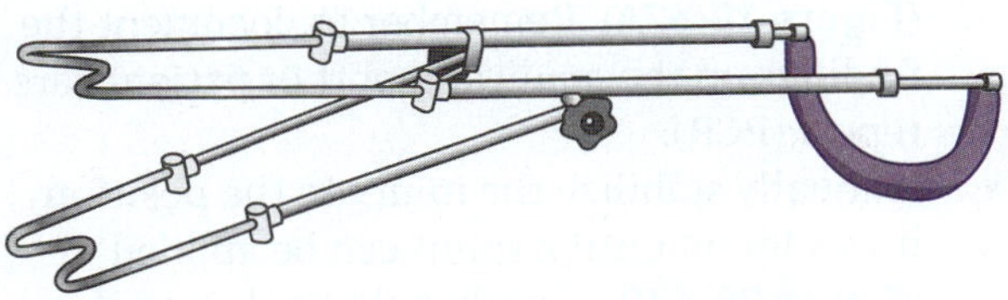

Figure 20-65 A Thomas splint.

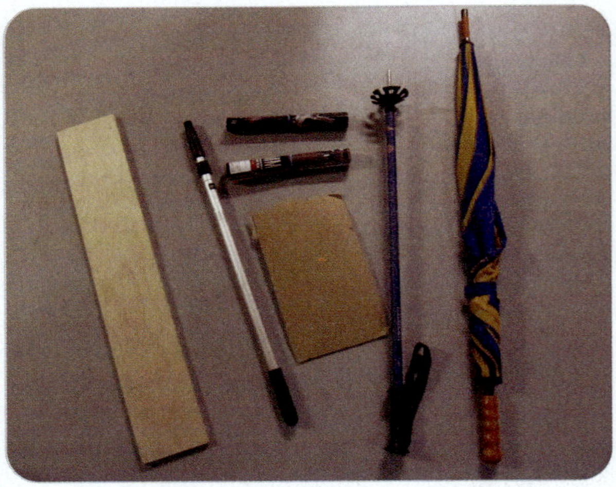

Figure 20-66 A variety of items can be used as splints.

encounter. Use an improvised splint only if the one commonly used for the injury is not available.

Principles of Splinting

Proper splinting requires a careful, methodical approach to prevent additional damage. As a rule, splint an injured extremity before moving the patient. The exceptions are the presence of an immediate hazard to the patient or rescuer, or when the patient's general condition demands *immediate* care and/or rapid transport for a life-threatening condition.

If the patient exhibits signs and symptoms of hypovolemic shock, first control bleeding. Next carefully attempt to align the injured limb(s) as close to normal anatomic position as possible. Place an injured arm to the chest and splint it anatomically, or an injured leg to the other leg and put the patient on transport device such as a toboggan and then treat for shock and provide rapid transport. You are not *reducing* a fracture of a limb but aligning the limb in a better position for transport.

The following list presents the key principles of splinting:

- Check distal CMS before splinting (**Figure 20-67A**). Remember to document the findings on the medical report or patient care report (PCR).
- Manually stabilize the injury in the position it was found until a splint can be applied (**Figure 20-67B**). Gently hold the bones above and below (proximal to and distal to) the suspected injury site.
- Select an appropriate splint.
- Properly size the splint (**Figure 20-67C**). The splint should span the joint above and the joint below the injury. If the fracture involves a long bone such as the radius, size the splint using the uninjured arm as a guide. If both arms are injured, use your judgment in sizing the splint. Malleable splints should be shaped to match the injured extremity (make all adjustments away from the injury so as not to accidently move the injured area).
- Pad the splint (if needed) to maximize the patient's comfort. This is especially important if the patient will be moved over rough or uneven terrain.
- Check distal CMS after splinting, and document the findings on the medical report or PCR.
- Position the splint. Place the splint next to the injured area or gently slide the splint under or around the extremity (**Figure 20-67D**).
- Secure the splint. Use roller gauze, or cravats, to secure the injured body part(s) to the splint (**Figure 20-67E**). Be careful not to make the wrapping too tight because doing so can affect distal neurovascular status. Ace bandages are not recommended to secure a splint.
- Reassess CMS, and adjust the splint if now compromised. Record your findings.

At times, placing an injured extremity into anatomic position before splinting may be difficult if not impossible. These circumstances include patients with open fractures, severely angulated fractures, dislocations, or fracture–dislocations close to a joint; patients or children who will not let you move the injured limb; and patients with an impaled object in the injured extremity. Elbow, shoulder, hip, and knee injuries with deformity may need to be immobilized using some creativity. When faced with these situations, remember the previously described principles, place the limb in the most comfortable, best immobilized position possible checking CMS before and after, and transport the patient.

OEC technicians should neither attempt to set (reduce) a fracture nor *force* exposed bone fragments of an open fracture back into their normal anatomic alignment, especially when the injury involves the femur. These procedures are the physician's responsibility. However, if bone ends do go

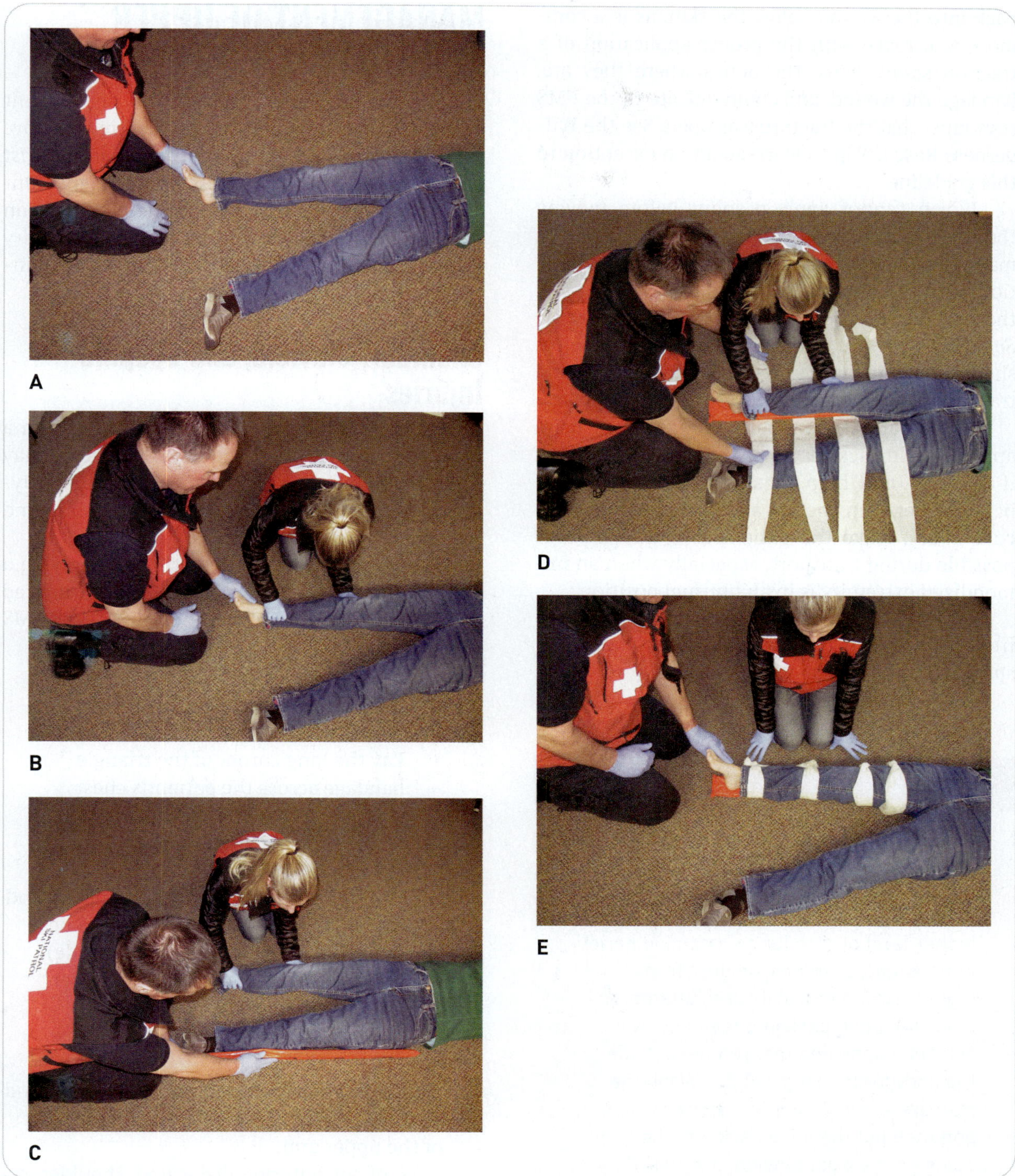

Figure 20-67 **A.** Assess circulation, motor, and sensory functions. **B.** Manually stabilize the injured limb. **C.** Measure the splint using the uninjured leg as a guide. **D.** Position the splint by sliding it next to or under the limb and then immobilize the joint above and below the injury. **E.** Secure the splint with gauze or roller bandage. Recheck CMS.

back into the wound below the skin, as is a common occurrence with the proper application of a traction splint, leave the bones where they are, bandage the wound, and communicate to the EMS personnel that the fracture was open. See the Wilderness Rescue Tip to learn about an exception to this guideline.

If you cannot apply a splint before moving the patient, such as one impaled on a fixed object, maintain manual traction or manual immobilization until the patient is free from the object, and then splint the injury. As described in Chapter 19, *Soft-Tissue Injuries and Burns*, an impaled object should be left in place unless it cannot be freed and transported with the patient.

If the patient complains of significant pain, applying cold packs or ice or snow in a plastic bag, if available, may help. Be sure to place a cloth or bandage between the ice and skin to avoid local cold injury. Make the patient as comfortable as possible during transport, especially when an immobilized extremity is in an unusual position.

Reassess neurovascular status of the limb frequently, and if it worsens, readjust bandages, splints, or other dressings as needed.

KEY POINT

Wilderness Rescue Tip

If you are unable to get a patient with a bone end protruding through the skin to a higher level of care for an extended period of time (approximately 4 hours from higher level of medical care), attempt to place the bone back into the body. The cells of a bone end that remain outside the body for too long will die. Wash the fracture site with sterile water or saline and then put the bone back into the body using gentle axial tension. If a sterile solution is not available, use clean water, boiled (and cooled) water, or disinfected water. Never use water from a pond or creek. This course of action may also be necessary on a cruise ship that is hours from port or hours outside of rescue helicopter range.

MANAGEMENT OF UPPER EXTREMITY INJURIES

When providing emergency care to any patient with an injured upper extremity, *be sure to remove rings, bracelets, and any other jewelry from the wrist or fingers* early in the process, before significant swelling occurs. Be sure to document this action on the patient care report and keep the jewelry safe. (If possible, put jewelry on the *other*, uninjured arm or hand.)

Shoulder, Clavicle, and Scapula Injuries

Nearly all of these injuries can be treated with a sling and swathe. During transport, patients may wish to remain partially sitting or may prefer lying on the unaffected side. To apply a sling and swathe, follow the steps in **OEC Skill 20-1**.

The following alternate method of applying a sling avoids placing any pressure on the injured shoulder or a fractured clavicle. Always check CMS before and after applying the sling.

1. Rescuer 1: Support the patient's elbow while it is bent to just under a 90-degree angle.
2. Rescuer 2:
   - Lay the long corner of the triangle bandage across the patient's chest and over the uninjured shoulder in the midclavicular line, as before (**Figure 20-68A**).
   - Bring the other corner of the sling up and around the forearm and under the near axilla (i.e., armpit of the injured side).
   - Tie this corner to the opposite upper corner *behind the patient's back* to keep pressure off the injured clavicle (**Figure 20-68B**).
3. Tie the swathe around the patient's chest and forearm rather than around the injured part of the upper arm.

Care of an anterior dislocated shoulder requires OEC technicians to use patience and sometimes creativity due to the position of comfort being away from the body. As a rule, OEC technicians do not attempt to reduce a dislocated shoulder. If you encounter patients who have a history of dislocated shoulders and ask you to assist in reducing their shoulder, do not do so. Instead, immobilize the patient's shoulder in a position of

OEC SKILL 20-1 Applying a Sling and Swathe

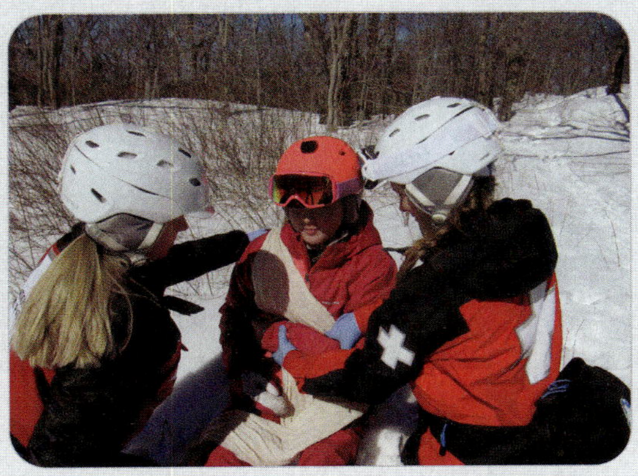

Assess CMS.

1 Rescuer 1: Support the patient's elbow while it is bent to about a 90-degree angle.

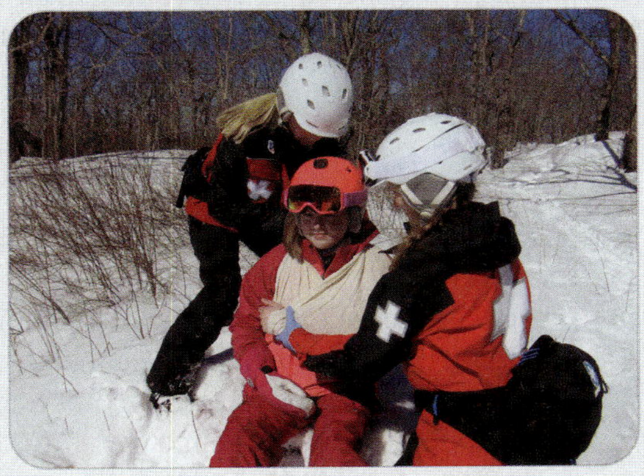

2 Rescuer 2:

- Place a triangle bandage on the patient's chest, under the injured arm.
- Position the long edge of the bandage so that it lies opposite the midclavicular line and just medial to the fingertips of the injured arm. The upper corner should pass over the opposite shoulder, and the apex of the triangle should be just beyond the elbow of the injured arm.
- Fold the lower corner of the bandage anteriorly around the forearm, and then up and over the shoulder on the injured side.
- Raise or lower the arm to an appropriate level at which it will remain.
- Tie the two long ends of the sling together at *the side of the neck* (to prevent pressure on the back of the neck); if the knot is placed over the midline of the neck, pad it for the patient's comfort.
- Bring the apex forward and pin it to the front of the sling or tie a knot in the apex.
- Reassess CMS.

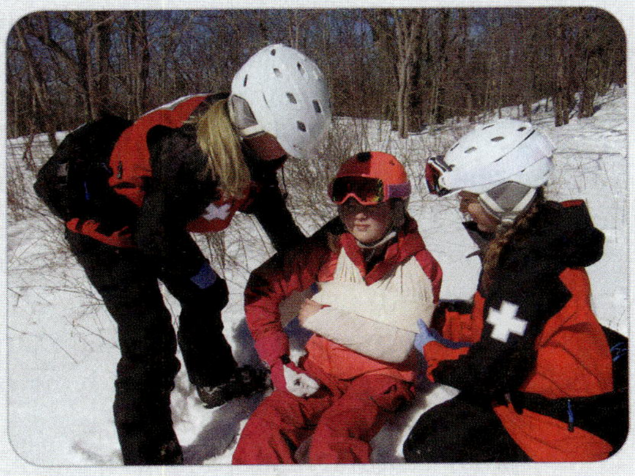

3 Make sure the tips of the fingers are visible to allow for CMS checks. Properly applied, the forearm should be cradled in the sling, with its weight evenly distributed.

To make the swathe:

- Fold a second triangular bandage to form a cravat that is 4 inches wide (or 6 inches, for humerus fractures).
- Wrap the cravat around the patient's chest, with the middle of the swathe over the injured arm that is resting on the side of the chest. Place the two ends of the swathe under the opposite arm.
- Tie the two ends snugly with a square knot.

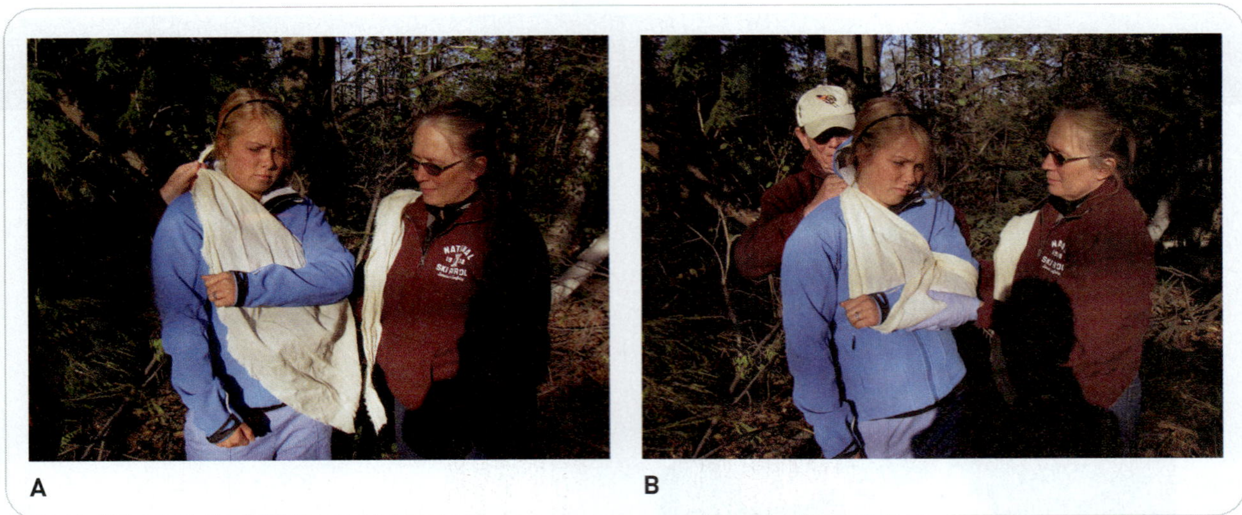

Figure 20-68 **A.** Lay one end of cravat across the patient's chest. **B.** Bring the other end of the cravat up around the forearm and under the axilla. Tie the corner to the opposite upper corner behind the patient's back.

comfort using a blanket roll or airplane splint and encourage the person to seek medical attention for reduction.

To apply a blanket roll splint to a shoulder, perform the steps of **OEC Skill 20-2**.

In the rare situation in which the patient's arm is unable to be brought down onto the blanket roll, stabilize the injured arm with cravats in the best way possible to avoid movement. The latter is best accomplished in a toboggan or on a litter with the patient in a semi-sitting position.

Humerus Fractures

Fractures involving the humeral shaft often need to be realigned by applying *gentle longitudinal tension* before they can be splinted. Tell the patient to expect some discomfort before applying tension, a splint, and a sling and swathe. If the patient resists your alignment effort, or if any movement to restore normal anatomic alignment is too painful, splint the arm in the position you found it using a rigid splint.

To realign a displaced fractured humerus:

1. Place the patient in a supine or sitting position if possible.
2. Assess CMS.
3. With the flattened palm of one hand, support the humeral shaft along the posterior surface of the humerus, just above the elbow.
4. Grasp the anterior surface of the distal humerus, just above the elbow, with the other hand.
5. Apply gentle longitudinal tension (not traction) down from the shoulder in line with the normal axis of the humerus while the upper arm is held along the side of the patient's body (**Figure 20-69**). The patient's forearm should be placed with the elbow at a 90-degree angle in contact with the patient's abdomen. You are not reducing the fracture but aligning it for better pain control and packaging.
6. Once normal length and improved alignment of the arm are achieved, continue to stabilize the limb by holding it in place with a sling and swathe using a *rigid splint* along the humeral shaft and forearm for stabilization.
7. Reassess CMS.

Follow the steps of **OEC Skill 20-3** to splint a fractured humerus using a rigid splint.

If there are no contraindications, place the patient in a high-Fowler position or lying on the uninjured side during transport.

If spinal motion restriction is needed, keep the patient supine and use the side of the patient's body as a splint. After tension is used on the arm at the side of the patient, place wide cravats around the arm above and below the elbow, tying them around the patient without affecting the alignment of the spine, holding the arm to the body.

Elbow Injuries

In the field, it is difficult to differentiate the types of elbow injuries, especially in children. Due to the abundance of blood vessels and nerves in the area,

OEC SKILL 20-2 Applying a Blanket Roll Splint to a Shoulder

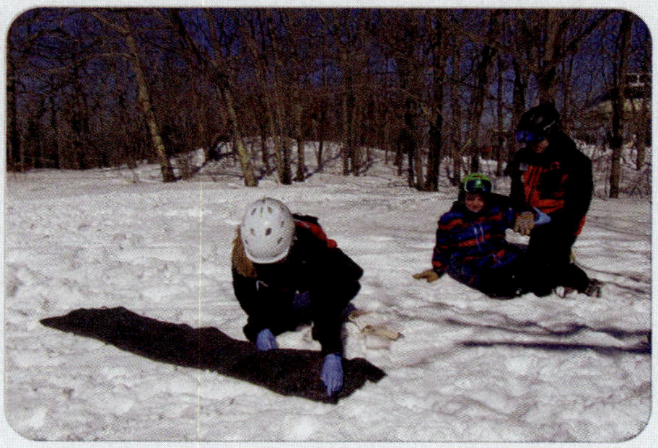

1 Rescuer 1: Place an open blanket on a flat surface. Fold it longitudinally in thirds or fourths lengthwise according to how large a splint you need based on the deformity of the injured shoulder.

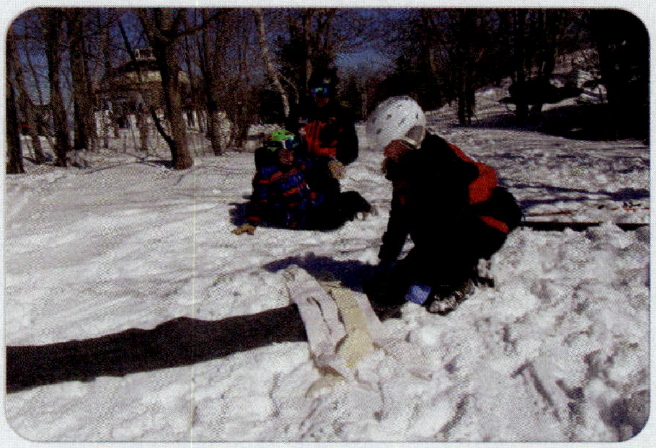

2 Place four cravats crosswise on one end of the folded blanket, then roll it up. For identification purposes later, you may tie knots in the ends of cravats (i.e., one in cravat 1, two in cravat 2, etc.) so that you will be able to identify the corresponding ends of the cravats when you go to tighten and then tie them.

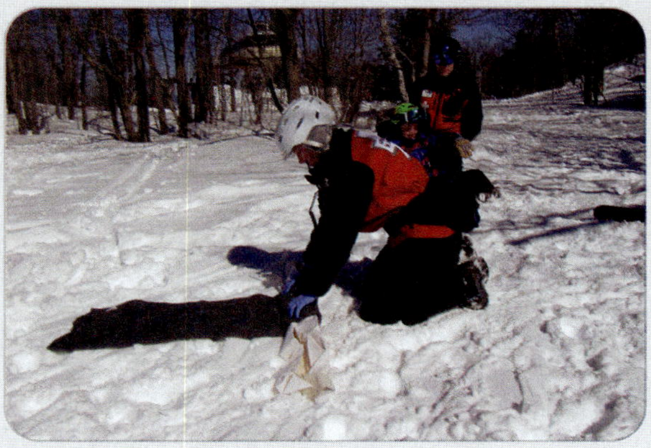

3 Roll the blanket firmly, including the cravats. Check CMS.

(continues)

OEC SKILL 20-2 Applying a Blanket Roll Splint to a Shoulder *(continued)*

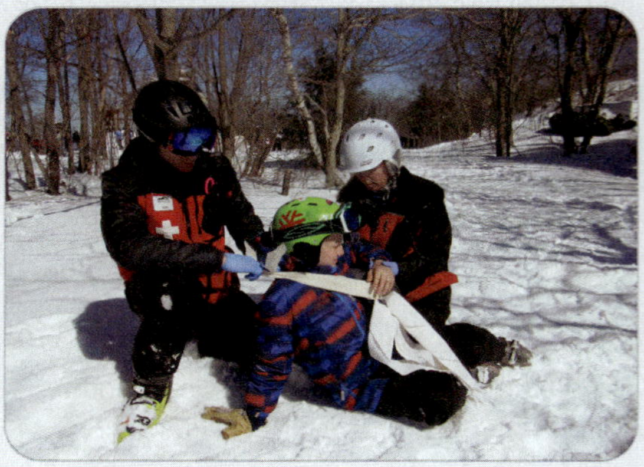

4 Position/place the roll snugly up in the axilla of the dislocated shoulder. Hold the roll in place. Rescuer 2: Tie one of the cravats over the opposite shoulder and around the neck.

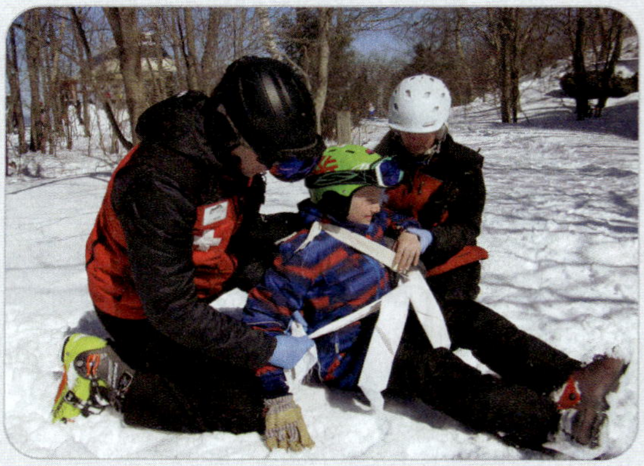

5 Tie the other cravat around the patient's waist.

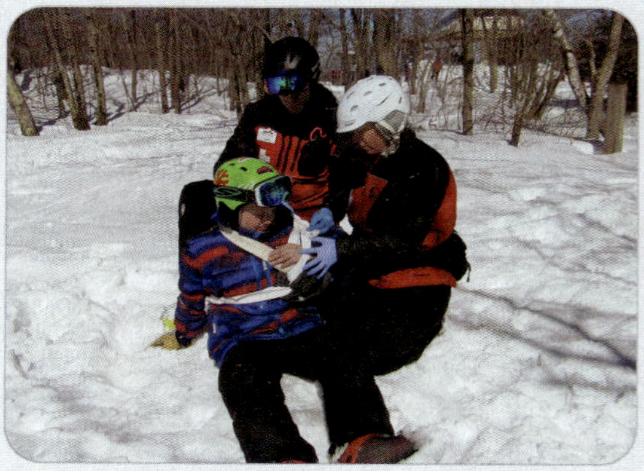

6 Stabilize the hand and forearm on the blanket with the other two cravats. Reassess CMS.

OEC SKILL 20-3 Splinting a Humerus Fracture

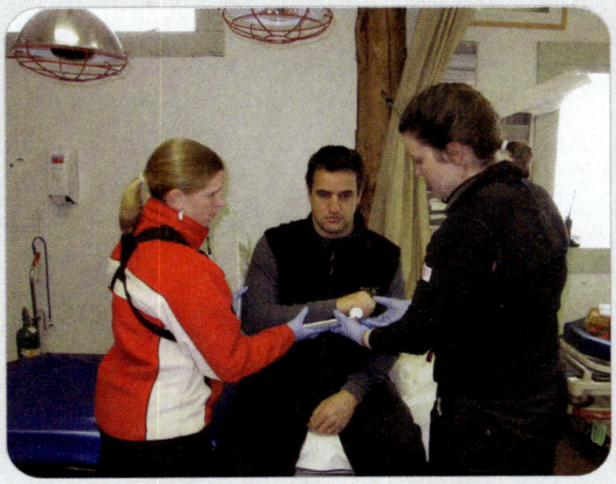

1 Select an appropriate splint (a wire, ladder, or malleable splint). Measure and form the splint using the opposite arm as a guide. The splint should be bent to hold the elbow at approximately a 90-degree angle and should be long enough to continue down the forearm to the distal palm crease, thereby immobilizing the wrist. Assess CMS.

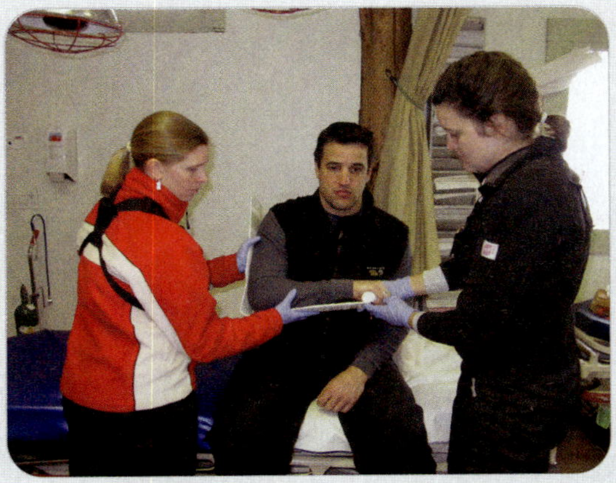

2 Gently place the splint under the arm.

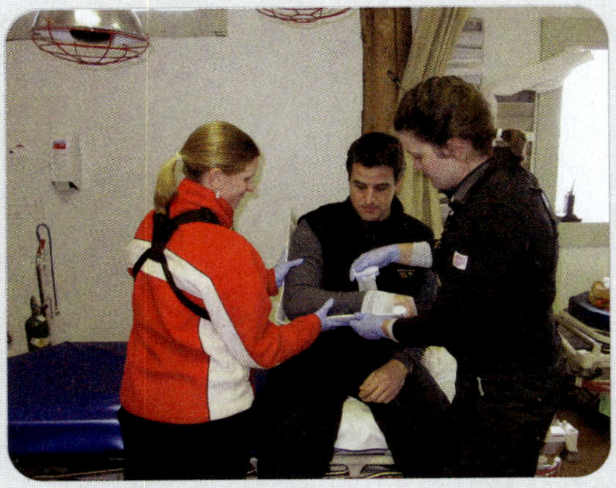

3 Secure the arm to the splint with roller gauze or cravats. The wrap should be "snug" but not tight. Never use elastic material, which can constrict blood flow. Gently place the upper arm against the patient's chest and the forearm on the patient's abdomen, and then apply a sling and a wide swathe, as previously described. Reassess CMS. Another option is to use a sugar tong SAM Splint: Use a sugar tong SAM Splint from the armpit around the elbow and back up the outside of the humerus to the top of the shoulder. Use a sling and swathe with this method. If the patient will not let you bend the elbow, a long rigid splint from the shoulder to the wrist can be applied. The arm is then strapped to the body.

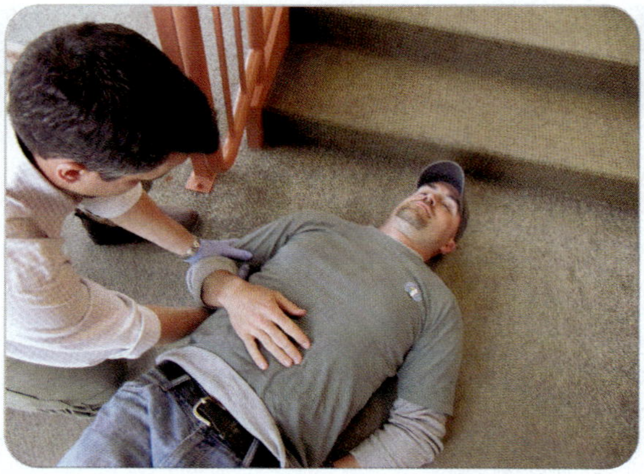

Figure 20-69 To align the humerus, place the patient in a supine position and apply gentle longitudinal tension.

KEY POINT

How to Tie a Square Knot?

A square knot is a very useful knot for securing a cravat. To tie a square knot, follow these instructions (**Figure 20-70**):

1. Cross end A over end B to form an "X."
2. Wrap end A around end B.
3. Cross end A over end B.
4. Wrap end A around end B and pull on both ends to tighten.

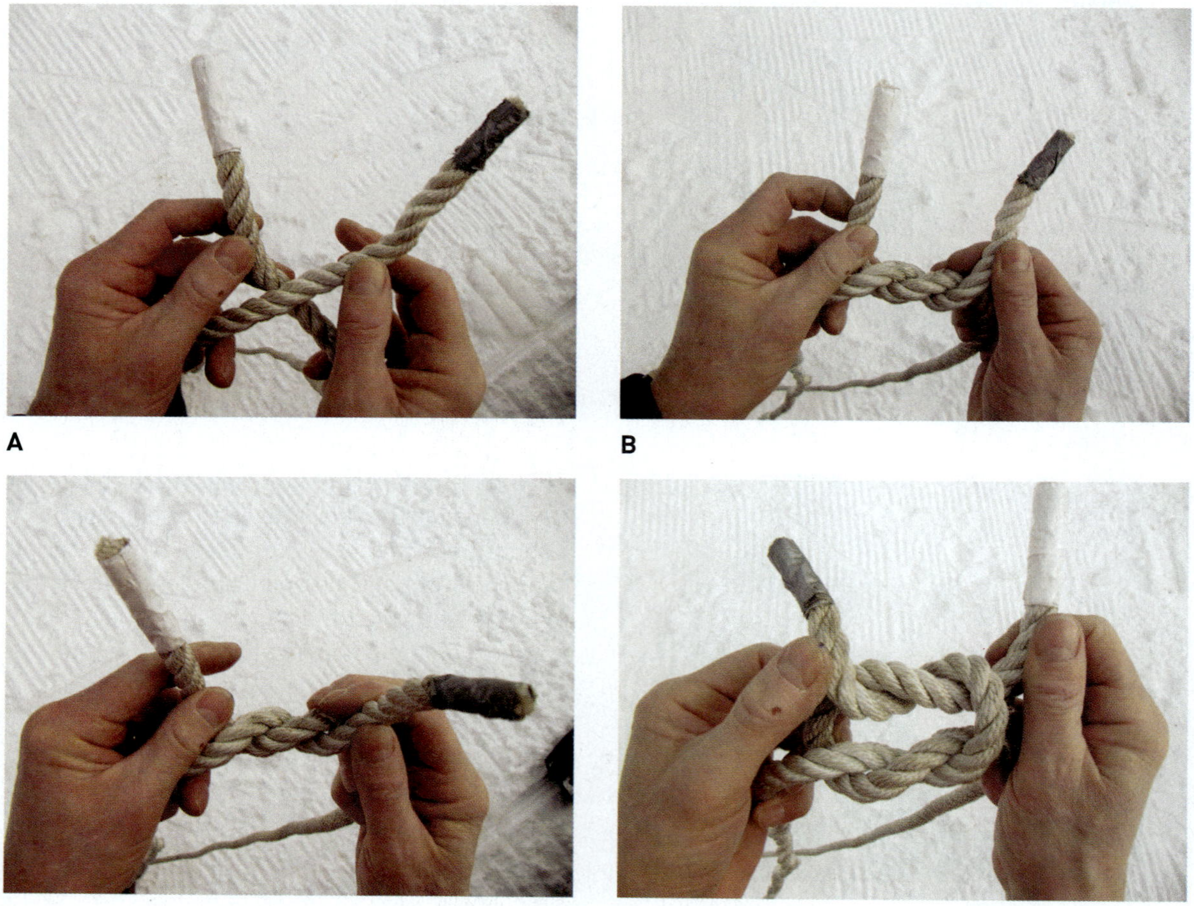

Figure 20-70 Tying a square knot. **A.** Cross end A (gray tip) over end B (white tip) to form an "X." **B.** Wrap end A around end B. **C.** Cross end A over end B. **D.** Wrap end A around end B and pull on both ends to tighten.

OEC SKILL 20-4 Alternate Method of Applying a Rigid Splint to an Injured Elbow

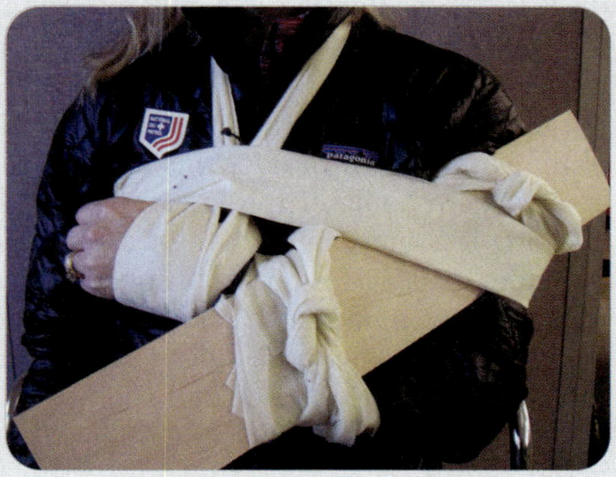

1. Rescuer 1: Stabilize the injured arm.
2. Rescuer 2:
   - Assess CMS.
   - Apply wooden splints to the medial and lateral aspects of the arm, extending past the wrist and past the upper third of the humerus.
   - Secure splints in place using three roller bandages or cravats:
   - Cravat 1 is applied around the splints and the upper arm.
   - Cravat 2 is applied around the splints and the forearm.
   - Cravat 3 is applied around both splints (but not the arm) in the hollow of the elbow.
   - Apply a sling and swathe.
   - Reassess CMS.

it is best to splint elbow injuries in the position found, apply a sling and swathe, and rapidly transport the patient to definitive care. The sling may be applied with the elbow at an angle greater than 90 degrees. Most elbow injuries are found in a bent position.

To immobilize an elbow injury, follow these steps:

1. Rescuer 1: Stabilize the injury above and below the elbow. Do not allow the elbow to bend more.
2. Rescuer 2:
   - Check CMS.
   - Select the appropriate splint (e.g., SAM Splint, wire splint).
   - Fold or bend the splint into the correct configuration to match the elbow's position and leave a pocket for the elbow.
   - Place the splint along the posterior aspect of the arm from the axilla to the hand (past the wrist).
   - Secure the splint to the arm with cravats or a rolled bandage, without putting pressure on the elbow. Do not use an elastic bandage.
   - Place the entire arm against the chest and abdomen.
   - Apply a sling and swathe.
   - Reassess CMS.

For an alternate technique to immobilize an elbow, follow the steps of **OEC Skill 20-4**.

If distal CMS is worsened by applying the splint or a sling and swathe, loosen them and reapply them with less pressure, or extend the elbow slightly. If CMS is still compromised, do not try to readjust again; instead rapidly transport the patient.

Splinting the arm of a patient who presents holding the injured elbow straight is a relatively easy task (**Figures 20-71**). Simply apply a malleable or other rigid splint from the axilla to the hand, along the entire length of the posterior arm, and secure the arm to the splint with roller gauze. Do not place pressure over the zone of injury. Then, splint the arm to the side of the body for transport with the patient supine on a litter or in a toboggan.

If during your assessment of a deformed elbow injury you determine the limb distal to the injury has a CMS deficit, it may be appropriate to gently attempt alignment to improve blood supply or

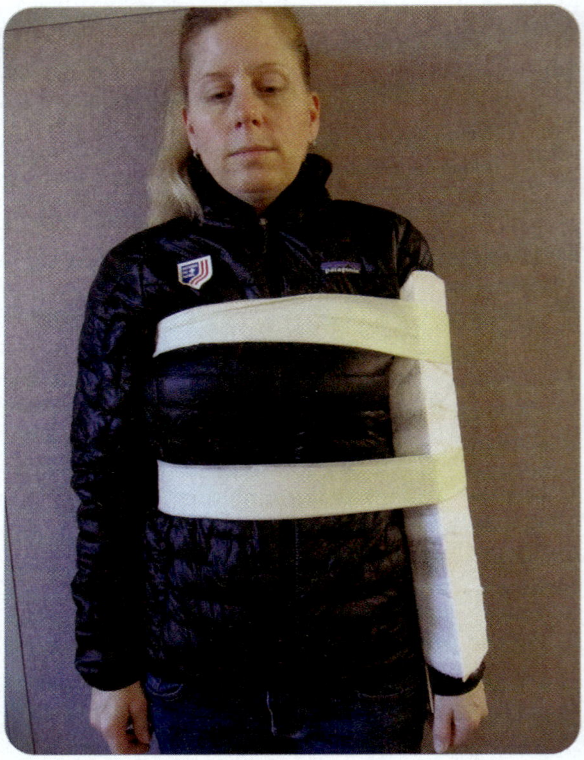

Figure 20-71 Application of a splint for a straight arm.

neurologic function to the distal arm by restoring normal anatomic appearance of the elbow. Always follow local protocol, preferably under medical direction, and do not attempt alignment if final definitive care by a physician is less than 2 hours away. The most common position of the elbow that restores CMS is extended just past 90 degrees. Have a finger where the radial pulse is located during gentle elbow extension, and when it returns, splint the arm in this position.

OEC technicians must be gentle and careful throughout this procedure because rough handling or excessive manipulation of the elbow joint may worsen neurologic or vascular compromise. If the pulse is restored after a single realignment attempt, splint the limb in the position where the distal pulse was restored. If no pulse returns after a single attempt, splint the arm in the position most comfortable to the patient. If possible, place the arm in a modified sling and swathe. Rapidly transport. If the elbow is straightened too much for a sling, secure the arm to the body with swathes.

Forearm Injuries

For fractures of the shafts of the radius and ulna, immobilize the elbow and the wrist. When the forearm is severely deformed (especially when there is CMS compromise), gently realign the arm if the patient will allow it; if not, splint the arm in the position found.

A sugar tong splint or long arm splint is one of the best ways to care for this fracture because it prevents *rotation* of the forearm at the elbow, allowing less movement at the fracture site and therefore causing less pain. A sugar tong splint is made using a malleable splint wrapped around a joint and covering both sides of the extremity, thereby preventing rotation of the joint.

To splint a forearm fracture, follow the steps of **OEC Skill 20-5**.

Alternatively, to immobilize a forearm fracture, use a *long* arm splint such as a ladder splint that starts at the axilla and proceeds posterior along the arm down to the palm crease along the arm. This method will also prevent rotation at the elbow.

Wrist Injuries

Generally, patients are most comfortable when an injured wrist and hand are placed in the "position of function" (**Figure 20-72**). If the patient resists this position, splint the injury in the most comfortable position.

Fractures of the distal radius and/or ulna can be managed by placing a SAM, cardboard, or wooden splint on the palm side of the forearm and securing it with a roller bandage or cravat. Alternatively, use a sugar tong splint or place splints on both the dorsum and palm side of the forearm and secure these in place with an appropriate bandage. Place padding in the palm to help immobilize the hand. A palm-side splint should extend beyond where the fingers attach to the hand and above the elbow. Leave the fingertips exposed to facilitate assessment of distal CMS.

Other injuries to the wrist (including carpal bone injuries) are treated the same way as a distal radius fracture: Place the hand in a position of function, splint the injury, and apply a sling and swathe. Encourage the patient to seek prompt follow-up care by a physician.

OEC SKILL 20-5 Splinting a Forearm or Wrist Injury

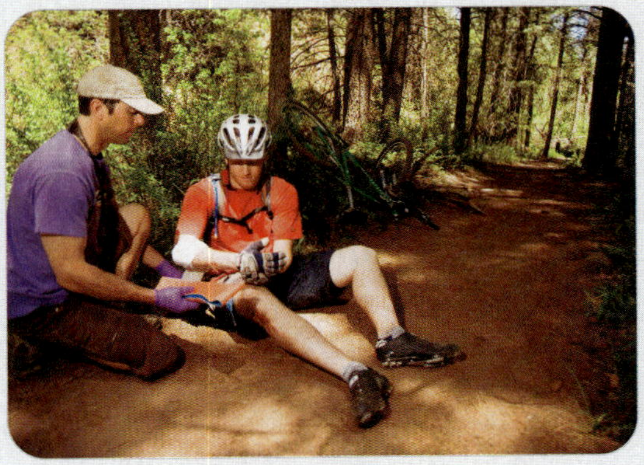

1 Rescuer 1: Stabilize the injury. Rescuer 2: Assess CMS. Select the appropriate splint (malleable, wire, or ladder splint). Form the splint into the shape of a sugar tong. Place a piece of padding into the palm of the hand so that it is in the "position of function." Gently move the splint into position. Apply the splint from where the fingers attach to the palm, then along the volar (palm-side) forearm, around the elbow so that rotation of the forearm is limited, and then on the dorsum of the forearm back to where the fingers attach to the back of the hand.

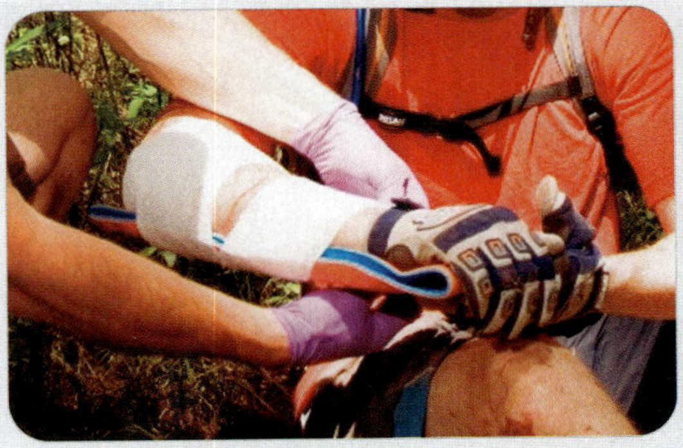

2 Secure the forearm to the splint using roller gauze or cravats.

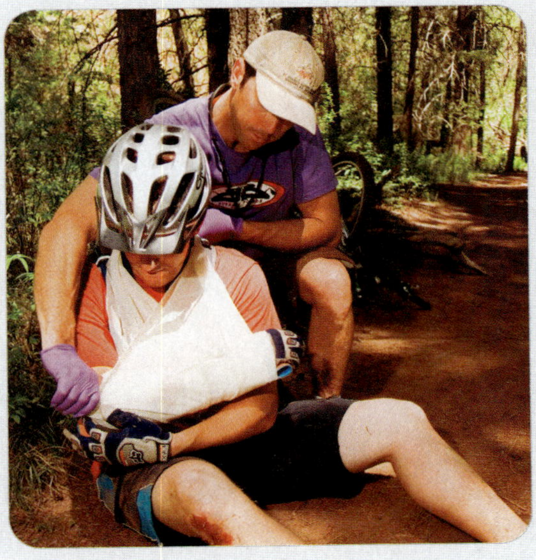

3 Apply a sling and swathe. Reassess CMS.

Hand and Finger Injuries

Splint a suspected fracture involving a metacarpal in a manner like that used for a wrist injury. Whenever possible, keep the hand in a position of function. For a fracture of the thumb or of the first metacarpal at the base of the thumb, immobilize the thumb and wrist as a unit. For suspected skier's thumb, splint the entire thumb (from tip to base) with a tongue blade, or use a small splint on the back of the thumb. Gently secure the thumb to the side of the hand with roller gauze to prevent the thumb from moving.

Splint other finger fractures using a tongue blade (or other small, stiff object) and tape (**Figure 20-73A**). An alternative is to tape the two fingers together with gauze between them (**Figure 20-73B**). Do not attempt to reduce dislocated fingers; instead, use a small splint to immobilize dislocated fingers in the position found

KEY POINT

Position of Function

The position of function, in which the wrist is slightly dorsiflexed (positioned upward) with the fingers slightly curled down, can be achieved by placing a soft roller bandage in the patient's palm (**Figure 20-74**). It can be used in conjunction with any method of splinting of the forearm or wrist for patient comfort. This is a good position to use when applying a splint.

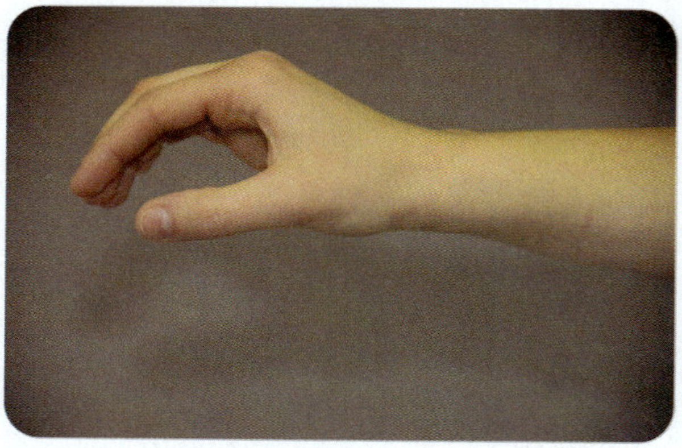

Figure 20-72 Hand in position of function.

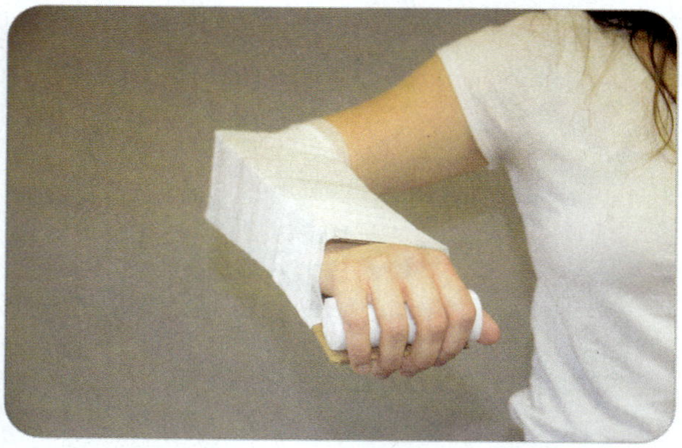

Figure 20-74 Forearm splinted with hand in position of function/comfort.

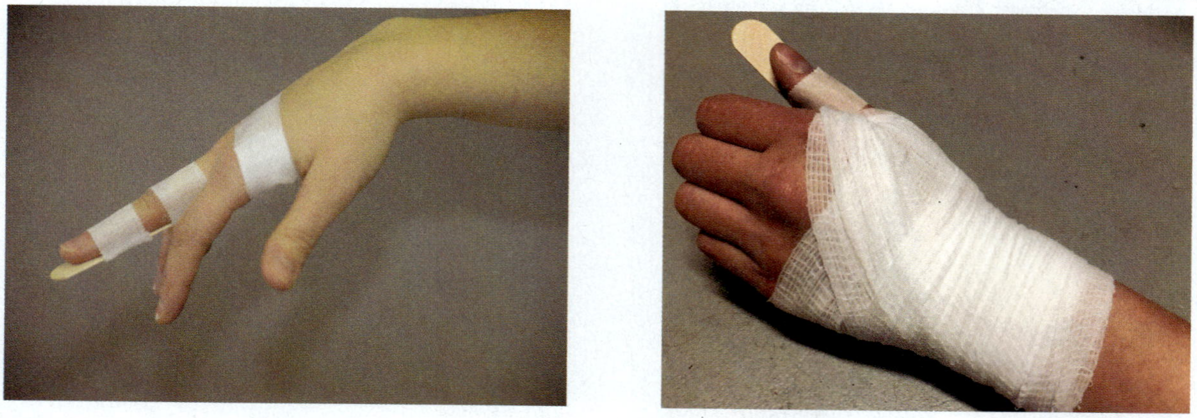

A

B

Figure 20-73 **A.** Use of a tongue depressor as a splint. **B.** Splint an injured finger to an adjacent finger.

OEC SKILL 20-6 Splinting to Immobilize the Hand

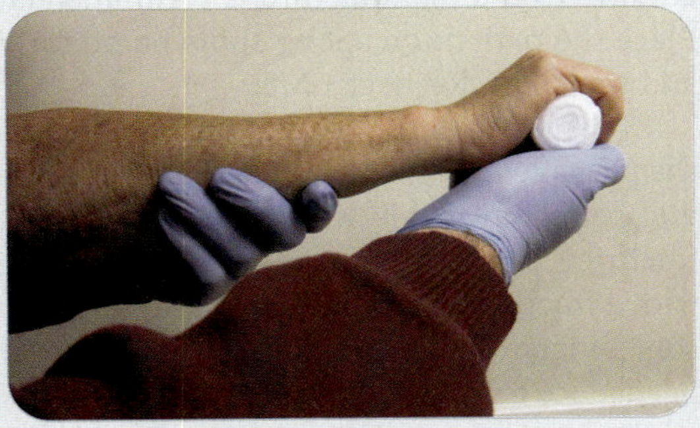

1 Rescuer 1 stabilizes the bones above and below the injury. At the same time, Rescuer 2 does the following:
- Assess CMS.
- Select an appropriate splint.
- Size the splint.
- Gently place the hand and fingers in a position of function.
- Place an unrolled roller gauze in the palm of the hand to maintain the position of function.

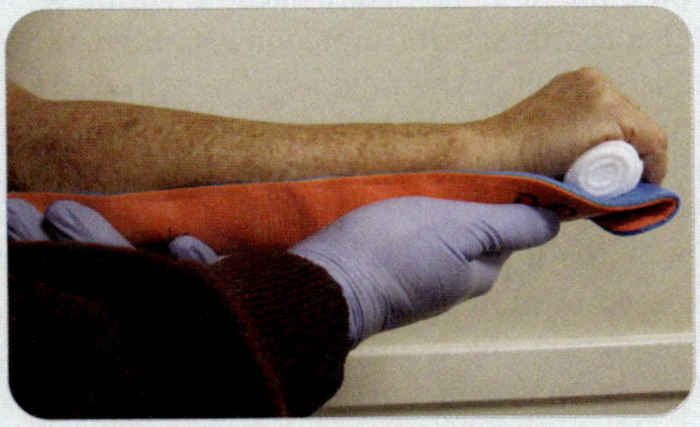

2 Place the palm side of the forearm, wrist, and hand on a cardboard, wooden, or SAM splint (the wrist should be slightly dorsiflexed).

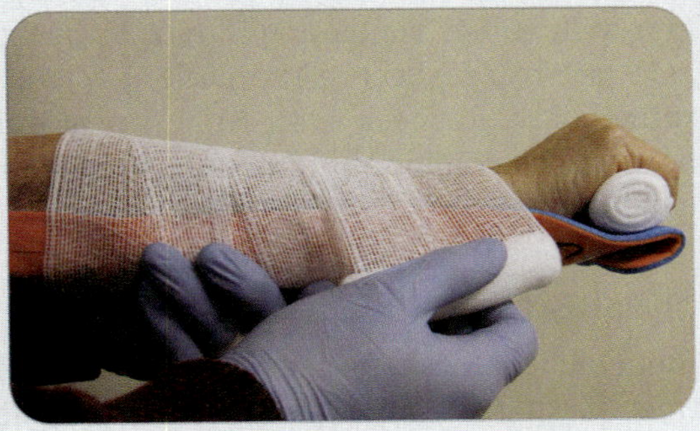

3 Secure the wrist and hand to the splint using soft roller gauze or cravats. Do not use elastic wrap. Leave the fingertips exposed. Apply a sling and swathe.

and recommend prompt follow-up care with a physician. Impaled objects that penetrate the hand or fingers should be stabilized in place. Amputated fingers should be managed as described in Chapter 19, *Soft-Tissue Injuries and Burns*, and transported with the patient. These patients should also seek prompt follow-up care.

To immobilize the hand using a forearm/hand splint, perform the steps of **OEC Skill 20-6**.

MANAGEMENT OF LOWER EXTREMITY INJURIES

Pelvis Fractures

It is best not to logroll a patient with a suspected pelvic fracture. Additional internal bleeding can occur when logrolling. It is more appropriate to use a bridge lift or another technique not involving rolling the patient when placing the patient on the transport device. Splint pelvic fractures using a pelvic binder, a sheet splint, or a SAM pelvic splint. The patient should then be immobilized using a long spine board or full-body vacuum splint. Because of potential significant blood loss, high-flow oxygen is needed in the field and later titrated to an oxygen saturation of greater than or equal to 94%. Due to the highly vascular nature of the pelvis and the potential for life-threatening bleeding, all patients with pelvic injuries should be transported to a hospital for evaluation by a physician. Pelvic binding is the treatment of choice for this injury. Be highly suspicious of possible spinal injuries and use spinal motion restriction when appropriate. Because this is usually a very painful distracting injury, spinal motion restriction with a collar is recommended.

Hip Fractures

Immobilize hip injuries, including fractures involving the proximal third of the femur, using a long spine board, a full-body vacuum splint, a double-pole splint (Hare), or a single-pole splint approved for hip fractures (Sager). Because of potential significant blood loss, high-flow oxygen is needed. The most commonly used method for immobilizing and transporting a patient with a hip fracture involves placing the patient gently on a long spine board, padding voids (especially the one under the knee), and strapping the patient to the board. Alternatively, place a full-body vacuum splint under the patient, wrap it around the torso, pelvis, and legs, and remove the air to form a rigid structure.

A single- or double-pole femur splint approved for hip immobilization may be used for a hip fracture, applying approximately 7 to 10 pounds of longitudinal *tension*, which is less than is used for a midshaft femur fracture. Have helpers stabilize the affected leg and apply the device according to the manufacturer's recommendations. Place the patient on a long spine board for lifting and transport. Recheck CMS.

Try to logroll the patient onto the board with the possible fractured hip side up. Try to have several people available when logrolling so that the fracture site is not moved. Rolling a prone patient with a fractured hip can be very difficult and takes some ingenuity. Transport with EMS is always needed for a possible hip fracture.

Full spinal motion restriction for an isolated hip fracture is not needed unless it is a distracting injury. However, if there are spinal findings that support spinal motion restriction, then this is necessary.

> **KEY POINT**
>
> **Injury to an Artificial Joint**
>
> If you encounter a patient with an injury to a limb that has an artificial knee, shoulder, or hip joint, care for the injury the same way you would for a limb that has a natural joint.

Hip Dislocations

Care for a dislocated hip focuses on stabilizing the affected leg and gently lifting or rolling and transferring the patient to a long spine board. Do not try to reduce the hip; most patients will not let you move it. Splint the hip in the position found by stabilizing the affected hip (and leg) with rolled blankets, pillows, or backpacks as a last resort. Secure the patient to the long spine board. Recheck CMS. Hip dislocations can occur more commonly in people with an artificial hip joint.

Midshaft Femur Fracture

Immobilize midshaft femur fractures with a traction splint, unless the patient has multisystem trauma and is rapidly deteriorating into a load-and-go situation. In that case, place a Quick Splint that has been reversed between the legs and several cravats around both legs, place the patient on a long spine board, and consider rapid transport the top priority (**Figure 20-75**). Because a large amount of blood (1,000–1,500 mL) can bleed into the thigh from a femur fracture, *anticipate shock*, especially if there are other significant injuries. Provide high-flow oxygen and, if possible, titrate to between 94 and 99%. A tourniquet is indicated only for *severe external* bleeding that cannot be controlled by direct pressure and is not indicated for a *closed* femur fracture.

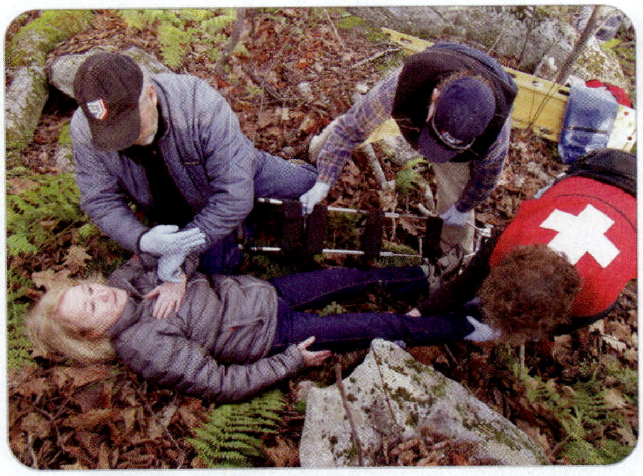

Figure 20-75 Immobilize midshaft femur injuries with a traction splint. If the patient's condition is rapidly deteriorating, forgo the traction splint, use "good leg splinting," and put the patient on a backboard to load and go.

> **KEY POINT**
>
> **Traction Splint Application**
>
> Use the following principles concerning the initial application of all traction splints, regardless of manufacturer: Have all resources available, fully prepare the splint for application, use proper axial alignment, provide continuous traction once traction is applied, avoid unnecessary movement of the injured leg, and secure the patient and splint to a long spine board.

Treat a suspected midshaft femur fracture as soon as is reasonably possible using manual stabilization and the application of in-line traction. In a snow sport setting, several factors should be considered before inline traction is applied:

1. If the ski or snowboard is still attached to the injured leg, leave it in place until "all is ready." A ski or snowboard can be a great "stabilizer" of the fracture site until the appropriate equipment and personnel are on scene.
2. If the ski/snowboard is no longer on the injured leg, leave the leg alone, perform a scene size-up and a primary assessment, and call for equipment/additional help.
3. Because the application of in-line traction can be very tiring, it should be performed for as short a time as is possible. Leave the ski in place, ensure that adequate personnel are present, expose the injury site, and have the traction equipment out, measured, and ready to be applied.
4. Apply the appropriate hitch and then apply manual traction.
5. Apply the splint according to the manufacturer's directions.

Ideally, two or more rescuers should be used to apply a traction splint. Depending on the terrain or slope angle, an additional rescuer or bystander may be needed to stabilize the patient to keep the patient from sliding in the direction that the traction is being pulled. Stabilize a patient by kneeling above the patient's head and grasping beneath both armpits. If a bystander helps you, direct the person's actions.

Among the most popular and effective commercial traction devices available to OEC technicians are the Hare, Slishman, Sager, and Kendrick Traction Device (KTD) splints. Learn the proper use of each device that is available to you.

Follow the steps of **OEC Skill 20-7** to apply a traction splint on a femur.

After the splint is applied, consider placing loosely rolled blankets or pillows between the patient's knees, and if time and the patient permit, splint the affected leg to the nonaffected leg with cravats. Logroll the patient onto the uninjured side or gently lift and secure the patient onto a long spine board. This step immobilizes the hip and helps with lifting the patient from the ground into the toboggan or onto a litter. Do not allow the patient to move to a sitting position because most traction splints will slide up the buttocks, rendering the splint ineffective. Place a folded blanket under the knee of the *uninjured* leg to keep it slightly flexed to relieve the muscle tension on the same side of the body as the broken femur.

OEC SKILL 20-7 Applying a Traction Splint to a Femur

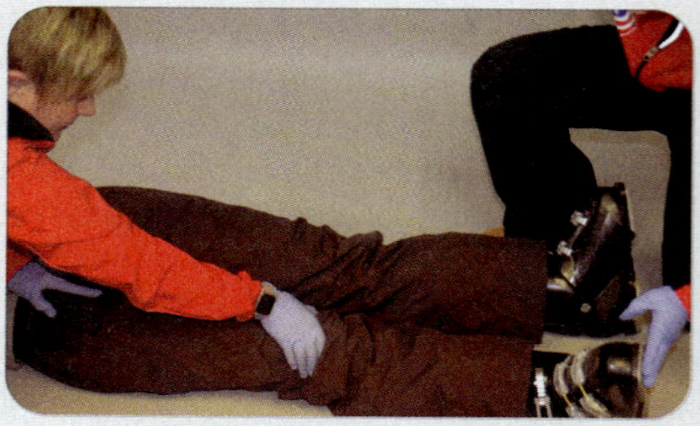

1 Rescuer 1: Use standard precautions. Assess the injury to determine its proximity to the hip or knee joint. Check for bleeding and treat it if present. If bleeding is present, remove overlying clothing by cutting or ripping along a seam. (Many ski pants have zippers that run the length of each leg.) Manually stabilize the fracture site both above and below the injury.

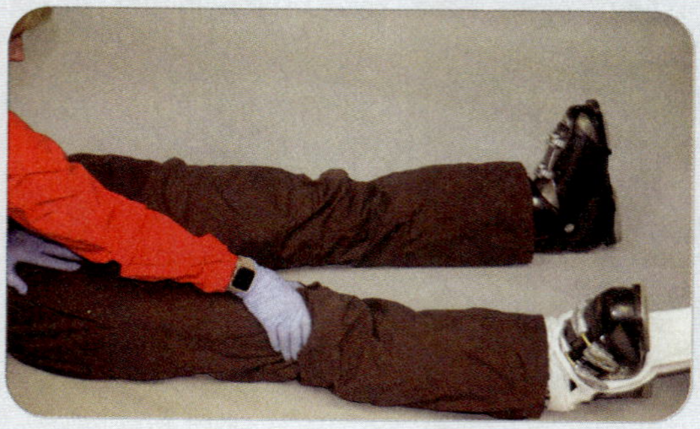

2 Rescuer 2:

- Use standard precautions. Check on distal CMS on the injured leg indirectly (e.g., tap on boot, ask the patient to wiggle the toes); remove the boot only when environmental conditions do not present additional hazards to the patient and your local protocols say you should do this.
- Prepare a traction splint and adjust it to the proper size according to the manufacturer's instructions; use the uninjured leg to measure the splint.
- Remove the ski or snowboard if present and then apply the ankle hitch while Rescuer 1 continues to manually stabilize the fracture site.

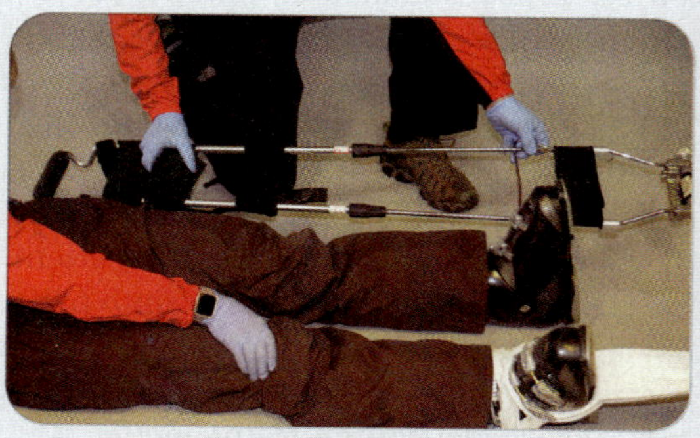

3 Rescuer 2: Firmly grasp the ankle hitch with one hand; place the other hand under the calf and cooperate with Rescuer 1 in using manual traction to straighten the leg into anatomic alignment. Maintain traction while Rescuer 1 releases the manual stabilization of the fracture site.

OEC SKILL 20-7 Applying a Traction Splint to a Femur (*continued*)

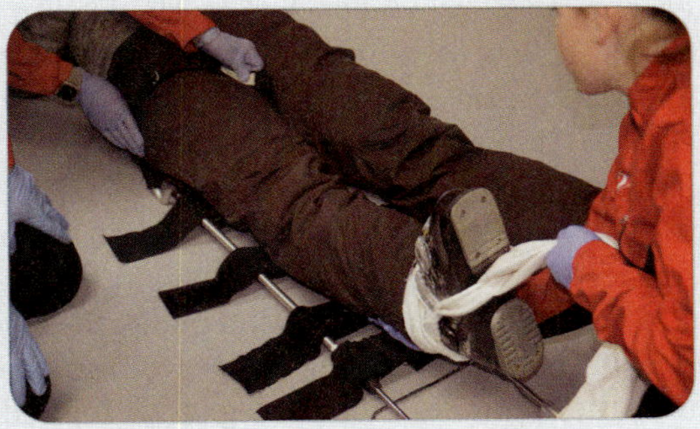

4 Rescuer 1:
- Position the splint snugly against the patient's ischial tuberosity.
- Secure the groin strap around the patient's upper thigh.

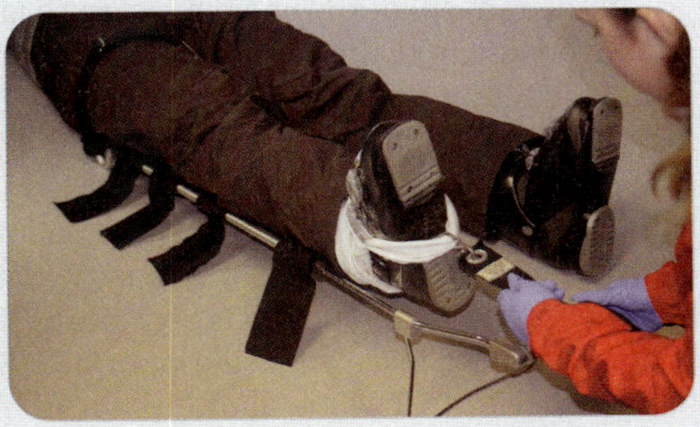

5 Connect the ankle strap of the hitch to the end of the splint and turn the crank/knob gradually to replace the manual traction of the splint with mechanical traction; as the mechanical traction is being applied, Rescuer 2 releases the manual traction. It may take some time for muscle spasms to ease off before the patient feels relief. Rescuers secure Velcro support straps per the manufacturer's instructions. (If needed, cravats can be used in place of Velcro straps.) Ensure that the limb is securely held in the splint. Reassess CMS in the injured leg. Treat for shock by keeping the patient warm and by providing high-flow oxygen.

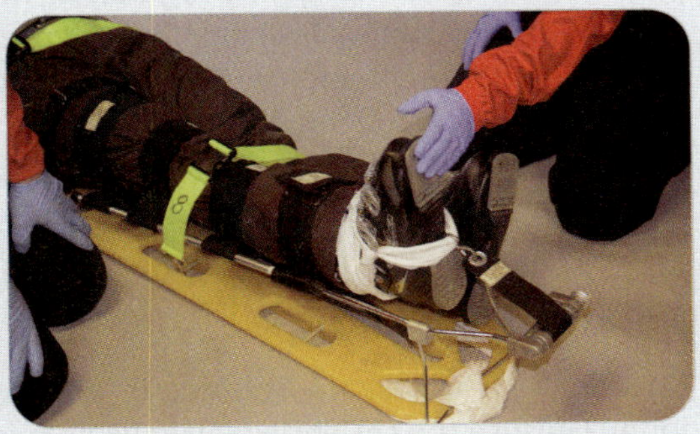

6 Strap the patient to a long spine board.

> **KEY POINT**
>
> **Traction Hitch**
>
> If the need arises, you can always improvise a traction hitch from cravats (**Figure 20-76**).

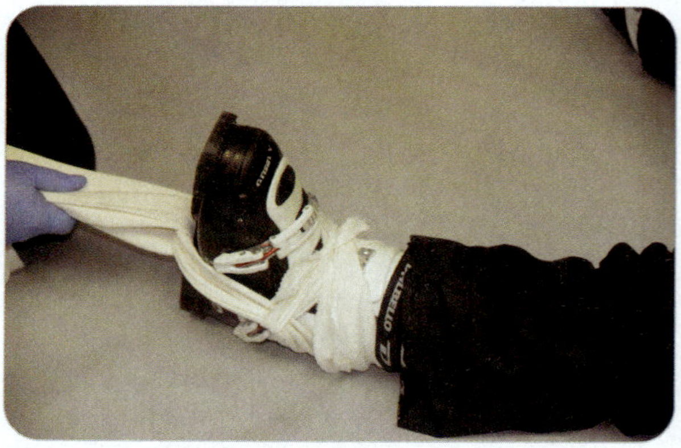

Figure 20-76 The use of a cravat to make an ankle hitch.

It is best to use a traction splint for *any* open or closed fracture of the middle third of the femur. If jagged bone ends sticking out of an open femur fracture cause additional pain as traction is applied, place a sterile bandage over any exposed bone, apply *tension* (not traction), and rapidly transport the patient. If a bone end retracts into the skin, leave it inside the body.

Some controversy exists regarding an open femur fracture and traction splinting. Generally, it is best to place the traction splint on correctly, even though the bone end may go back into the wound. This approach will slow bleeding, help with pain, and protect the bone ends. If the end of the femur sticking out is very dirty, you may wash it with saline or clean water before applying the splint. If the bone goes back in, always tell EMS personnel the bone was sticking out when transfer occurs. The doctor at the hospital should always open the wound over the fracture and clean the bone at the hospital.

A femoral traction splint should remain in place until the patient arrives at the hospital. However, it can be removed when mechanical traction is ineffective because of loosening or incorrect application, or when removing the footwear to assess CMS prior to transport to a hospital. Most EMS providers assess the bare foot for CMS prior to transport. If it becomes necessary to remove or replace the splint, provide and maintain manual stabilization and axial traction below the fracture site until mechanical traction is again established with the splint. If the lower leg is not injured, pull axially with both hands around the calf or ankle. If exposing the foot, it is best to do this in a warm environment.

In the rare situation where a patient has both femurs broken in the midshaft, taking the time to put two traction splints is usually not best. Blood loss from bilateral femur fractures can be life threatening. Immobilize one femur with a traction splint and the other femur with a Quick Splint that is placed as high as possible and then tie the legs together. If the patient exhibits significant shock, you may need to place an inside-out Quick Splint high between the legs, tie both legs together, secure the patient to a long spine board, and rapidly transport.

A traction splint should *not* be used for a distal femur fracture because the splint can force jagged bone ends posteriorly into the popliteal space, damaging the nerves and blood vessels there. The best splint for this injury is a rigid splint such as Quick Splint (sometimes in conjunction with an airplane splint). If the patient exhibits signs of distal CMS impairment and the total transport time to a definitive-care facility is greater than 2 hours, a single attempt to realign the leg (keeping the knee slightly bent) is appropriate.

Knee Injuries

Knee injuries are usually splinted in the position found because the patient will usually not want to straighten the knee. If the patient will straighten the knee out some, allow the patient to do so, as this makes immobilization easier. Splint the knee using either a Quick Splint (with or without a properly angled airplane splint or rolled blanket

CASE Update

You are concerned the teen has a dislocated knee. Since you are on the slope and it is cold, when help arrives, you splint the leg as it lies using a Quick Splint. A sling and swathe is placed on the injured shoulder. There is no other injury apparent, including no evidence of spinal injury by your evaluation. After immobilizing the shoulder and leg, you use a backboard as a litter and place him head downhill in the sled. Upon reaching the aid room, a paramedic has arrived. You explain to the paramedic what is wrong with the patient.

What should you do next?

KEY POINT

Gross Deformity of a Knee

If a distal pulse is present, do not attempt to align any major knee injury with gross deformity. Instead, splint the leg as found.

under the knee), two rigid board splints placed on each side of the knee with cravats, or a wire/ladder splint. If severe angulation is present, OEC technicians may need to use various types of padding and straps or cravats to immobilize the leg on a long spine board. Angulated knee injuries may also be immobilized using a vacuum splint or blanket roll.

Splint patella dislocations in the position found. Some patients may straighten out the knee themselves, reducing the dislocation. For a patella dislocation, even if the patella spontaneously reduces itself, splint the extremity and encourage the patient to go to the hospital for follow-up care. Inform receiving emergency personnel that the patella reduced spontaneously. Always apply intermittent cold packs to this injury because significant pain can occur.

A dislocated knee that has a distal pulse should also be splinted in the position in which it was found, because moving the joint could cause sudden distal neurovascular compromise (most notably, interruption of the blood supply to the foot). If there is no distal pulse and gross deformity, you may perform *one* attempt to axially align the knee joint with the help of other OEC technicians. If toboggan transport time to an aid room is short, spend a brief time splinting the leg outdoors and then attempt alignment indoors with two OEC technicians. One individual should apply manual stabilization above the knee and the second individual moves the limb slowly with gentle traction, extending the knee. Reassess the pulse on a bare foot as you move the leg. Stop as soon as you palpate a pulse in the foot and splint the leg in that position (usually straight in the frontal plane, with slight knee flexion). If the foot remains pulseless after alignment, splint the extremity and transport. All dislocated knees, even if they spontaneously reduce and have normal neurovascular findings, require immediate evaluation at a hospital because the popliteal artery can occlude several hours after the initial injury. Air transport may be appropriate for this injury in cases that involve prolonged land transport.

To apply an airplane splint, follow the steps of **OEC Skill 20-8**.

When splinting a bent knee, put the airplane splint behind the knee, attach it to the leg with cravats, and place both in a Quick Splint. This technique allows the knee to be placed in the Quick Splint without straightening it. Another way of dealing with this scenario other than using a Quick Splint, is to tie the two legs together after applying the airplane splint.

OEC SKILL 20-8 Applying an Airplane Splint

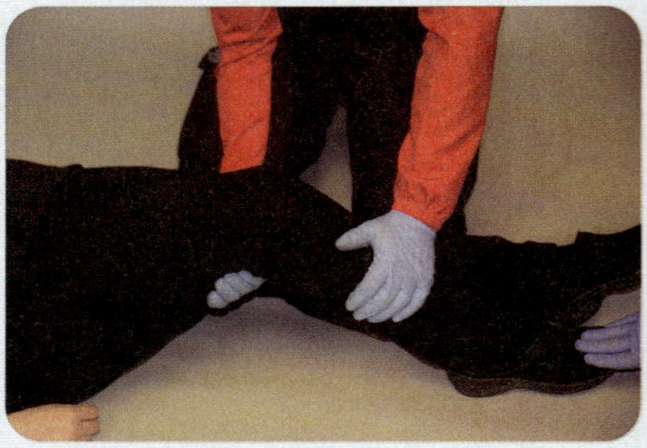

1 Rescuer 1: Manually stabilize the extremity. Rescuer 2: Check CMS.

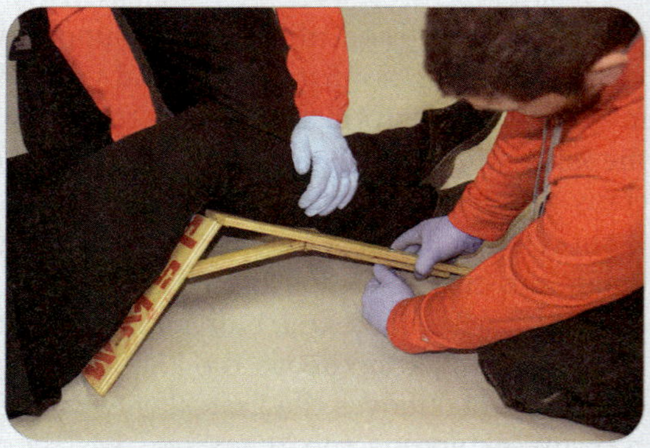

2
- Adjust the splint to the approximate correct angle.
- Turn the knob to lock the splint at the appropriate angle.
- Apply the splint to the extremity, and readjust the angle, if necessary.

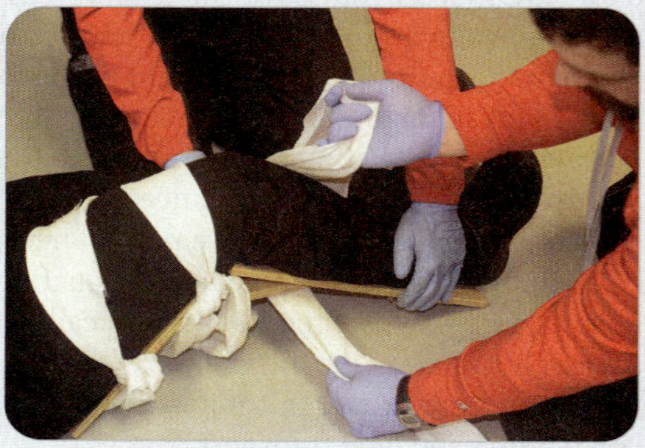

3 Rescuer 1: Hold the splint and leg in place. 4 Rescuer 2: Use cravats to attach the splint to the extremity—two above and two below the knee (not over the zone of injury).

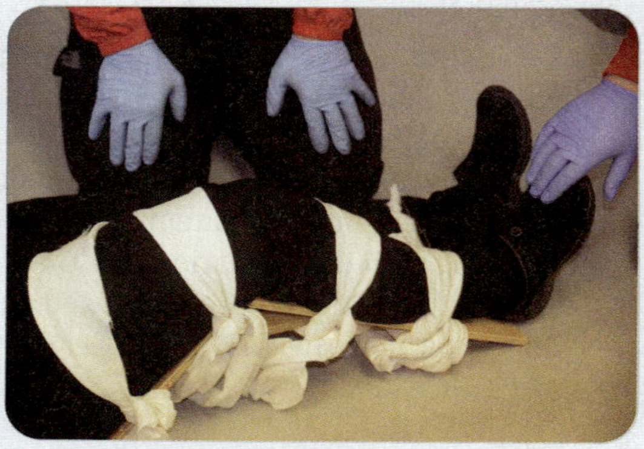

4 Reassess CMS after securing splint to leg.

OEC SKILL 20-8 Applying an Airplane Splint (continued)

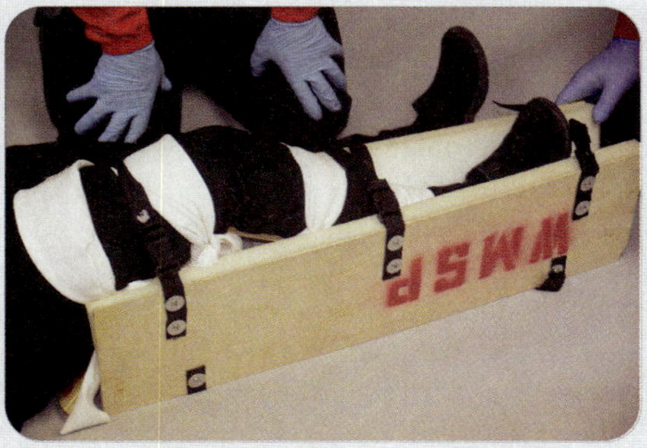

© Chris Pringle.

5 Secure the leg and airplane splint by applying a quick splint and reassess CMS.

To apply a Quick Splint on a knee, follow the steps of **OEC Skill 20-9**.

A Quick Splint that has been applied at the accident scene is often replaced by a disposable cardboard splint before sending the patient to the hospital. However, OEC technicians must use caution when considering the removal of a Quick Splint when there are serious multiple injuries, a very unstable fracture, a bandaged open fracture, or a fracture that is accompanied by advancing hypovolemic shock. In such cases, rapid transport takes precedence.

To perform the procedure for replacing a Quick Splint with a cardboard splint, follow the steps of **OEC Skill 20-10**.

Many knee injuries ultimately require surgical repair and rehabilitation. For this reason, any patient with a suspected knee injury should be advised to seek further medical care by a physician or orthopedist.

Tibia and Fibula Injuries

All suspected tib-fib fractures should be immobilized to prevent further injury. Expose the zone of injury if above the boot, control bleeding (if necessary), and cover the skin to prevent cold injury (if applicable). Cover open wounds with a sterile dressing to prevent contamination. Generally, the boot is left on until the patient is moved inside (see the discussion of boot removal in a later section). CMS can be assessed by tapping on the boot and asking patients if they can feel you tapping and then having them move their toes. Once the patient is inside, the boot can be removed using the technique described later in the chapter. The pulses, skin color, sensation, and movement of the foot and toes can be assessed inside, if not already done.

If the leg is angulated, it may need to be realigned before placement into a splint. As described previously, this procedure is best done with two rescuers. The principles of realigning a tib-fib fracture are like those used to realign a humerus fracture. If the patient will not allow you to move the injured leg, splint the angulated extremity in the position found. Often, this will require patience and ingenuity using blankets or pillows or using other methods.

Tib-fib fractures are best managed using a long ladder splint, two rigid splints, a vacuum splint, or a Quick Splint, which is the most widely used device for this type of fracture.

To immobilize a tib-fib fracture with two rigid splints, follow the steps of **OEC Skill 20-11**.

If a Quick Splint or other commonly used splint is not available, as a last resort a Hare or other double-pole traction splint may be used to cradle the fractured tibia. Support the fractures with Velcro straps and apply *tension* to the bones using the ankle hitch. Do not place straps over the zone of injury. This procedure is not appropriate for an ankle injury.

OEC SKILL 20-9 Applying a Quick Splint

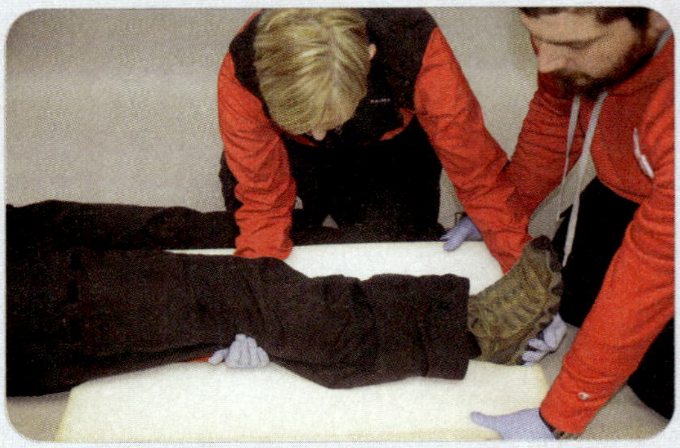

1 Rescuer 1: Open the splint flat, either parallel to the patient's injured extremity or in line with/ distal to the foot.

Rescuer 2: Take a position opposite Rescuer 1 if the splint is at the side of the patient's leg, or on either side of the leg if the splint is distal to the foot.

- Grasp the patient's foot with one hand, and place the other hand just below the knee or under the lower thigh to support the extremity. (The "pant leg pinch lift" is another useful method for lifting and supporting the injured extremity into a Quick Splint.)
- On the count of three, lift the extremity. Rescuer 1: Slide the splint underneath the leg from the bottom to the top or from the side. Rescuer 2: Gently lower the extremity into the center of the splint.

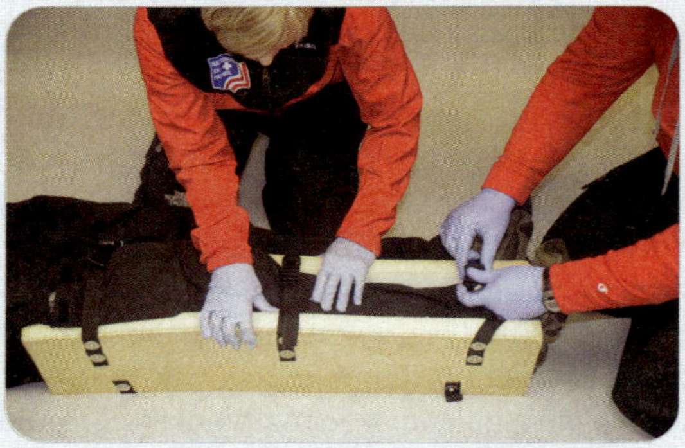

2 Rescuer 1: Close the sides of the Quick Splint like a clamshell, thereby holding the leg snuggly with the splint. Rescuer 2: Firmly secure the splint straps, rope, or webbing.

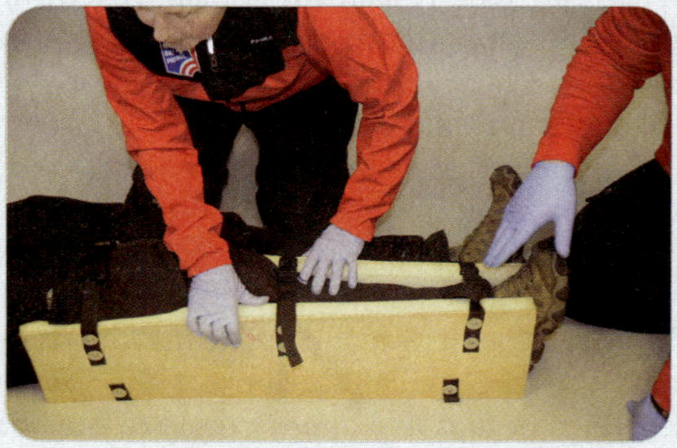

3 Reassess CMS.

OEC SKILL 20-10 Replacing a Quick Splint with a Rigid Splint

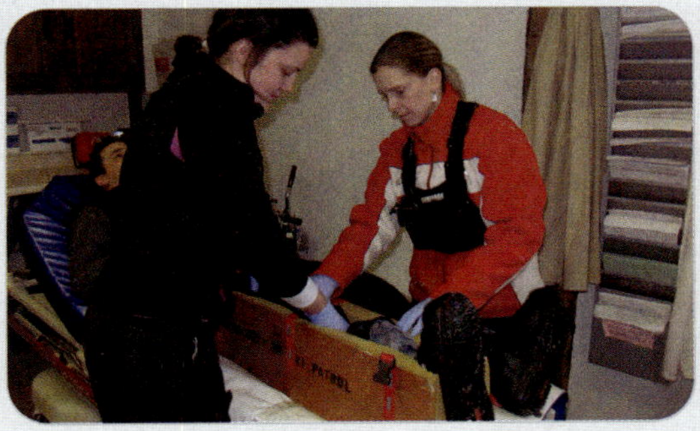

1 First manually stabilize the injury site.

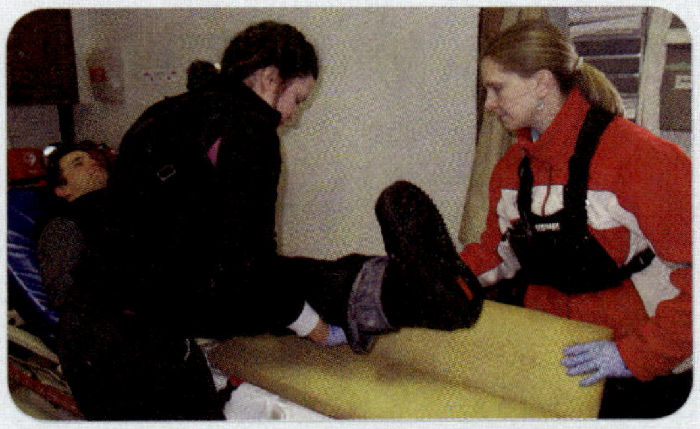

2 Detach and remove the Quick Splint.

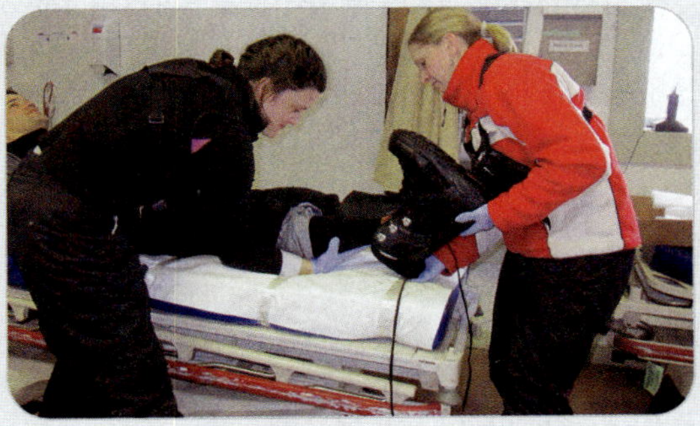

3 Remove the patient's boot in your emergency facility if appropriate and required by local protocol.

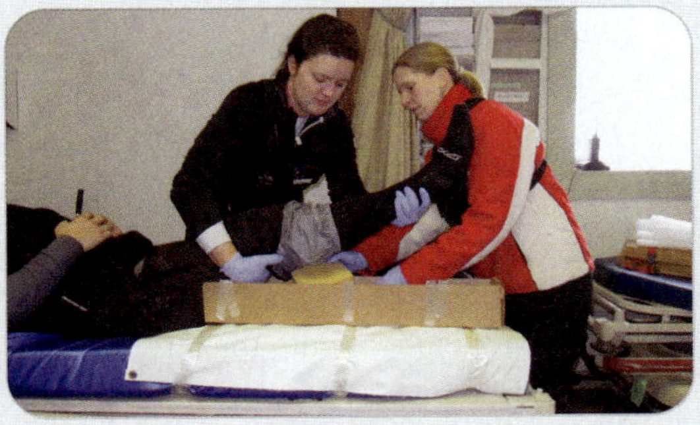

4 Carefully support and lift the injured extremity and then slide a preformed cardboard splint into position under the leg, in the same manner as you did when applying the Quick Splint.

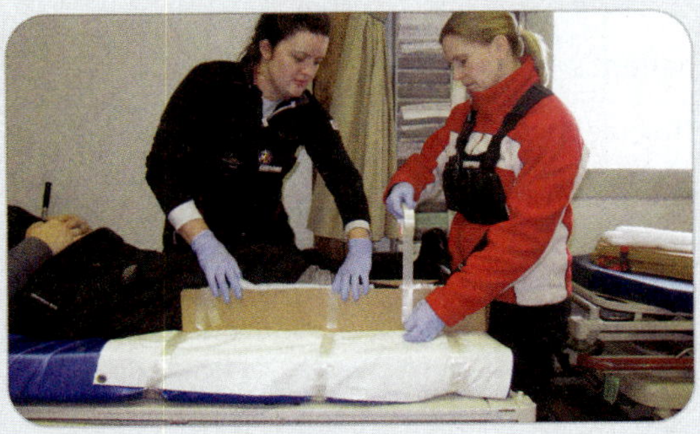

5 Lower the leg into the splint and pad all voids between the extremity and the cardboard. Pad under the knee to keep it slightly flexed. Tape the top of the pre-bent sides to hold the leg in place. Check CMS. Cardboard splints *do not replace traction splints* either at the scene or in the aid room.

OEC SKILL 20-11 Immobilizing a Tib-Fib Fracture with Two Rigid Splints

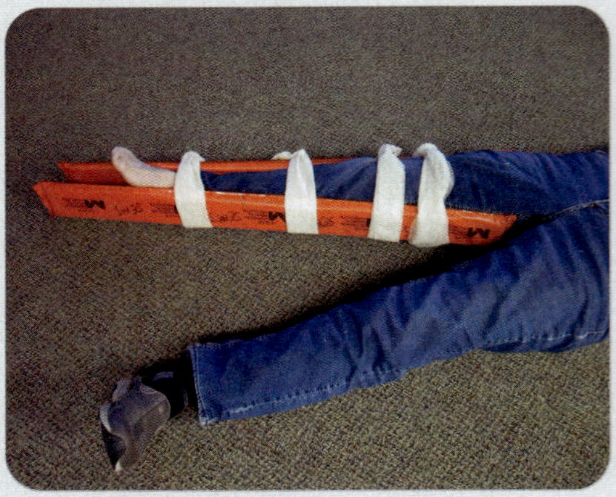

1. Rescuer 1: Stabilize the bones above and below the injury.

2. Rescuer 2:
   - Place one long padded splint on the *medial* aspect of the patient's leg such that it is above the knee and below the ankle.
   - Place a second, long padded splint on the *lateral* aspect of the patient's leg in the same relationship to the knee and the ankle.
   - Thread a cravat near the top of the splints and tie the two splints together. (Roller gauze may be used if cravats are not available.)
   - Thread a second cravat just above the knee (above the injury) and tie the two splints together.

3. Both rescuers:
   - Thread a third cravat below the injury and tie the two splints together.
   - Reassess CMS
   - Help the patient onto the stretcher or toboggan; use a long spine board as a lifting device, if needed.

Alternatively, perform the following steps to splint a tib-fib fracture using a vacuum splint (this procedure is best accomplished with two rescuers):

1. Rescuer 1: Stabilize the bones above and below the injury.
2. Rescuer 2:
   - Prepare the vacuum splint according to the manufacturer's instructions.
   - Place the splint next to the patient's leg.
3. Rescuer 1: Gently lift the patient's leg.
4. Rescuer 2: Slide the vacuum splint under the patient's lower leg.
5. Rescuer 1: Gently lower the patient's leg onto the vacuum splint.
6. Rescuer 2: Remove air from the splint following the manufacturer's instructions.
7. Reassess CMS.
8. Both rescuers: Gently lift and place the patient on a long spine board. Secure the patient's leg to the board.

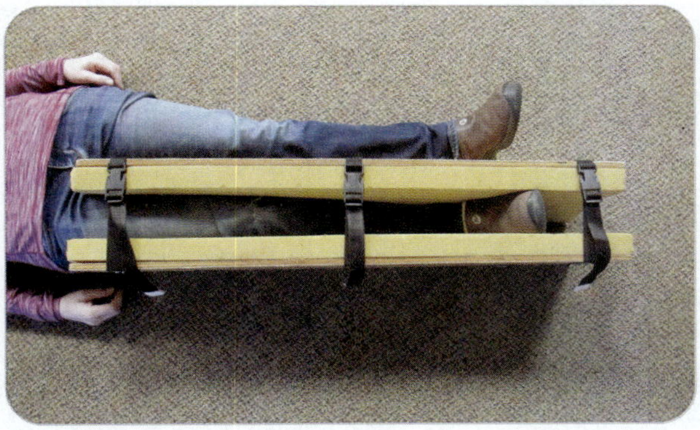

Figure 20-77 A Quick Splint can be used when injuries involve both the femur and the bones of the lower leg.

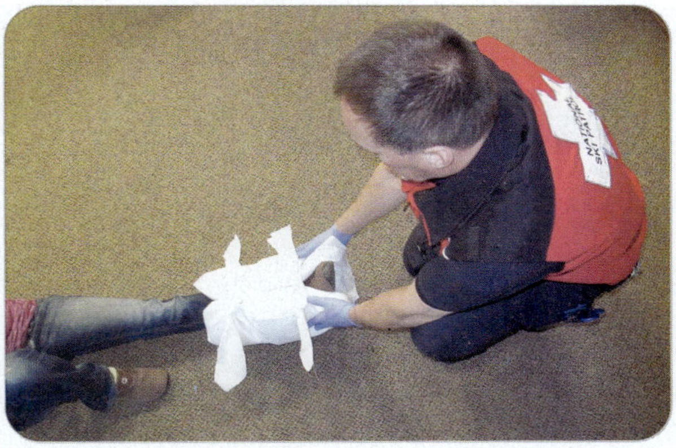

Figure 20-78 A pillow splint can be applied to an injured ankle.

Femur/Tibia Fracture in the Same Leg

Fractures involving the femur and tibia in the same leg disrupt the stability of the bones between the fractures, causing the knee to "float" between the two fractures. Patients with this type of injury often have other ABCD-related injuries that require attention first. While caring for the patient's more significant injuries, try to keep the affected leg axially aligned.

Immobilize a "floating knee" injury by applying a Quick Splint over the entire length of the leg (Figure 20-77). Another rescuer should provide tension and alignment, like the method used for an isolated tibia fracture. Splint the injured leg by tying it to the good leg after applying the Quick Splint.

Alternatively, apply a traction splint using only tension. A double-pole traction device such as a Thomas splint (or a Hare traction device with tension, not traction) may be used successfully.

Ankle Injuries

Ankle sprains are treated with immobilization using a splint, usually Quick Splint, and/or cardboard, elevation, and intermittent ice if painful. Since only an X-ray image can tell if an ankle is broken, recommend follow-up with a health care provider.

Ankle deformity generally indicates either a dislocation or (more frequently) a fracture–dislocation. OEC technicians should not attempt to align or reduce ankle deformities when CMS is intact. (Doing so is extremely painful.) If distal CMS is compromised or if the bone appears ready to come through the skin, *one* attempt to reduce the ankle may be tried. As with reducing other bones, apply *gentle* but firm tension by pulling on the heel (and the top of the foot) and put the ankle back into normal anatomic position. Regardless of whether the ankle is realigned, do not let go of it until it is immobilized. If the ankle becomes realigned and not immobilized, it could dislocate again. Because ankle sprains may be difficult to differentiate from ankle fractures, management of ankle injuries should include immobilization, splinting, and follow-up evaluation by a physician. A blanket roll or a pillow splint wrapped around the ankle is often best. Other splints such as a Quick Splint, a cardboard box splint, an air splint, or a malleable splint, may also be used but may be difficult to apply if the ankle is dislocated.

To apply a pillow splint, follow this procedure (Figure 20-78):

1. Rescuer 1: Stabilize the ankle above and below by holding the foot and the tibia at midshaft.
2. Rescuer 2:
   - Position a soft pillow under the ankle such that the foot rests in the middle of the pillow.
   - Gently bring the corner of the pillow over the dorsum (top) of the foot, molding the pillow to the shape of the foot. Leave the tip of the toes exposed to facilitate CMS reassessment.
   - Secure the pillow in place with roller gauze or tape.
   - Reassess CMS

CASE Update

The paramedic says he needs to examine the distal CMS in the injured leg. After the paramedic has started an IV and administered pain medication, you help remove the boot. The dorsalis pedis pulse is absent, and the patient cannot feel part of his foot. With your assistance holding the leg above the knee, the paramedic pulls axial traction on the foot and the knee "pops" back into place. The paramedic continues to gently provide traction while you place the Quick Splint back on. The dorsalis pedis pulse is now present, but the foot is still partially numb. Vital signs remain stable. The sling and swathe remain in place. You help the EMS personnel load the patient onto the ambulance stretcher, and he is transferred to the waiting helicopter.

What should you do next?

In wilderness settings, people with mild ankle injuries may need to self-evacuate. In this instance, it is important to firmly stabilize the zone of injury. Help patients walk by applying either cloth bandages, cravats, or tape wrapped in a figure eight pattern (**Figure 20-79**). Check CMS to the toes frequently because cravats or tape may become too tight as the foot swells. Using the "human crutch" may be helpful.

Boot removal may be very difficult in ankle injuries. During inclement weather, it is generally best to leave the boot on until the patient is inside, the ankle is elevated on an exam table, and more assistance is available. The procedure to remove a boot is discussed in the next section of this chapter.

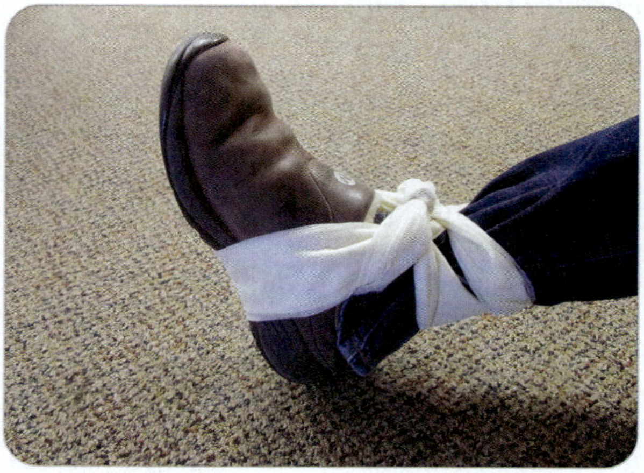

Figure 20-79 Using a bandage or a cravat to support an injured ankle.

Foot and Toe Injuries

Splint these injuries using a blanket roll, a pillow splint, or a rigid, well-padded splint. Be sure to leave toes slightly exposed so that distal CMS may be assessed. Foot and toe injuries, especially open injuries and puncture wounds, have a high rate of infection. For this reason, the patient should be encouraged to seek follow-up care.

CMS Compromise in a Leg

Any of the following findings of impaired CMS in a traumatized leg require immediate attention:

1. Impaired circulation presenting as a cold, pale foot
2. Absent dorsalis pedis *and* posterior tibialis pulses
3. Numbness of the foot or loss of motor function in the lower leg.

To realign a leg with distal CMS compromise, follow these steps:

1. Rescuer 1: Stabilize the thigh.
2. Rescuer 2:
   - Firmly grasp the posterior aspect of the top of the calf, just below the knee. If a distal injury is present, the ankle may be used instead of the calf.
   - Keeping the knee slightly bent, apply gentle but steady longitudinal traction to align the leg. Attempt this realignment *once only*.
   - Reassess CMS.

If distal pulses, sensation, or motor function return, or if the color of the foot improves, splint the extremity in the position where the improvement(s) are first observed. If the realignment attempt is unsuccessful, causes too much pain, or is met with resistance by the patient, splint the leg in the position of maximum comfort and transport rapidly.

MANAGEMENT OF OPEN FRACTURES

Open fractures require special care. When a bone is exposed to the outside environment, either by a jagged edge of a broken bone puncturing from the inside through the skin or from an object such as a stick puncturing through the skin damaging a bone, serious consequences can occur. Foreign contaminants such as dirt and bacteria can become attached to the end of the bone. The end of the bone sticking out has compromised blood supply. Any penetrating wound over a suspected fracture should be cared for as an open fracture, as the bone may have penetrated the skin and gone back in, or the penetrating object may no longer be present.

If an open fracture is not cared for promptly at a hospital, serious infection can occur. At the hospital, a doctor will thoroughly clean the bone, repair it as necessary, and replace the bone inside, leaving the wound open for drainage.

When a broken bone penetrates the skin and remains outside the body, the OEC technician should control bleeding and cover the exposed bone with sterile dressings. The injury should be immobilized in the position found, with the bone outside. Sometimes this requires "creative" splinting and padding with sterile dressings around the bone end. If the bone end goes back into the wound as you apply the splint, leave it inside the body. A midshaft femur fracture with a traction splint usually allows the bone sticking out to go back inside the body. This is preferred in this case.

When there is neurovascular compromise to an extremity with an open fracture (where the bone is outside the body) and definitive care is more than 2 hours away, it may be best to make one attempt to realign the bone, allowing it to go back inside the body, so neurovascular compromise is corrected. If there is no blood flow (pulseless, white extremity) to the distal part of the arm or leg, repositioning the fracture site once to obtain blood flow is appropriate. In this situation, before repositioning, if there is gross contamination, such as dirt or mud on the exposed bone end, pour sterile water over the bone end to clean it, but do not try to scrub it. If sterile water is not available, tap water may be used. It would be appropriate to clean and realign the extremity *inside* the aid room if this care is needed.

In a wilderness situation, where definitive care is not available for a long time and the bone is protruding and neurovascular status is intact, follow the same care for an open fracture with neurovascular compromise. Use potable (drinking) water to clean the exposed bone and reposition the bone inside the body. Do not use creek or pond water.

All open fractures require transport to a hospital for appropriate care. Always tell the transporting EMS personnel details about the injury and your care, including whether the bone was outside and went back into the body. Open fractures always need emergent transport and early definitive surgical care at a hospital.

BOOT REMOVAL

When a lower extremity injury occurs in snow sports, the decision whether to remove the individual's boot on the hill or in the aid room remains the subject of considerable discussion. The current recommendation of the National Ski Patrol is to leave the boot on in outdoor environments, unless local treatment protocols dictate otherwise. Because most transport times to the aid room are relatively short, leaving the boot on with better controlled removal inside as indicated makes sense.

Each area should develop a local protocol regarding boot removal. The formulation of this protocol must include input from the patrol medical advisor and should take into consideration the injury, environmental conditions at the time of the incident (temperature, precipitation, and wind), and transport times from the accident scene to the aid room and from the aid room to the hospital. Protocol considerations should also include the type of splint needed, probable or actual CMS status in the extremity distal to the injury, and the patient's comfort. Obviously, boot removal in the aid room with extra help is easier. Some patients require IV pain medication before removing the boot. An ALS paramedic can provide this, and then you may assist this provider with boot removal.

If the boot is unfamiliar to you, ask the patient how to remove it or remove the opposite boot first to learn how best to proceed. In general, do not use a saw on a ski boot. Hiking boots and other lace-up boots can be removed by completely undoing the laces.

To remove a boot, perform the steps of **OEC Skill 20-12**.

It is important to monitor the patient's perception of pain throughout this procedure. If resistance is met, stop and attempt to further loosen the boot. If necessary, stop the procedure and splint the ankle with the boot in place.

OEC SKILL 20-12 Removing a Boot

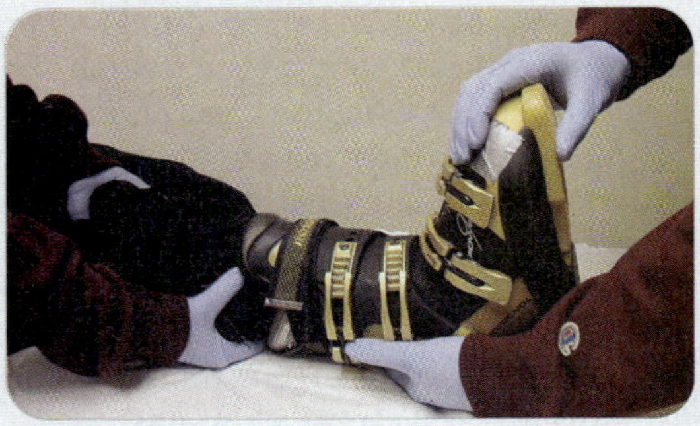

1 Rescuer 1: Stabilize the boot that is to be removed.

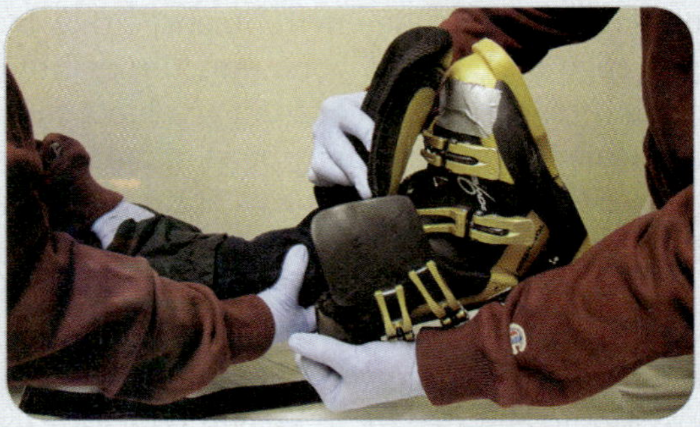

2 Rescuer 2:

- Unbuckle or unlace the boot completely.
- Spread the boot shell, pulling the tongue forward as far as it can go, or open a rear entry boot's back as far as it can go.

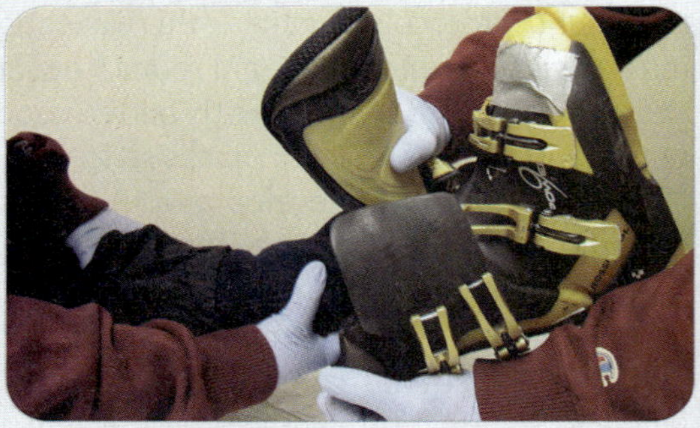

3 Rescuer 1: Stabilize the leg/ankle either by placing one hand on the front of the ankle and one hand on the back of the ankle, or by holding both sides of the ankle. Hold this position firmly as the boot is removed.

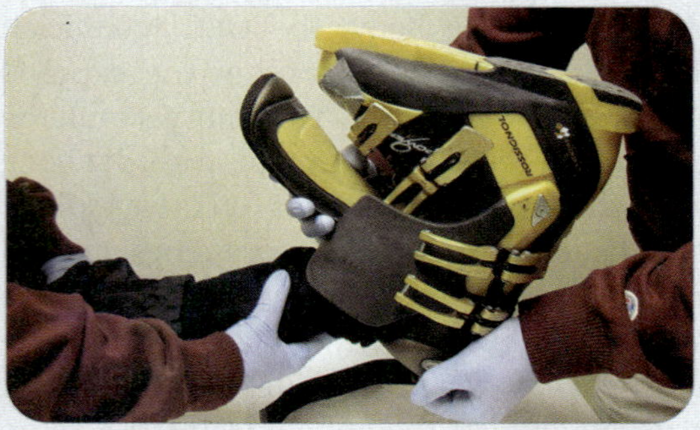

4 Rescuer 2:

- Gently remove the boot by sliding its heel away from the foot, followed by the toe.
- Assess distal CMS.
- Prepare and apply a splint.
- Reassess distal CMS.

OEC SKILL 20-12 Removing a Boot (*continued*)

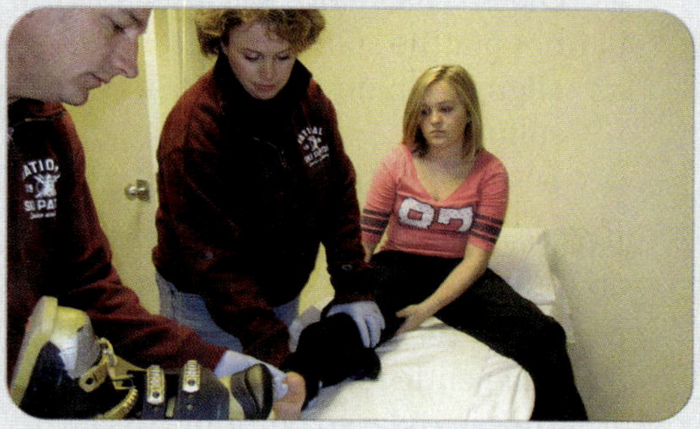

© Edward McNamara.

5 Assess distal CMS.
- Prepare and apply a cardboard splint as described previously.
- Reassess distal CMS.

CASE Outcome

Three weeks later, the teen, in a wheelchair, and his father return to thank you for saving the boy's leg. He had a complete dislocation of his knee, with three torn ligaments, and a proximal tibia fracture. His popliteal artery was compromised. After 4 hours of surgery, his leg's circulation and stability were restored. He said he faces a long rehab, but still has his leg. His shoulder has an A/C separation but should heal in a sling without surgery.

Section 3 Questions

1. Which of the following are the four main types of splints used by OEC technicians?
   a. Gauze, cravats, bandages, and improvised
   b. Traction, tension, improvised, and rigid
   c. Soft, rigid/semi-rigid, traction, and improvised
   d. Soft, traction, block, and improvised
2. Which of the following statements is *true*?
   a. Traction is approximately 15 pounds of force or 10% total body weight; tension is about 7 to 8 pounds of force or just enough to align the bone.
   b. Traction is approximately 10 pounds of force or 15% total body weight; tension is about 1 to 6 pounds of force or until the patient tells you to stop.
   c. Either traction or tension may be used when aligning a broken humerus.
   d. If necessary for pain relief, tension should be used on a broken femur, but traction should be used on a broken humerus.
3. When following the general principles of splinting, which of the following procedures is *not* accurate?
   a. Select an appropriate splint; properly size the splint; check CMS before and after; do not manually stabilize above and below the injury.
   b. Check CMS before and after; manually stabilize above and below; pad the splint; align the fracture; use an Ace bandage to secure the splint.
   c. Select an appropriate splint; pad the splint where necessary; check CMS before and after; align the injury where necessary.
   d. Select an appropriate splint; position the splint next to the injury, then gently slide it under or around the injury; secure the splint with an Ace bandage or cravats.
4. When placing the injured extremity in the splint in the anatomic position becomes difficult, the OEC practitioner should:
   a. check CMS before and after splinting.
   b. not put the splint on.
   c. align the injury so that it fits into the splint.
   d. Both a and b
5. If a gross deformity of the knee is found, and a distal pulse is detected, you should:
   a. adjust the knee to fit into the splint.
   b. pull gentle tension to straighten the knee in order to put it into a Quick Splint.
   c. leave the knee in the position found.
   d. use a traction splint and transport.
6. Which of the following findings of impaired CMS in a traumatized leg requires immediate attention?
   a. Numbness of the foot or loss of motor function in the lower leg
   b. Impaired circulation presenting as a cold, pale foot
   c. Absent dorsalis pedis and posterior tibialis pulses
   d. All of the above
7. When a forearm bone is protruding from the skin and there is no neurovascular compromise, you should do all of the following *except*:
   a. stop the bleeding.
   b. make one attempt to put it back under the skin.
   c. cover with sterile gauze.
   d. splint the extremity in the position found.

8. Which of the following statements regarding lower extremity injuries is *true*?
   a. You should never remove a boot outside.
   b. You should follow the local protocol on boot removal.
   c. You should always remove the boot while outside if the injury is from the knee down.
   d. You should never ask the patient how to remove the boot because you don't want the person to think you don't know what you are doing.

Answers: 1. c, Objective 20-3.2, p. 468; 2. a, Objective 20-3.3, p. 473; 3. b, Objective 20-3.4, p. 500; 4. d, Objective 20-3.4, p. 474; 5. c, Objective 20-3.6, p. 474; 6. d, Objective 20-3.5, p. 500; 7. b, Objective 20-3.7, p. 501; 8. b, Objective 20-3.8, p. 501

CHAPTER REVIEW

In Summary

- The musculoskeletal system allows movement and protects internal structures.
- OEC technicians may need to improvise splinting, all the while remembering the principle of "first do no harm."
- Immobilization decreases pain, slows bleeding, prevents further injury, and makes transport easier.
- During the assessment of extremity injuries, it is best to ask patients to point with one finger to exactly where it hurts.
- When immobilizing an extremity, OEC technicians need to remember to assess CMS, both before and after the application of the splint.
- A fracture is a disruption in the continuity of a bone.
- A dislocation is the disruption of a joint in which the bone ends no longer remain in normal contact with each other.
- A splint is a soft or rigid device applied to an injured extremity.
- The four basic types of splints are soft, rigid or semi-rigid, traction, and improvised.
- Open fractures require emergent care.
- A common upper extremity injury among skiers is skier's thumb.
- The clavicle is the most commonly broken bone in the body.
- For extremity injuries, remove all rings, bracelets, or other jewelry from the hand or foot immediately, before swelling occurs.
- Treat all threats to life first, and then manage musculoskeletal injuries.

Key Terms

Acromioclavicular (A/C) joint A joint of the shoulder in which the acromion (top of the scapula) and the clavicle articulate.

Angulation A sharp bend in a broken bone; a broken bone that is visibly crooked.

Articular cartilage The cartilage that is affixed to the end of a bone within a joint.

Articulation The site at which the ends of two or more bones come together to form a joint.

Bone crepitus A noise or palpable feeling of crackling when fractured bone ends rub together.

Cartilage A tough, elastic, fibrous connective tissue found in various parts of the body, including the joints, outer ear, and end of the nose.

Cortex The hard, outer layer of a bone.

Dislocation A separation or displacement of the bones of a joint.

Dorsal Toward the back of the body or of a body part.

Dorsiflex To move a part of the body dorsally (toward the back).

False movement Motion that occurs at the site of a fracture of a long bone that is not present when the bone is intact.

Fracture A break in a bone's cortex.

Guarding The act of holding an injured arm or leg in a protective position to prevent further injury.

Immobilization The process of holding an object in place, as for a fracture by a cast or internal orthopedic hardware.

Joints Sites at which two or more bones meet.

Joint capsule A sheet of fibrous connective tissue enclosing a synovial joint.

Ligaments Tissues that connect a bone to another bone; connective tissue that provides structure for a joint.

Meniscus A specialized cartilage found in some joints, such as the knee and the acromioclavicular joint.

Musculoskeletal system The combination of the bony skeleton, the voluntary muscles, and other supporting structures that gives the body form and enables movement.

Periosteum The thin vascular outer covering of the cortex of a bone.

Plantarflex Movement of the foot or toes downward, toward the sole of the foot.

Popliteal fossa The posterior part of the knee.

Skeletal muscle The type of muscle that attaches to the bony skeleton and is controlled voluntarily by the nervous system; functions to move joints to perform physical activities.

Sling and swathe A soft splint used to immobilize many upper extremity injuries.

Splint A mechanical device used to prevent a part of the body from moving, protecting it from further injury.

Sprain A stretched or torn ligament.

Strain A stretched or torn muscle or tendon.

Subluxation An event in which a joint partially dislocates and returns to its normal anatomic position.

Synovium The inner layer of the joint capsule whose cells make a viscous fluid that lubricates joints.

Tendons Dense tissues that connect muscle to bone.

Traction The amount of force required to straighten a limb and keep it in alignment; for a fractured femur, typically 10% of the patient's body weight, or approximately 15 pounds.

Traction splint A splint used on a lower extremity to align a fracture, such as a midshaft fracture of the femur.

Zone of injury The area that is close to or surrounding an injury of an extremity, such as a sprain or fracture.

Chapter Questions

1. What is the difference between a *strain* and a *sprain*?
   a. A strain happens to muscles and a sprain happens to ligaments.
   b. A strain happens to ligaments and a sprain happens to muscles.
   c. A strain can happen to either a ligament or a muscle.
   d. A sprain can happen to either a ligament or a muscle.

2. A gap under the skin is a sign of which of the following common musculoskeletal soft-tissue injuries?
   a. Fracture
   b. Ruptured tendon
   c. Sprain
   d. Strain

3. When assessing an A/C separation (shoulder separation), which sign or symptom would you *least* likely find?
   a. Point tenderness over the A/C joint
   b. Point tenderness just medial and inferior to the A/C joint
   c. Mild deformity at the distal end of the clavicle
   d. The arm "locked" in an outstretched position, away from the body

4. What is the term for a common skiing injury to the upper extremity in which a ski pole catches on the snow and bends the thumb laterally and dorsally (backwards), disrupting the ligament at the base?
   a. Skier's sprain
   b. Dumb thumb
   c. Skier's thumb
   d. Smith fracture

5. When assessing a skier complaining of pain in his knee, he tells you that he was "sitting back" on his skis when he felt and heard a "pop" and had immediate knee pain. This information leads you to believe that he injured his:
   a. anterior cruciate ligament.
   b. medial collateral ligament.
   c. meniscus.
   d. femur.

6. Which of the following is *not* a reason for splinting?
   a. Decreases the movement of bone ends to allow clotting and reduces muscle spasms
   b. Reduces pain, allowing the patient to return to skiing immediately
   c. Allows for easier transport and prevents sharp bone ends from penetrating the skin
   d. Decreases pain at the fracture site and prevents further damage to soft tissues

7. Application of a traction splint:
   a. reduces blood loss.
   b. prevents further soft-tissue damage.
   c. places in-line force in the direction of its normal alignment to regain bone length and reduce pain.
   d. All of the above

8. You come upon a patient complaining of pain in the right leg, approximately 2 to 3 inches below the hip joint. When treating this patient, you should do all of the following *except*:
   a. place the patient on a long spine board or a full-body vacuum splint.
   b. see if the patient can wiggle the toes.
   c. use a pelvic binder or sheet splint to secure the injury.
   d. fill the voids with padding or a blanket before strapping the patient to a backboard.

Answers: 1. a, Objective 20-1.3, p. 439; 2. b, Objective 20-1.5, p. 445; 3. d, Objective 20-2.1, p. 449; 4. c, Objective 20-2.1, p. 453; 5. a, Objective 20-2.1, p. 459; 6. b, Objective 20-3.4, p. 468; 7. d, Objective 20-3.4, p. 472; 8. c, Objective 20-3.6, p. 488

CHAPTER 21

SPINE, BRAIN, AND NERVOUS SYSTEM INJURIES

OBJECTIVES

Upon completion of this chapter, the OEC technician will be able to:

21-1 Identify and define the two major anatomic components of the central nervous system.
21-2 Define traumatic brain injury.
21-3 Describe traumatic injuries involving the spine.
21-4 Describe the signs and symptoms of spinal injuries.
21-5 Describe how to properly assess a patient with a suspected brain and spinal cord injury.
21-6 List the signs and symptoms of traumatic brain injury.
21-7 Demonstrate how to properly care for a patient with a brain and spinal cord injury.
21-8 Demonstrate how to maintain proper spinal alignment while placing a patient onto a long backboard from the following positions:
- Supine
- Sitting

21-9 Explain and demonstrate how to perform neutral head alignment.
21-10 Demonstrate how to size and apply a cervical collar.
21-11 Demonstrate how to perform an axial drag.
21-12 Demonstrate how to secure a patient to a long backboard.
21-13 Demonstrate how to place a patient on a full-body vacuum mattress.
21-14 Describe and demonstrate how to remove a helmet.
21-15 Explain and demonstrate the principle of "jams and pretzels."

KEY TERMS

Antegrade amnesia, p. 516
Axon, p. 512
Cerebral contusion, p. 517
Concussion, p. 516
Coup-contrecoup brain injury, p. 514
Cranium (skull), p. 513
Epidural hematoma, p. 517
Intracerebral hematoma, p. 517
Intracranial pressure, p. 515
Jams and pretzels, p. 535
Lucid interval, p. 517
Retrograde amnesia, p. 516
Stabilized extrication, p. 536
Subdural hematoma, p. 517
Traumatic brain injury (TBI), p. 515

WINTER EMERGENCY CARE WEC An Educational Program of the National Ski Patrol

HISTORICAL TIMELINE **1988.** Winter Emergency Care is published with Warren Bowman, MD, as the lead author.

CHAPTER OVERVIEW

Biking, trekking, rafting, skiing, equestrian activities, snowboarding, and other outdoor sports carry inherent risks for injuries, including serious injuries involving the brain, neck, or spine that range from relatively minor to immediately life threatening. Some have life-altering consequences. This chapter covers traumatic injuries to the nervous system. Stroke and other medical conditions that affect the central nervous system (CNS) are discussed in other chapters.

A person's ability to sense and react to the external environment depends on the coordinated functioning of the CNS and the peripheral nervous system. The CNS consists of the brain and spinal cord. The peripheral nerves connect to the spinal cord just inside the spine bones, or vertebrae, and go to the body (**Figure 21-1**). Proper prehospital care of nervous system injuries by an OEC technician can reduce the possibility of permanent disability or death. CNS injuries are among the most serious that OEC technicians encounter.

CNS trauma is associated with high mortality and morbidity rates, significant economic consequences, and serious effects on patient's quality of life. One of the most severe forms of CNS trauma

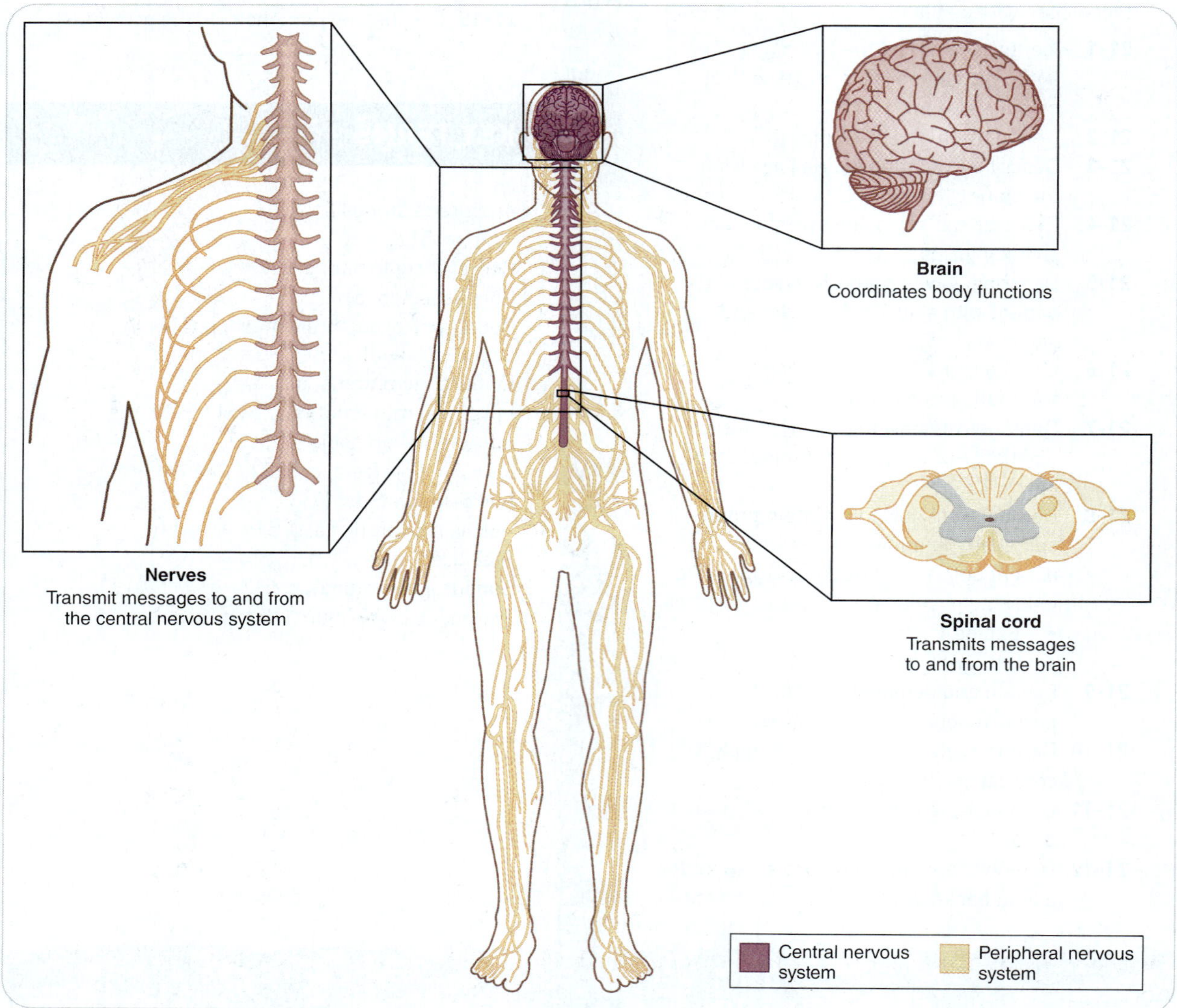

Figure 21-1 The nervous system is composed of the central nervous system and the peripheral nervous system.

CASE Presentation

You are dispatched to an accident where a skier has collided with a large tree. Upon your arrival, you find an unresponsive male skier, approximately 30 years old, lying on his back. After the scene is made safe, you prioritize by caring for life-threatening problems. There is no excessive bleeding. Next, you recognize the need for airway management. Using techniques to minimize injury to the spine (spinal motion restriction), you immediately open the airway with the jaw-thrust maneuver and simultaneously check for breathing and a carotid pulse. You find the patient is breathing and has a pulse. You immediately place an oropharyngeal airway. The individual is wearing a helmet that is cracked in two places. Blood and a clear fluid are leaking from the patient's nose and ears. The ski tracks indicate that the patient went straight into the tree.

What should you do?

is traumatic brain injury, a leading cause of traumatic death in individuals under age 45.

The US Consumer Product Safety Commission noted that during the 5-year period from 2007 to 2011, hospital emergency rooms treated the following numbers of sports-related brain injuries:

- Cycling: 221,150
- Winter sports (skiing, snowboarding): 32,643
- Hockey: 34,109

It is important for OEC technicians to understand the mechanisms responsible for traumatic CNS injuries and be able to quickly recognize the signs and symptoms of specific CNS injuries. They also must be able to safely manage patients with traumatic head and spine injuries, and minimize additional injury. By so doing, OEC technicians can help to reduce the morbidity and mortality associated with this devastating form of trauma.

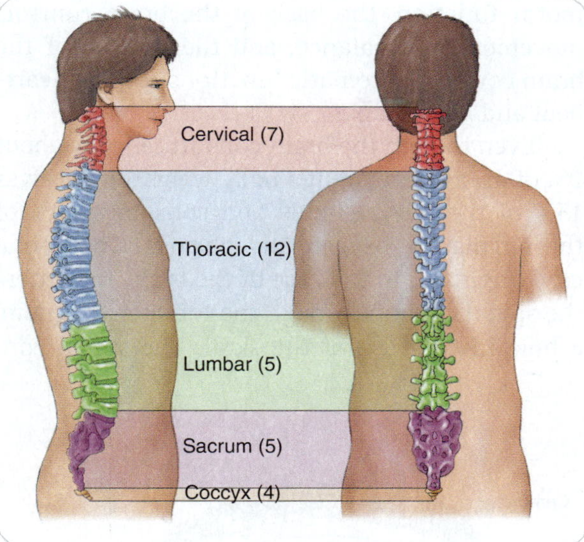

Figure 21-2 The spinal column is the body's central supporting system and consists of 33 bones divided into five sections. Injury to the vertebrae may damage the spinal cord, causing paralysis.

ANATOMY AND PHYSIOLOGY

The axial skeleton in humans consists of a skull and 33 vertebrae in the spine. The spinal cord consists of the cervical, thoracic, lumbar, sacral, and coccyx sections (**Figure 21-2**). The CNS has two major components, the brain and spinal cord. The brain is the central computer for the body. The spinal cord is the pathway from the brain to the rest of the body.

A highly specialized cell that conducts electrical impulses, called a neuron, is the functional unit of the nervous system. The body's millions of neurons transmit chemical and electrical signals throughout the body and collectively function as an organized and very complex wiring system. The largest collection of neurons, located within the brain, directs the functions of the other neurons.

An **axon** is the long, slender projection of a neuron that sends electrical signals away from the neuron.

Inside the skull is the brain, which has three parts: the cerebrum, cerebellum, and brainstem (**Figure 21-3**). The uppermost part, called the cerebrum, consists of an outer part, or cortex, which controls higher functions such as sense perception, voluntary movement, speech, thought, and memory, and an inner part, or hypothalamus, which is the major control center for the autonomic nervous system and controls body temperature, hunger, thirst, and fatigue (sleep). In the back, the cerebellum controls balance, motor coordination, movement, posture, and muscle tone. At the bottom, the brainstem is made up of the pons, thalamus, and medulla oblongata. The brainstem automatically controls basic body functions such as cardiac, respiratory, and other brain-processing functions. To summarize, the top of the brain controls thought, sensation, and motor function, the back of the brain controls movement and balance, and the bottom of the brain controls automatic functions such as heartbeat and breathing.

Even though the brain constitutes only about 2% of an average adult's body weight, it receives 15% of the blood supply and consumes 20% of the circulating oxygen and glucose. The spinal cord originates at the base of the brain and enters the spinal column through the foramen magnum, a hole in the base of the skull. The spinal cord travels inside the stacked vertebrae of the spinal column down to the level of the first lumbar vertebra; from there it becomes individual nerves down to the coccyx (**Figure 21-4**). The brain and spinal cord, which together make up the CNS, are covered by a three-layered membrane called the meninges. Circulating inside these protective membranes is cerebrospinal fluid (CSF) which provides a cushion and protection for the brain and spinal cord.

The spinal cord, which contains thousands and thousands of neurons, resembles an old-fashioned telephone cable containing many, many specifically organized wires. It serves as a pathway sending signals from the body to the brain and the brain to the body (arms and legs). If injured, both sensory and motor function below the level of interruption is lost.

The nerves that connect the rest of the body to the spinal cord make up the peripheral nervous system. The peripheral nerves that connect to the spinal cord in the neck send signals to and from the shoulders and arms, whereas the peripheral nerves that attach to the spinal cord in the low

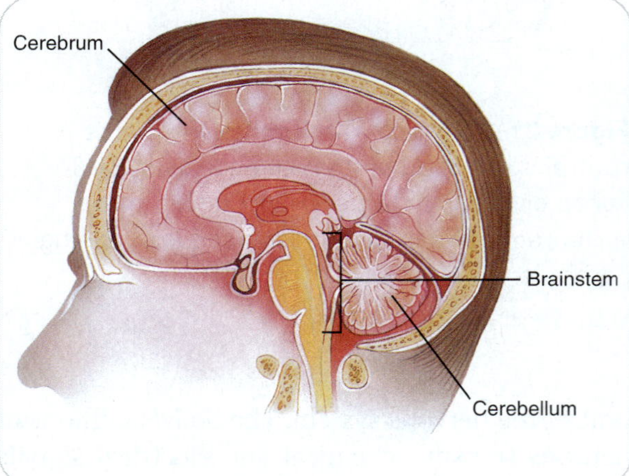

Figure 21-3 The major subdivisions of the brain: the cerebrum, the cerebellum, and the brainstem.

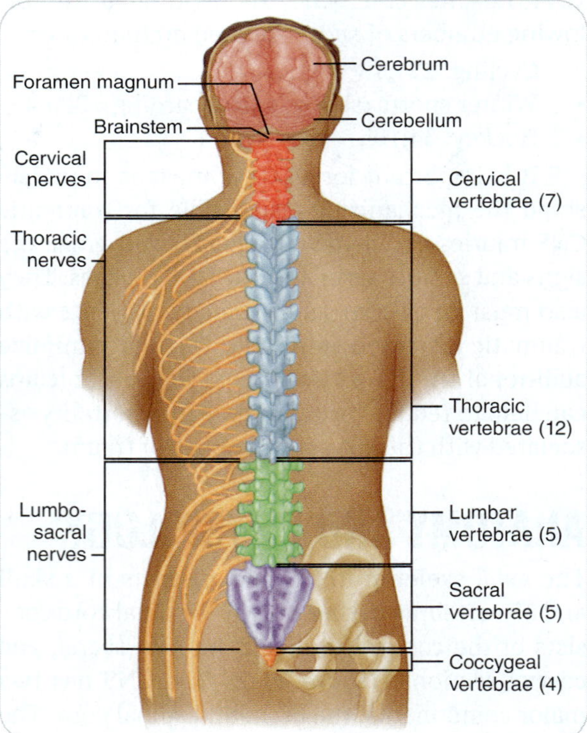

Figure 21-4 The spinal column is composed of 33 bones divided into five sections. Peripheral nerves are connected to the spinal cord at each level.

back (lumbosacral nerves) send signals to and from the buttocks, legs, and genitalia.

The peripheral nerves that connect to the spinal cord are divided into divisions like the vertebra. In the cervical region there are 8 cervical nerves, but only 7 cervical vertebrae, as the first nerve comes out above the C1 vertebrae, and nerve C8 comes out below the C7 vertebrae. All other regions have the same number of nerves as vertebrae.

All humans are "wired" by the peripheral nerves in the same way. Each of us has the same nerves in our arms and legs in generally the same anatomic location. These nerves contain both sensory neurons and motor (muscle) neurons. Peripheral nerves are responsible for both sensation and muscle activity in a very limited and specific area. In our arms and legs are specialized nerve endings called sensory receptors that sense the outside world, such as position, hot and cold, and pain. Sensory neurons attached to these specialized receptors in our arms and legs send messages from the body through peripheral nerves to the spinal cord and then on to the brain. The brain sends signals through the spinal cord to motor neurons to make muscles work. Sensory and motor neurons exist together inside each peripheral nerve.

KEY POINT

Open and Closed Injuries

Injuries to the CNS structures, the brain and spinal cord, can be divided into two broad categories: closed injuries and open injuries. Closed CNS injuries are those in which the integrity of the **cranium (skull)** and spinal column is not compromised to the outside environment. Open CNS injuries are those in which the brain or spinal cord is directly exposed to the environment, or in which CSF (or sometimes blood) is leaking from a wound or a cavity such as the nose or ears. When there is a break in the skin with a skull fracture underneath, it is an open injury.

HEAD SOFT-TISSUE INJURIES

Injuries to the head and neck include soft-tissue injuries, muscle or ligament strains, and fractures. Muscle strains of the neck and back are common sports injuries and are likely to be encountered by OEC technicians. Injuries involving the muscles near the spine are quite painful due to muscle spasms. Hyperflexion or hyperextension of the neck muscles may result in whiplash, a painful injury involving overstretching or tearing of the neck muscles and ligaments.

Injuries of the Scalp

The scalp is the thick skin that covers the skull. It is susceptible to a variety of soft-tissue injuries. Because the scalp has a generous blood supply, bleeding can be profuse in head injuries and in some cases can lead to significant blood loss if not treated quickly (**Figure 21-5**).

Skull Fractures

Skull fractures can result from blunt or penetrating trauma to the skull and are classified as linear, depressed, basilar, or open (**Figure 21-6**). A linear skull fracture has a single nondisplaced fracture line and usually presents with significant soft-tissue swelling and tenderness of the scalp. Conversely, a depressed skull fracture is a comminuted fracture with displacement which occasionally can be palpated as a "soft spot" or depression overlying the fracture with contusion and tenderness of the scalp. Depending on the force to the

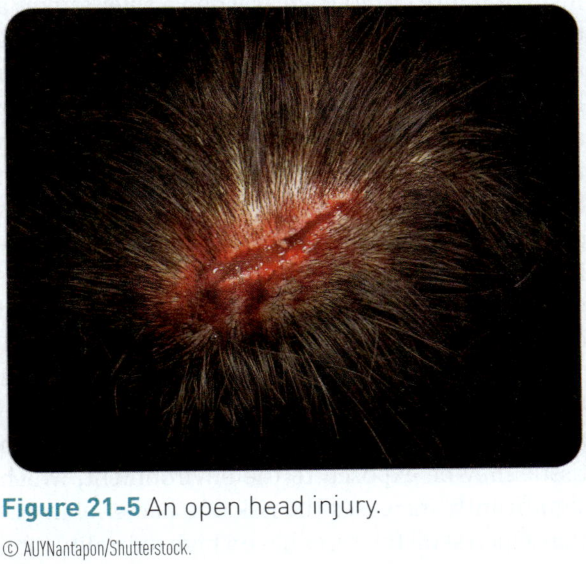

Figure 21-5 An open head injury.

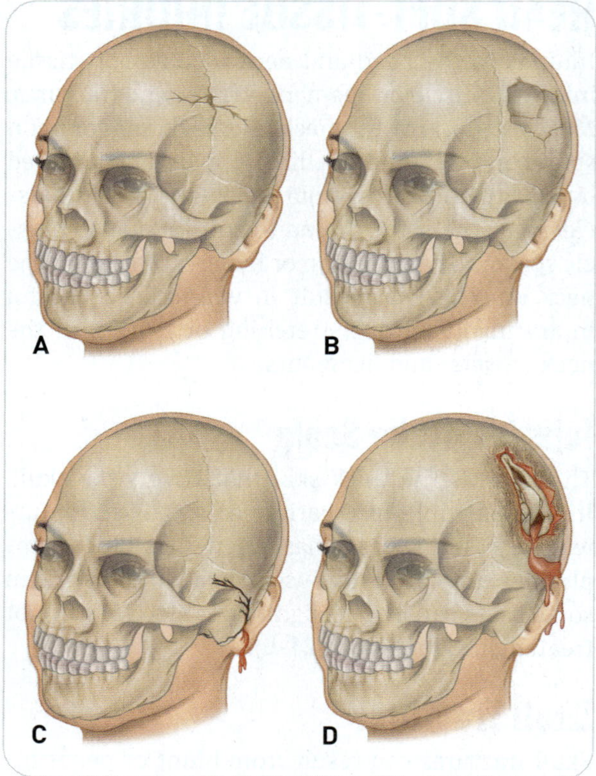

Figure 21-6 Types of skull fractures include linear **(A)**, depressed **(B)**, basilar **(C)**, and open **(D)**.

A-D: © Jones & Bartlett Learning.

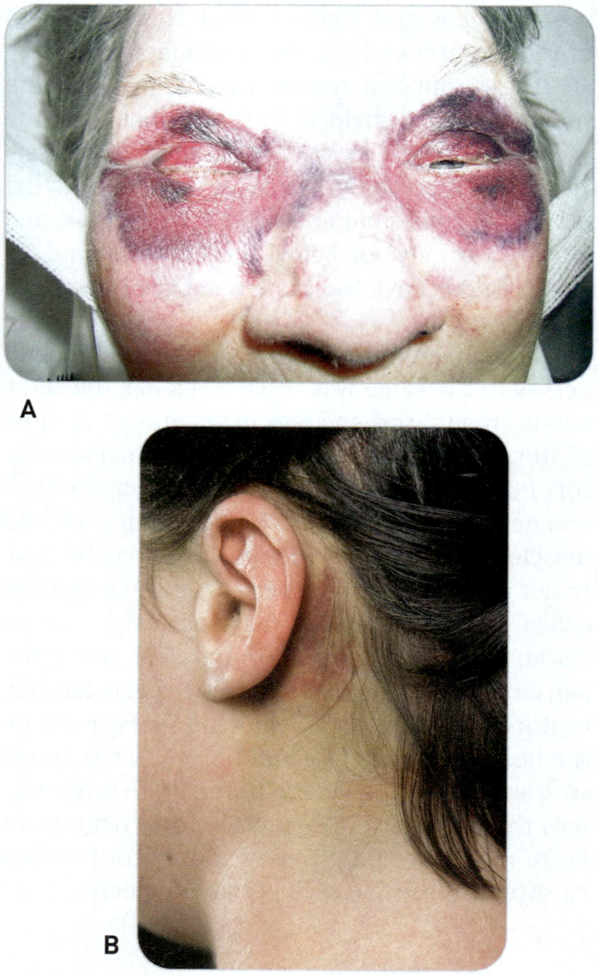

Figure 21-7 Signs of skull fracture. **A.** Ecchymosis under the eyes (raccoon eyes). **B.** Ecchymosis behind one ear (Battle sign).

A: © E.M. Singletary, M.D. Used with permission; B: © Medical-on-Line/Mediscan/Alamy Stock Photo.

skull, the fracture fragments may or may not intrude on the underlying brain tissue.

A basilar skull fracture is a fracture that occurs along the floor, or base, of the skull. This type of fracture is seen with a high-velocity blunt mechanism of injury (MOI) such as when a skier strikes a tree, when a climber strikes his or her head during a fall, or when a mountain biker crashes into a large stationary object. Fractures in this area can allow CSF to leak out of the cranial vault and into the ear canals, nasal passageway, or mouth. With basilar skull fracture after several *hours,* patients can develop one or both classic findings of a basilar skull fracture: ecchymosis (bruising) that develops under the eyes (racoon eyes) and behind one ear, called Battle sign (**Figure 21-7**).

An open skull fracture results when severe forces are applied to the head and is often associated with trauma to multiple body systems. Brain tissue may be exposed to the environment, which significantly increases the risk of a bacterial infection. Open skull fractures have a high mortality rate.

BRAIN INJURIES

Coup-Contrecoup Brain Injury

The brain "floats" in a layer of fluid (CSF) between the inside of the skull and the brain tissue. Although this fluid cushions and protects the brain, an impact or rapid deceleration to the head of sufficiently large force can cause the brain to strike the inside of the skull (**Figure 21-8**).

A **coup-contrecoup brain injury** is caused by rapid deceleration of the head, as can occur when a skier or a mountain biker strikes a tree or some other immovable object. Upon impact with the object, the brain keeps moving forward and strikes the inside of the skull ("coup") damaging the

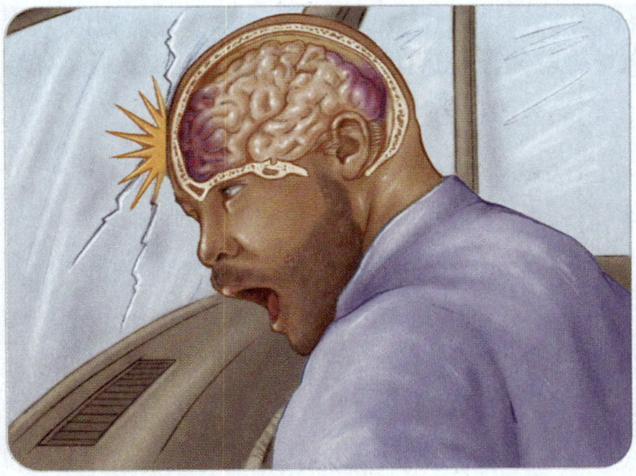

Figure 21-8 An impact or rapid deceleration to the head of sufficiently large force can cause the brain to strike the inside of the skull.

brain. The "contrecoup" portion of the injury occurs when the head stops and the brain rebounds in the other direction and strikes the inside of the skull on the opposite side, damaging the brain a second time. *Coup-contrecoup* is a French term meaning "blow-counter-blow."

In many instances, a coup-contrecoup injury is not immediately apparent because no external signs of trauma may be evident. This is especially true of deceleration injuries without impact. Depending on the forces involved, coup-contrecoup injuries can result in severe intracranial bleeding, swelling, and can compromise normal brain function.

Injury to the brain usually involve two events: a primary injury, such as a collision with a tree, a rock, or the ground, and a secondary (or delayed) injury, caused by inadequate oxygen delivery to the brain from systemic hypoxia and/or hypotension. Brain swelling or the development of a blood clot underneath the skull may result in elevated or increased **intracranial pressure** preventing the delivery of oxygen and glucose to the brain. The delayed injury may occur rapidly or take several hours to occur.

To maintain homeostasis, the body keeps a very narrow range of pressure on the inside of the skull and on the structures of the brain by making and absorbing the CSF. Because the volume within the skull is fixed, any increase in volume within the skull from bleeding or edema (swelling), increases the pressure inside the skull. After

Table 21-1 Long-Term or Lifelong Deficits of TBI

- Memory loss
- Reduced problem-solving capacity
- Stress and anger-management issues
- Emotional upset, including depression
- Job skill impairment
- Chronic seizure disorders
- Functional changes in thought, speech, learning, emotions, behavior, and sensation
- Increased risk of Alzheimer, Parkinson, and other brain disorders that become more prevalent with age

the initial traumatic injury to the brain, bleeding inside the skull or swelling of brain tissue from bruising creates increased pressure, a secondary injury. The result is compression of brain tissue, reduction in brain function, and ultimately death.

Many older people take anticoagulant medications, which delay blood clotting to decrease the risk or severity of heart attacks and strokes. Individuals taking these medications, which include warfarin (Coumadin), clopidogrel (Plavix), apixaban (Eliquis), aspirin, and many others, are at increased risk of intracranial bleeding inside the skull or in the brain from head trauma that can quickly result in a life-threatening problem.

Traumatic Brain Injury

Traumatic brain injury (TBI) is defined as a mechanical injury to the brain that results in short-term and/or long-term neurologic deficit (**Table 21-1**). The incidence of TBI has certain age and sex demographic differences (**Table 21-2**).

Recurrent TBI

A patient *must* fully recover from an initial TBI before resuming sports activities. If the first injury does not fully heal before a second injury occurs, the second injury, even if mild, may cause severe permanent brain damage or death, a term called second impact syndrome. Recurrent, mild TBIs that occur within hours, days, or even weeks can cause cumulative damage and can lead to severe long-term disability called chronic traumatic encephalopathy or can cause death. Patients exhibiting signs of a TBI are encouraged to cease the

Table 21-2 US Demographics of TBI (CDC Statistics, 2010)

- Males represent about 80% of all TBIs.
- Adults and elderly now are at the highest risk for TBI.
- Adults 60 years of age or older have the highest death rate from a TBI.
- Sports and recreational activities contribute to about 21% of all TBIs among US children and adolescents.
- Every year, 80,000 to 90,000 people experience the onset of long-term or lifelong disabilities associated with TBI.
- The mortality rate for TBI is 30 per 100,000, or an estimated 50,000 deaths in the United States annually. *Of those who die, 50% do so within the first 2 hours of their injury.*
- Deaths from brain injuries account for 34% of all traumatic deaths.
- TBI accounts for an estimated 2,685 deaths, 37,000 hospitalizations, and 435,000 emergency room visits in children ages 14 years and younger.

Data from Centers for Disease Control and Prevention. TBI data and statistics. https://www.cdc.gov/TraumaticBrainInjury/data/. Updated March 29, 2019. Accessed December 31, 2019.

activity that caused the injury and to seek medical care *with clearance* before resuming activities associated with the possibility of a second TBI. A second TBI could be fatal if the first one has not completely resolved.

Concussion

A **concussion** is a TBI caused by temporary disruption of coordinated brain function caused by trauma. Different scales are used to determine the severity of a concussion, but in general they are classified as mild, moderate, or severe. *Mild* concussion involves minor disruption of brain function and no loss of responsiveness but may include such signs and symptoms as confusion, dizziness, nausea, vomiting, headache, and visual and auditory disturbances. A *moderate* concussion is a brain injury involving a loss of responsiveness that lasts less than 5 minutes and more pronounced disruption of brain function. A *severe* concussion is a brain injury involving a loss of responsiveness lasting longer than 5 minutes and significant disruption of normal brain function. In both moderate and severe concussions, other signs and symptoms of brain injury are usually present.

Many patients who suffer a concussion exhibit some measurable memory loss, known as amnesia. The severity of amnesia depends on the extent of the concussion and can be classified as either retrograde or antegrade amnesia.

Patients with **retrograde amnesia** have no recollection of events *prior* to the injury, including the injury itself. **Antegrade amnesia** is characterized by no recollection of events occurring *after* the injury. Patients with amnesia often present with a distinctive speech pattern in which they repeatedly ask questions such as, "What happened?" or "Where am I?" or "Who are you?" sometimes for hours following the injury. This condition, known as perseveration, is indicative of both the confusion experienced by these patients and of antegrade amnesia.

KEY POINT

Retrograde and Antegrade Amnesia

Retro. Loss of memory before injury

Ante. Loss of memory after injury

Post-concussive syndrome is a complex set of symptoms ranging from permanent memory loss (usually limited to the event) to difficulty focusing and problem-solving to depression and behavioral disturbances. If antegrade amnesia lasts longer than retrograde amnesia, the prognosis is worse. Over time, many of these symptoms may disappear as the brain heals, although full recovery can take months or even years.

Cerebral Contusion

A **cerebral contusion** is a bruise involving the brain. This type of injury typically involves the rupture of small, superficial blood vessels and generally affects localized areas of the brain. A cerebral contusion is more serious than a concussion but may present with identical signs and symptoms.

Cerebral Hematoma

A hematoma is an accumulation of blood outside the vascular system. Because the skull or cranium is an enclosed space, a hematoma inside this space can compress the brain and result in serious, sometimes fatal consequences. There are three types of cerebral hematomas: an epidural hematoma, a subdural hematoma, and an intracerebral hematoma (Figure 21-9).

An **epidural hematoma** is a TBI that results in *arterial* bleeding between the skull and the dura mater. In most cases, the source of bleeding is the middle meningeal artery, generally as a result of blunt trauma that causes a skull fracture. This hematoma rapidly increases the pressure within the skull, which compresses the brain compromising blood flow and the delivery of oxygen and nutrients to the brain. The onset of signs and symptoms is rapid and consists of an initial period of unresponsiveness followed by a "**lucid interval**" in which the patient is relatively alert and then becomes increasingly less responsive and eventually unresponsive as blood accumulates inside the skull. This lucid interval only occurs in about 20% of all epidural hematomas. Without rapid surgical treatment, the patient can quickly die.

A **subdural hematoma** is a collection of venous blood between the dura mater and the brain. This type of injury is generally caused by rapid deceleration injuries. A subdural hematoma is often associated with underlying cerebral contusions and may resemble the signs and symptoms of an epidural hematoma. Because the source of bleeding is *venous* in origin and progresses more slowly, the onset of symptoms may not be appreciated for hours, days, or even weeks after the initial insult.

When a blood vessel inside brain tissue ruptures an intracerebral bleed occurs forming a hematoma inside the brain, called an **intracerebral hematoma**. This can happen spontaneously or from trauma. Such intracerebral bleeding can be life threatening because it can cause a rapid rise in intracranial pressure. The prognosis is very poor for individuals who take anticoagulants.

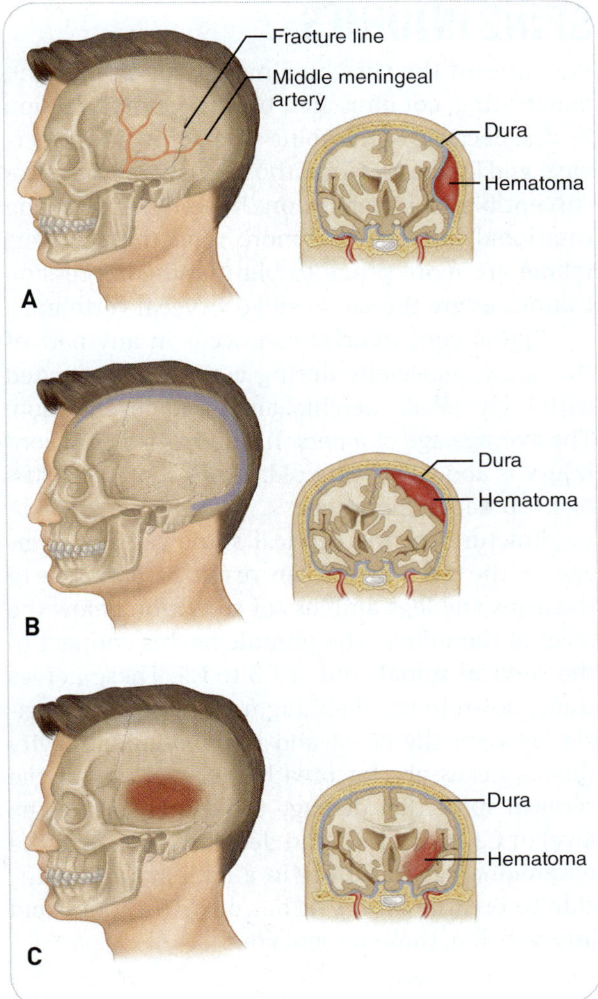

Figure 21-9 The three types of cerebral hematomas include the epidural hematoma **(A)**, subdural hematoma **(B)**, and intracerebral hematoma **(C)**.

Diffuse Axonal Injury

Diffuse axonal injury is a devastating TBI that results in widespread brain injury. It is caused by high-velocity rotational/deceleration mechanisms such as those experienced in high-speed ski, snowmobile, and bicycle crashes. Patients with diffuse axonal injury may be unresponsive at the time of injury, or become unresponsive later.

SPINE INJURIES

Fractures of the vertebrae may occur from blunt, penetrating, compression, twisting, or distraction forces. Because of the spine's flexibility in the cervical and lumbar regions, those vertebrae are more susceptible to hyperflexion, hyperextension, and rotational injuries. The more rigid thoracic vertebrae are more prone to blunt and compression trauma, as are the sacral and coccygeal vertebrae.

Spinal cord injuries can occur in any part of the spine, especially during activities associated with high speeds, heights, and rapid deceleration. The average age of a person who has a spinal cord injury is about 40 years old. Males represent 80% of all spinal cord injuries.

Fractures of the cervical spine causing damage to the spinal cord can result in paralysis of the arms and legs and loss of sensation below the level of the injury. The phrenic nerves connect to the cervical spinal cord at C3 to C5. These nerves travel down to the diaphragm, the large flat muscle between the chest and the abdominal cavity that is necessary for breathing. Fractures of the cervical spine that damage the spinal cord at the level of C3 through C5 can decrease signals to the phrenic nerves, resulting in a patient who is unable to breathe on his or her own. Without rapid intervention, these patients die.

KEY POINT

Damage to the Spinal Cord at C3 Through C5

One easy way to remember the nerves coming out of the spinal cord that control breathing is the phrase: "C3, C4, C5, keep the diaphragm alive."

The vertebrae of the thoracic spine are protected from rotational injuries by the rib cage. However, compression of a thoracic vertebra can occur from a fall or axial loading (force that is applied from one end of the spine to another) (**Figure 21-10**). Upper thoracic spine fractures are less common than fractures involving the cervical, lower thoracic, or lumbar spine.

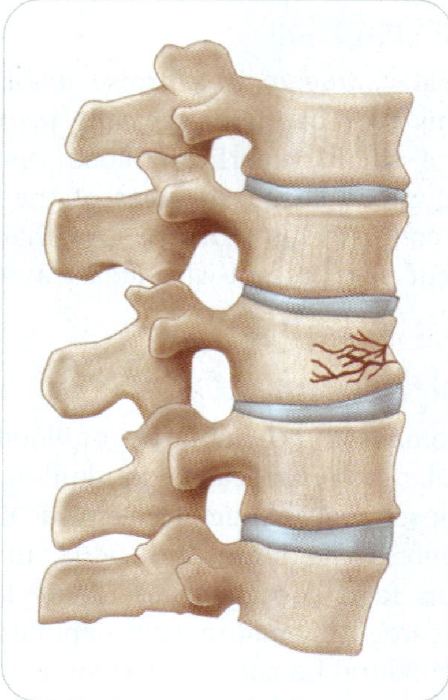

Figure 21-10 A compression fracture of a vertebral body looks like a stale marshmallow that has been squeezed between two hard surfaces.

The most common fractures of the spine occur in the lower-thoracic (mid-back) and lumbar (lower back) areas, or at the junction of the two (the thoracolumbar junction). Men experience fractures of the thoracic or lumbar spine from trauma four times more often than do women. Injuries involving the lumbar vertebrae are due to twisting forces and sudden axial loading, which can violently compress the vertebrae. Such injuries can also result from deceleration forces, as when deceleration flexes the lumbar spine in an individual restrained by a seatbelt. Injury of the sacral vertebrae is rare, whereas fracture of the coccyx is common and occurs when a person falls on the buttocks.

Neurologic injuries may result from direct or indirect injuries to the spinal cord. Direct or primary injury to the spinal cord can be caused by a broken or displaced vertebra putting pressure on the cord or by a laceration of cord nerve fibers by sharp bone ends. Indirect injury is caused by pressure from a hematoma inside the bony spinal canal which puts pressure on the spinal cord, or from traumatic swelling of the spinal cord, resulting in loss of blood supply to the cord called neural ischemia.

CASE Update

Since the patient is unresponsive, you immediately call for assistance. You instruct rescuers to bring a long backboard, a cervical collar, oxygen, and a trauma pack. You also request a toboggan and advanced life support. The supine patient's pulse is 62 beats per minute and regular. As you await help, you continue to maintain spinal motion restriction. At the same time, you begin to visually assess the patient's injuries. He has contusions on his right facial cheek and his forehead. Soon, several other OEC technicians arrive on scene.

What should you do now?

Neurogenic Shock

Neurogenic shock is a form of shock that is caused by disruption of the autonomic nervous system. As a result, peripheral blood vessels dilate, trapping blood in the capillary beds, which causes a precipitous drop in blood pressure. The most common cause of neurogenic shock is spinal cord injury. In addition to a low blood pressure, the condition is characterized by bradycardia (slow heart rate) and often a normal respiratory rate. Neurogenic shock is a potentially life-threatening complication of spine trauma that, although rare, must be considered. When caring for a patient with spine trauma, OEC technicians should always consider *other* causes of shock, especially hypovolemic shock, before attributing shock to neurogenic causes.

PATIENT ASSESSMENT FOR SPINE, BRAIN, AND NERVOUS SYSTEM INJURIES

After securing the scene, you begin the assessment of any patient by performing the primary patient assessment, looking for excessive bleeding and assessing the ABCDs (airway, breathing, circulation, disability). Investigate the chief complaint using SAMPLE (signs and symptoms, allergies, medications, past medical history, last oral intake, events leading up to the problem), and continue with the secondary patient assessment.

Evaluating the Brain for TBI

Look for the signs and listen for symptoms of TBI (**Table 21-3**). The OEC technician must realize that the signs and symptoms that may be attributed to a TBI can also be a result of other injuries or illness

Table 21-3 Signs and Symptoms of Traumatic Brain Injury
• Initial period of unresponsiveness • Altered mental status • Headache • Nausea, vomiting • Slurred speech • Pupillary dilation or unresponsiveness • Rise in systolic blood pressure and a widened pulse pressure • Slow pulse • Lucid period, after a period of unresponsiveness • Leakage of CSF from ears, nose, open wounds • Slow or irregular respirations • Amnesia • Dizziness • Seizures • Incontinence • Numbness, tingling, or paralysis in one or more extremities • Posturing • Paralysis • Raccoon eyes (a late sign, if seen at all) • Battle sign (a late sign, if seen at all)

to the nervous system such as a stroke, low blood sugar, low blood pressure, drug or alcohol ingestion, and others. Always consider other possibilities before saying the problem is a TBI.

Evaluating the Spine and Nervous System

Previously, many patients with neck or back pain were automatically strapped on a long backboard. This was referred to as "spinal immobilization." Many studies have shown this is not needed unless specific criteria are met. Since it is impossible to provide true immobilization to the spine in a prehospital setting, providers now use the phrase "spinal motion restriction" to describe decreasing the movement of the spine. Now many fewer patients need spine "protection" in the prehospital setting.

In unresponsive or altered mental status patients, if you *suspect* a spine injury in a trauma situation because of the possible catastrophic consequences of spinal cord injury, spinal motion restriction is maintained during the assessment and treatment. Conscious and alert patients can often be directed to simply limit movement of the spine allowing the OEC technician to complete an assessment and begin treatment. If you are alone, and CPR is necessary, begin one-person CPR as this takes priority. If two OEC technicians are available, one can provide spinal motion restriction while another performs the patient assessment or CPR if needed.

The assessment of a patient with a suspected brain or spinal cord injury should include an exam of the skull, spine, and nervous system. The first decision is whether or not to remove the helmet. It is recommended that you remove a helmet only if:

- The patient does not have a patent airway, is not breathing adequately, and the helmet prevents you from managing these problems.
- The helmet is too big or otherwise allows the patient's head to move while it is left in place.
- The helmet prevents you from properly placing a cervical collar due to its size or shape.
- The patient is in cardiac arrest.
- The helmet is broken and thus does not allow proper head and neck immobilization or visualization of injuries.

This assessment starts by palpating the head (skull) assuming you remove the helmet, each spinous process in the midline of the spinal column from the top of the posterior neck to the top of the sacrum. During this hands-on evaluation, look for pain and abnormalities such as a depression in the skull or misalignment or a step-off in the spinous processes of the spine. Look and feel for any evidence of trauma using the DCAP-BTLS mnemonic (deformity, contusions, abrasions/avulsions, punctures/penetrations, burns/bleeding/bruises, tenderness, lacerations, swelling).

Neurologic evaluation includes assessing responsiveness, looking for spinal fluid leakage, motor or muscle strength, sensation, and function of the eyes. It is recommended that OEC technicians use the AVPU scale (alert, verbal, pain, unresponsive) to determine the patient's level of responsiveness. Patients who have suffered neurologic insult may appear normal, confused, agitated, combative, or comatose. Assessment of the level of responsiveness must be repeated at least every 5 minutes because it can change rapidly.

Examine the eyes by performing a pupillary exam and an evaluation of extraocular movement. These tests were described in Chapter 7, *Patient Assessment*. Pay close attention to any abnormal findings such as pupils that are unequal, dilated, or unresponsive to light. Also make sure the patient can follow your finger with both eyes in all directions.

Examine the ears and nose for leakage of CSF, an indicator of a skull fracture. All skull fractures suggest a high-impact MOI, and almost always occur in combination with TBI. By itself, CSF appears clear and colorless and may be mistaken for sweat, rain, or melted snow. In the setting of neurologic trauma, CSF will likely be mixed with blood and may leak from the ear canals, nostrils, or mouth.

Damage to the spinal cord in the neck causes neurologic compromise to all four extremities. Injury to the spinal cord in the thoracic or lumbar region causes neurologic problems in just the legs.

Motor testing of nerves that come out of the spinal cord involves manually testing arm and leg muscle groups. In responsive patients, ask them to squeeze your index and long fingers, checking to see if strength is equal on both sides (**Figure 21-11**). Touch the fingers of both the patient's hands asking the person if they can feel it.

As you are performing your secondary patient assessment, obtain a SAMPLE history and take a complete set of vital signs. Attempt to determine the forces involved and whether the patient was

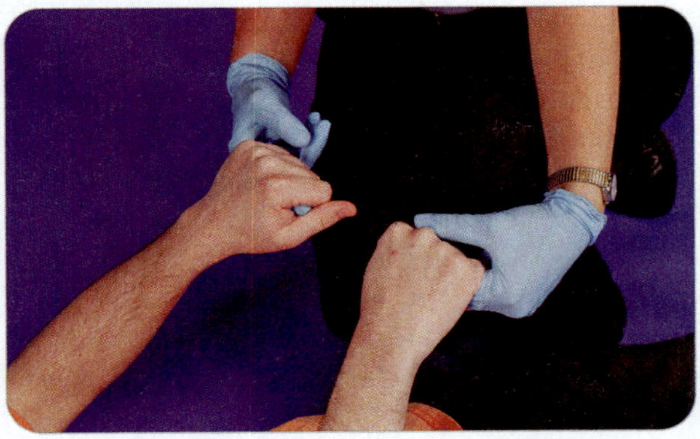

Figure 21-11 Assess the quality of strength in each extremity by asking the patient to squeeze your index and long fingers.

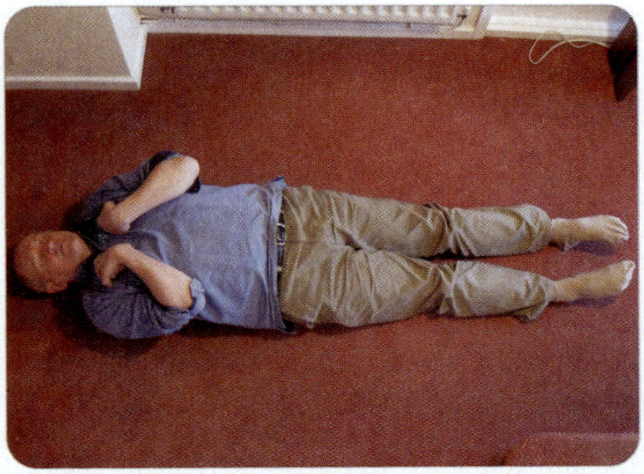

Figure 21-12 A patient exhibiting flexor posturing (decorticate).

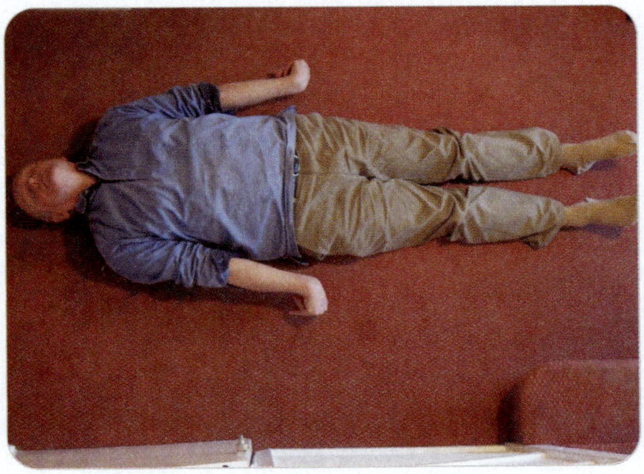

Figure 21-13 A patient exhibiting extension posturing (decerebrate).

rendered unresponsive, even if only momentarily. Be sure to ask the patient (or a friend or relative) if the patient has diabetes or a history of seizures, or if the patient used any mind-altering substances, including alcohol, legal and/or illicit drugs, because these can also alter neurologic findings. You may need to care for the patient for *both* a medical problem and the neurologic trauma.

Complete a head-to-toe exam noting any non-neurologic injuries, especially fractures of the scapula and posterior ribs. Patients with a suspected scapula or posterior rib fractures have a higher incidence of spinal injury. Many spinal injuries are not isolated, with extremity, chest, or abdominal injuries frequently present as well.

At the completion of the secondary assessment, and every 5 minutes thereafter, reassess the vital signs and carefully evaluate each value. TBI with increased intracranial pressure is associated with the following changes in vital signs:

- Increased systolic blood pressure
- Decreased diastolic blood pressure
- Tachypnea (abnormally rapid respiratory rate)
- Bradycardia (abnormally slow heart rate)

Other Findings

Posturing is an abnormal neurologic finding that indicates that the CNS has suffered a serious injury (**Figure 21-12** and **Figure 21-13**). Besides having loss of sensation and motor function below the injured level of the spinal cord, patients with a spinal cord injury often display a characteristic sign in which the skin below the level of the injury is *flushed*, whereas above the level of the injury the skin color is normal or pale. This response results from disruption of the nerve pathways. In most cases the impairment will be present on both sides of the body, but in rare instances it can be on one side only. As indicated previously, spontaneous breathing may be absent in a patient with a spinal cord injury at or above the level of C5. Males may have a persistent erection, called a priapism, due to CNS damage.

After you have completed the patient assessment, continue to monitor the patient's ABCDs, level of responsiveness, distal CMS (circulation, movement, sensation), and vital signs approximately every 5 minutes, documenting any changes you observe on your patient care report (PCR).

Spinal Motion Restriction

An OEC technician should always consider the possibility of injury to the axial spine and neurologic injury during the primary and secondary patient assessment. If spinal injury is found or suspected, it is necessary to provide careful transfer of the patient and spinal motion restriction to avoid further injury and to provide comfort. Spinal motion restriction means that all transfers should be done with careful attention to limiting spinal motion and may include the use of different devices such as a stretcher or a gurney, whole body vacuum splint, or backboard as transfer devices. When using spinal motion restriction, a cervical collar is necessary. Once the patient is moved to a transportation device, the spine should be protected against further movement with padding or bracing to fill voids and strapping to limit movement laterally and axially. Research has shown that securing an injured person to a backboard is not a benign procedure and subjects an individual to pain, apprehension, potential injury to skin, potential worsening of injury, and limited ability for the patient to protect the airway, so this should be avoided and done only for patients who need it.

KEY POINT

Spinal Motion Restriction

When a patient with spinal trauma is moved without taking spinal precautions using spinal motion restriction, damage to the spinal cord can occur. Unstable vertebrae or vertebral bone fragments may intrude into the spinal canal and may put direct pressure on the spinal cord.

The decision to institute spinal motion restriction involves three elements, as shown in **Figure 21-14**.

Spinal motion restriction is *required* when there is:

- Potential (MOI) for spine injury with normal patient mental status (*A* in AVPU) *and* actual exam findings associated with a spinal injury. In an alert patient, MOI alone should not dictate spinal motion restriction.
- Potential (MOI) for spine injury with an alteration of the mental status (less than *A* in AVPU) such that a reliable physical exam cannot be done.
- Any positive physical findings in the exam step.
- Potential (MOI) for spine injury in a patient with a distracting injury that makes evaluation impossible.
- An unresponsive patient (less than *A* in AVPU) involved in an unwitnessed trauma accident.

Spinal motion restriction is *not needed* for:

- Low energy incidents even with minor injuries.
- "Just in case" there is an injury (low level probability).
- A headache, brief loss of consciousness (a few seconds) or concussion in a now otherwise alert and oriented patient.
- Patients who are up and walking at the scene without physical findings or symptoms.
- Isolated penetrating trauma without spinal or neurologic deficit.

A distracting injury is *any* injury that makes your evaluation impossible to accurately determine. Not all serious injuries are distracting. You cannot make a list of distracting injuries. Even though the patient could have a broken hip or femur that is painful, this injury may not be distracting if you can have the patient concentrate and get an accurate evaluation and exam. However, someone with an open forearm fracture could be so fixated on this arm injury, that you may not get an accurate exam. The OEC technician needs to

KEY POINT

Distracting Injuries

A distracting injury is *any* injury that makes the patient focus on that injury instead of responding appropriately to your continued assessment.

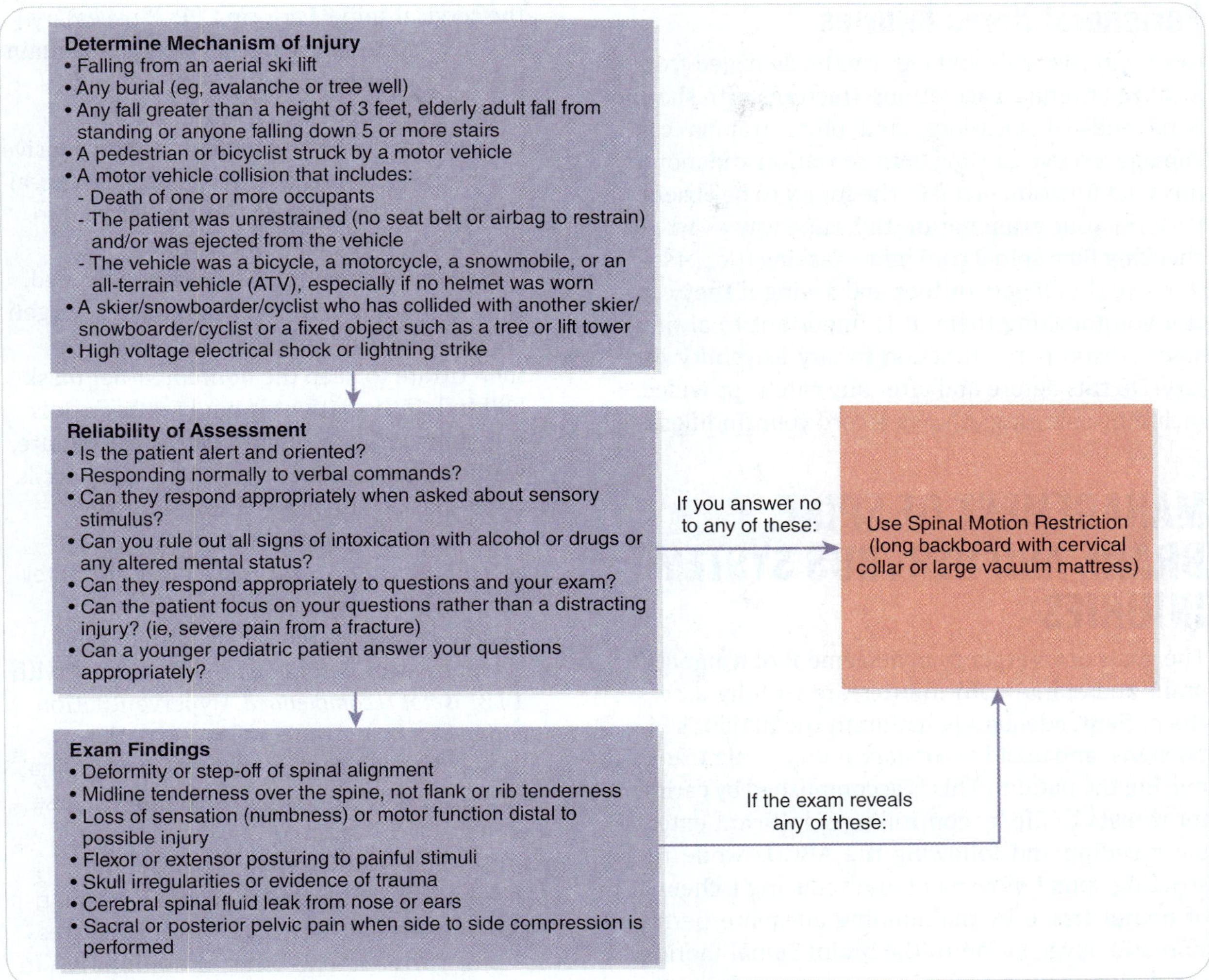

Figure 21-14 Spinal motion restriction algorithm.

decide if other injuries *distract* the patient from giving an accurate spine evaluation to determine if spinal motion restriction is needed. If you have any doubt that another injury is distracting the patient, err on the cautious side and use spinal motion restriction.

If you suspect a spinal injury in the field and you are in a situation where it is not possible to obtain an adequate exam or it is more important to get the patient inside as quickly as possible, for example, during severely inclement weather, use spinal motion restriction. Once you get the patient indoors and perform an adequate evaluation and exam, and if you find spinal motion restriction is not indicated, remove any materials used to restrict motion. This is *not* clearing the spine, but delaying your evaluation with restriction, until a proper evaluation can be done. This should not happen very often, as most patients can be adequately evaluated in the field. (Check if regulations in your state allow you to follow this guideline.)

Also, if the patient was not alert initially and later the mental status improves to normal and they are a solid *A* on the AVPU scale allowing you to accurately evaluate and examine the patient, if spinal motions restriction is not indicated, you can remove any materials or devices used to restrict motion. Again, this is delaying the evaluation until conditions permit, as now the patient has normal mental status allowing an accurate exam. When in doubt, continue spinal motion restriction until a higher-level EMS provider evaluates the patient. (If regulations permit you to do so within your state you may follow this recommendation.)

Peripheral Nerve Injuries

Nerves in the arms and legs can be damaged from localized trauma. Lacerations, fractures with sharp bone ends, dislocations, and blunt trauma can damage a nerve causing both sensation and motor (muscle) function distal to the injury to be absent. Perform your examination the same way as when checking for a spinal cord injury: asking the person to move the fingers or toes and seeing if they can feel you touching them. It is important to always assess distal nerve function in any extremity injury. Do this before and after any care is provided, including splinting. Always record your findings.

MANAGEMENT OF SPINE, BRAIN, AND NERVOUS SYSTEM INJURIES

The goals of emergency management of traumatic brain and spinal cord injuries are to fully assess the patient, adequately maintain the patient's vital signs, and avoid secondary injury while transporting the patient. This is accomplished by caring for threats to life by controlling significant external bleeding and following the ABCDs while restricting spinal movement and reducing ischemia of neural tissue by maintaining adequate perfusion and oxygenation to the brain. Spinal motion restriction is used to prevent secondary injury to the spinal cord.

Serious brain injuries are potentially life threatening and require rapid transport to a definitive medical facility, preferably a trauma center. OEC technicians are not expected to be able to differentiate between different types of serious brain injuries. It is, however, crucial that OEC technicians be able to identify patients with signs and symptoms of significant brain injuries and arrange appropriate transport to a trauma center capable of managing such injuries. One of the hardest decisions an OEC technician makes, is what to do with a head trauma patient when they are brought to the first-aid room. Always do a full evaluation, looking for subtle neurologic changes. When in doubt, EMS transport is best.

Care of patients with serious head or spine injuries consists of the following steps:

1. Correct any threats to life (ABCDs) that may be present while protecting the spine, especially the cervical spine. Perform CPR, if necessary. Control severe external bleeding and maintain blood flow to body tissues. Establish and maintain an adequate airway using the jaw-thrust maneuver. If the patient is unresponsive and has no gag reflex, insert an oropharyngeal airway or nasopharyngeal airway. Suction to keep the airway clear as needed.
2. Provide supplemental oxygen when needed. If the patient is breathing, administer oxygen via nonrebreather mask at 15 LPM, and then titrate to keep the nonrebreather mask half full. If the patient is not breathing or is breathing less than eight breaths per minute, ventilate the patient using a bag-valve mask, watching each breath so the chest rises normally, using supplemental oxygen *at a normal respiratory rate*. Use a pulse oximeter keeping the oxygen saturation between 94 and 99%. *Hyperventilation* with oxygen (oxygen saturation of 100%) of a patient with a TBI is *not recommended*. Hyperventilation can in fact be detrimental to the patient.
3. Protect the spine until assessment for spinal motion restriction has been completed. Use manual stabilization of the cervical spine, until spinal evaluation is done. If spinal motion restriction is needed, apply a collar, padding and backboard, or vacuum mattress.
4. If time permits, treat other minor injuries. In severe brain or spinal injuries, transport as soon as possible. If CSF is leaking from the ears or nose, do not attempt to stop the flow.
5. Transport the patient with the head uphill to prevent worsening of an intracranial head injury.
6. Continually monitor the patient. Check the patient's level of responsiveness and other vital signs every 5 minutes and record any changes later in the PCR.
7. Transport the patient to a definitive-care facility as soon as possible.

Manual Stabilization of the Neck

Initially manually stabilize the neck and spine of any patient with a significant mechanism for potential head or spinal cord injury. If findings do not indicate the need for spinal motion restriction after a quality spine and neurologic evaluation, manual stabilization can be discontinued. Put a cervical

KEY POINT

Oxygen Level for a TBI

Hyperventilation with oxygen of a patient with a TBI is *not recommended.* Use a pulse oximeter and titrate keeping the oxygen saturation between 94 and 99%.

collar in place if findings indicate the need for spinal motion restriction. To manually stabilize the neck and spine, follow the steps in **OEC Skill 21-1**.

Sizing and Applying a Cervical Collar

Manual in-line stabilization of the head and cervical spine is the first step in properly restricting motion in a patient with a spine injury. Because it is impractical to continue manual in-line stabilization during transport, use an adjunct device. Rigid cervical collars (also called C-collars or extrication collars) are designed to provide support for the head and cervical spine during transport, but they provide only partial restriction. Therefore, always use these devices in conjunction with a long backboard. The whole body vacuum mattress when applied correctly does not require a cervical collar.

OEC SKILL 21-1 Performing Neutral Head Alignment

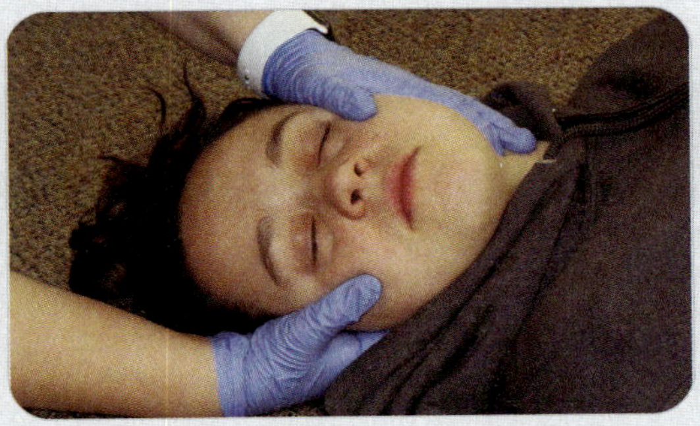

1 Kneel next to the patient's head, either to the side or at the top of the head. Place your hands on either side of the patient's head, with the palms adjacent to the ears and the fingers supporting the jaw and the back of the head.

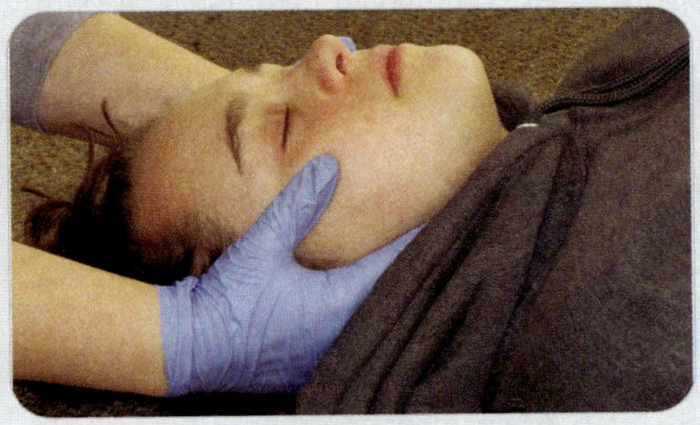

2 Gently move the head so that the patient's eyes are looking forward and the patient's nose and chin are aligned with the sternum. *Never force the head into alignment*. If the patient has muscle spasms in the neck or if your movement causes increased pain in the neck or numbness, tingling, or weakness in the extremities; or if alignment compromises airway or breathing, stop what you are doing and stabilize the patient in the position found. Continue to manually support the head while your partner applies a cervical collar around the neck. If the head cannot be moved into alignment, you may have to stabilize the head using a blanket roll. Do not allow the patient to move.

To be effective, a cervical collar must be properly sized to the patient. When properly sized, a cervical collar should rest on the shoulder and provide firm support under the chin, along both sides of the mandible, and at the occiput on the back of the head, without obstructing the airway (**Figure 21-15**). OEC technicians should always follow the manufacturer's directions.

In general, to properly size and apply a cervical collar, follow the steps in **OEC Skill 21-2**.

In general, a properly sized cervical collar will restrict motion of the head and cervical spine in neutral alignment without hyperextending the neck, and the chin will rest flush with the edge of the chin cup. Do not hyperextend or flex the neck. An improperly sized or applied cervical collar can compromise airway patency, cervical spine stability, and cause further injury. Therefore, if the appropriate size is not available, or if the cervical collar cannot be applied appropriately for any reason, do not use it. Instead, use a commercial head block, a tightly rolled towel against each side of the head as a head block, or place a horseshoe-shaped blanket over the top of the head, and then secure the patient's head to the long backboard using cravats (**Figure 21-16**).

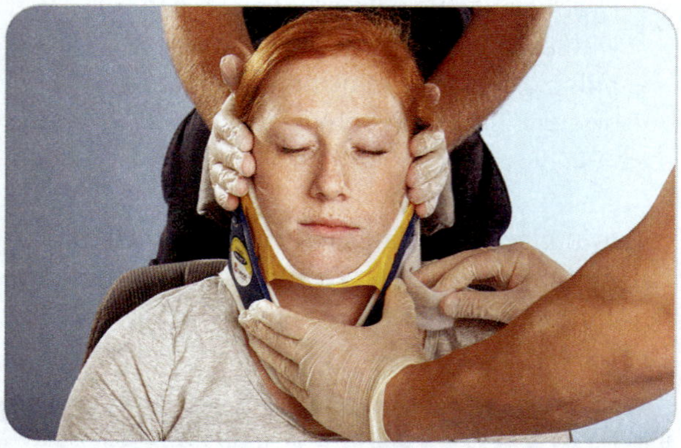

Figure 21-15 Some cervical collars can be adjusted to fit all sizes.

OEC SKILL 21-2 Sizing and Applying a Cervical Collar

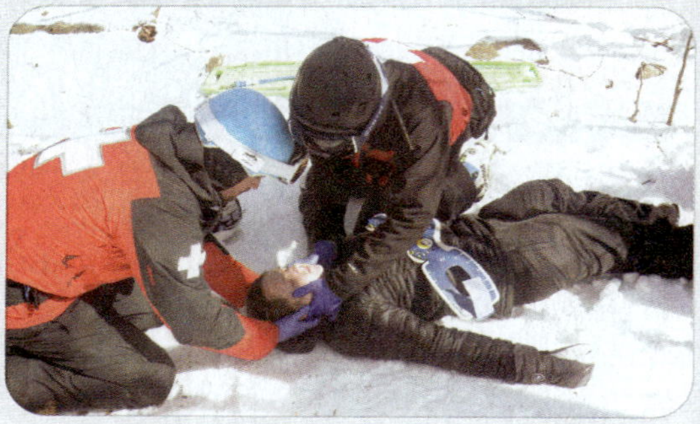

1. Maintain or establish manual stabilization of the head and cervical spine.

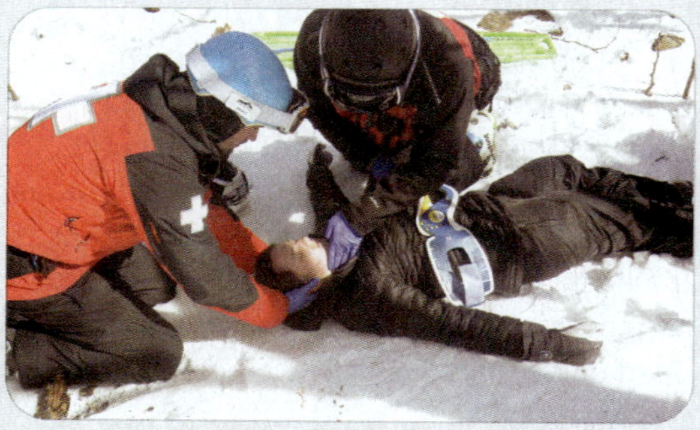

2. Measure the patient and the cervical collar. Be sure to follow the manufacturer's specifications for sizing for each of the different collar types.

(continues)

OEC SKILL 21-2 Sizing and Applying a Cervical Collar (*continued*)

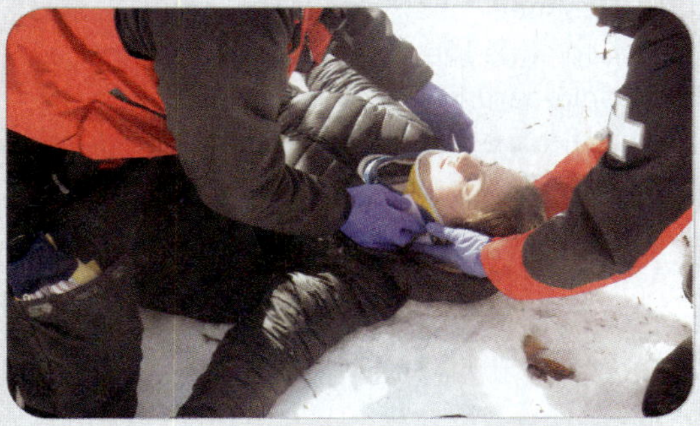

© Edward McNamara.

3 Apply the cervical collar.
- Open the patient's coat or shirt.
- Move any bulky clothing out of the way. Do not put the collar on over clothing.
- Slide the posterior neck portion of the collar behind the patient's neck.
- Swing the chin portion of the collar up over the patient's chest until it cups the chin.
- Secure the cervical collar using the Velcro closure and ensure a proper fit.

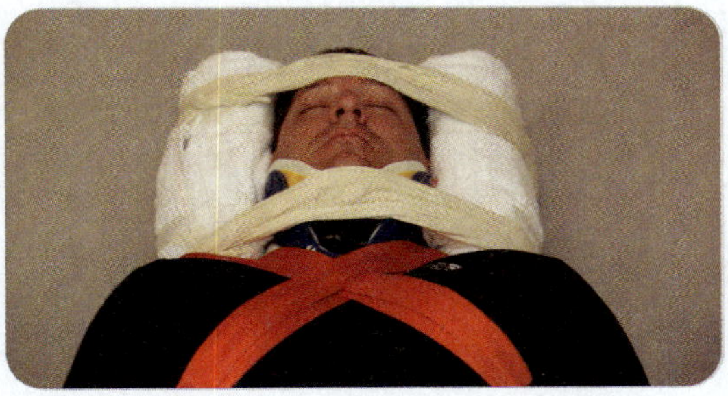

Figure 21-16 Head stabilization can be performed by using rolled towels or blankets placed on either side of the patient's head.

© Mike Halloran.

RESTRICTING THE MOTION OF THE SPINE

Placing a Patient on a Long Backboard

Supine Patient

For patients who are logrolled, the procedure must be carefully executed to prevent any twisting or excessive bending of the spine. Ideally, a logroll should be performed using at least four rescuers. Prior to beginning the logroll make sure a cervical collar has been applied. To logroll a supine patient onto a long backboard, refer to Chapter 5, *Moving, Lifting, and Transporting Patients* (OEC Skill 5-7).

As the rescuers continue to hold the patient, Rescuer 1 checks to make sure the patient is properly centered on the long backboard. If the patient is not centered on the long backboard, the patient must be centered by performing an axial drag. As discussed in Chapter 5, *Moving, Lifting, and Transporting Patients*, a drag is a method of pulling a patient on the ground to another location. An axial drag is used to center a patient on a backboard.

To center the patient on the long backboard using an axial drag, follow the steps in **OEC Skill 21-3**.

This procedure may be repeated as necessary until the patient is properly positioned on the long backboard. Alternatively, at the start of the procedure, place the long backboard with about a foot

KEY POINT

Vomiting

Vomiting is common with TBI. Have suction available and be prepared to turn patients who are placed on a long backboard onto their sides to prevent aspiration of the vomit.

OEC SKILL 21-3 Performing the Axial Drag

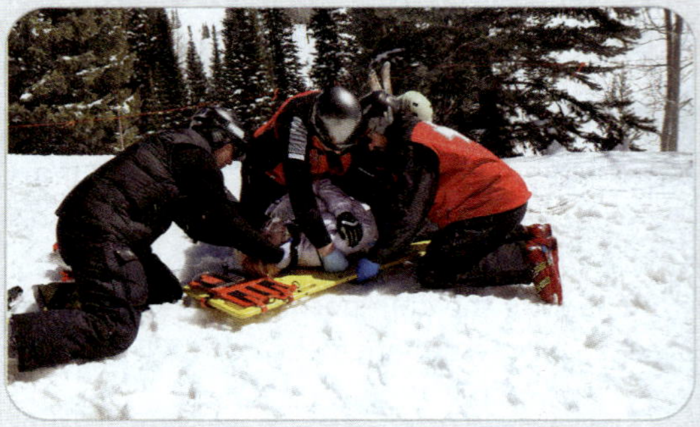

1 Rescuer 1 instructs Rescuers 2, 3, and 4 to slide the patient toward the foot of the backboard (toward the rescuers) on the count of three. Rescuers' hands should be at the hip area pulling the patient down to the foot of the board.

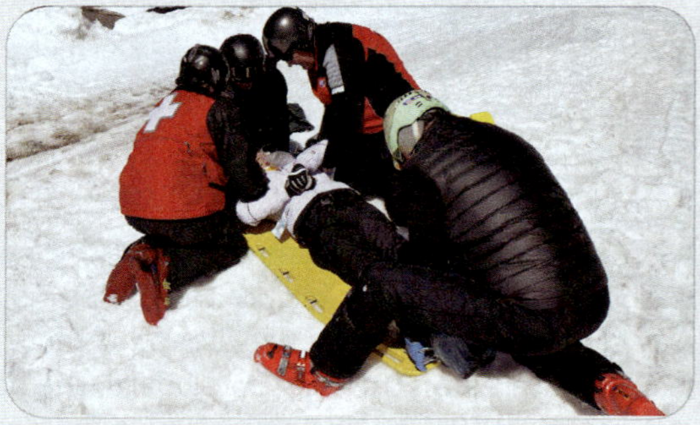

2 Rescuer 1 instructs rescuers to slide the patient into the proper position on the count of three. Pull the patient up toward the head of the long backboard with rescuers' hands under the armpits on each side and moving simultaneously.

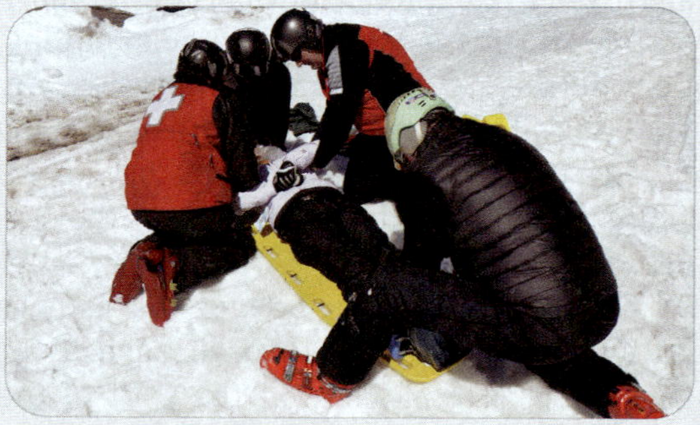

3 Repeat Step 2 until the patient is positioned on the board correctly.

and a half of it extending *above* the patient's head and then do an axial drag to center the patient. Once properly positioned on the long backboard, the patient is secured using straps, cravats, tape, or a commercial device.

Other types of emergency drags, including the shoulder drag, feet drag, blanket drag, and under-arm-wrist drag are covered in Chapter 5, *Moving, Lifting, and Transporting Patients*. To secure the patient onto the long backboard, perform the procedure presented in **OEC Skill 21-4**.

Sitting Patient

Not every spine injury patient you encounter will be lying down. Some will be wedged against a rock or tree, sitting in an automobile, or will sit down following their accident. Sitting patients who can move on their own volition and who are reliable, should be allowed to lay themselves onto a stretcher, toboggan, or vacuum mattress. Stabilize the head by placing a cervical collar prior to having the patient move. A sitting

KEY POINT

Pediatric Considerations

Because a child's head is larger in relation to its body than is the case for adults, pad beneath a child's shoulders to lift the thorax and allow the head and neck to assume a neutral position.

patient who has a neurologic deficit or is unreliable should be moved to a supine position after manually stabilizing the head and cervical spine and applying a cervical collar. The patient must be moved carefully to ensure axial alignment when moving from a sitting to a supine position. At that point move the patient to a long backboard.

Standing Patient

If the patient is standing and meets the criteria for spinal motion restriction, apply a cervical collar

OEC SKILL 21-4 Securing the Patient onto a Long Backboard

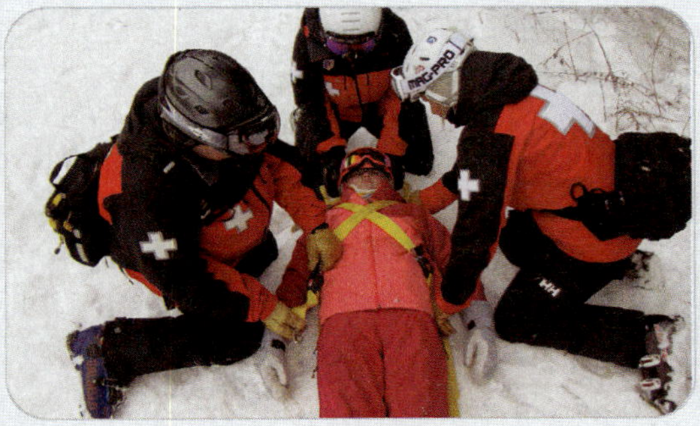

1 Secure the torso first. Cross the straps from over the shoulder to just above the opposite hip and tighten smoothly as the patient takes a deep breath. Do not tug or overtighten. (An appropriately tight strap should allow you to fit one finger between the strap and the patient and should never compromise the patient's ability to breathe.) If you are using a commercial device, follow the manufacturer's directions. Pad any voids using towels, blankets, or clothing to prevent movement or twisting of the spine and to improve the patient's comfort. There is usually a void under the knees that needs padding.

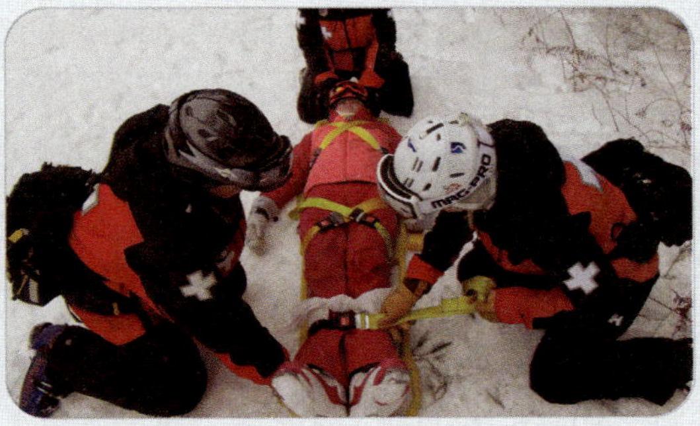

2 Secure the pelvis and the extremities next. Beginning where the torso straps end to prevent gaps, cross the pelvis straps from above the iliac crests (the patient's hips) to just below the level of the greater trochanter of each femur (the upper thigh). This ensures that the entire weight of the pelvis is contained within the straps and is properly immobilized. (Alternatively, a single strap can be placed across the pelvis at the level of the pubis bone.) An additional strap should be placed across the mid-thighs between the end of the pelvis straps and the knees. Place another strap across the lower legs. If the patient has a possible pelvis or hip fracture or an abdominal injury, you may need to place the straps just above or below the injury, but never place them tightly across the abdomen.

(continues)

OEC SKILL 21-4 Securing the Patient onto a Long Backboard (*continued*)

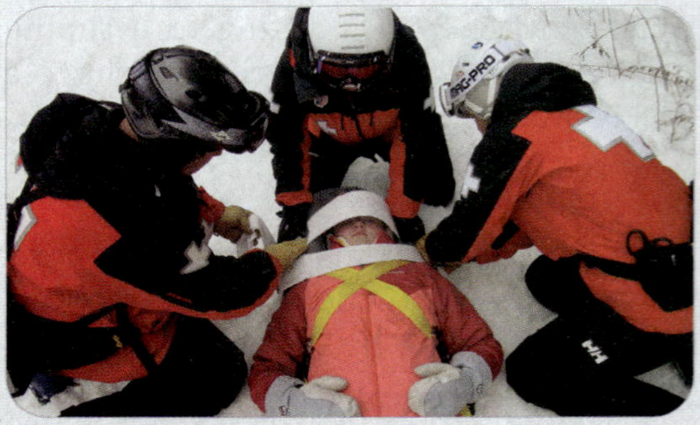

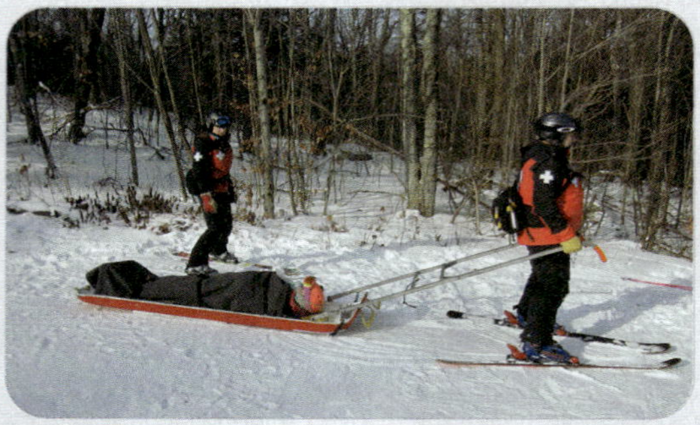

3 Secure the head last. If you are using a commercial head immobilization device (head blocks), follow the manufacturer's directions. If you are using towels rolls:

- Roll two standard towels and securely tape each roll.
- Place one towel on each side of the patient's head.
- Secure the head by placing a large piece of tape or a cravat over the patient's forehead. Be sure not to cover the eyelids. Place a second piece of tape over the C-collar just below the chin.

An alternative method is to place a rolled-up (horse-collar shaped) blanket around the patient's head and secure it at the chin and forehead.

If you have determined that the helmet should remain on the patient, use commercial head blocks or towels, and strap the helmet to the board.

4 Reassess the patient's airway and breathing. Also reassess distal circulation, sensation, and movement in each extremity. Document these CMS findings on the PCR. Monitor the patient throughout transport. Given that vomiting is common with TBI, have suction available and be prepared to roll patients who have undergone spinal motion restriction onto their sides while they remain strapped to the board.

and assist the patient in lying down on the backboard. Complete spinal motion restriction and transport the patient.

Placing a Patient on a Large Vacuum Mattress (Splint)

To get the patient onto the vacuum mattress use the same method as for a long backboard. The patient is logrolled onto their side, and the deflated mat is placed flat right next to the patient. The patient is kept in axial alignment as they are rolled onto the mattress. Then, with axial drags, the patient is centered on the mat. No straps are needed. The mat is rolled up on the sides, around the patient from head to toe, and the air is sucked out, forming a rigid construct around the patient, and providing spinal motion restriction.

To place a patient on a full-body vacuum mattress, follow the steps in **OEC Skill 21-5**.

OEC SKILL 21-5 Placing a Patient on a Full-Body Vacuum Mattress

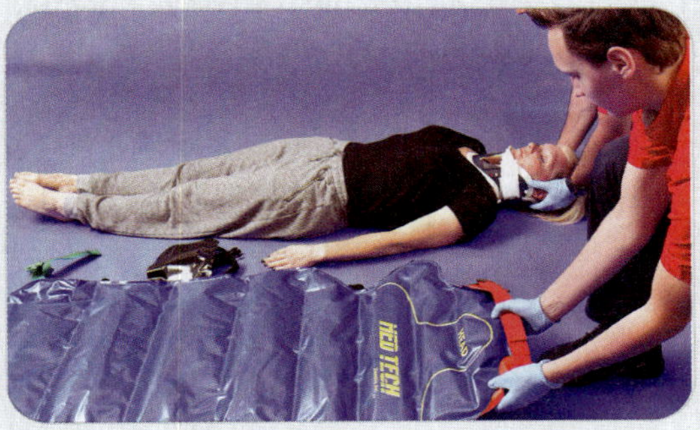

1 Place the mattress on a flat surface near the patient, with the head end of the mattress at the patient's head.

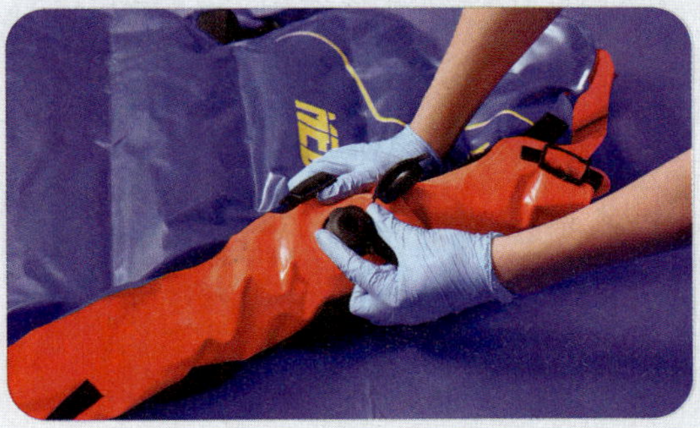

2 Allow air to enter the mattress. Keep the valve stem open until the mattress is soft and pliable.

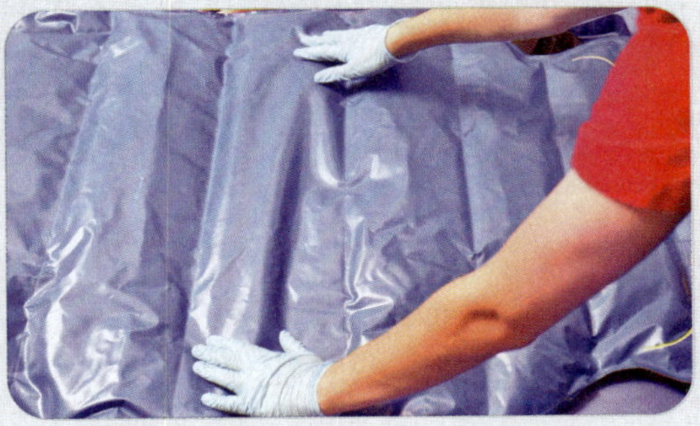

3 Smooth the mattress so it is flat and level.

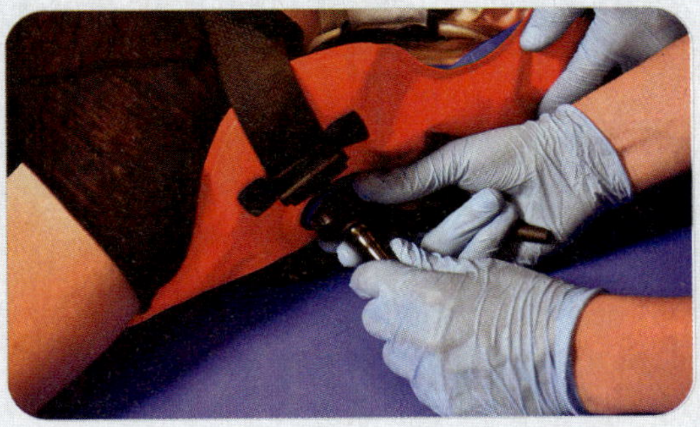

4 Connect the pump to the mattress.

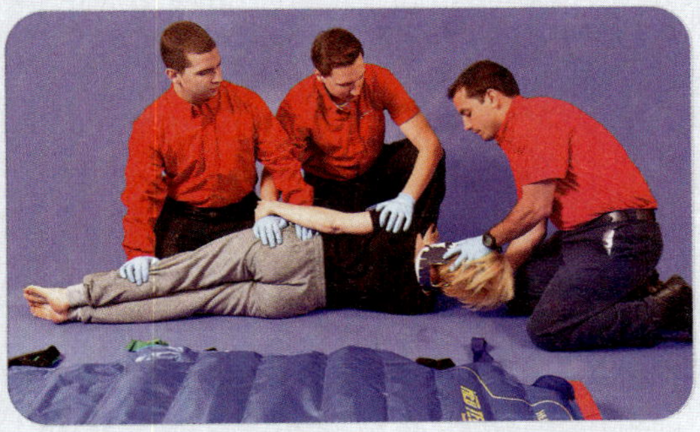

5 Determine which method you will use to move the patient onto the mattress. If you use the logroll, evacuate the mattress until it is partially rigid (this step is not needed if you are using the scoop stretcher method). The surface should be smooth and the beads should be spread out as evenly as possible.

(continues)

OEC SKILL 21-5 Placing a Patient on a Full-Body Vacuum Mattress (*continued*)

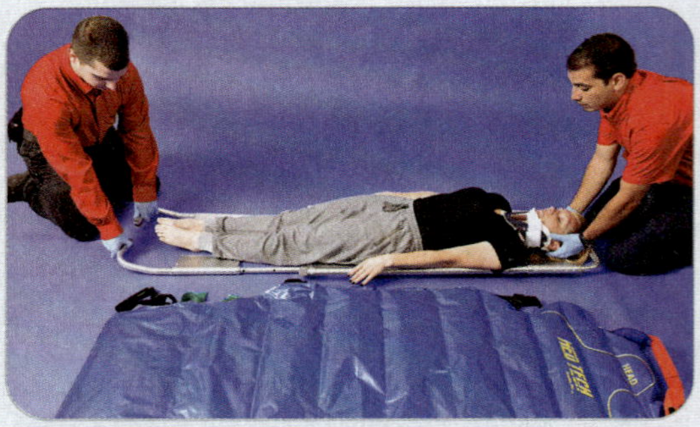

If using a scoop stretcher, you do not need to partially evacuate the mattress at this stage.

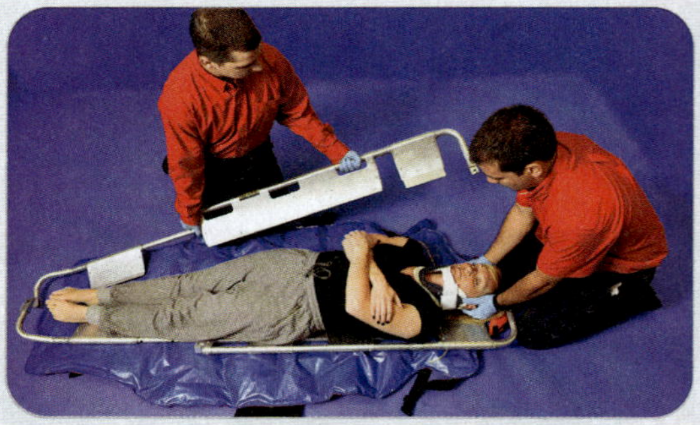

6 Move the patient onto the vacuum mattress using the method you determined during the previous step. Maintain spinal alignment.

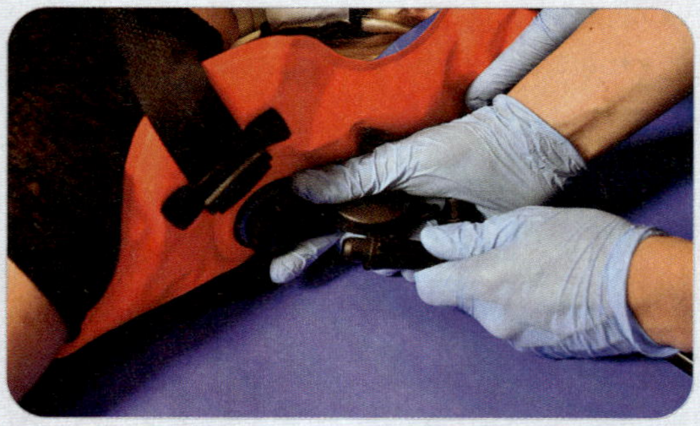

7 If the vacuum mattress is partially rigid, open the valve to allow air to enter. Keep the valve open until the mattress is pliable.

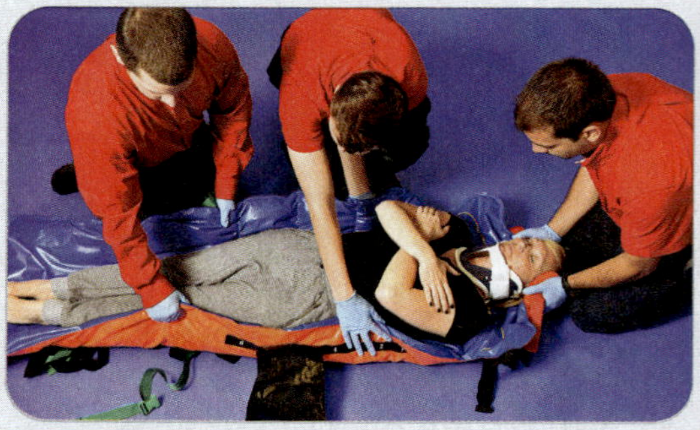

8 Conform the mattress to each side of the patient's head close to the shoulders, but not the top of the head. Continue to hold these "head blocks" that you have formed, and have a second person hold up the sides of the mattress to the patient's hips until the mattress is evacuated of air completely. Always form the mattress to meet the needs of the patient.

(continues)

OEC SKILL 21-5 Placing a Patient on a Full-Body Vacuum Mattress (*continued*)

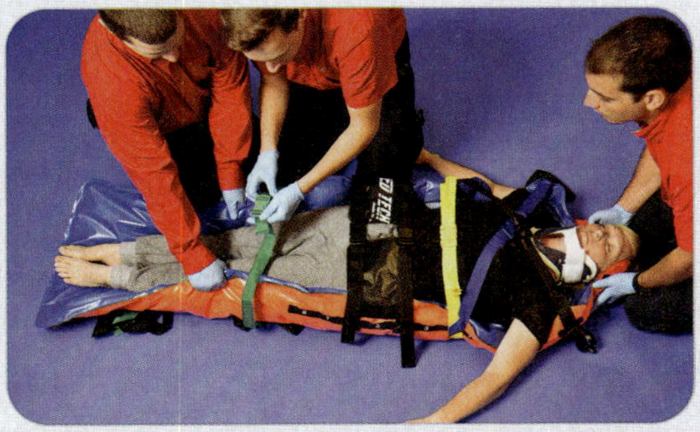

9 Secure the patient's chest, hips, and legs in the mattress.

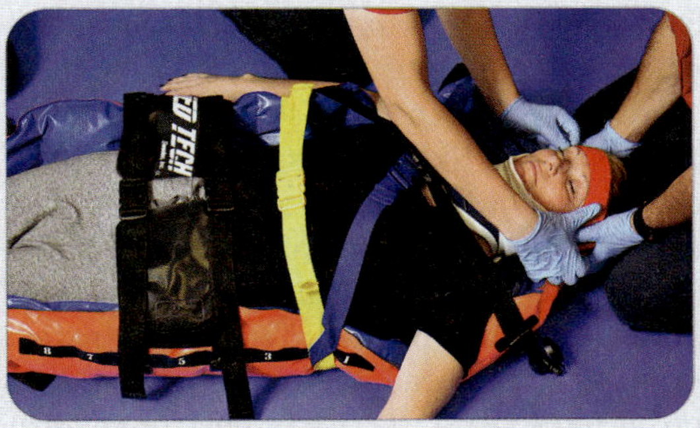

10 Secure the patient's head with medical tape. Pad any voids at the top of the shoulders.

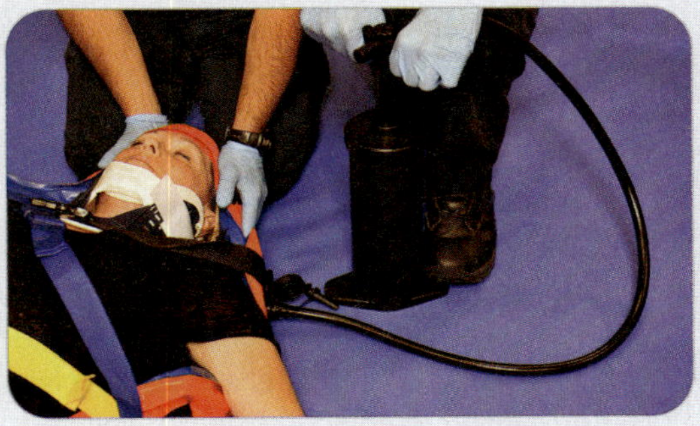

11 Ensure the patient is as comfortable as possible, then evacuate the remaining air to achieve immobilization.

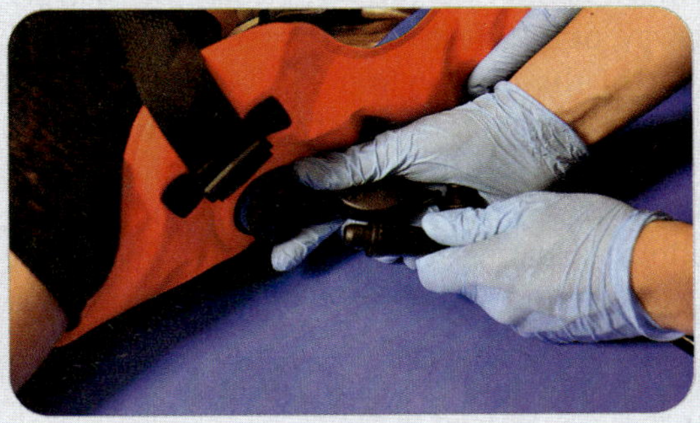

12 Disconnect the vacuum pump and ensure that the valve is closed or secured so the mattress is not accidently deflated.

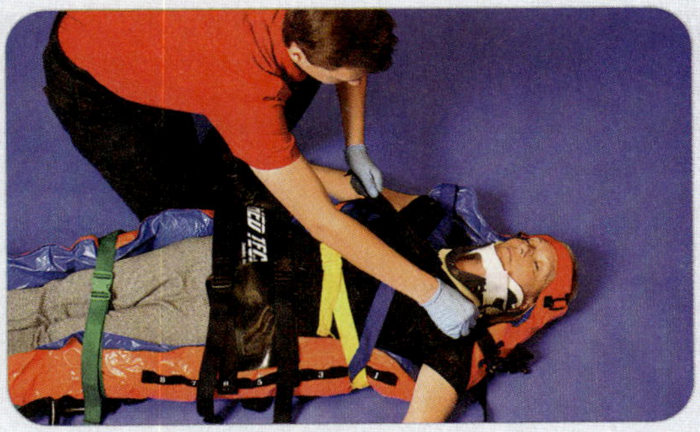

13 Reassess and adjust the straps around the chest, hips, and legs.

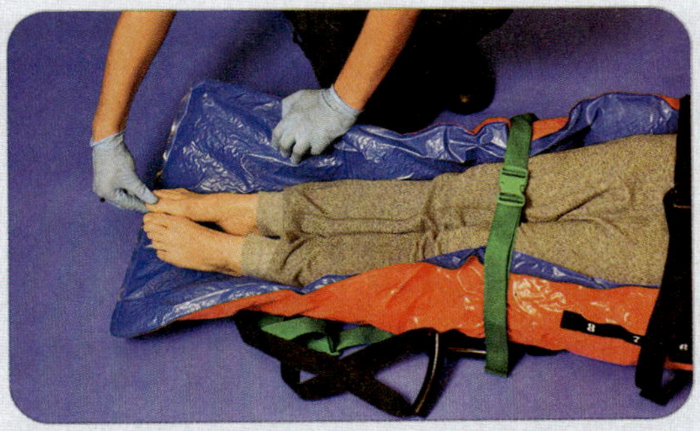

14 Check the patient's neurovascular status and recheck all straps prior to lifting or moving the patient.

Removing a Helmet

As a result of effective injury prevention efforts, most cyclists, all-terrain vehicle riders, snow machine riders, rafters, climbers, equestrians, and an increasing number of skiers and snowboarders and other outdoor enthusiasts, now wear helmets while participating in their chosen sports. According to the National Ski Area Association in 2019, 85% of skiers/snowboarders wore a helmet. The National Medical Committee of the National Ski Patrol recommends that anyone who participates in a snow sport wear a helmet to reduce the severity of injuries to the head. Wearing a helmet does not appear to increase the risk of neck or cervical spine injuries in adults.

Even though the presence of a helmet can complicate the management of the patient, you may not need to remove the helmet to care for the patient. If a helmet fits properly, does not obstruct the airway, or interfere with assessment and management of the airway, and can be incorporated into proper spinal motion restriction of the spine, it may be left on. If it is necessary to remove the helmet and the patient is sitting or standing, you may allow the patient to remove their own helmet if they are willing and able while you are stabilizing the head.

It is recommended that you remove a helmet only if:

- The patient does not have a patent airway, is not breathing adequately, and the helmet prevents you from managing these problems.
- The helmet is too big or otherwise allows the patient's head to move while it is left in place.
- The helmet prevents you from properly placing a cervical collar due to its size or shape.
- The patient is in cardiac arrest.
- The helmet is broken and thus does not allow proper head and neck immobilization or visualization of injuries.

To remove a helmet, follow the steps in **OEC Skill 21-6**.

KEY POINT

Removing a Player's Shoulder Pads

Current recommendations are not to remove shoulder pads but rather to pad under the head or shoulder to maintain neutrality. It is also recommended to not remove the helmet unless necessary.
If removing the shoulder pads from an injured football, lacrosse, or hockey player, do not pull them off over the head; instead, remove them by untying/unlacing/cutting them. This approach applies to any sports equipment, including helmets, whose removal causes hyperextension of the neck.

OEC SKILL 21-6 Removing a Helmet from a Patient

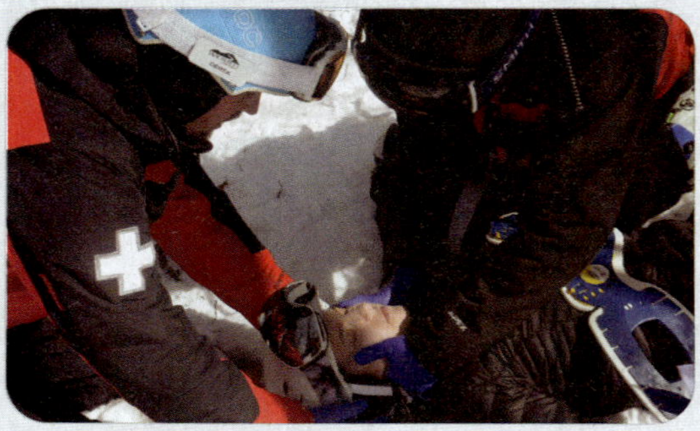

1 Align the patient axially. Rescuer 1: manually stabilize the head and cervical spine by placing one hand on either side of the helmet.

(continues)

OEC SKILL 21-6 Removing a Helmet from a Patient (*continued*)

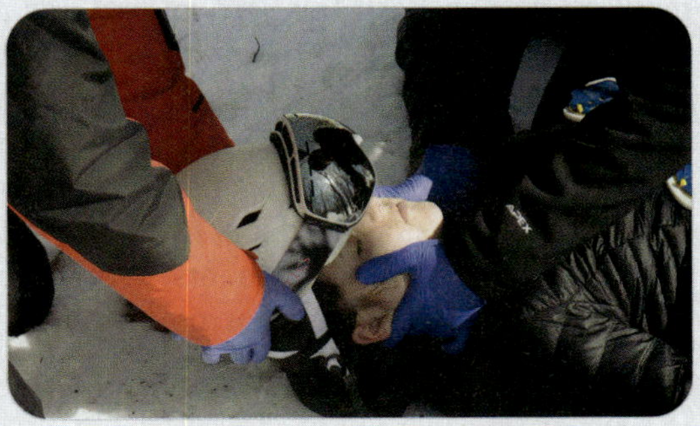

2 Rescuer 2: carefully open the face shield and/or remove goggles (if present). Unfasten the chin strap and place one hand at the occiput and the other at the chin. If blood is suspected, use standard precautions. As an alternative method, Rescuer 2 places one hand along either side of the patient's head sliding your hands inside the helmet, so that the fingers are in position to support each side of the face up over the ears. Either method is acceptable.

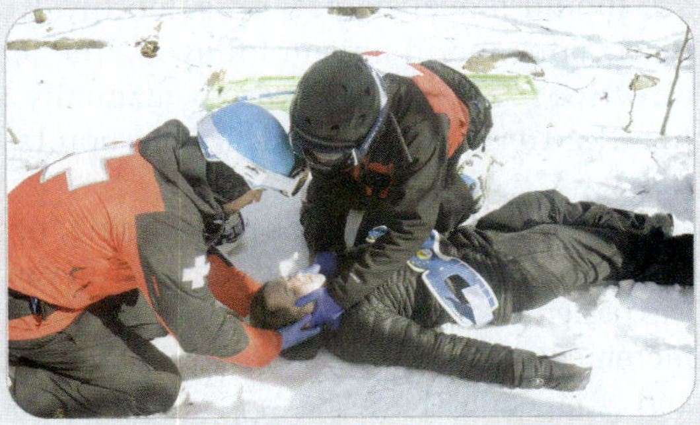

3 Remove the helmet.

- Rescuer 1 grasps the helmet straps or sides of the helmet and pulls them apart, spreading the helmet, then pulls the helmet axially away from the patient's head, providing forward rotation of the helmet to ease passage of the chin guard (plastic device that protects the mouth and chin area on some types of ski and other sports helmets) off the face.
- Rescuer 2 slides the fingers up to the occiput and chin (or on both sides of the head over the ears), ensuring that the patient's head and cervical spine remain immobilized. Continue to stabilize the head until a cervical collar is applied.

Stabilized Extrication and Transfer: "Jams and Pretzels"

Patients who incur serious injuries in the field often are found in a contorted position with severely angulated limbs. To effectively immobilize and transport these patients, it is often necessary to move them into an anatomically correct supine position so that they may be packaged with spinal motion restriction. This process is referred to as **jams and pretzels**. Always remember to apply a cervical collar prior to moving a patient when spinal motion restriction is necessary.

Rescuers encounter injured patients in one of six basic anatomic positions: three primary positions (1, 2, and 3) and three variations (1a, 2a, and 3a). These positions were popularized by Warren Bowman, MD, and were introduced to the NSP in

Outdoor Emergency Care, Third Edition under the general topic of "jams and pretzels." The following descriptions of positioning and the methods of moving patients are adapted from his descriptions.

- *Position 1.* Patients are supine, in a neutral anatomic position with the back straight and the eyes facing forward. The extremities are straight, with the palms against the thighs. Ideally, patients should be aligned in this position before transfer to a long backboard (**Figure 21-17A**).
- *Position 1a.* Patients are supine but their head, neck, back, and/or extremities are rotated, bent, or in some position other than an anatomically correct position (**Figure 21-17B**).
- *Position 2.* Patients are on their side, but in a neutral anatomic position with the back straight, the eyes facing forward, the extremities straight, and the palms against the sides of the thighs. Patients in this position should be rolled in one direction to Position 1 by using a logroll (**Figure 21-17C**).
- *Position 2a.* Patients are on their side, with the head, neck, back, and extremities in any position except a normal anatomic position (**Figure 21-17D**).
- *Position 3.* Patients are prone but in a neutral anatomic position, except that the head is usually turned to the side (**Figure 21-17E**).
- *Position 3a.* Patients are prone, with the head, neck, back, and extremities in any position except a neutral anatomic position (**Figure 21-17F**).

The goal of positioning an injured patient is to move the person, especially one with a suspected spinal injury, into Position 1, either on the ground or on a backboard, without causing any damage to the spinal cord or further neurologic injury. When a patient lies supine in the anatomic position, the back of the person's head (occiput), shoulders, buttocks, calves, and heels are all in the same line. In this position, the three important posterior reference points are the head, shoulders, and hips, and the three important anterior reference points are the nose, naval, and toes.

The process of placing a patient into anatomic alignment is termed **stabilized extrication**. The goal of stabilized extrication is to align the patient such that the three posterior reference points remain aligned in both the vertical and horizontal planes. The key to performing stabilized extrication, then, is to keep these three reference points both aligned and in the same plane while the patient is being moved. When this is accomplished, the spine will be stabilized and little or no motion will occur in the spinal segments. When properly positioned, the three anterior points should also form a straight line.

All movements should be coordinated by a lead OEC technician who, ideally, observes and directs the actions of the other rescuers. Rescuers should move the patient smoothly, without hesitation, and in unison following the leader's directions. The team needs to manually stabilize the three posterior reference points *at all times*.

Move the patient axially (by sliding) or vertically (by lifting and/or lowering), but never move the patient sideways. All movements should be in increments of 6 to 12 inches and should be started and stopped at the leader's command. When the patient's limbs, head, or neck need to be straightened, move only one joint at a time in only one plane at a time while manually stabilizing the three posterior reference points.

Align all body parts into Position 1, 2, or 3 as early as possible, unless major pain or resistance occurs. Begin with the head and neck so that the airway can be protected. Perform all maneuvers with confidence but not in a hurried manner. Try to keep the number of positions selected at a minimum, and generally try to progress from a higher numbered position to a lower numbered position. For example, a patient found in Position 2a should be manually aligned into Position 2, then logrolled into Position 1.

Moving a patient found in Position 3a with the head turned to the side is more complex. In this instance, the body and extremities are aligned into Position 3 while the head and neck are stabilized in the position found. The patient is then logrolled into Position 2a, with the head maintained as is until the body reaches Position 2. The head is then

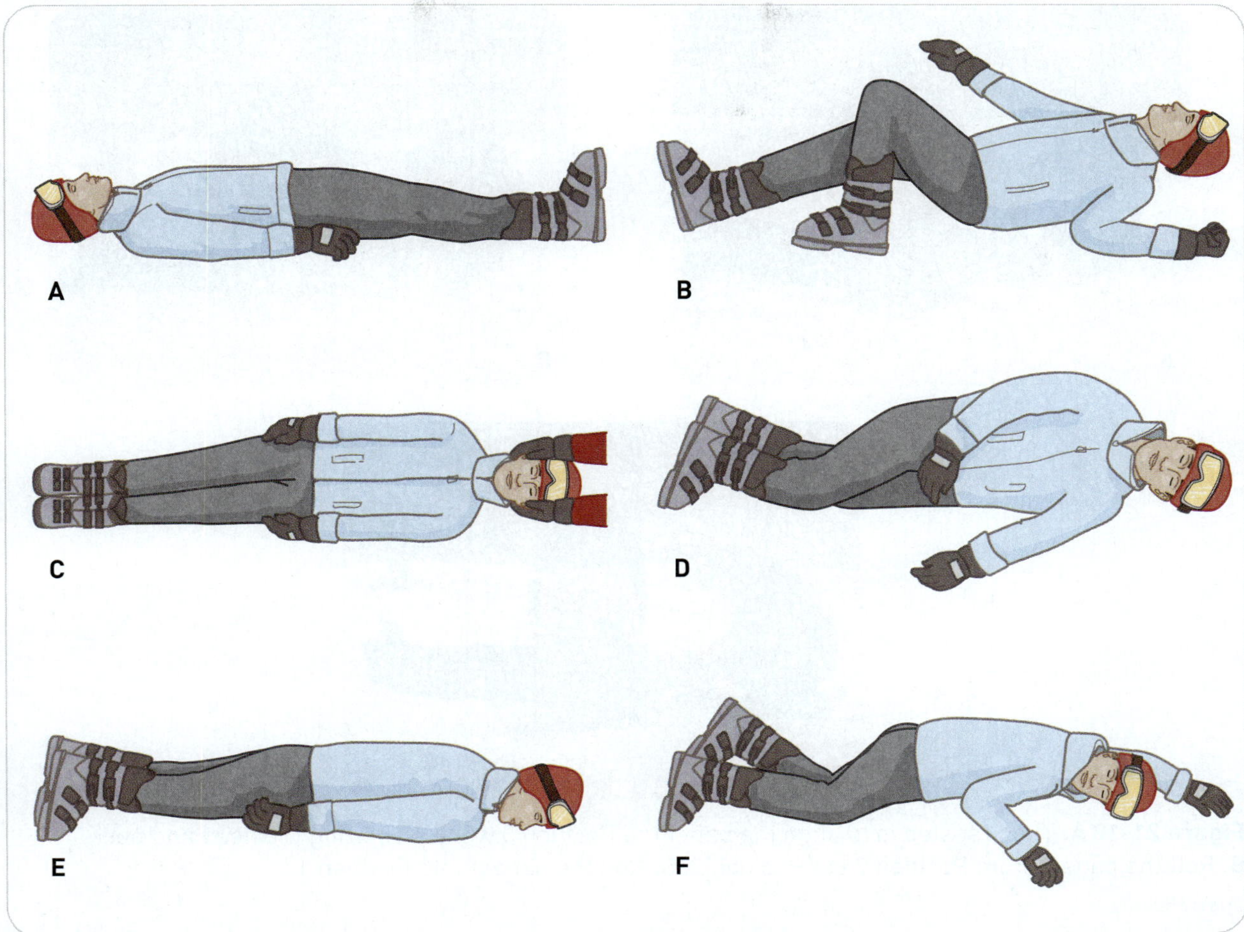

Figure 21-17 **A.** Position 1. **B.** Position 1a. **C.** Position 2. **D.** Position 2a. **E.** Position 3. **F.** Position 3a.

aligned to Position 2. Finally, the patient is logrolled into Position 1 on a backboard (**Figure 21-18**). If the patient is located in a confined area or is positioned awkwardly (for example, jammed against a tree), try to align the patient using the same method moving the patient *away* from the tree.

Rescuer safety is an important consideration when attempting to move a patient. To avoid injuring one's back or another body part, every rescuer should remember to lift with the hips and legs rather than with the back. Keep the back straight. Don't twist or bend forward or to the side, and hold the load (the patient) as close to the body as possible. You may wish to review the appropriate sections in Chapter 5, *Moving, Lifting, and Transporting Patients*.

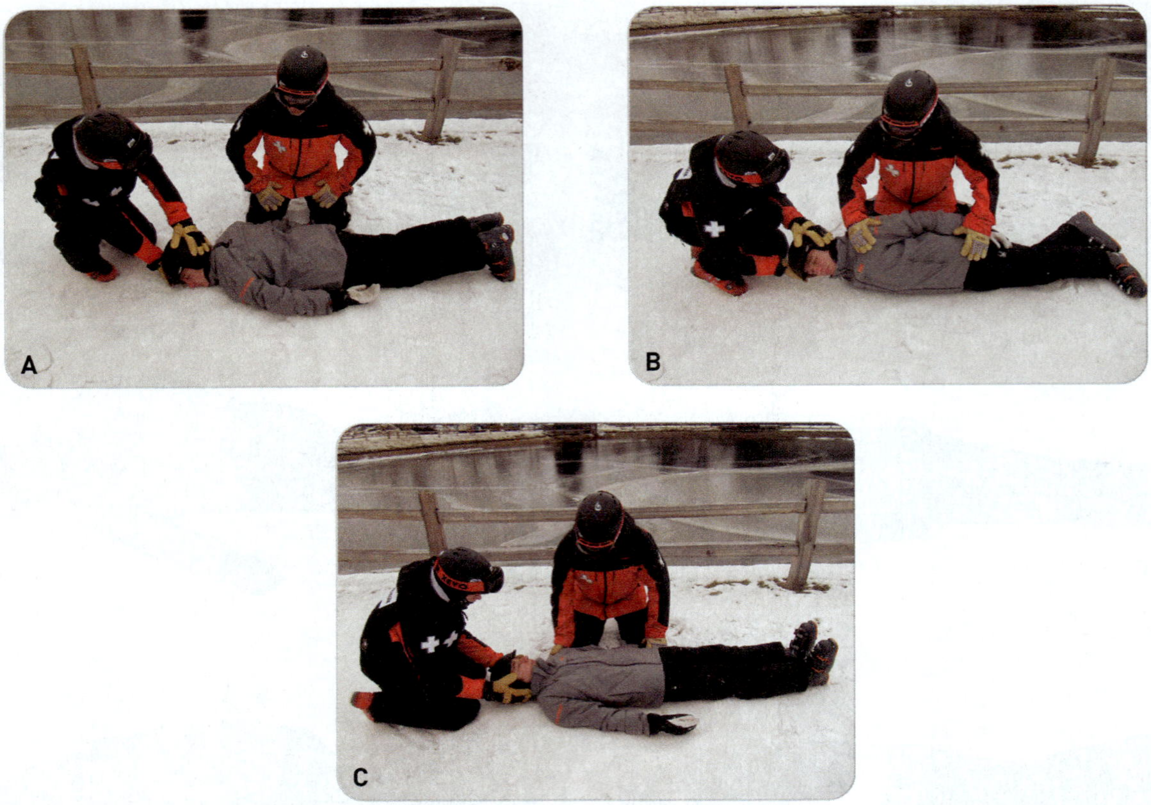

Figure 21-18 A. The first step is to align the patient to Position 3 while stabilizing the head and neck. **B.** Roll the patient from Position 2a to Position 2. **C.** Roll the patient into Position 1.

CASE Outcome

You instruct one OEC technician to take over manual in-line stabilization of the patient's cervical spine. You instruct another to place the patient on high-flow oxygen. You palpate the entire body and find no other injuries. You place a cervical collar on the patient, and with the assistance of other patrollers, carefully logroll the patient onto a long backboard for transport off the mountain. His vital signs remain stable. You provide spinal motion restriction with strapping, securing the patient's head to the long backboard last. You load him into a toboggan with his head uphill, and quickly transport him to a nearby landing zone, where his care is transferred to a helicopter's medical crew after giving them a brief but pertinent handoff report. The patient is then flown to the nearest trauma center.

During your monthly patrol meeting later that week, you learn that the patient had a linear skull fracture with an epidural hematoma, a fractured vertebra at C6, and neurogenic shock. Although the patient's condition is serious, he appears to be making progress and reportedly has a good chance of returning to a normal life. The neurosurgeon was very impressed with the care the patient received in the field and commends you and your team for recognizing the severity of the brain injury, protecting the patient's spine, and getting him to the hospital rapidly.

CHAPTER REVIEW

In Summary

- Brain and spinal cord injuries are potentially life altering or life threatening.
- In the setting of serious head or brain injury, always consider a spine injury.
- Spinal motion restriction is based on the mechanism of injury, the reliability of the exam, and the exam.
- "C3, C4, C5, keep the diaphragm alive." Injuries at or above C3, C4, C5 can result in loss of breathing.
- The treatment goals for neurologic injuries are preserving the ABCDs and minimizing spinal movement.
- All patients with a significant MOI or head, neck, and back injuries with positive physical findings should have spinal motion restriction on a long backboard.

Key Terms

Antegrade amnesia Loss of memory of events that occurred *after* a traumatic event to the brain; an inability to recall new information.

Axon Long, slender projection of a nerve cell (neuron) that conducts electrical impulses away from the neuron's cell body.

Cerebral contusion A bruise involving the brain.

Concussion Temporary unconsciousness (unresponsiveness) or confusion caused by a blow to the head.

Coup-contrecoup brain injury Dual-impacting of the brain into the skull; coup injury occurs at the point of impact; contrecoup occurs at the opposite side of impact, as the brain rebounds.

Cranium The skull.

Epidural hematoma a traumatic brain injury in which a buildup of blood occurs between the dura mater and the skull.

Intracerebral hematoma A hematoma inside the brain from bleeding inside the brain's tissue.

Intracranial pressure The pressure within the skull; can also be exerted on the brain tissue and cerebrospinal fluid.

Jams and pretzels A phrase that refers to the process by which someone who is injured and an awkward position is returned to normal supine anatomic position while maintaining spinal motion restriction.

Lucid interval A state in which the patient is relatively alert and then becomes increasingly less responsive and eventually unresponsive.

Retrograde amnesia Loss of memory of events that occurred before a traumatic event to the brain; an inability to recall old information.

Stabilized extrication Keeping a patient's spine anatomically aligned during removal from an accident, therefore preventing any neurologic damage.

Subdural hematoma An accumulation of venous blood between the outer covering of the brain (dura mater) and the surface of the brain.

Traumatic brain injury Physical trauma to the brain.

Chapter Questions

1. The two main components of the central nervous system are the:
   a. spinal cord and spinal fluid.
   b. brain and spinal cord.
   c. cerebrum and cerebellum.
   d. axons and neurons.
2. Traumatic injuries to the spine can occur from which of the following types of forces?
   a. Blunt
   b. Compression
   c. Twisting
   d. All of the above

3. Your patient was struck on the back of the head while exiting the chair lift. He is wearing a helmet and is unable to remember what happened. You are examining him within 10 minutes of the accident. What other signs and symptoms might you find on assessment?
   a. Headache
   b. Raccoon eyes
   c. Altered mental status
   d. Both A and C
4. Ski patrol is called to the area cafeteria to evaluate an 85-year-old man who is "not acting right" according to his family. He tells you he has a headache. Upon exam, you note a healing bruise on the right side of his head. His family states that he struck his head on a kitchen cabinet a few days ago. Based on your findings, what type of injury is most likely to have occurred?
   a. Diffuse axonal injury
   b. Subdural hematoma
   c. Intracranial hemorrhage
   d. Spinal cord injury
5. A person exhibiting loss of movement and loss of sensation in all four extremities has injured what part of the spine?
   a. Cervical
   b. Thoracic
   c. Lumbar
   d. Sacral
6. When assessing a patient with a suspected brain or spinal cord injury, you should check the:
   a. skull.
   b. spine.
   c. nervous system.
   d. All of the above
7. The following is *not* a sign of a traumatic brain injury?
   a. Incontinence
   b. Seizures
   c. Abdominal pain
   d. Posturing
8. Which of the following presentations indicates a need for spinal motion restriction?
   a. Patient has potential spine injury but normal mental status and no exam findings associated with a spinal injury.
   b. Patient is walking around at the scene of an accident.
   c. Patient complains of pain in the flank of his back.
   d. Patient has potential spine injury with an alteration of mental status such that a reliable physical exam cannot be done.
9. It is recommended that helmets should *not* be removed if:
   a. the patient needs airway assistance and the helmet is in the way.
   b. the helmet fits properly, holding the head in proper position.
   c. the patient is in cardiac arrest.
   d. the helmet prevents you from properly placing a cervical collar.
10. Your patient is found supine, with one arm over his head and one at his side, and one leg under the other. Using the principles of jams and pretzels, your goal is to get your patient to position "1." What position is your patient currently in?
   a. 1a
   b. 2
   c. 2a
   d. 3a

Answers: 1. b, Objective 21-1, p. 510; 2. d, Objective 21-3, p. 518; 3. d, Objective 21-5, p. 519; 4. b, Objective 21-5, p. 517; 5. a, Objective 21-4, p. 518; 6. d, Objective 21-5, p. 520; 7. c, Objective 21-6, p. 519; 8. d, Objective 21-9, p. 524; 9. b, Objective 21-14, p. 534; 10. a, Objective 21-15, p. 536

CHAPTER 22

FACE, EYE, AND NECK INJURIES

OBJECTIVES

Upon completion of this chapter, the OEC technician will be able to:

22-1 Describe the function of the eye.

22-2 Describe the assessment and management of ear injuries.

22-3 Describe and demonstrate the management of a patient with a penetrating injury to the eyeball.

22-4 Identify the important structures of the anterior neck.

22-5 List the signs and symptoms of traumatic injury emergencies of the neck and upper airway.

22-6 Describe the function of the lacrimal glands.

22-7 Describe the management of a dental injury.

22-8 List the signs and symptoms of emergent injuries to the face, eyes, and neck.

22-9 Describe and demonstrate how to assess face, eye, and neck injuries.

22-10 Describe and demonstrate the proper care of a face, eye, or anterior neck injury.

KEY TERMS

Anisocoria, p. 545
Blowout fracture, p. 546
Cornea, p. 544
Epistaxis, p. 546
External auditory canal, p. 546
Hyphema, p. 548
Lacrimal glands, p. 545
Mandible, p. 542
Maxillae, p. 542
Orbit, p. 544
Retinal detachment, p. 554
Sternocleidomastoid muscles, p. 545
Subcutaneous emphysema, p. 551

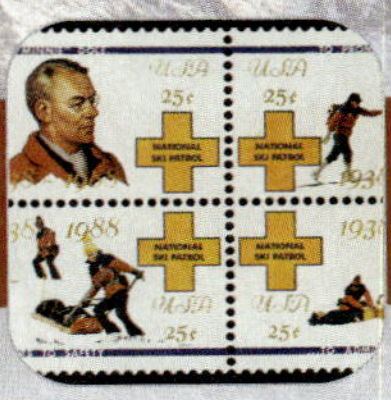

HISTORICAL TIMELINE 1988. U.S. postage stamp commemorates NSP 50th anniversary.

CHAPTER OVERVIEW

In individuals participating in outdoor recreational activities, the face and neck are typically exposed and thus are especially susceptible to direct trauma. Injuries to the face and neck can cause long-term disfigurement or be life threatening. The soft tissues of the upper airway can easily be affected, requiring immediate attention. Traumatic injuries involving the face or neck may bleed profusely due to the generous blood supply in these areas of the body. Serious injuries from blunt or penetrating trauma and environmental exposure can affect hearing, vision, and smell. Pain can be severe due to the abundance of nerves, especially in injuries involving the eyes. Facial and neck emergencies often result from mechanisms of injury that should alert OEC technicians to the possibility of coexisting injuries such as closed head and cervical-spine injuries. Cold-weather injuries to the face, especially frostbite to the nose and ears, are covered in Chapter 25, *Cold-Related Emergencies.*

ANATOMY AND PHYSIOLOGY

Facial Structures

The face contains numerous structures essential not only for sensing the environment, but also for survival (**Figure 22-1**). The sensations of sight, sound, smell, and taste all originate within the sensory systems of the face. The nose, mouth, and pharynx are parts of the upper airway. Sensory systems in the face are partially protected by the facial bones, whereas vital structures in the neck are relatively vulnerable. The trachea (windpipe) and great vessels of the neck are protected only by relatively thin layers of skin and muscle.

The face consists of 14 bones. The forehead, the most superior aspect of the face, is supported by the frontal bone, which protects the front of the brain. The zygomatic bones connect to the frontal bone to form the cheeks and the inferior rims of both eye sockets. These bones, along with the nasal bones and the **maxillae** (singular: maxilla) combine at the middle of the face to support the cartilage and soft tissues of the nose.

The maxillae, which are the largest bones of the face, form the upper jaw, the hard palate of the mouth, the floor of the nose, and the lower portion of each eye socket. The U-shaped **mandible**, or lower jawbone, hinges on both sides with the temporal bones at the temporomandibular joints, making the lower jaw the only movable bone of the face. The teeth are anchored in either the maxillae or the mandible. When brought together, the alignment of the teeth forms the bite or occlusion. The tongue, lips, gums, and palate constitute the rest of the oral structures.

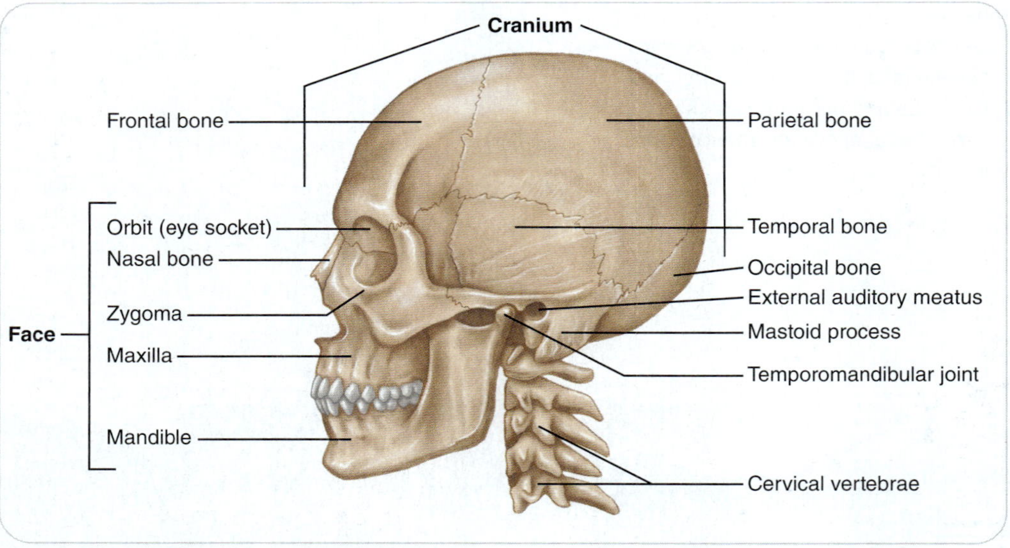

Figure 22-1 The cranium and facial bones.

CASE Presentation

You are checking boundary and trail closures when you see a snowboarder lying in the snow several feet beyond a yellow closure rope. As you approach, you notice that the rider's track goes underneath the closure rope. The rider is lying on his back, holding his face with both hands. He appears to be in considerable distress.

What should you do?

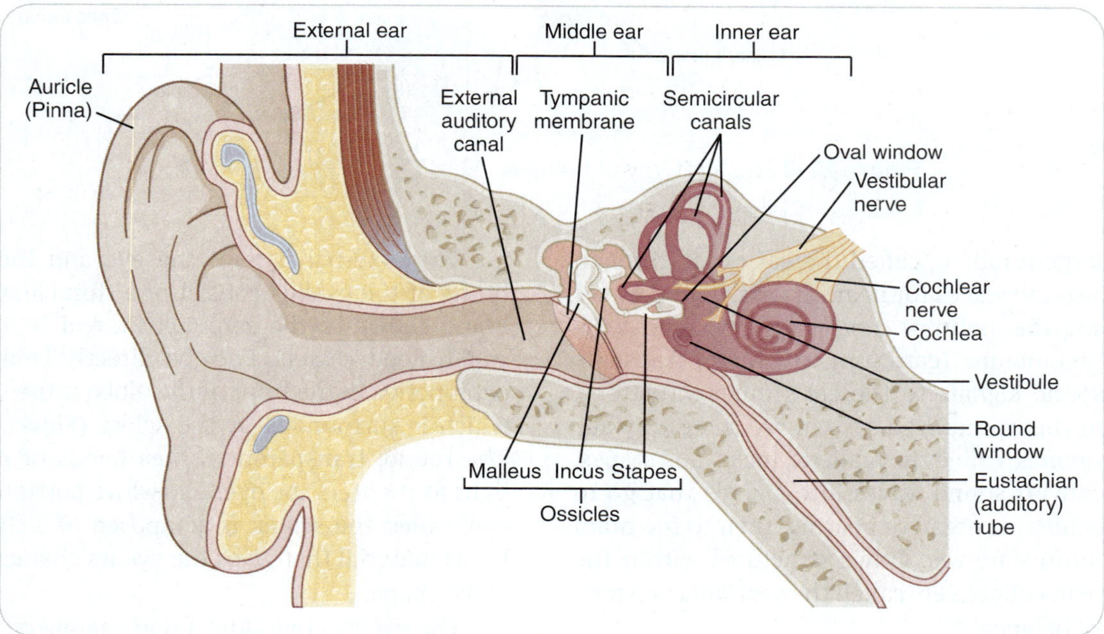

Figure 22-2 The anatomy of the ear.

The face and mouth are highly vascular, which explains why injuries to this region of the body typically involve significant external bleeding or internal bleeding that forms a hematoma.

The face contains cartilage that combines with the facial bones to provide overall structure to the face. The nasal septum is made of cartilage, as is the pinna, the cartilage of the external ear.

The face is interlaced with 43 muscles that control voluntary movement of the eyes and mouth and are responsible for facial expressions such as smiling and frowning. The facial muscles also are responsible for nasal flaring, which helps to bring more oxygen-containing air into the body in times of severe respiratory distress. The mastoid muscles connect to the mandible and facilitate the opening and closing of the mouth and chewing. The skull and facial bones have small openings, known as foramina, through which nerves and blood vessels pass to more superficial soft-tissue structures. Control of both the facial muscles and the sensory organs is provided by a vast network of nerves. One of the largest nerves, the facial nerve, traverses the zygomatic bones and controls the muscles of facial expression.

Auditory and Balance System

The external parts of the ear, known as the pinna, tragus, lobules (lobes), and helix, are positioned over the temporal bone on each side of the skull (**Figure 22-2**). Each temporal bone is penetrated

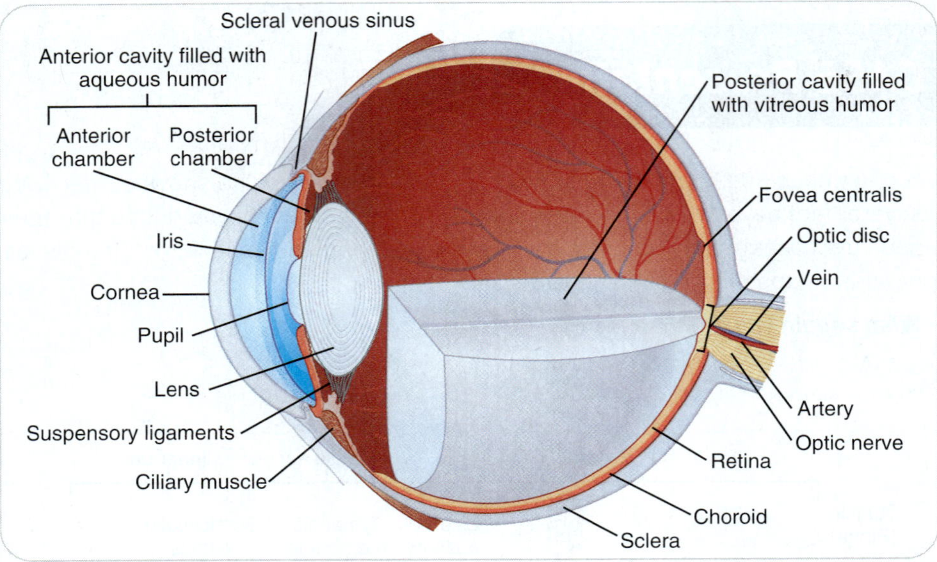

Figure 22-3 The anatomy of the eye.

by a large foramen, called the ear canal, through which sound waves for hearing pass. Sound waves entering the auditory canal cause the thin tympanic membrane (eardrum) to vibrate, transmitting sound signals to the ear's inner structures. Within this specialized system are three tiny auditory bones, called the malleus, incus, and stapes, that convert sound waves into signals that go to the cochlea, or organ of hearing, then to the brain via auditory nerves. Other structures within the inner ear, collectively called the vestibular system, control balance.

Visual System

The sense we call vision begins when light enters the globe-shaped eyeball. The eye captures light images that are then sent to the brain via the optic nerves. The eye is relatively well protected within a bony socket formed by the skull and facial bones. This socket, known as the **orbit**, protects much of the fluid-filled eyeball while simultaneously anchoring the muscles that go to the external surface of the eyeball and control eye movement. Although significant force is needed to injure the bones that make up the orbit, the front of the eyeball is relatively unprotected and therefore susceptible to injury. Six small muscles, known as extraocular muscles, attach to each eye and enable the two eyes to move in various directions at the same time. These muscles are controlled by nerves that come directly from the brain.

The external part of the eye and the inner lining of the eyelids consist of a thin clear membrane known as the conjunctiva, which contains small blood vessels. Located directly behind the conjunctiva in the front of the globe is the **cornea**, which is surrounded by the sclera (**Figure 22-3**). The round, transparent cornea bends or refracts light as it enters the eye. The white portion of the eye, called the sclera, is composed of a thick, fibrous material that gives the eye its characteristic globe shape.

The eye has two fluid-filled chambers: an anterior chamber and a posterior chamber. The anterior chamber is filled with a thin watery substance known as aqueous humor. This clear fluid can leak out of the eye in the event of a penetrating injury, but it is regenerated over time following repair of the eye. The anterior chamber begins behind the cornea and ends at the circular iris.

The iris works like a camera shutter to adjust the amount of light entering the eye. Pigment in the iris accounts for the color of the eye. In the center of the iris is the pupil, visible as a black circle. Constriction of the iris narrows the pupil and allows less light to pass through the lens of the eye, whereas dilation of the iris widens the pupil and allows more light to enter the eye.

Under normal conditions, the pupil very quickly becomes smaller in response to bright light. This is called the direct response. If you shine a light into only one eye, the other eye's iris (pupil) will also constrict if the visual system is functioning properly (indirect response). Under normal conditions, both pupils should be approximately equal in size. Unequal pupil size, a condition known as **anisocoria**, may be caused directly due to an insult to the eye, or indirectly due to a problem in the brain. In a small percentage of the population, approximately 20%, the pupils are normally unequal in size.

Between the iris and the lens is the posterior chamber. The lens of the eyeball is used to fine-tune the focusing of light at the back of the eye. Depending on the distance an object is from the eye, certain small muscles within the eye change the shape of the lens so that light is focused on the retina, which is like film in a camera. When the muscles contract, the lens becomes flatter; when they relax, the lens becomes rounder. Light then passes into the vitreous humor, a jelly-like fluid. Unlike aqueous humor, vitreous humor cannot be regenerated by the body if it is lost due to injury. It is the volume of these two fluids that fills the eyeball with enough pressure to maintain its globe-like shape.

Light entering the eye then strikes the retina, a sheet of light-sensitive nerve endings located in the back of the inside of the eye. These nerve endings transmit signals through the optic nerves to the brain, which then formats the information as a visual image. The sensation of depth perception is created because the brain receives slightly different signals from each eye when looking at a given object, especially close objects.

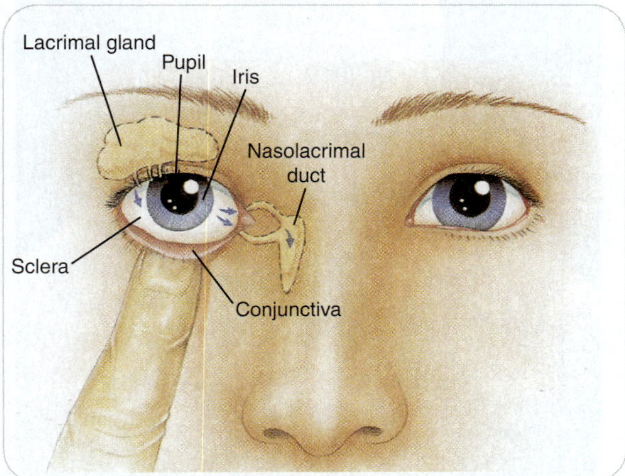

Figure 22-4 The anatomy of the lacrimal apparatus.

Tear glands, also called **lacrimal glands**, are positioned above each eye and provide constant irrigation in the form of tears (**Figure 22-4**). Tears and blinking flush away surface debris and clean the exposed surface of the eye. Tears drain toward the inner side of each eye and into the lacrimal (tear) ducts.

Neck Anatomy

The anterior part of the neck contains several unprotected vital structures: the carotid arteries, jugular veins, esophagus, trachea, and thyroid gland (**Figure 22-5**). Trauma to these structures can result in significant bleeding, swelling, and closure of the airway.

In the midline of the anterior neck, palpable just beneath the skin, is the thyroid cartilage of the larynx. This cartilage, called the Adam's apple, is more prominent in men than it is in women or children. Below the larynx (voice box) is the trachea (windpipe). The esophagus is situated directly behind the trachea. Approximately 1 to 2 cm on either side of the larynx are the large carotid arteries, which supply blood to the neck and head. The large jugular veins, which drain blood from the head, lie just beneath the skin in the anterior neck.

The **sternocleidomastoid muscles** are on the sides of the neck. In the posterior neck are the cervical vertebrae. Within the vertebrae is the spinal cord. The cervical spine and spinal cord are discussed in Chapter 21, *Spine, Brain, and Nervous System Injuries*.

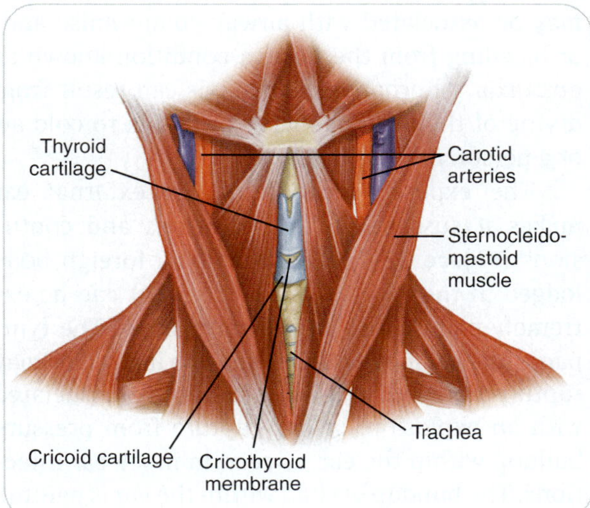

Figure 22-5 The anterior anatomy of the neck.

FACE, EYE, AND NECK INJURIES

Face Injuries

The face is exposed and thus susceptible to environmental injuries such as frostbite or sunburn, or to direct trauma, including fractures and a variety of soft-tissue injuries. Due to the vascular nature of the face and the proximity of major nerves to the surface of the skin, bleeding can be severe and can be accompanied by nerve damage. OEC technicians must make sure the airway remains open when caring for any facial injury.

Facial injuries seen by OEC technicians include lacerations from sharp objects or fractures from blunt or penetrating trauma. Blunt trauma with significant force to the front of the face can lead to multiple fractures involving the maxillae (bones around the nose and upper lip) and other bones in the face. These fractures often result in airway obstruction due to significant bleeding and swelling of nasal and oral structures. A mandible that is fractured may break in multiple locations and may produce significant bleeding inside the mouth.

A fracture that involves the bony socket of the eye, or **blowout fracture**, may either injure the eye or cause the muscles that attach to the eye to become trapped within the fracture. This injury can result in loss of normal eye motion and double vision (**Figure 22-6**).

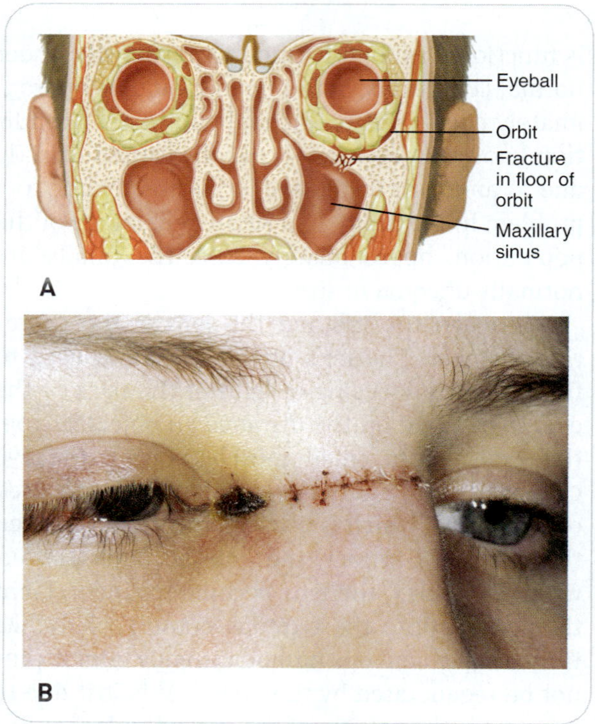

Figure 22-6 A. A blowout fracture of the left orbit. **B.** In a patient with a blowout fracture, the eyes may not move together due to muscle entrapment.

A: © Jones & Bartlett Learning; **B:** © DR P. MARAZZI/Science Source.

Direct trauma to the nose may result in a fracture of the nasal bone or damage to the cartilage at the tip of the nose. While nasal bone fractures do not typically require emergent treatment, they may be associated with airway compromise and/or bleeding from the nose, a condition known as **epistaxis**. Alternatively, epistaxis can result from drying of the mucous membranes due to cold air or a person picking the nose.

The exposed location of the external ear makes it susceptible to lacerations and contusions (**Figure 22-7**). Additionally, a foreign body lodged in the **external auditory canal** can be extremely painful and anxiety provoking. The tympanic membrane (eardrum) may be injured or may rupture from loud noises, such as those associated with an explosion, or can rupture from pressure buildup within the ear, as seen in inner-ear infections. The buildup of fluid within the ear is painful, but rupture of the tympanic membrane provides relief. Tympanic membrane rupture can also result

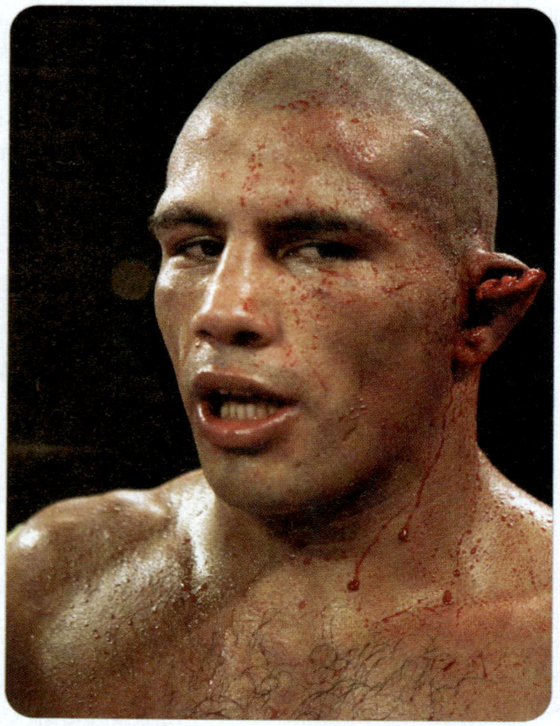

Figure 22-7 An injury to the ear.

© Ed Mulholland/Getty Images Sport/Getty Images.

from barotrauma incurred during deep-water diving.

Injuries to the teeth occur in outdoor activities when projectiles hit the mouth or when the person makes direct physical contact with another person or with a hard surface, especially when high speeds are involved. Chipping a tooth is the most common dental injury encountered, whereas a complete avulsion (a tooth knocked out) is a more serious dental injury. Teeth also may be fractured, leaving a jagged piece of tooth. When a tooth is bleeding, the nerves inside the tooth have been exposed, resulting in significant pain and an increased risk of infection. If a loose tooth becomes dislodged, airway obstruction can result. Direct trauma to the mouth can cause a dental appliance (e.g., dentures, a bridge, a retainer) to break, which can lacerate the gum or possibly obstruct the airway.

Eye Injuries

Light-related injuries are one of the most frequent sources of eye injury, especially if eye protection is not worn. Exposure to ultraviolet (UV) rays (from the sun or welding), chemicals, and various gases can cause eye damage. Injuries from overexposure to UV light, as commonly occur in snow sports, can range from a superficial burn to permanent damage to the conjunctiva or cornea. Often known as snow blindness, these injuries may not become apparent until several hours after the exposure. Additional UV light is reflected off the snow. UV light from an arc-welding lamp, a sun lamp, or sunlight reflected off water may cause the same condition with severe pain in association with conjunctivitis, swelling, and excessive tear production.

The eyes are especially vulnerable to abrasive and penetrating injuries, including impaled objects (**Figure 22-8**). Small particles such as blowing sand or rust particles getting into the eye when working on a car can get beneath the eyelid, abrading or scratching the surface of the eye. Patients may have the sensation that there is a foreign body in the eye and will likely be sensitive to bright light. In severe cases, particles can penetrate an unprotected eye. Work-related activities, such as grinding metal, operating a drill, performing high-speed sanding, or working around debris kicked up from helicopters, also can result in penetrating eye injuries from small particles. Objects such as tree branches, ice tools, ski poles, darts, and other pointed objects can also easily penetrate the globe. A ball or other smooth object can directly strike the globe, resulting in blunt trauma.

Regardless of the mechanism, globe laceration or rupture should be considered anytime the eye has suffered direct trauma or suspected penetration. Globe ruptures—conditions in which the integrity of the eyeball has been compromised—are a leading trauma-related cause of blindness (**Figure 22-9**).

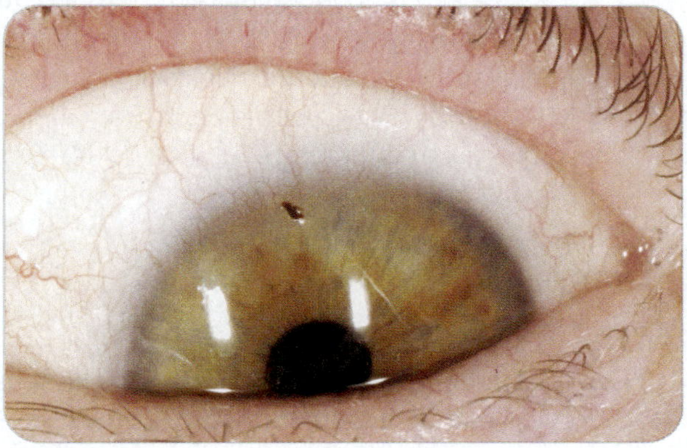

Figure 22-8 Unprotected eyes are susceptible to impaled foreign objects.

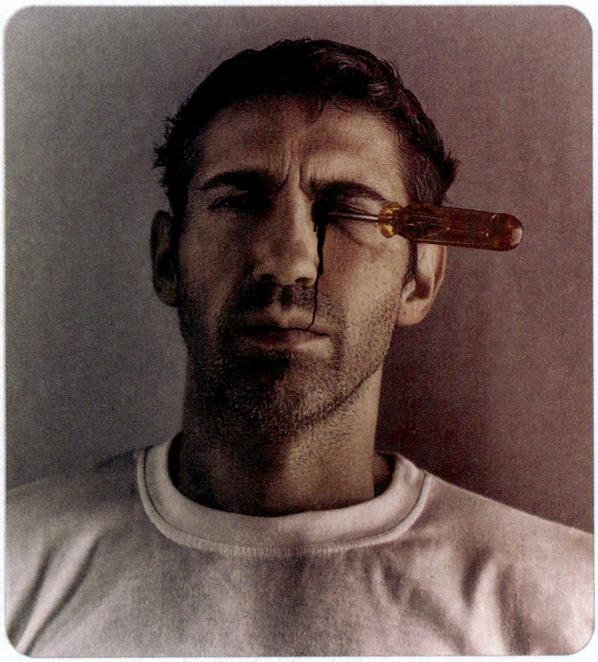

Figure 22-9 Penetration of the eyeball with a screwdriver.

CASE Update

Evaluating the scene as you approach the injured snowboarder, you look for fixed objects other than the closure rope that the patient may have hit. Evaluating the likely mechanism of injury, you suspect that the snowboarder could have serious neck trauma. Upon examination, you notice that the patient is clearly anxious and is having difficulty breathing. His respiration rate is 24 per minute with shallow inspirations, and as he tries to respond to your questions, he can speak only in a hoarse whisper. You note as well that the snowboarder cannot swallow his saliva and is drooling blood from his mouth. His pulse is 100 beats per minute. His jaw is crooked and his pupils appear equal. No trauma is apparent around his ears or scalp. When you examine the patient's neck, you notice a dark red abrasion and underlying swelling on the right anterior portion of his neck. Palpation of the posterior neck reveals no tenderness or deformities and there are no distal extremity neurological deficits. The jaw is swollen. You call for assistance.

What should you do?

Direct trauma to the eye can disrupt the lens of the eye, so that light cannot be focused correctly on the retina. Trauma can also cause the retina (film in the back) to become torn, which can lead to a retinal detachment and significant visual impairment. Lacerations to the upper or lower eyelid need attention by a properly trained physician. In both blunt and penetrating injuries to the eye, blood may accumulate in the aqueous fluid (anterior chamber) of the eye, resulting in **hyphema**. Usually seen in penetrating injuries, blood in the vitreous fluid (posterior eye) is a very serious problem.

Neck Injuries

Injuries involving the soft-tissue structures of the neck can be immediately life threatening. They are frequently associated with severe swelling or formation of a hematoma that can compromise the airway. Blunt trauma is a leading cause of neck and throat injuries that may damage not only the vital structures in the anterior neck but also the cervical spine. Injuries to the vertebrae and spinal cord are discussed in another chapter. Direct blows to the anterior neck and "clothesline" or ligature-type injuries can be deadly because the concentrated force can collapse the larynx or trachea. This type of injury also can cause deep lacerations and open wounds.

Neck injuries are usually difficult to manage in the field. Penetrating neck injuries are especially concerning because they often damage multiple structures, including the trachea and major blood vessels. Soft-tissue neck and throat injuries can be deceptive: Although they may initially appear benign, they are frequently associated with grave underlying trauma.

Open neck injuries are among the most serious injuries OEC technicians may encounter (**Figure 22-10**). Lacerations involving either a carotid artery or a jugular vein produce profuse bleeding that will result in life-threatening shock if not immediately controlled. In some instances,

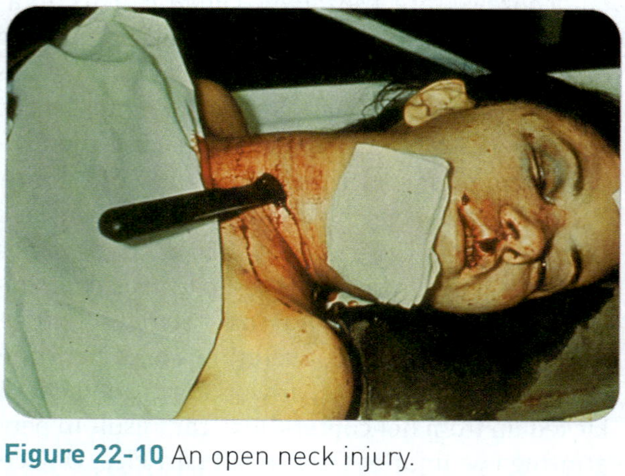

Figure 22-10 An open neck injury.

air may be sucked into the venous system through the damaged vessel, producing an air embolus. If large quantities of air reach the right atrium and right ventricle of the heart, cardiac air embolism causing cardiac arrest may follow. If the air passes through the heart, it can lodge in the lungs, causing pulmonary air embolism. Penetrating injuries to the trachea and esophagus can result in profound hypoxia, aspiration of gastric contents, and a host of other problems.

ASSESSMENT OF FACE, EYE, AND NECK INJURIES

Begin by controlling excessive bleeding and assessing the ABCDs (airway, breathing, circulation, and disability). Injuries to the face or neck frequently affect the upper airway. The rich vascular supply to the head and neck can result in profuse bleeding. Always use personal protective equipment (PPE). Disability from trauma to the brain or cervical spinal cord is likely. In a patient who has a significant head injury, the chances of having a significant injury to the cervical spine are greater than 10%.

After the initial primary assessment, OEC technicians should continually monitor the ABCDs, because over time the airway may become obstructed, bleeding can recur, or the patient's mental status or neurologic function may change.

If the initial primary assessment is unremarkable, OEC technicians should begin a secondary assessment by asking patients about their symptoms and their medical history in the normal fashion, using the SAMPLE acronym (signs and symptoms, allergies, medications, past medical history, last oral intake, events leading up to the problem) and the OPQRST mnemonic (onset, provocation, quality, radiation, severity, and time), respectively. As for all trauma patients, obtain a complete set of vital signs.

The physical examination already began with any observations made during the primary assessment. Continue the assessment by looking at the entire scalp and the face and neck for lacerations, abrasions, punctures, or other injuries. Look for facial asymmetry, such as a depressed cheekbone from a fracture.

Assessment of the Eye

Conducting an eye exam may be somewhat difficult, because patients may be reluctant to open a severely injured eye. *Gently* attempt to open a swollen eyelid. Never forcibly open an injured eye. If the patient can open the eyes, begin the ocular exam by asking patients if they can see normally, and if they can see normally with each eye. Hold up two fingers and ask how many they see? Ask if there is double vision. Next, look at each eye. Does each pupil appear round, or irregular? Patients who have had previous lens replacement surgery or cataract surgery may have irregularly shaped pupils, so be sure to ask about past eye surgery. Do they wear contacts or have a glass eye? Examine injured or painful eyes for the presence of foreign bodies, blood, or clear fluid that is leaking from the eye. If only one eye is injured, start the assessment by examining the other eye, noting its reaction to light. Then assess the injured eye by comparing it to the uninjured eye. Assess pupillary reaction and extraocular motion as described in Chapter 7, *Patient Assessment* (**Figure 22-11**). Remember that some patients may have different findings in each eye normally. Anisocoria (different-sized pupils) or different-colored irises of the eyes can be normal (**Figure 22-12**).

Assessment of the Midface and Nose

Examine the nose for bleeding, deformity, pain, or obstruction. Assess the cheeks for pain and deformity by looking at them and gently pressing on them. One or both cheeks could be deformed or depressed. Then, gently press on the bones between the nose and upper lip (maxillae).

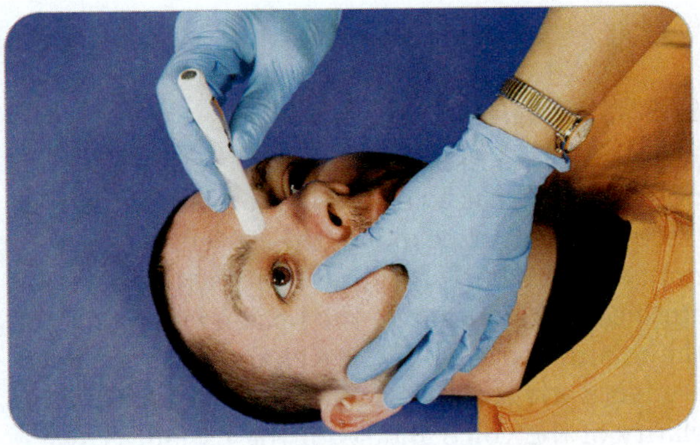

Figure 22-11 Check the pupils for size, equality, and reactivity to light.

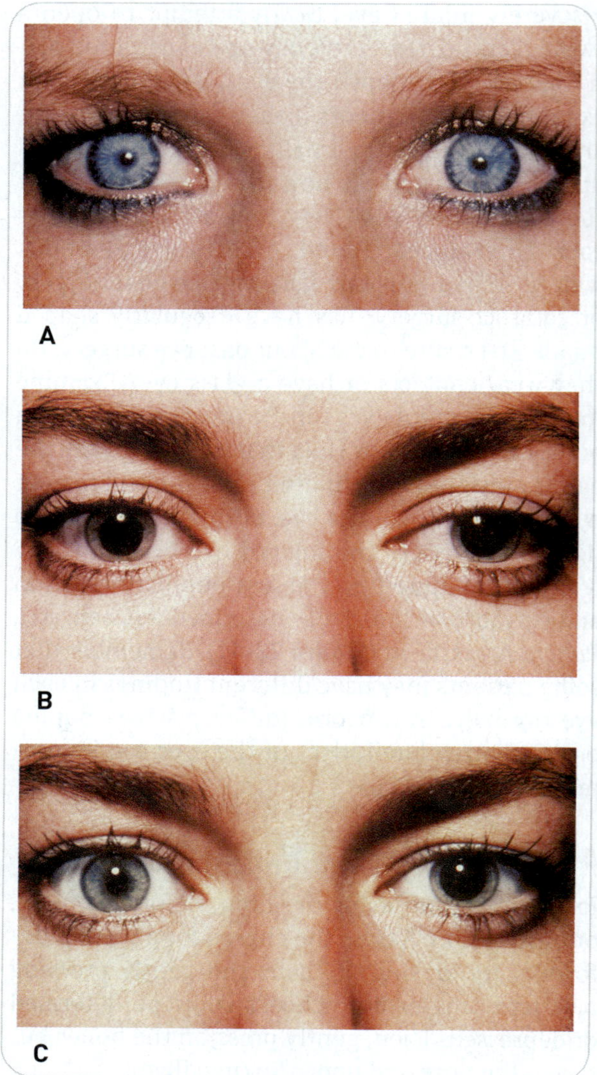

Figure 22-12 A. Constricted pupils. **B.** Dilated pupils. **C.** Unequal pupils.

Assessment of the Mouth

Ask the person to bite down. Then ask if this feels normal. If there is an offset due to a jaw fracture or fracture of the cheekbone, the patient will either not be able to bite or will say that the teeth do not close correctly. Examine the lips and the inside of the mouth for bleeding. Check for loose or missing teeth and lacerations of the tongue. Assess the clarity of the voice and see if the patient is swallowing normally. Difficulty or pain upon speaking or swallowing is a cause for concern and may indicate impending airway compromise.

Assessment of the Ear

Look at each ear for obvious evidence of trauma. If bleeding is present, try to determine whether the source is the external part of the ear, the ear canal, or a nearby site from which blood has flowed into the ear. Look for pink or *clear* fluid coming out of the ear; it may be cerebrospinal fluid leaking from a basal skull fracture.

Look for swelling or ecchymosis over the bony prominence of the mastoid process behind each ear; bruising to this area *hours* after head trauma, known as Battle sign, may indicate local trauma to the mastoid process or a serious fracture of the base of the skull. Examine the external canal of the ear for a foreign body, especially small toy parts in children and insects in both adults and children. Next, assess the patient's hearing by talking normally directly into each ear; use the same pitch and amplitude for each ear and then ask if your voice has the same quality and loudness in both ears. The patient may have preexisting deafness. In the event a patient has hearing aids, leave them in place unless you are caring for an injury to the ear that requires assessment and treatment.

Assessment of the Neck

The primary assessment using ABCD is important here. Make sure the airway is open and major bleeding is controlled. Provide inline manual stabilization of the head and neck for any face, eye, or neck injury, until an exam is done showing no evidence of spine or spinal cord injury. This exam includes assessing CMS (circulation, movement, and sensation) in all extremities. If spinal injury is apparent, use spinal motion restriction, which is further discussed in Chapter 21, *Spine, Brain, and Nervous System Injuries*.

Listen to the patient breathe and talk, noting any changes in voice quality, hoarseness, or audible breath sounds. Ask the patient to swallow, and observe the results. As when assessing the mouth, keep in mind that difficulty or pain upon speaking or swallowing is a cause for concern and may indicate impending airway compromise.

Look at and palpate the anterior and posterior aspects of the neck. Major bleeding from a laceration usually means a large carotid artery or jugular vein has been damaged. Carotid bleeding will spurt, while jugular venous bleeding flows freely. If no external bleeding is seen, look for symmetry between the two sides of the neck. Internal bleeding from a major blood vessel will cause a hematoma or palpable mass and could obstruct the airway.

Look to see if any midline structures appear to have shifted or if there is swelling or bruising. Look for air-filled bubbles that are palpable underneath the skin in the upper chest area and neck, called **subcutaneous emphysema**. These bubbles may sound like Rice Krispies cereal. This finding indicates an injury to an airway structure. Gently palpate the larynx and trachea for stability. Reassess the patient frequently, looking for airway compromise that occurs over time.

KEY POINT

Significant Facial Injury

A significant facial injury may be associated with a significant injury to the brain or cervical spine.

MANAGEMENT OF FACE, EYE, AND NECK INJURIES

Following the management of any safety issues, the primary assessment will include assessment of face and neck injuries. Control excessive bleeding of the face neck and scalp. Problems that affect the ABCDs (neurologic deficit) take precedence over secondary management concerns. If the airway is compromised, use the jaw-thrust maneuver to protect the cervical spine, not the head tilt–chin lift method. Suction the patient's mouth and nose as needed to keep the airway patent.

Because the face, mouth, and neck are highly vascular, and bleeding can be significant, it is always essential that standard precautions be observed. External bleeding usually can be managed with direct pressure; never use a tourniquet. If significant face or neck trauma is present and there are findings indicating the need for spinal motion restriction, restrict the motion of the patient's spine. If spinal injury is not suspected and bleeding of the face is present, lean the patient forward or place the patient on his or her side to prevent blood from draining into the airway and from being swallowed. Be prepared to suction the airway if necessary.

High-flow oxygen (if a pulse oximeter is available, keep oxygen saturation between 94 and 99%) should be provided to patients with airway or breathing compromise or when there is significant external bleeding. Reevaluation is needed frequently, especially during toboggan transports because these injuries can rapidly progress to life-threatening situations. ALS personnel should be notified to assist when appropriate.

Management of Facial Injuries

The primary goal when managing a patient with a facial fracture is to keep the airway open and clear. These patients often need aggressive airway management, including appropriate positioning, suctioning, oxygen, and occasionally ventilatory support.

Placement of an oral or nasal airway may be indicated. If the mouth or nasal area is severely injured or crushed, it may be difficult to insert an airway device. Assess the airway, and if you can easily place an airway device (oropharyngeal airway), this is usually best. Never force an airway device in the patient. If there are nasal injuries, a nasal airway device (nasopharyngeal airway) will not work.

Regardless of whether epistaxis (nosebleed) is mild or severe, direct pressure is the best way to control this type of bleeding. The nares (nostrils) should be pressed together just below the bony prominence of the nose (**Figure 22-13**).

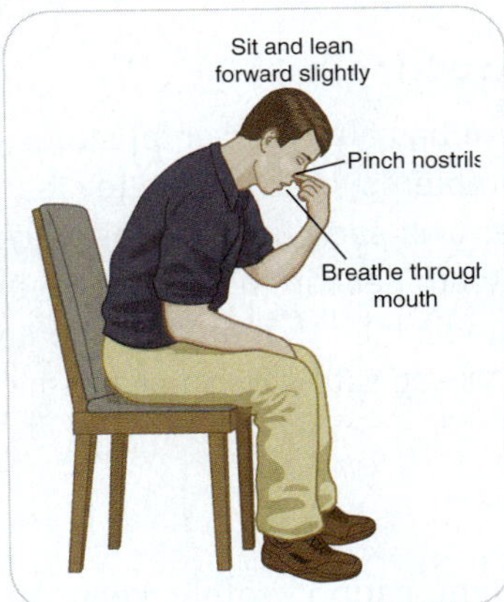

Figure 22-13 To control a nosebleed, have the patient sit down and lean forward, and pinch the nostrils together.

Hold pressure up to *15 minutes* before evaluating ongoing bleeding. Lean the patient forward to allow blood and other secretions to drain out of the nose and mouth. The most common mistakes in the management of epistaxis are removing the pressure too soon or having the patient lean the head backwards. If you are unable to control the bleeding with direct pressure, place a cloth- or bandage-wrapped ice pack on the bridge of the nose.

The focus of care for a mouth injury is ensuring a patent airway. Tongue lacerations are controlled with direct pressure. Remove any *broken* teeth that may be present. If a tooth is displaced but still in its socket and is at risk of falling out, causing airway obstruction, leave it in place and monitor the airway, if possible.

Pick up any tooth that has been completely knocked out of its socket (an avulsed tooth) by its crown (part that is exposed normally). Avoid touching the root (the part that was below the gum). *Do not wash or scrub an avulsed tooth.* If sterile saline or tepid tap water is available, rinse the tooth gently. If the patient is alert and has no airway problems, and if you do not anticipate transporting the patient over bumpy terrain, place the tooth back in the socket correctly or have the patient keep the tooth against the inside of the cheek. Remind the patient to not swallow the tooth.

KEY POINT

An Avulsed Tooth

If a patient has altered mental status, has airway problems, or is unable to clear his or her own secretions, never place an avulsed tooth back in the socket because of the significant risk that the patient will swallow or aspirate it during transport.

If a patient cannot safely keep an avulsed tooth in the socket or against the cheek, it should be preserved using other means. Ideally, the tooth should be placed in Hanks' solution, a product designed for tooth preservation. If this product is not available, place the tooth in either milk or sterile saline in a sterile or clean container. Doing so will allow reimplantation for up to 6 hours. Some patrols may have kits for avulsed teeth.

Management of Ear Injuries

Bleeding from a lacerated external ear and ear avulsions are controlled using direct pressure, a dressing, and a bandage. In both cases, the applied dressing should include bulky support between the pinna (external ear) and the scalp. If the external ear is completely amputated, preserve the part as described for an amputated finger in Chapter 19, *Soft-Tissue Injuries and Burns*. Many pinna-related injuries can be successfully repaired if they are attended to quickly. Any patient with a severe external ear injury should be transported to a physician for cosmetic repair.

Manipulation of a foreign body stuck in the external auditory canal can cause injury to the tympanic membrane and can be very irritating to the patient. When faced with this situation, turn the patient onto his or her side with the affected ear down to see if the object will fall out on its own. If it does not, the patient should be evaluated in a medical facility for removal and follow-up treatment. Tympanic membrane rupture, whether from trauma, diving, or infection, does not require an occlusive or pressure dressing. Instead, allow secretions to drain by having the patient tilt the head toward the affected side. If there are no other injuries, the patient may be transported in this position to a medical facility for further treatment.

KEY POINT

Eardrum Rupture

A ruptured tympanic membrane may produce sudden ear pain followed by no ear pain and is associated with varying degrees of hearing loss. Tinnitus, or ringing in the ear, is common with eardrum-related injuries. Dizziness and a bloody discharge from the external ear canal may occur. If an infection develops, the pain may develop slowly and be associated with ear drainage, fever, and pain.

Part of the inner-ear system controls balance. Symptoms of inner-ear balance problems are usually associated with chronic illness but may be caused by more serious problems such as a recent stroke. For this reason, any patient who reports dizziness, sudden balance problems, or a rapid onset of severe nausea should be evaluated by a physician.

Management of Eye Injuries

Because eye injuries can result in blindness, any patient with an eye injury should be transported for physician evaluation. Obvious penetrating injuries, massive orbital trauma, and suspected globe rupture require emergent referral to an eye specialist. Soft-tissue injuries around the eye should be managed with the utmost care to avoid applying pressure to the eyeball.

Small foreign bodies on the surface of the eye are a common problem. If the patient allows, carefully retract the upper and lower eyelids to examine for the presence of a superficial foreign body. The foreign particle could be present on the underside of the lid or on the globe. To examine the inside surface of the upper eyelid, pull the lid forward and up over a cotton swab (**Figure 22-14**). Inflammation—reddening of the conjunctiva, known as conjunctivitis—may be readily apparent. Pain may be aggravated by bright light. Send the patient for definitive care at a health care facility.

Objects that have adhered to the conjunctiva may penetrate the surface of the eyeball, especially when the injury involves metalwork, such as filing or hammering. These injuries require urgent consultation with an ophthalmologist. Larger foreign bodies impaled in the eye require eye stabilization prior to transport. Use a circular or ring dressing or cup to protect the eye and use a gauze bandage to stabilize the impaled object. Great care must be taken not to move the impaled object during transport, as described in **OEC Skill 22-1**.

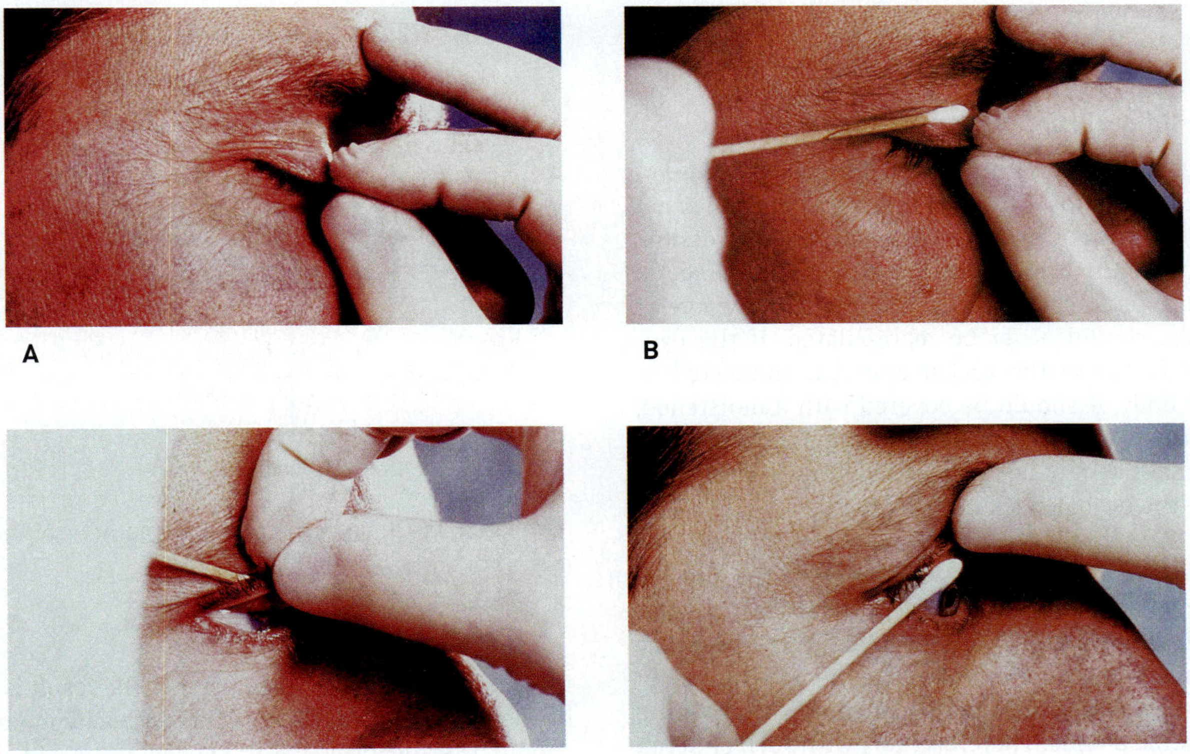

A B C D

Figure 22-14 **A.** To examine for a foreign body in the eye, grasp the eyelashes between the thumb and forefinger and instruct the patient to look down. **B.** Place a swab along the center of the upper eyelid. **C.** Pull the eyelid forward and up over the swab. **D.** Once the underside of the eyelid has been exposed, look for the foreign object. You may be able to gently dab with a cotton swab and remove the object.

OEC SKILL 22-1 Stabilizing an Impaled Object in the Eye

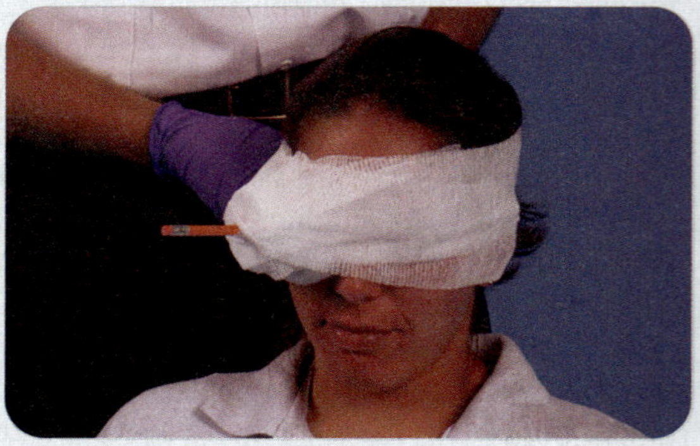

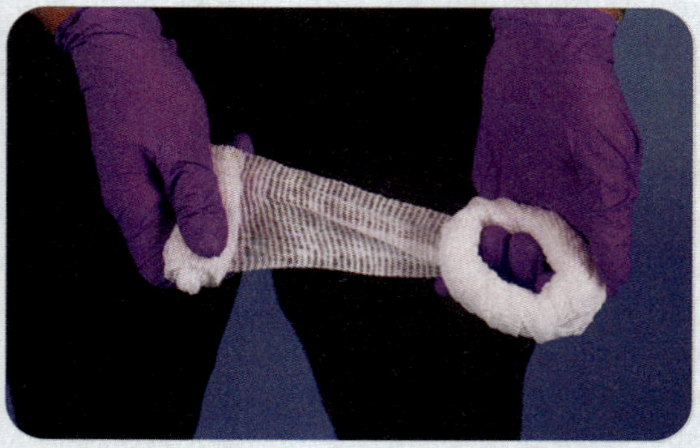

1 When an object has penetrated an eye, do not remove the object. Place padding around the eye, using a roll of gauze or cravat to create a "doughnut." An alternative is to place a paper cup over the eye.

2 Use a roller bandage to secure the doughnut or cup in place.

Eyelid and Eyeball Lacerations

Eyelid lacerations may bleed profusely because of the blood supply to this part of the face. They are commonly controlled with *gentle* direct pressure. Because the eyeball itself also may be injured, do not apply pressure to the eye's globe. The eye or globe should never be manipulated. If the eyeball is out of the socket and still connected to the body, it should be covered with a moistened, sterile dressing to prevent drying. Fully detached eyeballs cannot be reimplanted. Do not attempt to put the eyeball back in the socket.

When one eye is injured, cover both eyes to decrease synchronous movement of the injured eye when the uninjured eye moves. This is especially important in penetrating injuries. Note that bandaging both eyes will make the patient unable to see at all, which can be extremely frightening to some people. Therefore, stay with such patients and talk to them, guide them, and reassure them.

Blunt Trauma

Direct trauma to the eye or surrounding soft tissue can cause bleeding within the eye. If the bleeding fills the anterior chamber of the eye, the result is a hyphema (**Figure 22-15**). Patients with a hyphema should be transported with the head of the bed elevated 30 degrees if possible.

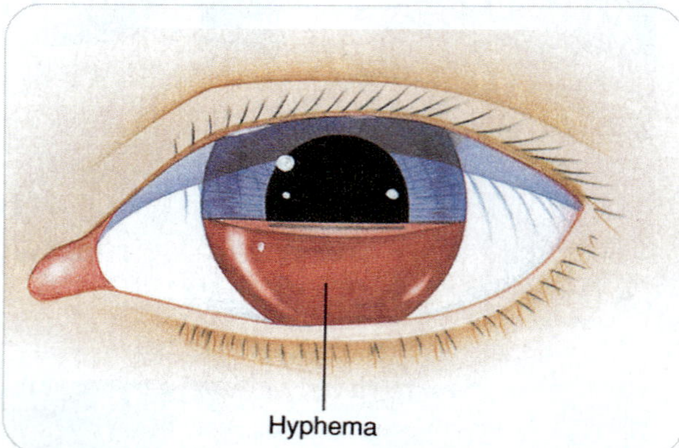

Figure 22-15 Blood in the anterior chamber of the eye is called a hyphema.

Any blunt trauma to the eye may also cause **retinal detachment**, the symptoms of which are seeing specks, flashing lights or "floaters" in the visual field, or decreased vision in that eye.

Patients reporting any of these symptoms require emergent evaluation by an ophthalmologist.

Burns to the Eye

Exposure to chemicals, heat, and UV or intense light can burn the surface of the eye. Such exposure often injures both eyes. Quick assessment and treatment of these injuries may allow OEC technicians to prevent further damage to the eyes.

Chemical Burns

Exposure to any chemical strong enough to irritate the eyes is an emergency. To minimize the injury, immediately gently open the eye and gently irrigate the eye with tepid sterile saline solution (or tepid tap water, if saline is not available). Do not use cold or hot water. Medical irrigation faucets may be available in commercial or industrial settings. In the absence of specialized equipment in outdoor environments, directly irrigate the eye with saline or clean water from a bag or bottle by pouring into the medial (inside) corner of the eye, letting fluid run across the eye to the outside. If available, a gently running shower or faucet also may work (**Figure 22-16**). Regardless of the flushing technique used, take care not to contaminate the unaffected eye. Put a shield up across the bridge of the nose to prevent the fluid from getting into the good eye.

To be effective, irrigation requires the use of copious fluids. Irrigate the affected eye for at least 5 minutes. If the burn was caused by a strong chemical, irrigate the eye for 20 to 30 minutes. If pain persists, continue the irrigation. It may be difficult for patients to keep their eyelid(s) open during irrigation, so they may require your assistance.

Damage from strong acids or strong bases can continue even after copious irrigation. Patients with such injuries should be transferred with ALS for emergency care. Assume that if the patient still has pain, then damage from the chemical remains ongoing. You may be able to reduce damage to the eye by continuing irrigation during transport. Be sure to note the chemical(s) involved using the material safety data sheet, which can often be provided by the patient's employer in an industrial accident, and include that information in your handoff report to subsequent rescuers or care providers. In the case of a chemical burn, any contact lenses should be removed prior to irrigating,

Patients who require eye irrigation will naturally want to keep their eyes closed, especially if they are experiencing pain. To facilitate irrigation, use PPE to keep the chemical off you, and if needed use gauze to help keep the slippery eyelids open. To irrigate the eyes, follow these steps:

1. Attach irrigation solution to intravenous tubing. If intravenous solution is not available, use *tepid* tap water. Place the water in a clean plastic bag and poke a small hole in the corner or pour slowly from a medicine bottle.
2. Gently hold the patient's eye open.
3. Direct the solution into the affected eye, so that it flows from the medial (nasal) side of the eye to the lateral (cheek) side of the eye.

Thermal Burns

When the eyelids or the surface of the eye is burned by the heat of a thermal accident, take immediate action to stop the burning. Then cover both eyes with a moist sterile dressing and immediately transport the patient for definitive care. Regardless of whether the burn is to the eyelid or the eye, specialist care and follow-up are required. The airway could also have burns when the eyes have been burned.

Ultraviolet Light Burns

Different sources of light burn different parts of the eye. Light from welders, UV light, snow blindness, and "black lights" can injure the eye. Depending on what part of the eye is injured, the patient may or may not have pain associated with the injury.

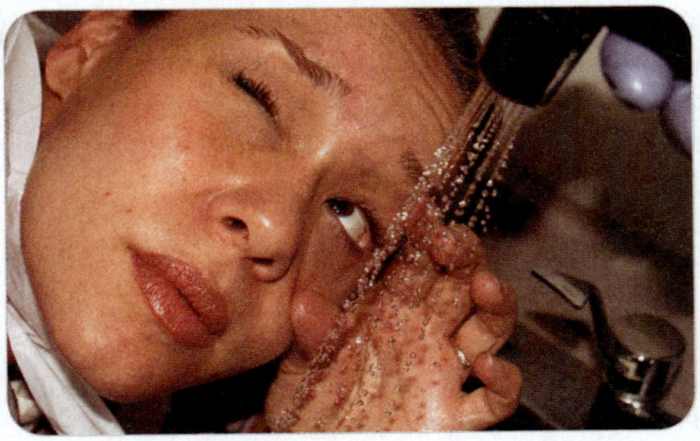

Figure 22-16 One method of irrigating the eye.

KEY POINT

Removing Contact Lenses

Ask the patient to remove his or her contact lenses. If the patient cannot or is unwilling, then follow these steps:

1. Put on gloves. Always remove the lens from the uninjured eye first.
2. Removing a soft contact lens: Instruct the patient to look up and then pull the lower lid down. Place your index finger on the lens and slide it down to the white of the eye. Squeeze the lens lightly with your thumb and index finger and remove it gently. Alternatively, you may be able to remove a soft contact lens by instilling one or two drops of saline or irrigating solution (**Figure 22-17A**).
3. Removing a hard contact lens: Put an index finger on the center of the upper lid and a thumb on the center of the lower lid. Press the thumb and index finger together to force the patient to blink. The contact lens will pop out. You may also use a small commercial suction device in order to remove the hard contact lens (**Figure 22-17B**).

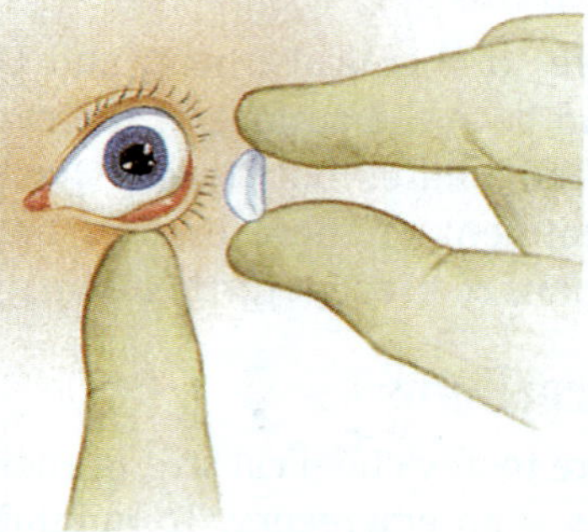

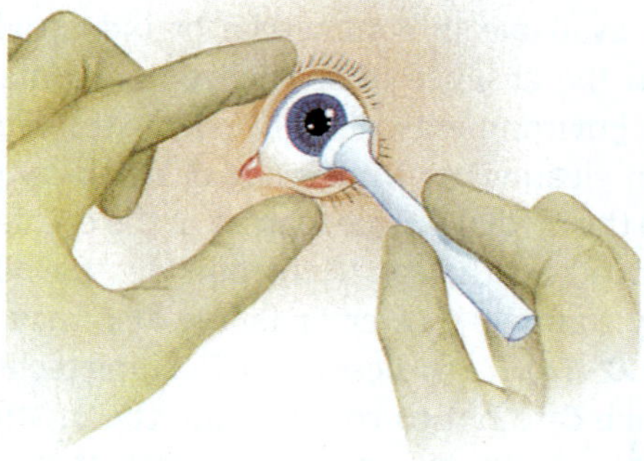

Figure 22-17 **A.** Removing a soft contact lens. **B.** Removing a hard contact lens.

Treat superficial burns to the cornea by applying a moist sterile dressing and an eye shield, and transport the patient for evaluation by a specialist as soon as possible. If you suspect a light injury as the cause of a loss of vision in the *absence* of pain, manage the injury as a retinal burn, which requires evaluation by a specialist.

Dealing with Contact Lenses

Contact lenses may be difficult to see upon physical exam. When evaluating patients for an eye injury, always ask them if they wear contact lenses. If the patient can remove their contact lenses by themselves, ask them to do so. Attempt to remove a contact lens only when a patient has suffered a chemical burn to the eye, when irrigating the eye, or when assisting someone who has requested your assistance in the removal of a lens. In other situations, the manipulation required to remove the lens may cause further damage to the eye. If the patient wore contact lenses during your eye exam, relay this information to the EMS provider who assumes care of the patient from you.

In a severely injured eye, do not attempt to remove contact lens.

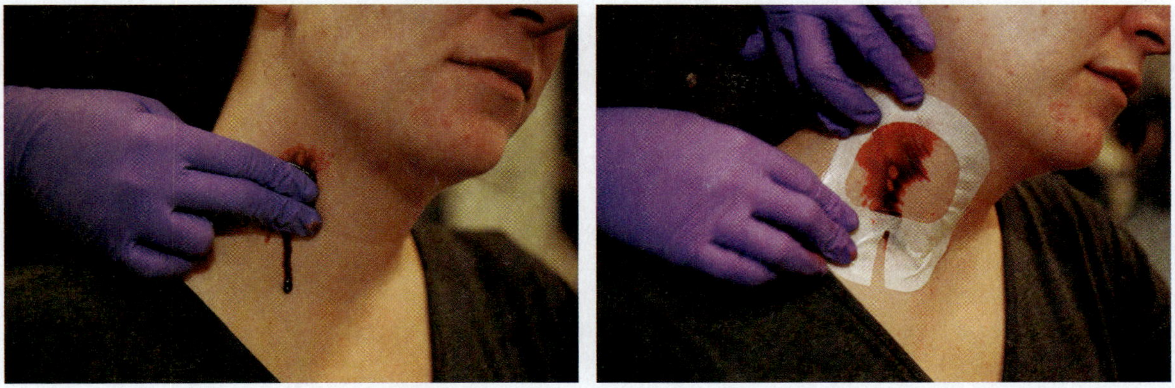

Figure 22-18 **A.** Treatment of a severed blood vessel in the neck begins with placing a gloved hand over the wound to control bleeding. Apply only enough pressure to control bleeding. **B.** Apply an occlusive dressing that extends beyond the wound; then cover with a regular dressing.

Dealing with Artificial Eyes

It may be difficult to distinguish a patient's prosthetic eye from a natural eye. Ask the patient if the eye is a prosthesis. The patient may have some ability to move the prosthetic eye using extraocular muscles, making any visible difference between the two eyes very subtle. A prosthetic eye will not have any pupillary response. If the eye is out of the socket, protect it, as prosthetic eyes are expensive.

Management of Neck Injuries

Injuries to the anterior neck can be life threatening, may be associated with cervical-spinal injuries, and should be considered an emergency by OEC technicians. Manage the ABCDs and the spine accordingly. Open neck injuries with severe bleeding usually can be controlled using the combination of an occlusive dressing and then sterile dressings and direct pressure (**Figure 22-18**). Keep patients with anterior neck bleeding lying down to help reduce the chances of air embolism. If the patient sits up, air can enter a large vessel in the neck.

Be careful not to apply direct pressure to both sides of the neck simultaneously because doing so can reduce blood flow through the carotid arteries to the brain. Likewise, do not wrap bandages around the neck because doing so can compromise both the airway and circulation. Instead, place an occlusive dressing over the wound and then secure a pressure dressing over the wound by wrapping roller gauze in a figure-eight pattern around the neck and around the arm and armpit of the opposite shoulder.

Immobilize impaled objects in place unless they compromise the airway.

Blunt trauma to the anterior neck can be more difficult to manage than penetrating neck trauma because structural damage may completely occlude the airway. Aggressively manage the airway, summon ALS assistance, and urgently transport the patient to the nearest medical facility.

CASE Outcome

As you wait for backup to arrive at the scene of the accident, you reassure the snowboarder, making sure the ABCDs remain stable. Upon the arrival of additional patrollers and equipment, you apply high-flow oxygen. The patient maintains *A* on the AVPU scale. You give clear instructions to your partners regarding your assessment of anterior neck soft-tissue trauma and a possible fractured jaw. Rapid transport to the emergency department is needed. During the brief transport, you reassess the patient's condition several times.

You give the ALS provider your handoff report, which includes your concern for possible compromise of the patient's airway. The ALS provider gives medications, so he can intubate the patient, as he is concerned that the airway could become obstructed. Following transport to the hospital, vascular studies show that the patient did not injure his carotid arteries, his jugular veins, or his cervical spine. His airway problem resolved over the first 24 hours of his 2-day hospital stay. He had surgery to repair a fractured jaw. One month later, the snowboarder stops at the patrol hut to thank you for the quality of care he received from you.

CHAPTER REVIEW

In Summary

- Facial and neck injuries can be associated with severe pain and anxiety.
- Facial and neck injuries can have significant internal or external bleeding.
- Facial and neck injuries can rapidly become life threatening.
- Assess the stability of the patient's airway by listening to the patient talk.
- Direct pressure applied to an injured globe of the eye may worsen the injury.
- Facial and neck asymmetry is a clue to traumatic injury.
- Facial fractures require a significant mechanism of injury, so associated closed head or cervical-spine injuries must be considered as well.
- Face and neck injuries require frequent assessment, especially the airway.
- Always assess the need for spinal motion restriction for any significant face, neck, or head injury.

Key Terms

Anisocoria Unequal size of the pupils.

Blowout fracture An injury caused by direct trauma to the eye or face that fractures the bony eye socket; can entrap the muscles that enable normal eye movement.

Cornea The clear but highly sensitive surface of the eye that refracts light entering into the visual system.

Epistaxis Nosebleed.

External auditory canal The passageway through the outer ear that ends at the tympanic membrane (eardrum).

Hyphema Blood in the anterior chamber of the eye.

Lacrimal glands The glands that produce tears, which irrigate the surface of the eye.

Mandible The jawbone.

Maxillae The bones of the midface that form the upper jaw.

Orbit The bony socket of the eyeball.

Retinal detachment Separation of the retina from the posterior wall of the inside of the eyeball.

Sternocleidomastoid muscles Powerful muscles at the sides of the neck that facilitate turning of the head.

Subcutaneous emphysema Air-filled bubbles that are palpable underneath the skin, indicating an injury to an airway structure.

Chapter Questions

1. The primary function of the iris is to:
   a. protect the retina.
   b. give the eye its globe shape.
   c. control the amount of light that enters the eye.
   d. act as a focusing lens.
2. Unequal pupil size is most likely the result of a problem in what part of the body?
   a. Chest
   b. Face
   c. Brain
   d. Neck
3. Your patient complains of pain and bleeding in his ear. Which of the following *might* be a source of his pain?
   a. Ruptured tympanic membrane
   b. Inner ear infection, causing a ruptured tympanic membrane
   c. Foreign body lodged in the ear canal
   d. All of the above

4. Your patient was skiing in a glade area and fell forward, colliding into a tree. A piece of tree branch has penetrated his right eye. Approximately 10 cm (4 inches) of the branch is visible, and the depth of penetration is unknown. Which of the following is *not* an appropriate action by the OEC technician?
   a. Bandaging both eyes to prevent excess movement
   b. Removing the branch to check his vision
   c. Using roller gauze, a paper cup, or a cravat "doughnut" to stabilize the branch
   d. Having a second OEC technician stabilize his head to prevent excessive movement
5. Which of the following are unprotected vital structures of the neck?
   a. Carotid arteries, jugular veins, esophagus, trachea, and thyroid gland
   b. Thyroid cartilage, esophagus, and spinal cord
   c. Jugular veins, carotid arteries, and cervical vertebrae
   d. Cervical vertebrae, thyroid gland, and jugular veins
6. Traumatic injuries affecting the neck and upper airway can be life threatening. Which of the following signs indicate that your patient is experiencing a potentially serious injury?
   a. External arterial bleeding from the neck
   b. Hoarse voice and difficulty speaking
   c. Air-filled bubbles that are palpable underneath the skin in the upper chest area and neck
   d. All of the above
7. The following are all acceptable means of safekeeping an avulsed tooth, *except*:
   a. placing it in the socket if patient is alert and oriented with no airway problems.
   b. placing it in Hanks' solution in a sterile container.
   c. placing it in milk or saline solution in a sterile container if Hanks' solution is not available.
   d. placing it in a bag of ice.
8. Which of the following injuries best represents an *emergent* problem with the face, eyes, or neck?
   a. Laceration to the exterior portion of the ear, with no hearing loss
   b. Chemical burn to one or both eyes
   c. Small branch impaled in the cheek, with no airway obstruction
   d. Epistaxis controlled with gentle pressure just below the bony prominence of the nose
9. Your patient is a mountain biker whose tire got caught between two rocks on a steep descent. While getting off the bike, your patient slipped and struck his eye on a tree stump. Upon your arrival, the patient is covering his eyes with his hands and moaning in pain. Which of the following actions is *not* appropriate?
   a. Forcibly opening the injured eye to check for any vision problems and to make sure the eye is not badly injured
   b. Asking the patient whether he is experiencing any double vision
   c. Evaluating pupil size in both eyes, if the patient can open the injured eye on his own
   d. Looking for any clear or blood-tinged fluid leaking from the injured eye

10. Your patient collided with another skier and fell just below the takeoff area of a jump. While your patient was on the ground, a third skier took the jump and collided with him. Upon arrival on scene, you find your patient supine with his gloved hand covering his neck. There is blood all over the front of his jacket and on the snow next to him. You can see more blood flowing between the fingers of his glove. Your actions should include which of the following?
    a. Keep him lying down.
    b. Control the bleeding with an occlusive dressing, sterile dressing, and direct pressure.
    c. Apply direct pressure to both sides of the neck simultaneously.
    d. Both A and B

Answers: 1. c, Objective 22-1, p. 544; 2. c, Objective 22-8, p. 545; 3. d, Objective 22-8, p. 552; 4. b, Objective 22-3, p. 553; 5. a, Objective 22-4, p. 545; 6. d, Objective 22-5, p. 550; 7. d, Objective 22-7, p. 552; 8. b, Objective 22-8, p. 555; 9. a, Objective 22-9, p. 549; 10. d, Objective 22-10, p. 557

CHAPTER 23

CHEST TRAUMA

OBJECTIVES

Upon completion of this chapter, the OEC technician will be able to:

23-1 List the major anatomic structures of the chest cavity.

23-2 Define and list the signs and symptoms of the following chest injuries:

- Contusions
- Fractures
- Rib fractures
- Flail chest
- Sternum fracture
- Aortic dissection and rupture
- Lower rib cage injury
- Pneumothorax
- Open pneumothorax (sucking chest wound)
- Tension pneumothorax
- Hemothorax
- Pericardial tamponade
- Commotio cordis
- Traumatic asphyxia

23-3 Describe and demonstrate how to assess the chest for trauma, including using the LAP method.

23-4 Describe the management of chest injuries.

KEY TERMS

Aneurysm, p. 568
Aortic rupture, p. 568
Closed chest injury, p. 566
Commotio cordis, p. 572
Flail chest, p. 567
Hemoptysis, p. 574
Hemothorax, p. 570
Myocardial contusion, p. 566
Open chest injury (sucking chest wound), p. 566
Paradoxical motion, p. 567
Pericardial tamponade, p. 571
Pulmonary contusion, p. 566
Tension pneumothorax, p. 569
Traumatic asphyxia, p. 573

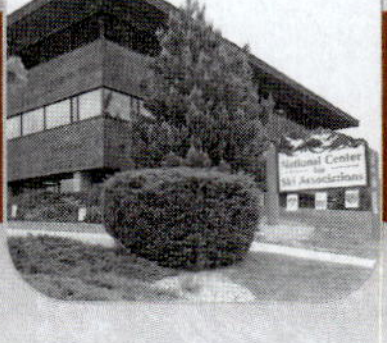

HISTORICAL TIMELINE **1990.** Office is consolidated with Professional Ski Instructors of America (PSIA) under management of the same Executive Director.

CHAPTER OVERVIEW

Many activities that involve traveling at a high rate of speed can allow the participant to hit an object causing serious bodily injury, including chest (thoracic) trauma. The chest (or thorax) contains such vital organs responsible for sustaining life as the heart, lungs, and great vessels. Trauma can cause superficial injuries that affect only the chest wall, or it can cause internal injuries to the organs and structures within the chest. Snowmobilers, off-piste travelers, rafters, skiers, snowboarders, Alpine climbers, bicyclists, and those who traverse avalanche-prone terrain have increased risk for chest trauma if there is an accident.

Even seemingly minor chest injuries can present numerous challenges because they can create breathing problems complicating other injuries or aggravate underlying medical conditions. For example, a nondisplaced rib fracture could make breathing difficult for someone who had to self-evacuate from the backcountry. Patients with chest trauma may appear to be stable at first, but if the injury is not recognized and treated quickly, consequences can rapidly lead to death.

Being familiar with the different mechanisms of injury that can produce a chest injury and the signs and symptoms of specific chest injuries will enable you to make better treatment decisions. Appropriate treatment and calling for urgent transportation in appropriate cases, will significantly reduce morbidity and mortality from severe chest trauma. The care for serious chest injuries includes controlling excessive bleeding and addressing the ABCDs (airway, breathing, circulation, disability), caring for the specific condition, proper positioning, providing oxygen if appropriate, and transporting rapidly to a higher level of care.

ANATOMY AND PHYSIOLOGY OF THE CHEST

The chest or thorax extends from the base of the neck to the lower edge of the rib cage or costal margin (**Figure 23-1**). It is enclosed by the bony rib cage, sternum, thoracic spine, and diaphragm. The ribs protect the thoracic organs and provide structural support through their connections to the thoracic vertebrae in the back and to the sternum through flexible cartilages in front. The chest cavity contains two major organs necessary for life: the lungs, which take in oxygen and excrete gaseous waste products, and the heart, which pumps the blood. The heart lies near the center of the chest beneath the sternum. Between the lungs above the heart is the area known as the mediastinum, which contains the heart, aorta, venae cavae, trachea, esophagus, thymus gland, and several important nerves.

The diaphragm, the primary muscle of respiration, separates the chest and abdominal cavities. This dome-shaped sheet of muscle attaches anteriorly at the xiphoid process, posteriorly at the lumbar vertebrae, and laterally at the lower ribs. It is the roof of the abdominal cavity and the floor

CASE Presentation

You are riding the chair lift when you observe a snowboarder entering the terrain park. He launches onto a rail and slams into the end of the rail. When he comes to a stop, you can see that he is lying on the snow and gasping for breath. You radio for someone to respond until you can get there. Upon reaching the summit, you hear another patroller at the scene requesting a trauma pack, and an ambulance with advanced life support (ALS). Grabbing the trauma pack that includes oxygen from the summit hut, you proceed to the scene. Upon your arrival, the patient is sitting up and is complaining of pain in the left chest and is having severe breathing difficulty.

What should the other patroller and you do?

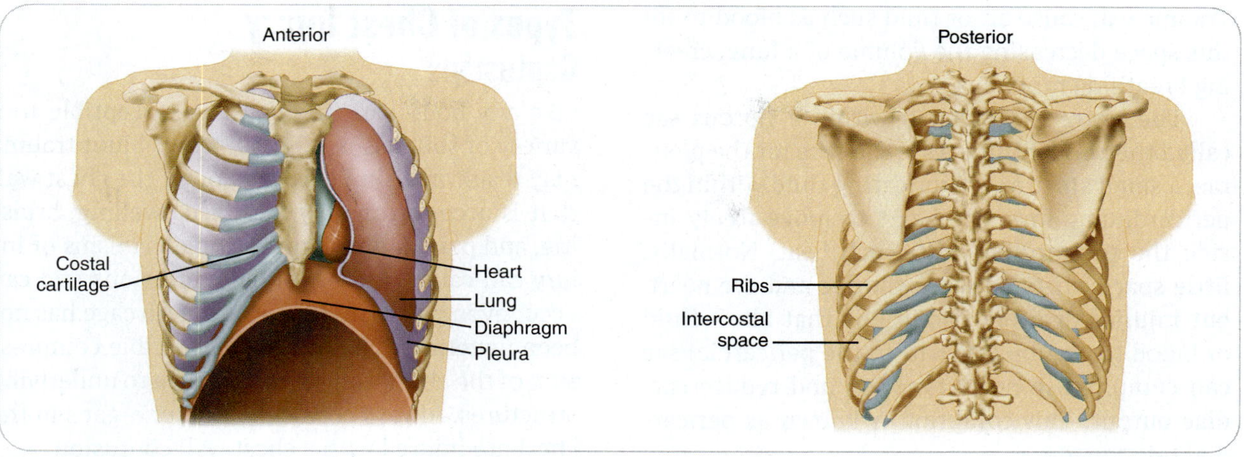

Figure 23-1 The anatomy of the chest cavity.

of the chest cavity. During inhalation, the diaphragm contracts and moves downward, enlarging the chest cavity and creating a negative pressure within the chest, which draws oxygen-containing air into the lungs through the mouth and trachea. During exhalation the diaphragm passively relaxes and returns to its resting position. This reduces the volume of the chest cavity and raises the internal pressure, expelling unused gases and carbon dioxide from the body.

The diaphragm is controlled by the two "phrenic" nerves that connect to the spinal cord at levels C3, C4, and C5 in the neck and travel to the diaphragm. Spinal cord injury at or above this level can impair respiration because the loss of signals through the phrenic nerves can affect diaphragmatic function (**Figure 23-2**). A respiratory arrest will occur if the spinal cord is completely transected at or above C3. The diaphragm is assisted in the work of breathing by the intercostal muscles, which are located between each of the ribs. Embedded within these muscles under each rib are the intercostal arteries, veins, and nerves that provide nutrients and innervation to these muscles.

The chest cavity contains two adjacent membranes called pleura. One membrane covers each lung, and one is on the inside wall of the chest. Between these membranes is a small amount of clear (serous) fluid, which acts as a lubricant that allows the lungs to move freely while they expand and contract. Normally there is little space except for the lubricant fluid between the two pleural layers.

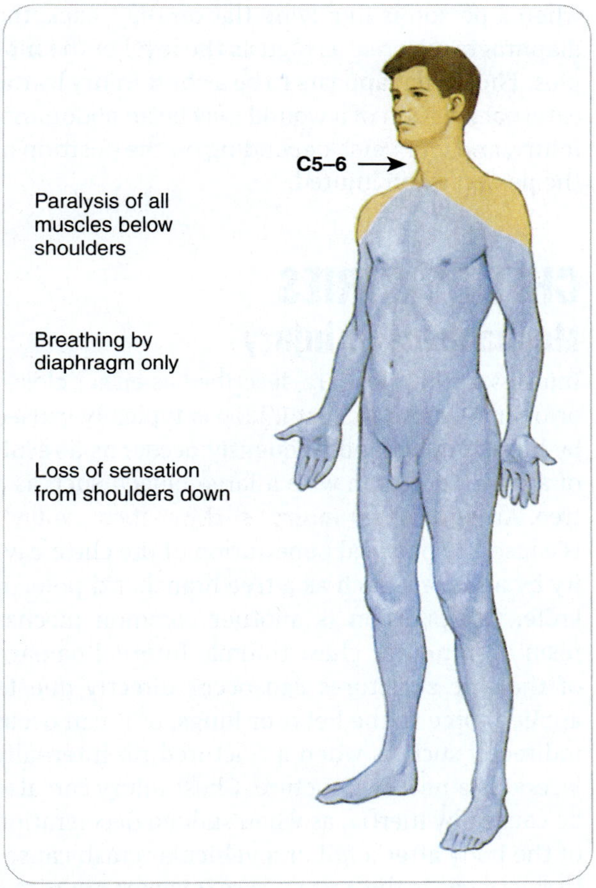

Figure 23-2 A patient who sustains a spinal cord injury below the level of C5 and is paralyzed can still breathe spontaneously because phrenic nerves, which cause the diaphragm to contract, originate at C3, C4, and C5 levels.

Trauma can cause air or fluid such as blood to fill this space decreasing the volume of a lung, creating breathing problems.

The heart is contained within a fibrous sac called the pericardium. As is the case for the pleurae, a small amount of lubricating fluid within the pericardium allows the heart to move freely inside the pericardium with each beat. Normally, little space exists between the sac and the heart, but injuries or other conditions that allow fluid or blood to accumulate within the pericardial sac can compromise heart function and reduce cardiac output. This condition is known as pericardial tamponade.

The chest cavity is unusual in that its overall size changes during each breath. Its size also can change due to the relative positions of the diaphragm or of the body as a whole. For instance, when a person is in a lying flat on their back, the diaphragm may rise as high as the level of the nipples. Thus, what appears to be a chest injury by the external location of a wound may be an abdominal injury, and vice versa depending on the position of the person when injured.

CHEST INJURIES

Mechanisms of Injury

Injuries to the chest are described as either closed or open. A **closed chest injury** is typically caused by blunt trauma and frequently occurs as a result of a fall or collision with a large object, such as a tree. An **open chest injury (sucking chest wound)** is caused by physical penetration of the chest cavity by an object such as a tree branch, ski pole, or knife. Compression is another common mechanism of injury for chest trauma. Internal damage of thoracic structures can occur directly due to applied force to the heart or lungs, or it can occur indirectly such as when a fractured rib internally lacerates a nearby structure. Chest injury can also be caused by inertia, as when sudden deceleration of the body after a fall or a vehicular crash causes tissues such as the aorta where it comes out of the top of the heart to move violently, tearing it away from its attachment. Regardless of the source, internal chest injuries are more difficult to assess, and sometimes to manage, than are more obvious external injuries, and they almost always require advanced care.

Types of Chest Injury

Contusions

Like any body part, the chest is susceptible to a variety of soft-tissue injuries. Minor blunt trauma may result in a simple contusion of the chest wall that is accompanied by localized swelling, bruising, and pain. More significant mechanisms of injury can cause internal organ contusions and can occur even when the skin over the rib cage has not been penetrated. In such cases, forcible compression of the chest wall causes damage to underlying structures. Always consider whether organs in the chest are injured with a chest wall contusion.

A **pulmonary contusion** is a bruise of the lung tissue that causes the alveoli to become filled with fluid and blood (**Figure 23-3**). As a result, gas exchange is compromised, which can cause hypoxia, the severity of which is related to the size of the contusion. A pulmonary contusion commonly occurs in patients who suffer rib fractures, even if the bones do not directly lacerate the lung tissue. Hemoptysis, coughing up blood, can also occur depending on the severity of injury.

A **myocardial contusion**, also called a cardiac contusion, is a bruise involving the heart that may cause heart contractions to become less effective. Severe bruising can result in an arrhythmia, reduced cardiac output, or cardiogenic shock.

Fractures

Impact-type injuries can cause fractures of the bones of the anterior and lateral chest wall, including the ribs, clavicle, and sternum. Crushing injuries can also cause fractures. The chest cavity is an anatomic marvel that can withstand relatively high amounts of energy while remaining intact.

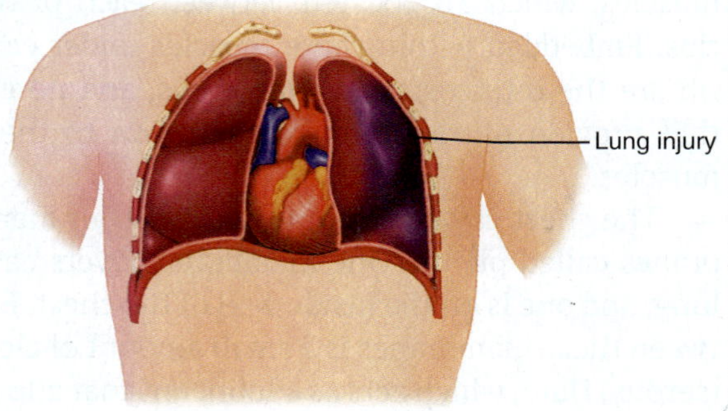

Figure 23-3 A pulmonary contusion.

When fractures occur, OEC technicians must have a high index of suspicion for internal damage because energy that is great enough to fracture a bone may be transmitted to underlying structures. Clavicle and rib fractures are among the most common chest injuries. Clavicle fractures are discussed in Chapter 20, *Musculoskeletal Injuries*. The thoracic spine can also be injured and discussed separately in Chapter 21, *Spine, Brain, and Nervous System Injuries*.

Rib Fractures

Rib fractures can impair breathing due to intense pain that is usually right over the fracture site. Breathing is often shallow because deep respirations increase movements of the fractured bone, intensifying the pain. To lessen discomfort, patients may "self-splint" or apply direct pressure over the injured site to keep the fractured bone ends from moving. In some instances, the sharp end of a displaced fractured rib can lacerate underlying lung tissue blood vessels, or both, causing additional problems. The elderly are at high risk for fractured ribs because their bones are more brittle than those of younger individuals. If multiple ribs are broken, a flail chest can occur.

Flail Chest

A **flail chest** is defined as fractures of two or more adjacent ribs, each of which is fractured in two or more places (**Figure 23-4**). Alternatively, two or more ribs could be separated off the spine posteriorly, or from the sternum anteriorly, and be broken in a separate place, and still be considered a flail chest. The resulting thoracic instability causes the injured segment of the chest wall to move independently of the rest of the rib cage. The isolated segment, or "flail" segment, moves inward upon inspiration and outward upon expiration, which is the opposite movement from that of the rest of the chest, a condition known as **paradoxical motion**.

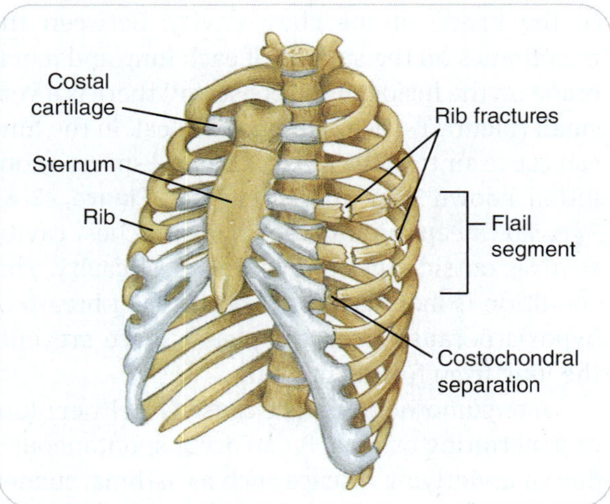

Figure 23-4 A flail chest is when two or more adjacent ribs are fractured in two or more places.

Patients with a flail chest usually complain of severe chest wall pain and shortness of breath. They may attempt to self-splint the injured area by firmly holding the flail segment in place as they breathe.

Be alert for other associated injuries, because the forces required to produce a flail chest may cause other serious internal injuries. The lung tissue directly beneath the flail segment is often contused or damaged and may not expand properly. This injury results in shallow breathing and can quickly result in the patient becoming hypoxic.

Sternum Fracture

Fractures of the sternum, although uncommon, can be associated with life-threatening injuries to underlying structures as well as other parts of the body. Due to the force required to fracture the sternum, injuries to underlying organs, including the heart, lungs, aorta, and other large blood vessels as well as upper abdominal organs should be considered. Rarely, the entire sternum can become a flail segment should the ribs on both sides become fractured or separated from the sternal cartilage. The most common cause of this is external chest compressions applied during CPR, even when performed properly. High-speed blunt chest trauma also can produce this type of injury. Seat belts help prevent this injury by preventing drivers from hitting the center of the steering wheel. If a patient has a sternal injury resulting from a very rapid deceleration, suspect an associated rupturing or tearing of the aorta, which is life threatening.

Aortic Dissection and Rupture

Rapid deceleration injuries such as hitting a tree while skiing or motor vehicle trauma are common sources of injury and can cause many serious problems that may not be immediately apparent. **Aortic rupture** is the most lethal of these hidden injuries.

The aorta is attached to tissue near the heart and rapid deceleration can cause the aorta to tear here, usually resulting in rapid death from massive internal bleeding. When the moving human body slows or stops rapidly and the chest hits a fixed object, the structures within the chest remain in motion for a short period of time. This inertia and the sudden stop inflict a tremendous shearing force on the internal organs and on the tissues that hold them in place. The upper aorta is especially vulnerable to deceleration injuries; the resulting rupture or tearing is usually followed by rapid internal hemorrhage, hypovolemic shock, and death. This can be seen when a skier's chest impacts a tree.

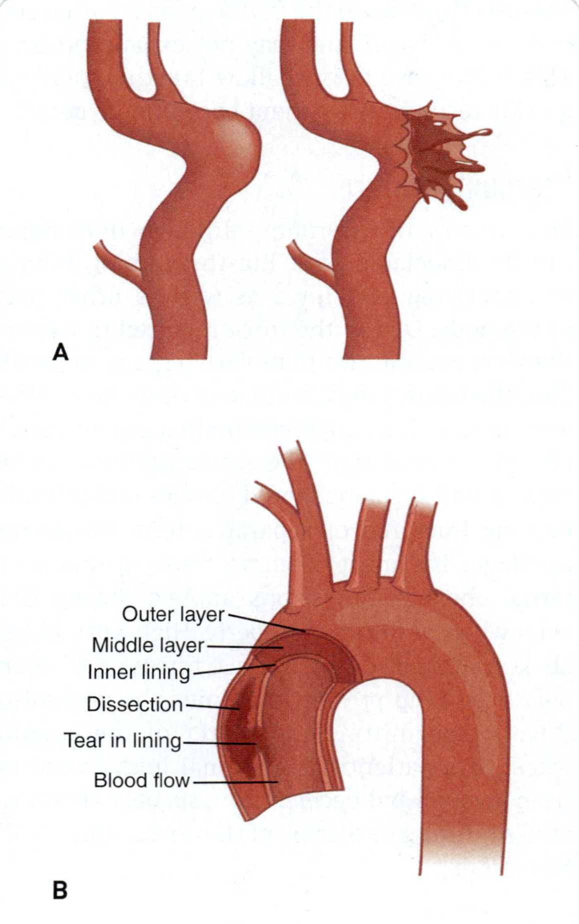

Figure 23-5 A. The progression of an aneurysm to rupture. **B.** Aortic dissection.

Only part of the thickness of the aorta's wall can be torn. This condition is not always immediately fatal, but it can cause other conditions, most notably an **aneurysm** (ballooning of the less dense outer layer of the wall of the aorta) or aortic dissection, in which blood leaks out between the layers of the wall of the aorta (**Figure 23-5**). This condition if unrecognized and left untreated, can eventually cause the vessel to rupture, causing massive and rapid internal bleeding and death.

Patients with an aorta-related injury usually present with severe acute chest pain or back pain, or a tearing or stabbing pain that radiates from the chest to the back between the shoulder blades. Such patients generally appear gravely ill, and if the aorta has ruptured, they exhibit signs of profound shock. If the tear in the aorta is between the large arteries that go to each arm the blood pressure can be different in the two arms. Rapid transport to a definitive-care center is necessary to prevent a lethal outcome.

Lower Rib Cage Injury

Cartilage along the bottom of the anterior rib cage can be torn, stretched, or separated from the bone, mimicking the signs and symptoms of rib fracture. This condition is usually benign but can be quite painful and may hinder breathing. In the field it is difficult to differentiate from a broken rib.

Pneumothorax

Under normal conditions, each lung lies very close to the inside of the chest cavity. Between the membranes on the surface of each lung and membrane on the inside of the chest wall there is a very small (pleural) space. Trauma or a leak in the lung can cause air to collect in this pleural space, a condition known as a pneumothorax (**Figure 23-6**). *Pneumo-* means air and *thorax* means chest cavity, so air is outside the lung in the chest cavity. This condition is manifested by shortness of breath or hypoxia because air in the pleura space prevents the lung from fully expanding.

A pneumothorax can be caused by either blunt or penetrating trauma. It can occur spontaneously due to underlying disease such as asthma, sudden changes in altitude, compressive forces on the chest, blast injuries, or other causes.

A common cause of a pneumothorax is penetrating trauma where a hole in the chest wall

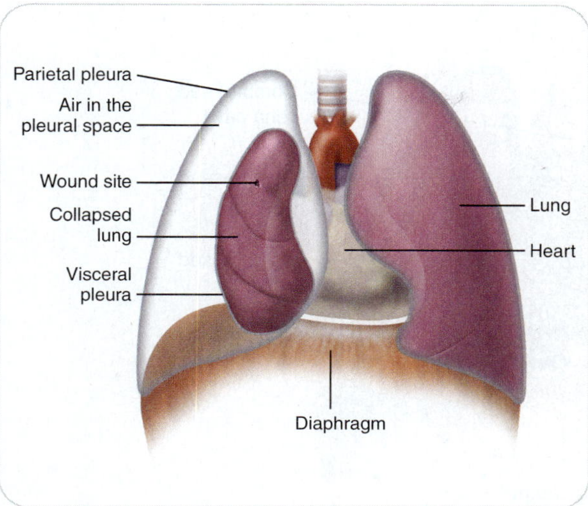

Figure 23-6 Pneumothorax occurs when air leaks into the pleural space.

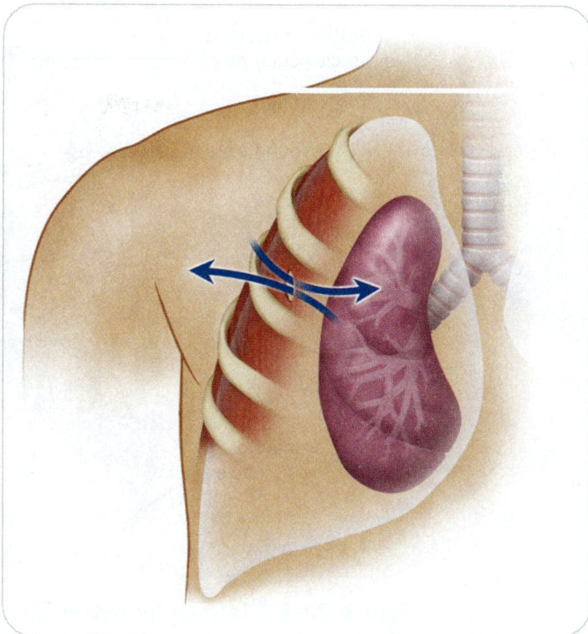

Figure 23-7 With a sucking chest wound or an open pneumothorax, air passes from outside into the pleural space and sometimes back out with each breath, creating a sucking sound.

allows external air to enter chest cavity. This may be referred to as an open pneumothorax. With each inspiration, the difference between the pressure within the thorax and the pressure in the external environment causes air to be sucked into the pleural space. If enough air enters the pleural space, the lung may partially or totally collapse, resulting in decreased gas exchange and hypoxia. With this type of injury, OEC technicians may hear a sucking noise each time the patient breathes. Air gets sucked through the hole in chest wall into the chest cavity. This situation is also known as a "sucking chest wound" (**Figure 23-7**).

Pneumothorax may occur as a result of blunt trauma. A direct blow that covers a large area of the thoracic wall at the peak of the inspiratory cycle can cause one or both lungs to burst. If air continues to accumulate within the pleural space, it can lead to an even more dangerous condition known as a tension pneumothorax.

A **tension pneumothorax** is defined as an accumulation of pressurized air within the pleural space that compresses the lungs (**Figure 23-8**). In this case there is no way for the air outside the lung to get out of the chest. Left untreated, this air will increase causing the organs within the chest cavity to become compressed, resulting in reduced lung capacity, severe respiratory distress, and eventually decreased cardiac output. With enough pressure from a lot of air in the chest, one lung will completely collapse. As more pressure builds, the heart, great vessels, and trachea within the mediastinum are pushed into the opposite side of the chest, sometimes collapsing the other lung. A rapid reduction in blood volume being pumped to the lungs occurs because the vena cava collapses, so no blood is returned to the right side of the heart. The collapse of both lungs from a tension pneumothorax is likely rapidly fatal.

A tension pneumothorax can develop in closed chest trauma when a sharp bone fragment of a fractured rib punctures a lung or bronchus. Air leaks out of the hole in the lung or bronchus into the pleural space. Pressure can build within minutes to a few hours, creating the same life-threatening situation. A tension pneumothorax can develop, or be made *worse*, by the application of positive pressure such as occurs in rescue breathing using a bag-valve mask. With each breath, more air passes through any internal airway hole into the pleural space, thereby changing a stable pneumothorax into an unstable tension pneumothorax. Therefore, when giving CPR with rescue breaths, you should not overinflate the lungs.

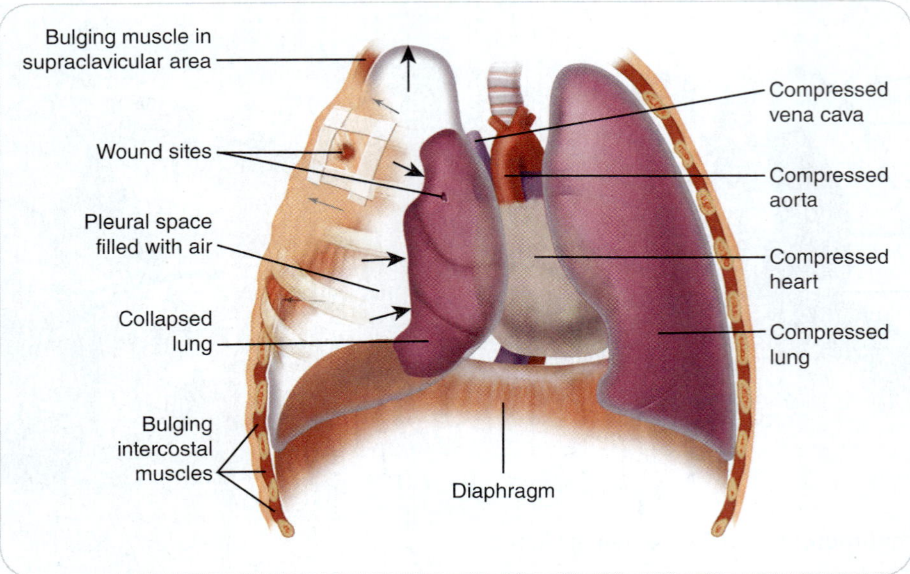

Figure 23-8 A tension pneumothorax can develop if a penetrating chest wound is bandaged tightly and air from a damaged lung cannot escape. The air then accumulates in the pleural space, eventually causing compression of the heart and great vessels.

The hallmarks of a tension pneumothorax are shortness of breath, distended (bulging) neck veins (known as jugular venous distention, or JVD), tachycardia, low blood pressure, and cyanosis. Advanced OEC technicians may detect decreased lung sounds in the lung that has deflated. Tracheal deviation, in which the trachea shifts away from the side of the tension pneumothorax, may be observed, but this is a very late sign.

Tension pneumothorax can lead to subcutaneous emphysema, or "sub-Q air." In this condition, pressurized air leaks out of the pleural cavity into the soft tissues and becomes trapped under the skin, causing a Rice-Krispies-like "crackling" sensation of the skin when pressed with the fingers. Because air rises, subcutaneous emphysema is typically found in the highest point of the chest cavity, so this condition is generally exhibited in the neck first but can spread to the shoulders, chest, or back, depending on the patient's position. Sub-Q air is usually benign, but the pneumothorax causing it can be life threatening.

Rarely, pneumothorax can occur spontaneously, typically in young adults or patients with chronic obstructive pulmonary disease. In this situation, no trauma occurs; however, a small defect, called a "bleb," on the lung surface ruptures, allowing air to escape into the pleural space. The signs and symptoms of this type of pneumothorax are identical to those previously described and can advance to become a tension pneumothorax should enough air enter the space. Patients often experience sharp pain in the chest and back.

Hemothorax

A **hemothorax** is like a pneumothorax except that instead of air, blood accumulates within the pleural space (**Figure 23-9**). This condition is caused by disruption of one or more blood vessels inside the chest and can be due to either blunt or penetrating trauma. Hemothorax due to arterial bleeding can be potentially lethal from hypovolemic shock; because the pleural space can hold 3 to 4 liters of blood. Blood can also compress or collapse one or both lungs, resulting in hypoxia and shock. As with other types of chest trauma, pain and shortness of breath are common complaints.

Both air *and* blood can leak into the pleural space simultaneously, producing a condition known as a hemopneumothorax. The mechanisms of injury that can produce hemopneumothorax are associated with multisystem trauma and have a high morbidity and mortality.

Pericardial Tamponade

Blunt or penetrating chest trauma can cause internal bleeding into the pericardial sac from a hole in the heart's muscular wall or the great vessels, causing the condition known as **pericardial tamponade** (**Figure 23-10**). The rupture of a cardiac blood vessel on the heart's wall can also cause this problem. Pericardial tamponade occasionally may be caused by various nontraumatic medical conditions in which fluid other than blood accumulates within the pericardial sac. In bacterial sepsis, pus may be the source of the tamponade. Viral infections around the heart can cause serous fluid to compress the heart.

As blood or other fluid accumulates within the fibrous pericardial sac around the heart, pressure constricts the heart from filling properly (**Figure 23-11**). Because the left ventricular wall is thicker than the right, the right ventricle becomes compressed first. This prevents the walls of the right side of the heart from expanding, impairing venous return of blood from the venae cavae. At the same time, blood backs up into the jugular veins in the neck causing them to bulge (JVD). With less blood being pumped to the lungs for oxygenation, cardiogenic shock and death occur rapidly.

Pain, shortness of breath, and distended neck veins are early signs of pericardial tamponade. If the problem is not immediately resolved, muffled heart sounds and a decrease in the pulse pressure develop. The pulse pressure is the difference between the systolic and diastolic blood pressure readings. The systolic and diastolic readings become close together. The combination of

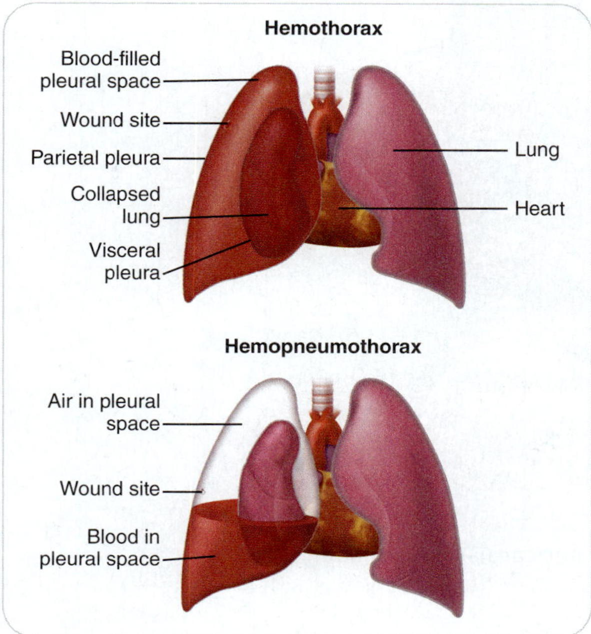

Figure 23-9 A hemothorax is a collection of blood in the pleural space.

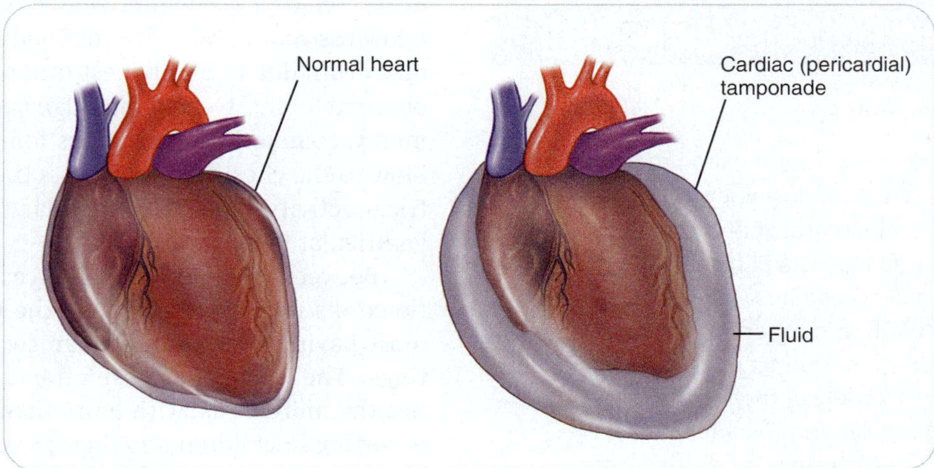

Figure 23-10 Pericardial tamponade is a potentially fatal condition in which fluid builds up with the pericardial sac.

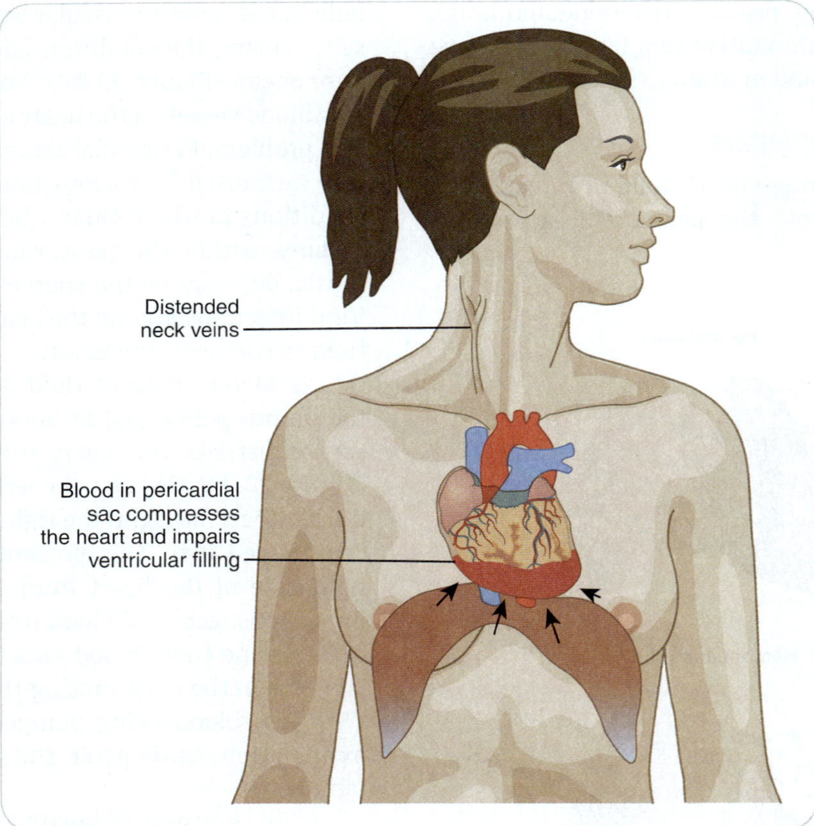

Figure 23-11 The physical findings of pericardial tamponade.

findings—distended neck veins, muffled heart sounds, and a pulsus paradoxus—is known as the Beck triad.

> **KEY POINT**
>
> **Pulsus Paradoxus**
>
> During every inspiration, blood pressure becomes reduced; during every exhalation, blood pressure increases. Pulsus paradoxus is a clinical sign in which a decrease in systolic blood pressure of 10 mm Hg or more occurs upon inspiration. Pulsus paradoxus is caused by a variety of thoracic injuries, including cardiac tamponade, and by such medical disorders as emphysema, pulmonary embolism, and left-side heart failure.

Commotio Cordis (Blunt Trauma to the Chest)

Blunt trauma to the chest, especially to the area over the heart, can cause lethal disruptions in the heart's electrical rhythm. One such condition is known as **commotio cordis**, defined as sudden cardiac death due to blunt chest trauma without any observable chest or cardiac damage. Most commonly, commotio cordis occurs following a direct blow to the chest that interrupts the heart's electrical activity causing ventricular tachycardia or ventricular fibrillation.

Between 1995 and 2017, 224 cases of commotio cordis were documented in the United States, most having occurred in urban recreational settings. The condition most often affects young, healthy individuals, with more than 90% of cases occurring in children less than 16 years of age. Of concern to OEC technicians is that as more young children flock to our nation's snow terrain parks and BMX bicycle parks, the potential for this injury is increasing. Although most reported cases involve direct anterior chest trauma from a baseball, a softball, or a lacrosse ball, one case involved a snowball, and in another case a child was hit in the chest by a snow sliding saucer.

Traumatic Asphyxia

Traumatic asphyxia, or crush asphyxia, is an injury in which external pressure on the chest wall prevents normal chest expansion for breathing, resulting in profound hypoxia or anoxia (**Figure 23-12**).

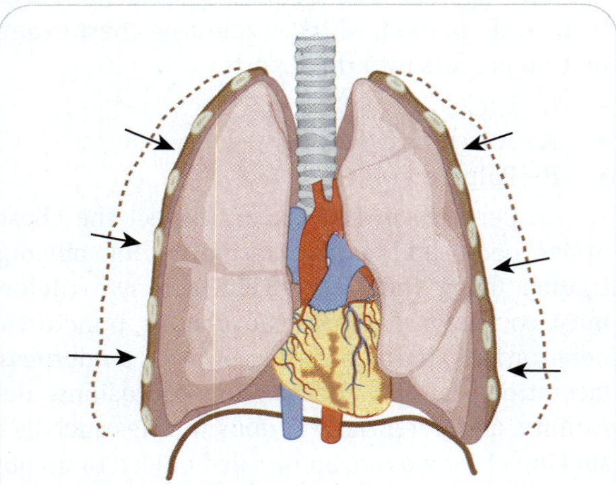

Figure 23-12 Traumatic asphyxia.

This injury involves compression that is typically caused by entrapment under a heavy object, such as a vehicle or avalanche debris. When buried in an avalanche, "concrete" snow packs around a victim's chest, making it unable to expand. Snow can also be packed into the airway, leading to the inability to exchange gas. In both cases, breathing cannot occur, so the person dies of asphyxia. Traumatic asphyxia also can result from massive thoracic cage fractures that render the chest wall unable to expand. Traumatic asphyxia may result in ruptured blood vessels, particularly in the face and neck, which can cause bulging eyes, ruptured blood vessels in the eyes, and an overall purplish discoloration of the face.

Environmental Factors

High altitude can complicate a chest injury due to the decreased partial pressure of available oxygen and lower barometric pressure (which expands gas volumes). This means less oxygen is available per breath the higher you go. Increased altitude may cause a pneumothorax to worsen. In one case report, a woman who had sustained an apparently mild chest injury boarded a commercial airliner. Even though the aircraft cabin maintained an atmospheric pressure equivalent to 8,000 feet, the relative change in air pressure caused a slight pneumothorax to worsen, resulting in severe difficulty breathing. A return to sea level relieved the patient's distress.

CASE Update

You calm the patient and convince him to allow your partner to maintain manual cervical spine stabilization while you perform secondary assessment. The patient's airway is open, there is no external bleeding, and circulation to all extremities is normal. The patient's mental status is also normal. His spine exam and neurologic exam are normal. He appears to be having severe difficulty breathing and is holding his left upper chest and side with both hands. He has shallow respirations at 28 breaths per minute that are unrelieved with high-flow oxygen via a nonrebreather mask. His pulse is 102 beats per minute and he is able to speak in only one- to two-word phrases. When you palpate the patient's left rib cage, he winces in pain. He states that his chest hurts "really bad" and that it is painful to breathe. Other patrollers arrive to assist.

What should you do now?

When at a high altitude, descent in elevation may improve breathing and oxygenation for many chest injuries. When you have a patient with a pneumothorax, take them to a lower altitude rapidly. The effects of altitude have direct implications for OEC technicians when considering the use of aeromedical evacuation of a patient with a suspected pneumothorax or other internal chest injury.

PATIENT ASSESSMENT FOR CHEST INJURIES

Assessment of patients with suspected chest injury is the same as for any other trauma patient. Begin with a scene size-up, evaluating and mitigating any hazards that may be present. Assess the mechanism of injury to determine the forces involved.

Take appropriate standard precautions and begin a primary assessment. Carefully assess the ABCDs and correct life threats such as severe bleeding if needed. Open and clear the airway as necessary. Next, assess the patient for adequate breathing and oxygenation, paying attention to the rate and quality of respirations. A patient with a chest injury may exhibit rapid breathing or other signs of respiratory distress, including the use of accessory muscles. Check the patient's pulse: Is it fast, normal, or slow? Is it bounding or weak? Are the pulses equal on both sides of the body? Assess the patient's mental status and neurologic condition. Mobilize additional resources as needed, including requesting advanced providers if the patient's condition warrants it.

Once the primary assessment is complete, and life threats have been corrected quickly move on to history taking as you begin the secondary assessment.

During the secondary assessment, note the patient's overall appearance and skin color. Does the person appear anxious? Is the patient pale or cyanotic? Quickly check the head, face, and neck. Do the patient's eyes appear bloodshot or bulge outward, which could indicate traumatic asphyxia? Are the neck veins distended, which could suggest pericardial tamponade or tension pneumothorax? Is the trachea deviated to one side? Is there **hemoptysis** (coughing up blood)?

Ask the patient to take a deep breath and then exhale and observe for any signs of discomfort such as grimacing or self-splinting. Also, observe the chest for equal and symmetrical movement. Advanced patrollers may have a stethoscope; use it to listen to each lung to make sure breath sounds are present bilaterally.

If major chest injuries are present or suspected, do not waste precious time identifying each individual injury. Instead, prepare the patient for rapid evacuation to a definitive-care facility.

Environmental or other conditions can make it impractical to perform a detailed chest assessment in the field. One approach that is often used is the LAP method, which divides the chest examination process into three parts:

- **L**—Look
- **A**—Auscultate (listen)
- **P**—Palpate

To perform an LAP exam, inspect the chest, upper back, and axillae (armpits) for obvious trauma using the DCAP-BTLS acronym (deformity, contusions, abrasions/avulsions, punctures/penetrations, burns/bleeding/bruises, tenderness, lacerations, swelling). *Look* for contusions, deformity, and potentially serious injuries such as a sucking chest wound, an impaled object, or an obvious flail segment. As the patient breathes, see if both sides of the chest expand fully and symmetrically. Look for paradoxical motion of the chest in which a portion of the chest wall moves inward during inspiration. If present, suspect a flail chest and impending shock.

Auscultate (listen) to the breath sounds. You may hear gurgling, gasping, wheezing, grunting, or other abnormal sounds, indicating breathing difficulty. Patrollers may listen to the lungs with a stethoscope both anteriorly and posteriorly to ensure that breath sounds are present, equal, and clear bilaterally. If breath sounds are absent or if any abnormal sounds are detected, suspect an internal injury to the pulmonary system or some underlying respiratory disease. OEC technicians need not understand all the different pathological breath sounds. OEC technicians can become familiar with normal breath sounds and should be able to identify abnormalities, such as diminished (difficult to hear) breath sounds, which may indicate the presence of a pneumothorax.

Palpate the entire chest, axillary regions, and upper back for tenderness and deformity. Be sure to "walk" the patient's clavicles with your fingertips, because a displaced clavicle fracture may cause a pneumothorax. Fractures involving the scapula are especially ominous because tremendous force is usually required to break this bone. Many scapular and sternal fractures are associated with internal chest injuries.

Next, assess the integrity of the sternum, again using your fingertips and then the flat side of your hand. As you palpate the chest, be alert for subcutaneous emphysema or any flail segments. If you do not detect any obvious injuries, use both hands to apply moderate inward pressure on the lateral walls of the rib cage and ask the patient to take a deep breath. Then, apply moderate downward pressure on the sternum, again asking the patient to take a deep breath. If the patient experiences pain with either of these tests, stop. These two tests are very helpful in identifying thoracic cage instability or rib fractures that may not be readily apparent.

Complete the remainder of your secondary assessment in the usual fashion and obtain a complete set of vital signs. Reassess the patient frequently, including vital signs and breath sounds. Document your findings on the patient care report. Serial vital signs are essential in any case involving suspected chest trauma because changes may be subtle and could indicate internal bleeding and decompensated shock. Pay close attention to the pulse pressure. Narrowing of the pulse pressure may indicate the presence of a pericardial tamponade. **Table 23-1** summarizes the signs and symptoms of chest trauma.

Table 23-1 Signs and Symptoms of Chest Trauma

- Pain at site of injury that can be aggravated by breathing
- Abnormal chest wall findings: punctures, contusions, unusual chest wall motion
- Dyspnea (shortness of breath)
- Tachypnea (rapid breathing)
- Absent or decreased breath sounds
- Cyanosis (blue skin color)
- Hemoptysis (coughing up blood)
- Tachycardia (fast heart rate)
- Falling blood pressure

MANAGEMENT OF CHEST INJURIES

When a pneumothorax is suspected, correct the ABCDs, provide high-flow oxygen, monitor the oxygen saturation level with a pulse oximeter if available, and call for transport with ALS. Consider transporting and caring for the patient in a sitting position which will provide ease of breathing. This may not be possible if there is a need for spinal motion restriction. In that case you need to raise the head of the backboard. The patient will demonstrate shortness of breath and need further care at a hospital.

Treat other soft-tissue injuries of the chest in the usual manner using standard bandages and dressings. Bulky pressure dressings may be needed to help control heavy bleeding.

Rib fractures can be very painful, especially upon inspiration or movement. Do not splint the chest as doing so will impair breathing. Although done in the past, it is now best to avoid placing a tightly constrictive bandage around the circumference of the chest because it can inhibit chest wall expansion during inhalation. Always consider the patient may have damaged internal organs when you suspect a rib fracture. The broken rib may puncture a lung, causing a pneumothorax.

Chest injuries are often associated with multisystem trauma and can very quickly progress to a life-threatening condition. Any chest injury that is associated with respiratory distress or hypotension is considered a "load-and-go" situation: Correct any life-threatening conditions, provide oxygen, immobilize the spine if necessary, and rapidly evacuate the patient to a definitive-care facility, preferably a designated trauma center.

Patients who have suffered commotio cordis will present in cardiac arrest and must be treated aggressively using current cardiopulmonary resuscitation techniques, including defibrillation. Likewise, patients with traumatic asphyxia must have the external pressure relieved from the thoracic cage quickly and then should be given aggressive ventilatory support.

If the patient has been caught in an avalanche, quickly remove snow or other avalanche debris from around the patient's chest. Ensure that the airway is open and clear, and that breathing efforts are effective. Use suction as necessary to ensure airway patency. If you suspect serious problems such as traumatic asphyxia, tension pneumothorax, or cardiac tamponade, summon additional assistance immediately. Call for transport and advanced care providers.

Apply high-flow oxygen via a nonrebreather mask if the chest-injured patient's breathing efforts are spontaneous and effective. When available, use a pulse oximeter and titrate oxygen keeping the oxygen saturation between 94 and 99%. If necessary, assist ventilations using a bag-valve mask and supplemental oxygen. Again, if the patient worsens while bagging, think of tension pneumothorax.

Any obvious sucking chest wound should be treated immediately to prevent the development or worsening of an underlying pneumothorax. Begin by covering the wound with a gloved hand to occlude the opening. Next, cover the wound with an occlusive dressing. Even if there is no obvious "sucking" sound, it is appropriate to cover any penetrating chest wound with an occlusive dressing. Among the several commercial products available for this purpose are Vaseline gauze, a Bolin chest seal, and an Asherman chest seal. If none of these products are available, an occlusive dressing may be improvised using plastic wrap, a plastic bag, aluminum foil, or other impermeable material. Tape the occlusive dressing in place on three sides, which will prevent air intake through the wound upon inspiration but will allow pressurized air within the chest cavity to escape (**Figure 23-13**). Monitor the patient closely for signs of tension pneumothorax and readjust the dressing so that air can escape if there is evidence of air buildup.

Remember that serious chest injuries are load-and-go situations. However, if a spinal injury is suspected, apply manual cervical spine stabilization and rapidly immobilize the entire spine (spinal motion restriction) using conventional procedures and equipment.

KEY POINT

Use of a Bag-Valve Mask

Use caution when using a bag-valve mask in patients with a suspected lung tissue injury and observe the results of your treatment closely. When there is a tension pneumothorax, using a bag-valve mask for ventilation may make the condition worse by forcing more air into the pleural space. In this situation, it may be better to allow patients who are still breathing on their own to breathe 100% oxygen using a high-flow rebreather mask without assistance. If the patient's respiratory rate and depth are not adequate, you may have no choice but to provide ventilations.

KEY POINT

ALS for Tension Pneumothorax

In most areas, ALS providers can provide needle chest decompression for tension pneumothorax in the field. The insertion of a needle into the pleural space allows the pressurized air in the chest to escape.

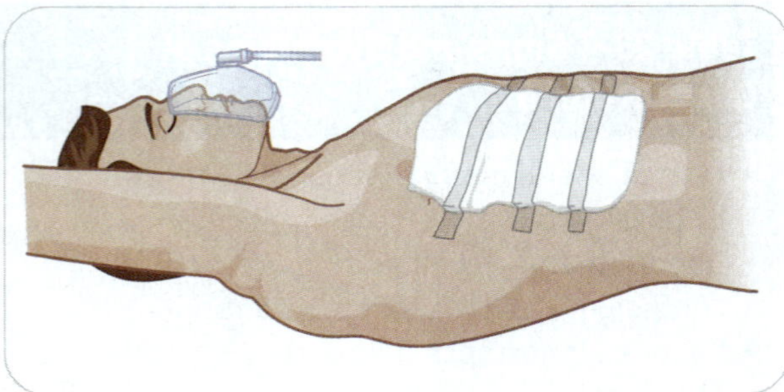

Figure 23-13 Treat flail chest by administering oxygen and gently splinting the flail segment with a blanket, a pillow, or pad.

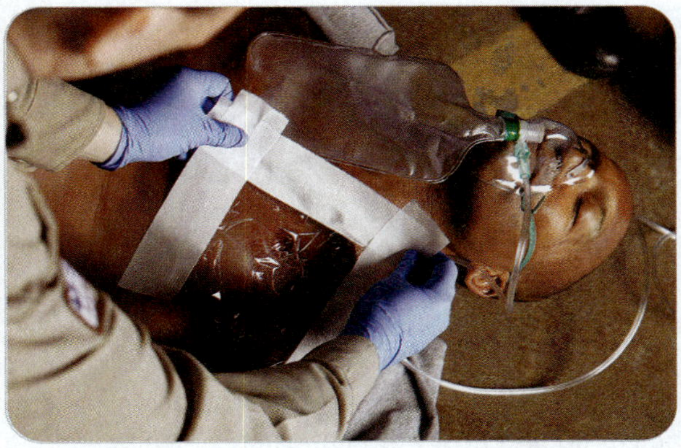

Figure 23-14 Taping an occlusive dressing on three sides of a sucking chest wound helps prevent a tension pneumothorax.

Splint flail segments above and below the fractured section in the same manner as for an isolated rib fracture. Do not use a tight circumferential bandage. If the flail segment is especially large, a large trauma dressing, pillow, folded clothing, magazine, or other material is often more effective in stabilizing the bones than are traditional dressings (**Figure 23-14**). If the patient can hold the splint in place, encourage him to do so and then secure the splint and dressing against the chest wall. If the flail segment causes severe pain or respiratory distress, it may be helpful to assist the patient's respirations using a bag-valve mask and oxygen. The positive pressure from the bag-valve mask will reduce the paradoxical motion of the flail segment. If the patient will not tolerate the bag-valve mask, it may be better to minimize distress by using a high-flow nonrebreather mask and allowing the patient to sit quietly. Put the patient in a position of comfort, which most likely will be sitting.

Impaled objects should be left in place and transport to a trauma center should be arranged immediately. Objects such as a tree branch, ski pole, or knife should not be removed because the object may be preventing hemorrhage, pneumothorax, or exsanguination. If the impaled object is large, you may need to shorten it (e.g., trimming a tree branch) to facilitate safe, efficient transport.

When shortening an impaled object, avoid causing further injury due to excessive movement of the object. Remove the impaled object from patients with rapidly deteriorating conditions *only* if the object is fixed (immovable) or if bringing in cutting equipment will take too long. In this situation, be ready to care for excessive bleeding, pneumothorax, or other threats to life once the object has been removed. It is always best to leave an impaled object in the patient if you can do so.

Give careful consideration when positioning the patient for transport. Patients who have a serious chest injury will benefit from being placed in a head-uphill position in a toboggan, which can reduce pressure on the diaphragm and thoracic organs and make breathing easier. A patient with dyspnea in the absence of trauma will benefit by sitting. However, many cases of chest trauma are accompanied by spinal injury requiring spinal motion restriction, which precludes transporting the patient in a seated position. In this case, consider elevating the head of the spinal immobilization device to ease breathing efforts.

When the patient is in shock and breathing is the primary concern, keep the patient warm and in a head-uphill position to assist with the breathing issue. Shock is no longer a determining factor in the placement of a patient in the toboggan for transport. Elevating the legs for shock is no longer recommended. Consideration for placement of the patient in the toboggan is based on their other injuries.

Table 23-2 summarizes the actions to take in managing serious chest injuries.

Table 23-2 Management of Serious Chest Injury

- Rapid care for ABCDs
- Support ventilation with bag-valve mask if needed
- Oxygen: 15 LPM via nonrebreather mask
- Use occlusive dressing on chest wounds, especially sucking chest wounds
- Immobilize spine if spinal injury is suspected
- Call for ALS if available
- Rapid transport to definitive care at a hospital
- Consider air medical transport

CASE Outcome

With the assistance of the other patrollers, you load him into a toboggan in a head-uphill position, place blankets behind the head and neck to assist with breathing, and transport him to the first-aid room at the base lodge. Once inside, you take a full set of vital signs; the pulse has increased to 114 beats per minute, the blood pressure is 100/70 mm Hg, and the respiratory rate is 28 breaths per minute. On high-flow oxygen, the oxygen saturation level using a pulse oximeter is maintained at just above 90%. As you deliver your handoff report to the paramedic, you show them a large bruise on the left upper chest wall that extends beneath the patient's armpit. The paramedic uses his stethoscope and does not hear breath sounds suggesting a complete pneumothorax on the left side.

Several days later during a patrol meeting, your medical advisor informs you that the patient was admitted to the hospital with a displaced rib fracture that had punctured the lung. The patient had a significant pneumothorax that required inserting a chest tube for several days. He compliments you on the care you and your team provided and states that the patient is expected to recover fully.

CHAPTER REVIEW

In Summary

- Injuries to the chest are described as either closed or open.
- Maintain a high index of suspicion for chest injury based on the mechanism of injury.
- Assessment of patients with suspected chest injury is the same as for any other trauma patient. Begin with a scene size-up, evaluating and mitigating any hazards that may be present. Assess the mechanism of injury to determine the forces involved.
- Chest injuries are often associated with multisystem trauma and can very quickly progress to a life-threatening condition.
- Any chest injury that is associated with respiratory distress or hypotension is considered a "load-and-go" situation: Correct any life-threatening conditions, provide oxygen, immobilize the spine if necessary, and rapidly evacuate the patient to a definitive-care facility, preferably a designated trauma center.
- If the condition of a hypoxic patient with chest trauma worsens, consider a tension pneumothorax.
- Call early for advanced life support, which is needed during transport for serious chest injuries.
- Look for a pneumothorax when you suspect a broken rib.
- Severe chest injuries may require prompt surgical intervention.

Key Terms

Aneurysm Ballooning of an artery that weakens it and predisposes it to rupture.

Aortic rupture Development of a leak in the largest blood vessel in the body; results in massive bleeding that is usually fatal.

Closed chest injury A chest injury without penetration of the chest cavity.

Commotio cordis Sudden cardiac death due to blunt chest trauma without any observable chest or cardiac damage.

Flail chest A condition in which two or more adjacent ribs are fractured in two or more places, causing a free-floating segment (paradoxical movement) of the chest wall.

Hemoptysis Coughing up blood.

Hemothorax An accumulation of blood in the pleural space.

Myocardial contusion A bruise of the heart muscle.

Open chest injury (sucking chest wound) A chest injury that involves penetration of the chest wall.

Paradoxical motion Inward movement of a flail chest segment upon inhalation.

Pericardial tamponade The accumulation of blood or other fluid within the pericardial sac.

Pulmonary contusion A bruise of the lung tissue.

Tension pneumothorax The accumulation of pressurized air within the pleural space; causes the displacement of the great vessels, tracheal deviation, distention of the jugular veins, and compression of the other lung.

Traumatic asphyxia The inability to breathe and hypoxia that results from the inability of the chest wall to expand due to external pressure or massive crushing trauma.

Chapter Questions

1. What are two major organs in the chest cavity necessary for life?
   a. The rib cage and sternum
   b. The heart and lungs
   c. The esophagus and spleen
   d. The diaphragm and liver

2. Which of the following describes the diaphragm?
   a. Separates the chest and abdominal cavities
   b. Is the primary muscle of respiration
   c. Is controlled by two "phrenic" nerves that connect to the spinal cord
   d. All of the above
3. There are two membranes in the chest cavity; one covers the lungs and the other lines the inside wall of the chest. What is normally found between these layers?
   a. A small space that contains only air
   b. A small space that contains only a clear fluid lubricant that allows the lungs to move freely while they expand and contract
   c. A small space that contains only blood
   d. All of the above
4. Which of the following describes flail chest?
   a. Is defined as fractures of three or more adjacent ribs, each of which is fractured in three or more places
   b. Is defined as fractures of two or more adjacent ribs, each of which is fractured in two or more places
   c. Results in the injured segment of the chest wall moving independently of the rest of the rib cage
   d. Both b and c
5. A 42-year-old patient skied off a trail at a high rate of speed and struck his anterior chest on a large tree. Which of the following findings would cause you to suspect the patient may have pericardial tamponade?
   a. Narrowing pulse pressure (systolic and diastolic readings getting closer together)
   b. Tracheal deviation toward the affected side
   c. Distended neck veins (jugular venous distention) and shortness of breath
   d. Both a and c
6. Classic signs and symptoms of a tension pneumothorax include:
   a. shortness of breath.
   b. low blood pressure and fast heart rate.
   c. distended neck veins (jugular venous distention).
   d. All of the above
7. You arrive and find a 25-year-old male who fell while skiing and has removed a ski pole that was impaled into his anterior chest. You suspect he has a sucking chest wound because:
   a. his wound is an open chest injury.
   b. you hear a "sucking" sound each time the patient breathes.
   c. his wound is now a closed chest injury.
   d. Both a and b
8. Management of a patient with a sucking chest wound includes:
   a. immediately covering the open wound with an ungloved hand.
   b. applying an occlusive dressing taped on three sides.
   c. applying a nonocclusive dressing taped on three sides.
   d. Both a and c

9. What is the three-step process that OEC technicians should use when assessing patients for chest trauma?
   a. Listen, act, and palpate
   b. Look, auscultate (listen), and palpate
   c. Listen, act, and percuss
   d. Look, auscultate (listen), and percuss

10. Management of a patient with a flail chest includes:
    a. splinting flail segments above and below the fracture in the same manner as for an isolated rib fracture.
    b. applying a sling and swathe.
    c. applying high-flow oxygen by nonrebreather and allowing the patient to sit quietly.
    d. Both a and c

Answers: 1. b, Objective 23-1, p. 564; 2. d, Objective 23-1, p. 565; 3. b, Objective 23-1, p. 565; 4. d, Objective 23-1, p. 567; 5. d, Objective 23-2, p. 571; 6. d, Objective 23-2, p. 570; 7. d, Objective 23-2, p. 576; 8. b, Objective 23-4, p. 576; 9. b, Objective 23-3, p. 574; 10. d, Objective 23-4, p. 577

CHAPTER 24

ABDOMINAL AND PELVIC TRAUMA

OBJECTIVES

Upon completion of this chapter, the OEC technician will be able to:

24-1 Identify and locate the major anatomic structures within the abdominal and pelvic cavities.

24-2 List and describe at least six abdominal and pelvic injuries.

24-3 Describe and demonstrate how to assess a patient with abdominal or pelvic trauma.

24-4 Describe and demonstrate how to manage a patient with abdominal or pelvic trauma.

24-5 Describe and demonstrate how to manage an abdominal evisceration.

24-6 Describe and demonstrate how to manage an impaled object in the abdomen or pelvis.

24-7 Describe and demonstrate how to manage a pelvic fracture.

KEY TERMS

Abdominal evisceration, p. 587
Straddle injury, p. 588
Symphysis pubis, p. 588

HISTORICAL TIMELINE **1992.** New senior program is implemented, and the manual is published.

CHAPTER OVERVIEW

You have learned the anatomy and physiology of the abdominal and pelvic cavities and how to manage various basic gastrointestinal medical emergencies. Assessing and treating trauma adds another dimension to your skills. As you learn to assess and manage abdominal and pelvic trauma, the goal is not to determine the exact cause of the problem, but rather to identify a potentially serious emergency, render emergent care, and quickly move the patient toward definitive treatment.

Organs in the abdominal cavity are less well protected than those in the chest or pelvic cavities. Though better protected, the structures within the pelvis can also be injured. Both cavities are served by a vast network of blood vessels that, when injured, can lead to life-threatening internal bleeding. Damaged organs can bleed internally, or they can leak contents that cause internal abdominal inflammation. When the bowel ruptures, bacteria can enter these cavities, causing infection that can proceed to sepsis and death. If the abdominal aorta is damaged, massive bleeding can be rapidly fatal.

This chapter will explain how to evaluate these injuries and provide field care as needed. Understanding which patients need prompt transport is one of the skills you will learn.

ANATOMY AND PHYSIOLOGY

The anatomy of the abdomen is shown in **Figure 24-1**. The abdominal cavity is separated from the thoracic cavity by the diaphragm, the muscle that contracts to expand the lungs. The inferior margin of the abdomen is the pelvic brim, which is an imaginary plane formed by the top of the pelvic bones. The pelvic cavity is encased by the pelvic bones. Together, the abdomen and pelvis constitute the largest cavity in the human body. Just posterior (behind) the abdominal cavity are the kidneys and abdominal aorta. Although these structures are not in the abdominal cavity, they can be injured from abdominal trauma.

Organs in the pelvic cavity are relatively protected from trauma by the bones of the pelvis—the ilium, the ischium, and the pubis. This is not the case with the abdominal organs, which are protected posteriorly by the spine and anteriorly and laterally only by the abdominal muscles and a layer of fat.

Some of the organs in or just behind (retroperitoneal) the abdominal cavity are involved with processing blood: The kidneys remove toxins from the blood, the liver processes nutrients and chemicals in the blood, and the spleen helps to fight overwhelming infections and removes old red blood cells. The aorta, the largest blood vessel in the body, and the companion inferior vena cava lie just in front of the vertebral column in the upper abdomen.

The abdomen is divided into four quadrants (**Figure 24-2**). Injuries in each involve different organs, can have markedly different outcomes, and call for different management strategies. Right upper quadrant trauma should make you consider liver injury, whereas left upper quadrant trauma should heighten your suspicion for spleen injury. Trauma to the midline of the upper

CASE Presentation

On an intermediate ski trail you see a young woman go off the edge of the slope. You note that she is trying to stop by sticking her poles into the snow ahead of her. Suddenly, the tip of a pole catches in the snow and the handle jams into her abdomen. She immediately falls to the ground. When you reach her, she is lying on the snow, gasping for air, and clutching her abdomen.

What is your first step in assessment?

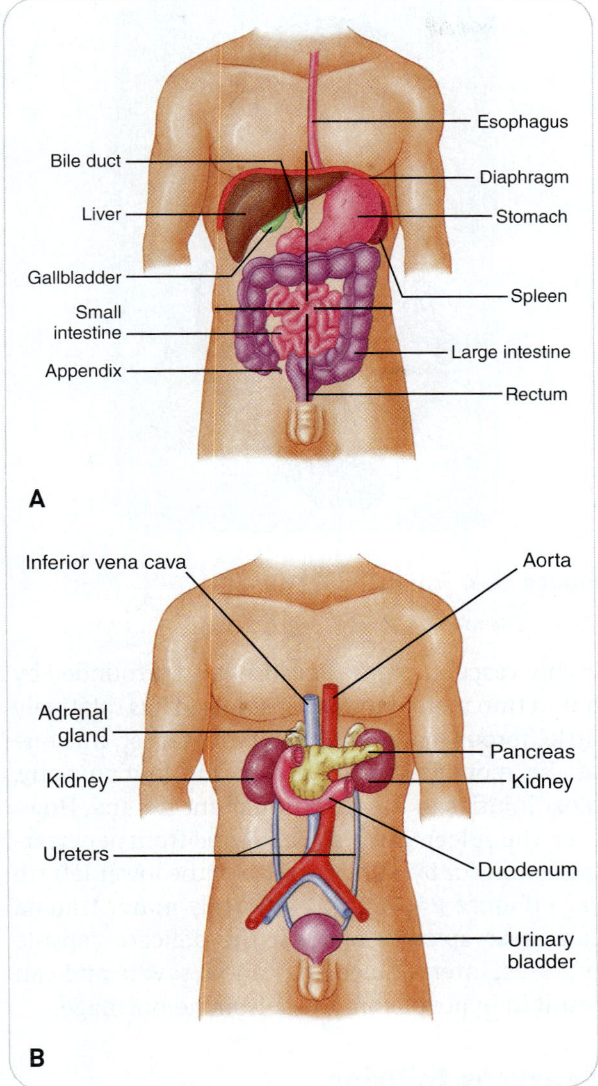

Figure 24-1 **A.** The organs of the abdominal cavity. **B.** The retroperitoneal organs lie behind the abdominal cavity.

abdomen should cause concerns for injury to the aorta, bowel, pancreas, spleen, or liver.

COMMON ABDOMINAL AND PELVIC INJURIES

The mechanism of injury can provide valuable information for identifying the nature of a patient's problems. Blunt trauma tends to cause injury to solid organs, whereas penetrating trauma may affect solid or hollow organs. Because blunt trauma is more common than penetrating trauma, it is more common to find solid organ injuries than hollow organ injuries. Trauma can injure more than one structure or organ in the abdominal and pelvic cavities.

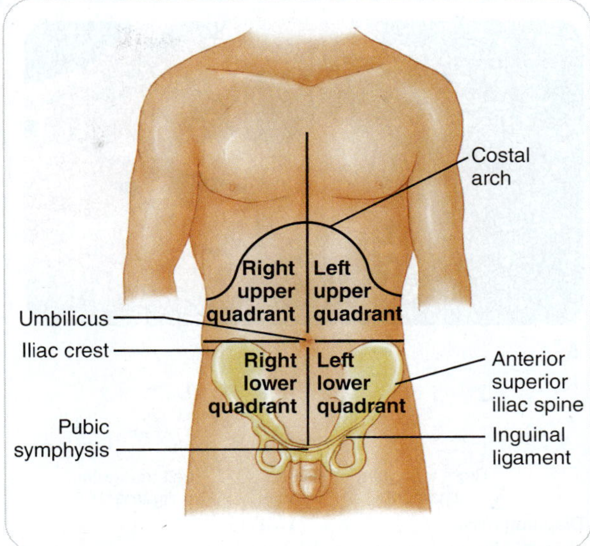

Figure 24-2 The four quadrants of the abdomen.

Abdominal Wall Contusion

Any trauma to the abdominal wall can cause bruising of the skin and superficial abdominal muscles. Most *mild* blunt trauma to the abdomen does not cause internal injury, but OEC technicians should be aware that any trauma can cause internal injuries. Careful assessment of the patient is important, and any concerns should be evaluated at a higher level of care.

Liver Injuries

The liver, in the right upper quadrant, is the largest solid organ in the abdomen, and injuries to it are not uncommon. Even though most of the liver is protected by the rib cage, it is vulnerable to both blunt and penetrating trauma (**Figure 24-3**). The liver's fibrous tissue and tough surrounding capsule enable it to withstand some trauma. However, because it is a highly vascular organ, injuries to it frequently cause internal bleeding.

Spleen Injuries

The spleen in the left upper quadrant and flank is partially protected by the lower rib cage and is a

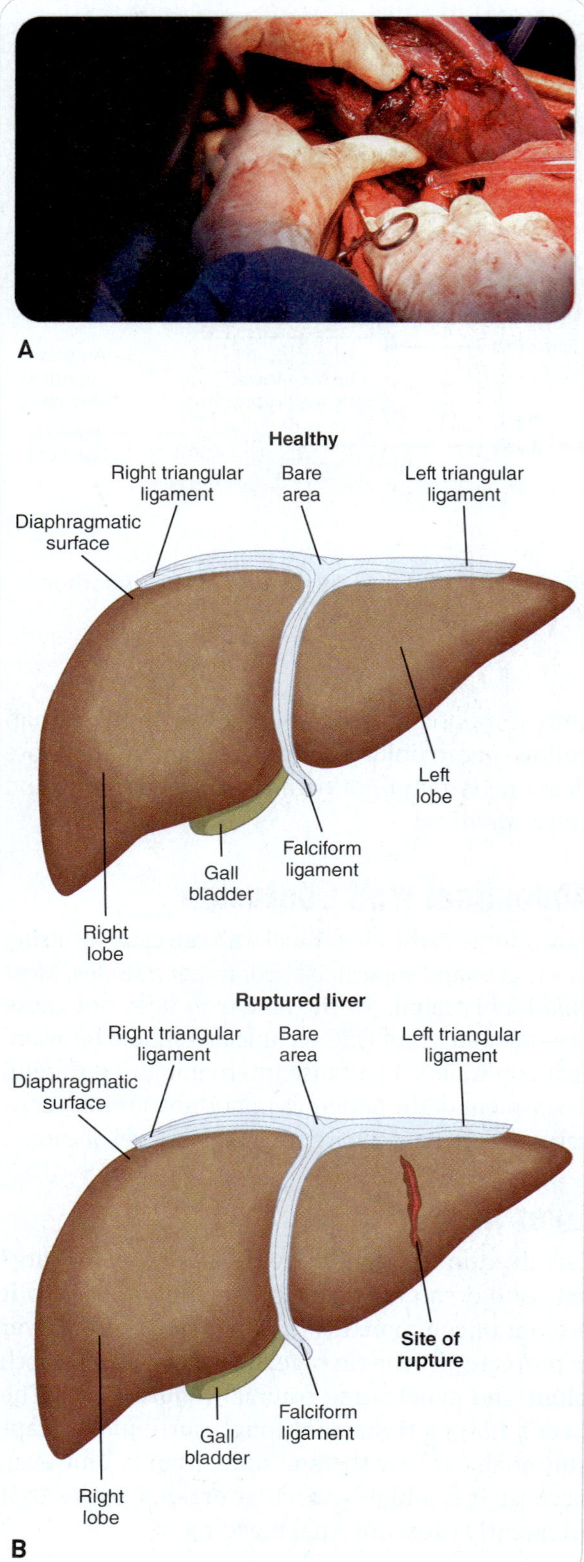

Figure 24-3 A rupture of the liver may be caused by blunt trauma or penetrating trauma.

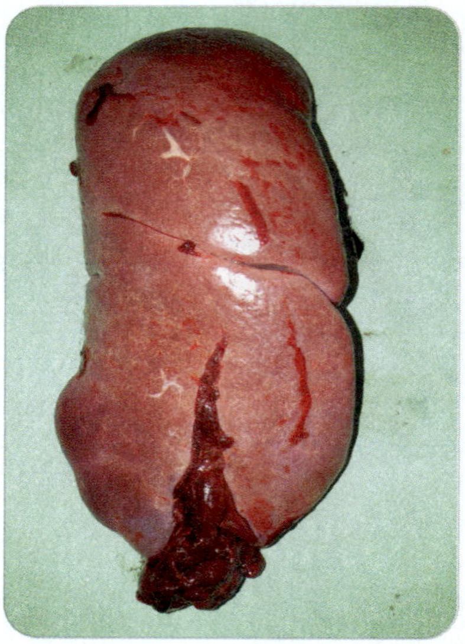

Figure 24-4 Trauma to the spleen.

highly vascular organ. Because it is surrounded by only a thin membranous capsule and has relatively little fibrous material holding it together, it is one of the more fragile organs in the human body. Most injuries to it occur from blunt trauma. However, the spleen can also be injured from penetrating trauma or by a fractured rib of the lower left rib cage (**Figure 24-4**). Even relatively minor trauma can cause splenic injury. If the delicate capsule ruptures, internal bleeding can be severe and can result in hypovolemic shock from hemorrhage.

Pancreas Injuries

The pancreas, a solid organ, can rupture or tear. Such injuries can cause digestive enzymes to leak into the abdominal cavity, which can destroy the pancreas and other surrounding structures and cause severe inflammation inside the abdomen. Abdominal impact such as falling on handlebars is a common cause of pancreas injury. Pancreas injuries are becoming more common as a result of collisions in outdoor sports, including bicycling, snowmobiling, snowboarding (striking a terrain park rail), and kayaking (striking the front deck). Any injury to the middle of the abdomen above the navel can damage the pancreas.

Vascular Injuries

The abdomen and pelvis contain numerous arteries and veins, both large and small. Among the larger vessels are the abdominal aorta, inferior vena cava, hepatic vessels, renal vessels, and iliac arteries and veins. Rapid deceleration that results when the body hits a fixed object is the most common cause of vascular injury, although penetrating trauma also can damage blood vessels. Bleeding can be severe and may be immediately life threatening, depending on the size of the vessel, number of vessels damaged, whether it is an artery or a vein, and the extent of vessel damage.

Diaphragm Tear/Rupture

The diaphragm is vulnerable to both blunt and penetrating trauma. Severe blunt abdominal trauma can cause increased intra-abdominal pressure, causing the diaphragm to tear away from its attachments or causing holes in the diaphragm. The most common diaphragmatic injury is a diaphragmatic hernia, which occurs when one or more abdominal organs pass through (herniate) the diaphragm at the site at which the esophagus penetrates the diaphragm from the left side of the chest cavity. Penetrating objects can directly cause holes in the diaphragm. Regardless of the mechanism of injury, tears or holes in the diaphragm allow structures within the abdominal cavity, mainly the intestines, to migrate into the thoracic cavity. An injury to the diaphragm or the presence of abdominal organs in the chest cavity can compromise the patient's breathing.

Intestinal Tear/Rupture

Some portion of the large intestine or the small intestine is in every quadrant of the abdomen. Many intestinal injuries are due to penetrating trauma, which can cause undigested food and fecal matter to leak into the abdominal cavity, resulting in severe pain, inflammation, and infection. Significant bleeding can also occur if a vessel in the intestinal wall is damaged. Blunt injuries to the intestines can also be concerning and sometimes have a more delayed presentation.

Impaled Objects

An impaled object that enters the abdominal or pelvic cavity can result in a variety of life-threatening injuries, depending on the structures that are damaged (**Figure 24-5**). Objects such as ski poles, tree branches, fence posts, knives, or pipes are common impaled objects. They may enter the body on one side and protrude from the other side, or they may lodge within the abdomen or pelvis without exiting. Many impaled objects in the abdomen or pelvis miss important organs or blood vessels, allowing the patient to do quite well with timely definitive care. Major complications are bleeding (initially) and infection (later).

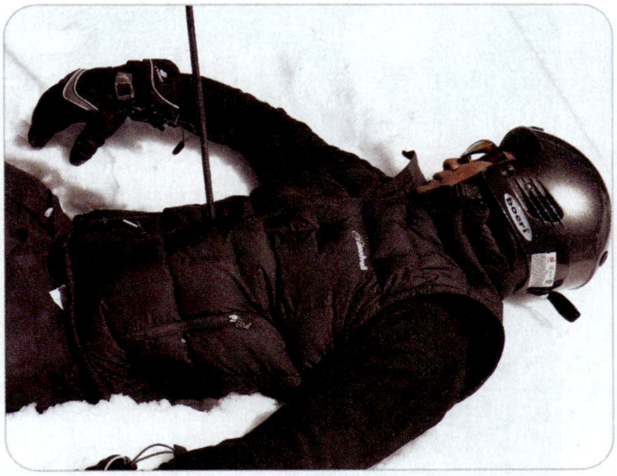

Figure 24-5 An impaled object.

Abdominal Evisceration

Abdominal evisceration occurs when a tear in the abdominal wall exposes the intestines and/or other organs to the external environment (**Figure 24-6**). Most often in the field, evisceration is caused by a penetrating injury that tears an opening through the abdominal wall and peritoneum. It presents many problems, including severe bleeding, rapid heat loss, and the risk of infection. Evisceration is an uncommon (but certainly upsetting and challenging) injury for the patient, rescuers, and bystanders.

Pelvic Fractures

Even though the pelvic bones are among the sturdiest bones in the body, the pelvis and the structures within the pelvic cavity are not immune to blunt or penetrating injury. Fractures involving the pelvic bones usually require great force and should be suspected in high-speed collisions, falls, motor vehicle crashes, pedestrian-vehicle collisions, pelvic gunshot wounds, or any other type of direct or blunt trauma. Because the pelvis is such a sturdy protector of the organs within it, forces needed to fracture the pelvic bones may result in

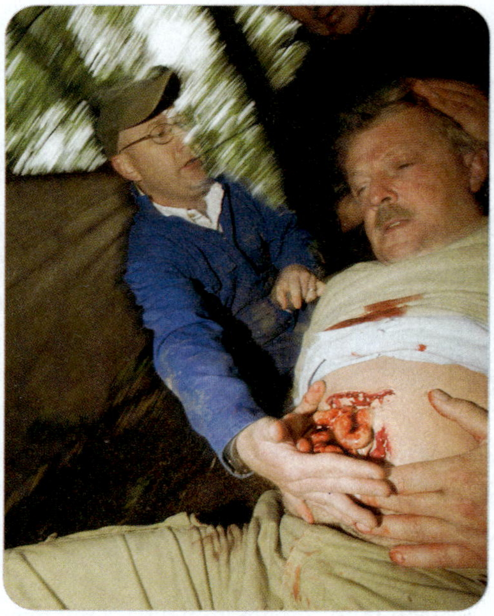

Figure 24-6 An abdominal evisceration.

Jonathan Kingston/National Geographic Creative.

injuries to internal structures such as the urinary bladder and blood vessels. The most significant complication of a pelvic fracture is acute internal bleeding. Because the pelvis forms a ring, it is likely to fracture in more than one location.

Lower Urinary Tract Injuries

The urinary bladder is located behind and is protected by the **symphysis pubis**. If the symphysis fractures, bone fragments can lacerate the bladder. Most commonly this occurs from direct blunt trauma to the symphysis. Falls and straddle injuries are common sources of this type of trauma. In addition, blunt trauma can cause the bladder to rupture, which is much more likely to occur when the bladder is full. The pressure of a seat belt at the end of a rapid deceleration also can rupture a full or distended bladder. If the forces are large enough, the urethra can be torn from the bladder. Injuries to the bladder or urethra can result in internal bleeding or in urine leaking into the pelvic cavity.

Genital Injuries

Genital trauma is generally not life threatening but can be a challenge for both the patient and the rescuer. In outdoor settings, most genital injuries are caused by a **straddle injury**, which occurs when the patient's groin strikes an object such as a ski pole, a rail, or the top bar of a bicycle. In general, genital injuries in females are limited to external structures because the uterus and ovaries are well protected within the bony pelvis. The labia, however, are very vascular, and external injuries to them can cause profuse bleeding. Injuries to the male genitalia are often more serious, can be very painful, and can result in long-term complications.

The external genitals can receive blunt or sharp trauma. In males, blunt trauma to the testicles can result in a hematoma in the scrotum. Lacerations can occur to the penis or scrotum and are seen most commonly when the genitals are caught in a zipper. In women, genital trauma causing a hematoma to the external labia can be quite painful and can cause a lot of mental anguish for the patient. When evaluating genital injuries, always consider the patient's modesty.

PATIENT ASSESSMENT OF THE ABDOMEN AND PELVIS

Abdominal and pelvic injuries are often difficult to assess because the initial presentation can be relatively benign and then the patient's condition can deteriorate. The assessment process follows the same guidelines described in previous chapters. Emphasis is on recognizing that an abdominal or pelvic injury exists rather than identifying exactly what organs have been injured. However, if OEC technicians are aware of the locations of the abdominal organs, a higher degree of suspicion can be maintained for such injuries as a splenic rupture.

As with any incident, begin by ensuring that the scene is safe. Next, look for excessive external bleeding and assess the patient's ABCDs (airway, breathing, circulation, disability), and provide immediate treatment if needed. A SAMPLE history (signs and symptoms, allergies, medications, past medical history, last oral intake, events leading up to the problem) with mechanism of injury is important, as is a good secondary assessment. Ask patients whether they have consumed alcohol or ingested any drugs. This information is important because the symptoms of abdominal and pelvic trauma may be masked by these substances.

As part of the history, be sure to ask the patient about any falls or collisions over the past few days, because some injuries may have gone unrecognized for several days.

As you perform the physical exam, note the presence of the following signs and symptoms that are consistent with an abdominal or pelvic injury:

- Pain
- Tenderness
- Visible external wounds
- Abdominal distention
- Abdominal rigidity
- Unexplained shock

If the patient is in pain, ask where the pain is located and assess its nature using the OPQRST mnemonic (onset, provocation, quality, radiation, severity, and time). Have the patient point with one finger where it hurts the most. The location of pain, especially early on, is helpful to determine which organs might have incurred injury. Early pain is often experienced where the initial impact occurred. Serious internal bleeding is not always obvious. Pain resulting from abdominal trauma is often initially localized in the place where the patient was injured and later becomes more generalized if blood, bile, or intestinal contents have leaked into the abdominal cavity and caused peritonitis (painful inflammation of the lining of the abdomen).

Inspect the abdomen for abdominal distention (bulging). If the abdomen is enlarging over time, this can be an indication of severe intra-abdominal bleeding. Note any discoloration of the abdominal wall. You may detect a large band of bruising across the lower abdomen, an area of discoloration known as the "seat belt sign." This sign may take several hours to appear (**Figure 24-7**). Although more commonly associated with rapid deceleration during vehicular crashes in which the abdomen slams against a seat belt, the seat belt sign also may be encountered if the abdomen strikes a fixed object such as a terrain park rail or a metal fencing cross bar. Also, be sure to inspect both flank areas for discoloration.

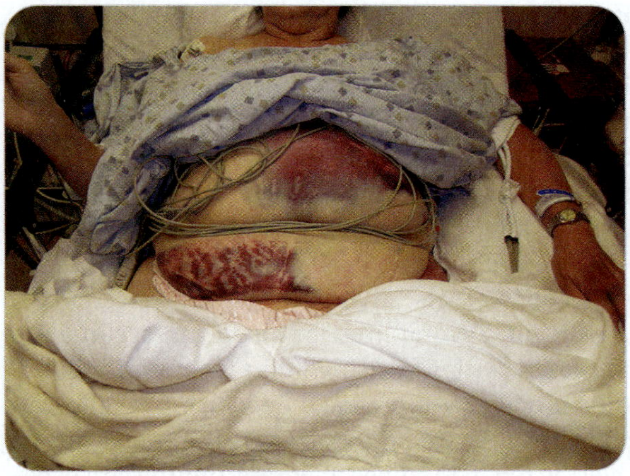

Figure 24-7 Bruising of the abdomen is a sign of blunt trauma and possibly internal bleeding, which can be a life-threatening condition.

Use the standard DCAP-BTLS assessment (deformity, contusions, abrasions/avulsions, punctures/penetrations, burns/bleeding/bruises, tenderness, lacerations, swelling), and palpate all four quadrants of the abdomen and the lower rib cage. Rib tenderness and crepitus are signs of rib fracture. Remember, the organs beneath a broken rib may be injured as well—usually the liver on the patient's right and the spleen on the patient's left. Carefully palpate the abdomen, beginning in the quadrant farthest from the site of pain.

When the spleen or liver is injured and bleeding from the organ irritates the underside of the diaphragm, pain can be referred to the shoulder on the same side as the injured organ, a finding known as the Kehr sign. Patients who complain of left shoulder pain in the absence of an actual shoulder injury may have a ruptured spleen. A lacerated liver may present with right shoulder pain.

Assess the integrity of the pelvis by placing your palms on the iliac crest on each side and applying *gentle* but firm inward (medial) pressure. Bone crepitus, increased pain, or tenderness suggests a potential pelvic fracture. Palpate the pubic bones *gently*, but do not press down hard or outward on any pelvic bone because doing so can worsen the fracture and/or cause more bleeding from ruptured pelvic blood vessels. Assess the front of the pelvis by placing the patient's hand on the pubic bone and then gently pushing on the patient's hand. Only one rescuer should examine a patient for pelvic fracture. If the pelvis is fractured, multiple examinations may lead to potentially life-threatening bleeding by disturbing the blood clot that has formed at the fracture site.

Genital injuries can be very painful and may be associated with pelvic fracture. The examination of potential genital injuries requires discretion on the part of rescuers. If injury is suspected, a brief exam is warranted. However, unless active bleeding is suspected, you may wish to wait to perform this exam in a more controlled environment such as the aid room. Preferably this exam should be performed by one OEC technician with a second in attendance that is the same gender as the patient.

If the patient is a child, ideally a parent or guardian should be present throughout the examination. However, while it is important to approach examinations of the pelvic region with care, do not delay an examination of a potentially life-threatening injury. If an examination is indicated, inspect the area for bleeding, discoloration, or soft-tissue injury.

The abdomen and pelvis are filled with numerous blood vessels, so monitoring for shock is very important. Several liters of blood can accumulate in these cavities. A rising pulse rate, a falling systolic blood pressure, and a decreasing level of responsiveness are ominous signs that must not be overlooked. Left upper quadrant injuries are especially worrisome because splenic injuries are especially prone to bleeding. So are pelvic fractures, although any injuries in the abdominal and pelvic cavities have the potential for serious blood loss.

The importance of follow-up exams and serial sets of vital signs cannot be overemphasized. If a patient with minimal symptoms develops abdominal distention, pain upon examination, an elevated pulse rate, or decreasing blood pressure, initiate management for shock and transfer to definitive care.

MANAGEMENT OF ABDOMINAL AND PELVIC TRAUMA

After ensuring that the scene is safe and putting on personal protective equipment, focus initial treatment on correcting excessive external bleeding and ABCD-related problems. Activate EMS for transport to definitive care as soon as a serious injury or threat to life is identified. Once life threats have been addressed, place the patient into a position of comfort, which typically is supine with the knees slightly flexed, reducing strain on the abdominal muscles. Place a small amount of padding under the patient's knees while maintaining spinal alignment and protect the cervical spine if spinal motion restriction is needed. Next, if the patient is having trouble breathing, place the patient on high-flow oxygen by nonrebreather mask to maintain oxygen saturation between 94 and 99%. Open wounds should be dressed and bandaged.

If during your assessment of the ABCDs the patient is having significant breathing difficulty, you may need to assist the patient with ventilations. The patient may also have a pulmonary problem or, if there is an abdominal injury, could have abdominal contents in the chest cavity from a ruptured diaphragm.

Impaled Objects

Impaled objects should be secured in place. First, expose the wound, manually stabilize the object, and control bleeding. Then further stabilize the object with a bulky dressing. If the length of an impaled object compromises transport or rescue operations, you may need to cut the object to allow for transport. However, do not remove the object unless absolutely necessary to transport; doing so could lead to life-threatening hemorrhage. Keep the impaled object stationary when shortening it, as movement could cause additional internal injury.

CASE Update

You ask the patient if she is OK, and she replies, "No, help me." You confirm that the patient's ABCDs are intact and that she does not have any serious external bleeding, spine pain or neurologic deficit. During your secondary assessment, the patient complains of severe pain in her "stomach." Examination of the abdomen reveals tenderness to palpation in the left upper quadrant. The patient's radial pulse is 124 beats per minute and her respirations are 20 breaths per minute. She says that she has no medical problems, is not taking any medications, has no allergies to medications, and last ate at breakfast approximately 3 hours ago. She denies any possibility that she could be pregnant. After 5 minutes, she appears to be breathing more easily but states that her "stomach really hurts." Pulse is now 108 beats per minute, and respirations are 16 breaths per minute.

What is your care and transport plan?

Abdominal Evisceration

It is acceptable to put abdominal contents back into a large wound so the organs do not dry out and the blood vessels are not stretched. This is more beneficial than leaving the organs out. If possible, clean off any gross contamination first. If there is a small hole, leave the contents out. Do not force the contents back in. If the transport time to definitive care is short, you may consider leaving the contents out. Cover the area with a sterile dressing moistened with sterile water or saline solution, if available. If you do not have access to sterile fluids, then keep the area moist with water that is clean enough to drink. Do not use pond or stream water, which could have bacterial contamination. Do not allow the eviscerated abdominal contents to dry out. In the event you are in an area where clean water is not available, use a dry sterile dressing. Keep the patient warm because evisceration can cause rapid, significant heat loss.

Fractured Pelvis

Apply a pelvic binder for a fractured pelvis, which will slow down the internal bleeding. Move any patient with a possible pelvic fracture as little as possible. More movement means more internal bleeding. Commercial binders are better than a "homemade" sheet binder, but if only a sheet is available, use a sheet. Studies published in 2019 show the commercial SAM pelvic binder may be superior.

Before or after applying a pelvic binder, it is best to not logroll a patient with a suspected pelvic fracture. Logrolling not only is very painful for these patients, but also can cause more bleeding, with resulting hypovolemic shock. In 2019 there were several reports in the medical literature of patients developing hypovolemic shock rapidly following logrolling in hospital emergency departments. The blood clots around the fractured bone ends of the pelvis were disturbed, causing greater internal bleeding.

It is best to use a carefully performed bridge lift for a broken pelvis. This procedure may be difficult to do with limited personnel, so do not unnecessarily delay transport for a patient with a fractured pelvis who is developing shock if more trained personnel are not immediately available. If responsible bystanders are present, they may be able to help you perform a bridge lift.

The best procedure for pelvic stabilization is described in **OEC Skill 24-1**.

OEC SKILL 24-1 Stabilizing the Pelvis

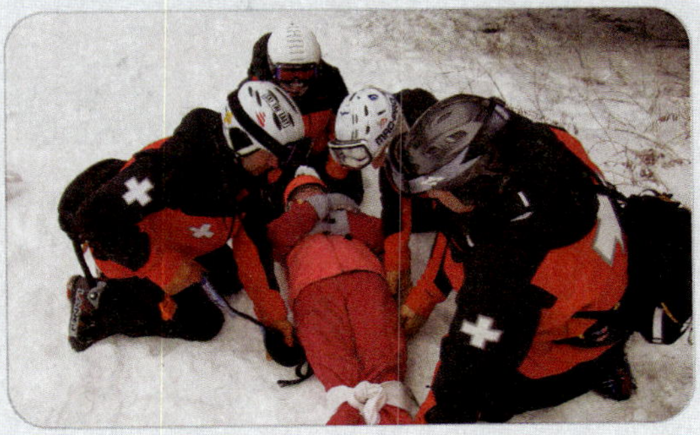

1 Prepare the commercial pelvic binder or folded sheet and place it beside the patient on the backboard, or stretcher, that is being used as a litter. Place it where the supine patient's pelvis will be. If possible, dig out the snow or material under the pelvis and slide the device under the patient and apply.

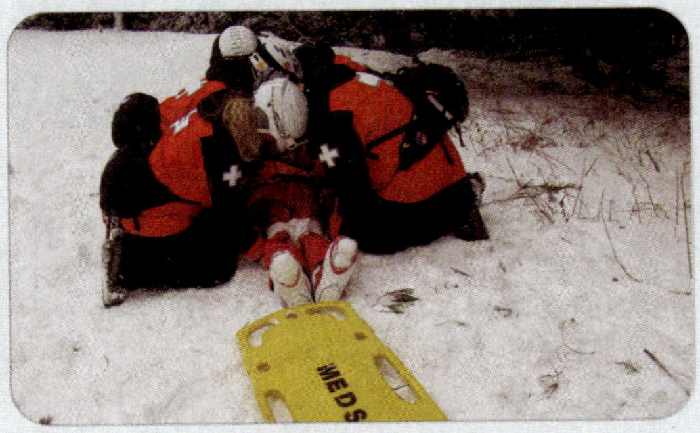

2 Perform a bridge lift. Place the patient on top of the sheet or the commercial binder so it is 1 to 2 inches below the iliac crests. Logroll only if absolutely necessary since doing so can cause more internal bleeding.

(continues)

OEC SKILL 24-1 Stabilizing the Pelvis *(continued)*

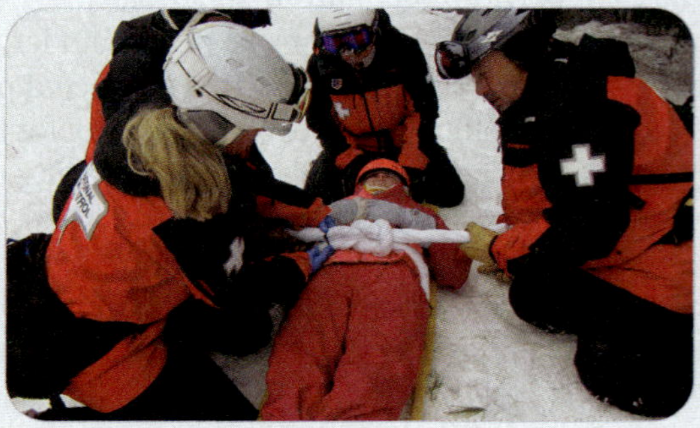

A

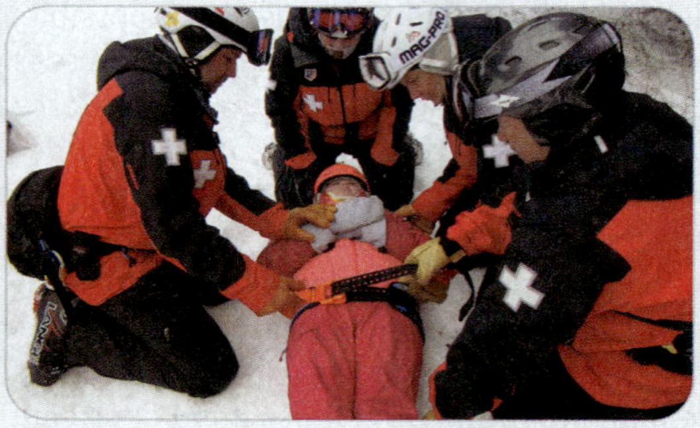

B

3 Fasten the binder:

a. *If using a sheet*, draw the two ends of the sheet together over the symphysis pubis, compressing the hips (greater trochanters) together. Then tie the sheet ends together snugly using an overhand knot. Plastic ties are in some cases better than using an overhand knot if available

b. *If using a commercial binder*, pull the two ends together snugly in a similar way and Velcro or belt the binder per the manufacturer's directions.

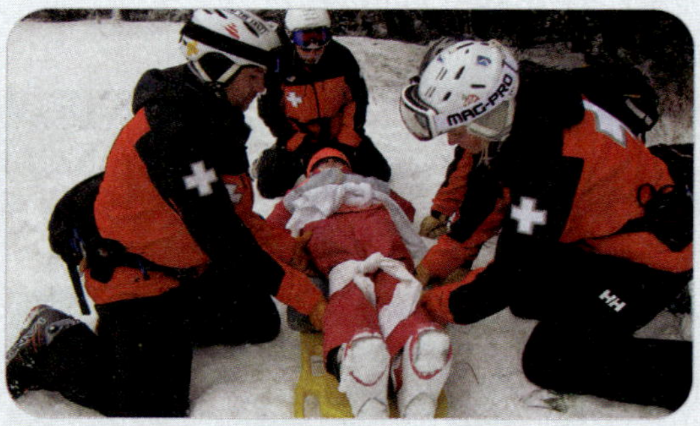

4 Lift the knees approximately 6 to 8 inches or to a position of comfort and place a blanket or other padded material under the knees prior to strapping the patient down.

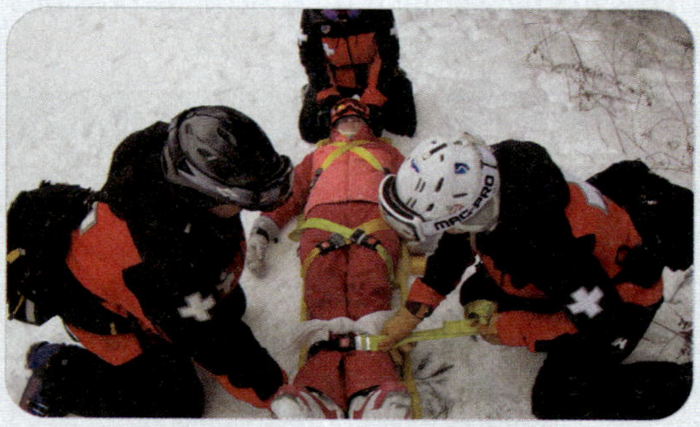

5 Finish securing the patient to the backboard or stretcher.

OEC SKILL 24-1 Stabilizing the Pelvis (*continued*)

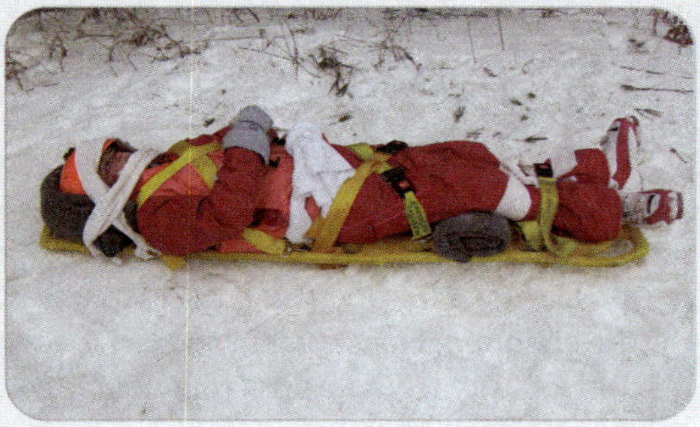

6 Because this is a distracting injury, apply a collar and head blocks and use spinal motion restriction (with the padding under the knees).

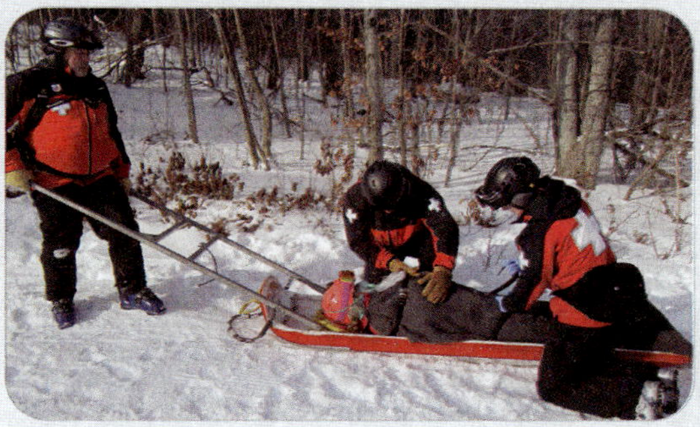

7 Lift the patient carefully into the toboggan or transport device outside. Again, a bridge lift is best.

KEY POINT

Caution About Logrolling

It is best to perform a direct lift for any patient movement, rather than logroll, if the patient has a suspected pelvic fracture.

Shock is common in abdominal and pelvic trauma and is treated in the usual manner. Patients who are in shock should not be given anything by mouth. As with any serious trauma, ALS should be requested if available, and patients should be rapidly transported to a definitive-care facility (ideally a trauma center). Overall management for abdominal injuries includes early recognition, specific care for the injury, treatment for shock, and rapid transport to a trauma center.

CASE Outcome

Other patrollers arrive. You administer oxygen to the patient on scene using a high-flow nonrebreather mask. Because she has significant left upper quadrant abdominal pain, you radio for ALS transport. The woman is transported in a toboggan in a head-uphill position because of breathing difficulties. In the first-aid room, the patient says, "I don't feel good." Further assessment reveals more generalized abdominal tenderness, and she tenses when you palpate her abdomen. There is no abdominal distention, but she is very nauseated. Her pulse is now 132 beats per minute, and blood pressure is 98/50 mm Hg. Keeping the patient supine, you add blankets, allow her to bend her knees, and help load her into an ambulance. You later find out the patient was admitted for an injury to her spleen. Following surgery to remove a badly ruptured spleen, she returns to thank you for saving her life.

CHAPTER REVIEW

In Summary

- The abdominal and pelvic cavities contain numerous solid and hollow structures and a vast network of blood vessels.
- The initial presentation for an abdominal injury may be relatively benign; shock may develop over time.
- Always consider the mechanism of injury when caring for abdominal injuries.
- Assessment of abdominal trauma includes examining all four quadrants and taking serial sets of vital signs.
- Do not give a patient with abdominal trauma anything by mouth.
- It is best to lift a patient with a fractured pelvis and logroll only if necessary.

Key Terms

Abdominal evisceration A tear in the abdominal wall exposing the intestines and/or other organs to the external environment.

Straddle injury An injury to the pelvis and the internal organs between the genitals and anus that results when a patient forcefully straddles a fixed object.

Symphysis pubis The site on the anterior pelvis at which the two pubic bones are joined together.

Chapter Questions

1. Trauma to the left upper quadrant of the abdomen may result in injury to the:
   a. spleen.
   b. appendix.
   c. liver.
   d. urinary bladder.
2. A patient complaining of pain in the right upper quadrant of the abdomen may be suffering from complications to the:
   a. spleen.
   b. appendix.
   c. liver.
   d. stomach.
3. Your patient has received blunt force trauma to the abdomen. The resulting intra-abdominal pressure causes the muscle used for breathing that separates the abdominal cavity from the chest cavity to tear away from its attachments. This injury affects the:
   a. lower urinary tract.
   b. pancreas.
   c. spleen.
   d. diaphragm.
4. Your patient has straddled a metal terrain park feature. The resulting direct, blunt force to the symphysis pubis may have caused injury to the:
   a. urinary bladder.
   b. pancreas.
   c. spleen.
   d. diaphragm.
5. When assessing the abdomen, you ask the patient to point with one finger to the area that is painful. The patient indicates pain in the right lower quadrant. You then gently palpate all four abdominal quadrants, beginning with the:
   a. quadrant farthest from the pain.
   b. quadrant closest to the pain.
   c. left lower quadrant.
   d. right upper quadrant.
6. When assessing the integrity of the pelvis, palpate the iliac crests by:
   a. applying gentle pressure inward.
   b. applying gentle pressure outward.
   c. applying gentle pressure downward.
   d. having multiple rescuers apply gently pressure.

7. Emergency care of a patient with abdominal pelvic trauma should include:
   a. placing the patient in a position of comfort.
   b. placing a small amount of padding under the patient's knees.
   c. evaluating the need for spinal motion restriction and supplemental oxygen.
   d. All of the above.

8. Emergency care for an abdominal evisceration should include:
   a. keeping the patient cool.
   b. gently placing eviscerated structures back into the abdominal cavity.
   c. covering the area with a sterile dressing moistened with sterile water or saline.
   d. Both a and b.

9. Your patient has an impaled object in the abdomen. You know that if you remove the object there is likelihood of:
   a. infection.
   b. life-threatening hemorrhage.
   c. fractures.
   d. evisceration.

10. Emergency care of a patient suffering from a suspected pelvic fracture should include:
    a. applying a pelvic binder.
    b. logrolling the patient and placing him or her on a spine board.
    c. placing the patient in the recovery position.
    d. placing the patient in a prone position.

Answers: 1. a, Objective 24-1, p. 584; 2. c, Objective 24-1, p. 584; 3. d, Objective 24-2, p. 584; 4. a, Objective 24-2, p. 588; 5. a, Objective 24-3, p. 589; 6. a, Objective 24-3, p. 589; 7. d, Objective 24-4, p. 590; 8. c, Objective 24-5, p. 591; 9. b, Objective 24-6, p. 590; 10. a, Objective 24-7, p. 591

CHAPTER 25

COLD-RELATED EMERGENCIES

OBJECTIVES

Upon completion of this chapter, the OEC technician will be able to:

25-1 Explain the wind chill index and how it applies to temperature.

25-2 List the signs and symptoms of frostnip and frostbite.

25-3 Explain the two types of hypothermia.

25-4 Define afterdrop.

25-5 Describe the assessment of a patient with cold injuries.

25-6 Describe the four categories of cold exposure.

25-7 Demonstrate the management of a patient with cold injuries.

25-8 Describe and demonstrate the emergency care of an avalanche victim.

KEY TERMS

Afterdrop, p. 602
Frostbite, p. 600
Frostnip, p. 600
Hypothermia, p. 601
Thermoregulation, p. 598
Wind chill, p. 599

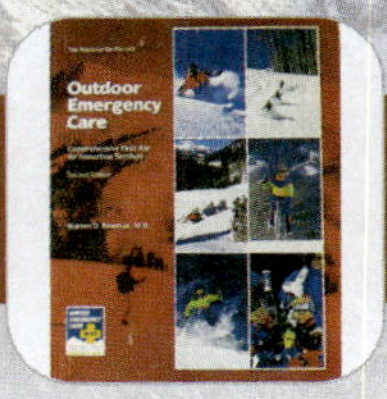

HISTORICAL TIMELINE 1993. *Outdoor Emergency Care, Second Edition* (formerly *WEC*) is published.

CHAPTER OVERVIEW

Cold temperatures, in combination with inadequate preparation including necessary clothing, food, and shelter can overwhelm the body's mechanisms for regulating temperature. A variety of medical emergencies can result from exposure to cold, particularly during recreational activities in wilderness and high-altitude environments. These emergencies include localized injuries (e.g., frostbite) and systemic illnesses (e.g., hypothermia and related problems). As an OEC technician, you can save lives by recognizing and responding properly to these emergencies.

This chapter describes how the body regulates its core temperature. Also discussed are various forms of cold emergencies and how to assess and treat victims of frostbite, hypothermia, and an avalanche.

ANATOMY AND PHYSIOLOGY

Humans evolved in tropical climates, making them much more adept at cooling (losing heat) than warming (reducing heat loss). As previously discussed, normal body temperature is 36.1–37.2°C (97–99°F), with a median of 37°C (98.6°F). When the body's core (internal) temperature decreases, sensors located throughout the body send signals to the brain. In response, the brain sends messages to various body systems that reduce heat loss, generate heat (energy) production, or both. The process of maintaining normal body temperature is called **thermoregulation**. Body temperature is controlled by the hypothalamus, a small area of the brain located just above the brainstem. This area of the brain, in combination with the skin, blood vessels, muscles, and other organs such as the heart, lungs, and kidneys, work together to maintain homeostasis. The exact effects depend on how much core temperature changes.

When core temperature decreases, the body initially responds by constricting peripheral blood vessels. By reducing blood flow in the extremities, the body reduces heat loss. Therefore, the fingers and toes get cold first. The brain, heart, and other vital organs are protected continuously receiving warm blood. The surface temperature of the skin becomes colder, so the body halts sweat production, allowing the skin to dry. In addition, body hairs stand on end to form a thin layer of trapped, warm air. If the core temperature continues to decrease, shivering begins.

Shivering is an involuntary response that generates heat through repeated muscular contractions. Shivering is an effective means of heat production, but it ceases when core body temperature drops significantly. Shivering also may be inhibited by traumatic injuries or certain drugs. Once shivering stops, the body's metabolic rate (use of energy) decreases as does the body's oxygen demand. For a while, this decline in oxygen

CASE Presentation

It is a beautiful spring day, with temperatures in the low 40s. A healthy 45-year-old woman and her 18-year-old son set out for a day of skiing. Two hours later, she falls through some soft snow into a shallow creek. Uninjured, she is easily able to extricate herself from the water, but not before getting wet up to her chest. The two skiers continue skiing. Riding the lift, she begins shaking uncontrollably. They decide to stop outside and drink what is left in their Thermos: hot chocolate and schnapps. They can make it to the gondola to ride to the base area. Halfway through the 20-minute ride, she is no longer shaking, appears sleepy, and closes her eyes. At the base area, her son is unable to wake her up. You are standing at the off-load ramp when the son yells out that he needs your help. He quickly briefs you while you conduct an initial assessment.

What should you do?

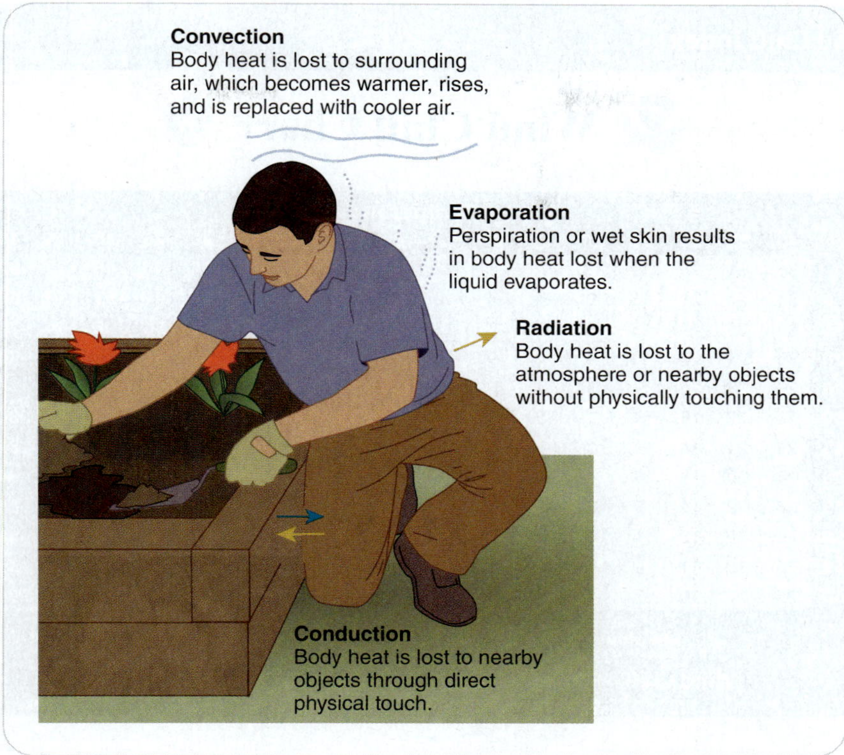

Figure 25-1 The different mechanisms of heat loss.

demand protects the body's organs and tissues from the low-oxygen (or poor-perfusion) environment that often occurs with cold injuries.

As previously discussed in Chapter 3, *Rescue Basics*, the body can lose heat through four mechanisms: conduction, convection, evaporation, and radiation (**Figure 25-1**):

- *Conduction.* Body heat is lost to nearby object through direct physical touch.
- *Convection.* Body heat is lost to surrounding air, which becomes warmer, rises, and is replaced with cooler air.
- *Evaporation.* Perspiration or wet skin results in body heat lost when the liquid evaporates.
- *Radiation.* Body heat is lost to the atmosphere or nearby objects without physically touching them.

Wind can make one more susceptible to cold weather injury. As the wind speed increases the "relative" temperature can become much worse as noted in (**Table 25-1**). **Wind chill** is the apparent temperature felt on exposed skin. It is a function of the air temperature and wind speed.

Two factors that can predispose a person to a cold injury are alcohol and age. Alcohol, one of the most common predisposing factors, causes peripheral vasodilatation of blood vessels in the skin. This leads to increased heat loss as more warm blood to reaches the skin surface with heat lost to the environment. Alcohol also depresses the central nervous system, which can impair both the shivering response and judgment. Impaired judgment can lead to such irrational behaviors as not seeking appropriate shelter or not wearing appropriate clothing in a cold environment. The body's ability to self-regulate temperature adequately decreases with advanced age. In older individuals, both body fat (needed for proper thermal insulation) and peripheral blood flow decrease. These factors, plus any chronic or underlying illnesses, put the elderly at high risk for cold injury.

Other factors that predispose a person to cold injury include:

- Freezing temperatures
- High winds
- High altitude
- Drug use
- Previous frostbite injury
- Overexertion, which produces fatigue and sweat

Table 25-1 Wind Chill Index

Wind Chill Chart

Temperature (°F)

Wind (mph) / Calm	40	35	30	25	20	15	10	5	0	-5	-10	-15	-20	-25	-30	-35	-40	-45
5	36	31	25	19	13	7	1	-5	-11	-16	-22	-28	-34	-40	-46	-52	-57	-63
10	34	27	21	15	9	3	-4	-10	-16	-22	-28	-35	-41	-47	-53	-59	-66	-72
15	32	25	19	13	6	0	-7	-13	-19	-26	-32	-39	-45	-51	-58	-64	-71	-77
20	30	24	17	11	4	-2	-9	-15	-22	-29	-35	-42	-48	-55	-61	-68	-74	-81
25	29	23	16	9	3	-4	-11	-17	-24	-31	-37	-44	-51	-58	-64	-71	-78	-84
30	28	22	15	8	1	-5	-12	-19	-26	-33	-39	-46	-53	-60	-67	-73	-80	-87
35	28	21	14	7	0	-7	-14	-21	-27	-34	-41	-48	-55	-62	-69	-76	-82	-89
40	27	20	13	6	-1	-8	-15	-22	-29	-36	-43	-50	-57	-64	-71	-78	-84	-91
45	26	19	12	5	-2	-9	-16	-23	-30	-37	-44	-51	-58	-65	-72	-79	-86	-93
50	26	19	12	4	-3	-10	-17	-24	-31	-38	-45	-52	-60	-67	-74	-81	-88	-95
55	25	18	11	4	-3	-11	-18	-25	-32	-39	-46	-54	-61	-68	-75	-82	-89	-97
60	25	17	10	3	-4	-11	-19	-26	-33	-40	-48	-55	-62	-69	-76	-84	-91	-98

Frostbite Times: 30 minutes; 10 minutes; 5 minutes

$$\text{Wind Chill (°F)} = 35.74 + 0.6215T - 35.75(V^{0.16}) + 0.4275T(V^{0.16})$$

Where, T= Air Temperature (°F) V= Wind Speed (mph) *Effective 11/01/01*

Courtesy of the National Weather Service/NOAA.

- Poor fitting, inadequate, or wet clothing
- Dehydration
- Impaired circulation from chronic disease (such as heart disease or diabetes)
- Poor nutrition

COMMON COLD-RELATED EMERGENCIES

There are several common cold-related injuries that OEC technicians need to understand. These include frostnip, frostbite, and primary and secondary hypothermia. Afterdrop, which occurs when warming a hypothermic patient, and windburn, are topics that are also important to emergency medical responders in cold climates.

Frostnip and Frostbite

Frostnip is a relatively minor, local cold injury that results from local vasoconstriction of blood vessels in response to cold. It does not involve freezing or permanent damage of the tissues. The ears, tip of the nose, fingers, and toes are prone to local cold injury such as frostnip. Also known as chilblains, frostnip can cause itching, red patches, swelling and blistering on your hands and feet. It usually clears up within 1 to 3 weeks. Frostnip may be called superficial frostbite.

Frostbite is the actual freezing of body tissue. The same parts of the body that are affected by frostnip are most susceptible to frostbite. Frostbite injury most commonly affects the fingers, toes, nose, ears, cheeks, and the male genitalia. It may involve only superficial tissues, or it may extend to deep tissues and even bones in severe cases. Although frostbite generally occurs at temperatures below freezing, severity is not always related to absolute temperature, but instead is determined by the extent and duration of the freezing of the tissues (**Figure 25-2**).

Tissue injury from frostbite is produced in two ways. First, the actual freezing of the tissue forms ice crystals from within and between cells, extracting water from them. This leads to dehydration and chemical imbalances in the cells and damages proteins. The second and more significant mechanism of tissue injury is loss of blood supply to cells as capillaries and other small blood vessels are damaged. Additionally, damage to surviving

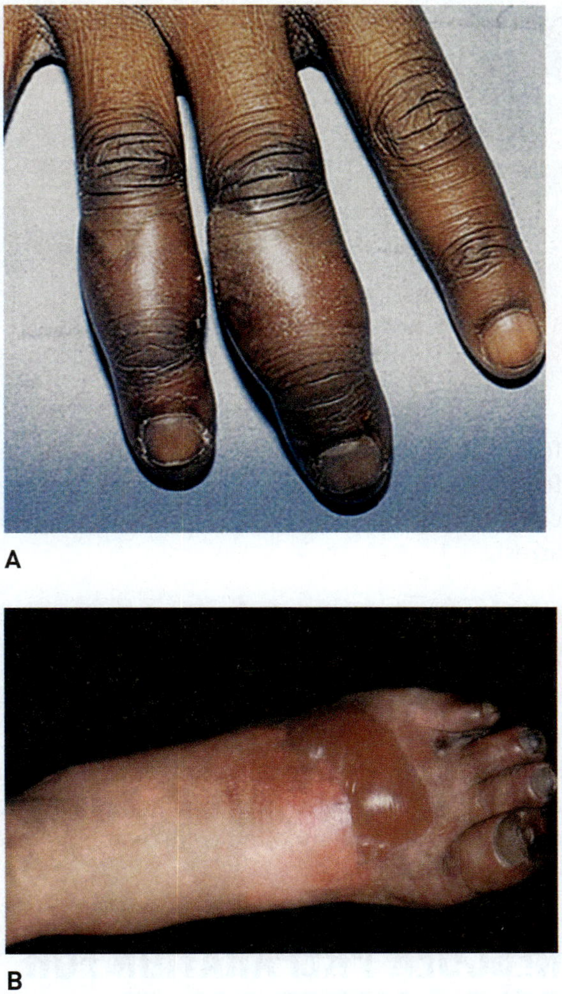

Figure 25-2 Frostbite. **A.** Superficial. **B.** Full thickness.

A: Courtesy of Neil Malcom Winkelmann; B: © Clinical Photography, Central Manchester University Hospitals NHS Foundation Trust, UK/Science Source.

capillaries and veins results in leakage of the liquid part of the blood (serum) out into the tissue. This causes sludging or thickening of the blood, making it semisolid. The blood eventually clots and forms blockages, further restricting blood flow. The lack of blood supply causes tissue death.

Obviously, the earlier the freezing is discovered and reversed, the less severe the overall injury will be. As with burns, the extent of damage caused by frostnip or frostbite is determined by how deeply the cold injury penetrates the skin and underlying structures. The conditions are categorized as follows:

- *Superficial (frostnip).* Affects the first or top layer of skin; no permanent damage to the tissues results.
- *Partial thickness (frostbite).* Affects the upper layers of skin; minor damage to the tissues results.
- *Full thickness (frostbite).* Affects all the layers of skin plus muscle and may even affect bone; and cause severe damage to the tissues

Hypothermia

Hypothermia is an abnormally low body temperature. Clinically, it is defined as a body temperature below 35°C (95°F) according to the American Heart Association (AHA). Hypothermia occurs when heat loss exceeds metabolic heat production and heat conservation. The condition can occur at temperatures well above freezing, especially when a person is in contact with flowing cold water or wind. As body temperature initially drops (mild hypothermia), metabolism initially increases, causing shivering, which serves to warm the body. As core temperature drops further (moderate to severe hypothermia), body systems slow, causing clumsiness, stumbling, mental confusion, removal of clothing, and eventually unresponsiveness. The patient is often unaware of what is happening, further exacerbating the seriousness of the condition.

Factors that predispose an individual to hypothermia include decreased heat production (due

KEY POINT

The Right Boot Fit

Tight fitting ski or hiking boots apply pressure to the top of the foot, constricting the dorsalis pedis artery on the top of the foot. This decreases blood flow to the toes and can exacerbate cold injury. If your feet get cold, loosen the buckle on the top of your ski boots or loosen the laces of your hiking boots to allow better blood flow to the toes.

to insufficient food and decreased metabolism), impaired thermoregulation (causes include reduced shivering due to exhaustion, plus alcohol, drugs, critical illness, and trauma), and increased heat loss due to environmental exposure (resulting from inadequate insulation in cold temperatures or immersion in cold water). In addition, the elderly and young may be susceptible to hypothermia in the home environment.

Hypothermia is commonly divided into two types: primary hypothermia and secondary hypothermia.

Primary Hypothermia

There are two types of primary hypothermia: immersion hypothermia and non-immersion hypothermia.

Immersion hypothermia occurs when the body is submerged. In cold-water immersion, body core cooling rates are fast, but hypothermia does not occur as quickly as might be thought. It takes more than 30 minutes for individuals to become hypothermic after falling into very cold water while wearing winter clothing, if the person is wearing a personal flotation device or can somehow hold his or her head above the water. The problem is that without a life jacket, the person must tread water, but muscle function in the arms and legs will be lost after 10 to 15 minutes, and drowning can occur.

Non-immersion hypothermia, or accidental hypothermia, occurs more slowly but may be accelerated by wind, rain, or snow if the person lacks adequate insulation. It does not involve immersion in water.

Secondary Hypothermia

Secondary hypothermia occurs with systemic disorders and is frequently associated with traumatized or critically ill patients. In this situation, an injury or illness is the primary problem, and hypothermia is an associated secondary problem. Secondary hypothermia still can be severe and even life threatening.

Afterdrop

Afterdrop is defined as a continued drop in core body temperature after removal from exposure to the cold. Typically, afterdrop occurs for a limited time, even *after* warming measures are initiated. It is thought to be caused by the return of cold blood from the extremities to the heart, resulting in a further drop in core body temperature. In severe cases, afterdrop can result in shock and cardiac arrest.

> **KEY POINT**
>
> **How to Convert Temperature**
>
> Fahrenheit to Centigrade: Subtract 32 from degrees Fahrenheit and then multiply by 5/9.
>
> Centigrade to Fahrenheit: Multiply degrees Celsius by 9/5 and then add 32.

Windburn

Windburn is an irritation of the skin that resembles superficial sunburn. It is partly due to the drying effect of low humidity. It can be prevented to some extent by wearing a facemask or by applying a greasy sunscreen. Although windburn is not a cold injury, it can compound cold-related injuries, especially frostbite.

RESCUER PREPARATION FOR COLD WEATHER RESCUE

Do not become the victim! Prevention of a cold-related injury centers on protecting oneself from the mechanisms of heat loss. Convection, conduction, radiation, and evaporation all play important roles in frostbite. Because the nose and ears are frequently exposed to cold weather, wet conditions, and wind, they are especially vulnerable to convective and radiant heat losses. These areas are easily chilled and therefore susceptible to freezing if not adequately protected. Because OEC technicians spend considerable time outdoors, they are at increased risk for cold injury. For more information about how to prepare yourself adequately for outdoor rescue operations, refer to Chapter 3, *Rescue Basics*.

To reduce your risk:

- Know your environment and be prepared.
- Bring adequate appropriate clothing for the environment and use a strategy of layering

CASE Update

You and another patroller move the patient from the gondola and into the aid room at the base building. Her clothes are wet, and she appears to be dead. Her skin is pale and cold to the touch, and she is unresponsive. You immediately check her carotid pulse for 10 seconds, and you identify that it is very slow. There are no signs of trauma.

What should you do now?

insulation, with inner synthetic "wicking" insulating layers and an outer shell layer.
- Be attentive to yourself and your companions.
- Maintain adequate nutrition and hydration.
- Stay dry. Pace yourself to avoid sweating and overexertion. Remove or add layers of clothing as appropriate. Keep your feet dry.
- Avoid tight and restrictive clothing and boots.
- Change your socks often (at least daily, and never sleep wearing wet socks).
- Avoid alcohol, caffeine, and drugs, because they predispose you to cold injury.

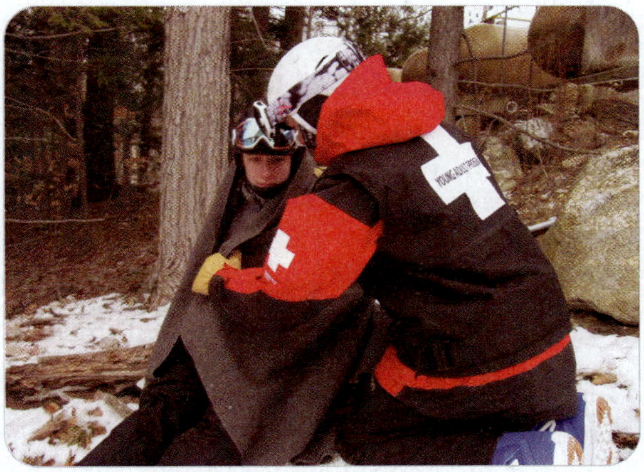

Figure 25-3 Patrollers should have a blanket available as the first method to help keep a patient warm.

PATIENT ASSESSMENT OF COLD INJURIES

Overall assessment of cold injuries begins with scene safety. First and foremost, rescuers must not become patients because this can jeopardize the safety of everyone on scene. In the past some OEC technicians have placed their jackets or clothing on a cold patient. If this will jeopardize the rescuer, it should not be done. It is better to rapidly transfer the patient to a warm environment. The OEC technician should be prepared by having a blanket available for the patient (**Figure 25-3**). Most ski patrols pack blankets in the rescue pack in a toboggan.

Once the scene is considered safe, control excessive bleeding and assess the patient's ABCDs (airway, breathing, circulation, disability) just as you would any patient. However, some adjustments may be needed because pulse rate and respirations can be very difficult to detect in a patient who is cold. For a patient with generalized hypothermia, when *no* pulse or respirations are detected, start CPR immediately. Performing inappropriate chest compressions because you failed to realize the patient had a very slow pulse can worsen the patient's condition by inducing cardiac arrhythmias such as ventricular fibrillation.

Many patients will have an injury that caused them to be caught out in the cold, resulting in hypothermia as a secondary problem. Once the primary assessment is complete, perform a secondary assessment looking for other injuries. Because cold injury patients may have coexisting injuries and/or illnesses, be sure to examine the patient fully using the DCAP-BTLS mnemonic (deformity, contusions, abrasions/avulsions, punctures/penetrations, burns/bleeding/bruises, tenderness, lacerations, swelling) and obtain a complete SAMPLE history (signs and symptoms, allergies, medications, past medical history, last oral intake, events leading up to the problem). Excessive exposure of the body surface while performing a physical examination promotes further heat loss. Make every effort to limit the surface area exposed.

As part of the physical examination, look for signs of cold injury, such as frostbite. Because the signs and symptoms of hypothermia may be exacerbated by alcohol, diabetes, altitude sickness, overdose, exhaustion, and other conditions, a rapid thorough assessment of the patient is warranted.

Patient Assessment of Frostnip

When frostnip occurs, an individual's skin appears cool and pale. While frostnip can be a painful injury, tissues remain intact. The skin is still pliable, and there is no permanent tissue damage unless it escalates into frostbite. Frostnip is occasionally called "superficial frostbite."

Patient Assessment of Frostbite

The earliest symptom of frostbite is pain at the involved site, although this is variable. This symptom is followed by numbness without pain, because as the tissue freezes, sensation and pain stop. The easing of pain is often mistaken for improvement of the condition.

Frostbite should be suspected if a painfully cold body part suddenly stops hurting but is not getting warmer. The affected part may initially feel soft but over time may become firm or woody to the touch. The affected area is initially gray or waxy and then turns pale or red, depending on severity. If the area involved is the head or face, someone other than the patient may be the first to notice it. Color changes in the hands and feet generally go unnoticed until these areas are uncovered.

Following warming, redness may persist over several days, followed by the appearance of clear or blood-filled blisters. In severe cases, death of the affected tissue occurs. The dead tissue appears black, shriveled, and dry, a condition known as dry gangrene (**Figure 25-4**). **Table 25-2** lists the signs and symptoms of frostnip and frostbite.

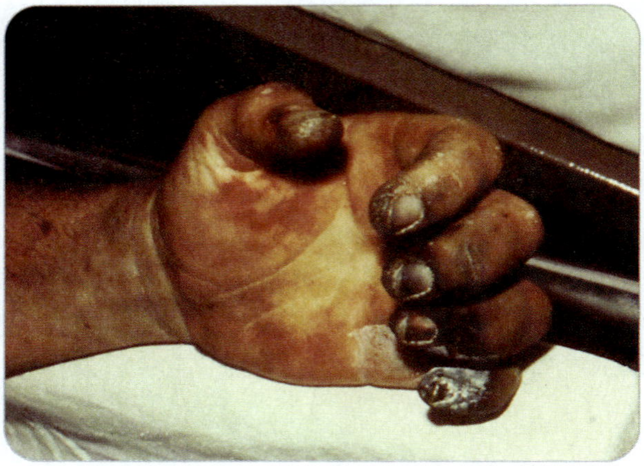

Figure 25-4 Gangrene occurs when tissue is frozen and destructive chemical changes occur in the cells.

Courtesy of Dr. Jack Poland/CDC.

Table 25-2 Signs and Symptoms of Frostnip and Frostbite

Superficial (frostnip)	Skin appears cool and pale and may be painful; tissues remain intact and pliable
Partial thickness (frostbite)	Skin has white- or gray-colored patches that are not painful; tissue may indent if pressed; tissue loss, if present, is minimal
Full thickness (frostbite)	Skin is cold and feels hard or woody; tissue is white or gray and will not rebound when pressed; the area is numb (no pain); no pulse can be detected

FOUR CATEGORIES OF COLD EXPOSURE

Cold patients are divided into four categories that are defined by core body temperature ranges. In the field, measurement of core temperature can be difficult or impossible. **Table 25-3** presents a system for estimating core body temperature and the severity of hypothermia based on the patient's presentation.

Cold Stressed

A person is considered cold stressed when the body temperature is below 36°C (97°F) but above

Table 25-3 Severity of Cold Exposure

Severity of Cold Exposure	Patient Presentation	Core Body Temperature
Cold stressed	Alert, starting to shiver, can help themselves	35–36°C (95–97°F)
Mild hypothermia	Alert but may be confused, shivering	32–35°C (90–95°F)
Moderate hypothermia	Drowsy, decreased level of responsiveness, not shivering	28–32°C (82–90°F)
Severe hypothermia	Unresponsive, may not be breathing	<28°C (<82°F)

35°C (95°F). When this occurs, heat is lost by the body, which in turn starts to compensate. Shivering usually begins when someone is cold stressed.

Mild Hypothermia

Generally, mild hypothermia first manifests as shivering, which can be vigorous. Shivering is an important mechanism that significantly increases muscle activity and heat production. It initially starts when the body's core temperature falls below approximately 35°C (95°F). Unless other factors are present, shivering should enable the patient to overcome heat loss and elevate core temperature. In fact, most patients with mild hypothermia can warm themselves through shivering alone, although they still require protection from further heat loss.

If core temperature continues to fall, uncontrollable shivering is observed until the core temperature reaches approximately 32°C (90°F). There are exceptions to this including exhausted patients who are unable to shiver and some cases of chronic exposure (several hours) in which exhaustion occurs and shivering stops. Such patients generally remain responsive, although they may be confused and exhibit both a loss of judgment and decreased fine motor coordination.

Moderate Hypothermia

The transition to moderate hypothermia (28–32°C, or 82–90°F) is characterized by *cessation of shivering* (usually at a core temperature of about, 32°C or 90°F). A progressive slowing of metabolism also occurs, as evidenced by a slow pulse and/or slow respirations. As the heart rate falls and peripheral vasoconstriction relaxes, hypotension results. In other words, the heart beats more slowly and the blood vessels in the arms and legs relax, allowing more blood into the extremities and causing blood pressure to fall. The level of responsiveness continues to decrease from slurred speech and a staggering gait to unresponsiveness. The surface temperature of the skin gets much colder.

Severe Hypothermia

As core temperature falls below 28°C (82°F), the heart is at risk of ventricular fibrillation, either spontaneously or in response to mechanical stimulation. For this reason, it is imperative to handle hypothermic patients gently and with great care. In severe hypothermia, mental status is severely depressed, resulting in coma. At core body temperatures nearing 25°C (77°F), the patient may appear clinically dead. Examination may reveal an unresponsive and comatose patient. The patient may be rigid, without palpable pulses or discernable respirations. The torso is cold to the touch. Pupillary eye reflexes and deep tendon reflexes are diminished or absent. Although apparently dead, the patient cannot be presumed dead unless those conditions persist after warming or obvious signs of fatal trauma are present. Suppression of energy-dependent processes markedly diminishes oxygen and metabolic demands. As cells become cold, they do not require as much oxygen and glucose. These decreased requirements explain the successful resuscitation of some hypothermic victims despite the appearance of death.

Measuring Core Body Temperature

Important in the diagnosis of hypothermia is knowledge of the body's core temperature, defined as the temperature of the vital organs in the *chest cavity*, including the heart, lungs, and large blood vessels. A special medical thermometer is needed to measure temperature in the chest cavity. Knowing the core temperature enables you to classify

> **KEY POINT**
>
> **Clinical Recognition of Hypothermia**
>
> OEC technicians should recognize the severity of hypothermia *clinically*. Using a thermometer in the field or in the aid room is much less important than observing patients and placing them in a "category" of severity. This will give a close enough approximation of how cold a patient is, allowing you to begin immediate care. Take an oral temperature in the aid room after warming has started.

hypothermia as mild, moderate, or severe. The aggressiveness of the treatment depends on the severity of hypothermia. Although multiple routes are available for assessing temperature, the most effective procedure is the use of a low-temperature rectal thermometer. This instrument provides the best approximation of core temperature obtainable without the more-invasive temperature probes used in a hospital. However, use of a rectal thermometer is usually not practical for the OEC technician. An oral thermometer (not containing mercury) used with the mouth closed although not perfect gives a reasonably close body temperature for an OEC technician in an aid room. Other methods such as axillary, forehead temperature patches, or infrared tympanic thermometers are not advised. Additionally, it is important to recognize that in non-steady state conditions of cooling or warming, temperature gradients exist in the body, and differences may be observed between core and peripheral temperatures.

MANAGEMENT OF COLD-RELATED EMERGENCIES

The general principles of OEC treatment apply to all cases of cold injury, regardless of cause or severity. As with any situation, rescuer safety is the top priority and is ensured by mitigating any hazards (scene safety) that may be present. Always correct any severe bleeding and correct any ABCD-related problems first.

Cold Stress and Hypothermia: Preventing Further Heat Loss and Warming the Patient

In winter weather, prevention of heat loss is important for the care of all patients. In the field, use insulating pads *beneath* the patient as a base; then add blankets while maintaining adequate exposure of the patient's airway and spine. This procedure will minimize convective and conductive heat loss while allowing for airway-related interventions, as needed. Place an insulating hat on the patient's head to decrease radiant heat loss. After caring for an injury, replace any clothing that was opened for the exam. A vapor barrier (e.g., a plastic sheet, space blanket, large trash bag) can be added to eliminate evaporative heat loss and to protect insulation from getting wet.

Move any injured or ill patient to a shelter and out of the wind. A heated building is best. In the backcountry, if the only heat available is from a fire, make sure adequate ventilation of the smoke and carbon monoxide occurs. Replace the patient's wet or cold clothing with dry insulating clothing. If shelter is not immediately available, protect the patient from the chilling effects of wind exposure and insulate the patient from the ground or other cold-conducting surfaces.

Once heat loss has been minimized, attention may be turned toward warming the patient. Warming methods are of two types: passive and active. Passive warming relies on retention of the patient's internal body heat, such as covering with a blanket (**Figure 25-5**). In addition to previously discussed heat loss prevention methods, shivering is the primary passive warming mechanism for patients in the field, and is often all that is needed to warm patients who are mildly hypothermic.

Active warming, which involves the application of heat, may be separated into external and internal modalities. A common active external warming method is the application of hot packs or hot water bottles to major superficial arterial sites (e.g., neck, armpits, groin), the periphery (e.g., hands, feet), and the trunk (e.g., chest, abdomen). This technique does not provide enough heat to warm moderately or severely hypothermic patients who are not shivering. Thus, the use of hot packs for these patients provides limited benefit and can burn the skin.

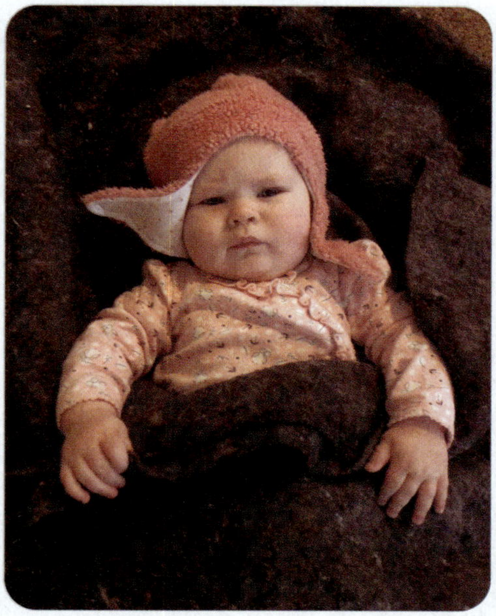

Figure 25-5 It is important to keep pediatric patients warm to prevent hypothermia.

© Ashley O'Rourke.

Inside aid rooms, electric blankets provide a good method for rewarming patients. A simple radio call to the aid room asking to have an electric blanket turned on prior to transport can prove incredibly beneficial. Upon arrival, offer warm beverages (provided there is not a reason to restrict oral intake). Warm, high-energy, nonalcoholic drinks and high-energy foods containing sugar are helpful, providing that the patient is responsive, can hold an object in the hand, and can swallow without choking. This provides fuel to the body, which enables the muscles to continue to shiver, thereby generating additional heat.

Management of Moderate to Severe Hypothermia

In moderate to severe hypothermic patients, aggressive warming such as whole-body warm-water immersion, should never be attempted because it may cause severe drops in blood pressure or ventricular fibrillation. Do not rub the extremities under any circumstances, as rubbing produces little frictional heat and may damage the skin and underlying tissue (especially if it is frozen). Rapidly transport the patient to a definitive-care facility as soon as possible.

If the patient is severely hypothermic and presents without any signs of life, begin treatment immediately. A cold, rigid, apparently lifeless patient who is hypothermic may not actually be dead. The apparent lack of pulse and apnea may be due to a very slow, faint heart rate and tissue rigidity. The time-honored tenet for caring for this type of patient is, "They are not dead until they are warm and dead!"

Open the airway. Check for breathing and a pulse. AHA recommends checking the pulse for 10 seconds, however new evidence in 2017 in the *Wilderness Medical Journal* states you should check the pulse (and respirations) for up to 1 minute in severe hypothermia. The cold effect may slow the heart rate considerably, so a pulse is hard to detect. If cardiac activity is not detected, initiate CPR in the usual manner. Although the cold slows metabolism, the patient still needs oxygen, and rescue breathing or using a bag-valve mask (with ambient air or compressed oxygen) poses no danger to the patient. Improved ventilation and oxygenation may strengthen cardiac activity and make the pulse detectable.

The specific procedure for providing CPR to a severely hypothermic patient should be confirmed with local medical advisors. Chest compressions should not be initiated on any hypothermic patient with signs of life (slow pulse or any respiratory effort) because this action may cause ventricular fibrillation. Additional treatment efforts should focus on heat loss prevention, warming, treatment of other injuries, and rapid evacuation and transport. Do not initiate chest compressions on a patient who has obvious fatal injuries, is frozen (e.g., has ice in the airway), has a chest wall that is so stiff that compressions are impossible, or if the rescuers are exhausted or are in danger.

Multiple case reports indicate survival from accidental hypothermia can still occur, even with prolonged CPR and downtimes. Thus, patients with severe accidental hypothermia and cardiac arrest may benefit from resuscitation even in cases of prolonged downtime and prolonged CPR. Patients should not be considered dead before warming has been provided (**Figure 25-6**).

Use of an AED may be beneficial, although the protocols concerning its use in this situation may vary. The temperature at which defibrillation should first be attempted in the severely hypothermic patient has not been established by AHA as of 2018. If an AED is available to be used, the 2018 AHA basic life support (BLS) guidelines

Assess cold patient
- Assess in order: Consciousness, Movement, Shivering, Alertness
- Assess whether normal, impaired, or no function
- The colder the patient is, the slower you can go, once patient is secured
- Treat all traumatized cold patients with active warming to upper trunk
- Avoid burns: follow product guidelines for heat sources; check for excessive skin redness

Conscious	Movement normal	Shivering	Alert	**Cold stressed, not hypothermic** 1. Reduce heat loss (e.g., add dry clothing) 2. Provide high-calorie food or drink 3. Move around/exercise to warm up
Conscious	Impaired movement	Shivering	Alert	**Mild hypothermia** 1. Handle gently 2. Have patient sit or lie down for at least 30 min. 3. Insulate/vapor barrier 4. Give heat to upper trunk 5. Give high-calorie food or drink 6. Monitor for at least 30 min. 7. Evacuate if no improvement
Conscious	Impaired movement	Not shivering	Not alert	**Moderate hypothermia** 1. Handle gently 2. Keep horizontal 3. No standing/walking 4. No drink or food 5. Insulate/vapor barrier 6. Give heat to upper trunk 7. Volume replacement with warm intravenous fluid (40–42°C) 8. Evacuate carefully
If cold and unconscious Assume severe hypothermia				**Severe hypothermia** 1. Treat as moderate hypothermia, and a) ***IF*** no obvious vital signs, ***THEN*** 60-second breathing/pulse check, or assess cardiac function with cardiac monitor b) ***IF*** no breathing/pulse, ***THEN*** start CPR 2. Evacuate carefully ASAP

Figure 25-6 Guide for the assessment and care of cold-exposed patients.

Data from Giesbrect GG. "Cold Card" to Guide Responders in the Assessment and Care of Cold-Exposed Patients. Wilderness Environ Med. 2018;29(4):499-503.

recommend up to three shocks if recommended by the AED in a patient with severe hypothermia and core temperature less than 30°C (86°F) as transport or rewarming is ongoing. Continue chest compressions in accordance with BLS protocol. The local medical director should provide input for your local protocol.

Attach an AED to the patient as soon as it is available. If the AED says shock advised defibrillation should be attempted. According to the AHA (2018) "It may be reasonable to perform further defibrillation attempts according to the standard BLS algorithm concurrent with rewarming strategies."

A patient with mild hypothermia who has been adequately warmed and has returned to normal mental status need not be emergently evacuated. Take care to prevent a recurrence of cold injury and monitor the patient to ensure resolution.

Any patient who does not respond to warming, who has moderate to severe hypothermia, or has severe frostbite must be evacuated as soon as possible and transported to a definitive-care facility. Evacuation must be as gentle as possible to prevent ventricular fibrillation or additional tissue damage/injury. During transport, continue to monitor the patient's vital signs, the skin underneath any applied heat sources (for potential burns), and distal circulation (e.g., hands and feet). Reexamine the patient frequently unless doing so could increase heat loss or cause tissues to refreeze. If this potential exists, limit the patient's exposure to the best of your ability.

Management of Frostnip

Frostnip is usually easily treated by seeking shelter and warming the affected area by simply placing a warm hand or applying a warm chemical heat pack covered in cloth (so that it's not too hot). Do not rub the affected body part. Various skin lotions may help itching and promote healing.

Management of Frostbite

The treatment for frostbite is rapid warming. Slow, gradual warming should be avoided because it is associated with greater tissue injury. Warming causes pain, sometimes severe pain, and this should be explained to the patient. Among the many factors to consider when rewarming frostbitten tissues are when, where, and how warming efforts should be performed.

When to Warm Frostbitten Tissue

Ideally, tissues should be warmed as soon as possible following initial discovery, and in some instances prior to transport to a medical facility. Doing so may avoid further injury. However, circumstances or the lack of proper resources may prevent prompt warming. Judgment is required when deciding when to warm frozen tissue. As a rule, warmed tissues must not be allowed to refreeze because in that case frostbitten tissue will become gangrenous, resulting in tissue death. If shelter and equipment are not available for thawing the part, then do not attempt to warm the tissue.

If you are in the backcountry and shelter and proper equipment are available, and if rapid warming is possible and there is no possibility of refreezing, then thaw the body part. If the decision is made not to warm frozen tissue in the field, great care must be taken to protect the area from additional injury. For patients who must self-evacuate, it is best to leave a foot frozen, because after it has thawed it will be too painful for walking.

Where to Warm a Frostbitten Body Part

Warming should be performed in a sheltered area where the patient's entire body can be kept warm. Additionally, proper equipment should be available to warm the patient adequately and prevent refreezing. This is best done in a medical facility. If you are in the backcountry and a shelter such as a cabin is available, you can build a fire to heat water, and if refreezing will not occur, a frostbitten body part may be thawed (**Figure 25-7**).

How to Warm a Frostbitten Body Part

Remove constrictive clothes, rings, or watches. Using a vessel large enough to accommodate the limb, prepare a warm water bath that is heated to 38.9–40°C (102–104°F). Ideally, use a thermometer to check the water temperature. If one is not available, you should be able to comfortably place your hand in the water. Suspend the frostbitten part in the center of the warm water bath, using caution to not contact the sides or bottom. Keep the affected area in the bath for 20 to 30 minutes. Stir the water to keep it at a constant temperature, adding warm/hot water as needed. Allow the affected part to air dry if further heat loss is preventable. *Do not* rub the tissues because this can cause sloughing and additional tissue damage.

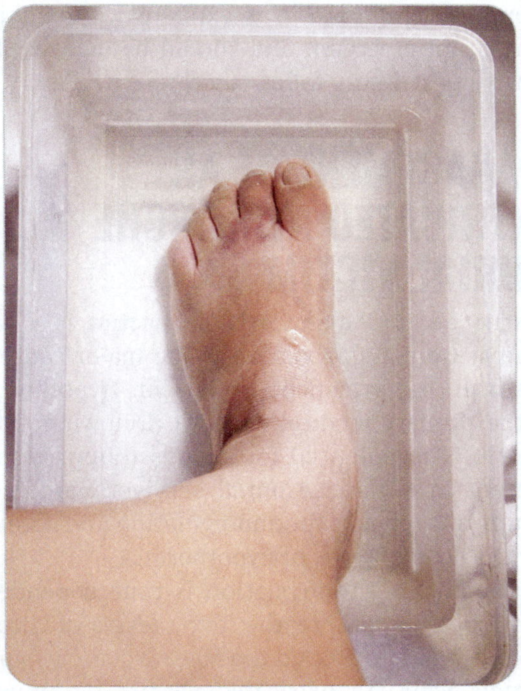

Figure 25-7 Warm the affected part by immersing it in warm water.

Once the area is warmed, aloe vera ointment and dry dressings may be applied. If available, the patient may self-administer ibuprofen or aspirin. Warming a frostbitten body part can cause severe pain that requires advanced life support (ALS) for narcotic pain management. Be sure to gently place dressings between the digits. Elevate the affected area to the level of the heart to reduce swelling.

Initially it is difficult to determine the full extent of the injury. In fact, it may take several days to weeks for the final demarcation of tissue damage. The damaged or dead tissue will eventually become gangrenous and mummify, and it may even auto-amputate. This explains why amputation is not emergent and should be delayed. Extensive post-injury follow-up care is needed.

MANAGEMENT OF AN EXTRICATED AVALANCHE BURIAL VICTIM

Rescue of an avalanche burial victim is a race against time. Asphyxiation is the major cause of death during avalanche burial, but hypothermia is the primary medical concern (following extrication). The potential for serious trauma also is present in avalanche burial survivors, and such trauma may impair thermoregulation and accelerate the development of hypothermia.

Death from asphyxiation is time dependent. If the person can breathe, toxic levels of carbon dioxide build up around the face. Avalanche burial victims who are extricated within 15 minutes have a greater than 90% chance of survival. The potential for survival is minimal when avalanche victims are buried for more than 35 minutes and have an obstructed airway and are in cardiac arrest on extrication. Survival beyond 35 minutes is usually dependent on whether the patient had an air pocket and could expand the chest for breathing.

The initial priorities in the emergency management of an extricated avalanche burial victim are the same as for other patients: open the airway, ensure adequate ventilation (by digging the chest out of the snow so it can expand), and control external bleeding. Provide supplemental oxygen while maintaining spinal motion restriction as defined by local protocol. The patient may have severe hypothermia, so follow the treatment for severe hypothermia, checking pulse and respirations for up to 1 minute.

The severity of hypothermia in an avalanche burial victim may be assessed by the level of responsiveness and the duration of burial. If the avalanche victim is responsive and the duration of burial is less than 1 hour, then mild hypothermia is most likely, and treatment consists of providing warm dry insulation and warm sugar-containing liquids. Warming will occur through shivering.

Development of hypothermia during avalanche burial does not occur as quickly as during cold-water immersion. It generally takes more than 35 minutes of burial in an avalanche to cause moderate to severe hypothermia, but moderate or severe hypothermia may occur in avalanche burial victims *after extrication* because of accelerated development of hypothermia during exposure to a cold, windy environment. Therefore, it is important in the emergency care of avalanche burial victims to handle them gently and package them quickly using warming wraps in order to minimize additional heat loss.

Avalanche burial victims who have a depressed level of responsiveness and are not shivering because they have progressed to moderate or severe hypothermia will require medical transport to a hospital for definitive warming. Unresponsive avalanche burial victims who are breathing are likely moderately to be severely hypothermic. Avalanche burial victims extricated after burials of 35 minutes or less who are pulseless have most likely died from asphyxiation. Although it is unlikely that resuscitation efforts will be successful, begin CPR. If CPR is unsuccessful after 30 minutes, usually the patient was already dead. However, you should continue CPR until higher-level medical personnel assume care. If burial time is greater than 35 minutes and core body temperature is less than 32°C (90°F), the victim may be severely hypothermic, and resuscitation efforts may be continued during transport to a medical facility.

KEY POINT

Avalanche Burial Statistics

Chances of survival:

- 77% survival if caught in an avalanche
- 48% survival if critically buried (burial that impairs breathing and may result in asphyxiation)
- 96% survival in partial burials

Cause of death:

- Asphyxia: at least 75%
- Trauma: up to 25%
- Hypothermia: very few

CASE Outcome

You decide from her clinical picture that the patient is severely hypothermic. You arrange for transport with ALS. You ensure an open airway, insert an OPA, and use a bag-valve mask for rescue breathing. Others help the patient gently remove her wet clothes. You then place her in a warm electric blanket.

The paramedics arrive, intubate the patient, and place her on a cardiac monitor, which shows that her heart has an organized rhythm with a very slow pulse. Additionally, the paramedics start intravenous lines and administer warm saline. They gently transfer her to the ambulance and take her to the hospital.

At the hospital her core body temperature initially is 26°C (79°F). The patient goes into ventricular fibrillation, an AED is used, and CPR is started. The patient has no response to initial defibrillation, or the drugs given. In the emergency department, the patient is aggressively warmed, and eventually her heart regains a normal rhythm. The patient remains in the intensive care unit for a few days and later is discharged from the hospital.

CHAPTER REVIEW

In Summary

- "They're not dead until they're warm and dead."
- Shivering ceases when body temperature falls to 32°C (90°F).
- Hypothermia is a common cold injury that can affect anyone almost anywhere and can occur at temperatures well above freezing, especially when water and wind are factors.
- Handle suspected hypothermia patients gently.
- Mild hypothermia can be treated with passive warming.
- Moderate to severe hypothermia must be treated with active warming.
- A slow, perfusing pulse is enough to sustain a severely hypothermic patient.
- Do not warm a frostbitten area if it will be reexposed to freezing.
- Frostbite requires rapid warming.
- The most important step in preventing cold injuries is preparation.
- Avalanche victims can have a multitude of problems, asphyxiation being foremost.

Key Terms

Afterdrop A continued drop in core body temperature after removal from exposure to the cold.

Frostbite Damage to tissues from freezing due to the formation of ice crystals between and within cells, rupturing the cells and leading to cell death.

Frostnip (chilblains) A relatively minor, local cold injury that results from local vasoconstriction of blood vessels in response to cold.

Hypothermia An abnormally low body temperature; below 35°C (95°F).

Thermoregulation The process of maintaining normal body temperature.

Wind chill The apparent temperature felt on exposed skin; is a function of the air temperature and wind speed.

Chapter Questions

1. As wind speed increases, the change in the "relative" temperature:
   a. decreases the risk of hypothermia.
   b. has no effect at all.
   c. increases the risk of hypothermia.
   d. always causes immediate patient injury.
2. Which of the following is *not* a sign of frostnip—also known as superficial frostbite?
   a. Pale, cool skin
   b. Pain
   c. Cold, hard skin that may be white or gray
   d. Intact, pliable skin
3. You are responsible for assessing a patient who was lost out of bounds and spent a cold, windy, and rainy night outside. What are some possible assessment findings that indicate full-thickness frostbite?
   a. White or gray patches on the cheekbones
   b. Patient's foot is hard, white, and cold
   c. Inability to palpate a pedal pulse
   d. All of the above
4. Hypothermia is generally categorized into two types: primary and secondary. Which of the following statements best describes *secondary* hypothermia?
   a. Hypothermia due to cold-water immersion
   b. Hypothermia that is accelerated by wind or rain
   c. Hypothermia that occurs in traumatized or critically ill patients
   d. Hypothermia that results from inadequate clothing or shelter on a cold day

5. Your patient is drowsy, with a decreased level of responsiveness, and is not shivering. This patient is in which category of cold exposure?
   a. Mild hypothermia
   b. Cold stressed
   c. Severe hypothermia
   d. Moderate hypothermia

6. Afterdrop is defined as:
   a. onset of pain during rewarming of an extremity.
   b. continued lowering of core temperature even after rewarming has begun.
   c. drooling.
   d. All of the above

7. For a patient with mild hypothermia, active warming is appropriate. Which of the following methods should be used?
   a. Apply hot packs or hot water bottles to the neck, armpits, and groin.
   b. Provide the patient with warm, high-energy, sugary drinks.
   c. Give the patient brandy and other "belly warming" alcoholic drinks.
   d. Both a and b

8. You are reviewing material for an upcoming avalanche class. What is the most likely cause of death for someone caught in an avalanche?
   a. Trauma
   b. Hypothermia
   c. Asphyxiation
   d. Frostbite

Answers: 1. c, Objective 25-1, p. 599; 2. c, Objective 25-2, p. 604; 3. d, Objective 25-2, p. 604; 4. c, Objective 25-3, p. 602; 5. d, Objective 25-4, p. 605; 6. b, Objective 25-4, p. 602; 7. d, Objective 25-5, p. 606; 8. c, Objective 25-8, p. 610

CHAPTER 26

HEAT-RELATED EMERGENCIES

OBJECTIVES

Upon completion of this chapter, the OEC technician will be able to:

26-1 Explain how to prevent heat-related illness.

26-2 Explain how the body adjusts to a hot environment.

26-3 List the signs and symptoms of a patient with the four types of heat-related illness.

26-4 Describe and demonstrate the assessment and management of a patient suffering from each of the four types of heat-related illness.

KEY TERMS

Ambient temperature, p. 616
Core body temperature, p. 616
Heat acclimatization, p. 617
Heat index, p. 617
Humidity, p. 616
Hyperthermia, p. 618
Thermoregulation, p. 616

HISTORICAL TIMELINE **1993.** First "Powderfall" is held at Snowbird, Utah.

CHAPTER OVERVIEW

Exercising or traveling in a hot environment may be part of everyday life for some people, and for others it may be part of a planned outdoor adventure. Being active in hot environments requires advance preparation and daily precautions to prevent heat-related illnesses (**Figure 26-1**). Insufficient preparation under hot conditions can lead to heat-related illness. Acute heat-related medical problems can be deadly. The mechanisms for adapting to cold by adding clothing are primarily behavioral. When exposed to heat the body can adapt to maintain homeostasis *over time* by mechanisms built into our bodies.

This chapter describes how to prevent heat-related illness. It explains how the body regulates its core temperature in hot environments. It then discusses the various forms of heat emergencies, including heat cramps, heat exhaustion, heatstroke, and sunburn, and how to assess and treat these conditions. OEC technicians must be able to recognize all heat-related illnesses and be prepared to care for patients when necessary.

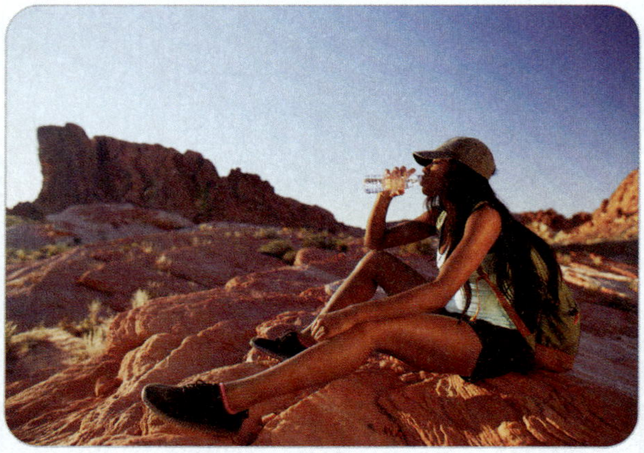

Figure 26-1 Your best defense against the dangers of hot environments is preparation and prevention. Be prepared for the weather you will be in.

ANATOMY AND PHYSIOLOGY

Normal **core body temperature** is 98.6°F (37°C). Regulatory mechanisms keep this internal temperature relatively constant, regardless of the temperature of the surrounding environment (**ambient temperature**). When these regulatory systems are no longer able to cool the body, heat-related illness occurs.

In hot environments or during vigorous physical activity (which causes excess heat production), the body discharges excess heat by sweating (evaporative heat loss) and dilation of the blood vessels in the skin (radiant heat loss). This process, known as **thermoregulation**, is an important part of maintaining homeostasis.

Sweating is the body's most important cooling mechanism. One must be adequately hydrated before sweating occurs. When sweat on the skin evaporates, heat is lost. In environments with high **humidity** sweating is less effective because sweat on the skin evaporates slower. In low-humidity environments sweating is a more effective mechanism of heat loss. Humidity is the amount of water as a gas, called water vapor, in the air.

Dilation of blood vessels in the skin brings warm blood to the skin surface, allowing heat to radiate directly into the environment. Remember heat transfers to cold. When ambient temperature

CASE Presentation

You are asked to patrol at a summer off-road bicycle race at your resort. The race starts at 10 AM and takes 3 hours. Morning temperatures are tolerable, but midday temperatures reach 90°F. You are stationed near the finish line. As one of the last bikers comes to the finish line, she collapses after getting off her bike. She stands, staggers over to you, and bends over panting. She asks for water and states she is hot and exhausted. Her face is flushed.

What should you do?

Temperature (°F)

Relative Humidity (%)	80	81	84	86	88	90	92	94	96	98	100	102	104	106	108	110
40	80	81	83	85	88	91	94	97	101	105	109	114	119	124	130	136
45	80	82	84	87	89	93	96	100	104	109	114	119	124	130	137	
50	81	83	85	88	91	95	99	103	108	113	118	124	131	137		
55	81	84	86	89	93	97	101	106	112	117	124	130	137			
60	82	84	88	91	95	100	105	110	116	123	129	137				
65	82	85	89	93	98	103	108	114	121	126	130					
70	83	86	90	95	100	105	112	119	126	134						
75	84	88	92	97	103	109	116	124	132							
80	84	89	94	100	106	113	121	129								
85	85	90	96	102	110	117	126	135								
90	86	91	98	105	113	122	131									
95	86	93	100	108	117	127										
100	87	95	103	112	121	132										

Likelihood of Heat Disorders with Prolonged Exposure or Strenuous Activity

Caution | Extreme Caution | Danger | Extreme Danger

Figure 26-2 The heat and humidity index risk scale.

Courtesy of the National Weather Service/NOAA.

exceeds body temperature, loss of body heat by radiation from the skin is not effective for cooling, and sweating becomes the major mechanism for heat loss. As discussed in Chapter 25, *Cold-Related Emergencies*, the body can lose heat through four mechanisms: conduction, convection, evaporation, and radiation.

This is the basis for the **heat index**, a measure of the risk for heat illness. The higher the temperature and the higher the humidity, the greater the risk of heat illness (**Figure 26-2**).

Adequate hydration is required for adequate heat loss from sweating. During exercise in hot environments, up to a liter of sweat can be lost each hour. Maintaining adequate hydration is essential to preventing heat illness. An individual must match hydration needs to the level of activity and the temperature of the environment, taking care to allow for adequate adjustment to the heat.

When cold, an individual will put on more clothes or go indoors. Adaptation to heat depends on physiological acclimatization (changes in the body to adapt to heat) rather than modifications in behavior alone.

Prior heat exposure lowers the skin temperature at which sweating occurs, which initiates cooling of the body by the evaporation of sweat at a lower skin temperature. Physical training improves heat tolerance through the same mechanisms, and it also improves the efficiency of the cardiovascular system. Poor physical fitness, obesity, lack of heat acclimatization, and dehydration decrease an individual's heat tolerance. Chronic medical conditions increase the risk of heat illness, and heat may exacerbate chronic medical conditions.

Heat-Related Illness Prevention

Adequate preparation is required to ensure that the body's heat-regulating mechanisms maintain normal body temperature in hot environments. To maximize tolerance to hot environments, a program for **heat acclimatization** is important. Individuals can improve their heat acclimatization before taking a trip to a hot environment by exercising daily in the heat for limited periods of at least 1 hour for at least several days, preferably for 1 week. If this is not possible before a trip, individuals should then limit periods of exercise during the warmest parts of the day for the first week of the trip.

During periods of exercise lasting several hours or more, salty snacks and adequate water intake are necessary. Urine that is a light-yellow color is a good indicator of adequate hydration status, whereas darker urine indicates dehydration. The color of urine may also be affected by certain medications, supplements, or liver disease.

In addition to the physiological mechanisms of heat loss—sweating and blood vessel dilation—behavior is important for maintaining normal body temperature in hot environments. Wearing loose-fitting, lightweight, sun-blocking, light-colored clothing and a wide-brimmed hat, avoiding exercise during the hottest part of the day, and resting frequently in the shade are all important measures for preventing heat illness.

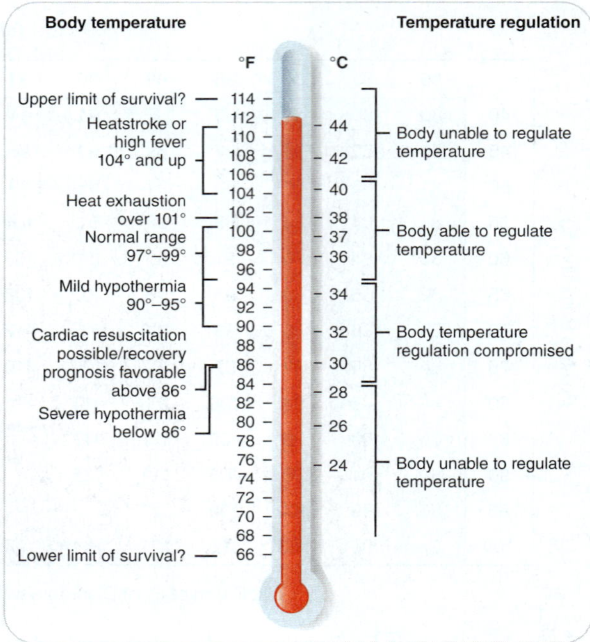

Figure 26-3 Core body temperatures for heat illnesses and the corresponding efficiencies of the brain's hypothalamic regulation.

COMMON HEAT-RELATED EMERGENCIES

Heat illness includes a broad spectrum of injuries caused by exposure to a hot environment and failure of the body's normal mechanisms for regulating body temperature, electrolyte levels, and body fluid status. An abnormally high body temperature, known as **hyperthermia**, is characterized by a high core temperature, usually 101°F (38.3°C) or more (**Figure 26-3**). Extreme or untreated hyperthermia can rapidly become life threatening.

Newborns, infants, the elderly, and the obese exhibit poor thermoregulation and are at greatest risk for heat illness. Newborns and infants are especially vulnerable if overdressed. Patients with chronic medical conditions like heart disease, lung disease, and diabetes are at increased risk of heat illness. Alcohol and drugs, which dehydrate the body or decrease the body's ability to sweat, make a person more susceptible to heat illnesses. Illicit drugs such as amphetamines or cocaine and some prescribed medications may cause dehydration or the loss of thermoregulation.

When the body's mechanisms for transferring heat to the environment are overwhelmed and the body is unable to tolerate the excessive heat, illness from heat exposure can ensue. While heat illness is a spectrum of injury, it is often categorized into four major phases:

- Heat-related syncope
- Heat cramps
- Heat exhaustion
- Heatstroke

Heat-related syncope and heat cramps usually precede the more serious conditions of heat exhaustion and heatstroke.

Heat-Related Syncope

Heat-related syncope is a condition that originates primarily in the cardiovascular system. Clinically, it is defined as a temporary loss of responsiveness or fainting due to a temporary loss of effective blood flow. Heat-related syncope occurs when the body is heat stressed and blood is diverted into the peripheral circulation (arms and legs) to allow heat to be lost at the body's surface. The blood does not return from the surface to the heart rapidly enough, which decreases brain perfusion and results in fainting. Although this condition may occur without warning while the patient is standing, it is often preceded by feelings of nausea or lightheadedness.

Heat Cramps

Heat cramps occur in large muscle groups after exercise in a hot environment and are caused by electrolyte disturbances and dehydration. Such cramps can be quite painful during the contraction (spasm) of the muscles. Stretching the muscles can alleviate the cramp(s), and rest, rehydration, and electrolyte replacement will prevent recurrence.

Heat Exhaustion

Heat exhaustion is characterized by exhaustion, dizziness, nausea, headache, leg cramps, excessive sweating, and decreased urine output, with a core body temperature that is greater than 101°F (38.3°C), but less than 104°F (40°C) and a level of responsiveness that is normal. When the body loses too much water and too many electrolytes through heavy sweating, the result is dehydration. Heat exhaustion is a common disorder resulting from dehydration to the point at which low body fluid volume (hypovolemia) causes signs and symptoms. The body responds rapidly to treatment, and changes in mental status do not persist or worsen.

Heatstroke

Heatstroke is a life-threatening emergency identified by a decreased level of responsiveness and a core body temperature greater than 104°F (40°C). It is associated with an elevated heart rate, a high respiratory rate, decreased sweating, and eventually a severe drop in blood pressure. The defining characteristic of heatstroke that differentiates it from heat exhaustion is altered mental status; a decreased level of responsiveness that persists or gets worse, which should prompt immediate treatment and evacuation.

Heatstroke is the most serious heat illness and can occur from either exposure to heat without exertion (classical heatstroke) or exertion in a hot environment (exertional heatstroke). In heatstroke, the body's normal mechanisms for shedding excess heat are overwhelmed. Core body temperature rises (above 104°F, or 40°C), and if untreated shock follows, it will cause damage to the brain, the heart and blood vessels, the liver, and the kidneys. Left untreated, heatstroke results in death.

MDMA (3,4-Methylenedioxymethamphetamine), commonly known as ecstasy, E, or Molly, has been implicated in causing heatstroke. MDMA can cause heatstroke by increasing heat production in the body and decreasing effectiveness of heat regulation mechanisms. The effects are made worse in hot environments, with reduced fluid intake, repeat drug dosing, use of other stimulants, crowded conditions, and physical activity.

Table 26-1 illustrates the signs and symptoms of serious heat emergencies.

Table 26-1 Comparing Conditions Resulting from Heat Stress

Variable	Heat Cramps	Heat Exhaustion	Heatstroke
Pathophysiology	Sodium and water loss	Sodium and water loss, hypovolemia	Failure of heat-regulating mechanisms
Mental and neurologic status	Normal	Normal and mild confusion	Altered, delirium, seizures
Temperature	May be mildly elevated	Usually mildly elevated	Usually > >40.0°C (104°F)
Skin	Cool, moist	Pale, cool, moist	Dry, hot, but sweating may persist, especially with exertional heatstroke
Muscle cramping	Severe	May or may not be present	Absent

CASE Update

You help the patient into the shade of the first-aid tent. Vital signs reveal her pulse is 120 beats per minute, her blood pressure is 100/60 mm Hg, and her oral temperature is 39°C (103°F).

What steps do you take now?

PATIENT ASSESSMENT OF HEAT INJURIES

OEC technicians should perform a scene size-up, address safety issues, perform a primary patient assessment, address life-threatening issues such as severe life threatening bleeding, obtain a SAMPLE (signs and symptoms, allergies, medications, past medical history, last oral intake, events leading up to the problem) history, and perform a secondary patient assessment, which should include assessing for injuries using DCAP-BTLS (deformity, contusions, abrasions/avulsions, punctures/penetrations, burns/bleeding/bruises, tenderness, lacerations, swelling) and obtaining a complete set of vital signs. For any heat emergency, address any threats to life and provide adequate protection from direct exposure to the sun for both patients and rescuers. The sections that follow describe assessment findings for several heat-related injuries.

Patient Assessment of Heat-Related Syncope

Patients who suffer from heat-related syncope are warm to the touch, may be lightheaded and have tachycardia, and may be hypotensive initially (**Figure 26-4**). Look for traumatic injuries especially significant bleeding resulting from falling after fainting. As with all unresponsive patients, ensure that you open their airway and simultaneously check for breathing while checking for a carotid pulse. If there is no pulse or breathing, follow current CPR standards. If the patient has a pulse and is breathing, maintain the airway while conducting the secondary assessment. Patients receiving prompt care usually rapidly regain responsiveness.

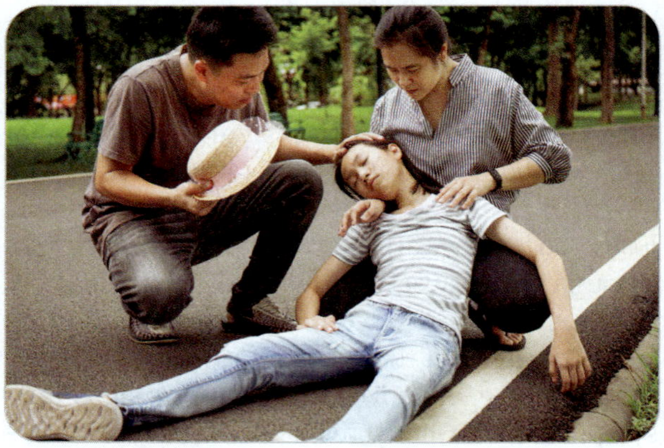

Figure 26-4 This person is suffering from heat-related syncope.

Patient Assessment of Heat Cramps

The hallmarks of heat cramps are intense, painful muscle spasm and painful cramping in affected extremities. Abdominal cramping also may occur and can be quite severe. Most cramps are self-limiting and resolve after a minute or two.

Patient Assessment of Heat Exhaustion

Depending on the severity of their condition, patients experiencing heat exhaustion exhibit a variety of signs and symptoms that include the following:

- Weakness
- Inability to work or participate in an activity
- Headache
- Anxiety
- Nausea
- Faintness, lightheadedness
- Decreased appetite
- Tachycardia

- Normal or slightly elevated body temperature
- Warm skin
- Sweating (moderate to heavy)

Patient Assessment of Heatstroke

Heatstroke is a life-threatening emergency characterized by an altered level of consciousness and organ dysfunction. Patients have the signs and symptoms of heat exhaustion, but also have significant altered mental status. Without prompt emergency treatment, heatstroke can be fatal. Classically, patients have hot, dry, flushed skin because the body's sweating mechanisms have been exhausted. However, heatstroke should be suspected in any patient that has an altered level of consciousness and does not respond quickly to treatment for heat exhaustion, even if the person is still sweating.

MANAGEMENT OF HEAT-RELATED EMERGENCIES

In most cases of heat illness, move patients to a cooler location as soon as possible and/or shade patients from direct exposure to the sun (**Figure 26-5**). The nature of further care is based on the cause of the suspected heat-related illness. If you suspect heatstroke, attend to any threats to life identified in your primary assessment. Provide appropriate hydration and any needed supportive measures. If the patient's oxygen saturation is less than 94%, provide oxygen.

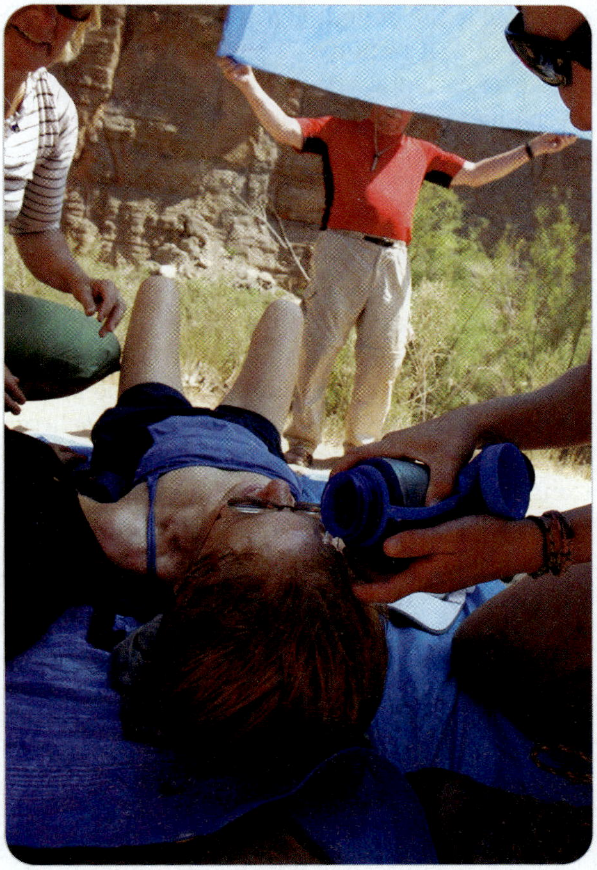

Figure 26-5 Remove patients from direct sunlight and begin to cool them immediately.

Management of Heat-Related Syncope

For heat-related syncope, remove the person from the heat source. Place the patient into a supine position with legs elevated 10 to 12 inches, which allows blood to flow to vital organs such as the brain. Provide supportive measures. For patients who can speak and swallow, give cool nonalcoholic liquids.

Management of Heat Cramps

Heat cramps generally respond favorably to oral electrolyte solutions such as commercial sports beverages. Sports drinks may need to be diluted to 50% water and 50% sport drink. If not available, mix 1/4 to 1/2 teaspoon of table salt into a quart of cool water and add some pleasant flavoring. This should be consumed slowly to prevent vomiting. Gentle stretching or massage of the cramped muscles is usually beneficial and can provide some relief. After recovery, activity may be resumed. However, if the cramps return, a 24-hour rest period is recommended.

Management of Heat Exhaustion

Treat heat exhaustion promptly to prevent it from developing into heatstroke by taking the following actions:

- Immediately move the patient to a location that provides shade and a cooler temperature.
- Place the patient in a position of comfort, usually supine with the legs elevated 10 to 12 inches.
- Remove clothing (or at least loosen it) and cool the patient by fanning (either manually or electrically).

- Provide the patient high-flow oxygen if oxygen saturation is less than 94%.
- If the patient can swallow, rehydrate the patient with cool water, a cool electrolyte-containing solution, or 1/4 to 1/2 teaspoon of table salt added to a quart of cool water. Never force oral fluids for patients who are not fully responsive because they could aspirate the liquid into the lungs.

In most cases, these measures will improve the patient's condition rapidly. Lack of improvement or a worsening of symptoms may be indications of heatstroke. *Because the distinction between heat exhaustion and heatstroke is not always clear*, transport to a hospital for further evaluation and treatment any patient for whom any of the following conditions applies:

- Symptoms that do not clear up promptly
- A decreasing level of responsiveness
- Body temperature that remains elevated
- The patient is very young, elderly, or has an underlying medical condition such as diabetes or cardiovascular disease

Management of Heatstroke

As previously indicated, heatstroke is a true emergency that requires immediate attention. Recovery from heatstroke depends on the duration of the hyperthermia and the speed with which treatment is administered. Emergency treatment should begin immediately in the field and has one objective: *lower the patient's body temperature by any means available.* Take the following steps when treating a patient with heatstroke:

- Notify EMS as quickly as possible for advanced life support (ALS) transport to a hospital.
- Move the patient promptly from the hot environment to a cool, shaded environment.
- Remove the patient's clothing.
- Provide supplemental oxygen only if oxygen saturation is less than 94%, and then monitor to ensure it remains between 94-99%.
- The most effective cooling mechanisms are convection and evaporation, which are accomplished by keeping exposed skin wet and having a continuous flow of air across the skin. Nearly naked patients may be sprayed with cool or room temperature water while a fan blows air across the skin, or if necessary while a bystander manually fans the patient with a towel or a jacket.
- Conductive cooling can also be effective, particularly if ice packs are applied to areas of high blood flow, such as the armpits and groin.
- The immersion of patients in cold water is the most effective treatment but is best done under direct medical supervision.

If possible, check the patient's temperature frequently to determine if core body temperature is cooling. Although a rectal temperature is best, an oral thermometer can be used. Forehead and tympanic "ear" thermometers are not accurate. When the body temperature reaches approximately 101°F (38.3°C), taper off the cooling efforts; rapid cooling below this point may lead to shivering (which will generate unwanted heat). If the patient returns to a level of responsiveness appropriate for oral hydration, give fluids. Do not give medications such as aspirin, ibuprofen, or acetaminophen. Rapid evacuation is indicated. Monitor patients carefully for a rebound increase in body temperature.

Differentiating Between Heat Exhaustion and Heatstroke

Heatstroke is differentiated from heat exhaustion by persistent profound mental status changes, hypotension/shock, and profound elevations in temperature. In heat exhaustion, mental status and blood pressure normalize rapidly upon rest in a supine position in the shade and oral rehydration. When there is doubt about whether a patient has heat exhaustion or heatstroke, treat as heatstroke and transport the patient with ALS to medical care as quickly as possible. **Table 26-2** lists the criteria that help differentiate between heat exhaustion and heatstroke.

Table 26-2 Differentiating Between Heat Exhaustion and Heatstroke

Finding	Heat Exhaustion	Heatstroke
Occurs in high environmental temperatures?	Yes	Yes
May be associated with exercise	Yes	Yes
Patient collapses	Possible	Yes
Level of responsiveness	Anxious	Significant altered mental status, progresses to coma
Elevated core body temperature	Yes, usually below 40°C (104°F)	Yes, may be higher than 40°C (104°F)
Pulse rapid	Yes	Yes
Breathing rapid	Yes	Yes
Responds to treatment in field or aid room	Yes, rapidly	Condition may worsen despite treatment
Shock, hypotension present	No	Yes
Action to take in the field	Treat in the field	Evacuate and initiate treatment
Treatment	Cooling, rehydration	Rapid cooling

CASE Outcome

Now that the patient is in the medical tent, you loosen her clothing and have her lie down with her legs elevated about 10 inches. Now her respirations are 20 breaths per minute and her pulse is 100 beats per minute. She is responding appropriately to questions. She drinks a diluted sports drink containing electrolytes, and once she lies down, she begins to look more comfortable. As you spray water on her, you fan her with a piece of cardboard. She continues to rest and sip liquids over the next 30 minutes, her breathing slows, and she becomes more talkative. Her pulse is now 80 beats per minute. Your findings suggest that she was suffering from heat exhaustion. Even though she has improved, the EMS personnel start an IV and recommend she go to the hospital for further evaluation.

CHAPTER REVIEW

In Summary

- Adequate preparation is required to ensure that body's heat-regulating mechanisms maintain normal body temperature in hot environments.
- Using preventive measures reduces the risk of heat-related injuries.
- Heat illnesses include a spectrum of disorders caused by exposure to a hot environment: heat-related syncope, heat cramps, heat exhaustion, and heatstroke.
- Heat-related syncope and heat cramps usually precede the more serious conditions of heat exhaustion and heatstroke.
- Patients who suffer from heat-related syncope are warm to the touch, may be lightheaded and have tachycardia, and may be hypotensive initially.
- The hallmarks of heat cramps are intense, painful muscle spasm and painful cramping in affected extremities.
- Patients experiencing heat exhaustion exhibit a variety of signs and symptoms that include weakness, inability to work or participate in an activity, headache, and mild confusion.
- Heatstroke is characterized by an altered level of consciousness and organ dysfunction.
- Move patients to a cool location, address life threats, and provide appropriate hydration and any needed supportive measures. If the patient's oxygen saturation is less than 94%, provide oxygen.
- Heatstroke is differentiated from heat exhaustion by persistent profound mental status changes, hypotension/shock, and profound elevations in temperature.
- Heatstroke is life threatening, does not respond quickly to treatment, and requires ALS transfer.

Key Terms

Ambient temperature The temperature in the immediate environment.

Core body temperature The temperature in the part of the body that contains the vital organs.

Heat acclimatization Adaptation of the body over time to a hot environment.

Heat index A measure of the risk for heat illness; combines the effects of increasing ambient temperature and increasing humidity.

Humidity The amount of water vapor in the air.

Hyperthermia Elevated core body temperature.

Thermoregulation The process of maintaining normal body temperature.

Chapter Questions

1. Preventive measures for heat-related illnesses include:
   a. adequate water intake and salty snacks.
   b. minimizing rest periods.
   c. exercising for an hour during the hottest part of the day.
   d. wearing dark colored, tight fitting, layers of clothing.
2. The body adjusts to a hot environment by:
   a. sweating.
   b. dilation of the blood vessels in the skin.
   c. a process known as thermoregulation.
   d. All of the above
3. Your patient has run several miles of a marathon and is found sitting on the side of the road complaining of intense, painful muscle spasm and cramping in her leg. You suspect that she is suffering from:
   a. heat-induced syncope.
   b. heat cramps.

c. heat exhaustion.
d. heatstroke.

4. Your patient is a gardener at a resort. He has been working in the gardens for several hours. His coworker says that he complained of being lightheaded and then fainted. You find that his skin is warm to the touch and his pulse is over 100 beats per minute. You suspect that he is suffering from:
   a. heat-related syncope.
   b. heat cramps.
   c. heat exhaustion.
   d. heatstroke.
5. Your patient is a mountain bike rider who is complaining of nausea, headache, and weakness. She is sweating profusely. You suspect that she is suffering from:
   a. heat-related syncope.
   b. heat cramps.
   c. heat exhaustion.
   d. heatstroke.
6. The outside temperature is 90°F. Your patient is a trail builder who has been working in the sun on the mountain trails for 8 hours. When you gently shake him, he responds by mumbling. His skin is hot and dry. You suspect that he is suffering from:
   a. heat-related syncope.
   b. heat cramps.
   c. heat exhaustion.
   d. heatstroke.
7. Your patient has suffered from heat-induced syncope. Your care will include removing the person from the source of heat, providing cool liquids and placing the person in a ____ position.
   a. supine
   b. prone
   c. lateral recumbent
   d. seated
8. Your patient is suffering from heat cramps. Your care will include stretching or massage of the cramped muscle and administering:
   a. a light meal.
   b. an electrolyte solution.
   c. an alcoholic beverage.
   d. syrup of ipecac.
9. Your patient is suffering from heat exhaustion. Your care will include:
   a. placing the patient in a position of comfort.
   b. moving the patient to a cool and shaded location.
   c. providing a diluted electrolyte solution.
   d. All of the above
10. Your patient is suffering from heatstroke. Your care will include:
    a. applying ice packs to the armpits and groin.
    b. activating EMS, with ALS.
    c. removing the patient's clothing.
    d. All of the above

Answers: 1. a, Objective 26-1, p. 618; 2. d, Objective 26-2, p. 616; 3. b, Objective 26-3, p. 619; 4. a, Objective 26-3, p. 618; 5. c, Objective 26-3, p. 619; 6. d, Objective 26-3, p. 619; 7. a, Objective 26-4, p. 621; 8. b, Objective 26-4, p. 621; 9. d, Objective 26-4, p. 622; 10. d, Objective 26-4, p. 622

CHAPTER 27

PLANT AND ANIMAL EMERGENCIES

OBJECTIVES

Upon completion of this chapter, the OEC technician will be able to:

27-1 Describe how plants and fungi can be harmful to humans.

27-2 Describe how mushrooms can be harmful to humans.

27-3 Describe and demonstrate how to assess a patient who has been injured following an encounter with a toxic plant, an animal, or marine life.

27-4 Describe and demonstrate how to manage an exposure to topical (on the skin) toxins.

27-5 Describe how to manage someone who has been bit by a poisonous snake.

27-6 Describe and demonstrate the proper management of wounds caused by animals, including reptiles, insects, and spiders.

KEY TERMS

Antivenom, p. 641
Envenomation, p. 639
Necrosis, p. 636
Poison, p. 629
Toxin, p. 629
Venom, p. 629

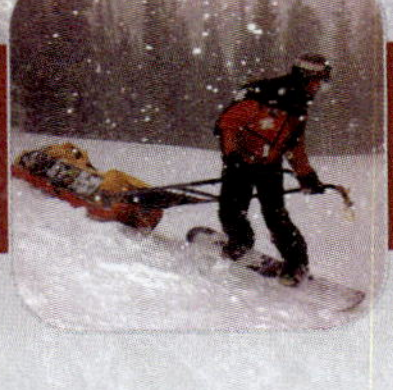

HISTORICAL TIMELINE 1994. Board approves a pilot snowboard patroller program.

CHAPTER OVERVIEW

Anyone who has spent time in the outdoors should be aware of the risks posed by avalanches, lightning, or flash flooding. Injuries stemming from these events, although dramatic, are rare. Much more common are injuries and problems resulting from exposure to plants and animals, including insects. With more ski resorts involved in summertime activities such as biking, a basic knowledge of these emergent medical problems is important.

Even though most encounters with plants and animals are benign, certain plants are highly toxic. Similarly, most animal sightings are enjoyable events; however, both large and small animals can inflict great injury. Maintaining the priorities of bleeding control, airway, breathing, circulation, and disability will help you assess and manage patients that have been injured by plants and animals. During the history and physical exam, OEC technicians should focus on determining what the patient's plant or animal exposure is.

This chapter discusses some common injuries resulting from exposure to plants and animals. Basic assessment considerations and treatment guidelines are also covered.

ANATOMY AND PHYSIOLOGY

The skin is composed of two major layers, the epidermis and the dermis. The outer layer, the *epidermis*, acts as a waterproof, protective barrier to invading organisms. Beneath it is the *dermis*, which contains hair follicles, blood capillaries, sweat glands, and nerve endings. The main functions of the dermis are sensation, temperature regulation, and fluid balance. Below the dermis is the *subcutaneous tissue* that contains many small blood vessels.

Injuries and topical exposures sustained from plants and animals nearly always affect the epidermis and dermis. Additionally, a forceful bite from a large animal through the subcutaneous layer can injure the underlying connective tissue, muscle, larger blood vessels, nerves, and bones. Not only can toxins from plants or animals cause local damage, but these poisons can enter the bloodstream affecting the cardiac, respiratory, and neurologic systems. In severe cases, respiratory or cardiac arrest may occur. Depending on the type of exposure, effects can be rapid or may evolve over hours or days.

CASE Presentation

You are at the mid-station of an off-road bicycle competition at a national park. A cyclist comes into the station and says someone was attacked by a bear about a quarter mile back. You and another patroller grab your packs, get on an all-terrain vehicle (ATV) with oxygen, medical equipment, and a stretcher, and head up the trail. A ranger with a rifle accompanies you on another ATV. A small crowd has gathered near the trail. You find a middle-aged man lying alongside the trail, bleeding and confused. You scan your surroundings for wild animals and ask others if any are near. None can be found. The ranger stands guard and keeps the crowd away from you but stays close in case the bear returns. The race is stopped further up the trail. You ask the injured man his name, and he replies, "Mike." You tell him you are here to help him. His right forearm has a large gash that is spurting bright red blood from severely damaged tissue. You control the bleeding with a pressure dressing. You notice he has a belt placed snugly around his upper right thigh, with a large amount of tissue missing from his lower right calf. You immediately radio for more help and EMS with air transport.

What should you do now?

POISONS, TOXINS, AND VENOM

It is important to understand the differences among a toxin, a poison, and venom. A **poison** is any substance that can cause severe organ damage or death if ingested, inhaled, injected into the body, or absorbed through the skin. Poisons can come from a living creature or from chemicals or substances that do not come from living creatures. A **toxin** is a poison made by a living creature, whether plant or animal. A **venom** is a specific toxin or poisonous secretion of an animal, most commonly from a snake, spider, or scorpion, usually transmitted by a bite or sting. After a toxin, poison, or venom enters the bloodstream, organs with more blood supply are affected first. Also, local necrosis (death of tissue) and infection can be seen at an injection site later.

ADVERSE EFFECTS AND EMERGENCIES FROM COMMON PLANTS AND FUNGI

While most toxic encounters from plants and fungi are topical in nature, outdoor enthusiasts may at times ingest vegetation or fruit that is harmful. When eaten, some plants can cause life-threatening systemic reactions. Common fruits and berries are rarely toxic. However, the ingestion of some plant material can cause severe illness and death.

The most common presentations of ingestion include nausea and vomiting. The body seems to know the substance that was eaten is toxic, so it tries to expel it. Some toxic plants may produce cardiac effects, resulting in rhythm disturbances, whereas others may have neurologic effects that produce hallucinations, confusion, or seizures. The onset of effects may occur within 15 to 30 minutes or over several hours. Do not ingest any plant material unless you are sure what it is.

Plants Toxic to the Skin

When plant toxins touch the skin (topical exposure) a localized skin reaction due to contact with plant material is a common occurrence (Figure 27-1). These reactions are typically a localized inflammatory response commonly called an allergic reaction. Chapter 14, *Allergies and Anaphylaxis*, contains details on allergic reactions. Plant toxins may cause itching only, or blisters and pain that can be severe enough to require evaluation by a physician and treatment with medications. In severe cases systemic effects may result in cardiovascular collapse or shock.

Poison Ivy, Poison Oak, and Poison Sumac

- **Description:** These plants can be found in many forms, from low-lying vines to tall shrubs (Figure 27-2). The vines may often be found growing on tall trees with no leaves visible on the vines. Poison ivy and poison oak characteristically have three leaves grouped together, whereas poison sumac has seven leaves grouped together.

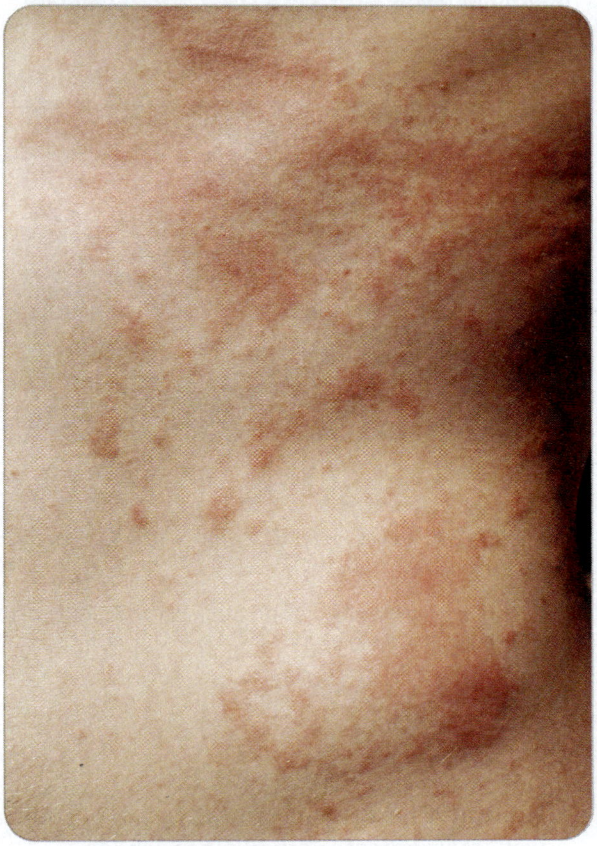

Figure 27-1 Rash from contact with a poisonous plant.

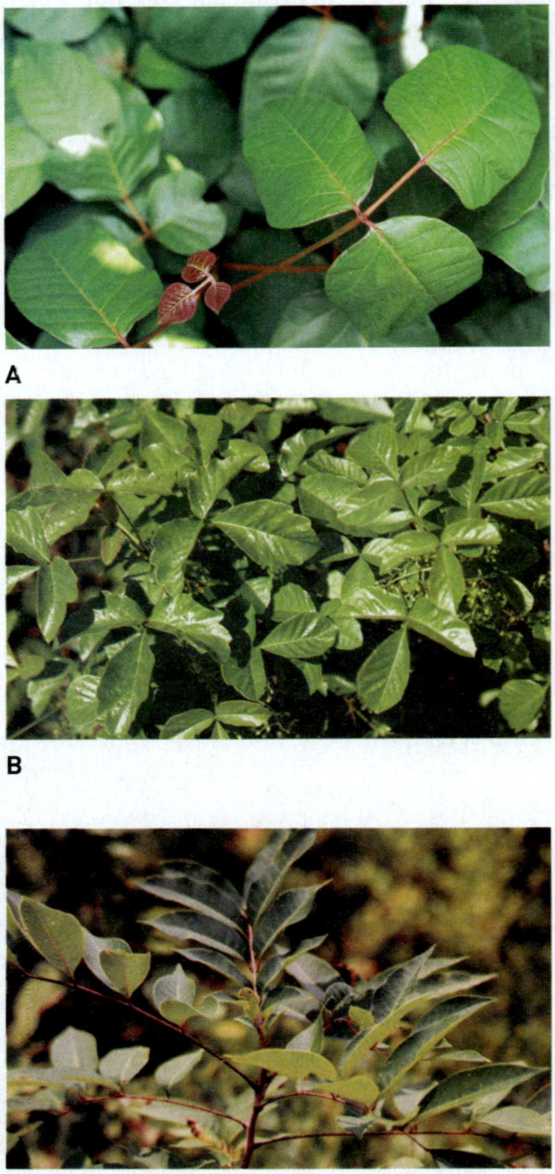

Figure 27-2 **A.** Poison ivy. **B.** Poison oak. **C.** Poison sumac.

A: © Thomas Photography LLC/Alamy Stock Photo; **B:** © Thomas J. Peterson/Alamy Stock Photo; **C:** Courtesy of U.S. Fish & Wildlife Service.

- **Habitat:** These plants typically grow in cool, wet environments with plenty of shade. Poison ivy and oak live throughout the United States, while poison sumac is in the eastern United States.
- **Toxic part:** All parts of the plant are considered toxic. The plants secrete a toxic oil, known as urushiol oil, that may remain active even after the plant has been dead for up to 5 years. The oil can also be released into the air if the plant is burned.
- **Toxic effects:** Urushiol oil acts primarily on the skin. When the oil contacts the skin, it leads to a red, itchy, irritating rash. The more oil and the longer it is in contact with the skin, the more severe the rash. In severe cases, blisters or bullae (large blisters) may form. In addition to skin contact, the oil can also be inhaled (especially when burned), causing inflammation of the airways, difficulty breathing, and respiratory distress.

KEY POINT

Poison Ivy, Oak, and Sumac Oils

Poison ivy, oak, and sumac oils remain active up to 5 years after the death of the plant and may be released into the air if the plants are burned.

Stinging Nettle

- **Description:** Stinging nettles have soft green leaves on a wiry stem that can be from 3 to 7 feet tall (**Figure 27-3**).
- **Habitat:** Stinging nettles grow in moist soil in forests with plenty of shade. They can be found in nearly all regions of the United States.
- **Toxic part:** The leaves and stem of this plant are covered with tiny hairs that can break off and become lodged in the skin.
- **Toxic effects:** Nettles that are stuck in the skin inject a chemical that causes a localized burning or stinging sensation. This burning may last from a few hours to up to a week.

Cactus

- **Description:** Cacti grow in many sizes and unique shapes and are typically covered in spines (**Figure 27-4**).

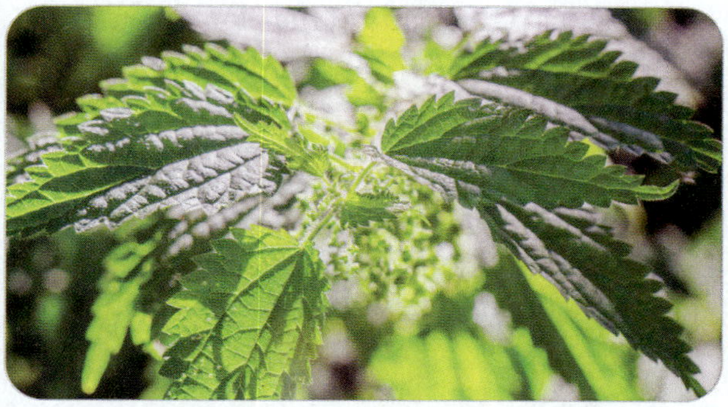

Figure 27-3 Stinging nettles.

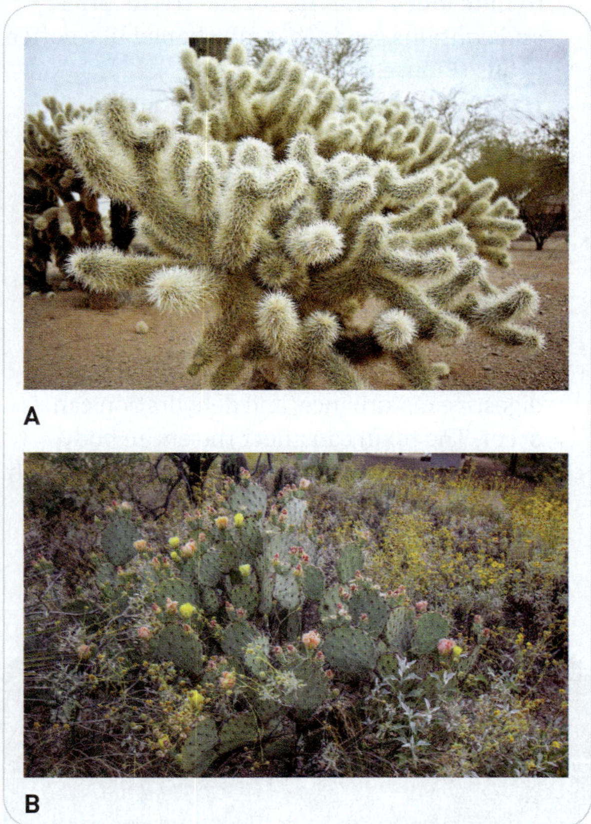

Figure 27-4 Various cactus plants.

- **Habitat:** Cacti grow in hot, arid environments characterized by plenty of sun and limited water. They are seen mostly in the southwestern United States.
- **Toxic part:** The cactus plant is covered by spines that can break off and become stuck in the skin.
- **Toxic effects:** The spines do not contain a specific toxin. However, when one gets stuck in the skin, a localized inflammatory response causes pain and redness in the affected area.

Plants Toxic upon Ingestion

While the majority of toxic encounters from plants are topical in nature, outdoor enthusiasts may at times ingest vegetation or fruit that is harmful. Most common fruits and berries are rarely toxic. However, the ingestion of many other plants can lead to illnesses ranging from mild nausea to death. The vast majority of toxic plant ingestions cause nausea and vomiting. Some toxic plants may produce cardiac effects, resulting in rhythm disturbances, whereas others may have neurologic effects that produce hallucinations, confusion, or seizures. The onset of effects may occur within 15 to 30 minutes or over several hours. It is best not to ingest any plant material unless you are absolutely sure what it is. Some toxic plants have medicinal purposes when the dose that is administered is small. Two of the more common of these plants are foxglove and the castor oil plant, which give us digitalis and castor oil laxative, respectively. Another is belladonna, which is used to treat diarrhea.

Lily of the Valley

- **Description:** The lily of the valley grows to about 12 inches high and has bright green leaves that appear to grow directly out of the ground. The leaves are approximately 4 inches long by 1.5 inches wide. The plant is also characterized by small, fragrant white flowers (Figure 27-5).
- **Habitat:** The plant is found within forested environments in partial shade. It is seen in the eastern and western United States.
- **Toxic part:** All parts of the plant are toxic when ingested.
- **Toxic effect:** When ingested, the plant causes nausea, vomiting, and headaches. Serious effects on the heart can cause fatal arrhythmias.

Foxglove

- **Description:** The foxglove plant grows to about 4 feet high and has many small thimble-shaped flowers (white, lavender, yellow, pink, red, and purple) (Figure 27-6).

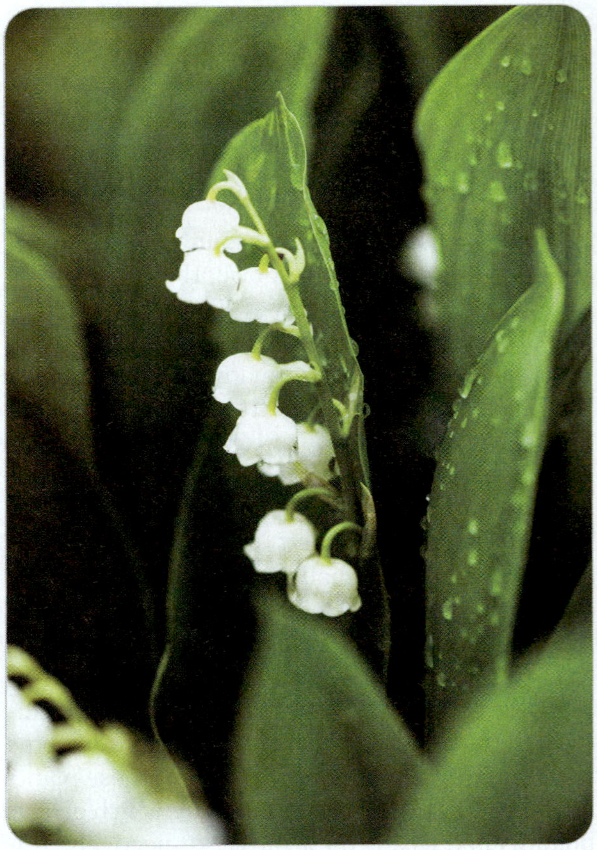

Figure 27-5 Lily of the valley.

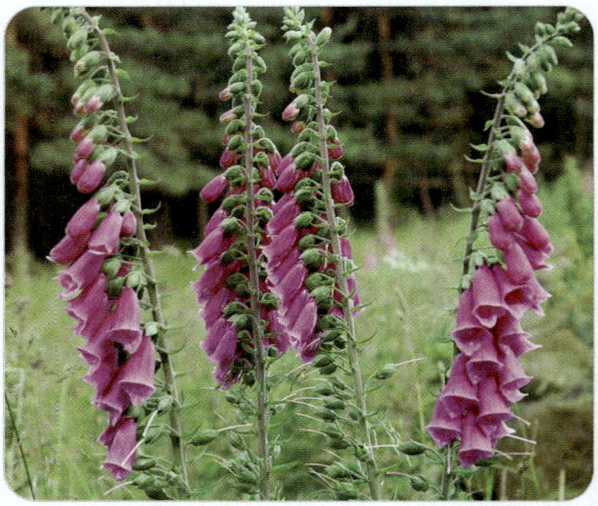

Figure 27-6 Foxglove.

- **Habitat:** The plant is commonly found in wooded areas and some gardens, both in sun and in partial shade. It is found in the western and northeastern United States.
- **Toxic part:** All parts of the plant are toxic when ingested.
- **Toxic effect:** The primary effects of ingestion of the foxglove plant are cardiovascular, resulting in arrhythmias that may be fatal. Although no longer used, historically when used in small amounts medicinally, this plant's toxin, digitalis, was beneficial to the heart.

Castor Oil Plant

- **Description:** The castor oil plant can grow to the height of a small tree up to 10 feet tall. Its large leaves are palm shaped and have seven to nine lobes. The fruit of the tree is prickly and contains seeds that are shaped like coffee beans (**Figure 27-7**).
- **Habitat:** The castor oil plant generally prefers warmer climates and is sensitive to cold temperatures. It is found in the eastern and western United States.
- **Toxic part:** All parts of the plant are toxic. The toxin, known as ricin, is especially concentrated within the seeds and is highly toxic, even in small doses.
- **Toxic effect:** Diarrhea, nausea, vomiting, digestive disturbance, and dehydration can occur. The toxin can affect the entire body, leading to multisystem organ failure and death. In very small doses, it is used as a laxative called castor oil. Historically, it can be made into ricin, and used as a chemical weapon.

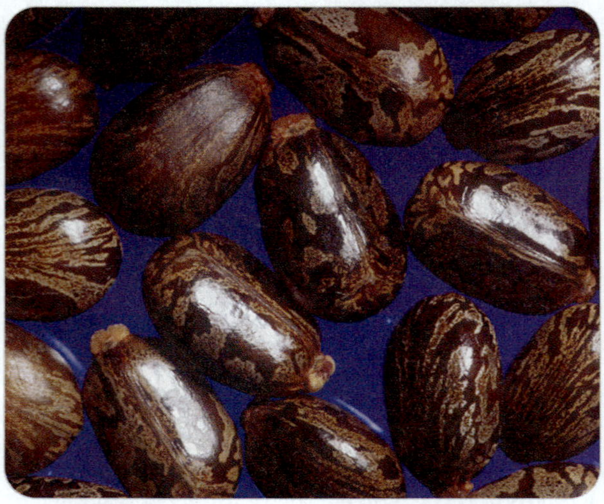

Figure 27-7 Castor bean.

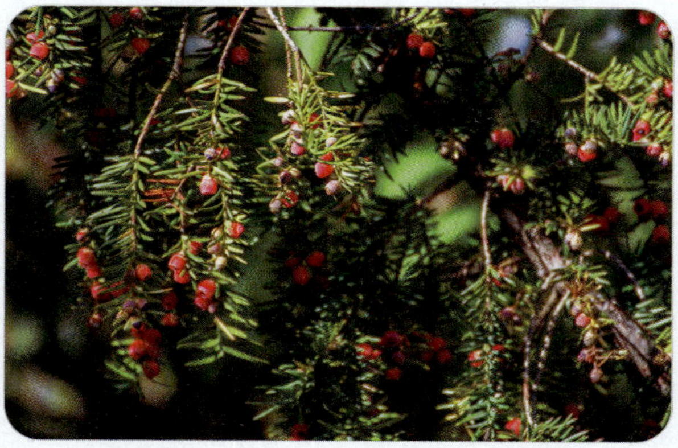

Figure 27-8 Yew.

Yew

- **Description:** The yew plant is an evergreen growing up to 100 feet high. The berries are a characteristic bright red and resemble hollowed-out grapes (Figure 27-8).
- **Habitat:** The yew grows in dense forests on mountainsides. It is found in the western and northeastern United States.
- **Toxic part:** All parts of the plant are toxic when ingested. The toxin is especially concentrated in seeds within the berries.
- **Toxic effect:** Harmful effects most commonly include nausea, vomiting, diarrhea. These can also cause neurologic symptoms and cardiovascular collapse.

Belladonna (Deadly Nightshade)

- **Description:** The belladonna plant grows as a branching shrub up to 5 feet in height. The bell-shaped flowers are typically a dark purple, and the berries are round and black (Figure 27-9).
- **Habitat:** The plant grows in moist soil in shaded areas. It is predominately found in the midwestern United States.
- **Toxic part:** All parts of the plant are toxic when ingested.
- **Toxic effect:** Harmful effects are quick in onset and include nausea, dry mouth, dizziness, visual disturbance, and agitation. The toxin also has cardiovascular effects that begin with a slowing of the heart rate and eventually lead to death. Medicinally, belladonna has been used in sedatives, stimulants, and antispasmodics (for the gastrointestinal system), but in recent years it has fallen out of favor.

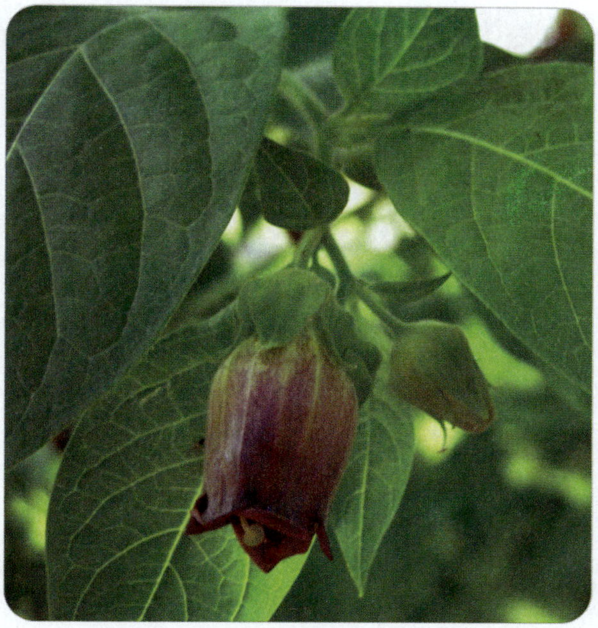

Figure 27-9 Belladonna (deadly nightshade).

Pokeweed

- **Description:** The pokeweed plant grows up to 10 feet with large green alternating leaves and a reddish stalk or stem. Berries grow in large clusters and are typically a dark purple or black (Figure 27-10).
- **Habitat:** The plant grows in warm, moist, tropical environments. It is found central and eastern United States.
- **Toxic part:** All parts of the plant can be toxic to various degrees. The most toxic parts of the plant are the roots and stem.
- **Toxic effect:** Effects include nausea and vomiting, shortness of breath, spasms, and bloody diarrhea.

Jimsonweed

- **Description:** Jimsonweed grows as a low shrub 3 to 5 feet tall. The leaves are a dark green and toothed, resembling the leaves of an oak tree. Berries are spiny and grow off the stem of the shrub (Figure 27-11).
- **Habitat:** Jimsonweed grows in moderate climates in partial sun. It can be found across the United States.

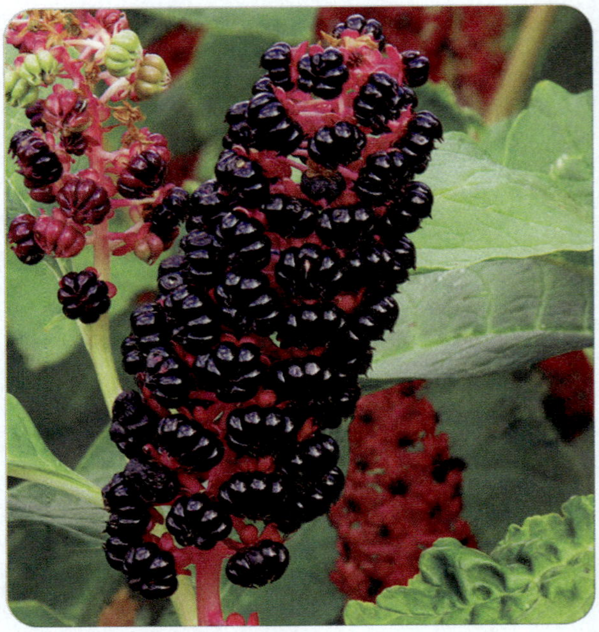

Figure 27-10 Pokeweed.

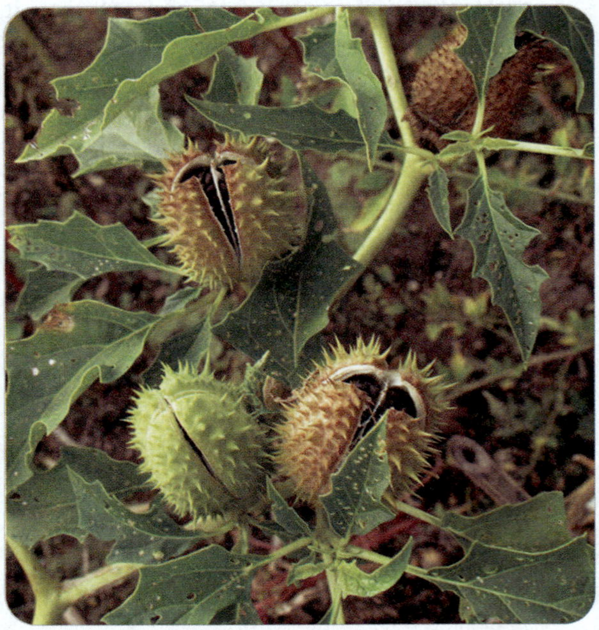

Figure 27-11 Jimsonweed.

- **Toxic part:** All parts of the plant are toxic when ingested.
- **Toxic effect:** Effects are primarily gastrointestinal, including nausea, vomiting, bloody diarrhea. Confusion and delirium are common, followed by a weak pulse, irregular breathing, hypothermia, and, in rare cases, respiratory arrest and death. This plant is particularly dangerous for children as very small quantities can be fatal.

Poisonous Mushrooms

There are three main groups of mushrooms (fungi) that are dangerous to humans: those within the *Amanita* genus, the false morels, and a catch-all category known as little brown mushrooms, often referred to as LBMs. Mushrooms in these groups are responsible for the fatal mushroom poisonings in the United States, with *Amanita* mushrooms alone accounting for 90% of mushroom-related deaths. Most victims are exposed by personal gathering and ingestion. Unless you are very knowledgeable about mushrooms, the safest place to find mushrooms is in the supermarket.

Hundreds of other mushrooms also cause problems ranging from a mild stomachache to severe physical distress, including vomiting, diarrhea, cramps, and loss of coordination. Two common poisonous mushrooms of this type are the jack-o-lantern and the green-spored lepiota. Although the effects of poisoning from these mushrooms may be startling, they usually pass in 24 hours or less with no lasting effects. Interestingly, the onset of symptoms provides a general guide to the lethality of the mushroom. The more benign species can cause gastrointestinal upset within the first 2 to 3 hours while the more dangerous types have delayed symptoms up to 8 hours after ingestion. In addition, some mushrooms, known as psilocybin, contain chemicals that can produce hallucinogenic effects in humans and animals. These can often be found in intentional ingestion as well as ceremonial events.

Amanita Mushrooms

- **Description:** Mushrooms belonging to the *Aminita* genus may be large with a brightly colored top that is typically speckled with a white warty material (**Figure 27-12**).
- **Habitat:** These mushrooms grow in large clumps in moist, shaded soil in woodlands. Found in the mountainous regions of the United States.

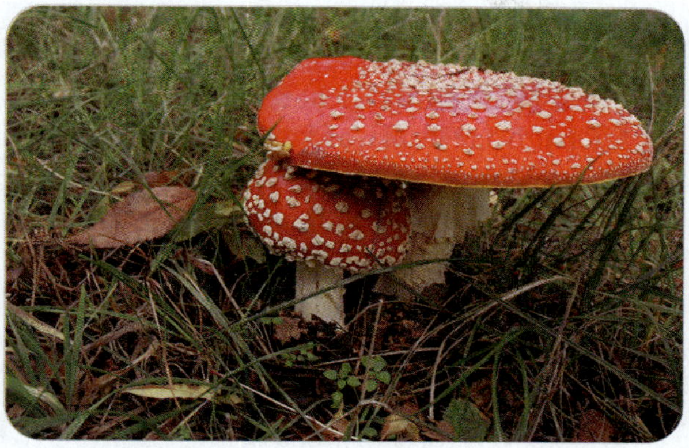

Figure 27-12 *Amanita* mushroom.

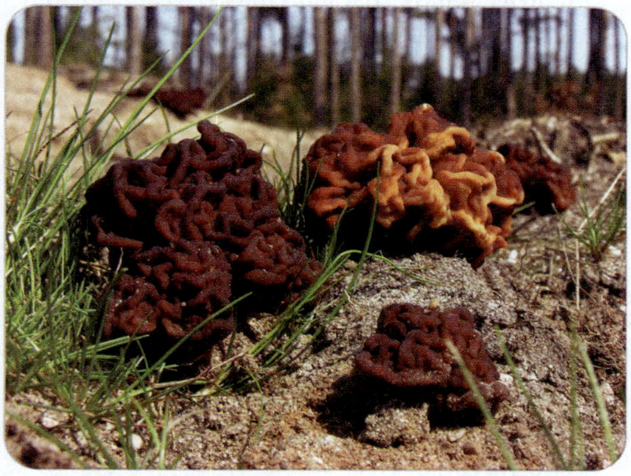

Figure 27-13 False morels.

- **Toxic part:** All parts of the mushroom are toxic.
- **Toxic effect:** Effects are difficulty walking, euphoria, gastrointestinal disturbances, drowsiness, confusion and then agitation, with liver failure over 1 to 2 days.

False Morels

- **Description:** False morels have a wrinkled, irregular cap that either is saddle shaped or resembles a brain (**Figure 27-13**). They may be black, gray, white, brown, or reddish.
- **Habitat:** False morels typically grow in moist soil around dead or dying trees.
- **Toxic part:** All parts of the mushroom can be toxic when ingested.

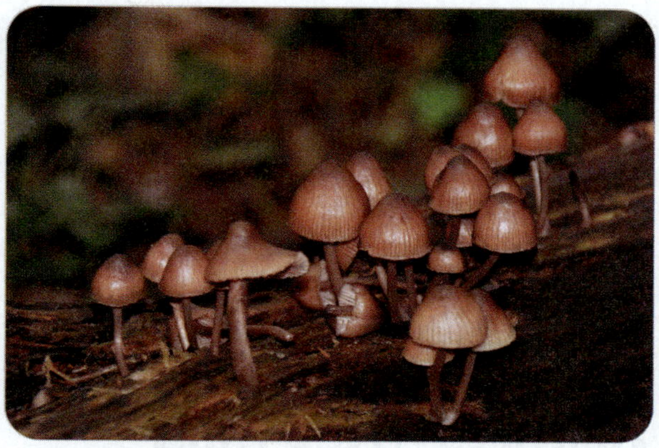

Figure 27-14 Little brown mushrooms.

- **Toxic effect:** Nausea, vomiting, diarrhea, and severe headaches occur. Ingestion can occasionally be fatal.

Little Brown Mushrooms

- **Description:** Literally hundreds of mushrooms belong in this category. All these mushrooms are small brown mushrooms that are difficult to identify (**Figure 27-14**).
- **Habitat:** These mushrooms live in varied habitats; most grow in moist soil.
- **Toxic part:** All parts of these mushrooms can be toxic when ingested.
- **Toxic effect:** Problems ranging from mild nausea to hallucinations can occur.

Jack-o-Lantern Mushrooms

- **Description:** The jack-o-lantern mushroom is a bright orange mushroom resembling a pumpkin. It is typically found in the fall.
- **Habitat:** These mushrooms generally grow in shaded habitats east of the Rocky Mountains.
- **Toxic part:** All parts of the mushroom are toxic when ingested.
- **Toxic effect:** Usually seen are mild to severe abdominal upset including nausea, vomiting and abdominal cramping. Ingestion of these mushrooms is generally not fatal.

Green-Spored Lepiota Mushrooms

- **Description:** The green-spored lepiota is a large mushroom with a tan parasol-shaped cap and a large ring on the stem. This mushroom has a greenish spore print (pattern and color produced after the cap of a

mushroom is pressed against a white piece of paper).
- **Habitat:** These mushrooms generally grow in open fields across the United States.
- **Toxic part:** All parts of the mushroom are toxic when ingested.
- **Toxic effect:** Ingestion of these mushrooms causes violent gastrointestinal upset, including nausea, vomiting, and abdominal cramping.

ADVERSE EFFECTS FROM INSECTS AND ANIMALS

Spiders

OEC technicians must be aware that spider bites can result in significant morbidity. Localized **necrosis**, infection at the bite site, and in some cases serious systemic illness can occur. The most harmful spiders in North America that bite are the black widow, brown recluse, hobo, and wolf spider.

Black Widow Spider

- **Description:** The black widow spider measures about 0.75 to 1.25 inches long. It has a jet-black body and a characteristic red hourglass on its abdomen (Figure 27-15).
- **Habitat:** The black widow spider lives in trees and shrubs above ground but may also be found under logs and stones in woods and fields. These spiders are found primarily in the Northeast United States. They may live as far south as Florida, as far north as Canada, and as far west as Texas.
- **Characteristics of bite:** Bites occur primarily between April and October and usually occur on the patient's hands and forearms. Most bites occur when the female spider is guarding her eggs. The bite site can resemble a "bull's-eye" or target and may sometimes become secondarily infected.
- **Toxic effect:** The bite is initially painful and is followed by swelling and redness that can spread over the entire limb. Systemic signs and symptoms may develop, including nausea, abdominal pain, fever, sweating, and (in some cases) paralysis.

Brown Recluse Spider

- **Description:** The brown recluse spider is light brown or dark brown and has a leg span up to 1 inch. It is identified by a characteristic violin or "fiddle" shape on its back, near the head (Figure 27-16).
- **Habitat:** The brown recluse spider typically is found under stones and in dark corners inside buildings. In the United States, the spider is found primarily in the Midwest and the Southwest.

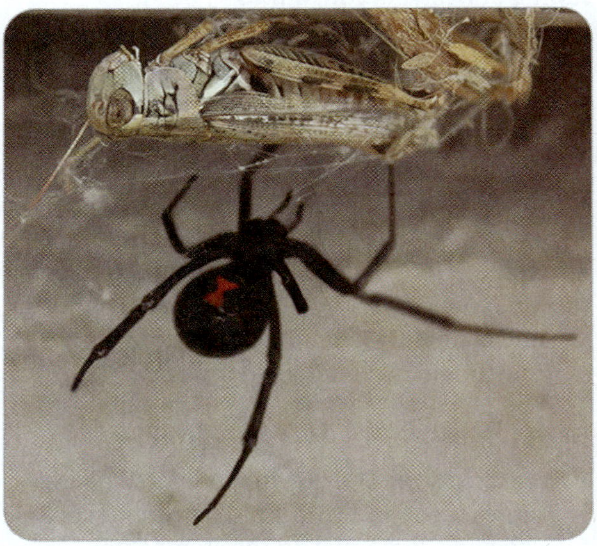

Figure 27-15 Black widow spider.

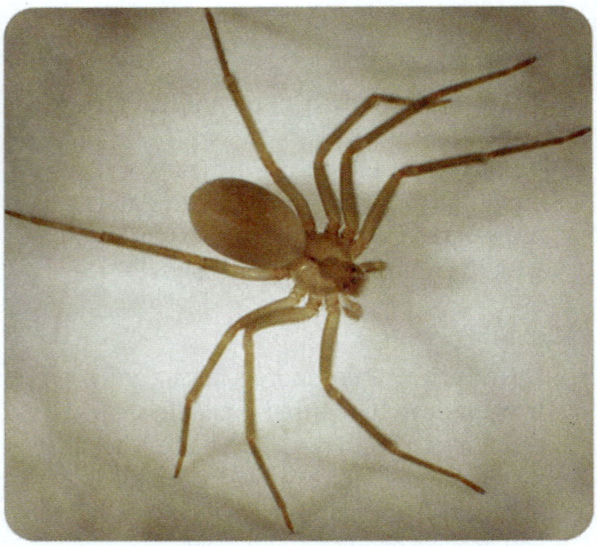

Figure 27-16 Brown recluse spider.

Courtesy of Kenneth Cramer, Monmouth College.

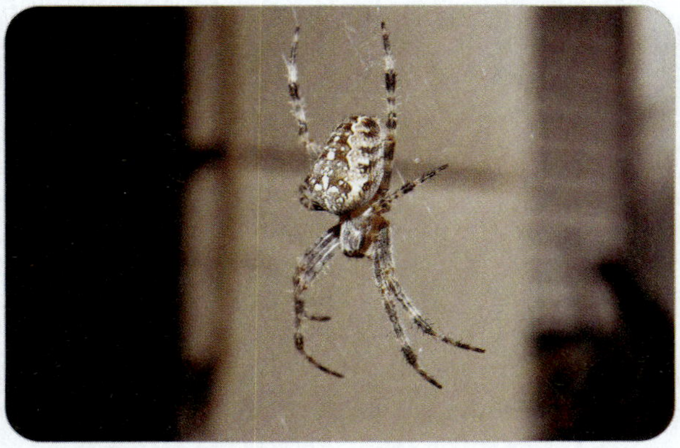

Figure 27-17 Hobo spider.

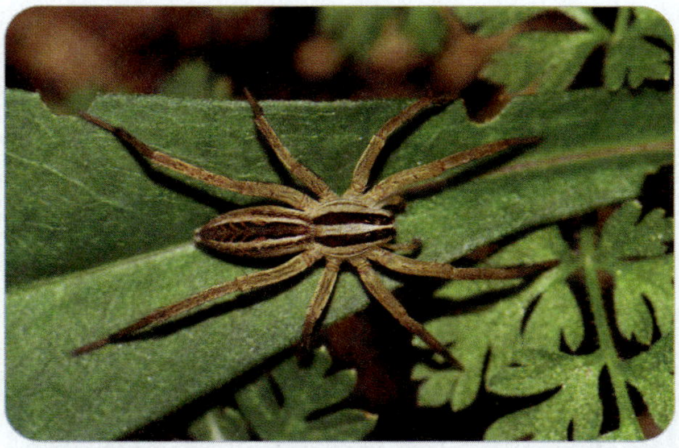

Figure 27-18 Wolf spider.

- **Characteristics of bite:** Local symptoms usually begin immediately after the bite. A sharp stinging sensation is possible, although a victim may be unaware of having been bitten. If there is stinging, it usually subsides in 6 to 8 hours.
- **Toxic effect:** The venom can destroy the tissue and blood vessels, resulting in localized tissue death and skin ulcerations. Fatalities have been reported from kidney failure.

Hobo Spider

- **Description:** The hobo spider is a small brown spider measuring about 0.5 to 0.75 inches in length. This spider has several V-shaped markings on the abdomen (Figure 27-17).
- **Habitat:** The hobo spider lives in damp locations such as wood piles and is found primarily in the Pacific Northwest.
- **Characteristics of bite:** This spider may or may not inject venom into its bite, which is often painless. The bite site initially appears red and then disappears over several hours. Over the next 24 hours, a blister may form that later breaks open, becoming an open lesion.
- **Toxic effect:** When venom is injected, an area of localized tissue death and skin ulceration often results.

Wolf Spider

- **Description:** The wolf spider ranges in size from very small to 1.5 inches. This spider characteristically carries its eggs and its young on its back (Figure 27-18).
- **Habitat:** The habitat of the wolf spider varies from coastal areas to woodlands across the United States.
- **Characteristic of bite:** The bite is initially painful.
- **Toxic effect:** Localized pain and swelling are typical. In fewer than 10% of cases, patients may also have systemic symptoms of nausea and/or headache.

Scorpions

Though fearsome in appearance, scorpions rarely bother humans unless provoked. When they do sting, most cases cause little more than local pain and discomfort.

Bark Scorpion

- **Description:** The bark scorpion is a small brown scorpion measuring up to 3 inches (Figure 27-19).
- **Habitat:** The bark scorpion lives in dark places during the heat of the day in arid environments. It is found in Texas, California, Arizona, and New Mexico.
- **Characteristic of sting:** The sting causes severe pain that lasts 24 to 72 hours.
- **Toxic effect:** The venom from a bark scorpion can cause severe pain, muscle jerking, nausea, vomiting, blurred vision, and occasionally disturbances of cardiac rhythm.

Ticks

There are many different varieties of ticks located throughout the United States. Two of the most common ticks are the deer tick and the wood (dog)

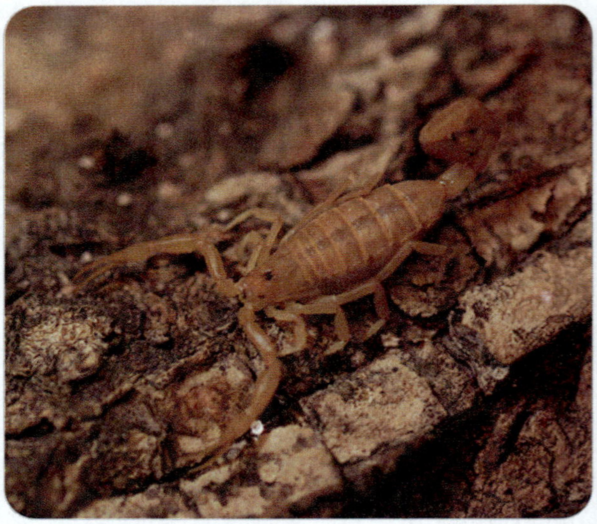

Figure 27-19 Bark scorpion.

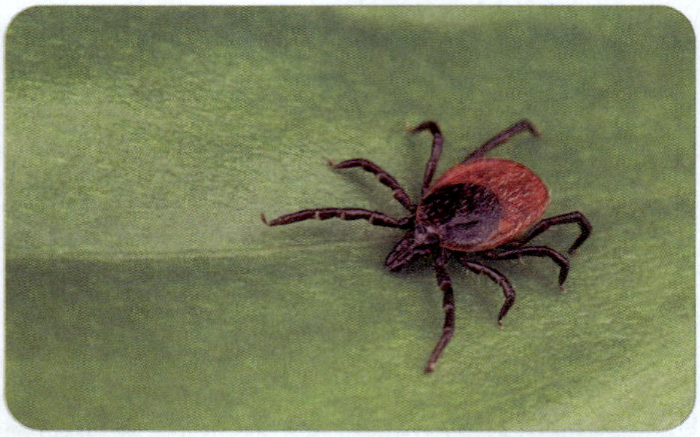

Figure 27-20 Deer tick.

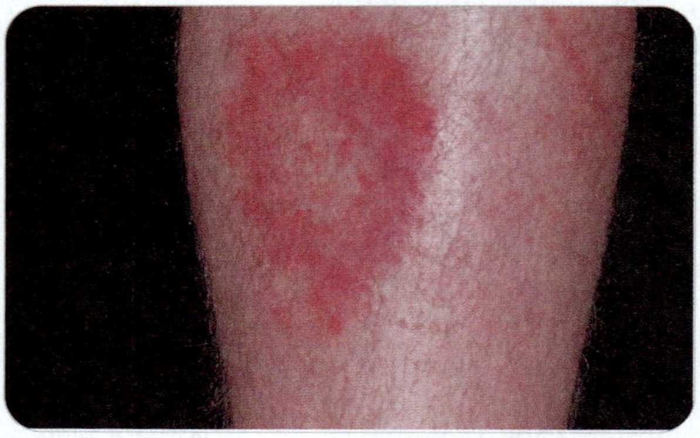

Figure 27-21 The target rash is typical of Lyme disease.

tick. There are many diseases transmitted by different ticks. Some are Lyme disease, Rocky Mountain spotted fever, anaplasmosis, babesiosis, rickettsia, and tularemia. Some of these can be very serious diseases. However, not all ticks transmit disease.

Transmission of tick-borne diseases occurs through the tick's saliva. The tick feeds on the blood of an infected animal, then transmits the disease by attaching to a human. Tick bites are typically painless, so the tick may stay attached to its host for 24 hours or more without the individual's knowledge. The best defense against tick bites is prevention by wearing appropriate clothing including long pants, long sleeve shirts, and shoes with socks in areas known for ticks. Less exposed skin means less risk of picking up a tick. Even proper clothing does not guarantee protection, so it is still important to check your skin regularly, especially in the evening before going to sleep. Tick repellant is also effective.

Deer Tick

- **Description:** The deer tick is a small tick. Nymphs measure about 0.04 inches, whereas engorged (recently fed) adults measure about 0.16 inches (about the size of a pencil point) (**Figure 27-20**).
- **Habitat:** The tick lives in wood piles and tall grasses, and on deer.
- **Characteristic of bite:** The bite is typically painless. When the tick leaves, a characteristic rash that is described as a red circle surrounding a blanched white center (a target lesion) may be visible at the bite site.
- **Disease transmitted:** The primary disease transmitted by deer ticks is Lyme disease. Lyme disease characteristically begins with a rash that is followed by flulike symptoms, including fever, nausea, and vomiting (**Figure 27-21**). As the disease progresses, patients develop generalized joint pain and may develop a facial droop. Sometime after the bite, people may develop both septic joints and meningitis. If not treated neurologic and cardiovascular problems may occur. Usually the tick needs to be attached for 2 to 3 days to infect someone.

Wood Tick (Dog Tick)

- **Description:** These large ticks measure up to 0.5 inch when engorged (**Figure 27-22**).

- **Habitat:** Wood ticks typically live in woods and open fields.
- **Characteristic of bite:** The bites of wood ticks are typically painless.

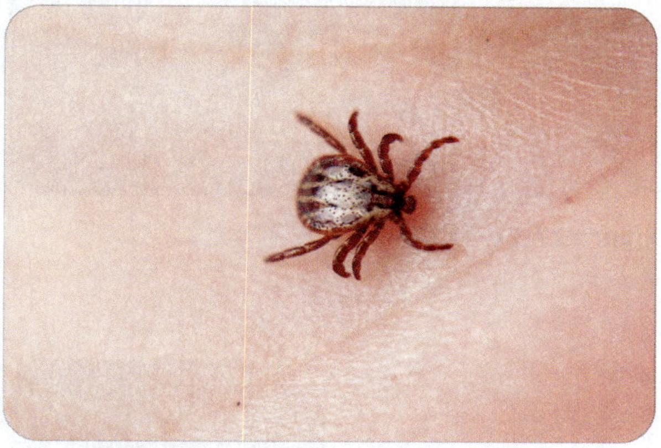

Figure 27-22 Wood tick (dog tick).
© Photopen/Shutterstock.

- **Disease transmitted:** Wood ticks can transmit Rocky Mountain spotted fever throughout the country. Despite the disease's name, more recent cases have involved ticks from forested areas on the East Coast. The disease is characterized by fever, nausea, vomiting, and a full-body rash consisting of small, red, raised areas. Usually the tick needs to be attached for 2 to 3 days to infect someone.

Bees, Wasps, Hornets, and Yellow Jackets

Bees, wasps, hornets, and yellow jackets cause the most instances of **envenomation** per year of any stinging creature (Figure 27-23). Most of the stings cause pain and swelling in a localized area of the skin and in the nearby joint. In severe cases,

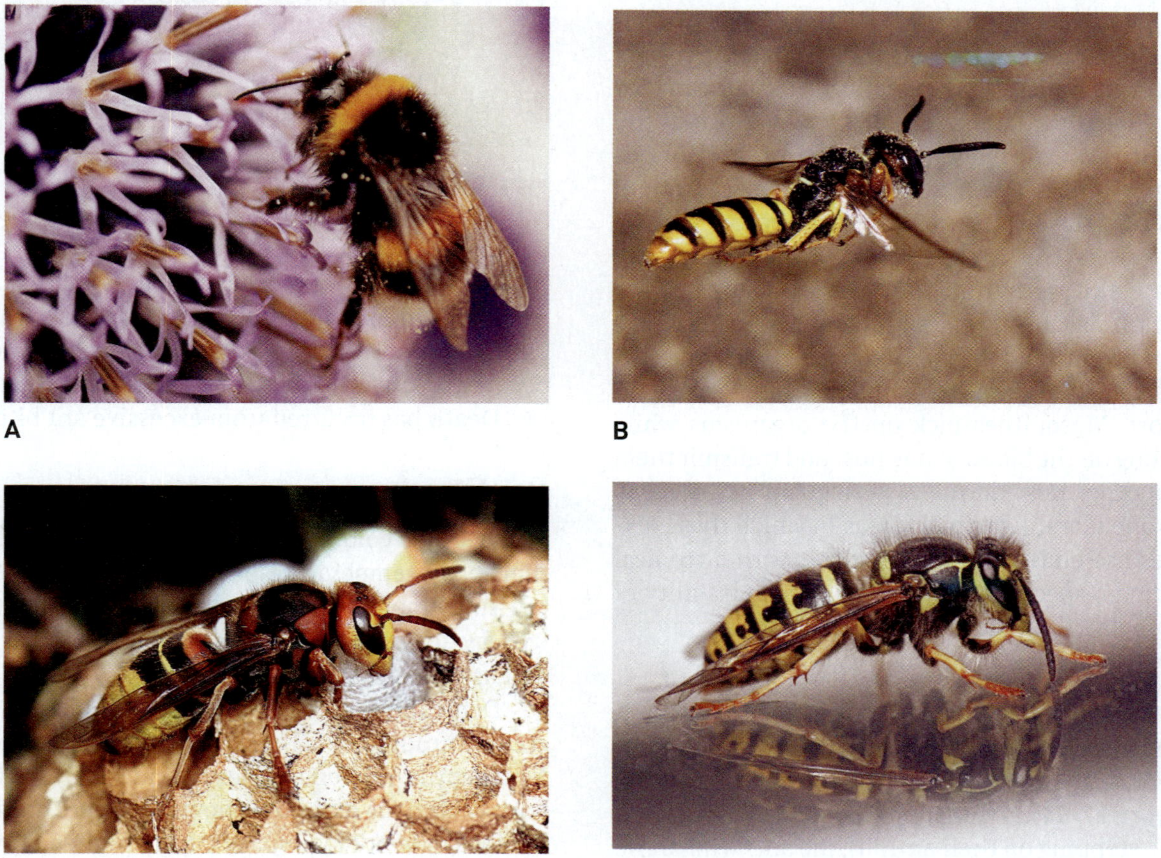

A

B

C

D

Figure 27-23 Most stings, whether bee (**A**), wasp (**B**), hornet (**C**), or yellow jacket (**D**), cause pain and swelling.
A: © Gudrunb67/Shutterstock; **B:** © Milan Vasicek/Shutterstock. **C.** © Ger Bosma Photos/Shutterstock; **D.**© Jim H Walling/Shutterstock.

anaphylaxis and death can occur (see Chapter 14, *Allergies and Anaphylaxis*). The Africanized honeybee, or so-called "killer bee," has recently extended its range into the southwestern United States and now exists as far north as southern Utah. A swarm of these bees can attack humans with deadly results.

Mosquitoes, Fleas, and Biting Flies

Although bites from mosquitoes, fleas, and biting flies typically do not cause serious illness in the United States, they do cause localized redness, itching, and swelling. Occasionally, a delayed reaction can lead to worsening edema and severe itching. Insect repellents containing DEET (N, N-Diethyl-meta-toluamide) are often quite effective in the prevention of bites.

West Nile virus (WNV), first seen in the United States in 1999, is transmitted by mosquitoes. People who contract WNV usually have mild or no symptoms. Those with symptoms may have fever, headache, body aches, a skin rash, or swollen lymph glands. If WNV enters the brain, the resulting encephalitis (inflammation of the brain) or meningitis (inflammation of the coverings of the brain) can be deadly. Eradication of mosquitoes from swamps and from standing water around homes is the best prevention strategy for WNV.

For travelers outside of the United States, the greatest concern from mosquitoes is the transmission of diseases, including malaria, dengue fever, yellow fever, and encephalitis. Like ticks, mosquitoes transmit disease organisms while feeding on a host. Mosquitoes pick up the organisms while feeding on the blood of one host and transmit them to another host during a subsequent blood meal. Anyone planning to visit areas in which these diseases are endemic should consult with a tropical medicine specialist concerning the advisability of prophylactic medication or a vaccination.

Ants

Fire ants, a grouping of ants that includes five different species, are known to bite and cause pain (**Figure 27-24**). If threatened by direct provocation (e.g., stepping on their anthill), the ants will swarm and many sting simultaneously. Most stings are painful at the injection site; in some cases, blisters, or bullae later develop (**Figure 27-25**). Aside from severe itching and pain, most bites do not cause further complications. Some sensitive individuals may have an allergic reaction much like that to a bee sting or a wasp sting. In addition, ant bites can become secondarily infected by excessive scratching. Death has occurred from excessive ant bites.

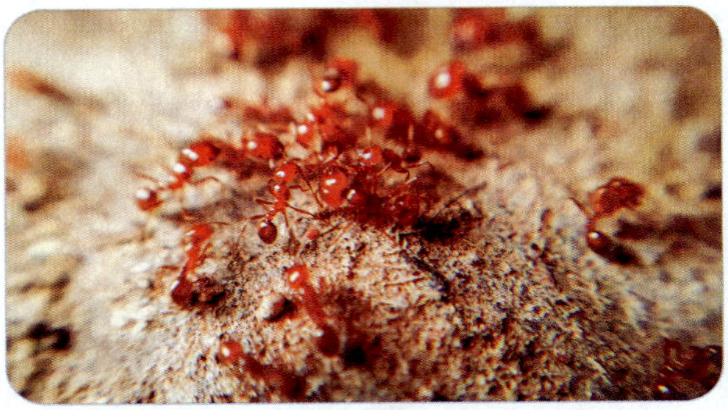

Figure 27-24 Fire ants.

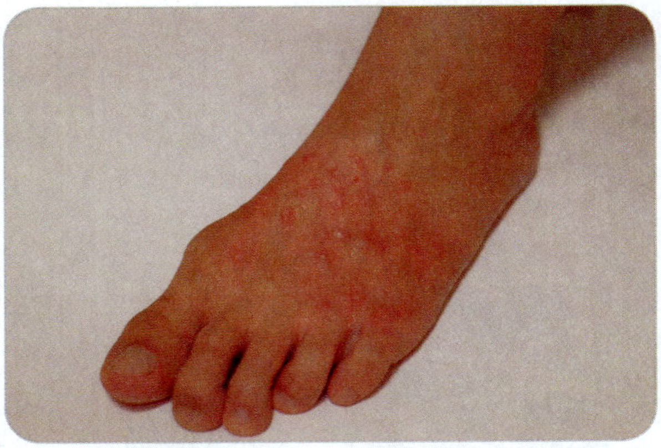

Figure 27-25 Fire ant bites.

Reptiles

Reptiles are cold-blooded animals that regulate their body temperature by moving in and out of the sunshine. These animals are also characterized by scales. Some reptiles produce venom for defense and for hunting prey.

Depending on the animal, venom may be secreted through its skin, saliva, or through a bite. Most reptile-related injuries are caused by snakes, both venomous and nonvenomous. There are two families of venomous snakes in the United States: pit vipers and coral snakes. Pit vipers have small depressions ("pits") between their nostrils and eyes that are used for detecting heat. In addition, they have movable fangs through which venom

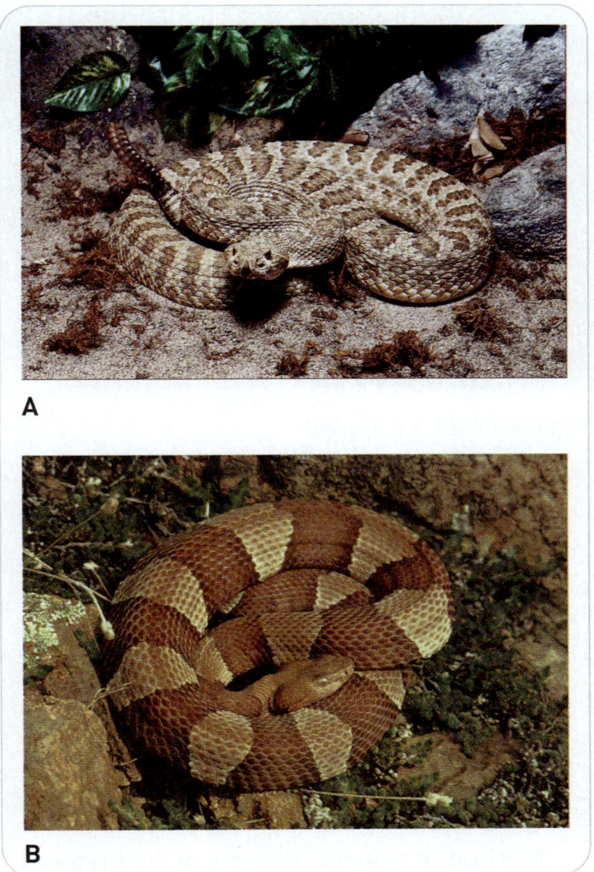

Figure 27-26 Common pit vipers in the United States include the rattlesnake (**A**) and copperhead (**B**) Copperheads bite more people annually in the US but the venom is less toxic than a rattlesnake.

A: © Photos.com/Getty Images; **B:** Courtesy of Ray Rauch/U.S. Fish & Wildlife Service.

can be injected. Within the United States, the most common pit vipers of concern are rattlesnakes, copperheads, water moccasins, and massasaugas (**Figure 27-26**). Coral snakes tend to be more reclusive (**Figure 27-27**).

Rattlesnake

- **Description:** There are approximately 30 species of rattlesnakes. Often brown with a checkered or diamond skin pattern, they have a rattle at the end of the tail that is composed of modified scales. Rattlesnakes use their rattles as warnings and usually do not attack humans unless provoked.
- **Habitat:** Rattlesnakes live in varied habitats, from arid environments to rocky outcroppings in forests.

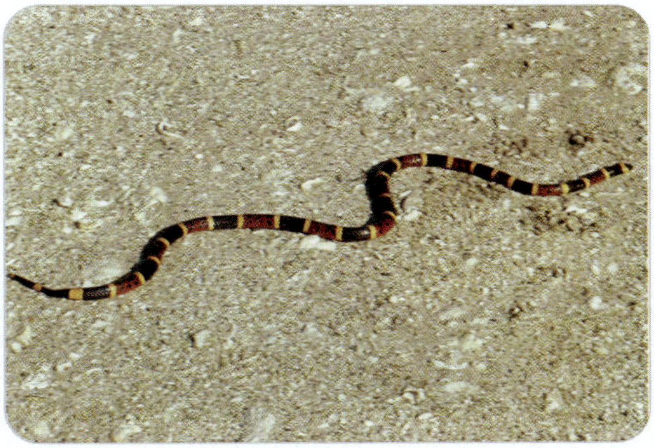

Figure 27-27 Coral snakes tend to be reclusive.

Courtesy of Luther C. Goldman/U.S. Fish & Wildlife Service.

- **Characteristic of bite:** Rattlesnake bites are typically very painful. There may be one or two puncture wounds or only a simple abrasion.
- **Toxic effects:** Rattlesnake venom destroys tissue near the bite wound. Severe bleeding can occur as this venom disrupts normal blood clotting mechanisms. Without treatment and **antivenom**, these bites are potentially fatal.

Coral Snake

- **Description:** These snakes are covered with brightly colored bands. Coral snakes in North America are most notable for their red, yellow/white, and black colored banding, with the red and yellow touching. Remember the expression, "Red and yellow kill a fellow."
- **Habitat:** The coral snake lives in grasslands and dry desert regions.
- **Characteristic of bite:** Coral snakes tend to chew more than strike at their prey.
- **Toxic effects:** The venom of the coral snake is a potent neurotoxin that can lead to paralysis and respiratory failure. Its venom is the second strongest of any snake.

Alligator and Crocodile

- **Description:** These animals are large lizards with strong jaws that can open wide and easily crush bones. Ranging in size from 8 to 15 feet, these animals can weigh up to 1,000 pounds or more and are covered with thick scales. Alligators have a wide, rounded u-shaped snout while crocodiles have a long pointed v-shaped snout. (**Figure 27-28**).

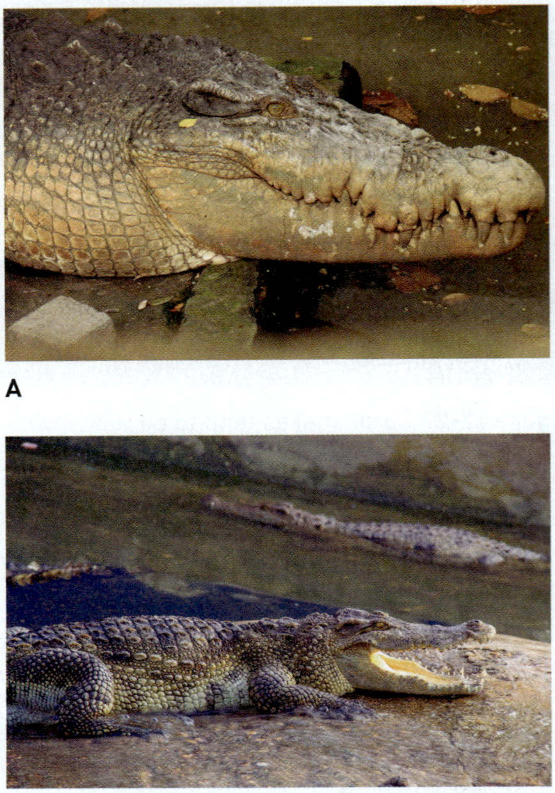

Figure 27-28 Alligators (**A**) and crocodiles (**B**) have strong jaws that can open wide and easily crush bones.

A: © Komarudin270975/Shutterstock; **B:** © aimpol buranet/Shutterstock.

- **Habitat:** These animals live in warm environments in swamps and shallow water but will also climb onto land. Crocodiles live in fresh, brackish, or saltwater, whereas alligators live in fresh water.
- **Characteristic of bite:** The bite typically results in massive soft-tissue damage, amputations, fractures, and severe internal bleeding.

Marine Creatures

Many species of marine creatures can cause injuries in humans, either through localized soft-tissue injuries or venom injection.

Moray Eel

- **Method of injury:** Injuries occur from the bite, which typically occurs when humans stick their hands into the eel's hole or when fishermen remove eels from a net.
- **Habitat:** Moray eels live in hollow openings in coral and rock formations.
- **Injuries:** Moray eel bites are rarely fatal, but local tissue damage can be extensive. Partial arm amputations have been reported, and severe soft-tissue injuries are common.

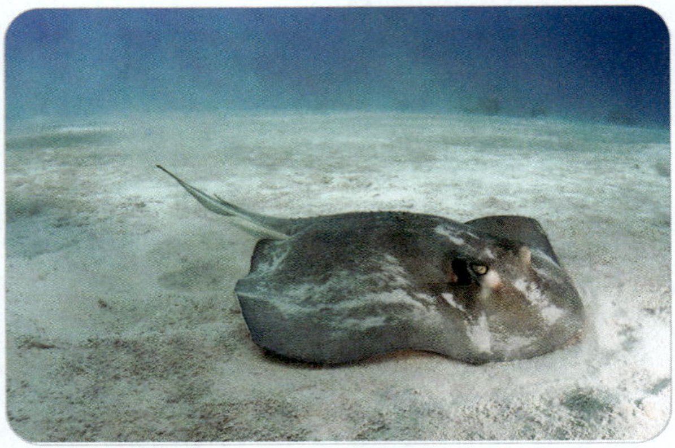

Figure 27-29 A stingray.

© Eric Carlander/Shutterstock.

Stingray

- **Method of injury:** Stingrays are not typically aggressive. However, threatened stingrays can cause injury by striking with their barb-tipped tails (Figure 27-29).
- **Injuries:** Injuries are generally local soft-tissue wounds. If the barb hits the chest or abdomen, internal injuries and potentially death can occur.

Jellyfish

- **Method of injury:** The tentacles of the jellyfish are covered with cells (nematocysts) that contain stinging chemicals used to kill their prey. When a jellyfish's tentacles encounter a human, these chemicals are injected onto the skin (Figure 27-30).
- **Injuries:** Jellyfish stings cause localized skin reactions. In addition, if the chemical is absorbed into the circulation, neurologic and cardiovascular effects that lead to paralysis, respiratory failure, and cardiovascular collapse can occur.

Sharks

- **Method of injury:** Sharks generally cause injury through their bite. Fortunately, shark

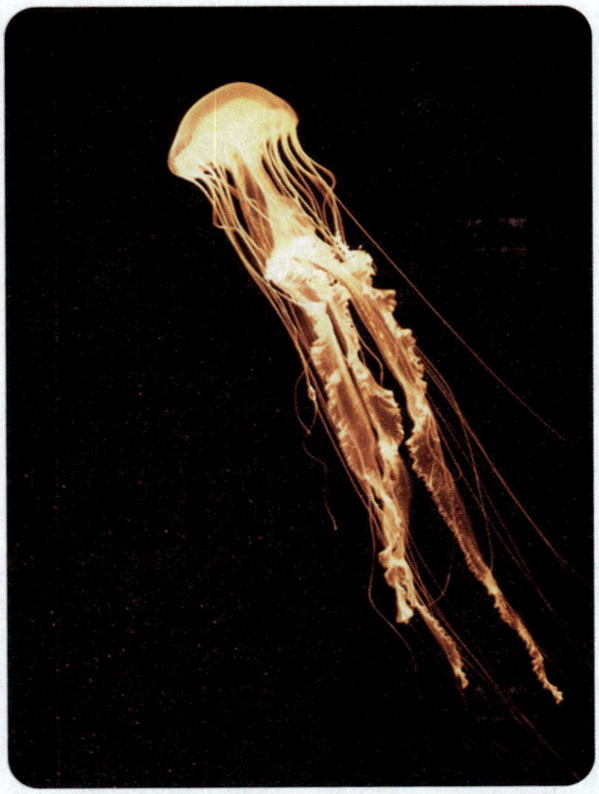

Figure 27-30 A jellyfish.

attacks are rare, with fewer than 75 reported worldwide each year. Common shark species known to have attacked humans are great white, tiger, mako, bull, white tip reef, and black tip reef.

- **Injuries:** Shark bites cause soft-tissue injuries, fractures, and amputations. Death usually results from hemorrhage.

Other Biting Fish

- **Method of injury:** Several other fishes have been known to bite humans, including piranha, catfish, northern pike, muskellunge, and barracuda.
- **Injuries:** Injuries are generally local soft-tissue wounds that range from minor to severe. Fish may occasionally cause fractures of the fingers or enough soft-tissue injury to result in massive hemorrhage.

Spiny Aquatic Animals

- **Method of injury:** Numerous freshwater and saltwater fish and marine creatures have spines that can easily puncture or become imbedded in human skin. Sunfish, blue gill, bass, walleye, swordfish, and sea urchins are examples.
- **Injuries:** Injuries are generally local soft-tissue wounds that range from minor to severe. Occasionally, spines may break off in a wound and result in a local infection. Some sea urchins have poison that can cause death.

Mammals

Mammals are warm-blooded, vertebrate animals whose females have mammary glands for feeding the young. These animals are covered with hair and have bones in the inner ear that are used for hearing. Most injuries caused by mammals result from bites or the animal's claws. Because many mammals have powerful jaws, bites can cause soft-tissue damage, broken bones, and localized soft-tissue infections. They can also transmit diseases.

Domestic and Wild Dogs, Wolves, Coyotes, and Foxes

- **Method of injury:** Most members of the dog family (canids) cause puncture or tearing-type soft-tissue injuries (**Figure 27-31**). The extent of injury is largely dependent on the size of the animal, the strength of its jaws, and the disposition of the animal. Occasionally, a tooth may break off and become lodged within the wound. Wild dogs, wolves, coyotes, and foxes rarely attack

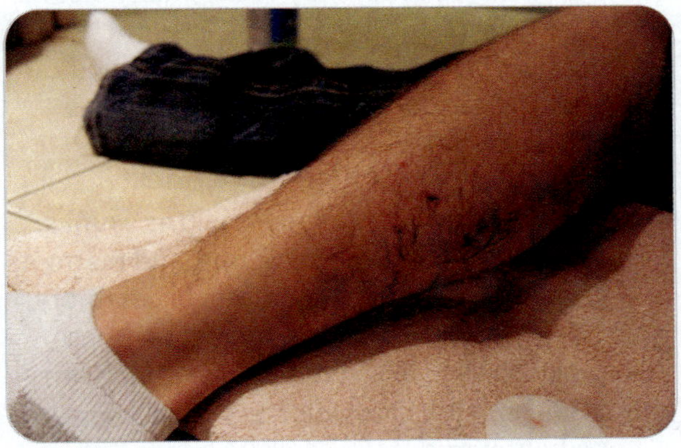

Figure 27-31 A dog bite.

humans unless they are sick, provoked, or protecting their young.

- **Injuries:** Canine bites cause localized soft-tissue wounds, bleeding, occasional retained foreign bodies, fractures, and infections. Whenever a wild animal has bitten a human, assume that the animal is sick until proven otherwise, which raises the index of suspicion for diseases such as rabies.

Domestic and Wild Cats

- **Method of injury:** Cat bites can cause deep puncture wounds. Domestic cats may also inflict scratches that inoculate bacteria into the skin.
- **Habitat:** Most wild cats (e.g., mountain lion, bobcat, lynx) are solitary creatures that live in forested areas and avoid human contact. However, with habitat encroachment and diminishing food supplies, wild cat attacks do occur.
- **Injuries:** Domestic cat bites are prone to becoming infected because the depth of the puncture wound prevents the wound from draining. Local tissues may become reddened and swollen; pain and fever may also occur. Bites on the neck and arms are common. Bites from larger wild cats can cause serious soft-tissue injuries and massive bleeding. Scratches from domestic cats can result in bacterial infection, called cat-scratch fever.

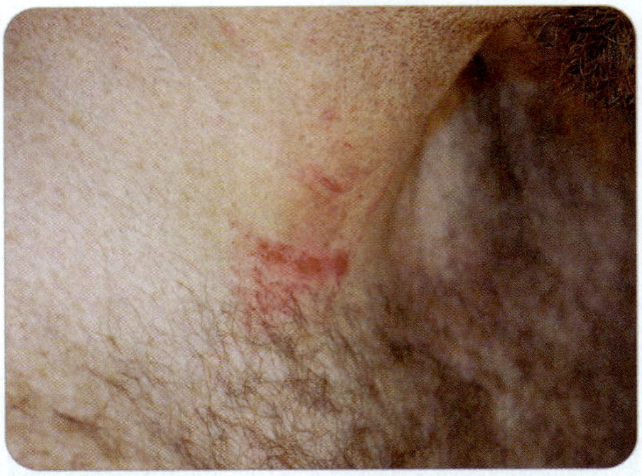

Figure 27-32 A horse bite.

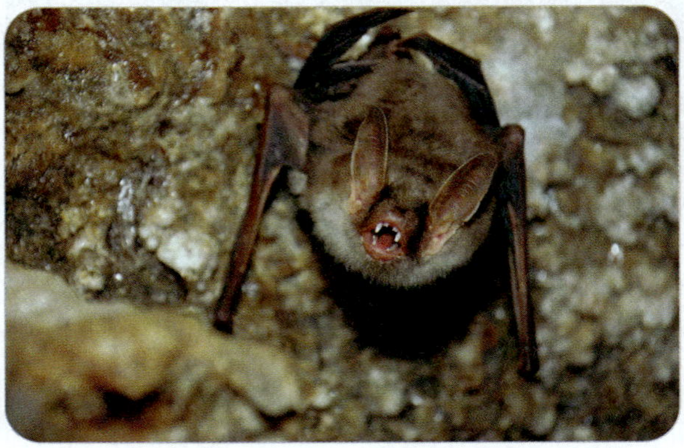

Figure 27-33 A bat.

Pack Animals

- **Method of injury:** Pack animals (e.g., horses, mules, llamas, alpacas) used on wilderness adventures are typically tame and harmless to humans, but they may occasionally bite or kick (**Figure 27-32**).
- **Injuries:** Bites or kicks can be severe and can result in soft-tissue injuries and fractures.

Rodents and Other Small Mammals

- **Method of injury:** Animals such as skunks, rabbits, rats, squirrels, raccoons, and marmots generally attack only when provoked. Injury is typically caused by bites, although these animals may also scratch. Rodents may carry pathogens that cause diseases such as plague and hantavirus.
- **Injuries:** Bites from these animals can cause local soft-tissue injury and localized infections. Scratches are usually superficial but can quickly become infected, especially if they are not promptly cleaned. Skunk, bats, fox and other mammal bites can transmit rabies, and infected rabbits can transmit tularemia.

Bats

- **Method of injury:** Bats typically do not attack humans unless provoked (**Figure 27-33**). Injury is caused by a bite.
- **Injuries:** Bites result in local soft-tissue injury and localized infections. Bats can transmit rabies, plague, and tularemia. In addition, even without a bite, the saliva of a bat can also transmit infections, usually rabies. From 1960-2018, a total of 125 human rabies cases were reported in the U.S. Roughly 1/4 of the cases resulted from dog bites

during foreign travel. Of the infections in the U.S., 70% were from bats (Centers for Disease Control and Prevention).

Moose, Elk, Deer, and Bison

- **Method of injury:** Most injuries occur when an inexperienced or unsuspecting hiker stumbles into the path of or foolishly attempts to touch one of these animals. Many injuries are caused by the animal charging the hiker who is knocked down or impaled on the animal's antlers (for moose, elk, and deer) or gored by the animal's horns (bison). Females will protect their offspring, so avoid a mother and its babies. Additionally, injuries may be caused by the animal's hooves or their sheer weight. Most injuries and deaths to humans occur from collisions that result when the animal walks into the path of an oncoming vehicle.
- **Injuries:** Incidents involving these animals cause soft-tissue injuries that range from minor to severe. Puncture wounds from antlers and horns are common. Internal injuries can also occur, as can head and spine injuries.

Bears

- **Method of injury:** Most bears do not attack humans unless provoked or defending their young. The exception to this involves grizzly bears, which have been known to attack unsuspecting hikers, fishermen, and other outdoor sports enthusiasts (**Figure 27-34**). Bears are great foragers and may wander into human camps looking for food. The best defense against bear incidents is to keep food away from tents and to store food in bear-proof containers. Most injuries are caused by the bear's powerful jaws and claws.
- **Injuries:** Most encounters with bears produce soft-tissue injuries, but large wounds, hemorrhage, broken bones, internal injuries, and head or facial injuries can also occur.

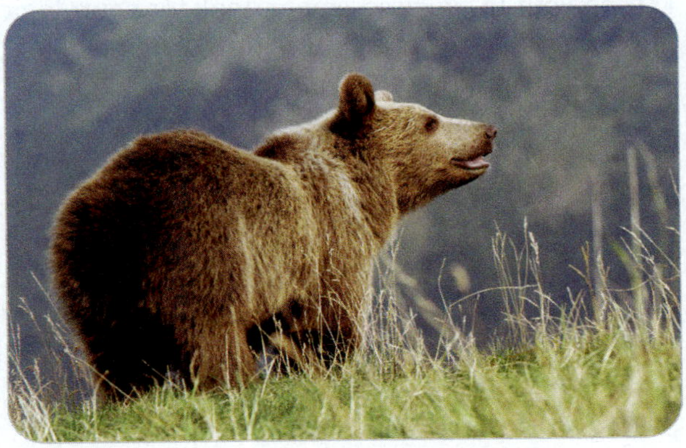

Figure 27-34 A grizzly bear.

CASE Update

More patrollers arrive and put on personal protective equipment (PPE). You take out the commercial tourniquet and place it and snug it down about 4 inches below the knee above the wound. The very narrow belt is removed. Bleeding is controlled. The times the tourniquet was placed is recorded. His pulse is 120 beats per minute, respirations are 18 breaths per minute, and blood pressure is 110/90 mm Hg. No other signs of trauma are evident. His mental status is now *A* in the AVPU (alert, verbal, pain, unresponsive) scale. He reports no medical problems, no medications, and no allergies. He has a normal spine exam. Sensing this is a load-and-go situation, you strap him onto the stretcher attached to the ATV.

What do you do now?

PATIENT ASSESSMENT FOR PLANT AND ANIMAL EMERGENCIES

In any harmful exposure to a plant or animal, OEC technicians must first determine whether the scene is safe. The same animal or plant can also harm the rescuer, creating a second patient. Control major bleeding and assess the ABCDs (airway, breathing, circulation, disability), first checking to see if the patient is responsive. If the patient is not responsive, simultaneously open the airway and check for effective breathing while feeling for a carotid pulse. If the patient has no pulse and is not breathing, immediately initiate CPR. If the patient has a pulse but is not breathing, begin rescue breathing. During your initial assessment, look for neurologic impairment, life-threatening external hemorrhage, signs of shock, and other serious trauma.

Once life threats have been managed, perform a secondary assessment using the SAMPLE acronym (signs and symptoms, allergies, medications, past medical history, last oral intake, events leading up to the problem) and the DCAP-BTLS mnemonic (deformity, contusions, abrasions/avulsions, punctures/penetrations, burns/bleeding/bruises, tenderness, lacerations, swelling), paying close attention to any known allergies. Begin by attempting to determine if the problem was a bite or sting, exposure to a plant (either contact or ingestion), or trauma from a large animal. Trying to identify the source of a plant or animal-related problem can be very challenging. A person walking in the woods, for example, could be exposed to poison ivy without knowing it. If the patient has a known environmental allergy (e.g., an allergy to yellow jacket stings) and has signs of anaphylactic shock, find out whether the patient has an epinephrine auto-injector.

For animal or insect injuries, expose and assess the affected area for findings such as rash, pale or discolored skin, and general swelling. Closely examine the mouth and nose for evidence of swelling. Look for bite or fang marks (**Figure 27-35**). Assess the patient for nausea and vomiting. Carefully assess the cardiovascular, respiratory, and neurologic status. Reevaluate the patient frequently, because vital signs may deteriorate quickly, depending on the source of the problem.

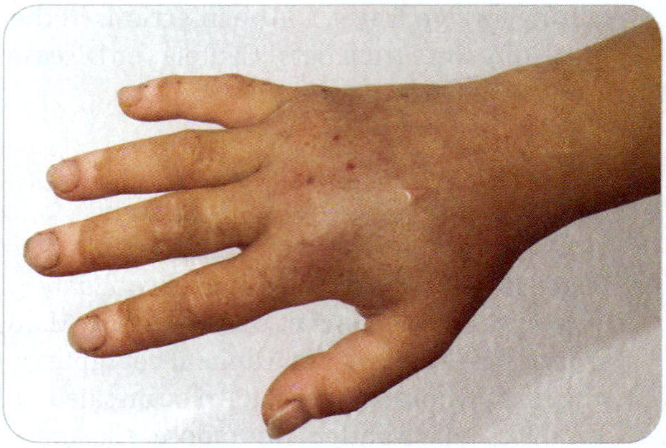

Figure 27-35 A snake-bite wound.

> **KEY POINT**
>
> **Epinephrine**
>
> Anaphylaxis is a major concern for anyone exposed to plant toxins or animal venom. Be prepared to assist in the administration of an epinephrine auto-injector if necessary.

Plant and Mushroom Poisonings

Skin contact with certain toxic plants can cause serious skin-related problems, allergic reactions, localized inflammation, or trauma from spines and needles. Evaluate the skin for signs of rash or trauma.

Gastrointestinal upset, abdominal pain (sometimes severe), muscle aches, and generalized weakness are common with the ingestion of toxic plants and mushrooms. Monitor the patient's vital signs frequently, and carefully evaluate for shock. Certain plants (e.g., deadly nightshade, cannabis) and certain mushrooms (e.g., peyote, psilocybin mushrooms) can produce hallucinogenic effects, including auditory and visual hallucinations.

Spider Bites and Scorpion Stings

The site of a spider bite or scorpion sting is usually very painful. Severe localized soft-tissue injury and later, tissue necrosis occur (**Figure 27-36**).

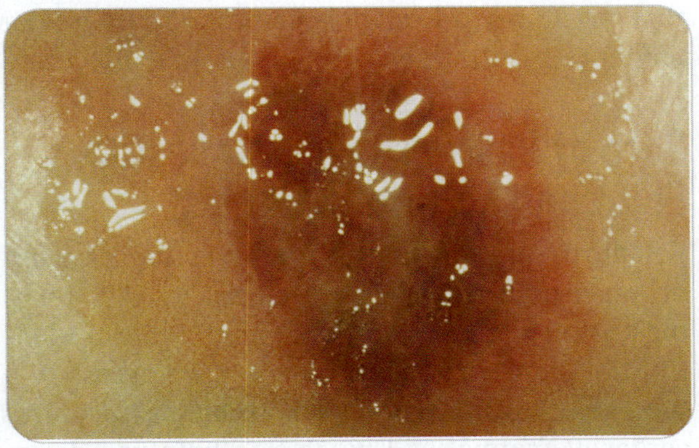

Figure 27-36 A late-stage brown recluse spider bite.

Courtesy of Department of Entomology, University of Nebraska.

Tick Bites

It takes several days to a few weeks for systemic illness to result from a tick bite, although a localized infection at the site may occur sooner. Ticks usually remain on a host's body for an hour or two before attaching, so it is important to look for them and remove them as soon as they are discovered. Have the patient monitor the attachment site for signs of a developing rash.

Stings from Bees, Wasps, Hornets, Yellow Jackets, and Red Ants

Monitor the site of the sting for localized inflammation and generalized signs of an allergic reaction. Since an allergic reaction can be severe, closely monitor the patient's vital signs, paying attention to swelling in and around the airway, change in voice, difficulty breathing, and instability of the patient's blood pressure. Multiple stings are especially concerning and increase one's risk for serious reactions causing anaphylaxis with airway swelling, difficulty breathing, and shock. Remember, even if the person says they are not allergic to a bee sting, there is always a *first* time.

Injuries Caused by Mosquitos and Biting Flies

Assess the affected area(s) for localized inflammation, which, in most cases, should be minor. Insect-transmitted diseases typically take several days to weeks to manifest themselves. Given that mosquitoes can transmit serious diseases, advise the patient to watch for signs of fever and systemic disease.

Reptile Bites

Snake bites can be life threatening. Assess the ABCDs and continue to monitor the patient. Snake venom can cause severe systemic bleeding, neurologic paralysis, hypotension, and delayed necrosis at the bite site. Monitor the patient's vital signs, paying close attention to any signs of shock. Large reptiles such as alligators and crocodiles generally cause major tissue damage, fractures, and amputations.

Injuries Caused by Marine Animals

Most injuries from marine animals cause local soft-tissue damage, but some injuries can cause cardiovascular or neurologic instability. Evaluate the severity of any soft-tissue injuries and monitor the vital signs.

Injuries Caused by Mammals

For injuries caused by large animals, pay close attention to excessive bleeding and the ABCDs, and perform a complete secondary patient assessment. Assess all soft-tissue injuries for the degree of external bleeding. Carefully evaluate the patient for evidence of internal injuries and head or spine injuries. Later, evaluate each soft-tissue injury for redness and swelling that may indicate a developing infection.

MANAGEMENT OF PLANT AND ANIMAL EMERGENCIES

As for any incident, ensure that the scene is safe with no plants or animal life that could further harm patients or rescuers. Observe standard precautions to prevent contact with plant toxins or animal-transmitted diseases. Next, control excessive bleeding and manage the ABCD-related problems. If the patient is unresponsive, immediately open the airway and simultaneously check for breathing and for a carotid pulse. If there is no pulse, immediately begin CPR using the latest guidelines. Request EMS assistance as needed. If an encounter with a large animal has resulted in trauma, evaluate to see if spinal motion restriction is needed. In the absence of significant trauma, place the patient in a position of comfort. Place patients who are in shock in a supine position and keep them warm. If indicated for breathing difficulties, apply high-flow oxygen by nonrebreather mask and titrate the oxygen saturation level with a pulse oximeter between 94 and 99%.

Further management of almost any serious animal-related injury, envenomation, or toxic ingestion should include urgent evacuation and transport to a definitive-care facility. Base your choice of transport (i.e., by ground or by air) on the length of transport, the severity of the injury, and local protocols. Given that the effects of many toxins take time to become evident, assume that patients have a life-threatening condition and plan accordingly. Descriptions of care for specific plant-related and animal-related problems follow.

Care of Cases Involving Plant Toxins

Patients with plant toxins on the skin need skin decontamination first. Remove contaminated clothing. Protect yourself from contamination (PPE), and remove any obvious resin or plant material that may be present. Next, vigorously wash the affected area with cool water and soap. Include cleaning under the patient's fingernails because toxins picked up from scratching may be present. If available, use commercial cleansers such as Tecnu or Oak-N-Ivy, which may help decontaminate the skin and medical equipment. If unavailable, use soap and water. Depending on the severity of the rash, the patient may need to be evaluated and treated by a physician. Severe rashes require a physician prescription of steroids. Itching and rash-related symptoms may be treated with diphenhydramine (Benadryl) and topical calamine lotion. Clean all exposed clothing, equipment, and supplies by washing with hot water and soap.

Patients who have inhaled smoke from a fire involving a poisonous or toxic plant such as poison ivy, poison oak, or poison sumac should be transported immediately to medical care due to the risk of severe respiratory problems.

If the injury is caused by a spine-bearing plant, remove large spines with tweezers as soon as possible. Smaller needles may be more challenging to fully remove and may require more specialized equipment. A physician should evaluate any area that continues to swell or becomes red, hot, and/or tender to the touch because of possible infection.

Care of Cases Involving Ingested Plant and Mushroom Toxins

For most cases involving the ingestion of plant or mushroom toxins, management by OEC technicians involves supportive care. If you can identify the plant or mushroom and have access to a telephone, call 9-1-1 and ask for a poison control center. Personnel will be able to help you determine if the plant or mushroom is toxic, whether to induce vomiting, and whether emergent transport is indicated. They can also provide other valuable care-related information. If the person is ill, rapid EMS transport to definitive care is necessary. Place the plant or mushroom in a plastic bag using PPE.

Care for Cases Involving Biting and Stinging Creatures

If a stinger is present, scrape the stinger off the skin using the edge of a firm flat object such as a credit card (**Figure 27-37**). Clean the bite area using soap and water. For spider bites or scorpion stings, immobilize (splint) the area to slow the spread of venom. Do not use a tourniquet unless there is severe bleeding. Continue to provide supportive care and arrange for transport. If the patient has a known allergy to certain insects, such as bees, they may have an epinephrine auto-injector. If indicated and authorized by your medical director and local protocols, you may need to assist the patient in administering an injection of epinephrine, following the procedure described in Chapter 14, *Allergies and Anaphylaxis*. Use the patient's own medication only.

Care of Tick Bites

To properly remove an attached tick, perform the following steps:

1. Grasp the tick as close to the surface of the patient's skin as possible, preferably with fine-tipped tweezers while using medical gloves (**Figure 27-38**). Do not apply fingernail polish, isopropyl alcohol, or a hot match head to the tick, because doing so can cause the release of toxins into the bite wound.

2. Pull the tick out with gentle, steady pressure, *taking care not to crush the tick's body.* The tick may release infected saliva into the skin when crushed.
3. After the tick is removed, disinfect the skin with isopropyl alcohol or another disinfectant.

Care of Snake Bites

Nonpoisonous snake bites initially need only local care. Follow-up medical evaluation is advised because delayed infection or skin necrosis can occur. One must make sure the snake was not a poisonous type. For all poisonous or non-identified snakes, make the scene safe by removing the person beyond striking distance of the snake. Call for immediate transport with ALS. Prompt evacuation and evaluation in a definitive-care facility in 30 minutes if possible are the primary focuses for a poisonous snake bite. Have the person lie down, keep the person calm, and place a limb below the level of the heart to slow the spread of the venom. Remove any jewelry from the area that was bitten. Remove shoes if the leg or foot was bitten. Allow the wound to bleed if its oozing and not arterial. Cover the wound with loose, sterile bandage. Apply a splint to avoid motion of an extremity. Because physical exertion should be avoided, do not allow the patient to hike over a great distance because doing so will enhance the spread of the poison.

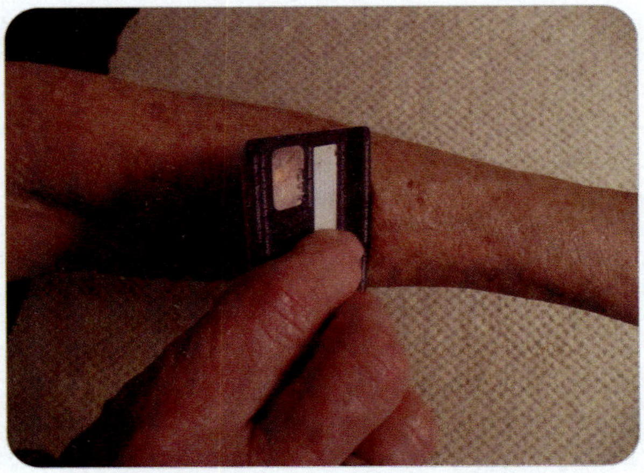

Figure 27-37 If an intact stinger is still in place, remove it by scraping it off with the edge of a credit card.

Never follow the outdated recommendation to "suck the poison out" or cut the wound to make it bleed; not only do these methods not work, they can worsen the envenomation. Also, *do not* apply a tourniquet, ice, or water to a snake bite. Do not give the patient alcohol, caffeinated beverages, or other medications. Antivenom may be indicated but should be administered by a physician or qualified person only.

Care of Alligator and Crocodile Bites

Treat for excessive bleeding and ABCD problems immediately. Large reptiles such as alligators and crocodiles generally cause crush injuries resulting in major tissue damage, fractures, and amputations. Treat massive bleeding with compressive dressings, tourniquets, or hemostatic dressings

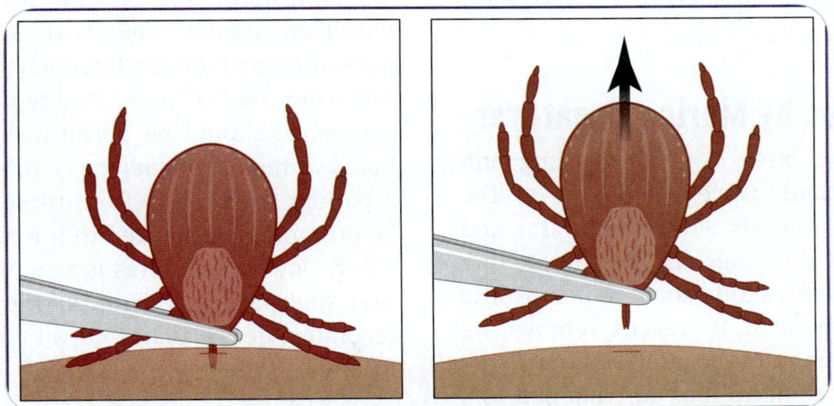

Figure 27-38 The proper removal of a tick using fine-toothed tweezers.

KEY POINT

Snake Bites

While waiting for an ambulance, here is how to care for a snake-bite patient.

- Don't raise the bite area above the level of the heart, because blood containing rattlesnake venom will reach the patient's heart more quickly.
- Keep the patient as still as possible, as movement will increase blood flow and the venom will circulate faster.
- Remove any tight clothing or jewelry.
- Let the wound bleed; bleeding may allow some of the venom to be released.
- Place a clean bandage on the wound.
- Try to keep patient calm, as anxiety and panic can increase the heart rate, which will cause the venom to spread.
- If you see signs of shock, lay the patient down on the back, raise the feet slightly, and keep the patient warm.
- Don't cut the wound; doing so doesn't help and could cause an infection.
- Don't suck the venom from the wound.
- Don't use a tourniquet or apply ice or water.

and splint fractures using standard precautions. Monitor the patient's vital signs and treat for shock if needed.

Care of Injuries by Marine Creatures

For marine animal bites, control bleeding and transport the patient. Once safely out of the ocean, irrigate all wounds with fresh water and apply appropriate dressings. If life-threatening hemorrhage is present, a tourniquet or hemostatic dressing is recommended. If present, remove the spines and decontaminate the affected area. X-ray imaging is usually done to look for retained foreign bodies, and antibiotics are routinely administered at the hospital.

For jellyfish stings, there are two important actions: preventing further nematocyst discharge and pain relief. To inactivate the nematocyst venom, liberally wash off the nematocysts from the affected area of skin with vinegar (4% to 6% acetic acid solution) as soon as possible for at least 30 seconds. Check with local authorities concerning frequently encountered species as this has been shown to work for only certain types of jellyfish. After the nematocysts are removed or inactivated with vinegar, the pain is treated by immersing the affected part in *hot* water (45°C, or 113°F) for at least 20 minutes or longer if the pain persists. Patient with a more systemic reaction should be emergently transported to a hospital.

To remove the sea urchin spines from your skin, first immerse the affected area for 30 to 90 minutes in hot water or vinegar to help smoothen or dissolve the spines. Next use tweezers to remove all spines stuck in your foot, hand, or body. Apply shaving cream to the injured area and remove the pedicellaria (moveable stalked structures with jaws) by scraping with a razor. Scrub the wound with soap and water. Rinse the injury with fresh water.

Care for Animal Bites

Care by an OEC technician for animal bites includes bleeding control, wound care, and shock management. The mouths of all animals contain multiple types of bacteria that can enter a victim's tissues through a bite. Wash bites with sterile or clean water, or a saline solution. Apply a sterile dressing. Immobilize suspected fractures in the usual manner. Recommend further medical care.

Although larger wounds often require thorough cleaning and closure with sutures by a physician, smaller wounds (less than 2 cm) and punctures are typically left open to allow drainage. Any wound debridement and repair, which may be extensive, should be performed by a physician. Because many rodents carry infectious diseases, a patient with a bite from these animals should be promptly transported to the hospital for treatment. Dog and cat bites pose a high risk of infection, and prophylactic antibiotics are sometimes recommended. If indicated, a tetanus booster will be given at the medical facility.

Trauma Caused by Large Animals

Injuries caused by large animals are treated according to the signs and symptoms present. For instance, a large bite or kick requires the same type of care as that indicated by similar trauma caused by any other mechanism. Control external bleeding, splint possible fractures, and provide spinal motion restriction if indicated. Bandage wounds as indicated to prevent further contamination.

Because an attack from these animals can result in massive injuries, monitor the vital signs carefully for signs of shock. Treat massive bleeding with compressive dressings, tourniquets, or hemostatic dressings using standard precautions.

KEY POINT

Rabies

Even though rabies can be lethal, only two or three people die of rabies each year. The rabies virus is transmitted when the saliva of an infected animal is introduced through a bite. The most common carriers of the rabies virus are bats, raccoons, foxes, and skunks, though the total number of infected animals is extremely low. Many regions of the country have not had a documented case of a rabies-infected animal in years. If not treated, the virus causes neurologic disease and ultimately death. Signs and symptoms include a flulike illness that is followed by hallucinations, confusion, severe neurologic pain, agitation, swallowing difficulties, partial paralysis, and death. It is best to advise anyone who has been bitten by an animal to seek medical care.

KEY POINT

Have Questions or Need Information About Poisoning?

The National Poison Center can provide valuable information regarding toxic plants and animals. This service is available 24 hours a day, 7 days a week by calling 1-800-222-1222 toll-free.

CASE Outcome

A landing zone has been set up near the administration building. As you approach the landing zone, a helicopter is about to land. After landing, a paramedic evaluates your patient, starts an IV line, provides medications, and then loads him into the helicopter. Later you discover the patient spent several hours in surgery, having his wounds cleaned and repaired. He received a blood transfusion for shock. A long road to recovery is needed, but his life was saved. The park ranger later finds a den 200 yards from the bicycle trail, with two bear cubs. The female bear was protecting her young.

CHAPTER REVIEW

In Summary

- Most skin rashes from contact with toxic plants are not life threatening.
- The ingestion of some plants can lead to illnesses ranging from mild nausea to death. When ingestion of a poisonous plant is suspected, obtain an exposure history.
- Unexplained altered mental status or severe nausea/vomiting may be associated with ingestion of a plant or mushroom toxin.
- Always be prepared for anaphylaxis in patients who have an exposure to insect or animal bites.
- Bites and scratches by certain wild animals warrant evaluation for rabies.
- Manage large bites and injuries as you would any traumatic wound.
- Many stings, whether by insects or marine animals, can be managed with localized treatment.
- Observation of signs of systemic involvement requires transport to a medical-care facility.

Key Terms

Antivenom A biological material (antibodies) administered to a patient to counteract exposure to a specific kind of venom; produced by injecting the venom into an animal and then harvesting the antibodies that the animal makes against the venom.

Envenomation Poisonous effects caused by bites or stings.

Necrosis Death of most or all the cells in an organ or tissue due to disease, injury, or failure of the blood supply.

Poison Any substance that can cause severe organ damage or death if ingested, inhaled, injected into the body, or absorbed through the skin.

Toxin A poison or venom of plant or animal origin.

Venom A specific toxin or poisonous secretion of an animal, most commonly from a snake, spider, or scorpion, usually transmitted by a bite or sting.

Chapter Questions

1. After hiking through a wooded area, you notice blisters on your lower leg. You realize that you may be having an allergic reaction caused by:
   a. venom from a plant or fungus.
   b. topical exposure to a toxin.
   c. ingestion of a poison.
   d. venom from an insect sting.
2. Topical exposure or ingestion of some plants can cause:
   a. anaphylaxis.
   b. cardiac problems.
   c. neurologic problems.
   d. All of the above
3. When ingested, poisonous mushrooms can cause:
   a. gastrointestinal upset.
   b. hallucinations.
   c. death.
   d. All of the above
4. When assessing a patient who has been injured by an encounter with a toxic plant or animal, it is important to:
   a. expose the affected area.
   b. ask about known allergies.
   c. attempt to identify the source of the injury.
   d. All of the above
5. Your patient presents with itching and rash-related symptoms after being exposed to poison oak. Your emergency care should include:
   a. removing contaminated clothing.

b. removing any resin or plant residue.
c. washing the affected area with soap and water.
d. All of the above

6. Your patient has been bitten by a rattlesnake. Your emergency care should include:
   a. lowering the bite area below the level of the heart.
   b. applying a tourniquet.
   c. applying an ice pack.
   d. cutting the wound to make it bleed.

7. Your patient has been bitten by a dog. You expose the injury site and find a large laceration. Your emergency care should include:
   a. cleaning the area with clean water or a saline solution.
   b. applying a sterile dressing and bandage.
   c. immobilizing any suspected fractures.
   d. All of the above

Answers: 1. b, Objective 27-1, p. 629; 2. d, Objective 27-1, p. 629; 3. d, Objective 27-2, p. 634; 4. d, Objective 27-3, p. 646; 5. d, Objective 27-4, p. 648; 6. a, Objective 27-5, p. 650; 7. d, Objective 27-6, p. 650

CHAPTER 28

ALTITUDE-RELATED EMERGENCIES

OBJECTIVES

Upon completion of this chapter, the OEC technician will be able to:

28-1 Define altitude.

28-2 Explain what happens to oxygen as altitude increases.

28-3 List risk factors for the development of altitude illnesses.

28-4 Describe strategies to prevent altitude illness.

28-5 List the signs and symptoms of the following altitude illnesses:
- Acute mountain sickness (AMS)
- High-altitude pulmonary edema (HAPE)
- High-altitude cerebral edema (HACE)

28-6 Describe how to assess a patient with altitude illness.
- Acute mountain sickness (AMS)
- High-altitude pulmonary edema (HAPE)
- High-altitude cerebral edema (HACE)

28-7 Describe the treatment of a patient with altitude illness.
- Acute mountain sickness (AMS)
- High-altitude pulmonary edema (HAPE)
- High-altitude cerebral edema (HACE)

KEY TERMS

Acclimatization, p. 657
Acute mountain sickness (AMS), p. 659
Altitude illness, p. 656
Ataxia, p. 660
Gamow bag, p. 665
High-altitude cerebral edema (HACE), p. 659
High-altitude pulmonary edema (HAPE), p. 659
Hypoxemia, p. 657
Khumbu cough, p. 661
Sleeping altitude, p. 658

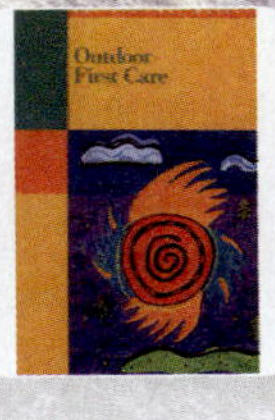

HISTORICAL TIMELINE 1994. A new first-aid program, *Outdoor First Care*, is introduced.

CHAPTER OVERVIEW

The mountains have provided many tourists and sporting participants great recreational opportunities (**Figure 28-1**). Snow sports enthusiasts, hikers, and sightseers have many opportunities to enjoy high-altitude activities. However, some unsuspecting or unprepared people can quickly have the adventure of a lifetime turn into a miserable or even life-threatening event that includes intense headaches, breathing difficulty, coughing spells, pulmonary edema, coma-inducing brain swelling, or even death. These illnesses are not caused by being "out of shape" but are due to high altitude, which can punish anyone who is not acclimatized to the thin air. Even hardy recreationalists are at risk. Altitude illness can affect up to 30% of visitors to the high-altitude resorts of the Rocky Mountains. Fifty percent of all hikers and climbers in the Himalayas suffer from some form of altitude illness.

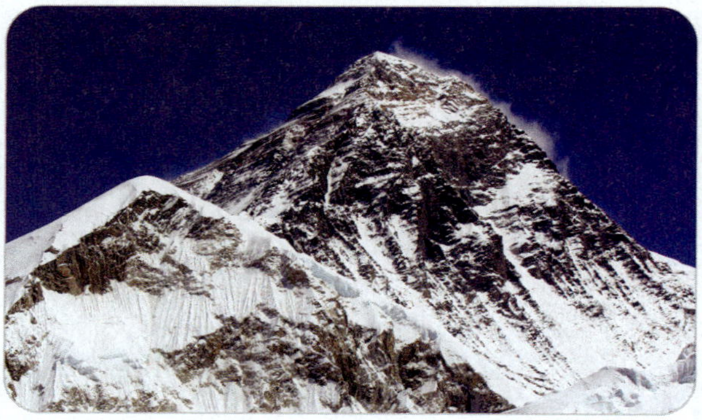

Figure 28-1 Mt. Everest stands at over 29,000 feet.

OEC technicians who work in high-altitude mountain resorts may encounter patients who are suffering from an altitude-related illness. You need to learn to recognize the signs and symptoms of acute altitude illnesses and know how to provide prompt, appropriate treatment.

This chapter discusses high altitude, how it affects the human body, and how the body attempts to adapt to it. It also describes how to distinguish among the different types of altitude illnesses, the signs and symptoms associated with each type, and techniques for managing specific altitude-related disorders. Because prevention is an essential component for reducing morbidity and mortality for any medical problem, the chapter also presents strategies for preventing altitude illness. This chapter will prepare you by providing a fundamental understanding of altitude illness, including its causes and its overall management.

ALTITUDE PHYSIOLOGY

The body's ability to preserve homeostasis includes the ability to adapt to changes in altitude. Here we define *altitude* as the height or vertical elevation above sea level, which is "0 feet" (**Figure 28-2**).

Although most **altitude illness** occurs at elevations higher than 8,000 feet above sea level, it can also occur at altitudes as low as 6,500 feet. The *rate of ascent* is very important in determining the probability of developing altitude illness;

CASE Presentation

You are working first-aid duty in the patrol room at a resort that is at 11,000 feet above sea level when a 28-year-old woman slowly walks in complaining of shortness of breath. Noticing that she does not look well and is slightly cyanotic around her lips, you help her to the nearest stretcher. She tells you that she hasn't felt great since arriving after her flight and driving up from sea level yesterday. She denies any chest pain but says she has a bad headache, is tired, becomes short of breath "just walking to the bathroom," and has had a dry cough. She has no significant past medical history, has not suffered any recent trauma, and is not currently taking any prescribed medications. She appears very concerned and says, "I have never experienced anything like this in my life."

What should you do?

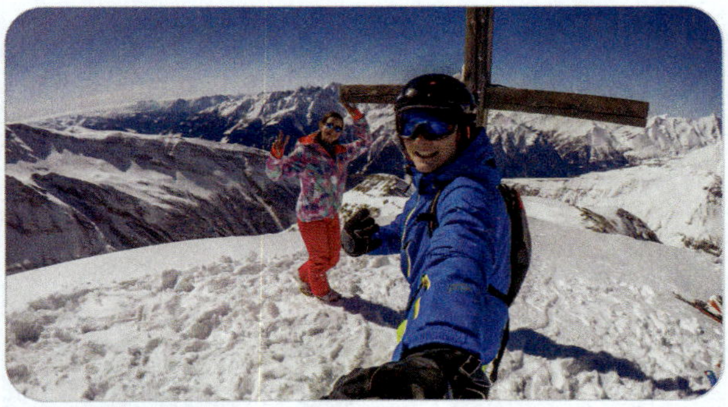

Figure 28-2 High altitude is defined as 8,000 to 12,000 feet above sea level. Altitude illness is most likely to occur within this range of elevation.

KEY POINT

Definition of Altitude

Altitude is defined as the height or vertical elevation above sea level (0 feet).

a rapid ascent is more likely to cause problems than a slower ascent (**Figure 28-3**). Even though the deadliest forms of altitude illness occur more frequently at extreme elevations, they can occur at intermediate altitudes as well. Scientific evidence suggests that the genetic makeup of some individuals helps them avoid altitude illness and acclimate to high altitudes more easily than other individuals.

High altitude dramatically affects the amount of oxygen available to the body's cells, which can have a profound effect on normal body function. Low blood oxygen content is called **hypoxemia**. As altitude increases, the atmosphere contains less air. At a high altitude, oxygen remains at the same percentage, 21% of air. However, since the atmosphere is less dense, there are fewer molecules of oxygen inhaled with each breath. The amount of oxygen contained in one cubic foot of air at a high altitude is less than in one cubic foot at sea level. So, each breath at a high altitude takes in fewer oxygen molecules. At 10,000 feet, oxygen taken in with each breath is only 69% of that taken in at sea level.

KEY POINT

Speed of Ascent

The more rapid the ascent (climb), the more likely it is that individuals will develop altitude illness.

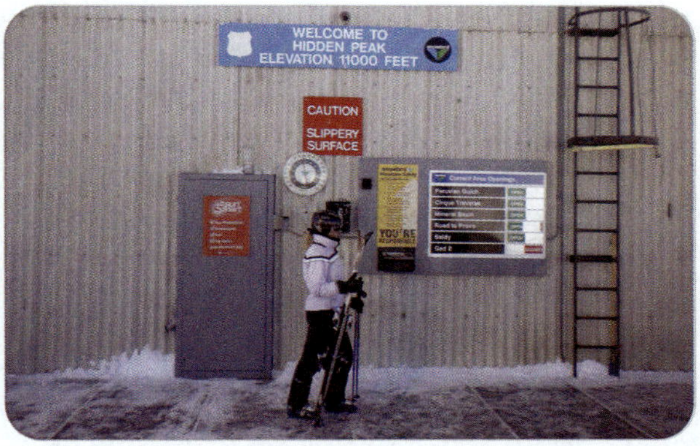

Figure 28-3 If this woman rose to this elevation (11,000 feet) too rapidly, she could experience altitude illness.

KEY POINT

Oxygen Concentration at High Altitude

As we go to a higher elevation, the oxygen concentration in the air is reduced, resulting in a lower oxygen intake per breath.

Altitude Acclimatization

The serious medical consequences of ascending to a high altitude can be prevented through **acclimatization**, which is the body's process of *gradual* adjustment to changes in altitude. This ability to adapt has allowed humans to travel to and inhabit some of the most inhospitable places on earth at high elevations. If a person who lives at sea level were to go directly to the top of Mt. Everest (over 29,000 feet high), the person would quickly lose consciousness and die.

With less oxygen available, the body must adjust to improve the delivery of oxygen to the tissues and cells. When traveling to high altitude too rapidly, altitude illness may occur because the body may not adjust fast enough to keep up with the body's oxygen demand. This insufficient oxygen supply results in problems that can range from mild annoyance to life-threatening conditions. The keys to preventing altitude illness are knowing when to expect it, how to avoid it, how to identify it, and what to do if symptoms arise.

In the process of acclimatization to altitude, the body makes a series of physiological adjustments that increase the delivery of oxygen to the body's cells. This gradual adjustment to hypoxia allows a person to temporarily endure extreme altitudes. These physiological adaptations that help preserve homeostasis include the following:

- *Increased rate and depth of respiration.* This change helps bring more oxygen into the body and is the result of a mechanism called the hypoxic ventilatory response. The degree of this response depends on the individual's genetic makeup.
- *Increased heart rate.* This adaptation allows more blood and oxygen to be pumped throughout the body and may result in a mild elevation in systolic blood pressure.
- *Increased red blood cell production.* This mechanism increases the amount of oxygen that can be carried to the tissues.
- *Constriction of pulmonary blood vessels.* The blood vessels that go to and from the lungs constrict, increasing resistance to blood flow through the lungs.
- *Increased urine production.* The body rids itself of excess fluid.

The ability to acclimatize varies from person to person and has nothing to do with how physically fit someone is (**Figure 28-4**). Some people can adapt quickly to altitude changes without any apparent discomfort, whereas others develop varying degrees of altitude illness. A few individuals fail to acclimatize, even with gradual ascent, and develop a life-threatening condition. The degree of hypoxia, the rate of ascent, and the individual's physiological makeup are the primary factors that determine whether the body successfully acclimatizes or becomes ill.

While acclimatization is a process that varies among individuals, there are steps all people can take to decrease the adverse effects of ascending to high altitudes. Mountain climbers who are advancing up a mountain over several weeks climb to an altitude higher than where they will camp each day. They "climb high and sleep low." By climbing up 1500 feet and then sleeping 500 feet below the greatest ascent, they can acclimate more effectively.

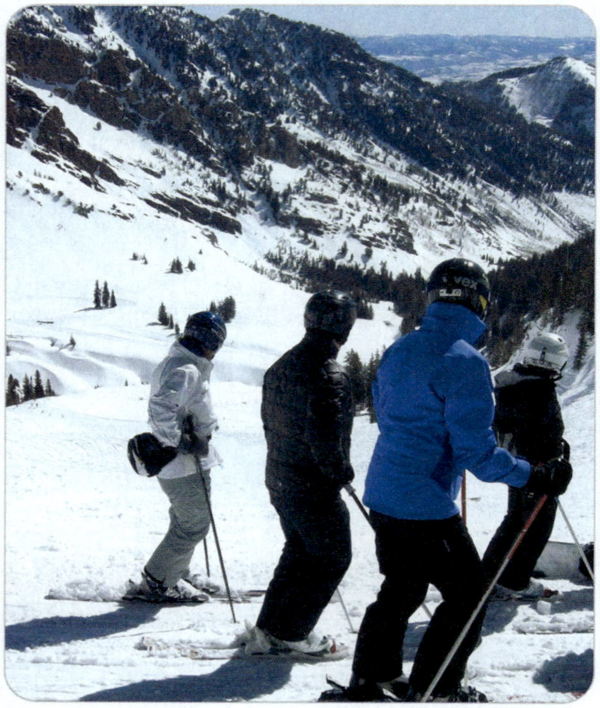

Figure 28-4 Some individuals acclimatize more quickly than others. The rate of acclimatization is not based on physical conditioning alone.

KEY POINT

Factors in the Severity of Altitude Illnesses

The development and severity of altitude illnesses depend on several factors, including:

- Rate of altitude ascent
- Ultimate elevation attained (more importantly, the **sleeping altitude**)
- Time spent at high altitudes
- Level of exertion
- Genetic susceptibility

Altitude illness is a spectrum of physical problems that begins with milder signs and symptoms and progresses to life-threatening medical illness if not reversed.

ALTITUDE-RELATED PROBLEMS

OEC technicians should be familiar with altitude-related problems they may encounter. This section reviews acute mountain sickness, high-altitude pulmonary edema, high-altitude cerebral edema, and some other altitude-related problems.

Acute Mountain Sickness

Acute mountain sickness (AMS) affects many outdoor enthusiasts each year. AMS is defined as a medical condition caused by exposure to high altitude. It usually occurs within *several hours to 1 day* after ascending to a higher altitude. It occurs when the rate of ascent outpaces the body's ability to adjust to the change in altitude. AMS rarely occurs at altitudes below 6,500 feet and is more often encountered at altitudes greater than 8,000 feet. It is especially prevalent among individuals who rapidly ascend to high altitude from elevations below 2,000 feet. For example, AMS affects 25% of all visitors who sleep above 8,000 feet in Colorado.

AMS is characterized by mild to moderate headache accompanied by one or more of the following symptoms: dizziness, fatigue, dyspnea on exertion, loss of appetite, nausea, and a general feeling of malaise (**Figure 28-5**). A headache usually develops in 2 to 12 hours. The other symptoms, which many patients compare to the feeling of an alcoholic hangover, commonly develop within 12 to 24 hours after arrival at a higher altitude but can appear in as few as 4 to 6 hours in susceptible individuals. If the person can acclimatize successfully, the symptoms decrease in severity by about the third day. Because there are no specific diagnostic signs for AMS, it is often misdiagnosed as a viral flulike illness, a hangover, exhaustion, dehydration, or a drug-related effect.

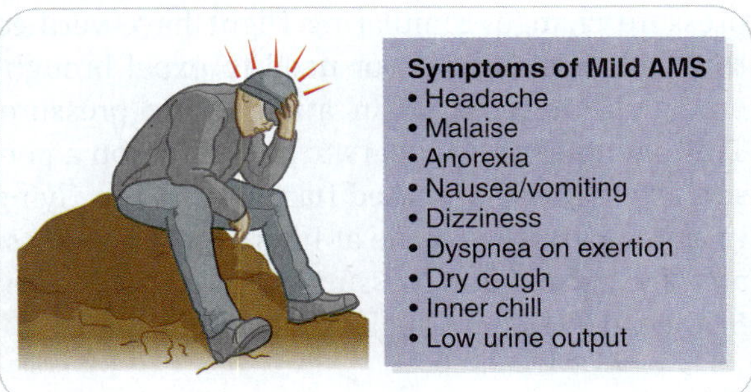

Figure 28-5 Signs and symptoms of acute mountain sickness.

High-Altitude Pulmonary Edema

High-altitude pulmonary edema (HAPE) is a condition in which fluid accumulates in the lungs of an individual at high altitude. Unlike some other forms of pulmonary edema, HAPE is not due to a preexisting cardiac disorder. In cardiac pulmonary edema, fluid builds up in the lungs because the heart is not pumping correctly. In HAPE, fluid buildup is caused by excessive blood pressure in the pulmonary artery. The elevated blood pressure causes extracellular fluid to leak into the alveoli, which reduces gas exchange and oxygenation and results in cellular hypoxia. When at high altitude, it is thought that the body is stressed by cold, exertion, and anoxia, causing HAPE.

HAPE is the most common cause of altitude-related death and rarely occurs at elevations below 8,000 feet.

Like AMS, HAPE develops as a result of several factors, including individual susceptibility, ascent rate, altitude reached, physical exertion, and certain underlying medical conditions. HAPE usually occurs within the first 2 to 4 days of ascent to altitudes above 8,200 feet and is heralded by the onset of marked fatigue during exercise. Untreated, fatigue is soon accompanied by severe dyspnea upon exertion, such as walking uphill or upstairs. About half of HAPE patients have symptoms of AMS first, but one can get HAPE without having AMS first. Patients may also complain of a persistent dry cough during the early stages, and their nail beds and lips may become cyanotic. The condition typically worsens at night. Labored breathing at rest and audible chest congestion herald the development of a serious, potentially life-threatening condition (**Figure 28-6**). HAPE may strike abruptly, especially in a sedentary person who may not notice the early stages. Pink (blood-tinged), frothy sputum is a very late finding and is accompanied by profound hypoxia.

Untreated, HAPE can be fatal within a few hours. Fortunately, it can be completely and easily reversed if recognized early and treated properly.

High-Altitude Cerebral Edema

High-altitude cerebral edema (HACE) is a potentially deadly condition in which the brain swells.

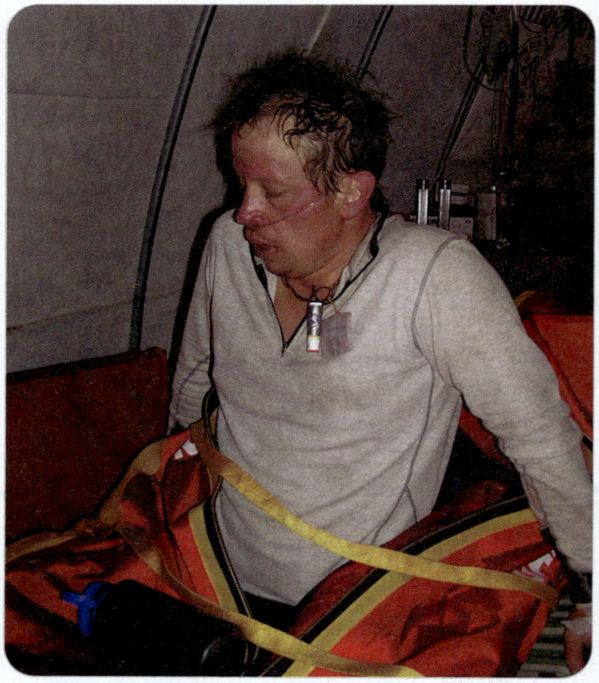

Figure 28-6 High-altitude pulmonary edema, a condition in which fluid accumulates in the lungs of individuals at high altitudes.

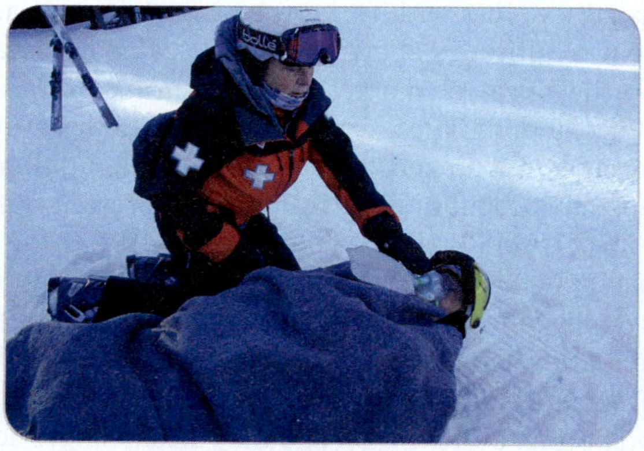

Figure 28-7 High-altitude cerebral edema, a potentially life-threatening condition and the most dangerous form of altitude illness.

HACE is the most severe form of altitude illness and is most commonly encountered at elevations over 9,600 feet. HACE or HAPE may be preceded by AMS. About 3% of patients who develop AMS go on to develop HACE.

HACE is a true medical emergency that can rapidly lead to death if not recognized and quickly treated (**Figure 28-7**). It is characterized by a progression of symptoms that usually begins with headache and nausea and progresses to **ataxia** plus any of the following signs and symptoms: altered mental status, fatigue, drowsiness, difficulty speaking, paralysis, coma, and death. Hallucinations and psychotic behavior also are commonly observed. Although uncommon, seizures can occur. The progression from AMS to HACE-induced coma may be as fast as 12 hours but usually requires 1 to 3 days. Recovery can be very quick, especially if treated early, but recovery can also be very slow and result in long-term complications, including decreased brain or neurologic function.

High-Altitude Flatus Expulsion

High-altitude flatus expulsion (HAFE) is a gastrointestinal syndrome involving the spontaneous passage of increased quantities of rectal gases at high altitudes. First described by Joseph Hamel in about 1820, a landmark study of this phenomenon was published in 1981 by Paul Auerbach and York Miller. Although mostly benign, except for abdominal discomfort, certainly people around you are affected by this condition.

The condition is produced by the differential in atmospheric pressure and is directly correlated with how often the person has experienced high-altitude conditions, as a person's metabolism tends to adjust with repeated exposure. As the external pressure decreases, the difference in pressure between the gas within the body and the atmosphere outside is higher, and the urge to expel gas to relieve the pressure is greater. Consistent with the principle of Boyle's law, controlling for dietary variance, the amount of gas produced is constant in mass, but the volume increases as the external pressure decreases. So, the person has increased flatulence.

Studies involving military pilots subjected to pressure changes simulating flight have verified this feeling of fullness or need to expel brought on by the differential in atmospheric pressure. This phenomenon appears to be the reason a person experiences increased flatulence when flying in a commercial airplane at high altitude, as most airplane cabins are pressurized to only between 6,000 and 8,000 feet of altitude.

Other Altitude-Related Problems

A decrease in available oxygen at high altitudes can complicate preexisting conditions, especially

CASE Update

Upon examination of the patient, you notice that her breathing is labored, even at rest. The patient appears physically fit, which she confirms by saying, "I run more than 50 miles a week." Her heart rate is 116 beats per minute, blood pressure is 132/80 mm Hg, and respirations are 36 breaths per minute. A pulse oximeter measures the patient's oxygen saturation at 84%. The rest of the physical assessment is negative for any abnormal signs or signs of trauma.

What do think is wrong with the patient? What should you do?

those involving the cardiovascular or respiratory systems, such as angina, congestive heart failure, and chronic respiratory conditions. Reduced oxygen availability can complicate pregnancy because of a reduction of oxygen delivered to the fetus.

In addition, altitude can adversely affect some medical equipment, most notably inflatable air splints, vacuum splints, and other pneumatic-based devices. The use of air splints at high altitude is not recommended.

Other medical conditions associated with altitude include Khumbu cough, peripheral edema, high-altitude retinal hemorrhage, radial keratotomy blindness, solar keratitis, and sunburn.

Khumbu Cough

Khumbu cough, also known as high-altitude bronchitis, is a dry, persistent cough that affects nearly all people who spend time at altitudes above 14,000 feet. The condition is named after the Khumbu region in Nepal, near Mt. Everest, where it was first observed. Khumbu cough is caused by prolonged exposure to cold, dry air, which dries out the lower respiratory passages. The resulting severe bronchial irritation and constriction cause a cough that can become so severe that it can break ribs.

Peripheral Edema

Mild to moderate edema of the face, hands, or feet is common among travelers at altitudes above 8,000 feet and is often seen without signs of AMS. Altitude-related peripheral edema is noncardiac in origin and results from fluid leakage into the surrounding tissues. The condition is usually self-limiting and is not a sign of illness.

High-Altitude Retinal Hemorrhage

High-altitude retinal hemorrhage is a condition in which small blood vessels in the back of the eye rupture. The condition is encountered most often at elevations above 8,000 feet. Symptoms, if present, can include blurred vision and small blind spots. High-altitude retinal hemorrhage usually resolves spontaneously and seldom has any long-term effects.

Radial Keratotomy Blindness

People who have had radial keratotomy, an older surgical method to correct nearsightedness, may become blind at high altitude. This condition, which is not generally seen below 9,000 feet, begins with blurring of vision due to reduced refraction of light. Lasik, a newer procedure for vision correction, does not seem to cause the same effect.

Solar Keratitis

Exposure to the increased amount of UV radiation in sunlight at higher altitudes can cause solar keratitis, or snow blindness, in individuals who wear inadequate or no protective eyewear. UV light may be reflected off snow-covered terrain or water surfaces and can cause eye burns like those suffered by welders. Solar keratitis starts several hours after overexposure to UV light and begins with intense eye pain and a gritty feeling in the eyes. Ideally, protective eyewear should be a "wraparound" type of sunglasses or glacier goggles to prevent light reaching the eyes from the side, and the addition of a visor helps deflect light entering from above (**Figure 28-8**).

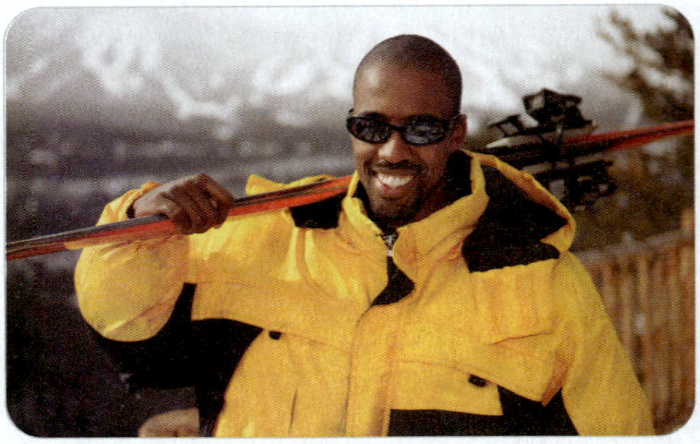

Figure 28-8 Wraparound sunglasses with UV protection help block UV light that causes solar keratitis (snow blindness).

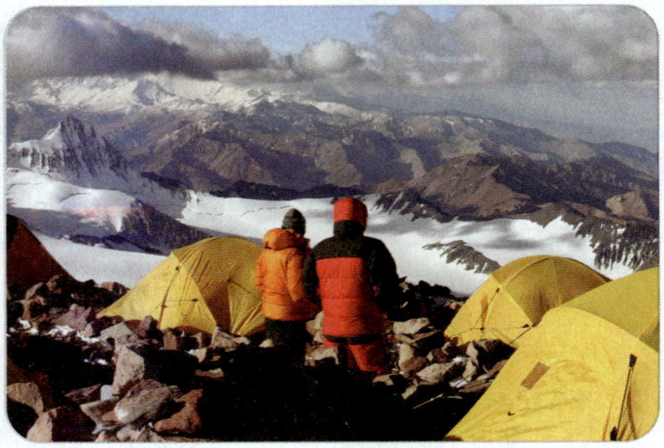

Figure 28-9 Proper acclimatization, such as a 2- to 3-day rest period at intermediate altitude (8,000–10,000 feet), can reduce the likelihood of altitude illness.

Sunburn

Sunburn is more prevalent at higher altitudes because the decreased air density increases one's exposure to the penetrating effects of the ultraviolet rays in sunlight.

PREVENTION OF ALTITUDE ILLNESSES

With proper precautions, the incidence of altitude illnesses can be significantly reduced. However, as indicated previously, exceptional health or physical fitness does *not* render one immune to altitude illness. Thus, the prevention of altitude illness depends on proper acclimatization. Follow these guidelines to achieve proper altitude acclimatization:

- Gradual ascent is the most effective way to prevent altitude illness, especially if you begin at sea level and continue above 10,000 feet.
- Incorporate a layover of 2 to 3 days at an intermediate altitude—that is, between 8,000 feet and 10,000 feet. For individuals traveling from sea level, a 1-day layover at 6,000 feet can dramatically decrease the risk of becoming ill (**Figure 28-9**).
- Once above 10,000 feet, limit increases in altitude to 1,000 feet per day. Then, for every 2,000 feet of elevation gained, take 1 or 2 extra rest days.
- As you reach higher altitudes, more rest and a smaller altitude gain per day may be necessary.
- Avoid heavy physical exertion for the first 24 to 48 hours at high altitudes.
- Stay hydrated. Altitude acclimatization is often accompanied by fluid loss, so drink lots of liquids (sometimes 3 to 4 quarts per day) to remain properly hydrated. Electrolyte drinks provide good hydration; however, it is recommended that they be diluted with water. As the respiratory rate increases at higher elevations, the amount of fluid lost during exhalations increases. Urine output should be copious and straw colored.
- Avoid alcohol and other depressant drugs (including most sleeping pills) because they decrease the respiratory drive during sleep, which can worsen symptoms and cause AMS. Additionally, alcohol promotes diuresis and can lead to excessive fluid loss. Also avoid tobacco, which reduces peripheral circulation by constricting peripheral blood vessels.
- If you begin to show symptoms of altitude illness, do not go higher until the symptoms resolve.
- People acclimatize at different rates, so if you are traveling in a group, make sure everyone is properly acclimatized before going higher.
- "*Climb high and sleep low.*" This common mantra among climbers helps to reduce the adverse effects of climbing at high altitudes. If you are feeling well, climb during the day and then descend to a lower altitude to sleep at night.

> **KEY POINT**
>
> **Prophylactic AMS Medications**
>
> Ask high-altitude patients if they have taken any prophylactic AMS medications; if they have, find out what they took, when they took it, and how much they took.

Several prescription and over-the-counter medications can reduce or even prevent altitude illness. OEC technicians should specifically ask high-altitude patients during the SAMPLE history whether they have taken one of these medications.

Medications for Altitude Illness

Acetazolamide (Diamox) is a prescription medication that often is taken prophylactically to prevent AMS. The drug improves the body's ability to acclimatize to altitude by forcing the kidneys to excrete bicarbonate. The resulting drop in blood pH stimulates hyperventilation and increased oxygen absorption. If taken early after the onset of AMS, acetazolamide can terminate AMS. Its effects may be delayed, so it is advisable to begin use 24 hours before ascent to altitude and to continue use for 48 to 72 hours at the maximum altitude attained. The prophylactic dose is 125 mg twice each day. Temporary side effects may include tingling of the lips and fingertips, blurred vision, and alteration of taste sensation (carbonated beverages have a metal taste).

Acetazolamide is a sulfonamide drug, so individuals who are allergic to sulfa drugs should not take it without prior testing. Because it is known to cause severe allergic reactions in people with no previous history of allergies, it is advisable to take a trial course of the drug before going to a remote location, where a severe allergic reaction could prove difficult to treat.

Dexamethasone is a prescription steroid that decreases swelling in the brain and in other structures and may reverse the symptoms of AMS. Dosage is typically 4 mg twice each day for a few days starting at the beginning of the ascent. Dexamethasone should be used with caution because it can mask signs of progressing disease. For this reason, it is recommended for prophylaxis in rare circumstances only.

Interestingly, sildenafil (Viagra) and tadalafil (Cialis) seem to prevent altitude illness. These medications seem to help prevent HAPE by dilating the pulmonary arteries. People who take nitrates (nitroglycerin) for cardiac disease should not take sildenafil or tadalafil.

Nifedipine (Adalat) has also been used in the prevention of HAPE in people susceptible to high-altitude illness.

PATIENT ASSESSMENT FOR ALTITUDE-RELATED EMERGENCIES

As has been stated throughout this text, the role of OEC technicians is not to diagnose the underlying cause of a given problem, but instead to recognize patients who have signs and symptoms of an emergent condition and quickly initiate lifesaving treatment, if needed.

As with any patient, the assessment process begins with a careful examination of the ABCDs (airway, breathing, circulation, and disability). If a potentially emergent condition exists, initiate lifesaving treatment instead of performing a complete physical examination and refer the patient to a higher level of care. The primary assessment is followed by a secondary assessment, which includes a thorough history, a physical exam, and an assessment of the patient's vital signs.

OEC technicians should ask patients about their medical history and symptoms using the SAMPLE acronym (signs and symptoms, allergies, medications, past medical history, last oral intake, events leading up to the problem) and the OPQRST mnemonic (onset, provocation, quality, radiation, severity, and time), respectively (**Figure 28-10**). Note whether patients have any underlying cardiac or respiratory conditions that could be worsened by altitude. Individuals with sleep apnea may become severely hypoxic at high altitudes. Ask patients about this condition during your evaluation. For patients who are experiencing shortness of breath, ask if it is associated with any pain or persists during rest. Ask patients if they have ever had problems like this on previous visits to high altitude. Also ask patients if they have any AMS-related symptoms such as a headache, difficulty sleeping, nausea, vomiting, or excessive fatigue.

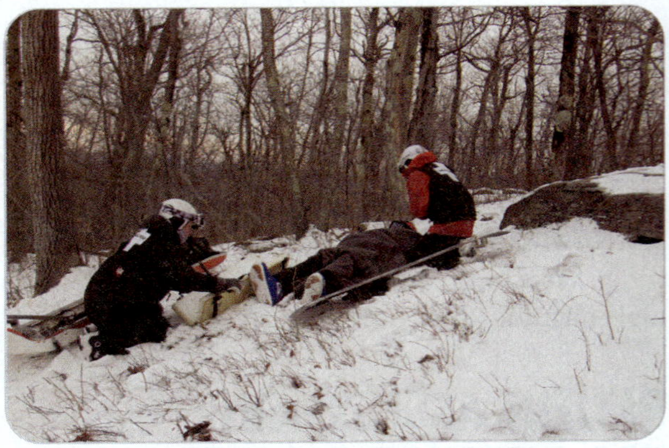

Figure 28-10 Ask the SAMPLE and OPQRST questions as an integral component of your assessment to fully understand what may be happening to the patient.

Physical examination of patients is best accomplished using the LAP exam, which involves looking, auscultating, and palpating. If possible, the exam may need to be deferred until patients have been moved inside because environmental conditions can make examining patients especially challenging.

Begin the physical exam by allaying the patient's fears by explaining what you will do. Then place the patient into a position of comfort, which may well be an upright position that allows the person to breathe more easily. Note whether the patient appears short of breath at rest. Inspect the conjunctivae, lips, and nail beds for discoloration or cyanosis, and the face, hands, ankles, and feet for edema. Examine the inside of the mouth for any pink (blood-tinged) saliva or sputum. If a stethoscope is available and you have been trained to do so, auscultate the lungs for any abnormal sounds that could indicate the presence of pulmonary edema. See if there are any visual problems, especially a decrease in acuity.

Complete the physical exam by thoroughly palpating the body for areas of tenderness or swelling, and by assessing distal skin temperature, circulation, movement, and sensation. For patients who are complaining of symptoms that suggest AMS or HACE, attempt to assess them for ataxia by asking them to walk a straight line, heel to toe. Evidence of unsteadiness or an inability to maintain balance at high altitude suggests HACE, which requires immediate treatment. Perform reassessments, including serial sets of vital signs, as needed.

MANAGEMENT FOR ALTITUDE-RELATED EMERGENCIES

The treatment of patients who present with a suspected altitude-related disorder is generally supportive in nature, and early recognition is the key to a successful outcome. *The fundamental treatment for all cases of altitude illness is to descend to a lower elevation*. Depending on the severity of symptoms, descent may need to be done urgently. Serious illnesses such as HAPE and HACE require more aggressive therapies, but OEC technicians can begin effective early treatment. As with any emergency, scene and rescuer safety take precedence over everything else. Do not risk yourself or others in a rescue. Be sure to remove potential hazards or move patients to a location where their conditions can be safely managed.

General Management

Initial treatment for all altitude-related illnesses includes correcting any problems involving the ABCDs and placing patients into a position of comfort. If there was trauma, control excessive bleeding and provide spinal motion restriction if indicated. Immediate administration of high-flow oxygen via nonrebreather mask keeping the oxygen saturation between 94 and 99%, especially when combined with rapid descent to a lower elevation, can be lifesaving. Keep patients warm by using jackets, blankets, reflective blankets, or sleeping bags as necessary, because cold stress elevates pulmonary pressures, decreases peripheral blood flow, and can worsen shock (**Figure 28-11**). Anticipate vomiting and be ready to clear the airway by removing the oxygen mask and turning patients onto their sides. Suction the airway as needed.

KEY POINT

Descent Is Key

The fundamental treatment for all types of altitude illness is descent to a lower altitude.

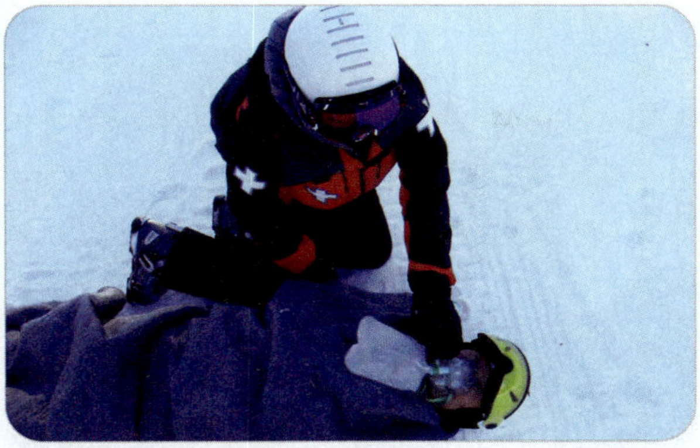

Figure 28-11 Besides descent, treatment of altitude illness includes keeping patients warm and administering oxygen.

© Edward McNamara.

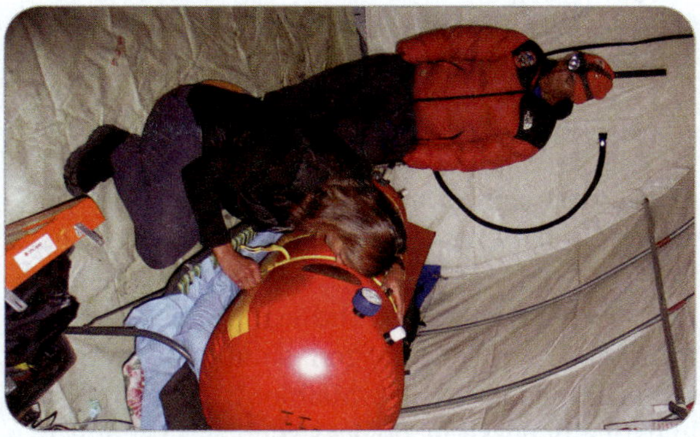

Figure 28-12 Use a Gamow bag if unlimited oxygen is available and descent must be delayed.

© Leanne Freer, MD.

Continue to monitor vital signs and prepare for transport because all patients with serious altitude illness require further evaluation and treatment at a definitive-care facility. Treatment of specific altitude-related disorders varies according to the underlying cause and the severity of symptoms.

AMS Treatment

Treatment of AMS centers on treating symptoms, halting ascent, and waiting for altitude acclimatization to improve, which can take 12 hours to several days. In all cases, minimize exertion to prevent the worsening of symptoms. High-flow oxygen, keeping the oxygen saturation between 94 and 99%, is particularly effective and can ease other symptoms such as headache and nausea. All other treatment is symptom based. For headache, which is a tell-tale sign of AMS, patients may self-administer conventional analgesics such as acetaminophen or ibuprofen. If acetazolamide has not been taken and the patient has a prescription for this medication, 250 mg twice a day may help treat AMS. If symptoms do not resolve, descent is indicated.

HAPE Treatment

The treatment of HAPE depends on equipment availability and other resources. If oxygen is scarce or unavailable, the emergent treatment for HAPE is rapid descent to an elevation that is at least 1,500 to 3,000 feet lower than the elevation at which symptoms were first observed. Unless there is no other way, avoid self-evacuation because it increases respiratory demands. Patients should be transported in a sitting position to a lower elevation as rapidly as possible. Rescue groups should make delivery of oxygen to the patient a top priority.

> **KEY POINT**
>
> **Gamow Bag**
>
> A Gamow bag functions as a mini-hyperbaric chamber. The patient is placed into the bag, which is then inflated to a pressure that simulates a temporary descent to a lower altitude.

If unlimited oxygen is available, descent may be delayed *for rescuer safety,* at least for a while, because oxygen immediately reduces pulmonary arterial blood pressure. In severe cases, the use of specialized devices such as a **Gamow bag** can be lifesaving (**Figure 28-12**).

Following evacuation to a lower altitude, patients should be transported to a hospital for further evaluation and treatment, which typically consists of rest and supplemental oxygen. In many cases, medications that reduce pulmonary blood pressure may be administered. Upon release from the hospital, patients are advised to resume normal activities gradually and are warned that it can take up to 2 weeks to recover their strength completely.

HACE Treatment

At the first sign of ataxia or a change in responsiveness, patients should be transported to a lower altitude, at least 1,500 to 3,000 feet below the elevation at which the symptoms were first noticed. High-flow oxygen should be administered immediately, if available. If descent is not logistically possible, devices such as a Gamow bag can "buy time" until descent is possible and can significantly decrease morbidity and mortality. All other care is supportive in nature. Patients should be transported immediately to a hospital for definitive evaluation and treatment, which often includes the administration of steroids to reduce cerebral swelling.

HAFE Treatment

Usually treatment is not necessary for this unfortunate medical condition. A diet with no beer, no beans, and no flatulence-producing vegetables may help. The person may wish to carry a small aerosol room freshener to help manage odor for others nearby.

Khumbu Cough Treatment

Khumbu cough is treated by placing a mask, a balaclava, or other cloth material over the mouth and nose to warm and humidify the air before it is inhaled into the lungs (**Figure 28-13**). Warm beverages also can help keep the airway passages warm and moist. If available, inhaled steam can be both soothing and preventive.

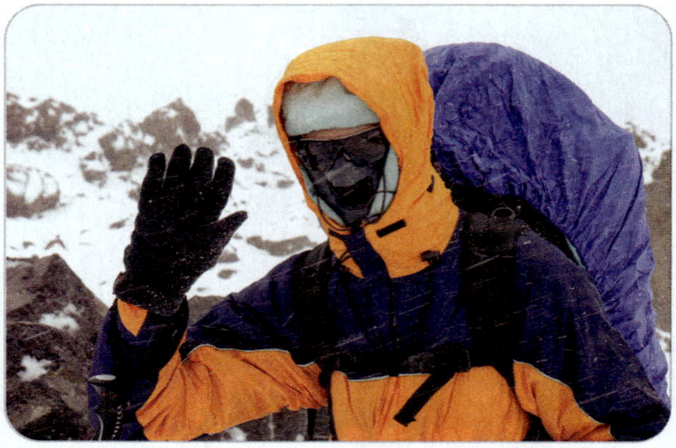

Figure 28-13 Treatment of Khumbu cough includes using a balaclava, a mask, and/or warm drinks to warm and moisten the air before it enters the mouth and nose.

Treatment of Other Problems

Other medical problems that may be aggravated by high altitude are treated in the usual manner but may not resolve with conventional therapies until the patient is transported to a lower altitude. Patients experiencing visual problems need to descend with the help of "a guide." They should seek care from a physician, preferably one trained in pathological conditions of the eye.

CASE Outcome

You are concerned that the patient has early signs of HAPE. You place her on high-flow oxygen, keep her comfortable, and mobilize resources to transport her to a hospital that is approximately 1,500 feet lower than your present location. Her oxygen saturation remains at 98% by pulse oximeter. Two days later, the patient's husband stops by the patrol room and thanks you "for taking such great care of my wife." He reports that her symptoms completely resolved within a day after descent and administration of supplemental oxygen. He further states that his wife was advised to either avoid going to a high altitude or to ascend more slowly on her next trip to a high elevation. She also was encouraged to speak with her private physician about using a prophylactic medication that can help prevent future episodes of HAPE.

CHAPTER REVIEW

In Summary

- Altitude illness can become life threatening.
- Once symptoms of AMS develop, do not ascend further until symptoms completely resolve.
- *Prevention* of altitude illness, when climbing to high altitude, is always preferred to treatment.
- Suspect HACE in the presence of headache and ataxia when at high altitude.
- Descent and supplemental oxygen almost always improve the symptoms of altitude illness.

Key Terms

Acclimatization The body's physiological process of *gradual* adjustment to changes in altitude. (Term also can be used for adjustment to light or temperature.)

Acute mountain sickness (AMS) A medical condition that is caused by exposure to high altitude.

Altitude illness Any type of illness caused by exposure to high altitude.

Ataxia Uncoordinated muscle movements; at high altitudes, it is associated with high-altitude cerebral edema.

Gamow bag A portable hyperbaric chamber that is used to treat altitude illness.

High-altitude cerebral edema (HACE) A potentially deadly condition in which the brain swells in individuals at high altitude.

High-altitude pulmonary edema (HAPE) A condition in which fluid accumulates in the lungs of individuals at high altitude.

Hypoxemia Insufficient oxygenation of the blood.

Khumbu cough A dry, persistent cough caused by inhaling excessively cold, dry air that is typical at high altitude; also known as high-altitude bronchitis and "dry hack cough."

Sleeping altitude The altitude to which a climber *descends* to sleep when climbing at high altitude; typically 500 to 1,000 feet below the highest elevation of that day's ascent.

Chapter Questions

1. Altitude is defined as:
   a. the height or vertical elevation below sea level (zero feet).
   b. the height or vertical elevation above sea level (zero feet).
   c. the height or horizontal elevation below sea level (zero feet).
   d. the height or horizontal elevation above sea level (zero feet).
2. As altitude increases, oxygen concentration in the air:
   a. decreases, resulting in higher oxygen intake per breath.
   b. increases to 50% at high altitudes.
   c. decreases, resulting in a lower oxygen intake per breath.
   d. B and C only
3. You are more at risk of developing altitude illness if you:
   a. rapidly ascend from sea level to 6,500 feet or higher.
   b. are genetically less likely to acclimate to changes in altitude.
   c. "climb high but don't sleep low."
   d. All of the above
4. Which of the following is *not* a strategy to prevent altitude illness?
   a. Ascend gradually, especially if you begin at sea level and continue above 10,000 feet.
   b. Perform heavy physical activity for the first 24 to 48 hours before going to high altitude.
   c. Stay hydrated by drinking lots of liquids (sometimes 3 to 4 quarts per day).

d. Avoid alcohol and other depressant drugs because they decrease the respiratory drive during sleep.

5. Acute mountain sickness is characterized by which of the following sign(s) and symptom(s)?
   a. Pink (blood-tinged) frothy sputum
   b. Hallucinations and psychotic behavior
   c. Mild to moderate headache accompanied by dizziness, fatigue, dyspnea on exertion, and nausea
   d. Increased flatulence
6. Classic signs and symptoms of a patient experiencing high-altitude pulmonary edema include:
   a. marked fatigue during exercise.
   b. severe dyspnea on exertion, progressing to labored breathing at rest with audible chest congestion.
   c. pink (blood-tinged) frothy sputum.
   d. All the above
7. Which of the following finding(s) during your assessment would suggest your patient is experiencing acute mountain sickness?
   a. During the SAMPLE history, the alert and oriented patient tells you she started taking Diamox 24 hours prior to ascending to a high altitude.
   b. The patient has headache, nausea, dizziness, and loss of appetite.
   c. During the SAMPLE history, the patient states she has a mild headache, fatigue, loss of appetite, and nausea, but denies shortness of breath.
   d. A and C only
8. Besides descent, treatment of altitude illness includes keeping patients warm and:
   a. laying all patients flat.
   b. administering oxygen at high flow by nonrebreather.
   c. administering your prescription for Diamox because the patient does not have his own prescription.
   d. withholding fluids.

Answers: 1. b, Objective 28-1, p. 656; 2. c, Objective 28-2, p. 657; 3. d, Objective 28-3, p. 658; 4. b, Objective 28-4, p. 662; 5. c, Objective 28-5, p. 659; 6. d, Objective 28-5, p. 659; 7. b, Objective 28-6, p. 659; 8. b, Objective 28-7, p. 664

CHAPTER 29

WATER-RELATED EMERGENCIES

OBJECTIVES

Upon completion of this chapter, the OEC technician will be able to:

29-1 Define drowning.

29-2 Explain the following water-related emergencies:
- Arterial gas embolism (AGE)
- Decompression sickness (DCS)

29-3 Discuss spinal injuries in submersion incidents.

29-4 Explain swimmer's ear, including assessment and care.

29-5 Explain how to assess a patient with one of the following water-related emergencies:
- Drowning
- Descent emergencies
- Ascent emergencies

29-6 Describe how to manage a patient who has suffered one of the following water-related emergencies:
- Drowning
- Descent emergency
- Ascent emergency

29-7 List multiple ways in which a water-based emergency may be prevented.

KEY TERMS

Arterial gas embolism (AGE), p. 673
Barotrauma, p. 672
Decompression sickness (DCS), p. 673
Drowning, p. 672
Laryngospasm, p. 672
Mammalian diving reflex, p. 671
Squeeze, p. 673

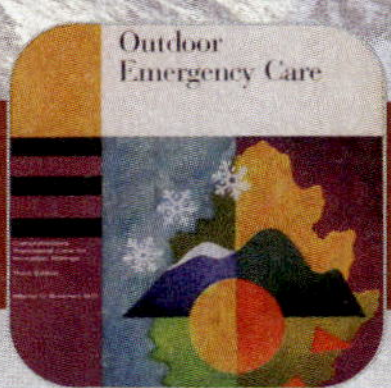

HISTORICAL TIMELINE 1998. *Outdoor Emergency Care, Third Edition*, is published.

CHAPTER OVERVIEW

Water-related injuries occur at any time and nearly anywhere (**Figure 29-1**). When people think of a water emergency, the image that usually comes to mind is of someone drowning in a recreational body of water, such as a swimming pool, a lake, or the ocean. But drowning can also occur in a bathtub, a well, or a creek. In fact, a person can drown in as little as 2 inches of standing water, in a bucket, or in a puddle like those found in any ski resort's parking lot (**Figure 29-2**).

Worldwide, an estimated 388,000 drowning deaths occur each year. However, this estimate is likely too low due to underreporting; nor does it include deaths caused by cataclysmic events such as natural disasters (e.g., tsunami, flood) or boating accidents (**Figure 29-3**). Drowning ranks second only to driving as a cause of accidental death. Moreover, it is the leading cause of death

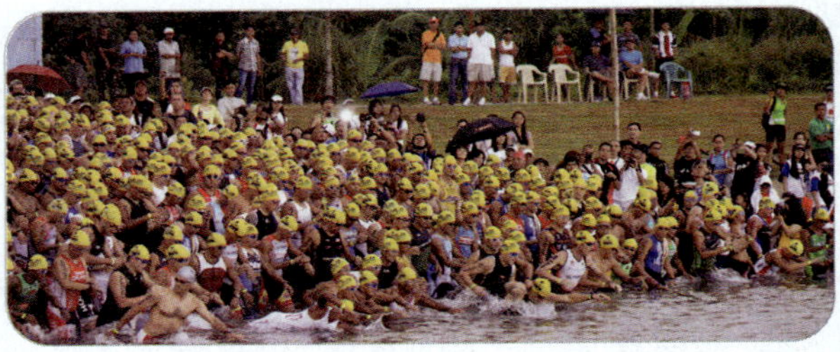

Figure 29-1 People gravitate toward water activities throughout the year. A water-related emergency may happen at any time.

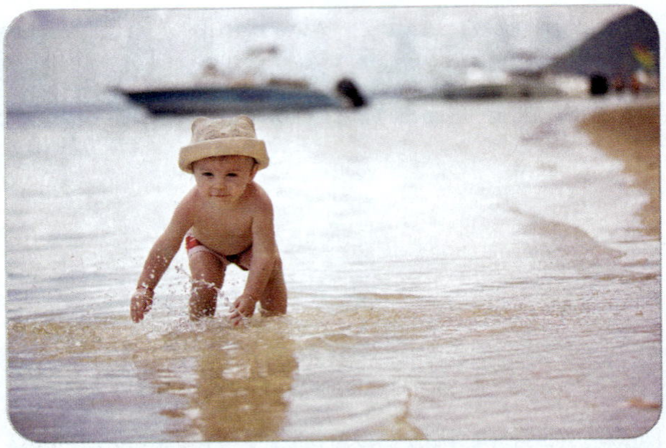

Figure 29-2 Drowning can occur in as little as 2 inches of water. This child is in more than 2 inches of water.

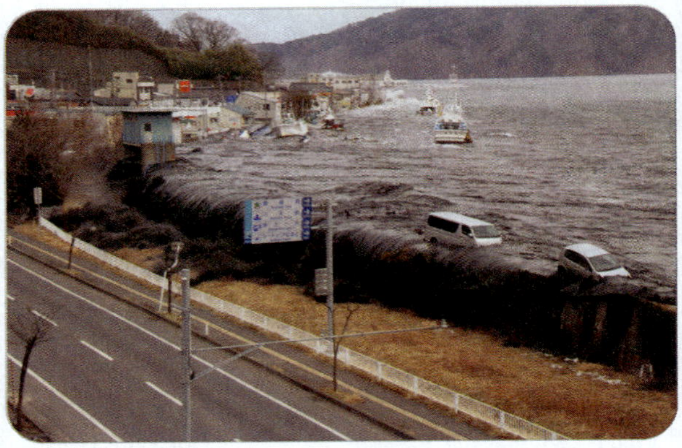

Figure 29-3 Statistical measures of drowning deaths do not include deaths caused by cataclysmic events.

CASE Presentation

You and several friends are at the ski resort's heated outdoor swimming pool when you hear shouts for help. As you near the scene in street clothes, you come upon bystanders who tell you someone is drowning. You see a teen-aged girl floating facedown in the water just under the diving board. You have someone stop people from using the diving board. There is a cervical collar and spine board nearby. You enter the water and with help quickly remove the girl from the water, protecting her neck. She is unresponsive and cyanotic. You notice that she has a large gash on the top of her head.

What should you do?

for infants and toddlers. According to the Centers for Disease Control and Prevention, an average of 10 people die in the United States from accidental drowning each day. For every one drowning death, an estimated 500 drowning victims survive but are injured.

OEC technicians will likely face a water-related emergency at some point in their career. In general, the assessment and initial stabilization of a patient with a water emergency are like those performed for other seriously injured patients. Understanding water-related emergencies and their complications will enable OEC technicians to more rapidly identify the problem and to render appropriate treatment in preparing patients for definitive care.

ANATOMY AND PHYSIOLOGY

Under normal conditions, the process of breathing is automatic. Air enters the nose or mouth, passes through the vocal cords into the trachea and bronchioles, and down into the alveoli. From there, oxygen molecules diffuse into the blood and are transported by red blood cells throughout the body. When a person's airway is submerged under water and an attempt is made to breathe, this process is interrupted, which can quickly lead to death by drowning.

A submersion injury is any injury that occurs when a person's airway is under water. A person submerged under water reflexively holds his or her breath. Depending on a person's overall health and conditioning, the person can hold off breathing for only a few seconds or up to several minutes, after which the body's internal increase in carbon dioxide and need for oxygen overrides any further attempts at breath-holding.

A person who must actively swim or "tread water" to remain above the water's surface will eventually become exhausted and give up, becoming submerged. The person will inhale water, which is aspirated into the bronchial tree and other airways. More water is brought into the lungs. Oxygenation of red blood cells becomes impossible, and the person suffocates, develops asphyxia, eventually suffers cardiac arrest, and dies.

Water temperature plays a significant role in morbidity and mortality of drowning victims. The survival rate is slightly higher for cold-water submersions than for warm-water submersions. Hypothermia has a cooling effect that slows tissue metabolism, slowing the death of tissue.

When the body is immersed or submerged in extremely cold water, peripheral blood vessels tightly constrict, which shunts warm blood away from the body surface, sending more to the heart and brain. At the same time, the body's metabolic and heart rates slow significantly, reducing oxygen demand and conserving oxygen. This very effective protective response, known as the **mammalian diving reflex**, helps to *temporarily* protect the heart and brain. Some patients have survived under cold water for more than 60 minutes due to this reflex. The mammalian diving reflex is most prominent in young children and, for reasons that are not fully understood, appears to diminish as a person gets older.

Even though cold-water submersion can occur at any time of year, most incidents occur during the winter and are typically associated with falling through ice.

PREVENTING WATER EMERGENCIES

As with other sports, water-based activities carry certain inherent risks of injury. Fortunately, many of these risks can be mitigated or prevented altogether by heeding the following recommendations:

- Avoid alcohol and other drugs when around water.
- Use proper safety equipment, including approved personal flotation devices (PFDs).
- Place fencing and self-closing gates around swimming pools.
- Never swim alone.
- Monitor the activities of anyone (*especially children and autistic people*) who is in or near the water.
- Never enter swiftly moving water.
- Confirm water depth before diving; never dive into water that is not deep enough.
- Check the thickness of the ice before traversing it.
- Scuba dive conservatively; ascend slowly while breathing normally.
- Watch for rip currents (currents that go *out* into the ocean).

COMMON WATER EMERGENCIES

Drowning

Drowning is defined as the process of respiratory impairment caused by submersion or immersion in a liquid. In other words, it is suffocation by submersion in water. Alcohol consumption, pre-existing seizure disorders, unsupervised children, and autistic people near water are major risk factors. Children younger than 1 year tend to drown in bathtubs and small swimming pools because they cannot get out by themselves when they fall into the water. Children aged 1 to 4 years drown in larger swimming pools, while those aged 5 to 14 years tend to drown in lakes, ponds, rivers, and oceans. In adults, males are four times more likely to drown than are females.

Drowning typically progresses in the following sequence:

1. Panic, struggle with breath-holding, and submersion
2. Gasp, swallowing of water with or without **laryngospasm**
3. Hyperventilation, then hypoventilation
4. Unresponsiveness, then apnea
5. Relaxation of laryngospasm (The passive aspiration of water causes decreased gas exchange in lungs.)
6. Cardiopulmonary arrest

If a person initially survives a drowning incident, secondary effects can cause more problems. Pathogens such as bacteria or parasites may be aspirated deep into the delicate lung tissues, resulting in local or systemic infections. Following resuscitation, patients still have significant breathing problems from injury to the lungs, requiring intensive care at a hospital.

Scuba Diving Emergencies

There were approximately 3 million scuba sport divers in the United States between 2006 and 2017. Medical emergencies related to diving are occurring more frequently, both to experienced and novice divers (**Figure 29-4**). The injuries are separated into the three phases of the dive: descent, bottom, and ascent.

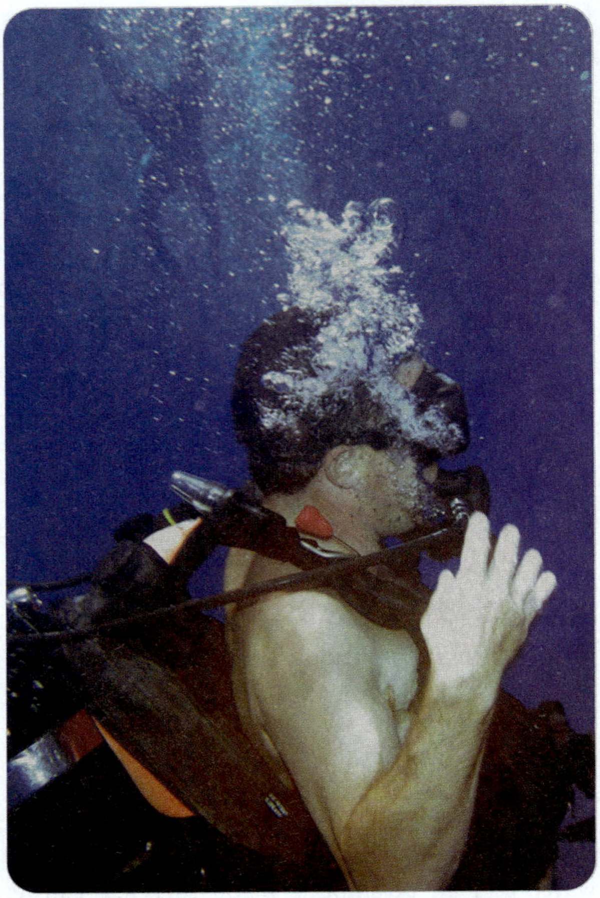

Figure 29-4 Medical emergencies may happen in scuba diving to both experienced and novice divers if participants are not careful.

Courtesy of Mass Communication Specialist 2nd Class Rebecca J. Moat/U.S. Navy.

Descent Emergencies

Barotrauma is a form of trauma that is caused by the difference in the pressure within air-filled structures of the body (e.g., sinuses, lungs, intestines, middle ear) and the pressure of the external environment. Such pressure differences result in the expansion or compression of the gas within those body structures. If the external pressure becomes too low, the unbalanced internal pressure within the structure can cause the structure to rupture. If the external pressure becomes too high, the internal pressure does not balance it and the organ is compressed.

There is severe pain as the pressure inside the organ or body cavity cannot adjust to the increased external pressure when diving to a depth. The resulting pressure is relieved by returning to the surface, thus equalizing the pressure, similar to how your ears "pop" when you rise in an airplane. However, if the person is very deep, rapid return to the surface may create other problems, described in the ascent section.

Squeeze is a generic term used to describe the effects of too much external pressure on various parts of the body. It is most commonly manifested in the ears. Squeeze can affect the ear if the canal between the middle ear and the nasopharynx (eustachian tube) is obstructed when descending to depth. The obstruction prevents the pressure in the middle ear from increasing to equalize with the pressure outside the eardrum. The resulting excessive pressure on the outside of the eardrum causes it to rupture. It is a more extreme version of the ear pain many people experience during descent in an airplane.

Emergencies at the Bottom

When scuba diving, the diver breathes air, not oxygen. Faulty equipment can cause poor mixing of oxygen and carbon dioxide, or other problems with breathing apparatus can cause drowning or problems when one rapidly ascends. These problems are rare, but usually very serious.

Equipment failures occurring during the deepest part of a dive can result in reduction or loss of air delivery to the diver. Depending on the depth, the diver may not have enough time to surface, even with rapid ascent, before the onset of anoxia and drowning. Some scuba systems, called rebreathers, filter out the diver's carbon dioxide, allowing the person's exhalations to be recirculated in order to minimize the amount of compressed air needed for a dive. Failures of this rebreather system can allow too little oxygen to be supplied as well as allowing carbon dioxide to be reinhaled, driving up carbon dioxide to dangerous levels in the diver's blood. In deep technical diving, the pressure is too great for compressed air to be used, so different gas mixes are used instead. Using an incorrect gas mix can result in hypoxia (too little oxygen supplied) or oxygen seizures (too much oxygen supplied). In some settings, contaminated air sources filling scuba tanks can also lead to underwater problems.

KEY POINT

The Term *Scuba*

Scuba is an acronym for *s*elf-*c*ontained *u*nderwater *b*reathing *a*pparatus.

Ascent Emergencies

Arterial gas embolism (AGE) is a serious, often life-threatening, medical problem caused by a rapid ascent during which a diver holds his or her breath and does not breathe (exhale) properly. When this occurs, the gas within the lungs expands too much and the alveoli rupture. The air from the ruptured portions of the lung then enters the bloodstream, resulting in air emboli. Air can get into the pleural space or mediastinum (the space in the middle of the chest between the lungs), resulting in a pneumothorax or pneumomediastinum. Approximately 6% of all diving problems involve AGE.

Decompression sickness (DCS), also known as "the bends," is a condition in which nitrogen bubbles develop within the blood vessels, obstructing blood flow. It occurs in scuba divers who stay at depth too long, ascend too rapidly, or do repeated dives without allowing enough time for the body to recover. It may also occur if a diver travels to high altitude (by either plane or car) too quickly after diving. DCS results when dissolved nitrogen within the blood and other tissues forms bubbles as nitrogen comes out of solution too quickly. Small bubbles combine, forming larger bubbles within the tissues, causing blood vessel blockage, severe pain, and major complications. Also called "the bends," the patient doubles up or bends over from joint and abdominal pain (**Figure 29-5**). This condition is like air embolism; however, generally air embolism occurs immediately on return to the surface, while DCS may not occur for several hours.

To illustrate this process, consider a bottle of carbonated soda. Dissolved within the liquid soda is carbon dioxide, a gas that gives the liquid its characteristic "fizz." The carbon dioxide cannot be seen because it is under pressure. Once the bottle is opened, however, the pressure within the bottle is rapidly released, causing carbon dioxide bubbles to form. In a diver who has ascended from a depth, dissolved nitrogen in the blood forms bubbles as the pressure of the water is reduced

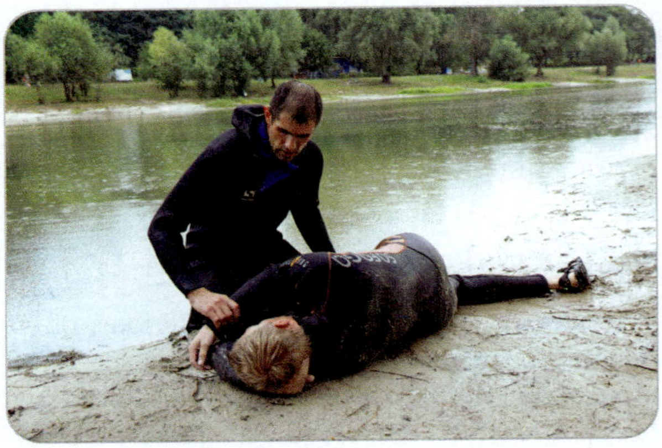

Figure 29-5 This person has decompression sickness ("the bends") and has been placed in the recovery position while awaiting transport to a medical facility.

by ascent. These bubbles then migrate from the bloodstream into the tissues, causing severe muscle and joint pain. Sometimes, large nitrogen bubbles can become emboli and block blood flow to critical organs.

DCS can be exacerbated by several factors, including, but not limited to, insufficient hydration, increased respiratory rate at depth, carbon dioxide retention, colder temperatures, cigarette and/or alcohol consumption, and exertion during the dive.

Although very rare, in "reverse" squeeze, during ascent, the eardrum can rupture from pressure in the middle ear pushing outward, as the external pressure decreases, resulting in severe ear pain. You may have experienced the sensation of pressure buildup or release (without the eardrum rupturing) during ascent or descent in an airplane flight or in a vehicle ride up or down a mountain road. This sensation is what makes some small children cry while flying, as they cannot equilibrate the pressure as well as adults can. More commonly, facial pain occurs as air expands inside the face's "unvented" sinuses.

Swimmer's Ear

Swimmer's ear is an acute bacterial infection of the external auditory (ear) canal that occurs when the skin of the external canal remains wet for a prolonged period (**Figure 29-6**). Patients usually present with severe ear pain, a yellowish discharge from the ear, and tenderness upon pushing on the tragus (the anatomic bump in front of the ear canal). Children and teenagers are more prone to this disorder, as are individuals with diabetes and immune system disorders. Most of the many preventive treatments available are mildly acidic or alcohol-based solutions that make the ear canal dry and inhospitable to bacteria.

Breath-Holding

To travel farther or deeper while under water, swimmers will sometimes intentionally hyperventilate to dramatically increase the amount of oxygen in their lungs and allow them to hold their breath longer. Unfortunately, hyperventilating also decreases the amount of carbon dioxide in the lungs, which removes the body's stimulus to breathe. As a result, *rarely* the person may pass out and drown. This condition most commonly affects children and young adults, and swimming pools are the most frequent setting.

CASE Update

You direct one of your friends to call 9-1-1 to get EMS help. The gash on the head and the shallow water suggest a cervical spine injury, so you protect the spine as you assess and correct the ABCDs. Using a jaw thrust, you open the airway, assess the carotid pulse, and look for breaths. She is not breathing. She has a weak carotid pulse, at 60 beats per minute, and her skin is cool to the touch. A cervical collar is applied to the patient's neck. A bystander says she knows CPR, so she begins rescue breathing with the pocket mask you have with you. You are holding the patient's neck in alignment.

What should you do now?

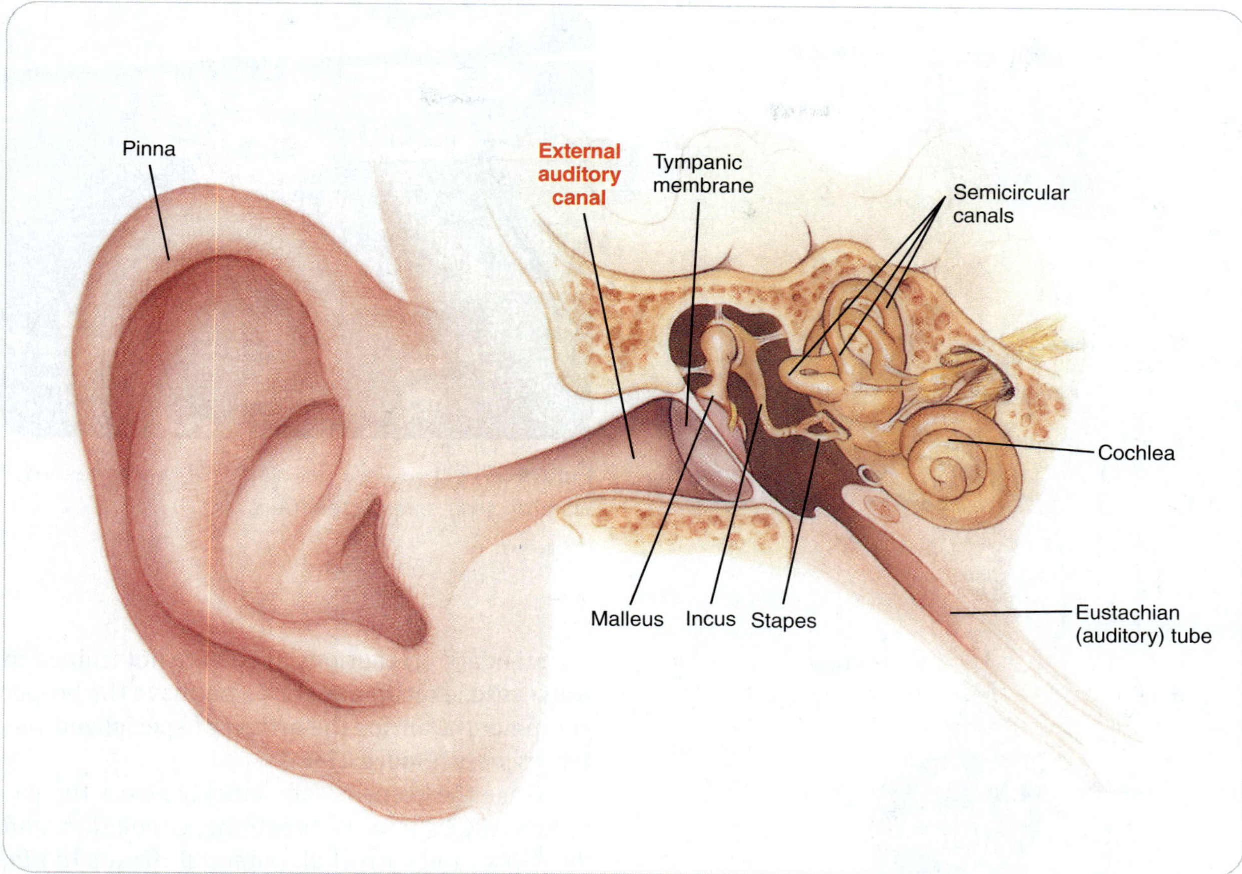

Figure 29-6 Swimmer's ear occurs in the external auditory canal.

KEY POINT

Water-Related Rescue Methods

For water-related rescues, try the following methods in the order they are presented here for alert victims (**Figure 29-7**):

1. *Reach* to the patient using a solid object such as a branch, an oar, or a pole.
2. *Throw* a rescue device such as a rope or a flotation device to the victim.
3. *Row* a boat to the patient.
4. *Go* (swim) to the patient (the last resort and the most dangerous option).

Many of these techniques, especially in-water rescues, require additional training. Carefully assess the conditions, your own abilities and training, available equipment, and support services before entering the water.

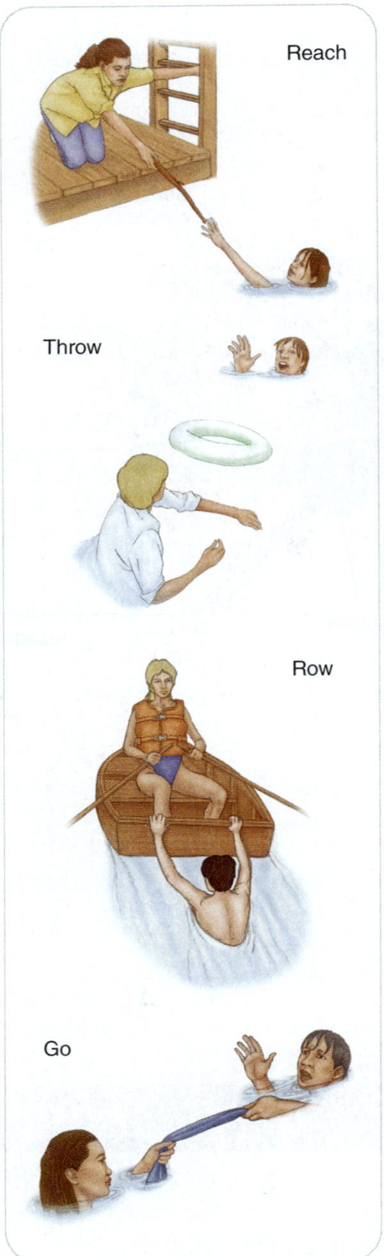

Figure 29-7 Basic rules of water rescue.

PATIENT ASSESSMENT FOR WATER-RELATED EMERGENCIES

The assessment of patients with a water-related emergency starts with ensuring the safety of yourself and others. Safety measures may include putting on a PFD, a helmet, and other safety equipment as the situation requires. When necessary, use standard precautions. If you are not trained in water rescue techniques or do not have the proper equipment, wait for the arrival of specialized water rescuers (**Figure 29-8**).

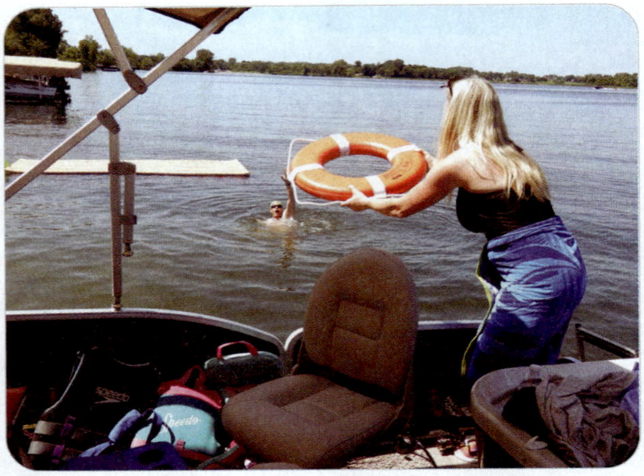

Figure 29-8 If you are not trained in water rescue, wait for professional rescuers.

Once the scene is safe, quickly assess the patient's ABCDs (airway, breathing, circulation, and disability) and correct all potential threats to life, including excessive bleeding before proceeding to a secondary assessment. Perform CPR if needed.

In any submersion injury, if necessary, carefully assess and protect the spine to prevent additional neurologic injury. Whenever possible, this should be initiated before the person is removed from the water. It may be easier to apply a cervical collar and place the patient onto a backboard in shallow water than to perform these procedures after you have removed the person from the water.

Spinal fractures and spinal cord injuries in submersion injuries may complicate the drowning. Spinal motion restriction may be needed. Spine trauma may be present if the following has occurred:

1. The submersion injury is associated with a diving mishap or fall from a height.
2. The patient is unresponsive, and there is no witness to the drowning, particularly in the ocean surf.
3. There is weakness, paralysis, or numbness in the arms or legs.

Unless the patient has serious or life-threatening injuries, perform a complete secondary assessment using the DCAP-BTLS mnemonic (deformity, contusions, abrasions/avulsions, punctures/penetrations, burns/bleeding/bruises, tenderness, lacerations, swelling). Additionally, perform a complete neurologic exam on all noncritical patients. Assess the vital signs, level of responsiveness, skin condition, and capillary refill frequently because each may provide early indications of the presence of a serious underlying injury. As part of the history, attempt to obtain as much information as possible about what has occurred, including how long the person was submerged, water temperature and salinity, and the person's appearance immediately after being removed from the water. If possible, determine if the patient has any preexisting medical conditions or is taking any medications.

The following are potential signs and symptoms of AGE, DCS, and swimmer's ear:

- AGE
  - Blotching or mottling of the skin
  - Frothy (sometimes pink) sputum
  - Severe pain in the muscles, joints, and abdomen
  - Shortness of breath and/or chest pain
  - Dizziness, nausea, and vomiting
  - Cough
  - Cyanosis
  - Vision problems
  - Paralysis or coma
  - Irregular pulse or cardiac arrest
- DCS
  - Pain, particularly near the joints
  - Numbness or paresthesia
  - Headache, lightheadedness, unexplained fatigue, malaise, nausea and/or vomiting, or anorexia
  - Dizziness or vertigo
  - Muscle weakness and discomfort
  - Cutaneous, or skin, problems—such as an itch, rash, or mottling
  - Impaired mental status
  - Breathing difficulties ("the chokes")
  - Impaired coordination
  - Reduced level of consciousness
  - Hearing problems, such as hearing sounds that are not there or having a hard time hearing
  - Swelling
  - Retention of urine
  - Compromised cardiovascular function
- Swimmer's ear
  - Foul-smelling purulent material in ear canal
  - Pain in the ear
  - Redness in the external ear canal
  - Difficulty hearing in that ear

MANAGEMENT OF WATER-RELATED EMERGENCIES

The treatment of a patient who has suffered a water-related injury depends on the nature of the injury and the severity of the patient's symptoms. Remove all patients from the water as quickly as possible, protecting the spine if needed. Victims with obvious clinical signs of injury, alcohol intoxication, or a history of diving into shallow water are at a higher risk of spinal cord injury. OEC technicians may consider spinal motion restriction for these victims. For these patients, initiate spinal motion restriction, preferably while the patient is still in the water (**Figure 29-9**). Rescue breaths may be given in the water; however, chest compressions are not practical in the water.

For any patient who has a submersion injury, after removal from the water, open the airway and simultaneously check for breathing and a carotid pulse. If there is no breathing or pulse begin CPR, *but start the cycle with 2 breaths*. This is a variation on the current CPR standards used for submersion injuries. If the patient has a pulse but is not breathing, immediately begin rescue breathing. There is no evidence that water in the respiratory system acts as an obstructive foreign body, so do not attempt to remove it. Maneuvers to relieve foreign-body airway obstruction are not recommended for drowning victims because such maneuvers are not necessary and can cause injury, vomiting, aspiration, and delay of CPR.

Call for advanced medical providers and transportation as soon as possible. When rescuing a drowning victim of any age, it is reasonable for the lone OEC technician to give 5 cycles (about 2 minutes) of CPR before leaving the victim to activate the EMS system. Victims with obvious clinical signs of injury, alcohol intoxication, or a history of diving into shallow water are at a higher risk of spinal cord injury, and OEC technicians may consider spinal motion restriction of the cervical and thoracic spine for these victims. For

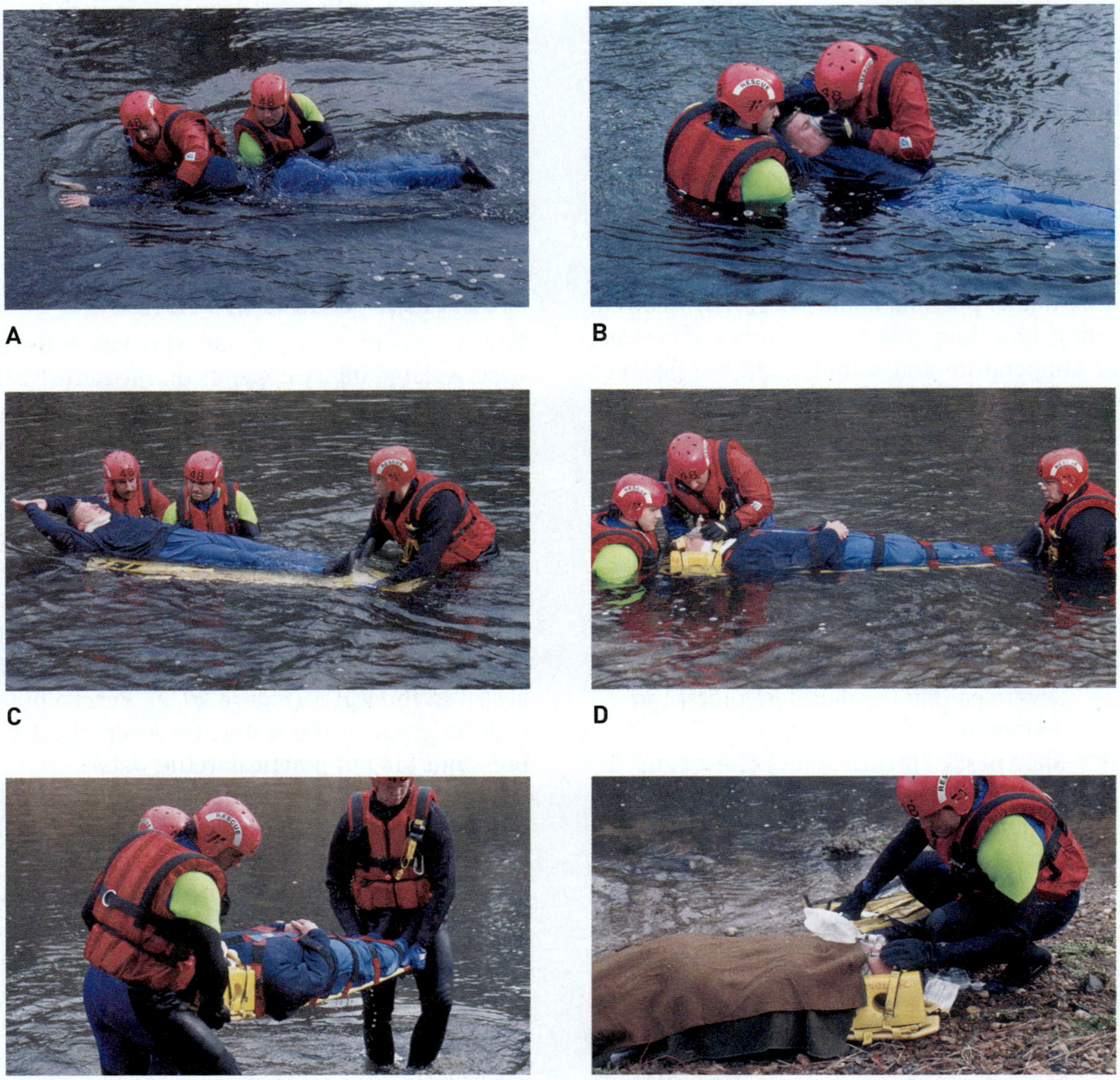

A B C D E F

Figure 29-9 Water rescue technique; note the precautions for a spinal injury. **A.** Step 1: Turn the patient to a supine position by rotating the entire upper half of the body as a single unit. **B.** Step 2: As soon as the patient is turned, begin artificial ventilation using the mouth-to-mouth method or a pocket mask. **C.** Step 3: Float a buoyant backboard under the patient. **D.** Step 4: Secure the patient to the backboard. **E.** Step 5: Remove the patient from the water. **F.** Step 6: Maintain the body's normal temperature and apply oxygen if the patient is breathing. Begin CPR if breathing and pulse are absent.

these patients, initiate spinal precautions, preferably while the patient is still in the water.

For a patient who has a pulse and respirations, if there is no concern for spinal cord injury, when on dry land place patients onto their sides to allow vomiting of gastric contents without aspiration and facilitate the drainage of water and debris from the upper airway. If spinal motion restriction is in place, tip the spine board to the side. Suction the airway as needed.

Thoroughly dry submersion patients and cover them with blankets, jackets, or a sleeping bag to reduce the risk of hypothermia. If breathing, place the patient on high-flow oxygen via a nonrebreather mask, and treat for shock, if present. When a pulse oximeter is available, titrate the oxygen to between 94 and 99%. Patients require ALS care and rapid transport, especially those who are not breathing or have a pneumothorax. In stable patients who are breathing, treat any soft-tissue or orthopedic injuries.

All patients who have suffered a submersion injury should be transported to the nearest hospital for further evaluation and treatment, *even if they seem to fully recover following appropriate field care.* Patients with suspected AGE or DCS require specialized care and should be transported by ground to a facility with a hyperbaric chamber because repressurization and the administration of supplemental oxygen are required to treat these disorders definitively. For additional information regarding the emergent treatment of diving injuries or barotraumas, contact the Divers Alert Network, available 24 hours a day, 7 days a week at 1-919-684-9111.

All patients who appear to be dead after removal from *cold* water should receive CPR and be transported to the hospital because the severe bradycardia induced by submersion in cold water can cause the heart rate to drop so low that the person appears pulseless. These patients can often be successfully resuscitated, even after an extended time under water.

Swimmer's ear is treated by keeping the external canal of the ear and the eardrum dry. Antibiotics are needed when infection occurs.

KEY POINT

Divers Alert Network

For immediate assistance concerning diving injuries or barotraumas, call the Divers Alert Network, available around the clock at 1-919-684-9111.

KEY POINT

When Is a Patient Dead?

Remember that *patients are not dead until they are warm and dead!* This is especially true in cold-water drowning.

CASE Outcome

Rescue breathing continues while others dry the patient off and cover her with towels. The head and neck are kept aligned. Within a few minutes, she starts to breathe on her own. Oxygen is provided, and full spinal motion restriction is applied. Vital signs improve. The patient is transferred to a trauma center, where she is diagnosed with a cervical spine fracture. Although her road to recovery will be long, she is expected to regain full neurologic function after spinal surgery.

CHAPTER REVIEW

In Summary

- Water emergencies can occur anytime and anywhere and may be life threatening.
- A person may be successfully resuscitated, even after being submerged in cold water for a long time.
- Spinal cord injury should be suspected in any patient with a submersion injury to which there was no witness.
- For all patients who have suffered a submersion injury, provide high-flow oxygen, titrating oxygen saturation to between 94 and 99% with a pulse oximeter, when available.
- In cold-water submersion, hypothermia may enable a person to survive prolonged submersion.
- All patients who suffer a submersion injury should be transported to the hospital for follow-up, even if they appear normal, because complications can arise several hours or even days after the incident and may be mitigated by prompt treatment.
- Patients are not dead until they are warm and dead in cold water drowning!

Key Terms

Arterial gas embolism (AGE) A condition that occurs immediately after rapid ascent in which air bubbles enter the bloodstream from a ruptured alveolus and lodge in an artery.

Barotrauma Trauma that is caused by differences in pressure between the body and the environment.

Decompression sickness (DCS) Formation of nitrogen bubbles in tissues from being underwater too long or ascending too rapidly.

Drowning The process of respiratory impairment caused by submersion or immersion in a liquid.

Laryngospasm Spasm of the vocal cords that prevents air movement through the respiratory tract.

Mammalian diving reflex A protective response when the body is immersed or submerged in extremely cold water whereby the metabolic and heart rates slow significantly, reducing oxygen demand and conserving oxygen.

Squeeze Severe pain when the pressure inside an organ or body cavity cannot adjust to increased external pressure.

Chapter Questions

1. Drowning is defined as impairment of what body system from submersion/immersion in a liquid?
    a. Cardiovascular
    b. Respiratory
    c. Circulatory
    d. Muscular
2. What water-related emergency results when dissolved nitrogen in the blood and other tissues forms bubbles, causing blood vessel blockage and severe pain?
    a. Swimmer's ear
    b. Bubble blocking drowning
    c. Decompression sickness
    d. Squeeze
3. Spine trauma may be present in a water emergency if which of the following has occurred?
    a. The submersion injury is associated with a diving mishap.
    b. The patient has "the bends."
    c. The patient becomes unconscious after hyperventilating.
    d. The patient has an arterial gas embolism.

4. Which of the following signs/symptoms would indicate to you that the patient may be experiencing swimmer's ear?
   a. Fever, itchy external ear
   b. Frothy sputum, dizziness, shortness of breath, and/or chest pain
   c. Foul-smelling purulent material in the ear canal, pain in the ear
   d. Both a and c
5. Upon entering the scene of a water-related emergency, you should begin by:
   a. quickly assessing the patient's ABCDs.
   b. assessing the spine and applying a spinal motion restriction device to prevent additional neurologic injury.
   c. ensuring your own and others' safety, using personal flotation devices as the situation requires.
   d. performing CPR, as necessary.
6. Sign(s) of an arterial gas embolism may include:
   a. frothy (sometimes pink) sputum, cough, cyanosis, and vision problems.
   b. skin problems (such as an itch, rash, or swelling) and impaired coordination.
   c. redness outside of the ear canal and puss (sometimes yellow) in the ear canal.
   d. cool skin and shivering/chattering.
7. You are called to assist a drowning victim. Witnesses say she hit her head on the diving board during a dive into the pool. She briefly lost consciousness and is now alert but is still in the water. The scene is safe, and you have completed your primary assessment. What is your next step?
   a. Complete a secondary assessment using the DCAP-BTLS mnemonic.
   b. Initiate spinal motion restriction in the shallow water by applying the cervical collar and placing her onto a backboard.
   c. Move her out of the water before spinal motion restriction to prevent further respiratory distress.
   d. Attempt to obtain as much information as possible about what has occurred, including water temperature and how long she was submerged.
8. Which of the following is *not* a precaution used to prevent a water-based emergency?
   a. Check the thickness of the ice before traversing it.
   b. Never enter swiftly moving water.
   c. Use proper safety equipment, including approved personal flotation devices.
   d. Avoid swimming up to 30 minutes after eating food.

Answers: 1. b, Objective 29-1, p. 672; 2. c, Objective 29-2, p. 673; 3. a, Objective 29-3, p. 676; 4. d, Objective 29-4, p. 677; 5. c, Objective 29-5, p. 676; 6. a, Objective 29-5, p. 677; 7. b, Objective 29-6, p. 676; 8. d, Objective 29-7, p. 671

CHAPTER 30

PEDIATRIC EMERGENCIES

OBJECTIVES

Upon completion of this chapter, the OEC technician will be able to:

30-1 List and describe the anatomic and physiologic differences between children and adults.

30-2 List and describe the six stages of child growth and development.

30-3 List the normal range of vital signs for each pediatric age group.

30-4 Explain and demonstrate how to communicate with a pediatric patient.

30-5 Describe the signs and symptoms of respiratory distress and failure in a child.

30-6 Identify the most common cause of cardiac arrest in pediatric patients.

30-7 List common causes of seizures in pediatric patients.

30-8 List indicators of potential child abuse and neglect.

30-9 Describe and demonstrate how to assess a pediatric patient.

30-10 Describe and demonstrate how to manage common pediatric illnesses and injuries.

30-11 Explain how to use the pediatric assessment triangle.

KEY TERMS

Child abuse, p. 696
Child neglect, p. 696
Epiglottitis, p. 691
Fontanels, p. 685
Meningitis, p. 693
Pediatric assessment triangle, p. 700
Shaken baby syndrome, p. 696
Sudden infant death syndrome (SIDS), p. 694

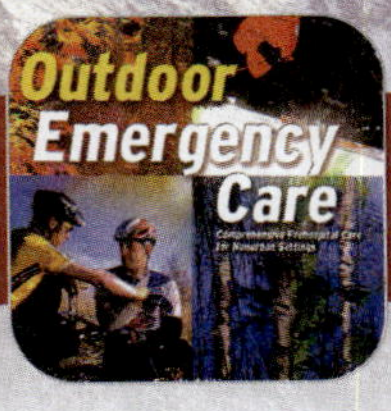

HISTORICAL TIMELINE 2003. *Outdoor Emergency Care, Fourth Edition*, is published.

CHAPTER OVERVIEW

Pediatric patients can be challenging for the OEC technician. There are different medical conditions, assessment challenges, and communication difficulties. Caring for a pediatric patient can be one of the most rewarding experiences an OEC technician can have; however, it can be stressful.

Children can present with different illnesses, problems, and patterns of trauma than adults (**Figure 30-1**). A child's unique physiology changes continually from birth to adulthood, which can make assessment and care difficult for OEC technicians. Problems such as respiratory distress, temperature regulation, or trauma can be more difficult to manage in young patients. Additionally, a child's ability to compensate for shock can cause a seemingly stable patient to deteriorate quickly.

This chapter defines medical conditions seen in the pediatric population. Variations in assessment, including age-related vital signs, are provided. It is essential that you can recognize the often-subtle clues that children may exhibit when they are ill or injured. The chapter describes strategies to help OEC technicians communicate with pediatric patients and their caregivers.

ANATOMY AND PHYSIOLOGY

Children are not miniature adults (**Figure 30-2**). The same basic anatomy and physiology is present, but differences in understanding, size, proportion,

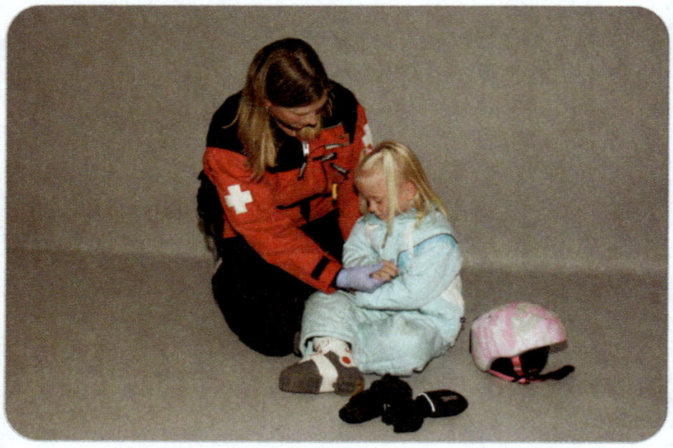

Figure 30-1 Children can present special challenges for emergency care providers because their medical needs differ from those of adults.

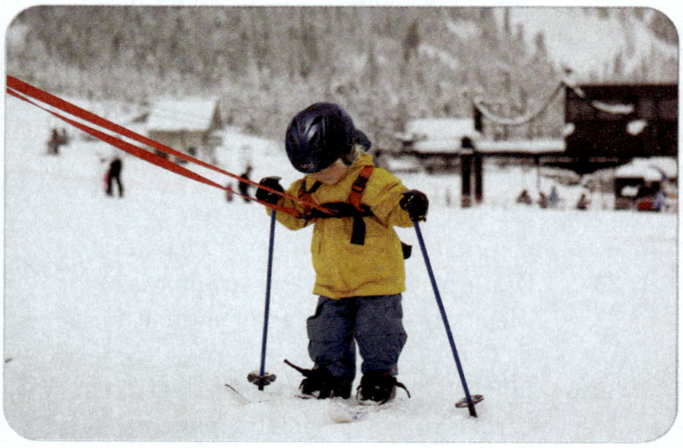

Figure 30-2 Many children participate in outdoor recreational activities, so OEC technicians need to know how to treat children. Remember: children are not "little adults."

CASE Presentation

You are skiing down an easy slope when you notice a woman frantically waving you down. She tells you that her 8-year-old granddaughter fell and landed with her arm outstretched. You find the girl sitting cradling her arm against her jacket. She is shivering. Her grandmother tells you that her upper arm and shoulder hurt. The girl is whimpering but screams and begins to cry when you approach.

What should you do?

and metabolism make pediatric patients unique. Large variations in behavior, vital signs, and the physical and emotional ability to cope with the stresses of injury and illness evolve as the child grows into a full-grown adult.

Two of the most important anatomic differences between children and adults are the size of the airway and the mechanism of breathing. These differences are especially relevant in infants and younger children, who have relatively small mouths and airways. Until approximately 8 years old, a child's tongue is proportionally larger in relation to the oral cavity, which increases the risk of airway obstruction by the tongue.

A child's trachea is shorter and smaller in diameter, and it is more flexible because the tracheal cartilages have not yet fully developed. For this reason, OEC technicians must be careful when opening the airway of an unresponsive child because hyperextension of the neck can cause the trachea to become compressed or even collapsed.

As children age, the oral cavity enlarges, the jaw elongates, and the tongue becomes proportionately flatter and smaller, allowing a relatively larger airway. The larynx sits higher and more anteriorly in the neck and is funnel shaped. Unlike an adult, the narrowest part of the child's airway is at the opening of the glottis (**Figure 30-3**). Because airway obstructions occur inferior to or below the vocal cords, the risk of foreign-body airway obstruction is increased in children.

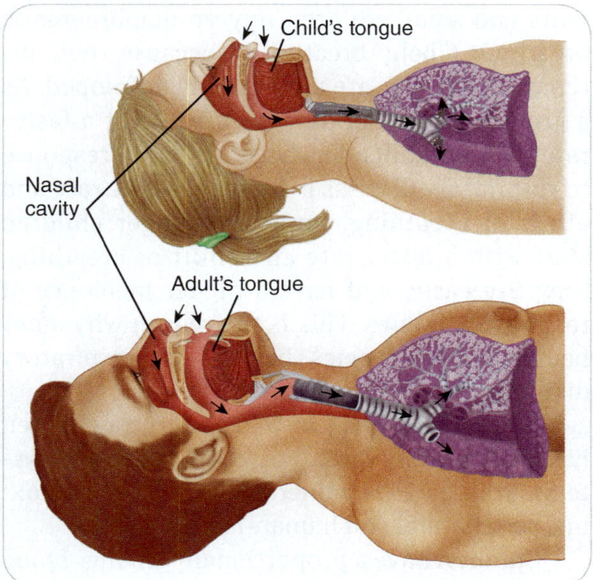

Figure 30-3 The respiratory anatomy of a child compared to that of an adult.

Anatomically, a child's head is proportionally *larger* and heavier in relation to the body than is an adult's head. This is more pronounced in younger children. As a result, young children are more susceptible to heat loss from the head, and during rapid deceleration the head is propelled forward first, before the body. A child's larger head also causes neck flexion when a spine board is used, which has implications for airway management and for maintaining a neutral cervical-spine alignment when a child's neck is immobilized.

Children also have a greater body surface area to mass ratio, thinner skin, and less muscle mass and body fat than adults. Thus, children are at greater risk for heat loss, faster absorption of toxins through the skin, morbidity from burns, and multiple organ injuries.

A child's musculoskeletal system is immature and grows rapidly, especially during the first year of life. The brain of an infant can grow because the cranial bones are not fused but instead are separated by gaps called **fontanels** (**Figure 30-4**). The larger of a newborn's two fontanels, the anterior fontanel, is in the front above the frontal bone; the posterior fontanel is in the back above the occipital bone. By approximately 18 months of age, both fontanels have closed, making the skull one continuous bony structure.

A child's bones, joints, and ligaments are softer and more flexible than those of an adult. The thoracic cage also is more pliable. As a result, a child's skeletal system generally can absorb more force without breaking. This is not entirely advantageous, however, because with trauma energy is transferred through the bones and muscles to the underlying structures, resulting in a higher rate of internal organ injury. A child's bones can bend without breaking (greenstick fracture).

Growth plates are found at the ends of long bones as well as within the bones, the pelvis, and the skull (**Figure 30-5**). With proper nutrition (especially an adequate supply of calcium), the growth plates produce cartilage, which later calcifies into bone, making the bone grow. The area of the growth plate is weak, and fractures at this site are common. Growth plates begin closing around age 12 years and usually disappear by age 16 years when adult size is reached.

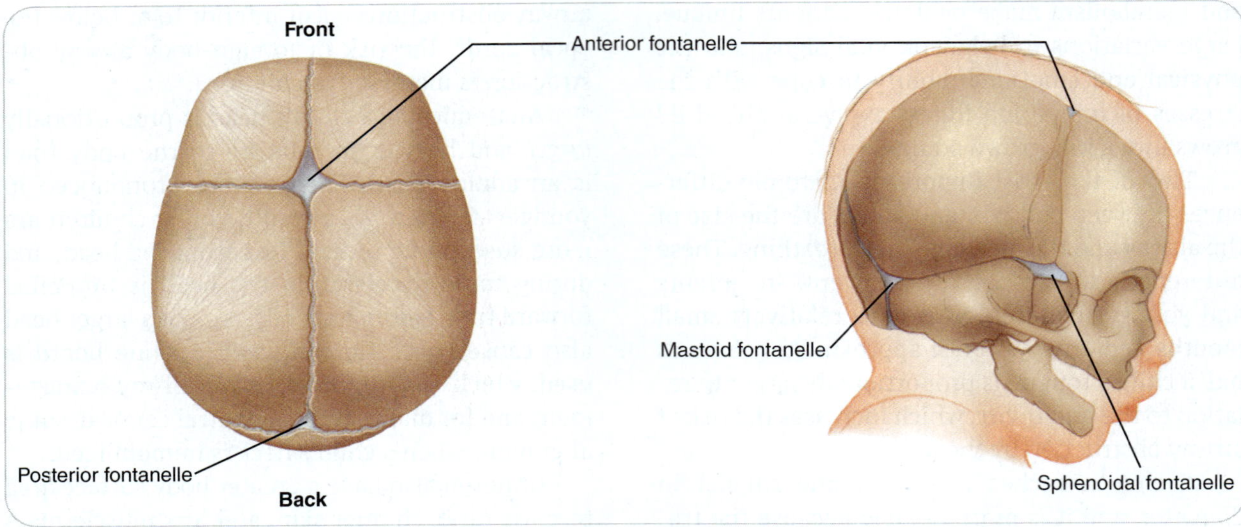

Figure 30-4 The fontanels.

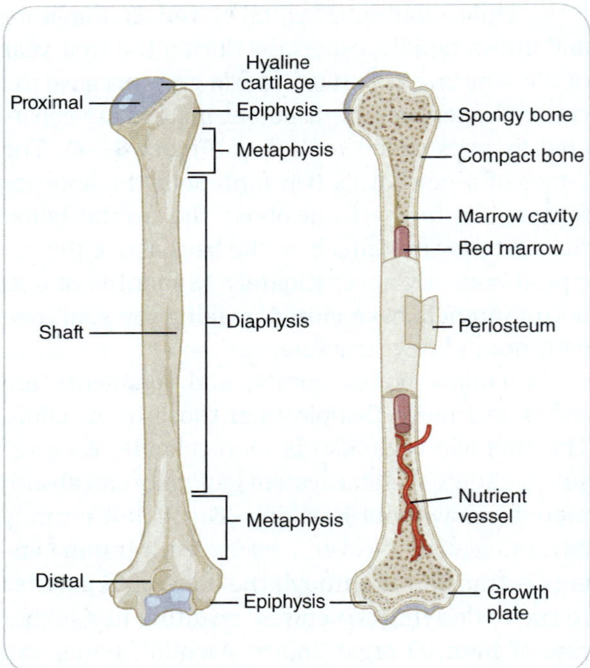

Figure 30-5 This shows the growth plate in children.

Compared to adults, children have a higher rate of metabolism (burn energy more quickly) and have fewer energy reserves. This explains why children exhibit great bursts of energy followed by sudden, profound fatigue. It also explains why children need regular meals and can consume enormous amounts of carbohydrates at once without ill effects. The younger the child, the more frequently meals are needed.

Children and adults also differ in how they breathe. With few exceptions, newborns breathe through their nose. If a newborn's nose becomes obstructed by mucus or a foreign body, breathing difficulty will occur quickly. Also, infants and small children rely on diaphragmatic breathing ("belly breathers") because their intercostal muscles are not yet fully developed. As a group, children of all ages breathe at a faster rate than do adults. The body's primary response to respiratory distress is to increase the rate and effort of breathing. Because younger children start with a faster rate and effort of breathing, they tire easily and have a higher incidence of respiratory failure. This is the reason why *many* pediatric emergencies begin with respiratory distress.

Unless born with a birth defect, most children have very healthy cardiovascular and nervous systems. Still, they are vulnerable to a variety of toxins, both natural and human-made.

Children have a proportionally smaller blood volume than adults yet can bleed at the same rate (**Figure 30-6**). They also have a higher heart rate and lower blood pressure. This combination enables a child to *initially* compensate better to

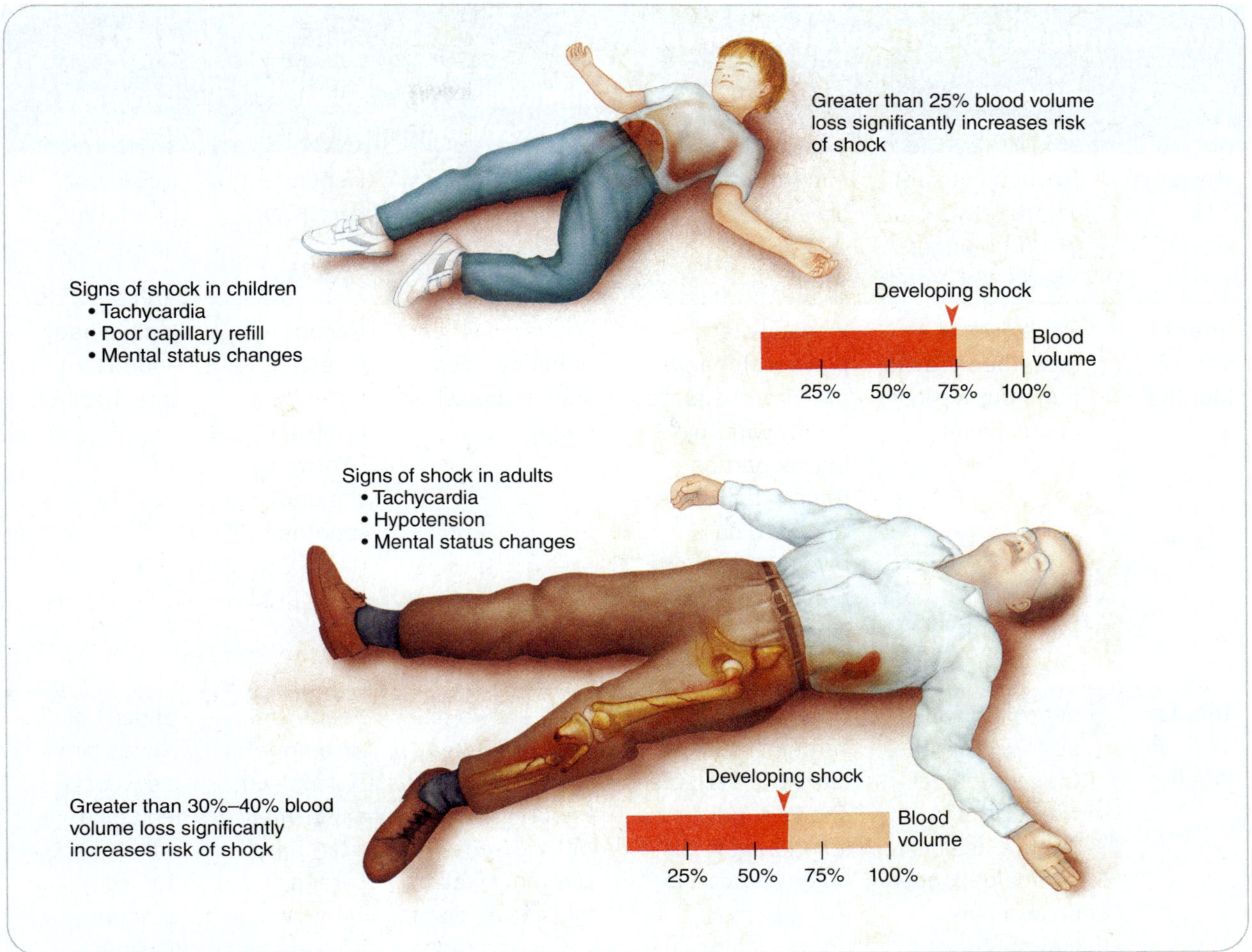

Figure 30-6 All children with abdominal injuries should be monitored closely for signs of shock. Although children may compensate for significant blood loss better than adults, shock develops in children after proportionally smaller blood losses.

shock. However, the compensatory mechanisms can fail quickly, which can cause an apparently healthy child to suddenly go into life-threatening shock, often with little or no warning. Hypovolemia, whether due to blood loss, vomiting, or diarrhea, can quickly lead to decompensated shock.

Due to an underdeveloped hypothalamus in the brain, children have difficulty regulating body temperature, which places them at high risk for both hyperthermia and hypothermia. A child's temperature can rapidly rise from illnesses to 40.6°C (105°F), creating an emergent condition. Equally important, the larger ratio of skin surface area to body mass in children (infants through school-age) can cause rapid cooling, which, when combined with a slow central nervous system response, can result in hypothermia.

HUMAN GROWTH AND DEVELOPMENT

Between birth and the age of 18 years, humans undergo a great variety of physical, intellectual, emotional, and social changes. Language evolves from crying and grunts to organized spoken words and written communication. The rate of change varies from child to child, but the pattern of development leading to adulthood moves through six identifiable but overlapping stages (**Table 30-1**).

1. Newborn (neonatal) stage
2. Infancy
3. Toddler
4. Preschool
5. School-age
6. Adolescence

Table 30-1 Human Growth and Development

Age	Physical Development	Intellectual Development	Emotional Development	Social Development	Language Development
Newborn 0 to 1 Month	Responds to light, temperature (cold or hot), hunger (taste), and sound	Minimum development	Cries if unhappy	Dependent on caregiver	Occasional unintelligible noise
Infant 1 to 12 Months	Rolls over at first, then crawls, pulls up; walks at about 1 year	Visually alert, plays with hands; at 6 months plays briefly with toys; learns names (mom, dad); learns to pinch; puts toys in mouth and laughs; laughs when a jack-in-the-box pops up	Still cries when unhappy, coos and smiles when happy	Recognizes parents; is unafraid of strangers until 6 months	Makes baby sounds, utters syllables
Toddler 12 to 36 Months	Learns to walk up to 14 months, then kneels; at 18 months to 3 years, learns to sit unaided, goes up and down stairs sitting, runs, and tries to throw a ball; spatial awareness increases; can play pat-a-cake	Opens and closes containers; learns to scribble; shows right- or left-handedness; holds a spoon to eat; can stack up 3 to 6 blocks; identifies people in photos	Early shows of affection; likes to look at books; explores more with no sense of danger; later role-plays; does not understand sharing; becomes clingy when upset; wants instant gratification, has tantrums and can be stubborn; does not like to be restrained	Feeds self with fingers; drinks from a cup with a lid; helps caregiver with getting dressed; is mischievous; is selfish, saying "mine"; begins toilet training	Understands simple words, including name but also screams if wants something; by 3 years, can speak 50 words and understands many more; starts simple three-word sentences
Preschool 3 to 5 Years	Develops balance; learns to climb stairs at 3 years; can skip; can pedal a tricycle	Very developed imagination; can understand directions; fantasies seem real; says, "I'm hurt because I was bad"; learns alphabet, numbers, and colors; understands concepts of past, present, and future	Understands humor; becomes very inquisitive; develops fantasies and a vivid imagination	Begins to share; can use the toilet; eats with utensils; can dress independently; can wash hands	Can answer simple questions; can have a conversation; starts developing vocabulary and grammar

Age	Physical Development	Intellectual Development	Emotional Development	Social Development	Language Development
School Age 6 to 12 Years	Learns to ride a bike around 6 years; learns specific skills for sports; muscles begin to develop	Learns to read; develops math skills; learns about more than one's immediate surroundings and about one's impact on others	Can differentiate emotional and physical pain; can make own decisions	Develops understanding of right from wrong; begins to develop team skills	Can answer more complex questions directly; becomes more efficient with communication skills
Adolescent 13 to 18 Years	Can lack coordination during growth spurt but later becomes efficient and very skilled at sports	Learns life skills; easily comprehends complex problems; understands government	Has first loving and emotional experience with individuals of the opposite sex; understands authority and laws	Joins clubs and sports teams; understands society	Develops vocabulary of words; can write a story with correct grammar

COMMON PEDIATRIC ILLNESSES AND INJURIES

Children suffer a variety of medical disorders and traumatic injuries. Although most of these conditions are similar in nature and frequency to those seen in adults, some are unique to the pediatric population. Moreover, some disorders occur more frequently in certain pediatric age groups than in others. Because infants and children have smaller airways and immature immune systems, respiratory emergencies are common.

Airway Problems

The most common upper airway conditions that cause respiratory emergencies in children are croup, tonsillitis, and foreign-body airway obstruction. Lower airway problems such as bronchiolitis, pneumonia, and asthma can also occur.

Croup

Croup is an inflammation of the larynx, trachea, and bronchi that typically results from an airborne viral infection that primarily affects children between the ages of 6 months and 3 years (**Figure 30-7**). Croup is characterized by sudden onset of a sharp, seal-like barking cough. Most cases of croup occur in the late fall and winter and are preceded by 2 to 3 days of "cold-like" symptoms (runny nose, increased mucus production, and fever). Although most cases are mild and resolve without complications, croup can produce severe respiratory distress. Younger children are generally more affected due to the smaller size of the airways.

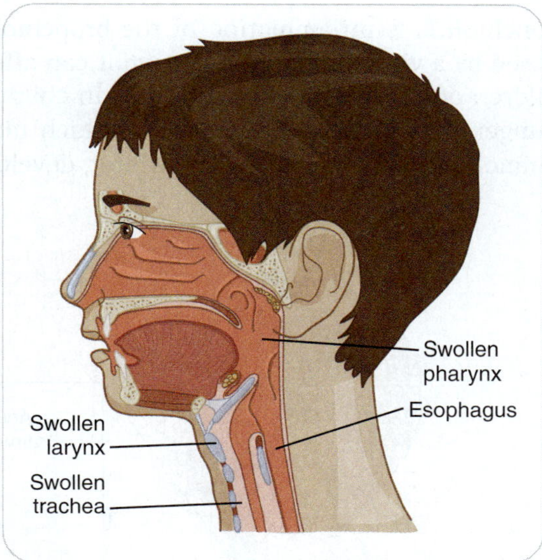

Figure 30-7 Croup, an inflammation of the larynx, can cause narrowing of the airway.

Tonsillitis

Tonsillitis, an inflammation of the tonsils, is a common childhood disease that primarily affects children ages 5 to 15 years. It usually results from a viral infection, but can also be caused from "strep throat," a bacterial infection. Tonsillitis is characterized by severe sore throat and difficulty swallowing. While painful, it rarely results in respiratory distress.

Foreign-Body Airway Obstruction

Because young children often explore their world by placing objects in their nose or mouth, small objects such as hard candy, toy parts, or coins can become lodged in a child's airway, resulting in partial or complete obstruction. Food is the primary cause of foreign-body airway obstruction in older children and is primarily due to either putting too much food in the mouth or not completely chewing food. Dislodged teeth or vomitus can also cause partial or complete airway obstruction.

Bronchiolitis

Bronchiolitis is inflammation of the bronchioles caused by a viral infection. Although it can affect children of all ages, most cases occur in children younger than 2 years. Bronchiolitis, which most commonly occurs in the fall and winter, develops over a period of 2 to 3 days and is characterized by fever, cough, and difficulty breathing, which in some cases can be severe.

Pneumonia

Pneumonia is a viral or bacterial infection of the lungs that is often preceded by an upper respiratory infection, a fever, and a cough. It can occur any time of year but is most commonly encountered during the winter and spring. Although pneumonia can occur at any age, children who have aspirated a foreign body or have a history of either recurring respiratory infections (e.g., bronchiolitis) or chronic illnesses are at greater risk for contracting pneumonia. Untreated, pneumonia can lead to respiratory distress, respiratory failure, and even respiratory arrest. A similar condition can occur when the lungs are exposed to certain chemicals.

Asthma

Asthma is a reactive disease of the small airways that is characterized by marked constriction of the bronchioles and wheezing (**Figure 30-8**). Among the most common triggers of asthma are viral

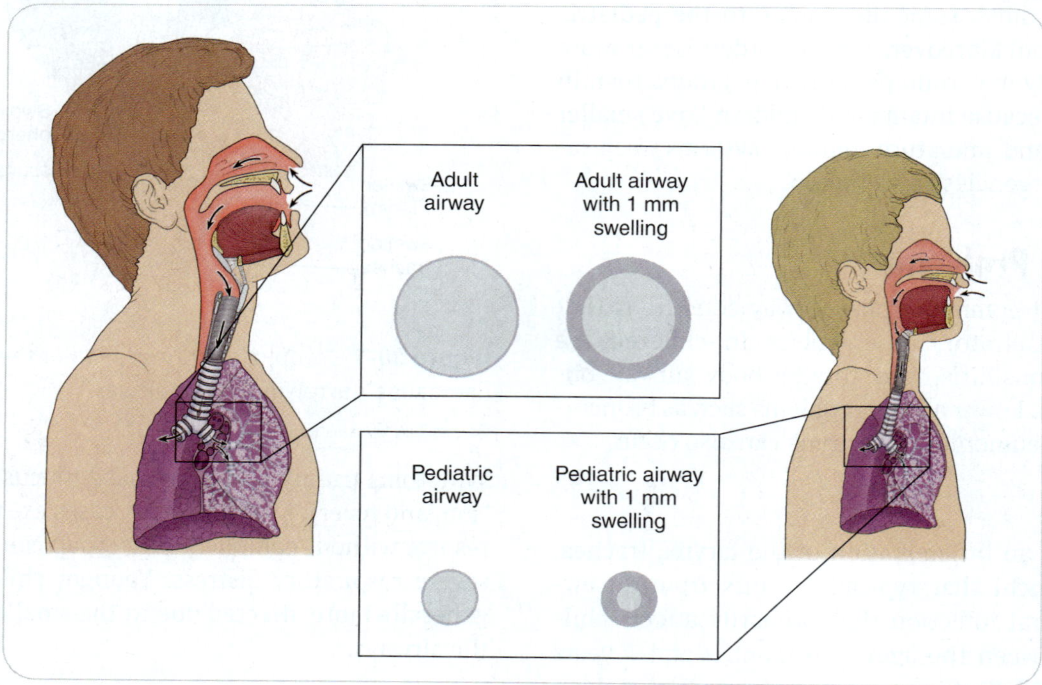

Figure 30-8 In asthma, inflammation of the airways reduces their diameter, causing respiratory difficulty.

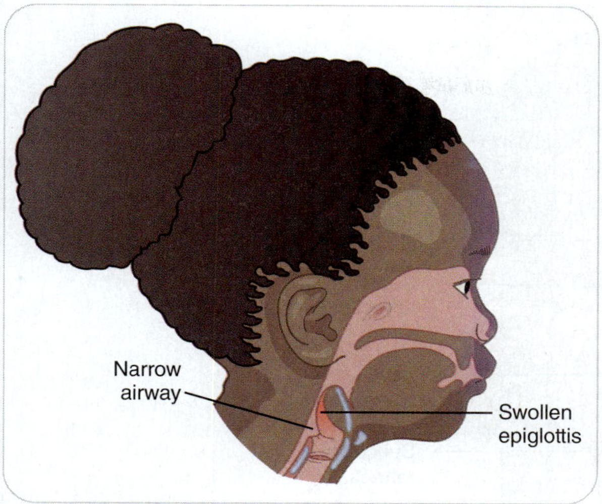

Figure 30-9 Epiglottitis can obstruct or completely block the airway.

illnesses, pollen, exercise, pet exposure, and contact with cold air. Asthma affects just over 8% of children in the United States. Children who suffer from childhood asthma usually have the condition by the time they reach 5 years of age. For more information on asthma, refer to Chapter 13, *Respiratory Emergencies*.

Epiglottitis

Epiglottitis is a true medical emergency that can produce life-threatening respiratory distress. This severe inflammation of the epiglottis can completely block the upper airway (**Figure 30-9**). Epiglottitis results from a bacterial infection and is characterized by high fever, sore throat, and an inability to swallow. The hallmark of epiglottitis is a patient who is sitting forward, is very still, and is drooling. If not treated quickly, epiglottitis can result in death. Although now a rare disease in children thanks to vaccination for *Haemophilus influenzae* bacteria, the disease most commonly affects children ages 1 to 7 years. It is still seen in nonvaccinated populations, including individuals immigrating from countries where the vaccine is not commonly administered.

Respiratory Failure and Cardiac Arrest

Respiratory failure is defined as the inability of the lungs to exchange gases properly. It is a true emergency that if not immediately corrected can be quickly fatal. Children, especially young children, are much more susceptible to respiratory failure than are adults. This is mainly because their immune systems are not fully developed, upper and lower airways are narrower and thus more easily obstructed by swelling or secretions, and the respiratory muscles are inefficient and become fatigued rapidly.

When a child has trouble breathing, the body compensates quickly by increasing the heart and respiratory rates. Although temporarily effective, this process has a potentially fatal drawback: as the heart rate dramatically increases, so do the heart's oxygen needs. The resulting increased effort to breathe can easily exhaust and overwhelm a child, resulting in respiratory distress and progressing hypoxia (**Figure 30-10**).

As exhaustion occurs, the respiratory rate continues to slow and can progresses to respiratory arrest. For this reason, most cases of cardiac arrest in children are preceded by respiratory arrest. The development of relative bradycardia in a child with respiratory distress is an ominous sign of impending respiratory and cardiac arrest.

Abdominal Pain

Abdominal pain is a common childhood complaint. Of the many causes of pediatric abdominal pain, the most common is constipation. This condition can occur due to changes in development, dietary habits, sleep patterns, and dehydration. When in outdoor settings or when simply confronted with an unfamiliar restroom, shyness about defecation may cause some children to intentionally withhold a bowel movement, sometimes for up to a week. The resulting accumulation of feces in the bowel causes constipation and pain.

KEY POINT

Understanding Cardiac Arrest in Children

Cardiac arrest in children usually is the result of respiratory arrest.

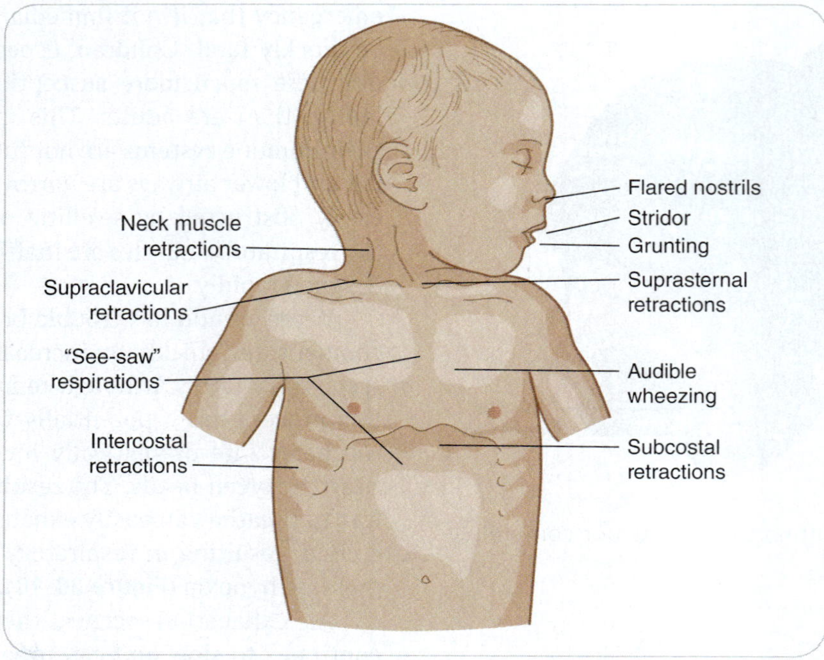

Figure 30-10 Some signs of respiratory distress.

Gastroenteritis and appendicitis are two other medical sources of pediatric abdominal pain that OEC technicians may encounter. Gastroenteritis with nausea, vomiting, and/or diarrhea can occur at any age, has numerous causes, and may mimic several very serious conditions. Appendicitis occurs much less commonly in children than in adults, but if unrecognized it can lead to peritonitis, shock, and death. Of the other conditions that cause abdominal pain in children, most are rare and beyond the scope of this text. As a rule, any child who presents with severe abdominal pain and appears ill should be evaluated by a physician.

Nausea, Vomiting, and Diarrhea

Nausea, vomiting, and diarrhea, sometimes referred to collectively as NVD, are among the most common complaints OEC technicians encounter in children and are associated with a variety of pediatric illnesses and injuries. This triad of complaints has many causes, including gastroenteritis, viruses, bacteria, parasites, tainted or unfamiliar food, lack of sleep, and overstimulation. Depending on the underlying cause, nausea, vomiting, and diarrhea can range in severity from mild to life threatening. Severe vomiting and diarrhea can lead to marked dehydration, hypovolemia, and shock.

Seizures

As described in Chapter 11, *Altered Mental Status*, a seizure is an electrical disturbance within the brain that results in alterations in awareness, attentiveness, responsiveness, behavior, and/or body movement. Seizures may be classified as either partial (affecting one part or side of the body) or generalized (affecting both sides simultaneously). The many causes of seizure include fever, hypoxia, diabetes, epilepsy, toxins, and head injury.

In children, febrile seizures are the most common type, accounting for approximately half of all seizures. Most febrile seizures occur in children between the ages of 6 months and 5 years and typically affect otherwise healthy children who have the combination of an infectious illness and an elevated temperature. Febrile seizures are generalized in nature, usually last less than 5 minutes, and have a postictal phase lasting several minutes. Most febrile seizures are harmless; there is no evidence that febrile seizures, *by themselves*, cause death, brain damage, epilepsy, mental retardation, decreased IQ score, or learning difficulties.

Children are susceptible to status epilepticus, a condition that is characterized by a seizure lasting more than 10 minutes, a prolonged postictal state, or three or more seizures in a row between which the patient does not return to normal mental status. Status epilepticus is a true emergency that requires immediate medical care.

A less serious type of seizure that may be seen in children is the "absence seizure," which lasts from a few seconds to a minute or more and is characterized by a period in which the child remains awake but is momentarily unresponsive to external stimuli. Usually benign, a child may experience multiple absence seizures in a single day. The cause of this type of seizure is unknown, and most children outgrow this condition by the age of 18 to 22 years.

Meningitis

Meningitis, inflammation of the meninges (the membrane that covers the spinal cord and brain), is a potentially life-threatening condition that is considered a true medical emergency and requires prompt medical care. Meningitis due to a bacterial or viral infection usually develops over 1 to 4 days and may be highly contagious. It is characterized by lethargy, high fever, severe headache, and a stiff, sore neck. In infants, the fontanels may bulge outward. Young children are especially vulnerable to meningitis, especially from birth to 5 years of age. Vaccinations have drastically decreased the cases of bacterial meningitis.

Poisoning

Toddlers and preschool children are at high risk of accidental poisoning due to their inexperience in distinguishing random items, candy from medications, or harmless plants from those that are toxic (**Figure 30-11**). Infants are at greatest risk because they constantly put things in their mouth. Unfortunately, many toxic substances smell good or taste good, and even small amounts of some toxins can make a child very ill.

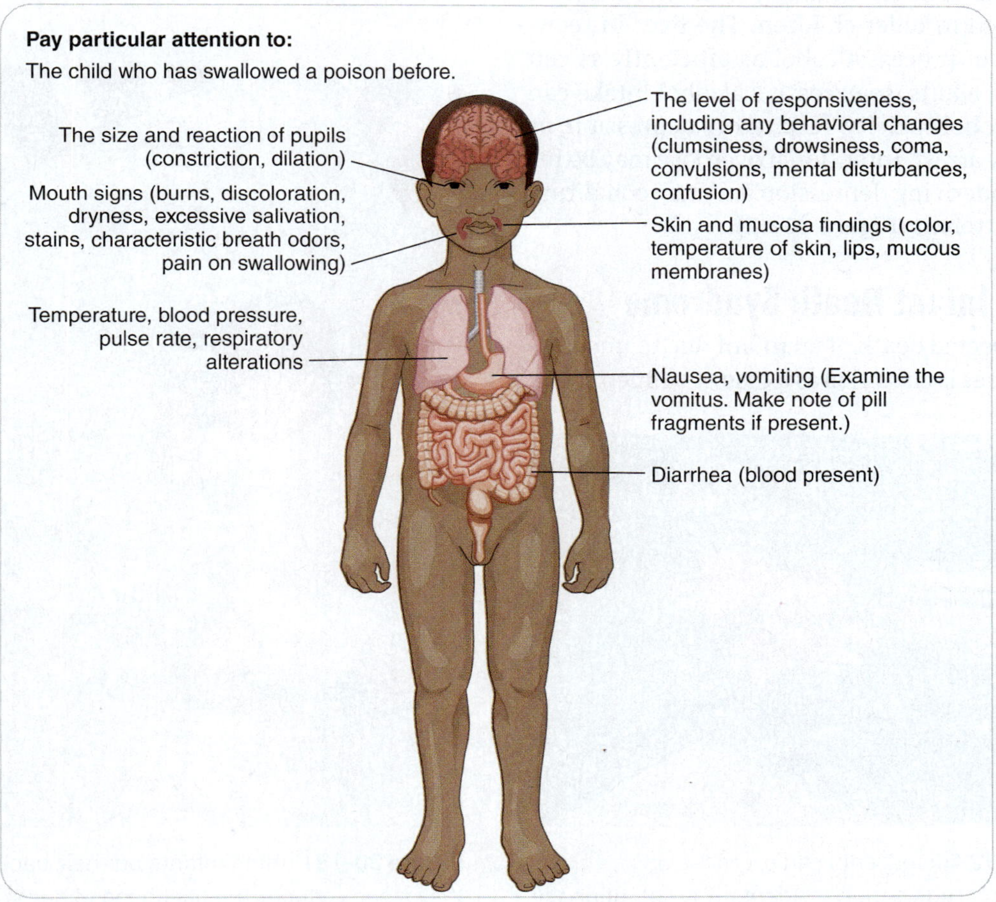

Figure 30-11 Possible signs and symptoms of ingested poisoning in children.

Children can be poisoned by medications, both prescription drugs and over-the-counter drugs such as aspirin or acetaminophen (Tylenol). Some medications, especially those formulated for pediatric patients (e.g., cough syrups, pain relievers, children's vitamins) taste like candy. If ingested in large amounts, overdose and toxicity can quickly occur.

Pediatric poisonings can also occur from petroleum-based solvents, rodent poison, antifreeze, or just about anything that is kept unlocked within a curious child's reach such as under the kitchen sink. Long-term lead poisoning can occur from eating lead-based paint on toys or on the railings of a staircase. Some items from China have been shown to have cadmium in the paint, which is also very poisonous. The ingestion of too many vitamin tablets can result in iron toxicity.

Adolescents also can be poisoned either accidentally or intentionally. Opioid medications, both prescription and street acquired, and other illegal drugs can easily lead to poisoning, respiratory depression, and death. Excessive alcohol consumption is another common type of poisoning encountered in older children. The liver in teenagers cannot process alcohol as efficiently as can the liver in adults, so excessive alcohol intake can lead to alcohol toxicity, respiratory depression, or respiratory arrest. Intentional overdose may be related to underlying depression and may constitute a suicide attempt (**Figure 30-12**).

Sudden Infant Death Syndrome

The unexpected death of an infant due to undetermined causes is classified as a case of **sudden infant death syndrome (SIDS)**. According to HealthCommunities.com, approximately 4,000 babies die from SIDS every year in the United States. It is the leading cause of death for babies between 2 and 4 months old in the United States. Males are affected slightly more frequently, and African Americans, Native Americans, and Alaska Natives are affected more frequently. Risk of SIDS increases if the mother is younger than 20 years, smokes, uses drugs, or drinks alcohol while pregnant.

The exact cause of SIDS is unknown; there is still no universally accepted reason why apparently healthy children die unexpectedly. It does not appear that SIDS is caused from suffocation, and research has shown that there is a tendency for SIDS to run in families. A reduction in the incidence of SIDS over the past 15 years is likely due to the recommendation of several practices, including (first and foremost) placing babies on their backs for sleep, avoiding redundant soft bedding and soft objects in the infant's sleeping environment, and avoiding having adults sleeping with an infant in the same bed (**Figure 30-13**).

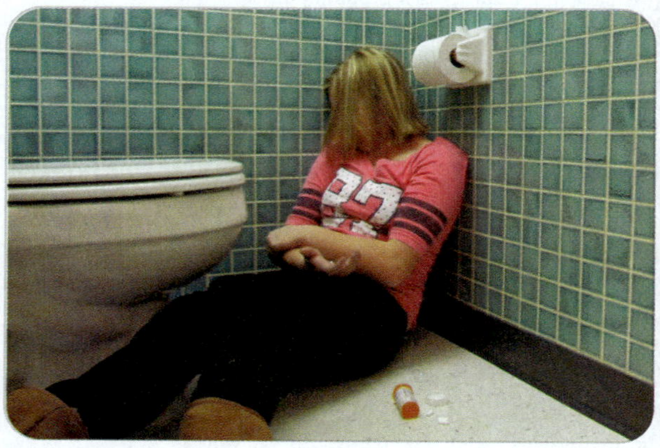

Figure 30-12 Adolescents can overdose on prescription drugs either accidentally or intentionally.

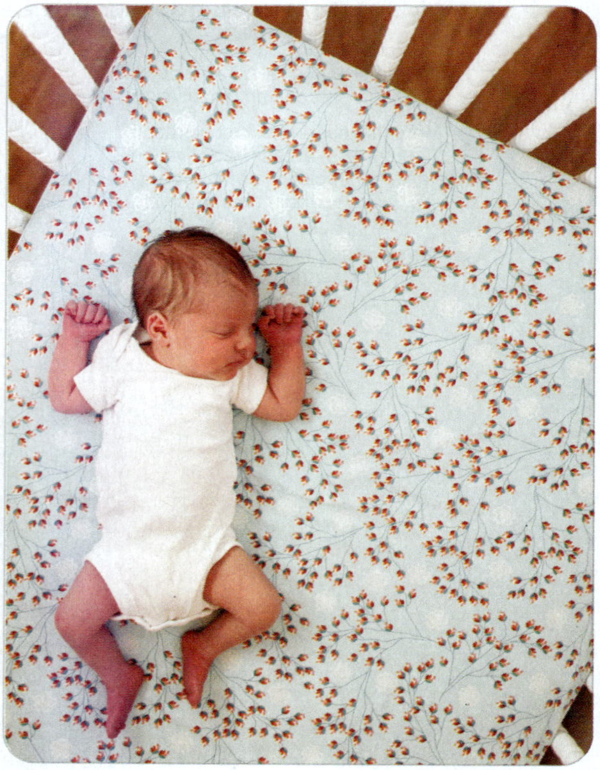

Figure 30-13 Putting infants on their backs while they sleep reduces the likelihood of death from SIDS.

In a typical SIDS case, parents will attempt to awaken the infant in the morning, only to find that their baby is dead. In addition to profound grief, many parents suffer severe guilt following the death of a child from SIDS.

Trauma

Children of all ages are inherently risk takers and frequently engage in activities that can result in serious bodily injury. Accidental trauma is the leading cause of death in children older than 1 year. The leading cause of death from accidental trauma is vehicle crashes, followed by firearm-related injuries and drownings (**Figure 30-14**). Blunt trauma is the leading mechanism of injury.

Head and Neck Injuries

Head injury is a common pediatric injury, and among infants and toddlers, the primary source of head injury is falls. Because infants and toddlers have a relatively large head, weak neck muscles, and flexible bones and ligaments, they have difficulty controlling head movement. As a result, the head tends to lead the way in a fall. Injuries occur to the surface of the head and face, to the skull, and within the skull. Due to the highly vascular nature of a child's head and the thinness of the skin, head injuries can result in significant bleeding.

In general, head injuries tend to be more severe in children. Small children with severe traumatic brain injuries can rapidly develop elevated intracranial pressure. The relatively small size of the brain compared to the skull allows blood to fill the inside of the skull, causing a cerebral hematoma that results in lethal pressure in the skull, often before significant symptoms are noticed. Among adolescents, motor vehicle collisions are the leading cause of head injuries, followed by trauma resulting from acts of violence.

Compared to adults, toddlers and preschoolers have a lower incidence of spine injury. However, spine injuries in children tend to be high cervical injuries and therefore are more lethal. During adolescence, the adult pattern of neck injuries is seen. Among teenage males, diving injuries are a common source of cervical-spine injury.

Chest and Abdomen Injuries

Because the chest wall in young children contains more cartilage, less bone, and less muscle than that of an adult, the transmission of the energy of blunt trauma to the underlying organs is increased. Since the ribs are more pliable, flail chest and displaced broken ribs due to blunt trauma are rare in younger children, but contusions of the lungs or heart, hemothorax, and pneumothorax can occur (**Figure 30-15**).

A potentially life-threatening pediatric chest injury is commotio cordis, the sudden death of a

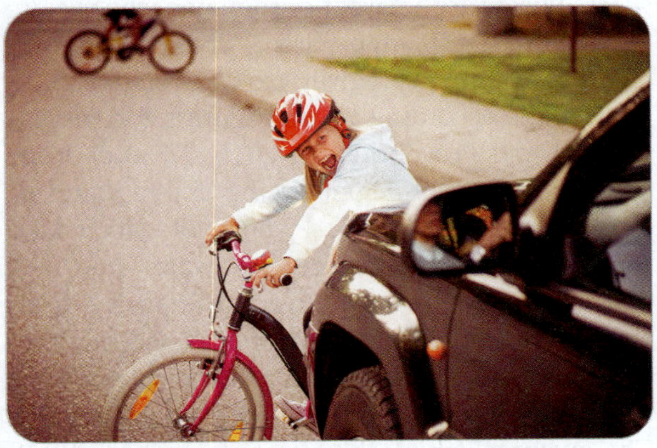

Figure 30-14 Accidental trauma is the leading cause of death in children older than 1 year.

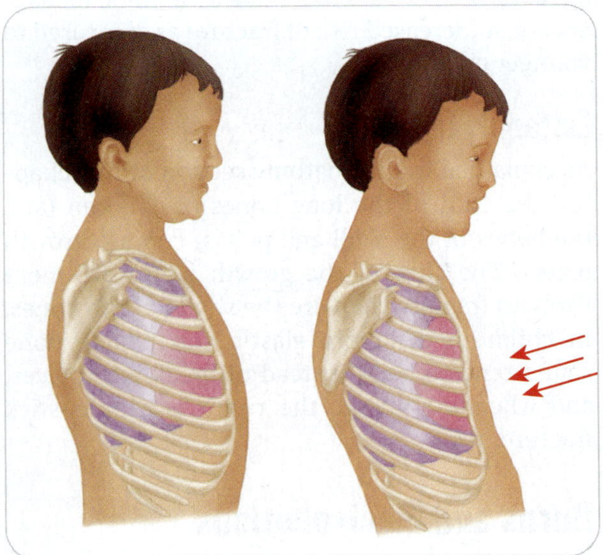

Figure 30-15 A child's ribs are softer and more flexible than an adult's. As a result, they may compress the lungs and heart if there is blunt trauma, causing serious injury with no obvious external damage.

healthy preadolescent who is struck in the chest by a hard object such as a baseball, or strikes a hard surface with the chest, such as might occur during snowboarding, skiing, or mountain biking. The transmission of the blunt force through the child's chest wall to the heart interrupts the normal electrical pattern of the heart, resulting in ventricular fibrillation and sudden cardiac death. If not immediately treated by defibrillation, resuscitation outcome is poor. Commotio cordis normally occurs in males between the ages of 8 and 18 years, 61% of whom were playing baseball at the time of the event.

Abdominal and Pelvic Injuries

Immature abdominal muscle provides less anterior and posterior protection to the abdominal organs. In blunt force trauma, more energy is transmitted to the intra-abdominal solid organs (liver and spleen) and to the kidneys. Injuries to these organs can result in significant internal bleeding, leading to hypovolemic shock. Hollow organ trauma in nonpenetrating injuries to the abdomen is less common in children than in adults.

Because the pelvic bones in younger children are softer and more flexible, fractures of the pelvis are less likely in children than in adults. Because a teenager's pelvis is more like an adult's, teenagers are at increased risk of fracture as compared to younger children.

Extremity Injuries

As explained in the anatomy section of this chapter, the ends of the long bones of children (and the bones of the skull and pelvis) contain growth plates. The sites of the growth plates are more likely to fracture than are the shafts of the bones. In children, the more elastic and pliable bone shafts tend to bend instead of break into pieces, and when they bend, the result is a greenstick fracture.

Burns and Electrocutions

In recent years, the incidence of burns in children has decreased; however, burns are among the most common childhood injuries. Scald-related burns are the most common type of burn, especially among toddlers and preschool children who pull hot fluids down onto themselves. Injuries involving open flames most commonly affect school-age children and adolescents. Chemical burns occur less frequently and affect older children more often than younger children.

Infants and toddlers are more susceptible to electrical burns than are older children due to their curiosity and lack of understanding of electricity. Electrical injuries most commonly occur when a toddler or preschooler sticks a metal object into a wall outlet or when a small child chews on a live electrical cord. Most burn and electrocution injuries occur within the home.

Child Abuse and Neglect

Child abuse is a legal term, not a medical diagnosis, and its definition can vary according to state or provincial law. **Child abuse** is defined as any act, or the failure to act, on the part of a parent, a caregiver, or any adult that results in serious physical or emotional harm, or imminent risk of harm to any child (**Figure 30-16**). As with adults, abuse can be physical, emotional, psychological, or sexual. **Child neglect** is more common than physical abuse and is defined as the failure to provide for the shelter, safety, supervision, and nutritional needs of a child.

Cultural norms concerning the treatment of children vary widely. What one culture may view as appropriate care and discipline of a child may be viewed in another culture as abusive. Child abuse is not a new phenomenon, but instead a painful part of human culture since parenting began.

Sadly, many children in the United States are abused or neglected. Child abuse is seen in all cultures, socioeconomic classes, races, and religions. Most abusers are a parent or someone who is close to the child (e.g., step-parent, divorced parent's significant other, caregiver, sibling, relative, family friend). According to the Centers for Disease Control and Prevention, in 2016, 1,750 children died from abuse or neglect in the United States.

One form of physical abuse of which OEC technicians should be acutely aware is **shaken baby syndrome**. Also known as abusive head trauma, shaken baby syndrome is a condition that results when a person picks up and *intentionally* shakes a newborn, an infant, or a young toddler. The ensuing "whiplash" effect causes the child's brain to forcefully contact the bones within the skull. Traumatic brain injury can result, often with fatal consequences. Studies show that most cases

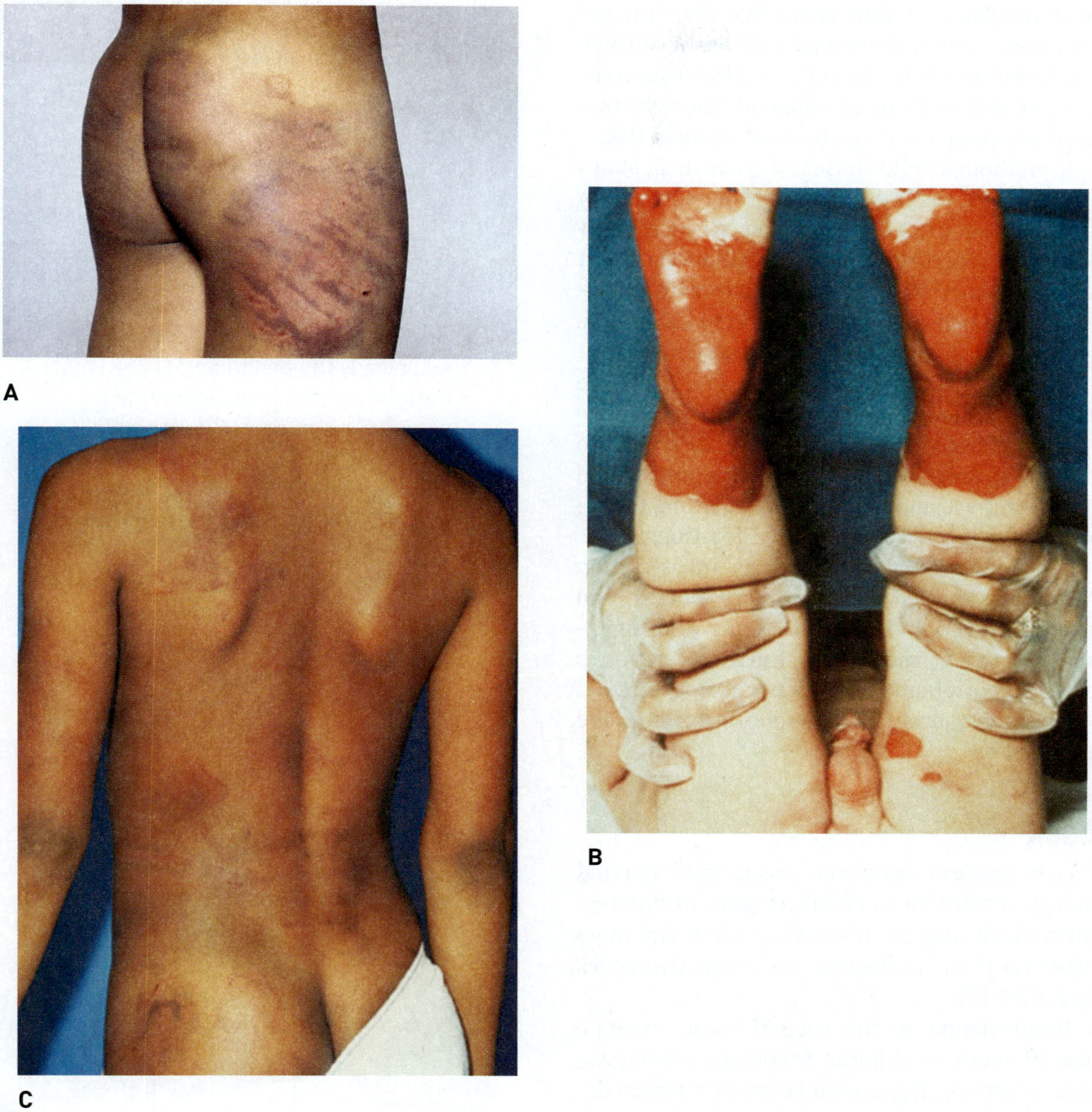

Figure 30-16 A. An injury that is in an unusual location, is not age appropriate, or cannot be logically explained can be a sign of child abuse. This child's buttocks were abused. **B.** A symmetric scald is a sign of child abuse. **C.** Multiple injuries at different stages of healing can suggest child abuse.

A: © Clinical Photography, Central Manchester University Hospitals NHS Foundation Trust, UK/Science Source; **B** and **C:** Courtesy of Ronald Dieckmann, M.D.

of shaken baby syndrome are perpetrated by the child's caregiver, babysitter, or someone close to the child. In the event of a pediatric head injury, shaken baby syndrome should be suspected if the child is younger than 1 year old and the caregiver cannot give a plausible explanation of what happened to the child.

Even though some adults may express their fear and genuine worry for an injured child by acting angry, it is prudent to suspect child abuse whenever a parent or caregiver becomes verbally abusive to a child or berates the child for getting hurt. Calling a child names such as "stupid" or "idiot" also may be an indicator of emotional or physical abuse. While it is common for a child to fear that a parent will be angry that the child got hurt ("Dad's going to be mad that we have to go home because I broke my leg"), children who completely withdraw from or cringe at the sight of a parent or caregiver should be considered at risk.

Even though child abuse is a crime in all states and provinces, the laws regarding the reporting of possible abuse vary. Most states and provinces allow anonymous reporting to prevent retaliation against the person who reported the suspected abuse. Generally, individuals who report suspected abuse are legally shielded from lawsuits, but only if they report suspected abuse to the proper agency. In some jurisdictions, medical personnel are required by law to report any suspicion of abuse and are subject to penalties if they do not. OEC technicians should determine the legal requirements regarding the reporting of suspected abuse in their locations.

The report of abuse starts an investigation by specially trained social workers, nurses, and physicians, who look for the signs and symptoms of abuse. In most cases, the investigation is stopped if corroborating evidence is not found. If abuse is substantiated, intervention services are implemented.

KEY POINT

When to Suspect Child Abuse

- Multiple injuries (mix of new, old, and/or partially healed injuries)
- Bilateral injuries (injuries on both sides of the body)
- Circumferential bruising (bruise extends completely around an extremity)
- Bruises located in unusual places (especially the genitalia)
- Pattern bruises (e.g., an outline of an adult's hand, a clear line of demarcation)
- Injuries that are not age appropriate (e.g., a skull fracture in a child who is too young to walk)
- Inconsistent histories from the child and caregiver or from two caregivers
- History that is vague or changes over time
- Older children who cannot or will not provide an explanation for their injuries

Shock

Shock is a state of inadequate tissue perfusion that can have medical or traumatic origins. In children, hypovolemic and distributive shock occur more frequently than cardiogenic or obstructive shock (**Figure 30-17**).

Hypovolemia is the second most common cause of shock in children following sepsis (systemic infection). Hypovolemia can occur from dehydration due to vomiting and/or diarrhea, from acute external blood loss, or from internal bleeding. Whereas most adults can easily tolerate the loss of a pint of blood (the amount typically removed during blood donation), a pint can equal 30% of the total blood volume of an infant or small child. It is important to remember that children may not become hypotensive until they have lost 30% of their blood volume. By that point the child is near death. Adults deteriorate slower or less dramatically than children. Be proactive if you suspect internal bleeding while managing shock. Don't wait to see if the blood pressure drops. It may be too late for a child!

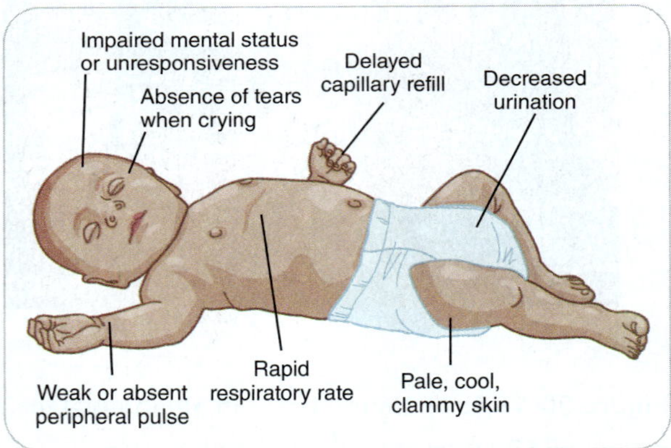

Figure 30-17 Signs of shock in a child.

Additionally, anaphylaxis resulting from an insect bite, a food allergy, or exposure to a poison also can cause shock. Cardiogenic shock is rare except in children who have a congenital heart condition. Obstructive shock can rarely occur and is usually due to blunt chest trauma that results in pericardial tamponade or a tension pneumothorax.

CASE Update

You make the scene safe and then approach the young patient, kneeling down beside her. You introduce yourself to her and to her grandmother and reassure both that you are there to help. You request and receive the grandmother's permission to examine the child. Sensing her fear and pain, you ask the child her name. Although the grandmother already told you what happened, you ask the girl, "What happened?" and "Where does it hurt?" In response to your calm, caring approach, she stops crying and points with her left index finger at her upper right chest.

What should you do now?

ASSESSMENT OF THE PEDIATRIC PATIENT

Assessment of a pediatric patient follows the same steps as that of an adult. However, you may need to modify the assessment based on the child's age and level of development.

When assessing a child, remember that the heart rate and respiratory rate can change very rapidly because of the child's emotional response to injury or fear of being approached by a stranger. A child's crying can make assessment very difficult. More importantly, the metabolic compensation mechanisms in a child's body can make the condition appear stable when, in fact, the patient is in shock. For these reasons and others, OEC technicians must not assume that all is well with a child who does not exhibit findings of serious illness or injury. OEC technicians need to carefully evaluate both the child and the mechanism of injury or nature of illness and use this information with the assessment findings; the child's history, age, and developmental stage; and the parent's knowledge of what is normal and abnormal for the child.

Scene Size-up, Mechanism of Injury, and Consent

As with any incident, the assessment process begins with a scene size-up. Remove all potential hazards. Especially for young patients, do not overlook seemingly innocuous objects such as a pencil, keys, or small objects that could become a hazard in the hands of a curious child. If numerous potential hazards are present, consider moving a patient who does not have a spinal injury and their caregiver to a safer, more secure location. If trauma is suspected, attempt to determine the mechanism of injury, and be sure to assess it carefully and in context with the child's anatomy and developmental stage. As with any patient, observe proper standard precautions.

If a parent is present, be sure to ask for permission (consent) to assess and care for children younger than 18 years (or under the age of majority in your state or province). If there are no contraindications (e.g., a suspected spinal injury), leave a young child in the caregiver's arms, which will help both to feel more secure and in control. Remember, to a young child, you are a stranger. Many children obtain cues from their parent or caregiver that may dictate their response. If the parent is comfortable with your approach and assessment, the child will likely be less afraid and more cooperative. If a parent or caregiver is not present, and the child needs care, implied consent takes effect (see Chapter 1, *Introduction to Outdoor Emergency Care*). Always kneel or sit at the child's level, as standing and looking down may cause anxiety for the child.

Primary Patient Assessment

As you approach the patient, begin to formulate a general impression of the patient's overall condition. Upon making physical contact with the patient, perform a primary assessment in the usual manner. Pay close attention to potential threats to life, especially severe bleeding, and correct any that may be present. Because cardiac arrest in pediatric patients is generally preceded by respiratory arrest, assess the airway and respirations very carefully. Also, because a child's condition can change quickly, frequently reassess the ABCDs (airway, breathing, circulation, disability). If there is any evidence of ABCD-related compromise, treat the problem, request ALS assistance immediately, and rapidly transport the patient to a definitive-care facility.

The American Academy of Pediatrics recommends the use of the **pediatric assessment triangle**, which enables rescuers to quickly assess a child's appearance, work of breathing, and circulation to skin (**Figure 30-18**). By evaluating these criteria, OEC technicians can quickly determine whether a child is "sick" or "not sick." In most instances, this exam can be performed in just a few seconds by simply looking and listening as you approach the patient.

KEY POINT

Signs of Complete Airway Obstruction

- Inability to cough
- Inability to speak or cry
- Respiratory arrest

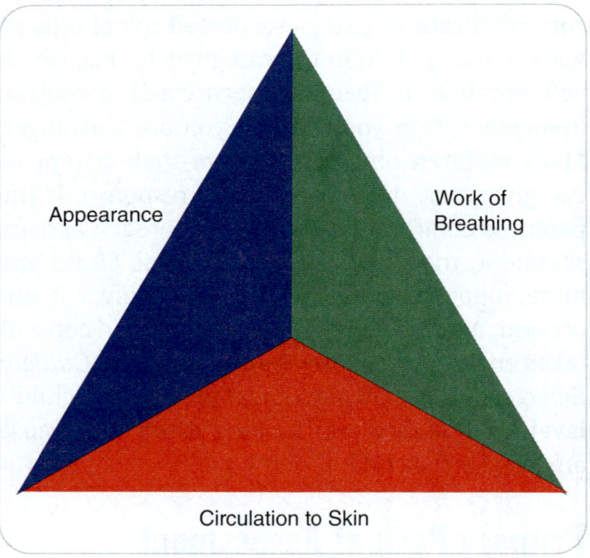

Figure 30-18 The pediatric assessment triangle.

The Pediatric Assessment Triangle: Accuracy of Its Application by Nurses in the Triage of Children. Horeczko, Timothy et al. *Journal of Emergency Nursing*, Volume 39, Issue 2, 182 - 189.

The Child's Appearance

As you approach the child, observe the patient's appearance (**Figure 30-19**). Is the child obviously injured or ill? Observing that a child is unresponsive, has labored breathing, is pale, and/or has major bleeding should cause you to suspect a possible life-threatening problem. Obvious limb deformities, "painful" crying, or an apparent decreased level of responsiveness are also signs of a serious condition. If there are no obvious findings of major illness or injury, continue to observe the patient for other clues, and ask yourself the following questions:

- *Is the child active and moving about, or is the child quiet and sitting still?* Children who are laughing or playful are not seriously ill. A child who sits still or is sitting forward and drooling is in a condition that warrants rapid transport.
- *Does the child make eye contact?* It is generally a good sign if a child immediately focuses on your face and can follow your movements. Likewise, toddlers or preschoolers who make eye contact with you, start crying, and then immediately seek their parent are probably not seriously ill. Such children are responding in an age-appropriate manner to a stranger.

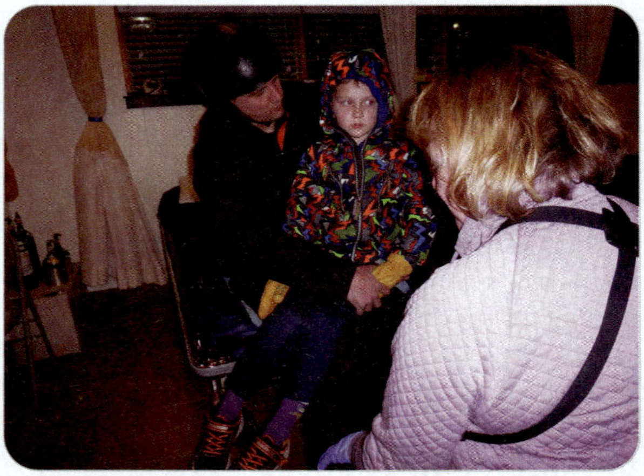

Figure 30-19 Remember to approach the patient on his or her level and include the parents as necessary.

Children who do not engage you or look at you and then refocus on themselves, have a weak cry, or are not moving should alert you to a possible serious medical condition.

- *Does the child appear irritable or agitated?* Under normal conditions, a parent or caregiver should be able to console and quiet a child. Children who are ill often cry or whine upon even small movements or changes in position and often cannot be comforted. An infant who is paradoxically irritable—that is, one who becomes quiet when left alone but is irritable when in the caregiver's arms—should be considered very ill.
- *Does the child respond to the caregiver's voice?* A child who quiets, smiles, or appropriately responds to a caregiver's voice is generally less ill than one who does not.

Work of Breathing

Observe children for signs of increased respiratory effort. In most cases, the appearance of a child in respiratory failure is striking. A child who is in respiratory distress is typically found sitting upright and may assume the tripod position (**Figure 30-20A**). Infants may also extend the head and neck into the "sniffing" position, with the nose in the air, which straightens the airway as much as possible to allow as much air as possible to reach the lungs (**Figure 30-20B**). Children with epiglottitis may also be drooling because swallowing is extremely painful.

Look for the use of accessory muscles and for nasal flaring. The child's head may bob up and down as the sternocleidomastoid muscles contract during inhalation and relax during exhalation. Paradoxical breathing, also known as see-saw breathing, may be present. With paradoxical breathing, the abdomen extends outward and the chest collapses inward upon inhalation. During exhalation, the opposite occurs: the abdomen sinks inward and the chest protrudes outward. If the patient is shirtless, look for retractions, where the soft tissues above the sternum and clavicles and between and below the ribs sink inward upon inhalation. Be aware that in older children, retraction becomes less obvious.

Listen to how the child is breathing. Respiratory sounds can vary greatly with the severity of

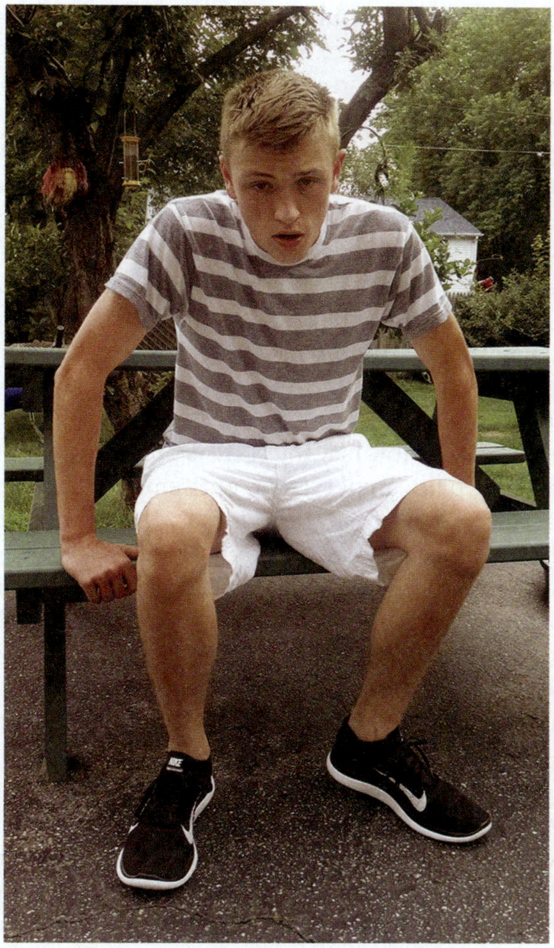

A

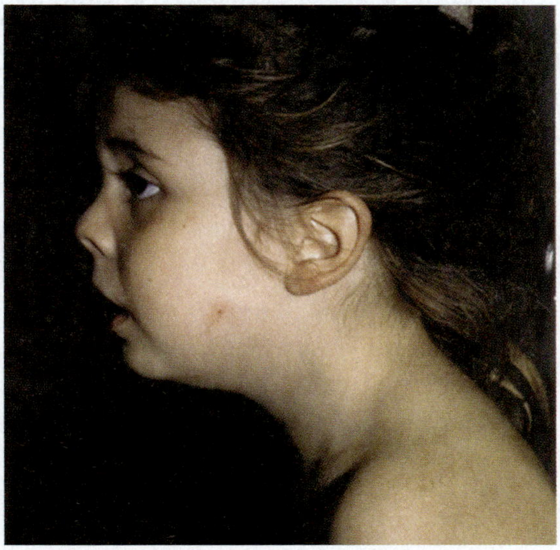

B

Figure 30-20 A. Tripod position. **B.** Sniffing position.

distress, ranging from an almost inaudible sigh to wheezing or grunting. Sounds can be heard during inhalation, exhalation, or both. Wheezing may be heard during inhalation or exhalation, whereas grunting is heard only during exhalation. In children, wheezing is a high-pitched whistling sound. Grunting is a low-pitched sound that may sometimes resemble a whimper. It is usually constant but can be intermittent. Grunting opens the smallest passages to the alveoli, maximizing gas exchange. Both wheezing and grunting indicate lower airway problems and severe respiratory distress. A high-pitched sound upon inspiration, called stridor, suggests croup.

Observe how fast the child is breathing, realizing that pain, anxiety, fear, excitement, and other factors can increase the respiratory rate, and that the normal rate of respiration depends on the age of the child. Even though crying can make it difficult to assess the rate of breathing, it generally indicates that air is moving in and out of the lungs well. When assessing breathing effort, ask yourself not only "Is air moving?" but also "Is air moving *well*?"

Circulation to the Skin

Assess the child's skin color for clues regarding the perfusion of the patient's tissues. If poor lighting, cold environments, or dark skin make assessment more difficult, assess the sclera of the eyes, the lips, or the palms of the hands. The skin should appear pink, not pale, mottled, gray, or blue. If the skin is pink, the child is generally well oxygenated and has good tissue perfusion. An exception to this rule is carbon monoxide poisoning, in which the skin may appear pink or red even though blood oxygen levels are very low.

Paleness suggests that either the blood is poorly saturated with oxygen or circulation is poor, as is seen with excessive blood loss, respiratory distress, or heart failure. Mottled skin (areas of red, purple, and white patches) or gray skin also indicates poor tissue perfusion. Cyanosis, a bluish tint to the skin and mucous membranes, is an ominous sign that indicates a serious respiratory problem or hypoxia. Use a pulse oximeter and make sure the oxygen saturation is greater than or equal to 94%.

KEY POINT

Questions to Be Asked Following a General Impression

- Is the child sick or not sick?
- Is the child having a problem breathing?
- What is the likely cause of the illness or injury?
- Are urgent interventions needed?
- Should rapid transport and EMS help be initiated?

The History

For toddlers or preschoolers, most (if not all) of the SAMPLE history (signs and symptoms, allergies, medications, past medical history, last oral intake, events leading up to the problem) will come from the caregiver, who thus becomes an integral part of both the assessment process and the child's caregiving team. Establishing trust with both patients and caregivers early on is critical.

Approach children slowly and gently, crouching beside them so that you are at their eye level. Smile. Introduce yourself to both caregiver and child (**Figure 30-21**). Ask for both of their names and ask children directly what they like to be

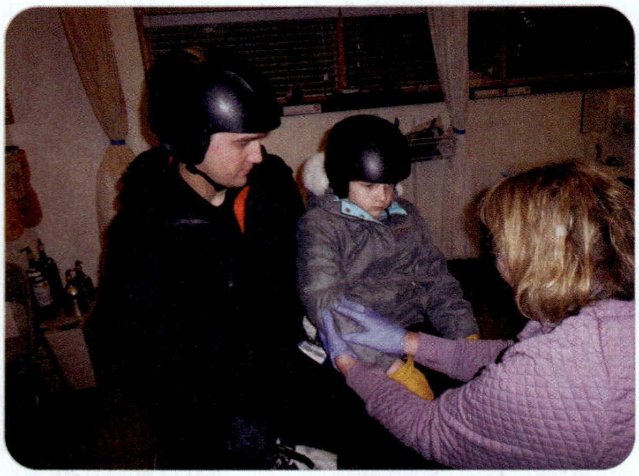

Figure 30-21 When performing an assessment on a child, you will need to stay at eye level with the child and may need to modify or simplify the terms you use. Engage the parents during the assessment process if they are present.

called. Speak in a normal, calm, and unhurried tone of voice, using words a child can understand. If the adult begins by telling you what happened, actively listen. Then, turn your attention to the child and paraphrase this information to the patient. For example, you might say, "It sounds like you took a pretty hard tumble on your arm! Can you show me where it hurts?" This acknowledges the information given by the caregiver and incorporates the child into the SAMPLE process. Alternate speaking and looking at the child and the caregiver, posing questions to both. Modify the words you use for body parts as appropriate. Use words such as "tummy" for preschoolers or younger school-aged children, and "belly" or "abdomen" for teens.

School-age children and adolescents should be treated as adults with respect to their need for respect and privacy. If you suspect possible substance abuse, pregnancy, or other privacy issues, have your partner interview the caregiver separately while you interact with the patient.

Honesty, Trust, and Communication

When caring for a child, always be honest. If something you will do will cause the child pain, say so in a kind way: "This may hurt some." Trust is essential when interacting with a pediatric patient. Once lost, it may be impossible to regain, and lost trust can affect other OEC technicians who may become involved in a patient's treatment. How you interact with children and caregivers can truly "make or break" events at the scene.

Explain to children (if old enough to understand) and to caregivers what you are doing, step by step, *before* you do it. Children younger than 6 years might not be able to explain what is wrong or localize pain. For example, a child with a fractured humerus might scream when touched anywhere on the body. Screaming or crying due to pain, fear, or the desire to block out the situation can make communication difficult or impossible. Although it may be difficult, understand that crying is a normal way for children to cope with a frightening or stressful situation. At all times, refrain from showing irritation or anger, even if it is difficult to do so.

Try gently placing a hand on the child's (uninjured) arm and make eye contact. Quietly ask children if they are afraid or in pain and acknowledge and accept what they tell you. Show understanding, such as nodding and saying calmly, "I'd be feeling scared too, if I fell and hurt myself." Offer honest reassurance such as, "We are going to do everything we can to make you better." Be careful not to promise something you cannot provide, such as a guarantee that nothing you do will cause pain. Never belittle or admonish the feelings of either a child or a caregiver; instead, show acceptance and respect and provide reassurance that you are there to help.

Also, be careful how you phrase questions to avoid placing yourself in a no-win situation. For example, asking a child, "Is it okay if we splint your arm now?" might land you in a trust-breaking impasse if the child answers "no." Instead, offer the patient or caregiver a choice, such as, "Can I help your mother (or father) put this splint on you?" while *you* apply the splint (with the parent's help). This empowers the child through choices and ensures the needed outcome (in this case, splinting the arm).

Nearly all children settle down and communicate with an OEC technician if they are made as comfortable as possible (**Figure 30-22**). Providing warmth—or better yet, moving an injured child indoors as quickly as the situation will allow—is a good first step in providing for the child's safety, comfort, and well-being.

When obtaining the SAMPLE history, be sure to ask when the child was last well. Parents will often state that the child was well when put to bed but awoke during the night complaining of symptoms. Ask about the child's normal appearance and behaviors, including eating habits; this information is essential, especially when

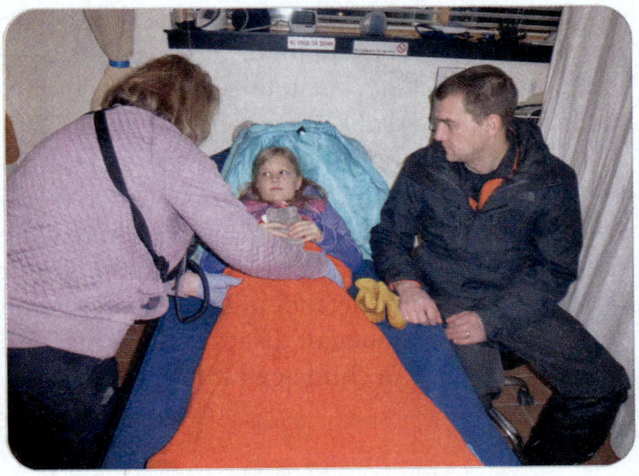

Figure 30-22 Make the child as comfortable as possible.

assessing young children who may not understand questions or be able to answer them. Have the caregiver describe any abnormal behaviors and explain what the corresponding normal behaviors are. If, for example, a parent reports that a child "spaced out for a while" or that an infant was grunting rhythmically while lying unresponsive in his crib, the problem could be related to seizure activity.

If the initial complaint is pain, assess the symptoms using the standard OPQRST mnemonic (onset, provocation, quality, radiation, severity, and time), using age-appropriate words and terms. Be sure to ask where the pain is located, because ear or throat pain may indicate the presence of an infectious disease such as tonsillitis or epiglottitis. Also ask if the pain is associated with nausea, vomiting, or diarrhea; if it is, ask how long the nausea, vomiting, or diarrhea has been present, and how many known episodes the patient has had.

Gastroenteritis usually presents with repeated episodes of vomiting and is frequently accompanied by five or more explosive watery stools per day. Although vomiting usually lasts approximately 12 hours, diarrhea may persist several days to a week. If the patient is very young, ask if the child has had episodes of crying, and if so, how many hours or days it has been occurring.

Ask the parents of young children about fluid intake and output. For newborns and infants, ask how many bottles or feedings the child has had in the past 24 hours. Ask if the feedings have been of a normal frequency and amount and if the child has experienced excessive urination or has had diarrhea.

Be sure to ask about any medications, vitamins, and nutritional supplements a pediatric patient may be taking, including over-the-counter medicines and herbal supplements.

Also ask if anything was done to help relieve the child's symptoms before your arrival on scene. For cases of croup, the parents may state that they placed the child next to a humidifier or took the child into the cool night air, whereupon the symptoms lessened or disappeared. They also may have given the child acetaminophen to control a fever.

Secondary Patient Assessment

Next, perform a secondary assessment. Depending on the child's age and stage of development, you may need to use a somewhat different strategy. The success of the secondary assessment often is directly related to an OEC technician's ability to effectively communicate and interact with the child and, when present, the caregivers.

The Physical Exam

The physical exam of a pediatric patient can be challenging. The order in which the exam is performed may need to be modified according to the child's age and the suspected severity of the problem. For instance, it is often more productive to assess newborns and infants using a toes-to-head approach, instead of the traditional head-to-toes approach. The exam for infants can often be made easier playing "peek-a-boo" during the exam. For preschool children, the exam may be facilitated by distracting the child with a toy or a tongue blade. Many emergency-care providers have toys that are used specifically for this purpose. Let the child play with the toy as you perform your exam. Additionally, involve the child in the exam process by allowing the child to assist. If appropriate (based on the medical problem), infants or small children will usually feel more secure if you allow them to remain in their parent's arms.

Children are naturally curious, and young children may be far more willing to allow you to listen to their lungs if you let them listen to their own lungs first. Some children may become frightened if you examine their head first. In this case, examine the trunk and extremities first, and the head and neck last. Be aware when performing a physical exam that many children are ticklish and may flinch when their bodies are touched.

Most school-age children have been examined by a pediatrician and understand the process of a physical exam. Some may be fearful you are going to give them a "shot." Acknowledge their fear and be honest and reassuring about what you will and will not do. For example, you might say something like, "I don't like shots, either! But don't worry, I don't give shots." Be careful not to make statements such as this if you know that other members of the care team or ambulance crew may later need to give them a shot.

Begin each physical exam by obtaining an initial set of vital signs (**Table 30-2**). At a minimum, include the pulse rate and the respiratory rate, the

Table 30-2 Normal Values for Pediatric Vital Signs

	Infants (Birth to 1 Year)	Children (1 to 8 Years)
Pulse	90–180 beats per minute	70–150 beats per minute
Respirations	25–60 respirations per minute	15–30 respirations per minute
Systolic blood pressure	50–95 mm Hg	80–110 mm Hg
Temperature	36.1–38.0°C (97.0–100.4°F)	36.1–38.0°C (97.0–100.4°F)
Pulse oximetry	≥94%	≥94%
Mental status	*A* in the AVPU scale	*A* in the AVPU scale

KEY NOTE

Tips for Examining Pediatric Patients

1. Identify yourself to caregivers (if present) and to pediatric patients who are old enough to understand. Talk to the child but include the parent or caregiver in the conversation. Use your first name, saying, "Hi, I'm David. What's your name?" Ask permission to care for the child if a parent or caregiver is present. In most states, implied consent takes effect when an injured or sick child is alone and you are giving appropriate aid.
2. If the parents are not present, tell the child in simple language that someone will find them as soon as possible. Assigning the task of finding the parents to another OEC technician in the presence of the child can reassure the child that the parents will be on the way as soon as possible.
3. If the patient is unresponsive or is severely injured or ill, control significant bleeding and then correct problems relating to the ABCDs. Call for help and transport rapidly. Move as quickly as possible without creating more anxiety for the child or caregivers.
4. If the child does not have life-threatening injuries, proceed at a calm, reassuring, relaxed pace. Include pediatric patients in the care by giving them a toy or an inflated glove, or by letting them listen to their own heart/lungs first.
5. Sit, kneel, or squat so that you are down at a child's level. Standing over small children can make them feel fearful or threatened. Try to avoid loud or distracting noises, including transmissions from your radio. Try to keep bright light out of a patient's eyes, and keep the number of rescuers who are interacting with the patient to a minimum.
6. Be friendly and include both the patient and caregivers when speaking. Try to alleviate any fears any of them might have. Acknowledge and accept each patient's feelings. Smile sincerely.
7. Allow smaller children to remain in their parent's arms, if possible. Doing so can be comforting and reassuring to both.
8. Always be honest with pediatric patients. Some may be fearful, for instance, that you are going to give them a "shot." Avoid telling them "this won't hurt" when you know it might. Acknowledge their fear and be honest and reassuring about what you will and will not do. Helping a patient breathe

(*continues*)

KEY NOTE (*continued*)

through pain can also facilitate getting a painful procedure done. When applying a splint to a child's broken arm, for example, try acknowledging that it might hurt and then suggesting that the child take in a deep breath through the nose and then blow it out hard through the mouth ("smell the roses, blow out the candle") while you manipulate the arm.

9. Ask pediatric patients where it hurts, or ask caregivers where they suspect it hurts, and examine that area *last*. Obviously, if a body part requires a life-supporting measure, do this first. If a child points to a wrist, for example, examine the rest of the child's body, then examine the rest of the injured arm, and only then gently palpate the wrist. If you touch the painful wrist first, you might have a difficult time examining the rest of the patient.
10. If you need to use any equipment for the exam or for care, explain what you are doing in language your patient can understand. Whenever possible, allow a child to touch or examine the equipment first. Ask patients if they have any questions, and then answer them honestly and simply.
11. Although most school-age children have been examined by a pediatrician and understand the process of a physical exam, young children might not understand what you mean by, "I'm going to examine you." Accordingly, explain each step of the examination as you do it. Be willing to stop to answer questions or to reassure the child.
12. Maintain good eye contact with patients, both to maintain their confidence and to pick up subtle clues, such as a small grimace that indicates that something hurts. Speak directly to pediatric patients in simple language and reassure them that you are there to help them.
13. Make sure pediatric patients understand what you are saying. Ask questions such as, "Do you know how to take a deep breath? Can you do it for me?" Or better yet, show them how to do it. Simple praise, such as, "Oh, that was a great deep breath!" can work wonders in gaining the cooperation of preschoolers.
14. Continually reassure anxious caregivers. Never lose your cool, and never get excited.

latter of which is the most important vital sign in young children. Because children have a more variable respiratory rate than that of adults, count breaths for 30 seconds and multiply by 2.

Assess circulation by measuring the peripheral pulse and blood pressure. Among the places to check the pulse are the brachial or femoral pulse in infants, the brachial pulse in small children, and the radial or carotid pulse in older children (**Figure 30-23**). Assess capillary refill (**Figure 30-24**). Use a pulse oximeter to assess oxygen saturation.

Measure blood pressure using a properly sized pediatric cuff (**Figure 30-25**). A standard adult-sized blood pressure cuff usually can be used for teenagers. Note that blood pressure can be very difficult to measure in children younger than 3 years. *Remember that because children can compensate well for shock initially, blood pressure is not a reliable indicator of shock.*

For school-age children and adolescents, perform a head-to-toe examination in the usual fashion. For preschoolers and younger children, after completing the primary assessment, begin the physical exam by gently palpating the extremities, leaving out any part that could hurt *until the end of the entire exam*.

Check distal sensation by gently scratching a child's hand or foot. Small children will withdraw the extremity if they have sensation, whereas older children can tell you they can feel you. Assess skin color. Examine the pelvis gently, in the same way you would for an adult.

Expose and inspect the abdomen, looking for any signs of injury using the DCAP-BTLS mnemonic (deformity, contusions, abrasions/avulsions, punctures/penetrations, burns/bleeding/bruises, tenderness, lacerations, swelling) (**Figure 30-26**). Gently palpate each abdominal quadrant, leaving until last the quadrant the child has identified as being painful. Watch each of the child's responses carefully, because even minor trauma can cause splenic or liver injuries in children due to the poor protection their undeveloped abdominal muscles provide. Assess the bony pelvis (**Figure 30-27**).

Expose the chest to look for evidence of trauma, again using DCAP-BTLS (**Figure 30-28**). Due to thoracic flexibility, children can receive significant injuries within the chest cavity with only minor external chest wall findings. Whenever children will tolerate it, listen to the lungs, noting any abnormal sounds. Always warm the stethoscope head before listening to the chest.

Palpate the entire spine (**Figure 30-29**). Be sure to watch the child's facial expressions for any

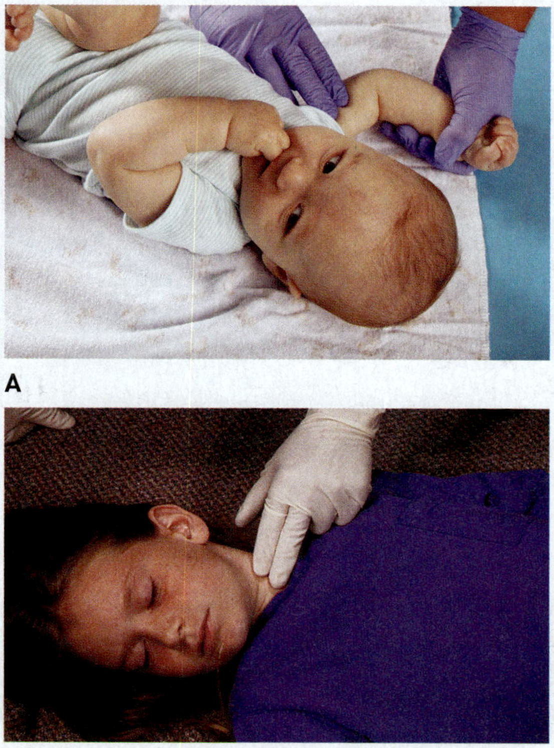

A

B

Figure 30-23 A. Checking the brachial pulse in an infant. **B.** Assessing the carotid pulse in an older child.

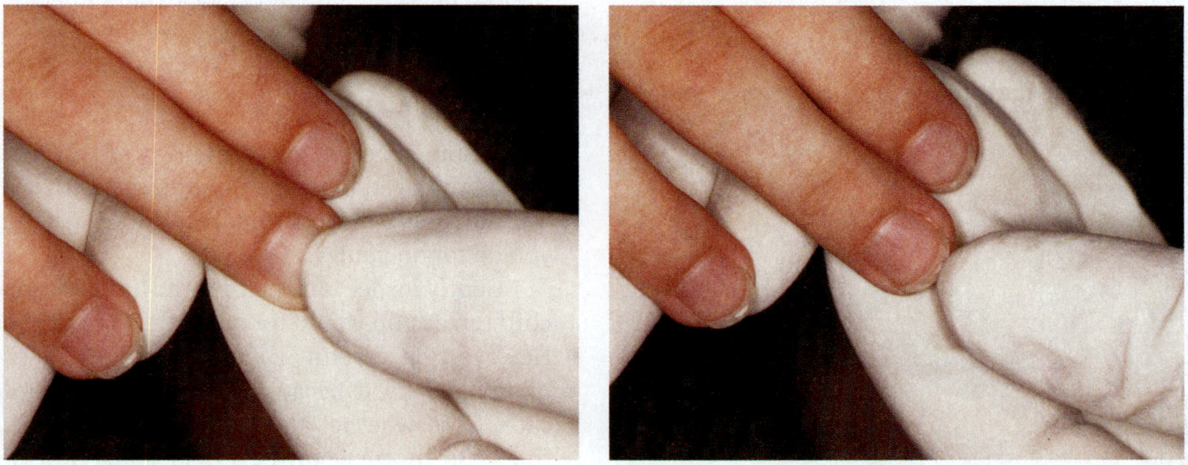

A B

Figure 30-24 A. To test capillary refill, compress the fingertip for 5 seconds using moderate pressure. **B.** Release the fingertip and count the number of seconds it takes for the normal color to return to the nail bed.

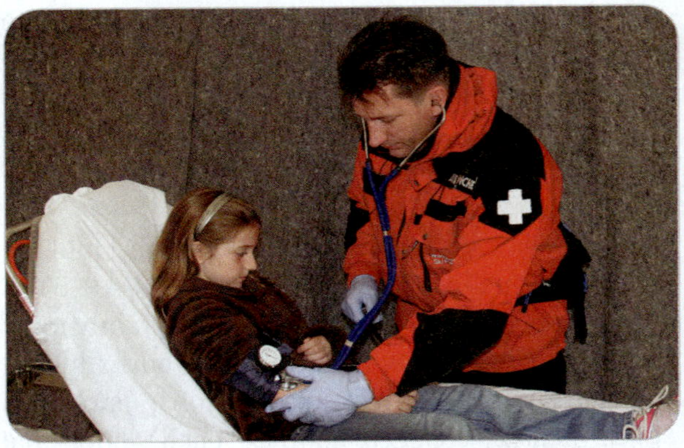

Figure 30-25 Take a child's blood pressure using a pediatric blood pressure cuff.

© Mike Halloran.

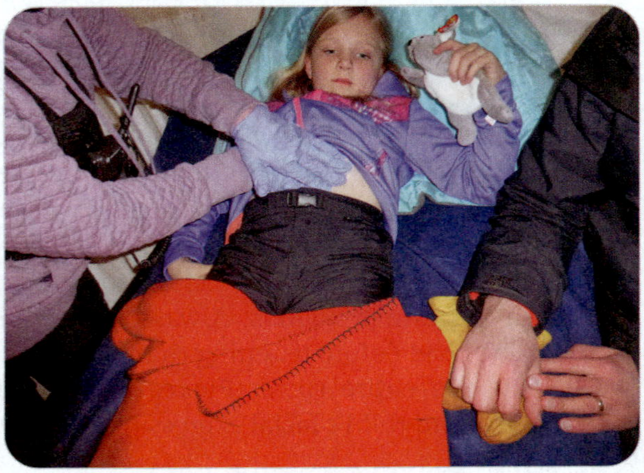

Figure 30-26 Expose and inspect a child's abdomen using the DCAP-BTLS mnemonic.

© Deborah Endly.

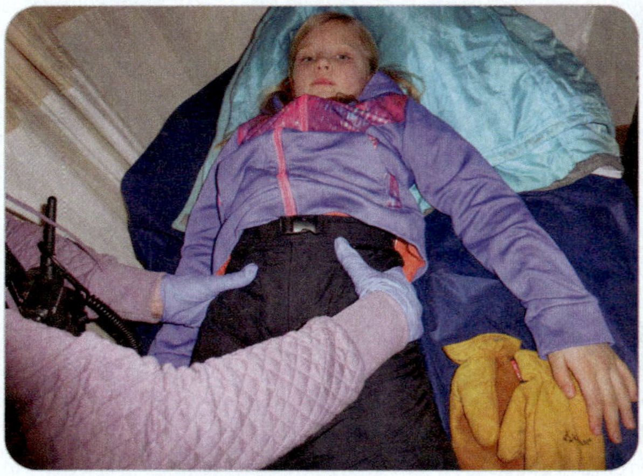

Figure 30-27 Assess the pelvis in a child gently, in the same way you would for an adult.

© Deborah Endly.

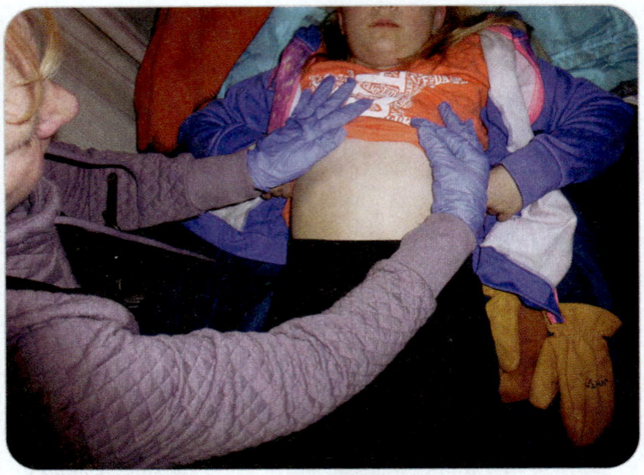

Figure 30-28 Expose the chest to look for signs of trauma.

© Deborah Endly.

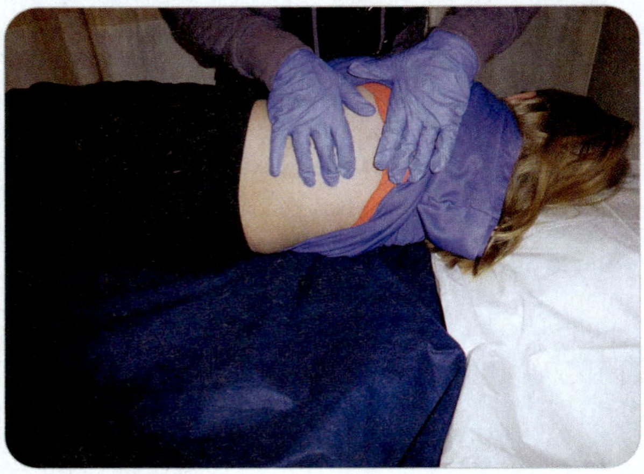

Figure 30-29 Palpate the child's entire midline spine.

© Deborah Endly.

indications of pain; such findings are an indication of the need for spinal motion restriction. Follow the same exam for spinal motion restriction as you do for an adult.

Gently inspect and palpate the head and face of children as you would for an adult (**Figure 30-30**). However, be careful when assessing a newborn or infant's head because the fontanels are delicate. Note whether the fontanels are level with the scalp (normal) or are either sunken or bulging (both abnormal). Look in the child's nose and ears for blood or fluid. Check the nose and mouth for excess mucus, swelling, or obstructions. Gently palpate the neck, again looking at the child's face for signs of discomfort (**Figure 30-31**).

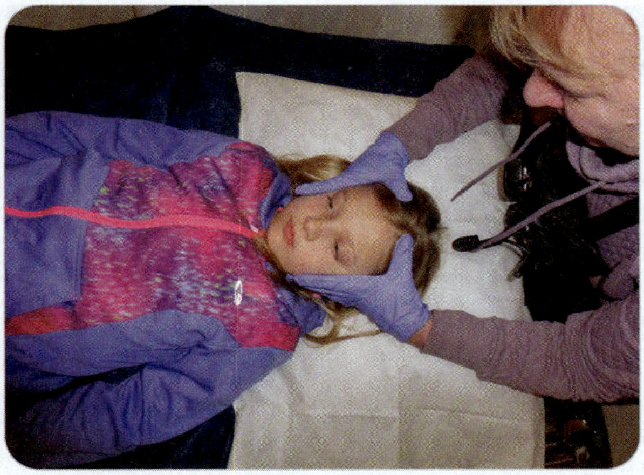

Figure 30-30 Inspect and palpate the child's head and face.

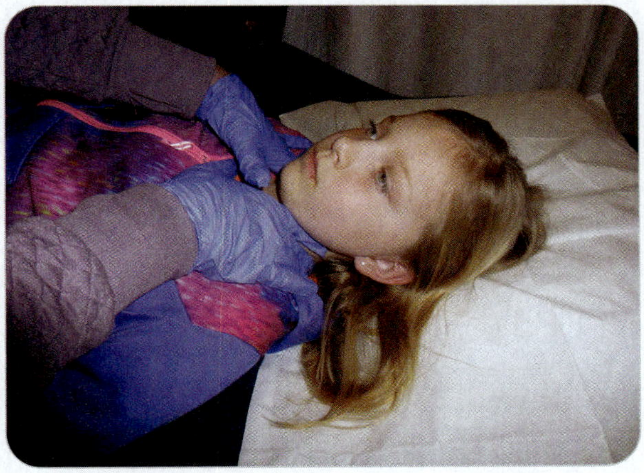

Figure 30-31 Examine the neck, watching the child's face for signs of discomfort.

Finally, assess any other area(s) that appear to be injured. Be gentle, take time to explain what you will do before you do it, and warn patients about any part of the exam that might produce discomfort. **Table 30-3** summarizes the approaches to examining the different age groups of pediatric patients.

Continue to monitor pediatric patients and perform frequent reassessments, including respiratory and circulatory status, level of responsiveness, skin color, and vital signs, for valuable clues concerning whether patients are responding to care. Because children can deteriorate quickly, never take your eyes off pediatric patients. Assess the vital signs every 5 minutes for children who are ill or injured, and every 10 minutes for pediatric patients with no apparent problems.

MANAGEMENT OF PEDIATRIC EMERGENCIES

The basic principles for treating pediatric patients are the same as those for treating adults: mitigate any hazards and correct any ABCD-related problems. CPR for children, infants, and newborns is discussed in your CPR/AED class. Because children have a smaller blood volume, control external bleeding aggressively; children easily can go into shock from a minor head laceration that is bleeding profusely. Even though children have vigorous compensatory physiological mechanisms that allow them to respond to serious illness or trauma, compared to adults

Table 30-3 Tip for Age-Based Assessment of Children

Infants: Ages 1 Month to 1 Year
• This child is aware of surroundings but has limited experience with being examined. • Examine the child in a caregiver's arms, if possible. • Engage the caregiver in the evaluation; if possible, have the caregiver assist whenever removing the patient's clothes is necessary. • Approach at the level of the child. • Move slowly and calmly during the exam. • Tell the caregiver what you are doing. • Examine the least painful body parts first and the painful body part last. • Inform the caregiver about possibly painful parts of the exam.

(continues)

Table 30-3 Tips for Age-Based Assessment of Children (*continued*)

Toddlers: Ages 12 to 36 Months • This child may be fearful of strangers. • Examine the child in a caregiver's arms, if possible. • Approach at the level of the child. • Move slowly and calmly, talking to both the child and the caregiver. • Address the child first. • Recognize that children can understand language that is 6 to 8 months more advanced than their speech. • Toddlers may push your hands away and be uncooperative. • Be gently persistent. The child's resistance will lessen. • Avoid asking any question to which the child can answer "no." • Perform the most painful part of the exam last, if possible. • Inform both the child and caregiver whenever pain could be associated with part of the exam.
Preschool Children: Ages 3 to 5 Years • These children can move between fantasy and reality and are magical thinkers. • They have good verbal skills and can be quite vocal. • History taken from them is not always accurate; may need to rely on the caregiver instead. • If very sick, preschoolers can regress to the level of a toddler. • Let patients decide whether they want to be examined in a caregiver's arms. • Before you do something, use simple language to explain what you are going to do. • Allow patients to examine equipment or listen to their own heart through a stethoscope first. • Limit a patient's options to two choices. • Praise good behavior in patients. • Because a preschooler's temperament can change rapidly and unexpectedly, expect "meltdowns" or regressions in behavior.
School-Age Children: Ages 6 to 12 Years • These children understand cause and effect and recognize authority. • Speak to children in simple terms and include caregivers. • Perform the physical assessment in a head-to-toes fashion. (Touch the painful part last, if possible.) • Respect each child's modesty and need for privacy. • School-age children may respond better to a same-sex examiner. • Inform school-age children what you are going to do before you do it. • Inform patients if some part of the examination might hurt. • If seriously injured children regress and become mute, involve caregivers in the examination.
Adolescents: Ages 13 to 18 Years • These children are rational and analytical. • Decision making and control skills are not as advanced as analytic and verbal skills. • Ask their permission to examine them. • Respect their privacy. • Evaluate and examine them apart from a parent's or caregiver's presence, especially if substance abuse or pregnancy may be involved. • Respect their independence. • Obtain the history directly from patients. • Assess adolescents as you would an adult. • Be direct and honest.

they have a smaller compensatory reserve and can go into shock quickly, often without exhibiting any external signs. Any child who looks sick and does not *appear* to be getting better with care is probably getting worse, even if the vital signs remain unchanged. For children who appear sick or injured, summon advanced life support (ALS) personnel and/or arrange for rapid transport to a definitive-care facility.

Pediatric shock, whether due to a medical or a trauma-related cause, can be extremely difficult to manage in the field due to the child's inability to compensate once initial compensatory mechanisms fail. If shock is suspected, immediately evacuate the patient by ALS transport to a definitive-care facility, preferably one that specializes in pediatric emergency care.

You may need to modify how you deliver care based on a child's developmental stage. For instance, if ventilations are required, avoid hyperextending the necks of young children, or the airway may collapse (**Figure 30-32**). For children younger than 1 year, open the airway by using the head tilt–chin lift maneuver to place the patient in a "sniffing" position (**Figure 30-33**). Administer any needed ventilations at the respiratory rate that is normal for that child's age group.

If spinal motion restriction is needed, apply a pediatric cervical collar and immobilize the child to a spine board. If a pediatric collar is not available, stabilize the head and neck with other means. Often infants, toddlers, and children can be effectively immobilized using a vest-style immobilization device. Padding may be needed to keep the spine straight and airway open (**Figure 30-34**).

Because respiratory-related problems are more common than cardiac disorders in children, administer high-flow oxygen using a pediatric mask if a child has an altered level of responsiveness, appears ill, or has obvious injuries, and titrate with a pulse oximeter, keeping the oxygen saturation between 94 and 99% (**Figure 30-35**). Because some children (especially young children) can become frightened by an oxygen mask, you may lessen their anxiety by applying brightly colored stickers of popular cartoon characters, superheroes, or animals to the mask before putting the mask on their face. Parents or caregivers can often help a child accept the use of an oxygen

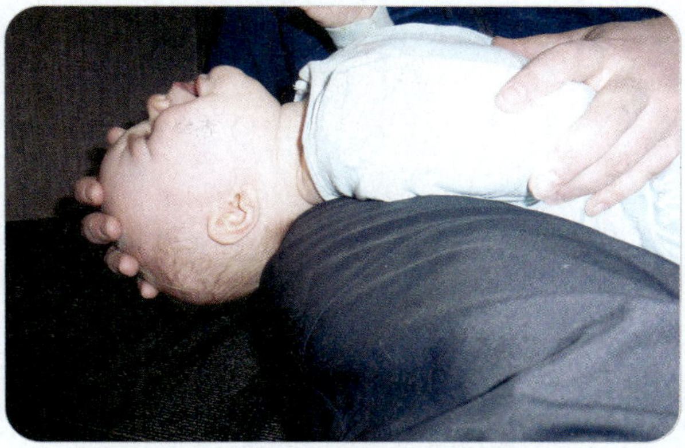

Figure 30-32 This child's neck is hyperextended, something you should avoid, or the airway may collapse.

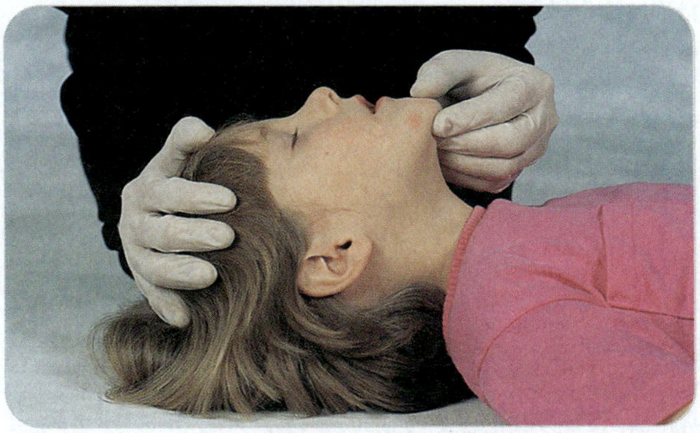

Figure 30-33 Use the head tilt–chin lift maneuver for children younger than 1 year. It is demonstrated here on an 8-year old.

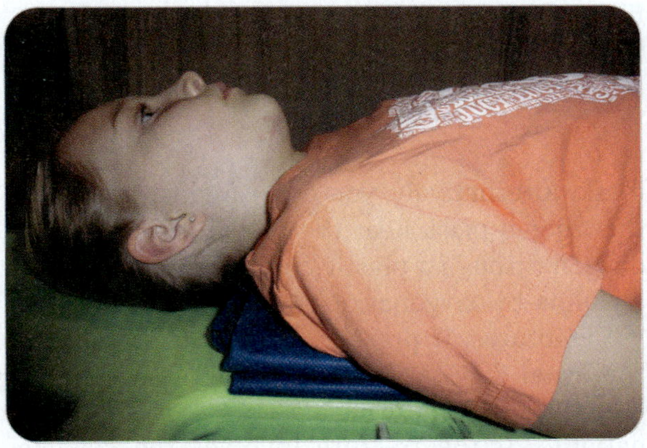

Figure 30-34 Padding beneath the shoulders of a child on a backboard helps keep the airway open.

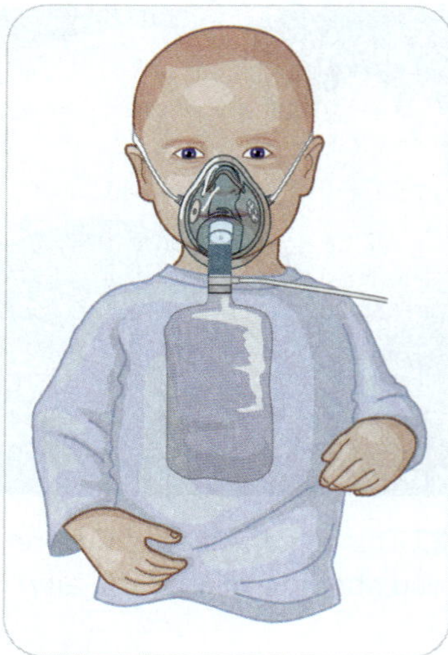

Figure 30-35 Administer oxygen to a child using a pediatric mask.

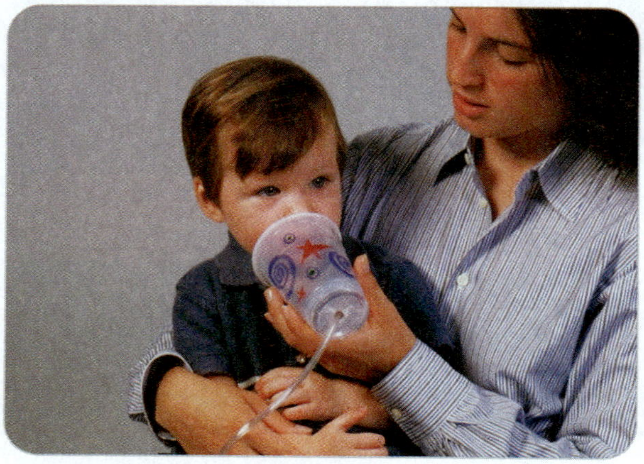

Figure 30-36 Consider using blow-by oxygenation with an infant.

mask. Alternatively, you or a caregiver may hold the oxygen mask near the patient's face or feed oxygen through a plastic cup in a process known as "blow-by oxygenation" (**Figure 30-36**).

Fractures, if present, should be splinted in the usual fashion. Malleable splints are highly effective for splinting fractures in pediatric patients. If the fracture involves the clavicle, shoulder, or upper extremity, be sure to apply a sling and swathe to decrease movement and to lessen pain. If available, use a pediatric traction splint for a midshaft femur fracture in a small child. For teenagers, an adult splint will usually work.

The symptoms of some pediatric airway-related disorders, such as croup, tonsillitis, and bronchiolitis, may be improved with cool and/or humidified air such as might be obtained by taking the child outdoors. Other problems such as asthma and epiglottitis are potentially life threatening and require more advanced care in a definitive-care setting. In these cases, rapid transport with ALS measures is the mainstay of field care. For a child with asthma, assist the older child or the caregiver in administering medicine from the child's own metered-dose inhaler.

Manage foreign-body obstructions according to current American Heart Association guidelines. Because a foreign body can become lodged beyond a child's vocal cords, aggressive airway management may be required to relieve the obstruction. In this case, continue BLS maneuvers while rapidly transporting the patient to ALS care.

Nausea, vomiting, and diarrhea are difficult to manage in the field. If severe, they could indicate the presence of an abdominal problem that might require surgery, so do not allow the patient to take anything by mouth, and rapidly transport to definitive care.

Manage seizures as described in Chapter 11, *Altered Mental Status*. Do not attempt to physically restrain a child who is actively seizing, and do not allow anyone to place anything in the child's mouth. Once the seizure has stopped, open and clear the airway as necessary. If no spine injuries are suspected, place the child in the recovery position and continue to monitor the child's airway and vital signs (**Figure 30-37**). Febrile seizures are managed by placing cool cloths in both axillae (armpits), in the groin, and on the forehead to reduce body temperature. An acetaminophen suppository can be inserted by a parent or a caregiver. Febrile seizures are usually benign; however, it is important to protect the child from trauma during the event. Focus on reducing the fever and attempting to determine the cause of the elevated temperature and the seizure.

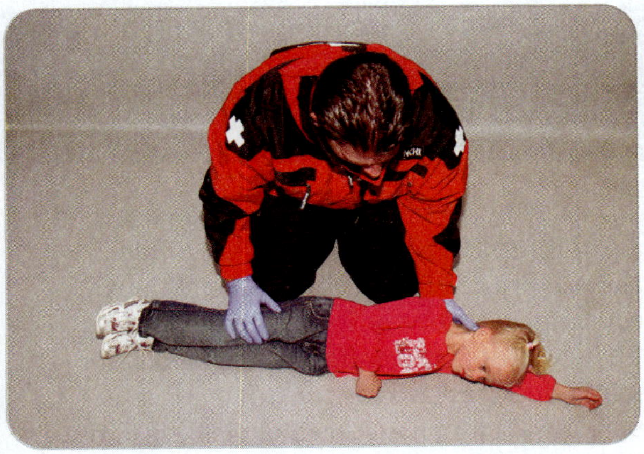

Figure 30-37 If no spine injury is suspected, place a child who had a seizure in the recovery position.

OEC technicians will rarely see a SIDS patient. There is little OEC technicians can do to help a SIDS patient. By the time the infant is discovered, advanced signs of death (i.e., rigor mortis, livor mortis) are often apparent. In such circumstances, OEC technicians should turn their attention to the parents or caregivers. Summon law enforcement if required in your state or province and comfort the family as best as possible.

Manage other pediatric medical conditions as you would for an adult, following the recommendations described in previous chapters. Trauma-related pediatric problems also are managed as described in other chapters; pay special attention to controlling external bleeding.

CASE Outcome

After confirming that there are no immediate threats to life, you perform a secondary assessment, which reveals an obvious deformity over the right clavicle. The girl begins to cry again, and you ask her why. She tells you she is afraid that you will hurt her, or worse, give her a shot. You reassure her that you don't give shots and tell her that you'd like to splint her arm, which will help take away some of the pain. You explain, however, to both the girl and her grandmother, that it might hurt when you move the arm into the splint and sling. The girl looks at her grandmother, who gives her an encouraging smile and tells you, "We'll both be big girls."

Other patrollers arrive, a blanket is placed underneath the patient and a second one around the patient to prevent hypothermia.

The grandmother holds the child's uninjured hand while you and the other OEC technicians prepare to carefully splint, sling, and swathe the girl's injury. You continue to talk to the girl quietly, telling her a story while you splint the arm. When you are done, she tells you it feels better.

You place the girl in a toboggan and take her to the aid room, keeping a close eye on the girl's respirations, appearance, and vital signs. The grandmother stays with the girl. Her vital signs remain stable. An ambulance takes her to the hospital.

The next day, the child's grandmother calls and tells you that her granddaughter did indeed suffer a broken clavicle. She thanks you for your calm, caring approach in helping the child.

CHAPTER REVIEW

In Summary

- Children are not miniature adults; they do not perceive or respond to the world as adults do.
- Children undergo six growth and development stages: newborn, infancy, toddler, preschool, school-age, and adolescence.
- Whenever possible, incorporate caregivers or parents into the assessment process.
- Be sensitive to an adolescent's need for independence, respect, and privacy.
- A child can maintain a normal blood pressure and appearance during compensated shock.
- Children can change rapidly from compensated shock to decompensated shock.
- Assume that the condition of a child who looks sick and is not improving with care is worsening.
- Report suspected child abuse to the proper authorities.
- Approach children slowly and gently. Smile and be friendly.
- A child who is crying or screaming has a patent airway.
- A slow heart rate in a child with respiratory distress is an ominous sign of severe illness and impending cardiac arrest.
- Cardiac arrest in children is nearly always preceded by respiratory arrest.
- Parents often demonstrate their fear by showing anger or irritation.

Key Terms

Child abuse Any act or failure to act on the part of a parent, a caregiver, or any adult that results in serious physical or emotional harm or imminent risk of harm to a child.

Child neglect A failure to act on the part of a parent, a caregiver, or other responsible adult to provide for the physical, emotional, educational, safety, or social needs of a child to the extent that emotional, developmental, or physical harm may occur.

Epiglottitis Inflammation and swelling of the epiglottis, the small, leaf-shaped structure that covers the larynx when a person swallows and prevents food from entering the trachea.

Fontanels The unfused sutures between the bones of the skull of a newborn that allow expansion of the growing brain; the fontanels have closed by approximately 18 months of age.

Meningitis Inflammation of the membranes covering the spinal cord and brain; may be caused by viruses or bacteria.

Pediatric assessment triangle An assessment tool that utilizes a pediatric patient's appearance (mental status, body position, and muscle tone), work of breathing (visible movement, effort, and audible sounds), and circulation (skin color) to assess the patient's well-being.

Shaken baby syndrome A condition in which an infant or toddler is picked up and violently shaken, causing a traumatic brain injury.

Sudden infant death syndrome (SIDS) The sudden, unexplained death of an infant in which a postmortem examination fails to determine the cause of death.

Chapter Questions

1. The pediatric airway differs from the adult in what way?
    a. It is shorter.
    b. It is more flexible.
    c. The tongue is larger in proportion to the oral cavity.
    d. All of the above

2. Which of the following explains why children compensate for shock differently than adults?
   a. Higher blood volume, higher heart rate
   b. Lower blood volume, lower heart rate
   c. Lower blood pressure, higher heart rate
   d. Lower blood pressure, lower heart rate
3. If your patient has a "meltdown," exhibits magical thinking, has good verbal skills, and needs to touch and examine your equipment, you are likely assessing a child from which age group?
   a. Toddler
   b. Adolescent
   c. School-age
   d. Preschool
4. For a 7-year-old, which of the following sets of vital signs is within normal limits?
   a. Pulse 90, respirations 25, systolic BP 100 mm Hg
   b. Pulse 130, respirations 50, systolic BP 70 mm Hg
   c. Pulse 40, respirations 10, systolic BP 120 mm Hg
   d. Pulse 80, respirations 40, systolic BP 110 mm Hg
5. What happens during respiratory failure in pediatric patients?
   a. Heart rate dramatically increases and the heart's need for oxygen increases.
   b. Exhaustion occurs due to efforts to compensate by increasing heart and respiratory rates.
   c. Hypoxia results from exhaustion due to compensatory mechanisms failing.
   d. All of the above
6. Cardiac arrest in pediatric patients is most often caused by:
   a. traumatic injury.
   b. respiratory arrest.
   c. an underlying genetic condition.
   d. a medical illness.
7. A pediatric seizure patient who presents with a history of infectious illness and a fever that developed rapidly most likely experienced what type of seizure?
   a. Status epilepticus
   b. Absence
   c. Partial
   d. Febrile
8. You are assessing a child who fell in ski school and is complaining of arm pain. During your assessment, which of the following findings suggest the child might be a victim of physical abuse?
   a. Multiple bruises in various states of healing
   b. Hypothermia
   c. Reluctance by the child to explain older injuries
   d. Both a and c
9. The pediatric assessment triangle is a good tool to quickly recognize whether your pediatric patient is seriously ill or injured. It is composed of which of the following three components?
   a. Blood pressure, pulse rate, and pupil reaction
   b. Respiratory function, blood pressure, and Glasgow Coma Scale
   c. Mental status, pulse rate, and skin color
   d. Work of breathing, circulation to skin, and appearance

Answers: 1. d, Objective 30-1, p. 685; 2. c, Objective 30-1, p. 687; 3. d, Objective 30-2, p. 710; 4. a, Objective 30-3, p. 705; 5. d, Objective 30-5, p. 691; 6. b, Objective 30-6, p. 691; 7. d, Objective 30-7, p. 692; 8. d, Objective 30-8, p. 698; 9. d, Objective 30-11, p. 700

CHAPTER 31

GERIATRIC EMERGENCIES

OBJECTIVES

Upon completion of this chapter, the OEC technician will be able to:

31-1 Describe physical changes that occur to six body systems with aging.

31-2 Describe effective methods for communicating with geriatric patients.

31-3 Describe the effects of the following illnesses and diseases on geriatric patients:

- Cardiovascular and respiratory disease
- Neurologic diseases
- Gastrointestinal diseases
- Altered mental status

31-4 Describe how medications can affect the results of an assessment of geriatric patients.

31-5 Explain why the following traumatic conditions/injuries are different in geriatric patients: falls, hip and pelvic fractures, traumatic brain injury, and cervical spine injury.

31-6 Explain how the management of geriatric patients is different than that of other patients.

KEY TERMS

Geriatric, p. 719
Kyphosis, p. 721
Lordosis, p. 721
Osteoporosis, p. 721
Polypharmacy, p. 725
Scoliosis, p. 721
Vital capacity, p. 720

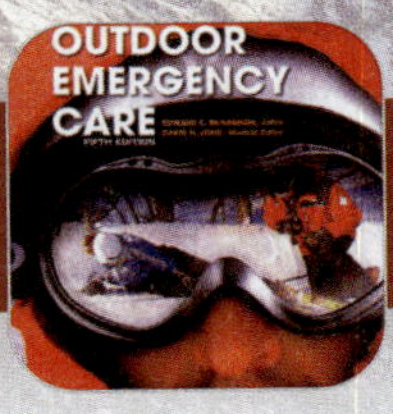

HISTORICAL TIMELINE 2011. *Outdoor Emergency Care, Fifth Edition,* is published.

CHAPTER OVERVIEW

Seniors represent a fast-growing population segment in the United States. This group is growing as the baby boomer generation retires. A senior is defined as a person who is 65 years of age or older.

The number of Americans ages 65 years and older is expected to more than double from 46 million today to over 98 million by 2060, and this age group's share of the total population will rise from 13% to over 24%. A larger number of seniors are enjoying outdoor activities during all seasons. Many seniors are bicycle and snow sports enthusiasts. Bicycling among adults ages 60 to 79 years increased over 300% between 1995 and 2007. According to the National Ski Area Association in 2018, seniors make up 5.2% of the 9.4 million total skiers in the United States. That is almost half a million people older than 65 years participating in snow sports. The percentage of snow sports enthusiasts older than 65 years has grown each year since 2008. Other seniors accompany their families on outings, engaging in nonrecreational activities, such as staying in the lodge and preparing a picnic lunch or babysitting young children while the family skis.

Despite improvements in their overall health and activity level, seniors cannot escape the inevitable changes that come with aging. As people age, they become physiologically different than when they were young. These differences make the health care needs of geriatric patients different from those of younger patients. Thanks to advances in medicine and technology, today's seniors are healthier, live longer, and are far more active than the elderly of the past (**Figure 31-1**). Seniors increasingly participate in activities that

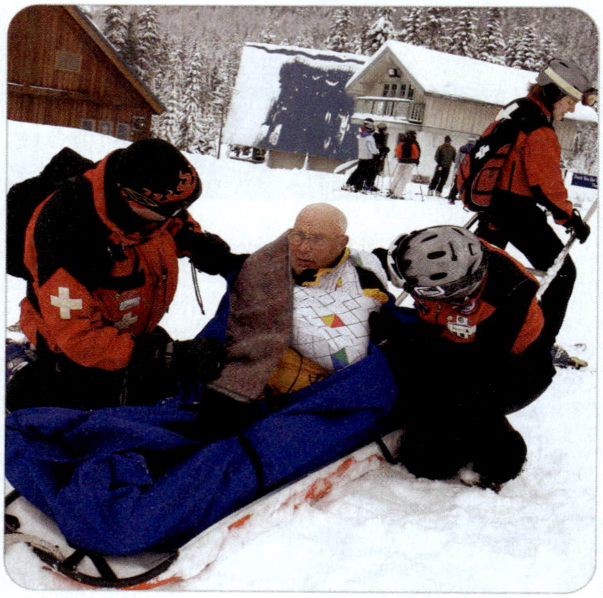

Figure 31-1 More seniors now enjoy outdoor activities, but the effects of aging increase their risk of injury.

CASE Presentation

You receive a call for a woman feeling ill in the lodge. Upon arrival, you find an elderly woman sitting at a table. She appears confused. Several family members are with her. The patient states that she was waiting for her family to come in for lunch and says, "I just fell and bumped my head." Upon questioning the patient, she tells you that she briefly "felt faint" before falling and now complains of feeling "a little dizzy" and having a headache.

A small hematoma begins to form on her forehead. She denies any cervical spine tenderness and has no other complaints. The woman tells you she is on medications for high blood pressure and "for a mechanical heart valve." Upon checking her radial pulse, you note that it is strong but slow and slightly irregular. The rest of the physical exam is unremarkable. The woman says she is embarrassed that her clumsiness has resulted in so much attention, insists that she will be fine despite the dizziness, and wants to eat lunch with her family. Something about the situation makes you uneasy.

What should you do?

bring them to the attention of ski patrollers and other OEC technicians.

A fundamental understanding of the aging process and geriatric physiology, knowledge of medications and their affects, and the ability to effectively communicate with this population will prepare you to address the unique medical needs of our nation's elderly. This chapter discusses the various medical problems and traumatic injuries seen in this population. Being able to modify your assessment and management techniques, looking for and reporting elder abuse, and understanding advance directives are important for an OEC technician.

PHYSIOLOGICAL CHANGES OF AGING

The aging process makes **geriatric** patients different from younger patients (**Table 31-1**). The changes that occur with aging can alter the body's response to various medical disorders and traumatic injuries (**Figure 31-2**). However, age-related changes do not always make the elderly frail or helpless. Many seniors maintain an active lifestyle that includes participating in and enjoying a variety of outdoor activities.

Neurologic Changes

As the body ages, changes within the nervous system make the brain and peripheral nerves less effective at processing data and transmitting impulses between various parts of the body. Such changes can seriously affect the body's ability to respond to disease or trauma. The total number of brain cells decreases, causing the brain to shrink in size. By age 85 years, total brain weight can be reduced by as much as 10%. Cerebral blood flow is reduced, which can decrease the amount of

Table 31-1 Physiological Changes with Aging

Effect of Aging	Result
Deposits of cholesterol within thickened arterial walls	Increased risk of heart attack, stroke, and high blood pressure
Decreased cardiac output	Diminished physical activity; reduced tolerance of physical stress; fatigue easily
Decreased elasticity and function of lungs	Decreased ability to clear foreign substances from lungs; higher risk of pneumonia and other respiratory infections
Fewer taste buds, less saliva; reduced acid production and slower movement along the digestive tract	Less enjoyment of eating; difficulty chewing and swallowing; early feeling of fullness when eating; difficulty digesting and absorbing food; constipation
Diminished liver and kidney function	Increased toxicity from alcohol and medications; diminished ability of blood to clot
Diminished thyroid function	Decreased energy; increased risk of hypothermia and hyperthermia
Decreased muscle mass, loss of minerals from bones	Decreased strength; falls more likely; minor falls more likely to cause fractures
The presence of multiple medical conditions	Use of many different medications, sometimes prescribed by different physicians; potentially harmful medication interactions
Loss of skin elasticity, shrinking of sweat glands	Thin, dry, wrinkled skin, that can tear or bruise easily; loss of sweating to cool body
Deaths of friends and family	Depression; loss of social support; increased risk of suicide

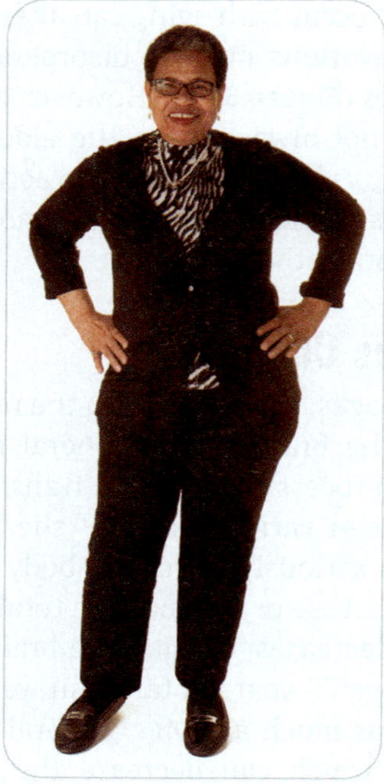

Figure 31-2 Changes that occur with aging can alter the body's response to illness and injury.

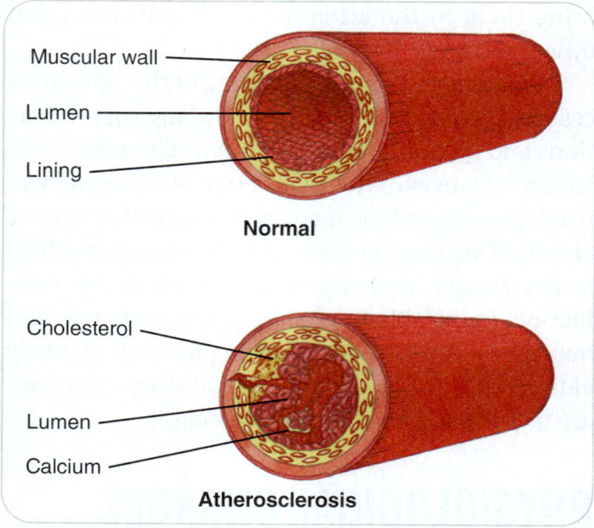

Figure 31-3 Blood vessels become stiffer from atherosclerosis.

glucose and oxygen that reaches brain cells. Nerve impulses are slowed, resulting in slowed reflexes, longer reaction times, and reduced perception of stimuli such as light, sound, and pain. As a result of reduced vision and hearing acuity, geriatric patients may not see hazards or hear warnings until it is too late. The inner ear balance organs may be less effective, causing older people to fall more easily. Additionally, the reduction of pain perception with age may lead seniors to underestimate the seriousness of their injuries.

Cardiovascular Changes

As the heart ages, the walls of the ventricles become less effective at pumping blood. Additionally, the heart rate may become irregular due to changes in electrical conductivity. In some cases, medications called beta-blockers are prescribed, which slow the heart rate intentionally and do not allow the heart rate to increase during stress caused by acute blood loss or shock. Blood vessels become stiffer from atherosclerosis, resulting in decreased elasticity and increased peripheral vascular resistance, both of which increase a geriatric patient's risk of hypertension, cardiac disorders, and cerebrovascular disease (**Figure 31-3**).

All these changes explain why a geriatric patient's cardiovascular responses to stress, illness, or injury are less effective than those of younger patients.

Respiratory Changes

Changes within the respiratory system of seniors include decreased elasticity of the lungs and changes in the way the body senses and responds to oxygen and carbon dioxide levels within the blood. The **vital capacity** is the maximum amount of air a person can take in in one breath. A healthy 90-year-old has approximately half the lung capacity of a healthy 30-year-old. These changes in respiratory function ultimately affect the way geriatric patients respond to stress to maintain a life-sustaining oxygen concentration.

Gastrointestinal Changes

The sense of smell and the abundance of taste buds decline with age, causing food to be less appealing. The gums and teeth deteriorate, increasing the risk of malnutrition due to the inability to chew food and the resulting disinterest in eating. The gag reflex decreases with age, increasing an older patient's risk of aspiration. This risk is especially heightened in patients with Parkinson disease or who have had a stroke. Throughout the gastrointestinal tract—from the esophagus to the large intestines—normal function slows, often resulting in constipation. Function of the liver and pancreas is reduced. Overall, the secretion of gastric buffers and digestive enzymes declines, causing a marked decrease in digestion that slows the rate of absorption of nutrients, water, and oral medications. Older patients are at higher risk for various gastrointestinal disorders, including obstruction, ulcers, diverticulitis, and perforations.

Changes in Kidney Function and Electrolyte Balance

With advancing age, the kidneys become less effective at filtering waste products, toxins, and medicines out of the blood. As a result, the effects of medications may be prolonged. Kidney function decreases by 30% to 40%, which can alter water balance and electrolyte levels within the body. Urine production and excretion are affected as well. By the time a person reaches 65 years, total body water can decrease by as much as 30%, making geriatric patients more susceptible to fluid loss and dehydration during physical activity and reducing their ability to respond to shock.

Musculoskeletal Changes

Bones lose density and muscle mass declines as the body ages. **Osteoporosis**, a disease that results in decreased bone density due to excessive mineral loss, affects 5% of men and nearly 25% of women older than 65 years. This condition predisposes seniors to fractures, especially of the hips, spine, and wrists (**Figure 31-4**).

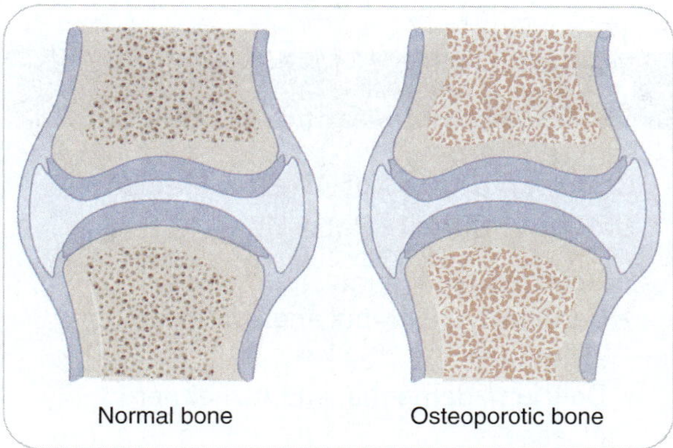

Figure 31-4 Loss of bone density due to osteoporosis makes bones less elastic and more brittle, thus more prone to breakage.

The alignment of the spine may become altered with increasing age, causing spinal curvatures. **Scoliosis** is an abnormal lateral curvature of the spine that causes the spine to curve in an "S" shape. **Kyphosis** is an abnormal curvature, usually in the upper thoracic spine, that produces a "humpback" appearance. Increased **lordosis** causes "swayback," or excessive inward curvature of the lumbar spine. Scoliosis and kyphosis can affect lung function, whereas lordosis causes lower back pain. Spinal motion restriction may be more difficult.

Aging also causes changes in ligaments, making them stiffer and less flexible, and predisposing the ligaments to rupture. Cartilage degenerates due to the loss of water, resulting in degenerative arthritis in the joints. Muscle tissue becomes more susceptible to injury, and muscles atrophy. The rib cage becomes stiff and the respiratory muscles lose strength, contributing to a decrease in lung function.

Integumentary and Endocrine Changes

With aging, the skin thins by as much as 20% and loses elasticity, with fat content under the skin decreasing. The resulting decreased insulation (from fat) predisposes the body to bruising and hypothermia. As the skin becomes less elastic, it is more susceptible to tearing and other dermatologic injuries. Because the body has fewer sweat glands with age, a patient's risk of hyperthermia is increased because the body is less effective at cooling itself.

Endocrine function also diminishes because the pancreas becomes less effective in regulating blood glucose. Half of all individuals older than 65 years have or will develop type 2 diabetes, especially if they are obese. Immunologic response also is decreased, making geriatric patients more susceptible to infections and increasing the time it takes them to heal.

COMMON GERIATRIC ILLNESSES AND CONDITIONS

Altered Mental Status

Among the many causes of altered mental status in elderly individuals are infection, head injury, transient ischemic attack and stroke, acute

KEY POINT

Common Causes of Altered Mental Status in Elderly Patients

- Head injury
- Cardiac dysrhythmia and acute coronary syndromes
- Delirium, dementia, and Alzheimer disease
- Seizure
- Infection
- Medication or drug toxicity
- Shock or severe dehydration
- Hypoxia and respiratory disorders
- Hypothermia or hyperthermia
- Stroke and TIA
- Blood glucose abnormality

cardiovascular conditions, hypoxia, and endocrine disorders such as hypoglycemia. OEC technicians also should consider environmental factors that change mental status, such as hypoxia due to high altitude, hypothermia, and hyperthermia. Toxicological ingestions, medications, stings, and envenomations also can alter normal thought processes. Additionally, the aging process increases an elderly individual's risk for such conditions as dementia and Alzheimer disease.

Hypertension

Hypertension is clinically defined as a systolic blood pressure greater than 130 mm Hg or a diastolic pressure greater than 80 mm Hg according to the 2018 American Heart Association guidelines. Blood pressure increases as we age, resulting in hypertension in many seniors. Physicians once believed that slight elevations in blood pressure were acceptable in elderly individuals. Today, however, most physicians urge older individuals to keep blood pressure below the recommended normal values. Seventy-five million people (one in three) in the United States have elevated blood pressure, but only 54% achieve adequate blood pressure control, according to the Centers for Disease Control and Prevention in 2016. Many of the individuals are older than 65 years. Nearly 1,000 people die every day in the United States from elevated blood pressure as a primary or secondary contributing cause. Untreated, hypertension is a serious medical disorder that can adversely affect other body systems, and it is a major risk factor for such diseases as myocardial infarction and stroke. Hypertension is generally not symptomatic; thus it has been nicknamed "the silent killer."

KEY POINT

The Dangers of Hypertension

High blood pressure increases your risk for dangerous health conditions:

- *First heart attack.* About 7 out of 10 people having their first heart attack have high blood pressure.
- *First stroke.* About 8 out of 10 people having their first stroke have high blood pressure.
- *Chronic (long-lasting) heart failure.* About 7 out of 10 people with chronic heart failure have high blood pressure.
- *Kidney disease.* High blood pressure is a major risk factor of this disease, too.

Source: Centers for Disease Control and Prevention. High blood pressure facts. https://www.cdc.gov/bloodpressure/facts.htm. Reviewed November 30, 2016. Accessed January 4, 2020.

Myocardial Infarction

The incidence of myocardial infarction (MI) increases with age and is aggravated by risk factors such as uncontrolled hypertension, high cholesterol, diabetes, smoking, obesity, and a strong family history of coronary artery disease. An MI can also be provoked by rigorous physical activity in susceptible individuals. Chest pain is the most common symptom of a heart attack and is often accompanied by pain or numbness in the jaw or left arm (possibly radiating to the right arm) and by shortness of breath. Symptoms can also include nausea and diaphoresis (heavy sweating).

KEY POINT

Signs of MI in Seniors

- Chest pain "with or without pain radiating to jaw and left arm" and shortness of breath
- Weakness
- General unease
- Neck pain
- Back pain
- Mild chest discomfort

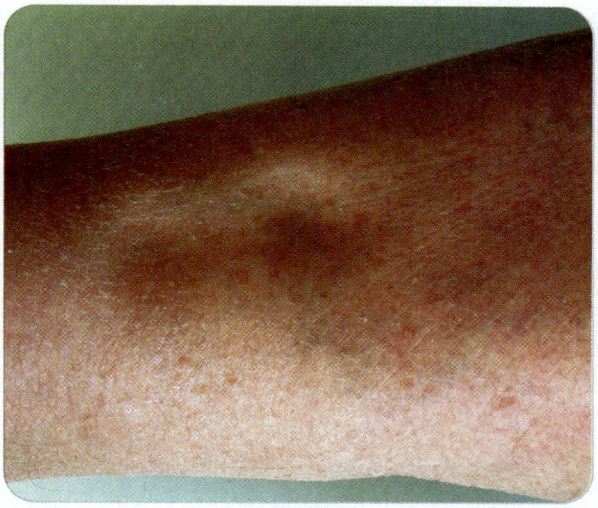

Figure 31-5 Swelling (edema) of the ankles is a sign of congestive heart failure. Removal of the pressure exerted by the examiner's finger may leave an indentation in the swollen tissue, a sign called "pitting edema."

In seniors, the signs and symptoms of an MI may not be straightforward. Geriatric patients may complain only of weakness or of a general feeling of unease. They also may complain of neck pain, back pain, upper abdominal pain, or mild chest discomfort. Such presentations, which are considered atypical for younger cardiac patients, appear to be more common for geriatric heart attack patients. Maintain a high index of suspicion for heart attack in older patients, and be vigilant for subtle symptoms of heart attack in seniors who have risk factors for coronary artery disease.

Congestive Heart Failure

Congestive heart failure is a condition in which the heart cannot pump enough blood to meet the needs of the body's other organs. As you learned in Chapter 15, *Cardiovascular Emergencies*, heart failure results from ineffective pumping by the right or left ventricle, or both, and is commonly caused by long-standing hypertension or by a previous heart attack that damaged the heart muscle. Seniors who have congestive heart failure typically take medications that improve the pumping strength of the heart, control blood pressure, or help reduce fluid levels and swelling in the body (**Figure 31-5**). Physical exertion can aggravate the condition, as can ascending to high altitude.

Syncope

A common disorder that affects millions of seniors each year is syncope, a brief loss of responsiveness due to an inadequate amount of oxygen reaching the brain. Even though most syncopal episodes in the general population are from simple fainting, syncope should be considered a life-threatening event in seniors until proven otherwise because it may stem from other medical conditions such as an irregular heart rhythm, a sudden drop in blood pressure, or a stroke or transient ischemic attack. Syncope in the elderly usually requires further medical evaluation to rule out any potentially serious underlying causes.

Stroke

A stroke is a reduction of blood flow to brain tissue resulting from narrowing, blockage, or rupture of a cerebral artery in the brain. The resulting neurologic dysfunction corresponds to the area and amount of the brain that is affected. Older patients have the highest risk for stroke and may initially present with only mild confusion or altered mental status. Typical neurologic deficits such as facial droop, slurred speech, abnormal behavior, or changes in limb function may not initially be present. Transient ischemic attacks, which are variants of stroke that are of short duration and are accompanied by complete resolution of symptoms, are also prevalent among seniors. Despite

KEY POINT

FAST Stroke Recognition

- **F** *Face.* Ask the person to smile. Does one side of the face droop?
- **A** *Arms.* Ask the person to raise both arms. Does one arm drift downward?
- **S** *Speech.* Ask the person to repeat a simple phrase. Is the person's speech slurred or strange?
- **T** *Time.* If you observe any of these signs, call 9-1-1 immediately.

an apparently normal appearance, patients with presumed transient ischemic attack require urgent medical evaluation because they are at increased risk for developing a serious stroke.

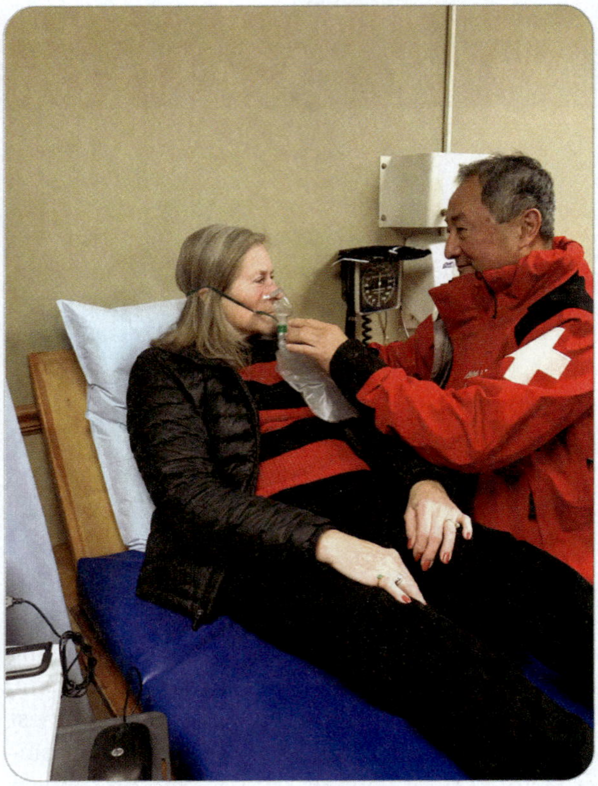

Figure 31-6 Low-flow oxygen may help a patient who is having respiratory difficulties.

Chronic Obstructive Pulmonary Disease

Chronic obstructive pulmonary disease (COPD) is any respiratory disease, including chronic bronchitis, emphysema, and asthma, that results in an increased obstruction to expiratory airflow (breathing out). Seniors are at greater risk for COPD due to long-term smoking, which is the leading cause of COPD, and various occupational exposures. Older patients with COPD are very sensitive to sudden changes in exertion and typically require low-flow supplemental oxygen therapy as well as inhaled bronchodilators to maintain homeostasis (**Figure 31-6**). This delicate balance in respiratory function can be compromised during even mild physical activity or as a result of a rapid ascent to a higher altitude.

Table 31-2 Causes of Abdominal Pain in Elderly Patients

- Abdominal aortic aneurysm
- Appendicitis
- Bowel obstruction
- Bowel perforation
- Cholecystitis/biliary colic
- Diverticulitis
- Gastritis and gastrointestinal bleeding
- Hernias
- Mesenteric ischemia
- Pancreatitis

Abdominal Emergencies

Elderly patients who present with an acute abdomen represent true emergencies because the underlying cause could be a life-threatening condition such as a rupturing abdominal aortic aneurysm, a bowel obstruction or perforation, gastrointestinal bleeding, or peritonitis (inflammation inside the abdomen) (**Table 31-2**). In fact, over 60% of the causes of abdominal pain in elderly patients require surgical intervention, nearly double the rate for younger patients. Due to the age-related reduction in pain sensation, even serious causes of abdominal problems may present with few or no signs or symptoms in seniors. Thus, because older individuals tend to have more serious conditions associated with abdominal pain, arranging rapid transport to a physician for evaluation is very important for geriatric patients.

MEDICATION USE IN THE ELDERLY

Longevity and quality of life in the elderly have improved greatly in recent decades thanks to new technology and many new medications created each year. In 2019, people age 65 years and older made up close to 13% of the US population but accounted for 34% of all prescription medication use and 30% of all over-the-counter medication use.

The average geriatric person, not in a nursing home, takes five or more medications weekly. The concurrent use of multiple medications, known as **polypharmacy**, is common among older patients because they often have multiple, coexisting medical conditions. Taking medications in combination can cause a host of adverse reactions and can significantly affect assessment findings. Always ask geriatric patients about their use of herbal supplements and over-the-counter medications; some seniors may not consider them true "medications" and may not mention them unless directly asked.

Ask elderly patients directly if they share medications with friends or family because they may not readily admit to this practice. Because of cost, many older patients do not take prescribed medicines, or take only part of the prescribed dosage (**Figure 31-7**). Obtaining a complete accounting of senior patients' past medical history and medications during the SAMPLE (signs and symptoms, allergies, medications, past medical history, last oral intake, events leading up to the problem) history can help you and higher-level providers provide better care for geriatric patients.

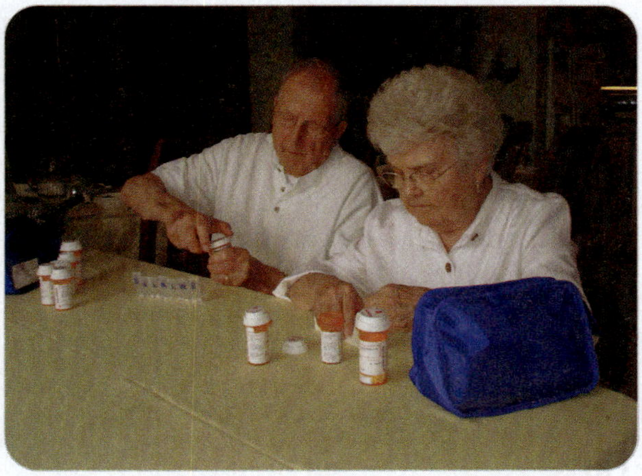

Figure 31-7 Seniors consume almost 34% of all prescription medications.

Unfortunately, elderly patients may not know the names of all the medications they take. They may be able to provide you with a list of their medications. If not, OEC technicians should ask what each medication is used for, because this information may well provide clues that may help identify the medication. For instance, a patient may say, "It makes me have to pee" or "It makes my heart beat slower."

Medications for treating hypertension are among the most commonly prescribed classes of medications among older patients. A few examples of these cardiovascular medications are beta-blockers, calcium channel blockers, and diuretics. Beta-blockers are used to manage cardiac arrhythmias. They make the heart contract more efficiently, decrease the blood pressure, and slow the pulse rate. These medications are highly effective in reducing the amount of stress placed on the heart and are commonly used to lower blood pressure. Unfortunately, they also can adversely affect the body's compensatory mechanisms when the body is stressed or in shock. For example, the expected increased heart rate in response to blood loss in a patient with traumatic internal bleeding may not occur if the patient's heart rate is being slowed by beta-blockers. Common beta-blockers include metoprolol (Lopressor), propranolol (Inderal), and atenolol (Tenormin).

Calcium channel blockers reduce heart rate, blood pressure, and (to a lesser degree) heart contractility. Like beta-blockers, calcium channel blockers can potentially counteract the normal compensating mechanisms during stress or trauma. Common calcium channel blocking agents include diltiazem (Cardizem), nifedipine (Procardia), verapamil (Isoptin), and amlodipine (Norvasc).

Diuretics decrease the volume of circulating fluid within the cardiovascular system in order to reduce blood pressure, treat heart failure, or help with pedal edema. By causing the kidneys to excrete more urine, diuretics alter the body's fluid

CASE Update

Upon examination of the patient, you find that she has a blood pressure of 180/92 mm Hg, a heart rate of 58 beats per minute, and normal respirations. Your partner reviews the patient's medications with a family member and reports that she is taking warfarin, Lopressor (beta-blocker), and aspirin. As you continue with your evaluation, the patient vomits and then says, "It must have been something I ate for lunch." Her mental status is unchanged: slightly confused but cooperative. You conduct a FAST exam and find a slight grip weakness in her right hand. You sense something is wrong with this patient.

What should you do?

and electrolyte balance. Elderly patients who take these medications are more susceptible to hypotension, dizziness, syncope, and slower heart rates and may exhibit shock faster due to a lower blood volume. Common diuretics include hydrochlorothiazide (HCTZ), triamterene (Dyazide), and furosemide (Lasix).

Blood "thinners" are another class of medications that deserve special attention. They are called anticoagulants because they stop blood from coagulating (clotting). These medications are commonly prescribed to patients with a history of mechanical heart valve replacement, an irregular heartbeat, or blood clots in the legs (deep vein thrombosis) or lungs (pulmonary embolism). Blood thinners can increase or prolong trauma-related bleeding. Even a nosebleed or a traumatic brain injury could have disastrous consequences due to uncontrolled bleeding. A patient with blunt abdominal trauma may have increased internal abdominal bleeding caused by a blood-thinning medication. Thus, any trauma patient who is on a blood thinner should be carefully examined, no matter how trivial the injury.

Common blood thinners include warfarin (Coumadin), clopidogrel (Plavix), dabigatran (Pradaxa), apixaban (Eliquis), rivaroxaban (Xarelto), and enoxaparin (Lovenox). Aspirin has blood-thinning properties also. Because of the increased risk of bleeding, many trauma systems recommend that patients on blood thinners who have any *significant* mechanism of injury be transported not to a local emergency department, but instead to a trauma center, where the large quantities of blood products often needed by such patients are available. Some antibiotics and herbal supplements can affect anticoagulants, prolonging bleeding time.

TRAUMA CONSIDERATIONS IN ELDERLY PATIENTS

For any type of trauma, geriatric patients have higher mortality rates compared with those of younger patients. The mortality rate of seniors from traumatic brain and spinal cord injuries, for example, is higher than that of patients younger than 65 years, and rises with age. As an independent risk factor, age presents the greatest increase in risk for a poor outcome of trauma cases. These statistics are important to OEC technicians because they will be increasingly likely to encounter older patients with a traumatic injury, whether from skiing, hiking, mountain climbing, or other activities.

Assessment of seniors can be particularly difficult. What may appear to be a relatively minor complaint could be a life-threatening injury. A trivial mechanism of injury can lull OEC technicians into thinking that nothing is wrong with the patient. Other factors, including underlying disease and medication use (especially "blood thinners"), must be considered in trauma.

Falls

The geriatric population has a higher incidence of inadvertent falls than do other age groups. Among the more common serious traumatic injuries from falls are pelvic and hip fractures, traumatic brain injury, rib fractures, and cervical spine injury. Wrist fractures, severe contusions, and other injuries may occur. Approximately 8% of adults 65 years and older visit the emergency department each year due to a fall-related injury, and about 25% of these patients ultimately require inpatient medical care. More importantly, falls cause 12% of all deaths in the geriatric population, both directly and indirectly.

Many falls are caused by an underlying medical condition that may be unknown to the patient. Although the outdoors presents numerous trip-and-fall hazards, OEC technicians should not automatically assume that a fall was due to clumsiness or inattentiveness. Instead, it is vital that OEC technicians evaluate not only the traumatic injuries related to a fall but also the *potential cause of the fall*. Some falls result from a medical issue, such as a syncopal episode. Red flags in the medical history that suggest this possibility include palpitations, chest pain, lightheadedness, or dizziness before the fall. The medical condition causing the fall could be more serious than the injury.

KEY POINT

The Significance of a Fall

When a geriatric patient falls and sustains an injury, always consider why the person fell. It could be from a serious unrelated medical problem.

Hip and Pelvic Fractures

Fractures to the hips and pelvis are common among elderly patients (**Figure 31-8**). Osteoporosis makes elderly patients more susceptible to these fractures. Common mechanisms of injury that can produce these fractures are trips and falls, low-speed collisions, bicycle crashes, equestrian and snow sports mishaps, and other forms of blunt trauma. Older patients have more bleeding complications from hip and pelvic fractures. Hip or pelvic fracture must be considered when evaluating hypotensive geriatric patients who have an altered mental status in the absence of obvious evidence of external bleeding, chest or abdominal trauma, or other long-bone fractures.

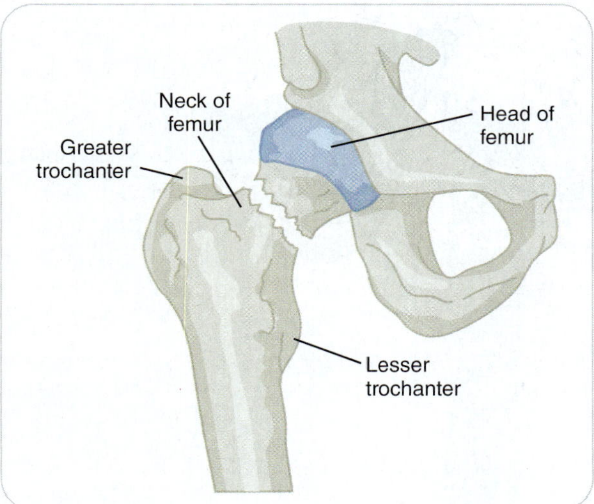

Figure 31-8 A displaced femoral neck fracture—commonly known as a fractured hip—is a common result of a fall among seniors.

Traumatic Brain Injury

Two major age-related changes put geriatric patients at greater risk of traumatic brain injury: the dura mater (lining around the brain) becomes more adherent to the skull, and the brain shrinks in size. The combination of these two changes increases the space between the outside of the brain and the inside of the skull, allowing for more brain movement within the skull. Deceleration head trauma, even with a relatively minor mechanism of injury, can cause brain injury. Additionally, the use of warfarin or other blood-thinning medications and the presence of chronic medical conditions such as hypertension or diabetes dramatically increase the risk of bleeding within the skull. These factors explain why an older person who experiences apparently minor head trauma may have a severe traumatic brain injury.

The typical symptoms associated with traumatic brain injuries may not be readily apparent in geriatric patients. Maintain a high level of suspicion of brain injury in any geriatric patient who has suffered a head injury; pay especially close attention to any changes in the patient's level of responsiveness.

KEY POINT

Cervical Spine Injury in Geriatric Patients

Devastating cervical spine injury and paralysis in geriatric patients may result from trauma during skiing or biking but are *also seen from simply falling from a standing or seated position*.

Cervical Spine Injury

Significant injuries to the cervical spine deserve special consideration among seniors because fracture patterns tend to involve more than one level of the spine, are frequently unstable, and often accompany head trauma. As a result of weakened neck muscles and osteoporosis, high cervical injuries at the C1 to C2 region are seen in geriatric patients. Devastating cervical spine injury and paralysis in geriatric patients have resulted from trauma during skiing or biking but are seen also from simply falling from a standing or seated position. OEC technicians should be alert to the possibility of cervical injury and assess geriatric patients following the spinal motion restriction guidelines in Chapter 21, *Spine, Brain, and Nervous System Injuries*.

ADDITIONAL CONSIDERATIONS

Several medical advancements have vastly improved the quality of life for seniors and have increased their ability to participate in various outdoor activities: joint replacement, implantable devices, and external ports and medical apparatus. OEC technicians must be aware of these developments because they can influence treatment decisions.

Artificial Joints

As a result of advances in orthopedic surgery techniques, geriatric patients can now undergo complete joint replacement, enabling them to continue their favorite outdoor activities (**Figure 31-9**). Commonly replaced joints include the shoulder, hip, and knee. Vertebral discs can also be replaced, and vertebrae can be fused. Artificial hip and shoulder joints dislocate more easily; however, patients should be treated the same as someone with a

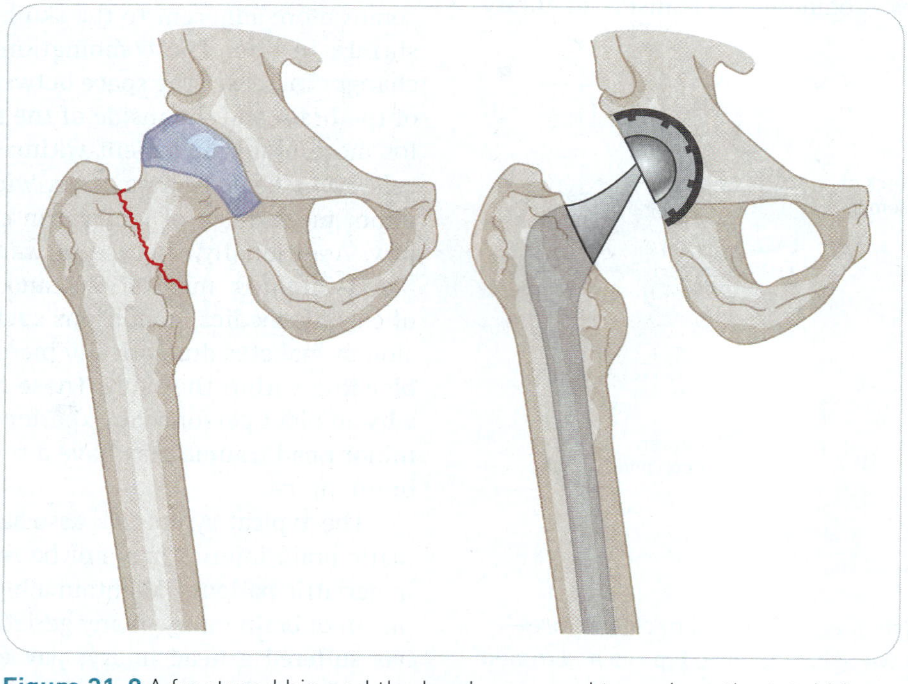

Figure 31-9 A fractured hip and the hardware used to replace the total hip.

dislocated natural joint. Additionally, patients who have had spinal surgery are more likely to have back or neck problems following a spinal insult.

Implantable Devices

The increased use of implantable devices—cardiac pacemakers, internal defibrillators, artificial heart valves, neurostimulators, cochlear devices, and internal drug pumps—has allowed seniors who could no longer participate in outdoor activities to again enjoy those activities.

Although each of these devices provides numerous therapeutic benefits, they also may cause or worsen many medical conditions. For instance, failure of a cardiac pacemaker can cause life-threatening arrhythmias or cardiac arrest and can override the heart's compensatory mechanisms in a patient in shock. Failure of an internal drug pain pump can lead either to life-threatening narcotic overdosing or to withdrawal when narcotic pain medicine is no longer being delivered properly. Failure of an implantable cochlear device affects hearing and can hinder communication.

Implantable devices also can be compromised by factors in the external environment. For instance, portable radios, microwaves, and magnetic objects may inactivate a cardiac pacemaker or an implantable defibrillator and can cause interference with cochlear devices.

External Openings, Ports, and Medical Apparatus

Many elderly patients with endocrine, gastrointestinal, or genitourinary disorders rely on an external port (opening) to assist with a normal body function or to facilitate a therapeutic intervention. A patient may have a urinary catheter to collect urine or an abdominal colostomy bag that collects feces from the large intestine. Some patients may have a temporary or permanent shunt or catheter placed into one of the large veins of the arm or chest for kidney dialysis or for the administration of medications such as chemotherapeutic drugs. Problems can arise with any of these openings or ports, and the most frequent problems involve clogging or infection.

OEC technicians also encounter portable drug infusion pumps and battery-operated oxygen devices. Portable infusion pumps are used to provide medications such as insulin in either a continuous dose or timed increments. External diabetic pumps, which have a catheter that is inserted into the skin, usually in the abdomen, can be as small as a digital pager and often are found in a shirt pocket or attached to the patient's belt. Malfunction can cause hyperglycemia or hypoglycemia. Inflammation may occur, usually from infection at the site where the catheter enters the body. Battery-operated oxygen tanks of various sizes are used to treat respiratory ailments. Even though most external medical apparatus units are hermetically sealed, problems can arise should dirt or other debris enter the system and interfere with the device's internal systems.

Advance Directives

The use of advance directives is increasing in the United States, especially among the elderly. Advance directives are legal documents that provide guidance regarding a patient's wishes in the event the patient is unable to communicate during a life-threatening medical emergency. A common form is called MOLST, which stands for medical orders for life-sustaining treatment.

Communicating with Elderly Patients

Effective communication is especially important in gathering the history and assessing geriatric patients (**Figure 31-10**). Always show the utmost respect for elderly patients and avoid being overly casual or too aggressive with them. Courtesy goes a long way.

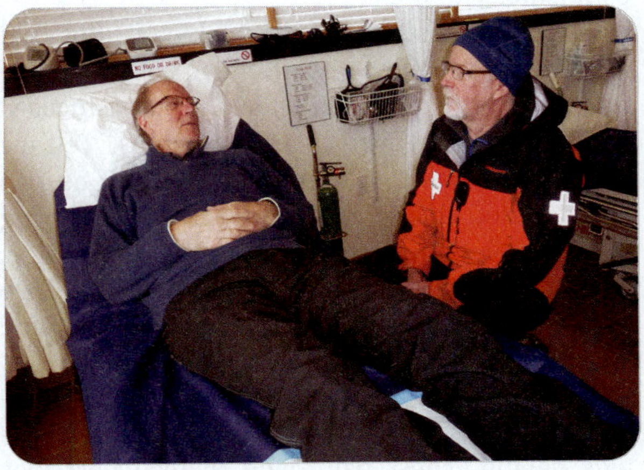

Figure 31-10 Effective communication with an elderly patient will reduce anxiety.

When evaluating an elderly patient at the scene, eliminate distractions such as music or other loud noises. Place yourself at the patient's level and maintain eye contact. Do not assume that all elderly patients are hard of hearing; use a normal speaking voice. If it becomes evident that the patient cannot hear you, increase the volume of your voice slightly and slow your speech until the patient can hear you. Speaking in a lower pitch may help the patient hear you better. You may also consider asking if the patient has one ear that hears better than the other.

Independence is very important to seniors. Allow elderly patients to remain in control of their bodies, and obtain their consent before assessing or treating them. When addressing seniors, always use "Mr.," "Mrs.," or "Ms." followed by their last name. Avoid using a nickname or a first name unless the patient requests it. As you build rapport, the interaction may take on a more casual tone, but you should not be the one to initiate it. Also avoid terms such as "hon" or "sweetie," because some seniors consider them offensive or demeaning.

Be clear and purposeful in your conversations with patients. Speak directly to the patient. To avoid confusion, have only one OEC technician speak with a patient, and ask only one question at a time.

Do not direct your questions to a patient's family or friends as if the patient were not there. If a patient is unable to speak or comprehend and family or friends are present, designate one person to speak on the patient's behalf. Having multiple people trying to answer for the patient is too confusing.

When obtaining a history, ask questions that are easy to answer, not open-ended questions. Patients may struggle to provide a prompt, focused answer to open-ended requests such as "Tell me about your pain." Closed-ended questions can be answered easily and are useful for clarifying specific points or obtaining specific information. Examples of closed-ended questions are, "Do you have pain?", "Is the pain sharp or dull?", and "Point to where it hurts."

Use good listening skills to understand a patient's complaints or symptoms. If a patient denies having "chest pain" and instead describes it as "discomfort," confirm your understanding by saying something like, "Is the discomfort like someone is sitting on your chest?" As your exam progresses, continue to refer to the symptom as "discomfort." Whenever possible, use lay terms instead of complex medical terminology. Using these strategies will increase the effectiveness of your interview and will allow you to obtain a more complete medical history.

ASSESSMENT OF THE GERIATRIC PATIENT

Assessment of geriatric patients is no different from assessment of any other patient (**Figure 31-11**). It includes a scene size-up, a primary assessment, history taking, a secondary assessment, and ongoing reassessment. However, you need to be aware of problems that are unique to the elderly, due to the aging process.

The scene size-up includes an evaluation of the surroundings for any potential hazards that may endanger you or others. In cases involving trauma in an elderly person, take an extra moment

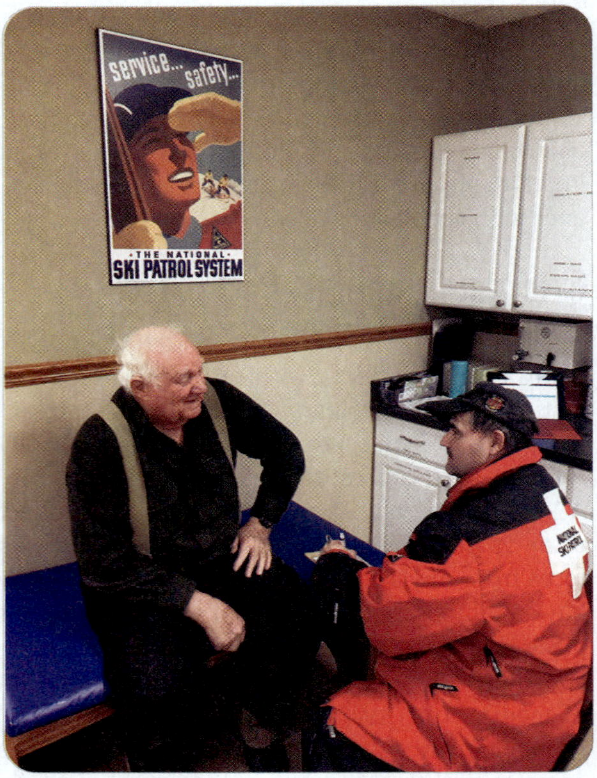

Figure 31-11 The assessment of a geriatric patient is the same as for any other age group. You may need to speak slowly and clearly and look directly at the patient.

to look for clues about what might have contributed to the patient's problem. For instance, loose rocks, slippery surfaces, uneven terrain, and exposed roots can all create trip-and-fall situations in outdoor environments, whereas loose rugs, torn carpeting, exposed power cords, benches, and other floor-level objects can cause indoor falls. Walking in rigid ski boots, hiking boots, or cycling shoes also can cause inadvertent stumbling, especially when combined with the less-acute senses and unstable balance of some elderly individuals.

Begin the primary assessment by looking for excessive bleeding and evaluating the ABCDs (airway, breathing, circulation, disability) to identify any life-threatening problems that require immediate attention. After you know the patient has an airway, is breathing, has a pulse, and is not bleeding, evaluate the patient's neurologic status. The response you get when you first ask a patient what happened or what is wrong will give you important neurologic information. Be suspicious of any apparent change in mental status, however minor, and do not assume that any behavioral abnormalities are simply "due to old age." Consult a family member or caretaker, if present, to determine whether a patient's mental status is normal or abnormal.

Next, begin a secondary assessment with a SAMPLE history. As you talk with the patient, use good listening skills. Be aware that an elderly patient may have multiple concurrent medical conditions, with signs and symptoms of one disorder overlapping or masking those of another disorder. Obtain a full accounting of the patient's current or recent medications, including all over-the-counter medications and herbal remedies. Obtaining information about past surgeries and current medical conditions may help explain the patient's current condition. If elderly patients do not volunteer information during the history-gathering process, ask specific questions to get the information you need. Be sure to ask patients when they last ate, because the patient may not have eaten, helping to explain altered mental status, fatigue, dizziness, or weakness. If pain is present, fully explore its extent and severity using the OPQRST (onset, provocation, quality, radiation, severity, and time) mnemonic.

Perform a thorough head-to-toes physical exam using the DCAP-BTLS mnemonic (deformity, contusions, abrasions/avulsions, punctures/penetrations, burns/bleeding/bruises, tenderness, lacerations, swelling). Obtain a baseline set of vital signs. Check the pulse for regularity and equality on both sides of the body.

Obtain vital signs every 5 minutes for unstable patients, looking for indications that the patient's condition is changing. Remember that a patient's medications can alter the vital signs. For example, patients who take a beta-blocker cannot generate a tachycardic response, even in response to hypovolemia or acute blood loss. If a patient has an implantable or external medical device, ask if it appears to be operating normally. Likewise, check any openings or ports for patency and proper functioning with the help of the patient or a family member.

MANAGEMENT OF GERIATRIC EMERGENCIES

Management of geriatric patients is typically more complicated than that of younger patients because of their complex medical histories, their use of multiple medications, and age-related physiological changes. Management may be different because of the effects of aging. For example, a greater tolerance for pain in elderly patients may mask serious injury. Changes in the curvature of the cervical and thoracic spine can make it much more difficult to immobilize an elderly person's neck and back using standard practices and equipment. Some medications can reduce the body's ability to compensate during stress or shock. Combinations of medications may cause drug interactions, further confusing the clinical picture. Finally, aging can present communication challenges by reducing the ability of seniors to hear, see, and process information.

Additionally, any delays in treatment may cause their condition to worsen more than would be expected for younger patients. As a result, geriatric patients often require more aggressive treatment to mitigate complications related to poor cardiac output, respiratory distress, blood loss, or shock. Maintain a high index of suspicion for injury and disease; if something does not seem right, refer or transport elderly patients to a higher level of care. Should you identify a life-threatening problem while your transportation is on scene, interrupt the secondary assessment, provide immediate appropriate emergent care for the problem, and transport the patient to a higher level of care. You must remember, as was discussed in Chapter 11, *Altered Mental Status*, that it is important to get anyone who is having a stroke to a hospital that provides urgent diagnostic care and treatment as soon as possible.

As for any patient, initial management of geriatric patients centers on correcting all life-threatening problems discovered during the primary assessment. Aggressively manage airway and breathing concerns as soon as they are identified. Control external bleeding using the techniques described in Chapter 19, *Soft-Tissue Injuries and Burns*. Even though blood thinners can make controlling hemorrhage more difficult in elderly patients, direct pressure (perhaps including a pressure bandage) is often all that is needed. The control of bleeding may take longer than normal. Use a tourniquet or hemostatic dressing for severe bleeding.

Because even minor alterations in a patient's level of responsiveness may indicate underlying cerebral hypoxia, especially at higher altitudes or as a result of rigorous physical activity, the use of supplemental oxygen can be very beneficial. Treat suspected hypoxia with the appropriate airway adjunct and high-flow oxygen, keeping the oxygen saturation between 94 and 99%. If hypoglycemia is suspected, treat as described in Chapter 11, *Altered Mental Status*.

Use the spinal motion restriction protocol, as described in Chapter 21, *Spine, Brain, and Nervous System Injuries*, and place the patient on a board with a collar when indicated. Take into consideration the fact that a spinal column abnormality, osteoporosis, or other degenerative spine disease can make cervical collar placement or long spine board immobilization difficult in elderly patients. Use towels, jackets, or other material to fill any voids (including the back of the head) and pad bony prominences to reduce overall movement, make the patient more comfortable, and reduce the incidence of pressure sores.

Treat the specific medical disorders encountered in the order of severity, giving precedence to those that negatively affect the ABCDs. If the patient has a history of asthma, is exhibiting signs of respiratory distress, and is in possession of a personal inhaler, consider assisting the patient in taking the medication if your state and local protocols allow it. Likewise, you may need to assist patients who have severe chest pain and a history of heart attack in taking their own nitroglycerin tablet or aspirin, if permitted within your jurisdiction.

Dress and bandage all soft-tissue injuries in the usual manner. Splint and stabilize obvious fractures. Stabilize pelvic fractures by carefully binding the pelvic girdle as described in Chapter 20, *Musculoskeletal Injuries*. Treat a dislocated artificial joint in the same way you would treat any dislocated joint. Aggressively manage hypotension and shock by placing the patient in a supine position. The classic signs of shock may not be evident due to the physiological changes of aging or medication use. Keep patients warm by covering them with a blanket. Transport patients who require further evaluation or additional treatment to an emergency care facility.

Because hypertension affects many seniors, it is important to recognize that any abnormally high blood pressure warrants further investigation. Patients with a systolic blood pressure reading of 200 mm Hg or more or a diastolic blood pressure of greater than 120 mm Hg require *urgent* evaluation by a physician.

ELDER ABUSE

Abuse of elderly individuals—called elder abuse—can be neglect (the most common), emotional and psychological abuse, physical abuse, sexual abuse, domestic abuse, or financial exploitation. When taking a history for an elderly patient for whom you suspect abuse, be simple, direct, nonthreatening, and nonjudgmental. Any history from an injured senior that is inconsistent with the observed pattern of injuries should raise suspicion for elder abuse. You may need to ask the patient about this without other people around; even then, elderly patients may be reluctant to share this information for fear of retribution.

The finding upon a physical exam of injuries at various stages of healing (e.g., older bruises, healing cuts, fresh bruises) in elderly patients should raise suspicion of elder abuse. Intentional burns, cord or rope marks, or cigarette burns on the thin skin of elderly individuals can provide clues to identify potential elder abuse.

It is impractical to address the issue of elder abuse at the scene; instead, treat all life-threatening injuries, arrange for transport to a hospital, and then immediately report your concerns about elder abuse to the appropriate authorities based on state requirements. In most states, mandated reporters include physicians, nurses, prehospital providers, and law enforcement officers.

CASE Outcome

You are concerned that the patient may have a head injury. You also are worried about the patient's high blood pressure. You are unsure if something medically could be causing the confusion. Your help arrives, and you place the patient on high-flow oxygen, keeping the oxygen saturation between 94 and 99%. You mobilize resources to transport her to the hospital. Although the patient initially refuses treatment, you tell her your concerns and gain her cooperation. Reluctantly, the patient goes by ambulance to the emergency department at a nearby trauma center.

The next day, the ambulance crew gives you an update on the patient. She became increasingly lethargic while en route. She was diagnosed with a stroke. The warfarin, or "blood thinner," she was taking increased the stroke's intracranial bleeding to a serious condition. She apparently fell, after having the stroke, and bumped her head. After hospitalization, she was placed at a rehab facility.

CHAPTER REVIEW

In Summary

- Beta-blocker and calcium channel blocker medications can alter the vital sign changes seen in shock, especially tachycardia.
- Aging causes physiological changes that increase a geriatric patient's risk for disease and injury.
- Polypharmacy can affect clinical findings.
- Speak directly and clearly to geriatric patients.
- Address seniors as "Mr.," "Mrs.," or "Ms." followed by their last names.
- Never assume that geriatric patients cannot understand you simply because they are elderly.
- "Atypical" complaints are normal for geriatric patients.
- Have a low threshold for advising geriatric patients to undergo further evaluation.
- Consider the underlying cause of a fall in geriatric patients.
- Elderly patients are at greater risk for mortality due to traumatic injuries.
- Elderly patients have low compensatory reserves and thus benefit from aggressive intervention.
- Never attribute altered mental status to old age alone.

Key Terms

Geriatric Pertaining to elderly persons or to the aging process.
Kyphosis Abnormally increased dorsal curvature of the thoracic spine.
Lordosis Abnormally increased anterior curvature of the spine (usually the lumbar spine).
Osteoporosis A disease process that leads to a reduction in bone mass, allowing fracture to occur more easily.
Polypharmacy The simultaneous use of several medications in combination.
Scoliosis Abnormal lateral curvature of the spine.
Vital capacity The maximum amount of air that can be expired following a maximum inhalation.

Chapter Questions

1. When spinal motion restriction is called for with a geriatric patient, consider:
   a. using towels or jackets to fill voids and pad bony prominences.
   b. laying the patient in a lateral recumbent position to reduce pressure on the spine.
   c. raising the patient's feet to increase blood flow to the head.
   d. placing the patient in a prone position to eliminate pressure on the spine.
2. Hypertension in geriatric patients:
   a. can adversely affect other body systems.
   b. is a risk factor for stroke and myocardial infarction.
   c. generally presents without symptoms.
   d. All of the above
3. Your geriatric patient presents with acute abdominal pain. You know that:
   a. the underlying cause could be life threatening.
   b. these conditions rarely require surgical intervention.
   c. transport to definitive care can be delayed.
   d. an increase in pain sensation often leads to misdiagnosis of the condition.
4. When communicating with geriatric patients, it is helpful to:
   a. speak loudly and in a higher octave.
   b. use terms of endearment such as "honey" to address the patient.

c. direct all questions to knowledgeable family members.
d. be clear and purposeful in your conversation.

5. Changes that occur to the respiratory system due to aging include:
   a. increased lung capacity.
   b. increased lung elasticity.
   c. changes in the way the body senses and responds to oxygen and carbon dioxide levels in the blood.
   d. increased oxygen reserve levels.

6. Your geriatric patient has slipped and fallen on the walkway at your resort. Due to the patient's age, you should:
   a. determine if the fall was caused by an underlying medical condition.
   b. assume the fall resulted from clumsiness.
   c. assume the fall resulted from inattentiveness.
   d. determine if the patient was having an allergic reaction.

7. Hip and pelvis fractures in geriatric patients differ from those in younger patients in which of the following ways?
   a. They have more bleeding complications.
   b. They are more likely to be cause by osteoporosis.
   c. They are more common.
   d. All of the above

8. Your geriatric patient has lost a large amount of blood. You control the bleeding and check his pulse, which you find to be 52 beats per minute. You know that external bleeding typically increases the heart rate. You suspect that your patient's pulse rate might be influenced by:
   a. medications he is currently taking.
   b. internal bleeding.
   c. regular exercise.
   d. a blood clot.

Answers: 1. a, Objective 31-6, p. 732; 2. d, Objective 31-3, p. 722; 3. a, Objective 31-3, p. 724; 4. d, Objective 31-2, p. 730; 5. c, Objective 31-1, p. 720; 6. a, Objective 31-5, p. 727; 7. d, Objective 31-5, p. 727; 8. a, Objective 31-4, p. 726

CHAPTER 32

ADAPTIVE ATHLETES

OBJECTIVES

Upon completion of this chapter, the OEC technician will be able to:

32-1 Define the following terms:
- Disability
- Handicap
- Impairment

32-2 List two disorders that cause physical disabilities.

32-3 List two disorders that cause intellectual disabilities.

32-4 List two disorders that cause sensory impairment.

32-5 Describe and demonstrate how to assess an adaptive athlete.

32-6 Describe and demonstrate how to care for an adaptive athlete who is injured or ill.

32-7 Describe some special considerations that should be followed for extrication, transport, and evacuation of disabled athletes.

32-8 Describe various special equipment that may be used by adaptive athletes to participate in outdoor recreation.

32-9 Describe how to effectively communicate with a person who has an intellectual disability.

32-10 Describe three ways to communicate with a deaf person.

32-11 List the signs and symptoms of autonomic dysreflexia.

32-12 Describe and demonstrate how to manage an above-the-knee amputee with a femur fracture of the same leg.

32-13 State the phone number to dial to allow you to talk to a deaf person.

KEY TERMS

Adaptive athlete, p. 740
Attention-deficit/hyperactivity disorder (ADHD), p. 746
Autonomic dysreflexia, p. 742
Bi-ski, p. 753
Bucket, p. 753
Cochlear implant, p. 749
Cognitive disabilities, p. 745
Dyslexia, p. 746
Expressive aphasia, p. 746
Four-track adaptive skier, p. 754
Guide, p. 739
Mono-ski, p. 753
Ostomy bag, p. 749
Outrigger, p. 740
Paraplegics, p. 742
Prosthetic, p. 749
Quadriplegics, p. 742
Sit-ski, p. 753
Ski bra, p. 753
Ski spreader, p. 753
Ski stander, p. 753

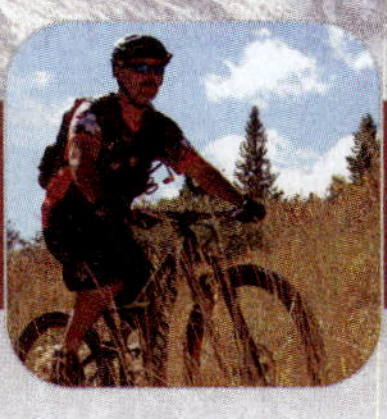

HISTORICAL TIMELINE **2017.** The National Board approves bike patrols as a specialized registration unit.

Sliding board, p. 752
Snow slider, p. 752
Stoma, p. 749
Tether, p. 753
Three-track adaptive skier, p. 754
Two-track adaptive skier, p. 753

CHAPTER OVERVIEW

Many athletes have an impairment but can participate and compete in sports events. However, the physical and social barriers these athletes may face while participating in outdoor sports can be profound. Just getting from the parking lot to the venue can include significant challenges.

Certain factors determine whether an impaired person can participate in a sport. Active participation usually requires mental ability equivalent to performing activities of daily living (e.g., dressing oneself, brushing one's teeth), while passive participation (e.g., sitting in a sit-ski) requires less physical and mental ability. Physical participation depends on the person's balance, muscle strength, coordination, and neurologic processes; impairment of one or more of these functions can make active participation difficult.

According to the Centers for Disease Control and Prevention, in 2018 there were 61 million people in the United States with a disability. This number is increasing each year. Much of this increase is due to our aging population. Neurologic impairment, amputations, and muscular disease are the most common conditions affecting athletes with physical impairments.

A person can have an intellectual impairment, a physical impairment, or both. Intellectual impairments can involve a learning disability, or psychological and personality problems. The inability to see, hear, or become aware of something using the senses makes life more challenging. These patients present unique challenges to the OEC technician during communication and while rendering care.

Participation in outdoor sports has become more popular for adaptive athletes due to improved access, trained helpers, and innovative equipment (**Figure 32-1**). In 1990, the US Congress passed the Americans with Disabilities Act (ADA), which prompted many facilities to open to the public to provide wheelchair access and remove physical building obstacles. For ski areas that use government-owned land, additional requirements regarding rentals, lessons, and lift access were initiated for adaptive snow sliders. Although not mandated by the government, today many privately owned ski resorts encourage adaptive skiers to participate (**Figure 32-2**). Incorporating new materials that are less expensive, stronger, and lighter into adaptive equipment has meant more independence for impaired athletes. Many young US military veterans with traumatic physical problems and/or brain injuries want to continue to be active in recreational sports. Outdated thinking regarding recreational opportunities appropriate for athletes with impairments has changed.

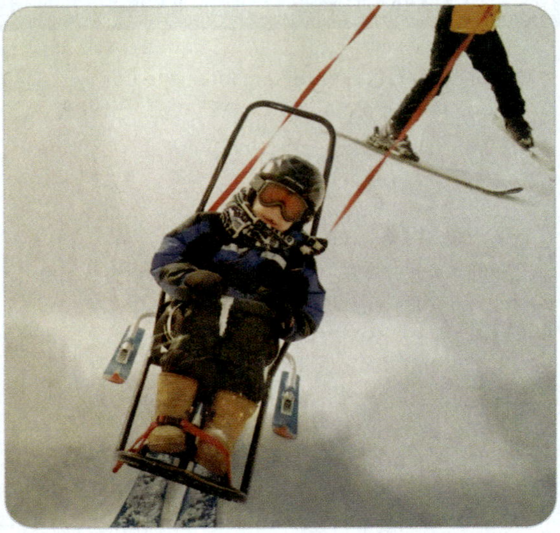

Figure 32-1 Advances in adaptive equipment allow more disabled persons to participate in outdoor sports.

CASE Presentation

You are stationed at your ski resort's recreational racecourse during a special event for disabled athletes when an adult coach calls you to her group. As you approach, you notice an adaptive competitor using skis and outriggers (a four-track adaptive skier) sitting on the snow wearing a helmet. Before reaching the skier, you talk with the coach. The coach explains that the 14-year-old girl has cerebral palsy and has not been acting normally since she finished racing about 10 minutes ago. The coach explains the athlete is usually much more interactive, and even though the skier just negotiated the racecourse without mishap, she had "a few falls" earlier that day.

Kneeling next to the girl, you begin your visual assessment and address her at eye level. She stares off in one direction, not making eye contact with you. She does not respond to your questions and is unable to follow verbal instructions. The coach repeats, "This is not her normal personality." Concerned that the patient's mental status has changed, you radio dispatch for equipment and assistance.

What should you do while you are waiting for assistance?

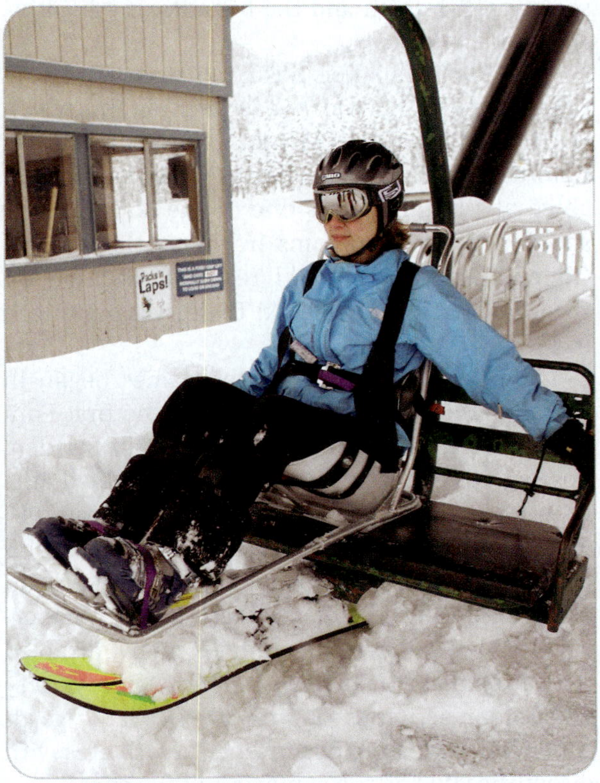

Figure 32-2 Buildings, facilities, and chairlifts on government lease areas must comply with ADA standards for accessibility.

As a result of these changes, OEC technicians must be prepared to care for sick or injured adaptive athletes. Patients with impairments may present unique challenges for assessment and management by OEC technicians. Specialized equipment may be required to evacuate these athletes from the scene. A **guide**, instructor, coach, or companion accompanying a disabled athlete may be required to assist during a rescue.

The terms used to describe a person with a limitation are important. The two terms used to describe a person who has a limitation are impairment and disability. An *impairment* is a loss of a specific physical, physiological, or psychological ability, while a *disability* is any physical or mental condition that prevents a normal function or daily activity. An individual can have an impairment and not have a disability. For example, someone who is missing two fingers could have an impairment, but not be disabled from riding a bicycle. However, they would have a disability if they tried playing the piano. Many people with impairments are not disabled from many activities.

A *handicap* is a condition that markedly restricts a person's ability to function physically, mentally, or socially. Individuals with disabilities, whether genetically inherited or acquired through

KEY POINT

Impairment or Disability

A person with one arm has a significant impairment in life but would have no disability with respect to reading a book, eating, or skiing down a slope. However, the same person may have a disability with respect to tying a shoelace.

trauma or illness, prefer the term disability to the term handicap. The National Ski Patrol has adopted the term **adaptive athlete** to describe any individual with an impairment who participates in a sport or an outdoor activity. The following terms are no longer acceptable and should be avoided: deaf, dumb, mute, retarded, crippled, or lame.

This chapter will review many of these disabilities, showing OEC technicians how to manage medical and traumatic problems for these patients.

HISTORY OF ADAPTIVE SPORTS

Physically impaired athletes began using adaptive equipment for winter sports in Europe when disabled combat veterans began skiing for rehabilitation and recreation. In 1942, leg amputee Franz Wendel, a German veteran of World War II, made the first **outriggers** (a crutch that is attached to a small ski and used to aid an impaired skier in balancing and steering) from crutches and short skis (**Figure 32-3**). By the late 1940s, the Austrian Ski Association had a program for disabled skiers. After World War II, there were many US veterans with lower extremity amputations who wanted to continue to be active outdoors.

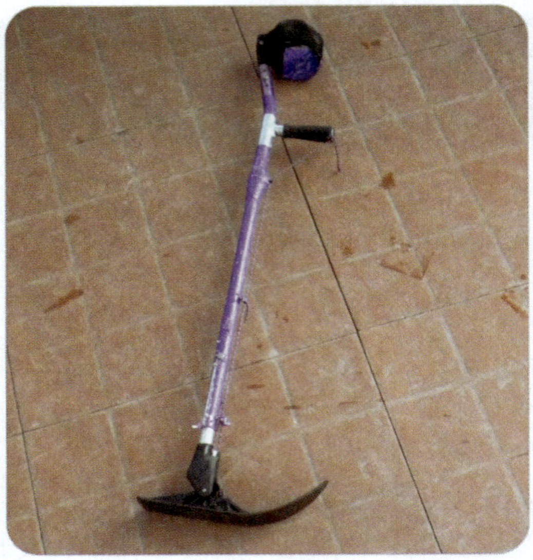

Figure 32-3 An outrigger.

Jim Winthers, a veteran of the famed US Tenth Mountain Division, began teaching veterans and others with leg amputations to ski on one leg. One of his students, Jim Graham, was a former skier who lost his leg to cancer. Graham began helping Winthers teach, becoming the first certified ski instructor with a disability. Interest in adaptive skiing grew, with the National Amputee Skiers Association being created in 1967. This program grew beyond just amputees, skiing, and winter sports, and in 1994 became Disabled Sports USA, which now has over 120 chapters overseeing more than 50 adaptive sports. The growth of the adaptive sports movement, both for recreation and competition, gave countless impaired members of society self-esteem and the benefits of a healthy, active lifestyle.

In 1968, Arapahoe Basin ski resort in Colorado started a handicapped ski program, which was moved in 1970 to Winter Park resort, also in Colorado. The National Sports Center for the Disabled at Winter Park is one of the largest snow sports adaptive programs in the world. The US Olympic Handicapped Ski Team, predecessor to the US Olympic Disabled Ski Team, was organized in 1974.

The Para Olympic Summer Games began in Rome in 1960 and was followed by the first Para Olympic Winter Games in 1976 held in Sweden, hosting athletes from 12 countries. Disabled athletes from all over the globe now participate every 2 years in various events following the regular Olympic Games. Improvements in equipment, along with the successes of these highly competitive athletes, have encouraged many disabled recreationalists to participate in a wide variety of outdoor activities (**Figure 32-4**). Many North American ski resorts host events for athletes with disabilities during the summer and the winter.

Originally conceived by Eunice Kennedy Shriver, the first summer Special Olympics was held in Chicago in 1968 and was followed by the first winter Special Olympics in Steamboat Springs, Colorado, in 1977. This program allows people

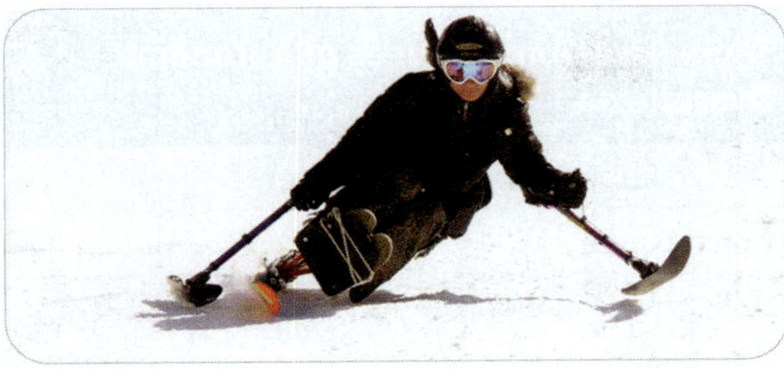

Figure 32-4 Team USA Para Olympic legend Sarah Will won gold medals in all four speed events at the 2002 Para Olympic Games in Salt Lake City, Utah.

© Jim Heath.

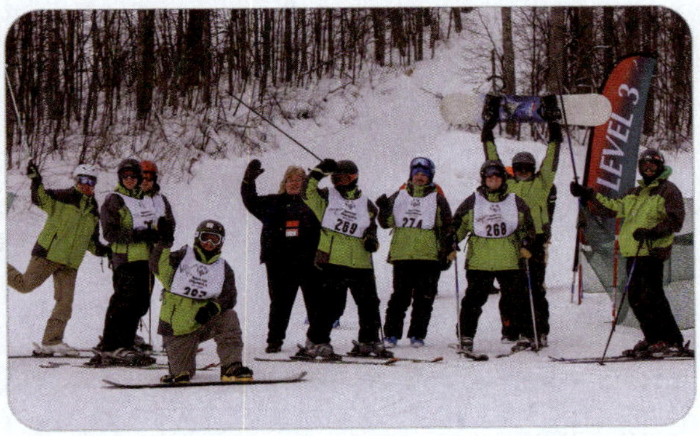

Figure 32-5 The Special Olympics offers athletes with intellectual and developmental disabilities the opportunity to compete in dozens of sports. Snow sports is just one of them.

Courtesy of Special Olympics Michigan.

with cognitive or intellectual disability, who may have additional physical impairment, to compete in many sports. In 2003, the Special Olympics began hosting events worldwide for disabled athletes with mental impairment (**Figure 32-5**).

IMPAIRMENT CATEGORIES

Athletes can have various impairments, including physical, intellectual/cognitive, or sensory. Some may have a combination of these, making participation more difficult. For athletes with multiple problems, passive participation may be the best way for them to enjoy sporting activities.

Physical Impairment

There are many adaptive athletes with physical limitations of different types. They are often able to overcome their disability using specialized equipment and/or assistance (**Figure 32-6**). The OEC technician should take note of the adaptive equipment used by the athlete, as this can often provide clues to the patient's underlying physical impairment and possible injuries.

KEY POINT

Popular Adaptive Sports

The following are just some of the sports enjoyed today by adaptive athletes, as recognized by Disabled Sports USA:

- Archery
- Basketball
- Boccia
- Canoeing
- Cross-country skiing
- Curling
- Cycling
- Alpine skiing
- Equestrian
- Fishing
- Golf
- Hand cycling
- Hiking
- Hunting
- Kayaking
- Martial arts
- Mountain biking
- Paddling
- Rafting
- Rock climbing
- Running
- Sailing
- Scuba
- Skateboarding
- Sled hockey
- Snowboarding
- Snowshoeing
- Soccer
- Strength training
- Surfing
- Swimming
- Tai chi
- Tennis
- Volleyball
- Water skiing
- Wheelchair racing
- Yoga

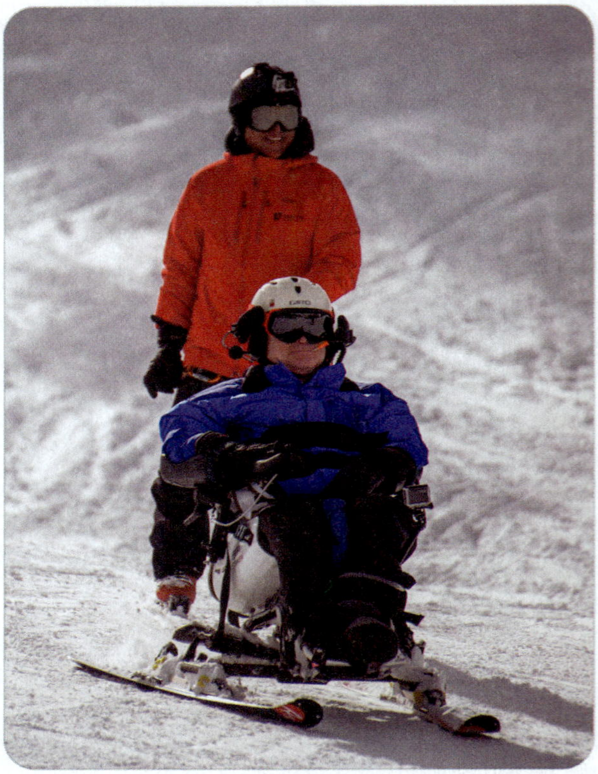

Figure 32-6 This adaptive athlete is using a blow tube and joy stick to control his sit-ski.

Spinal Cord Problems

Spinal cord problems can result from traumatic spinal cord injuries (SCIs), congenital malformations, tumors of or near the spinal cord, and other conditions. Nerve damage within the spinal cord typically affects sensory perception and motor control below the damaged level of the spinal cord. Above this level, the athlete usually will have normal sensation, muscle strength, and coordination. People who do not have use of their legs are called **paraplegics**, while people who have lost function in all four extremities are called **quadriplegics**. Adaptive athletes may not be able to "feel" new trauma or cold-related injuries below the level of their SCI.

Adaptive athletes with SCIs may have a loss of autonomic nervous system control of body function below the level of cord injury. Loss of this control can lead to blood pressure problems or possibly deep vein thrombosis with subsequent pulmonary embolus. SCI athletes who have lost temperature sensation and now cannot sweat or shiver below the level of injury are at increased risk of hypothermia or hyperthermia (depending on the season). These people are at increased risk of coronary heart disease and, depending on the injury level, may not perceive the pain of angina or acute myocardial infarction Although acute mountain sickness is not seen more frequently in adaptive athletes with SCIs, those with disabilities due to neurologic impairment have significantly worse acute mountain sickness than those without disabilities.

Table 32-1 Some Causes of Autonomic Dysreflexia
Blocked urinary catheter
Constipation
Constrictive clothing
Deep vein thrombosis
Distended bowel or bladder
Fracture or any pain below the level of a spinal cord injury
Hemorrhoids
Infection
Ingrown toenail
Kidney stones
Pin sticking in skin
Pinching of skin
Pressure ulcer
Scrotal compression
Sexual arousal
Sunburn
Urinary tract infection

Autonomic Dysreflexia

Autonomic dysreflexia is an abnormal function of the nervous system that can lead to dangerously high blood pressure. It is a potentially life-threatening emergency in a patient with a previous SCI due to *a new problem below* the level of the preexisting midthoracic or higher SCI. Autonomic dysreflexia may be triggered by a variety of causes, including pinching of skin, sunburn, distended bladder or bowel, sexual arousal, or constipation (**Table 32-1**). Autonomic dysreflexia may initially present with feelings of panic or anxiety. It can cause a rapid increase in blood pressure to dangerously high levels, possibly resulting in a stroke. Seizures and cardiac arrest may also occur.

Symptoms may include a pounding headache, dizziness, nausea, altered mental status, and/or blurry vision. Physical findings commonly include skin changes such as sweating or flushing, dilated pupils, fluctuations in body temperature, a slow pulse below 60 beats per minute (bradycardia), and severe high blood pressure.

Look for a cause and correct it. Take off tight clothes, unblock the urinary catheter, or look for other irritants. Have the patient urinate to relieve a full bladder. When autonomic dysreflexia occurs, have the patient sit up. Sitting upright helps move blood to the lower body and eases the high blood pressure. Arrange transport with ALS as soon as possible. Even if you find the problem and correct it, allowing the patient to regain normal vital signs, you should still transfer the patient for further medical care.

Spina Bifida

Spina bifida results from a congenital malformation of the spine and spinal cord, often at the lumbar level. Adaptive athletes with spina bifida frequently have sensory or motor deficits below the level at which the spinal cord is affected (**Figure 32-7**). *Allergies to natural latex rubber in spina bifida patients can cause anaphylactic shock and death.* Some spina bifida patients also have abnormal cerebrospinal fluid circulation, which can cause a damaging increase in pressure on the brain and spinal cord. A surgically implanted drainage tube under the skin, known as a shunt, allows excess cerebrospinal fluid to flow from inside the skull into the abdomen. If this tube becomes blocked, the additional accumulation of cerebrospinal fluid around the brain can cause life-threatening pressure to build up within the skull affecting the brain. Although infection is a leading cause of shunt malfunction, trauma can damage the drainage system. Therefore, any patient with a shunt who reports a worsening headache or has changes in mental status requires emergent physician evaluation.

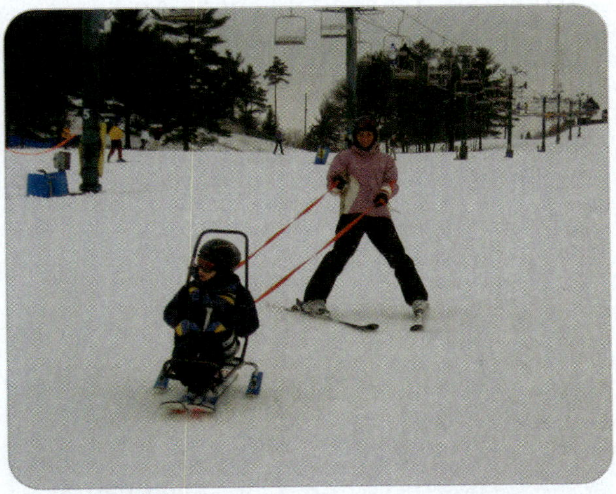

Figure 32-7 A bi-ski with fixed outriggers and guided with tethers allows adaptive athletes with severe disabilities such as spina bifida to participate in skiing.

Cerebral Palsy

Cerebral palsy (CP) is caused by brain hypoxia (lack of oxygen) just before, during, or right after birth. The subsequent brain injury typically results in impaired voluntary motor function and coordination in one of three patterns. *Spastic CP*, the most common form of CP, is characterized by intermittent or repetitive involuntary muscle contractions in one or more extremities, causing jerking body movements and impaired balance. *Athetoid CP* causes slow, involuntary movements and contractions, which also impair balance. *Dystonic CP* is characterized by rigidity in one or more extremities. Half of people with CP will have mild intellectual compromise, while 20% will have profound mental compromise.

All adaptive athletes with CP are at increased risk of extremity injury during falls. They may not be able to protect or relax an extended extremity during an accident. Trauma may worsen spasticity, making field treatment with splinting of the injured extremity difficult. Among individuals with CP, those with athetoid or mild spastic CP are most likely to ski. Individuals with dystonic CP have the most problems skiing because their rigid muscles make it difficult to accommodate them in a sit-ski.

Seizure Disorders

Seizures are discussed in Chapter 11, *Altered Mental Status*. According to the Epilepsy Society, the incidence of any type of seizure disorder in developed countries is approximately 50 per 100,000 persons per year. Regular participation in physical activity can improve psychosocial outcomes for persons with seizure disorders. Seizure activity often is reduced in patients who regularly exercise. Persons with seizure disorders are discouraged from driving motorized vehicles and from participating in scuba diving and skydiving. When riding a chair lift, a person with a known seizure disorder should consider riding with another person.

Multiple Sclerosis

Multiple sclerosis is an intermittently progressive disease that causes degeneration of both central and peripheral nerves. Each progression is associated with a rapid onset of motor and sensory deficits. Impairments vary widely but typically include paralysis, balance problems, reduced stamina, and visual deficits. Mood changes and slurred or slowed speech may also occur making assessment more difficult. Although individuals with multiple sclerosis generally function at a high mental capability initially, their intellectual condition usually deteriorates if the disease progresses.

Muscular Dystrophy

Muscular dystrophies affect the skeletal muscles of the arms and/or legs, and around the spine. Patients with muscular dystrophy have spinal curvature, lax joints, and weak and wasted muscles. They are easily fatigued but have normal mental status. The most common form of childhood muscular dystrophy affects males more commonly than females, and many of these children die young (average 25 years). Most adaptive athletes with muscular dystrophy will use a bi-ski (discussed later in the chapter).

Spinal Muscular Atrophy

Spinal muscular atrophy is a genetic disease affecting the part of the nervous system that controls voluntary muscle function. The arm and leg muscles are affected because they do not receive signals from spinal nerve cells. All the body's muscles get smaller from disuse (atrophy). The age at which spinal muscular atrophy symptoms begin roughly correlates with the degree to which motor function is affected: the earlier the age of onset, the greater the impact on motor function.

Peripheral Neuropathy

Peripheral neuropathy refers to many conditions that involve decreased function of the peripheral nervous system. According to HealthCommunities.com, more than 20 million people in the United States have been estimated to have some form of peripheral neuropathy, and many seek to be involved in adaptive sports despite their impairment. Diabetes is the leading cause of neuropathy in the United States.

Symptoms vary depending on the type of nerves—motor, sensory, or autonomic—that are damaged. Sensory nerve damage decreases the ability to feel pain and changes in temperature, especially in the hands and feet. Motor nerve damage is most commonly associated with muscle weakness. Autonomic nerve damage results in an inability to coordinate complex movements like walking, fastening buttons, or maintaining balance. Other symptoms include excess sweating, heat intolerance, inability of the small blood vessels that regulate blood pressure and blood flow to expand and contract, and problems eating or swallowing.

Amputations

Individuals with amputations are one of the largest groups of adaptive athletes. Amputations can be congenital, traumatic, or surgical in origin, and some people have more than one amputated extremity. A below-the-knee amputation is known as B/K amputation, whereas an above-the-knee amputation is an A/K amputation (**Figure 32-8**). The relative impairment resulting from amputation depends on whether the amputated extremity is an arm or a leg and how much of the extremity was lost. People who have a limb missing from birth adapt early in life to the loss of the limb.

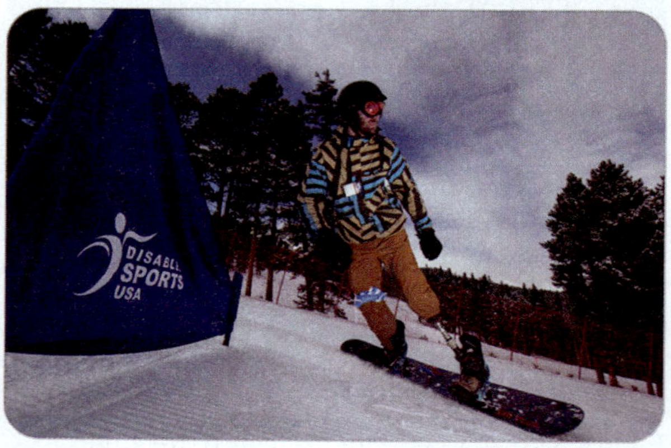

Figure 32-8 An adaptive athlete may be missing all or part of a limb due to either an accident or a congenital deformity.

Photo courtesy of Disabled Sports USA.

These individuals use a wide variety of adaptive equipment and prosthetics to overcome physical impairments. Loss of an upper extremity affects the ability to participate in many activities but has little effect on participation in snow sports or cycling.

Congenital Deformities

Adaptive athletes may have a wide variety of congenital physical deformities that may interfere with some normal body functions. These individuals will have adapted to their situation over their lifetime and have acquired strategies for overcoming their disability, sometimes using adaptive equipment. It is important for the OEC technician to discuss the patient's condition with respect, especially if the injured area involves their preexisting congenital deformity.

Artificial Joints

Some athletes have artificial shoulder, hip, knee, and ankle joints. The new joint is surgically inserted to help correct an impairment. Although it is up to the individual person and their surgeon whether they continue a sport, some continue to participate in more strenuous sports. Breaking a bone near an artificial joint presents very difficult reconstruction and rehabilitation for the patient. Also, trauma can loosen these joints, or they can break. Artificial shoulders and hips can dislocate the same as a natural joint. Many orthopedic doctors allow their more athletic patients to continue to ski or snowboard, but at a reduced level or with specific limitations, provided the risk is understood.

Intellectual/Cognitive Impairment

OEC technicians will provide care to patients with intellectual or cognitive disabilities. Cognitive ability refers to conscious mental activity such as thinking, reasoning, or remembering. These disabilities include a wide range of conditions, including learning disorders, attention-deficit/hyperactivity disorders, dyslexia, autism, mental illness (psychotic and emotional), and post-traumatic stress syndrome. **Cognitive disabilities** result from any loss of brain function that limits the ability to process information. Sensory perception, coordination, movement, and communication can all be affected. Seizures and other physical impairments can be associated with cognitive disabilities. Because many of these individuals often have coordination problems, they may use equipment for daily life that helps them with balance and muscular control.

Caring for patients with cognitive disorders where mental perception is altered (i.e., the person cannot acquire knowledge and understanding through thought, experience, or the senses) can be challenging.

An OEC technician's ability to meet the emergent medical and emotional needs of these

CASE Update

The adaptive athlete remains sitting on the snow as you establish that airway, breathing, and circulation (of ABCD) appear to be intact. There is no excessive bleeding. However, you are concerned that *D* for disability may not be her baseline response. You introduce yourself and ask if you can help. During your assessment of the patient, the coach lists the patient's medications and describes her known seizure disorder. Two other patrollers arrive with a fully loaded toboggan. The patient begins to have a tonic-clonic (grand mal) seizure.

You direct one of the other patrollers to maintain the airway. You consider the possibility that she has sustained a head injury. The patient's seizure activity stops spontaneously after about a minute and she becomes postictal.

What should you do now?

athletes depends on understanding the unique features of each disability. Not all athletes with a specific syndrome or category of disability have the same degree of impairment or the same types of behaviors. Remember that broad descriptive terms such as "not right" or "mentally retarded" are neither useful nor acceptable.

OEC technicians must realize that people with lifelong intellectual and social development deficits need understanding, patience, and kindness during the assessment and treatment processes in outdoor environments. These patients may be frightened or disoriented. Always try to communicate with these patients in the same manner as with other patients, even though this may not always be possible. Often it is possible to use a patient's caretaker to help you communicate with these patients. Patients with intellectual impairments may exhibit anxiety, hyperactivity, apathy, bad judgment, or impulsiveness. They are also easily distracted, which can hinder both assessment, first-aid management, and transportation.

Learning Disorders

People with learning disorders typically have one of two conditions: attention-deficit/hyperactivity disorder and dyslexia. **Attention-deficit/hyperactivity disorder (ADHD)** is characterized by a short attention span. Some individuals with this condition may have a genetic predisposition. Hyperactivity, impulsive behavior, and restlessness are also commonly seen in association with ADHD.

Dyslexia is another learning disorder where individuals have difficulty processing information, especially visual images. It is characterized by difficulty in reading, memorizing, and identifying words, and delays when learning a new skill or sport.

Learning disorders are not necessarily associated with below-normal intelligence, but they may impair an athlete's ability to communicate with or respond to a rescuer.

Autism Spectrum Disorder

Autism spectrum disorder (ASD) is a developmental disability with a variety of manifestations that affect communication and behavior. Individuals with ASD—which includes autism, Asperger syndrome, and atypical autism—are challenged by participating in normal day-to-day social interactions and activities. According to the US Centers for Disease Control and Prevention, ASD constitutes the fastest-growing group of developmental disabilities in the United States. Individuals with ASD often have both learning and language impairments that limit effective communication. Unfamiliar environments or strangers may cause repetitive movements, fear, or aggression. Moving away from a rescuer or appearing to ignore a stranger are two examples of ways in which an athlete with ASD may respond to an OEC technician. Many people with ASD do not exhibit outwardly visible signs of this disability until they are stressed. People with ASD are prone to wander and are attracted to bodies of water (e.g., lakes, pools), a combination that explains why drowning is a leading cause of death for people with ASD.

Mental Illness

Mental illnesses also manifest as a wide variety of symptoms and behaviors. Schizophrenia and bipolar (manic-depressive) disorder are examples of impairments that can cause sudden personality changes or bizarre behaviors. Emotional illness with mania or depression can be very disabling. OEC technicians should be able to differentiate among the various types of mental illnesses. Communicating with people who have mental illness can be very difficult. For more information about mental illness, refer to Chapter 33, *Behavioral Emergencies and Crisis Response*.

Post-traumatic Stress Disorder

Post-traumatic stress disorder (PTSD) is a long-term anxiety disorder that develops following frightening, stressful, or distressing life events. Characterized by intense fear, helplessness, and stress, PTSD affects normal life and functioning of the patient. Many military veterans have this condition and can demonstrate bizarre behavior. An OEC technician must be patient when caring for a person with PTSD.

Aphasia

Aphasia refers to difficulty talking or expressing ideas, understanding everyday language, or reading and writing secondary to a brain problem. Types of aphasia include receptive aphasia, which involves difficulty understanding the spoken word, or **expressive aphasia**, which means the patient knows what they wish to say but is unable to get the words out. The severity and scope of the problems depend on the extent of damage and the area of the brain affected. Patience, the use of gestures, note writing, and the assistance of caregivers will be important strategies for the OEC technician to use when communicating.

Intellectual Disabilities

A multitude of genetic and environmental factors can cause lifelong intellectual disabilities. "Mental retardation" is an outdated general label that implied a below-average intelligence quotient, or IQ. Among the prenatal causes for impaired intellectual function are inherited genetic conditions (e.g., Down syndrome), fetal alcohol syndrome, and syndromes that affect embryonic brain growth. Birth or infant asphyxia, brain trauma, brain tumors, lead or mercury poisoning, and meningitis can also affect mental development and intellect.

Combined Physical and Intellectual/Cognitive Disability

People who have both physical and intellectual/cognitive impairments are usually a challenge when caring for them (**Figure 32-9**). For these individuals, the OEC technician needs to use knowledge for both the physical *and* intellectual impairments.

Down Syndrome

Down syndrome is caused by the presence of an extra chromosome that results in physical and intellectual disabilities that vary widely from one individual to another (**Figure 32-10**). The characteristic facial features, body appearance (including short stature), and pleasant nature of individuals with Down syndrome are not predictive of the degree of intellectual impairment. Because adaptive athletes with Down syndrome are often highly competitive and less likely to complain about an injury or illness, they should be carefully evaluated to avoid dismissing a potentially serious injury. These individuals are at increased risk of musculoskeletal injuries due to general hypotonia (an abnormally low level of muscle tone) and lax ligaments. In the neck, the ligament that stabilizes C1 to C2 can be torn, causing instability of the upper cervical spine.

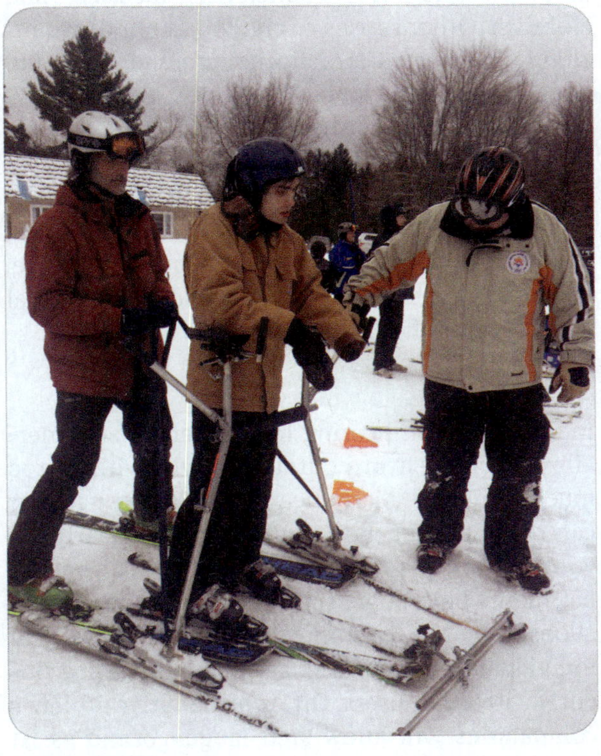

Figure 32-9 A ski stander is being used by this athlete who has a severe intellectual/cognitive impairment affecting balance and control. The athlete can steer independently, and the guide can help with speed modulation using tethers.

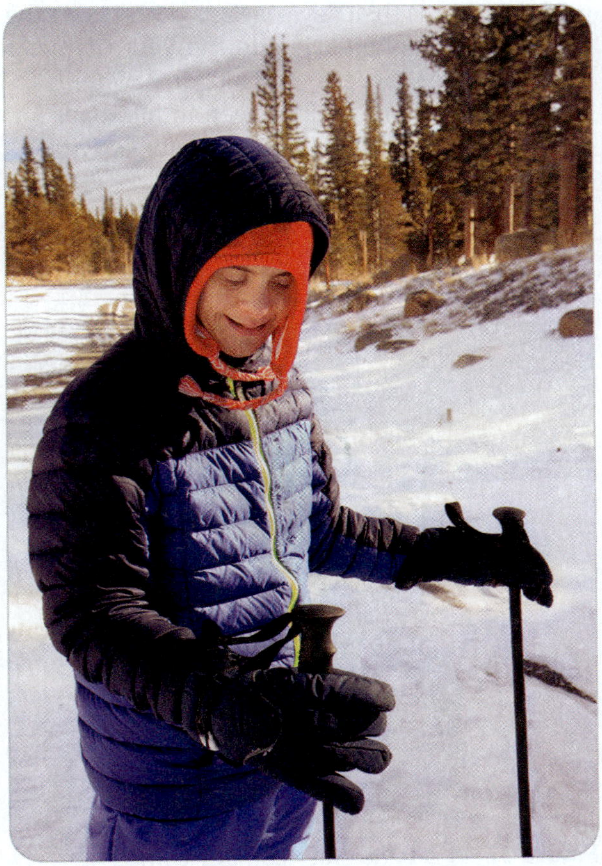

Figure 32-10 The physical and intellectual abilities of adaptive athletes with Down syndrome can vary widely among individuals.

Traumatic Brain Injury

Traumatic brain injury usually results from a violent blow to the head or body, an object that penetrates brain tissue, or the brain tissue being deprived of oxygen following trauma, allowing brain cells die. The long-term symptoms of traumatic brain injury can be divided into several categories, including physical changes, cognitive effects, sensory effects, perceptual effects, social-emotional changes, or a combination of these. Traumatic brain injury is discussed in more depth in Chapter 21, *Spine, Brain, and Nervous System Injuries*.

Sensory Impairment

Outdoor enthusiasts who are visually or hearing impaired represent a large percentage of adaptive athletes. The age of onset and the severity of their impairment will affect the level of their disability.

Blindness

Blind skiers are seen often on gentle slopes with guides acting as their "eyes" (**Figure 32-11**). At the other extreme, blind skiers in the Para Olympics regularly exceed speeds of 50 mph in downhill racing. The pattern of injuries seen in blind participants in snow sports is the same as participants with normal vision.

There are many different definitions of the terms *blind* and *visually impaired* that are used for different purposes. The word *blind* generally refers to the total absence of vision or to the ability to determine only the existence (not the source) of light. A visual impairment is any vision problem that is severe enough to affect an individual's ability to carry out the tasks of everyday living. People are said to have *low vision* if they have a severe visual impairment even after the best possible correction (with eyeglasses, contact lenses, or surgery) but still have some usable vision. People with vision acuity that is worse than 20/200 with glasses or contact lenses are considered "legally blind" in the United States.

Visual impairments take many forms and exist in varying degrees. Visual acuity (sharpness of vision) alone is not a good predictor of a person's vision problems. There are also levels of visual impairment based on visual field loss (loss of central or peripheral vision.) A person with a loss of vision in their central visual field who has no peripheral vision, may be able to read with accommodations, but not be able to drive.

Common causes of blindness in children include congenital cataract, retinopathy of prematurity, vitamin A deficiency, measles, and albinism. Other causes of childhood blindness include uncorrected strabismus (crossed eyes) and uncorrected amblyopia (lazy eye). Around 60% of children born with vision impairments have other impairments and are classified as multiply disabled. Older adaptive athletes may be visually impaired due to glaucoma, head or eye injuries, diabetic retinopathy, cataracts, corneal disease, macular degeneration, optic nerve disease, retinal damage, or multiple sclerosis.

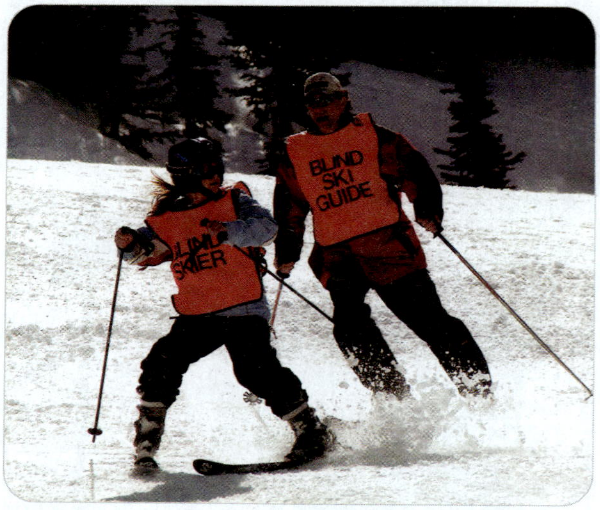

Figure 32-11 A blind skier can overcome this sensory impairment and participate in skiing through the use of a guide.

Deafness

Individuals with hearing impairments can generally participate in any outdoor activity without too much difficulty. Many hearing-impaired patients can read lips, but they must be able to clearly see your mouth. Most individuals with hearing impairments have some speech problems, and many choose not to communicate verbally. Some deaf individuals use sign language communicating fluently with other users. Often, an adaptive athlete's companions will know sign language and assist and act as "translator" for the OEC technician. American Sign Language (ASL) and British Sign Language (BSL) are two distinct languages with their own unique alphabets, sounds, and grammar (**Figure 32-12**).

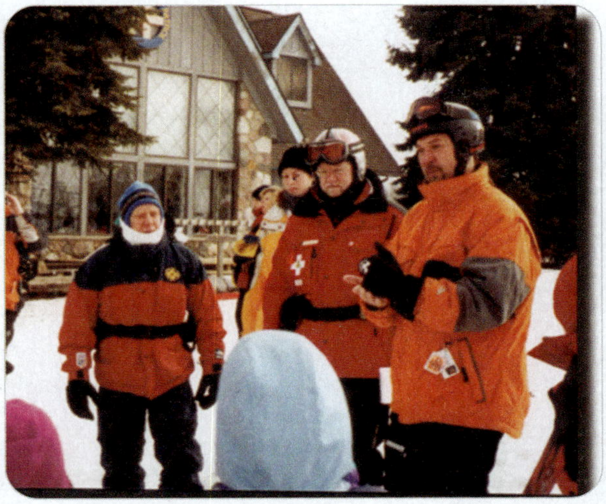

Figure 32-12 A deaf ski group leader signing "help you" in American Sign Language.

People who are hearing impaired may be able to hear some of the speech and sounds around them. If they can barely hear any sound at all, they are "profoundly" deaf. Deaf people may be able to hear a few environmental sounds but can't understand speech, even with assistive technology. Hearing problems at birth (congenital hearing loss) are rare: fewer than 3 out of 1,000 newborns have a moderate or severe hearing problem. These can be caused by inherited neurologic disorders, premature birth, or birth trauma. Hearing loss can also develop in childhood following an illness, such as meningitis, tumors, medical reactions, consequences of medications, or repeated or severe middle ear infections. Although hearing loss and deafness affect people of all ages, these problems are particularly common in older people due to age or accumulated lifetime environmental noise exposure (loud machinery or rock music). The use of hearing aids and or a **cochlear implant** can assist many hearing-impaired people, although they may not always wear these devices while participating in outdoor sports (**Figure 32-13**).

MEDICAL EQUIPMENT AND AIDS

The medical equipment used by adaptive athletes with physical impairment can be generic or custom. Many have generic devices such as catheters, collection bags, and special clothes. A catheter inserted into the urethra or lower abdomen just above the pubic area connected to an outside bag may be used to collect urine. Patients may have an **ostomy bag**, a clear plastic bag that enables the collection of feces through a surgically created port (**stoma**) in the abdominal wall. Another example is a urostomy, a surgically created port in the anterior abdomen or near the kidneys that drains the urinary system. Compression stockings may help with swelling in the legs. Some athletes have stool and urinary incontinence and wear diapers.

Although many devices can be used by different adaptive athletes, some have custom equipment, from specialized wheelchairs to custom tricycles. Because OEC technicians will increasingly encounter adaptive athletes and their equipment, it is important that they have a basic understanding of the types of equipment these individuals use, both for recreation and for activities of daily living.

An artificial part that substitutes for a missing or impaired body part is a **prosthetic** (**Figure 32-14**). These devices can be functional, cosmetic, or both. Even though prosthetics can replace any body part, from a heart valve to a leg, only musculoskeletal parts are considered in this chapter. Due to the expense of the prosthetics and the risk of damage, many adaptive skiers or snowboarders do not wear a daily cosmetic prosthetic device while participating, but instead use a specialized athletic prothesis.

Prosthetic legs come in many designs and can have only an ankle joint or both a knee joint and an ankle joint, depending on where the leg was amputated. Many have electronic components today. Some prosthetic legs are designed for a specific sport. For example, some track athletes when running use legs that function like springs to run quite fast in some sprinting events. Amputee skiers that ski on one leg and use two outriggers may wear a brace on their "good" leg to decrease the risk of strain and injury Although arms may be amputated at any level, most prosthetic arms have a hook-shaped pinching device that enables objects to be grasped and manipulated. A strictly cosmetic nonfunctioning hand can replace the hook on some prosthetic arms. Newer prosthetic arms may have a hand controlled by computer chips that can open and close and look and function very much like a real hand.

Some people use a cane while walking, either to help with balance or to partially unload one leg. By acting as an extension of one arm, a cane

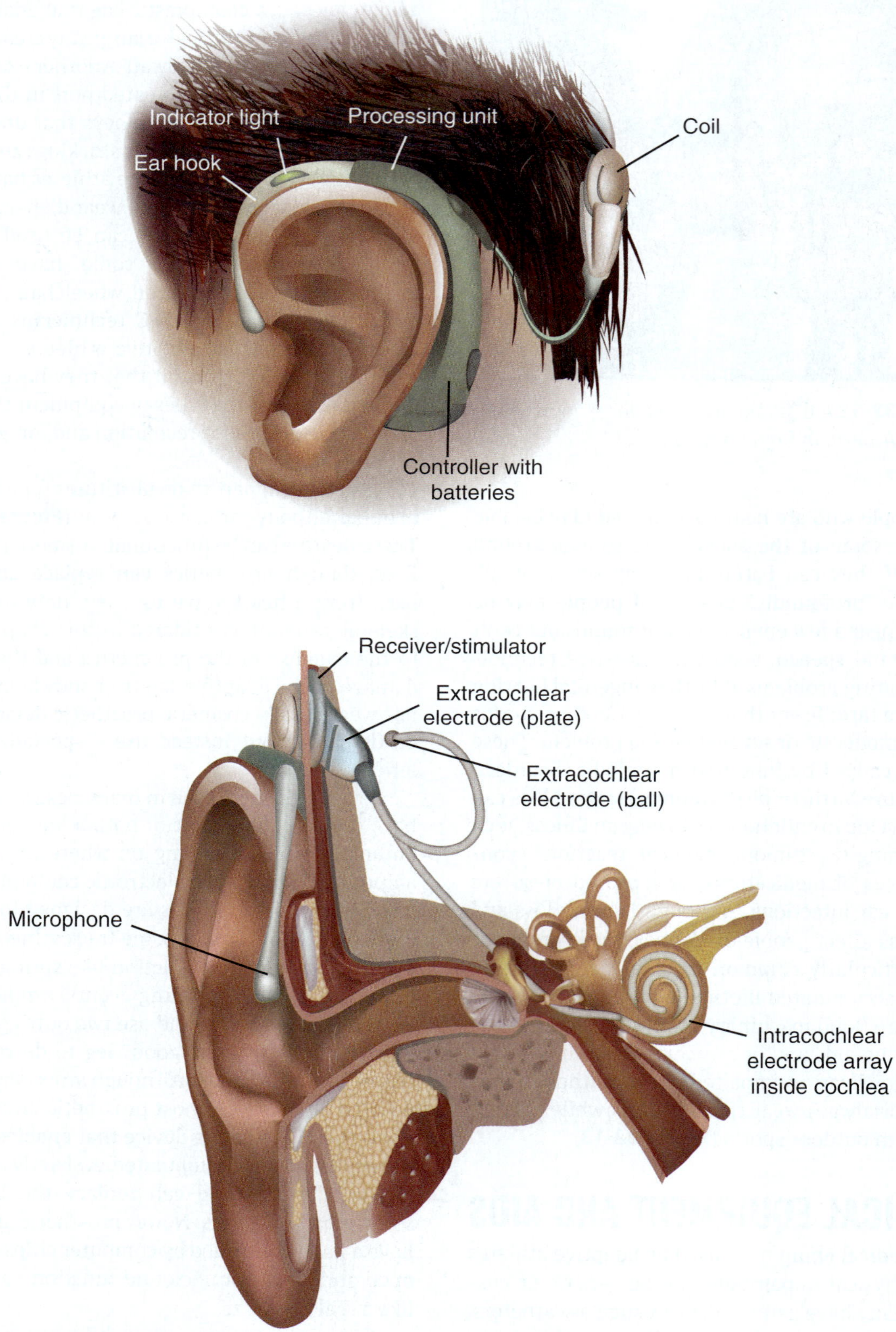

Figure 32-13 Cochlear implants can allow hearing-impaired persons to hear more effectively by capturing and processing environmental sounds and speech, which then directly stimulate the cochlea in the inner ear.

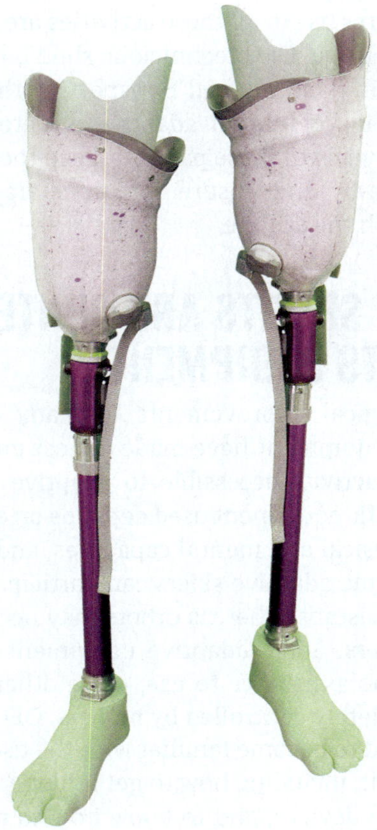

A

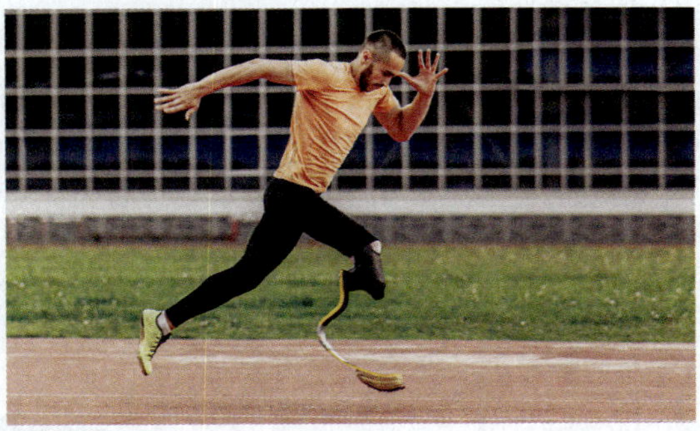

B

Figure 32-14 Artificial legs come in a variety of shapes, sizes, designs, and functionality.

A: © Vereshchagin Dmitry/Shutterstock; B: © sportpoint/Shutterstock.

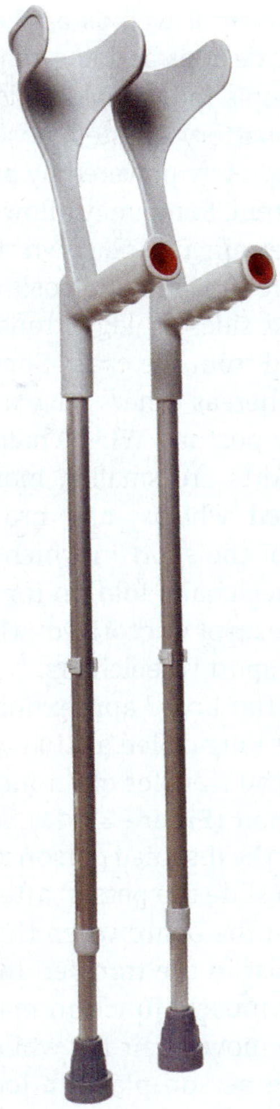

Figure 32-15 Crutches come in many shapes, sizes, and materials and are used for a variety of purposes. Most crutches used in adaptive sports are modified versions of the Lofstrand-type crutches shown here.

© IgorZD/Shutterstock.

aids balance by giving its user a third point of contact with the ground. Although most people with a balance problem hold a cane in the hand on the opposite side from the affected leg; a cane can be used on the same side as the affected leg to allow some weight to be transferred from the leg to the cane. Standard crutches transfer some body weight to the armpits, but most of the body's weight is borne by the hands and wrists and transferred through the arms to the shoulders. To use crutches effectively, a person must have good upper body strength. Other types of crutches, including the Canadian and Lofstrand crutches, are made of aluminum or another lightweight metal and are designed to transfer body weight from the hands/wrists to the shoulders only with no weight transferred to the armpits (**Figure 32-15**). Most adaptive sport crutches, such as ski outriggers, are modifications of these crutches. Outriggers aid mostly with balance and some weight transfer.

The primary alternative mode of transportation for those who cannot walk is a wheelchair, which comes in many designs and has countless features to meet a person's individual needs. They may be self-propelled, battery assisted, pushed by another person, or completely powered by an onboard battery/motor system. Some may allow for movement across severe terrain, up and down stairs, and allow patients to move to a standing position. Many come with removable sides or leg extensions that ease transfers to and from the chair. Some come with a padded seat, whereas others have a bucket seat to aid upper body posture. Wheelchairs designed especially for sports are smaller, more lightweight, have specialized wheels, and are built for the unique needs of the sport in which they are used. All modern wheelchairs fold up for easy transport in a vehicle, except motorized wheelchairs and some specialty sport wheelchairs.

A smooth, flat board approximately 12 inches wide and 3 feet long called a **sliding board** may be used to assist the transfer of an individual to and from a wheelchair (**Figure 32-16**). A sliding board may be used by the disabled person alone, or others may use one to slide the person after performing a "total lift" onto the board when the disabled person cannot assist in the transfer. Individuals with little or no leg muscle function may opt to use a sling device to move their leg while sitting. With this device, the person places a loop around the foot and, keeping the leg straight, uses the arms to move the leg to the desired position such as into a wheelchair, sit-ski, handcycle, or kayak.

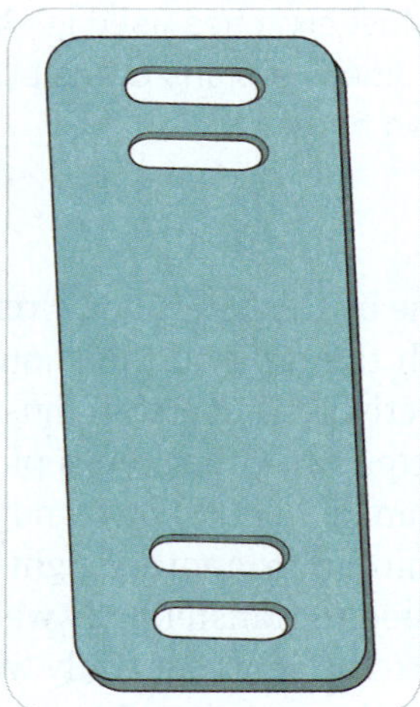

Figure 32-16 A sliding board can be used to transfer an adaptive athlete to or from a wheelchair or a sit-ski.

The equipment and prosthetic devices adaptive athletes use in all these activities are typically very expensive. OEC technicians should take special care in handling and transporting the equipment of ill or injured adaptive athletes. When caring for each of these patients, keep their equipment nearby and ensure that it is transported safely with the athlete.

SNOW SPORTS AND WINTER SPORTS EQUIPMENT

Technological improvements in many different types of equipment have made almost any winter sport or activity accessible to adaptive athletes. The specific equipment used depends on each athlete's physical and mental capacities, and specific needs. Some adaptive skiers can participate without an assistant, whereas others may need one or two helpers. Some adaptive equipment requires little or no assistance to use, while other devices are completely controlled by helpers. OEC technicians need to become familiar with the use of such equipment, including how to get athletes into and out of the devices, and to know how to remove a handicapped person from a ski lift using specialized adaptive equipment.

One of the simplest ways an adaptive athlete can participate in winter sports is to use a snow slider. A stand-up **snow slider** is like a walker with ski tips attached, allowing the athlete to stand on skis and to move forward on a flat surface by sliding one ski in front of the other, usually with the help of an assistant (**Figure 32-17**).

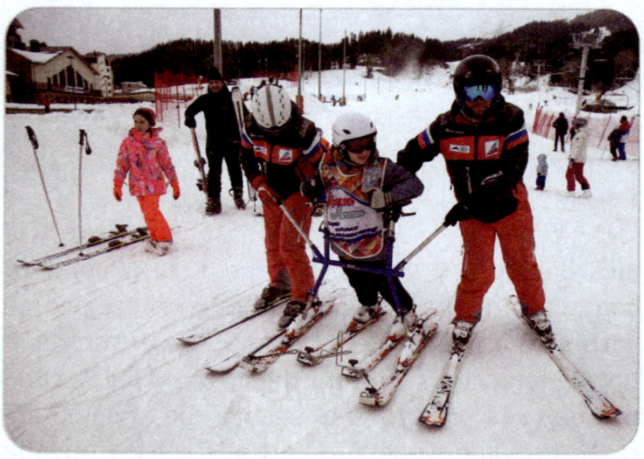

Figure 32-17 A snow slider helps the athlete to ski on a flat surface.

A more advanced version, known as a **ski stander**, assists an adaptive skier in keeping an upright posture; with the help of an assistant, it can be used to ski down a hill. A snowboard version is also available.

Other adaptive alpine skiers with physical impairments can be categorized into groups: sit-down skiers (who use a sit-ski, either a mono-ski or a bi-ski), and stand-up skiers (two-, three-, and four-track skiers). A **sit-ski**, which allows a person to ski in a seated position, consists of a **bucket**, or seat on which the athlete sits, plus one or two skis attached to the bucket (**Figure 32-18**). The adaptive skier's feet are strapped into extensions of the frame to which the bucket is attached, and the skier turns the sit-ski by shifting the weight of their head, shoulders, and arms and steering with handheld outriggers. A sit-ski with two skis, called a **bi-ski**, can be skied independently or skied using stabilizing outriggers and/or a tether controlled by an assistant (**Figure 32-19**). The presence of two skis provides a relatively stable platform, so many beginning adaptive skiers use a bi-ski first. Bi-skis are used for both downhill and cross-country skiing. A **mono-ski**, which has only one ski under the bucket, is more difficult to use than a bi-ski but offers more performance for expert adaptive skiers. Sit-skis may include a shock absorber and/or a hydraulic mechanism to raise or lower the bucket for getting onto a chairlift. Some adaptive athletes are now attaching a snowboard to their bucket, producing a sit-board.

Individuals of each group use unique equipment. Important aids used in conjunction with major snow sport equipment include tethers and outriggers. A **tether** is a strap (or pair of straps) that is attached either to the sit-down device or to the skier's waist and is held by a helper skier, who both guides the adaptive skier and prevents the buildup of too much speed. An outrigger is essentially a lightweight metal crutch that is attached to a small ski and used to aid a stand-up or sit-down skier in balancing and steering. Commercial outriggers come with hinged skis that can be folded upward to convert the outrigger into a crutch.

Any skier who can stand and maintain balance while in motion without outriggers can engage in two-track skiing, with or without the aid of tethers, ski bras, ski spreaders, and/or traditional ski poles. A **two-track adaptive skier** uses two skis. A **ski bra** is a device that attaches to the front of each ski and holds the skis a fixed distance apart, so that the tips do not cross or spread apart (**Figure 32-20**). A **ski spreader** is a piece of wood or pipe that fits between the heels of ski bindings; in conjunction with a ski bra, it can keep

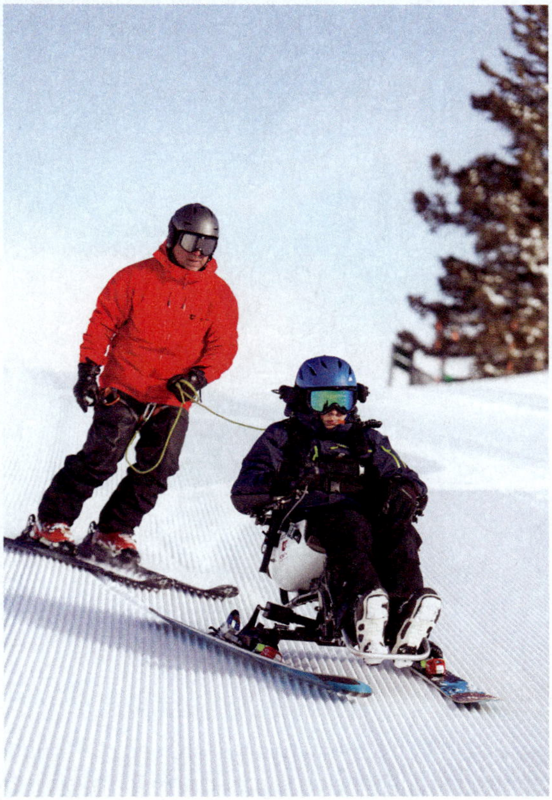

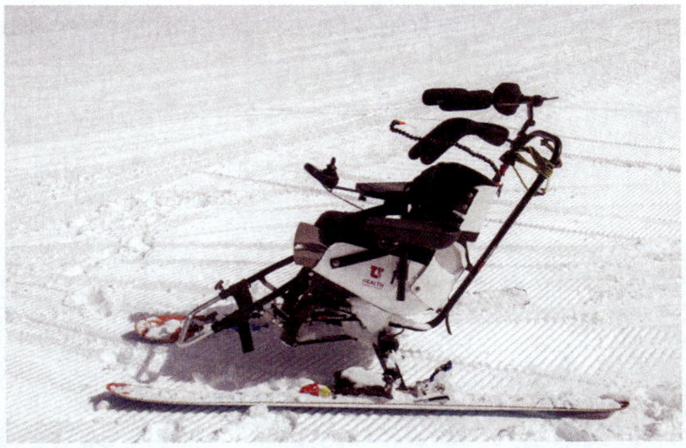

Figure 32-18 A Tetra-ski is a specially constructed sit-ski that can be steered by an adaptive athlete through the use of a joystick or "sip and puff" controls.

Courtesy of Tetradapt.

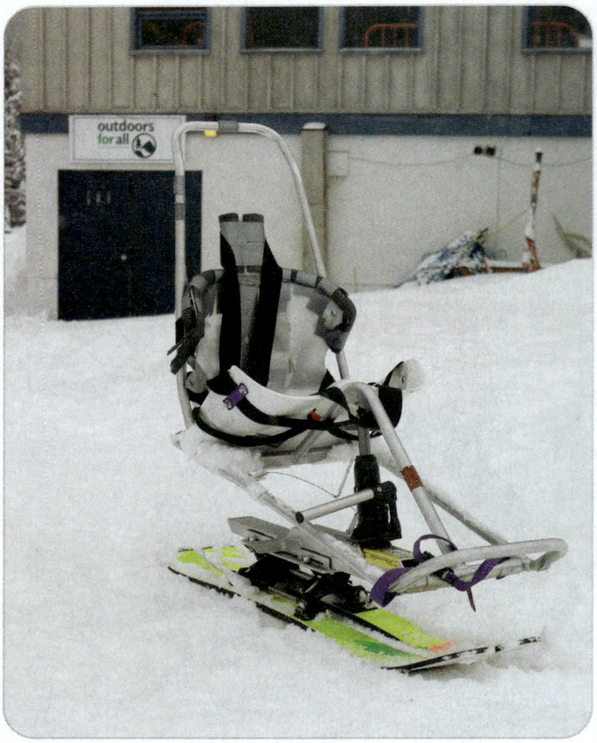

Figure 32-19 This bi-ski has two shaped skis, rubber bushings for suspension, a pump arm for raising the chair for loading onto a chairlift, an aluminum alloy frame, and several straps for securing the skier into the molded polyurethane bucket.

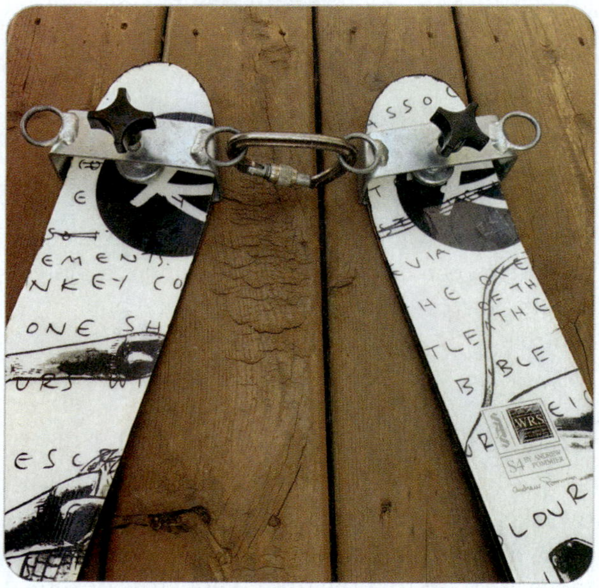

Figure 32-20 A Ski Bra.

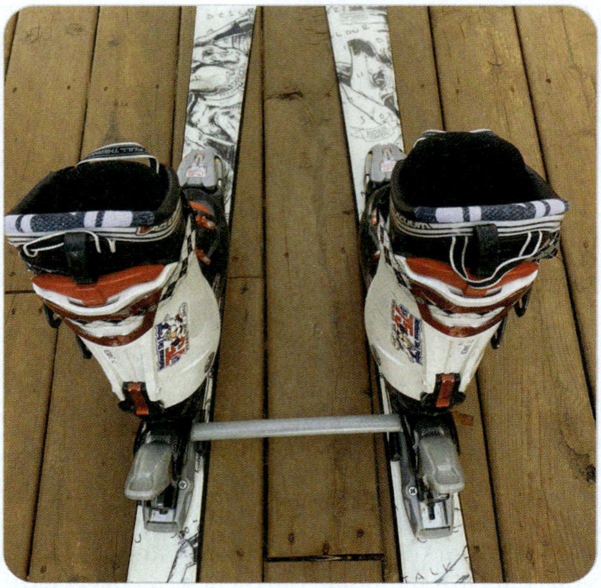

Figure 32-21 A ski spreader

an adaptive skier's skis in a fixed wedge position for balance and control (**Figure 32-21**). Two-track skiing is best suited to athletes with developmental and cognitive disabilities, and novice skiers with visual impairment.

A **three-track adaptive skier** uses two outriggers plus one ski or a snowboard, whereas a **four-track adaptive skier** uses two outriggers plus two skis (**Figure 32-22**). Some may initially require a tether, but these skiers can be independent once they have learned to use the equipment. A person with one leg may three-track, leaving an artificial leg off, or four-track with the artificial leg in place. Athletes with leg problems other than an amputation may also four-track.

Sledge hockey, or sled hockey as it is called in the United States, is a sport that enables adaptive athletes to play a slightly modified version of ice hockey while sitting in a sled that has two large parallel skate blades under it (**Figure 32-23**). The athletes propel themselves around an ice rink using a pair of special hockey sticks, each of which has a standard blade on one end for handling the puck and small "picks" on the other end for propelling the sled. An inline roller skate version of this sport allows the same game to be played off the ice, using two rows of inline wheels under the bucket seat.

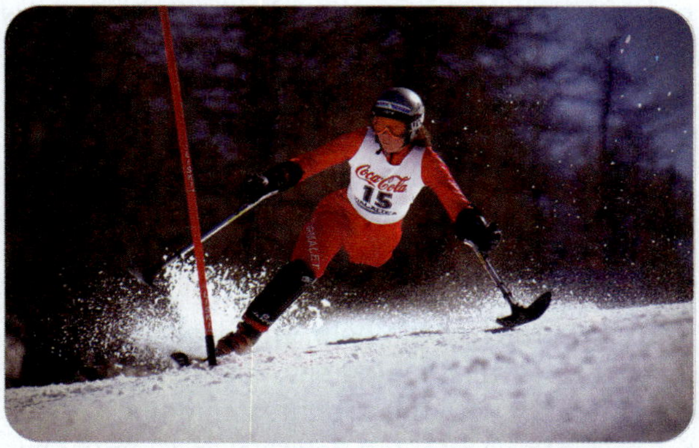

Figure 32-22 A person with one leg may three-track, leaving the prosthetic leg off

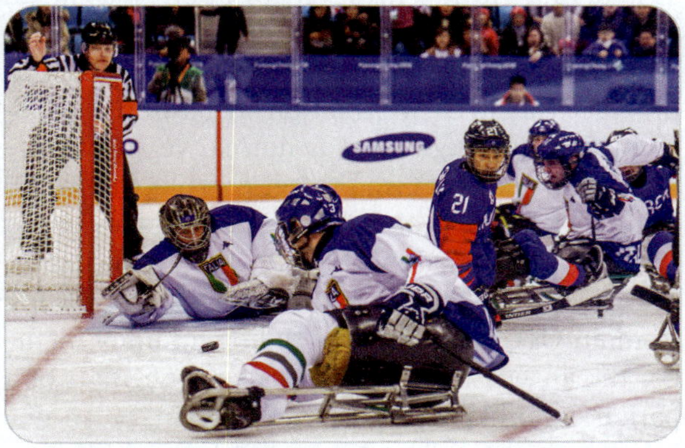

Figure 32-23 Sled or sledge hockey enables adaptive athletes to play ice hockey.

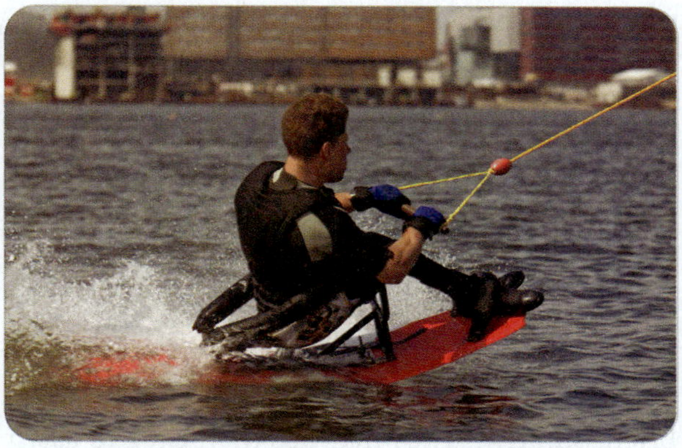

Figure 32-24 Wakeboarding can be adapted for athletes who have use of their arms (such as a person using a manual wheelchair) and for those who do not have upper body control or strength (such as persons with quadriplegia or neuromuscular disorders).

OTHER ADAPTIVE SPORTS EQUIPMENT

Many different types of equipment are available to assist adaptive athletes who wish to participate in a variety of warm weather sports, including water sports, cycling, horseback riding, basketball, hiking, running, and climbing (**Figure 32-24**). Athletes who participate in water sports should wear a properly fitting US Coast Guard–approved life jacket. Many paraplegics are accomplished swimmers who use only their arms for propulsion. Adaptive sailors who have little or no mobility can use specialized seats and rigging and "puff technology," which enables even quadriplegic sailors to use their mouths to "puff" or "suck" on tubes to activate computerized motors that control the rudder and sails. Canoeing and kayaking can be accomplished using specialized seats, paddles, backrests, and pontoons for stability. Water skiing, too, can be done with sit-down water skis, special booms and ropes, twin skis, and other devices.

Cycling is a highly popular sport among adaptive athletes, and many different types and styles of adaptive bikes are available. Tandem, recumbent, and hand-powered bikes enable persons with a wide range of disabilities to power a cycle. Special "trident" and "quad" hand cycles enable many participants with balance problems to ride in comfort and with confidence. Other adaptive features include special seats, gearing, pedals, and controls.

Adaptive horseback riders can choose among many different types of saddles, bridles, and bits for use in specialized riding programs. Wheelchair basketball is very popular today and features special competition chairs that are easy to maneuver. A variety of adaptive equipment is also available for adaptive hikers and climbers.

Cognitively/intellectually impaired athletes may not need any special assistive equipment for participation in outdoor activities. Adaptive athletes with cognitive impairments affecting balance or control, and ones with concurrent physical impairments, may use devices such as a ski or snowboard stander, ski bras and spreader bars, tether lines with a waist band, and long poles held by a guide for balance, direction, and control. Some cognitively impaired athletes require specialized equipment like tricycles for warm weather sports.

Visually impaired athletes will not likely have any special assistive vision technology on the hill other than eyeglasses. They may wear occluded goggles during the day to avoid the distraction of bright sunlight. They may use their cane to assist them in navigating about the lodge. Guide dogs are trained to be alert to their owners and are "on duty" whenever in their harness. Do not allow the guide dog to be distracted by petting or feeding. The ADA allows guide dogs in ski lodges and in the first-aid room. Blind skiers, snowboarders, bicyclists, and runners will always be accompanied by a guide, who helps guide them to, from, onto, and off of the lifts and down the ski hill through verbal commands. Usually, the blind skier and the guide will be identified with high-visibility vests while on the mountain. Novice blind skiers may also have tether straps attached to their waist and manipulated by the guide. Alternatively, the blind skier or snowboarder and the guide may both hold a long pole for direct physical assistance with guiding.

Deaf and hard-of-hearing athletes may or may not wear their hearing aids or cochlear implants while participating in outdoor recreation. This is because the devices are small, easy to dislodge and lose, and expensive and time consuming to replace. Should you need to remove these devices on the ski hill (and only with the patient's permission), it is recommended that you place them immediately in one of their zippered pockets.

COMMUNICATION STRATEGIES

Adaptive athletes with physical impairments such as amputations, spinal cord trauma or impairment, or peripheral neurologic conditions generally communicate as any other individual would, but their level of anxiety may be higher. They should not present the OEC technician with any specific communication challenges, unless in addition to their physical condition, they have secondary cognitive or sensory impairments. As indicated in Chapter 8, *Communications and Documentation*, good communication provides the basis for understanding and is one of the hallmarks of a highly trained rescuer. Effective communication includes addressing the patient at an appropriate level for eye contact. You should consider sitting or kneeling to speak with a wheelchair or sit-ski athlete. OEC technicians can gain the confidence of injured or ill adaptive athletes if they ask how they can help, and how best to care for them and their equipment. Finally, if unable to communicate with the patient, communicate with the patient's companion, relative, or caregiver because they may have important information that guides your care.

Impairments caused by intellectual disabilities are likely to affect communication between an adaptive athlete and OEC technicians to varying degrees. Always attempt to talk to the adaptive athlete first. However, a severe disability may mean that an OEC technician must rely on the athlete's companion to answer history-related questions, provide valuable information regarding assessment findings (e.g., what is normal versus abnormal for the patient), and to get complete SAMPLE information (signs and symptoms, allergies, medications, past medical history, last oral intake, events leading up to the problem). Withdrawing from an OEC technician or telling a family member the answer to your questions may be part of a patient's normal reaction to fear, pain, or an unfamiliar face. Intellectual disabilities may slow an adaptive athlete's ability to understand or respond to questions or appreciate the importance of scene safety, including the need to move quickly to a safer location. Use simple, direct, polite sentences.

Using clear and concise communication when managing an adaptive athlete's injuries is an OEC technician's greatest asset. *Present one question, instruction, or statement at a time.* Avoid using phrases that have more than one meaning or include difficult medical words. Open-ended questions may be too difficult for an intellectually impaired adaptive athlete to understand in a stressful situation, so ask questions that can be answered *yes* or *no*. Avoid frightening patients by making sudden movements or by speaking in a loud voice. On-scene stimuli, such as noise from snowmaking equipment, may distract patients. Direct other rescue team members to manage any distractions in and around the scene. These adaptive athletes may be extra anxious that your treatment will cause further pain, so be gentle. Establishing personal space boundaries or understanding the need for a physical exam may be very difficult and stressful for adaptive athletes with an intellectual disability. Lastly, always be honest.

Adaptive athletes with learning disorders or cognitive disabilities may not be able to process questions normally or understand what you are doing without explanation. Mental illness may cause a personality or behavior change that impairs an adaptive athlete's ability to follow instructions. Try to address the patient directly, even if his or her cognitive capacity is diminished. Gain the person's respect and attention. Sit in front of and at the same level as him or her and maintain eye contact. Rescuers should expect that some athletes will have unpredictable reactions to treatment. A patient with an intellectual disability, for example, may panic when wrapped in the weatherproof tarp of a toboggan. First demonstrating what you need to do next is a good way to communicate your intentions and may relieve anxiety and build confidence in your care. One of the most difficult situations could be strapping an intellectually impaired patient to a spine board during a "load and go." Since this patient has a critical injury, the explanation may need to be cut short, creating severe anxiety for the patient.

It may be difficult to establish whether a patient with an intellectual impairment such as preexisting aphasia has altered mental status as a result of a new injury. A relative or caretaker may be able to help you determine if something new has happened regarding the patient's mental status.

When initiating a conversation with a blind adaptive athlete, greet as you would any other person and be sure to *reassure them that the scene is safe*. Always ask their permission before touching them and avoid having multiple rescuers touching them at the same time. Introduce to the athlete to *all* patrollers and others who are present at the scene. Explain the scene for them: who is there, what their role is, what equipment may have been brought to the scene. Also explain the source of any distracting noises nearby. Speak directly to the blind person, not through the person's guide. The patient is blind, not deaf, and should not have any trouble understanding you. When inside, verbally close a conversation and announce if you are leaving the room. As on the hill, explain who is in the room and what their role is, announce when others arrive or leave the room. Your voice substitutes for their eyes.

> **KEY POINT**
>
> **Speaking to a Deaf Person on the Phone**
>
> Call 7-1-1 to enable you to speak to a deaf person on the phone.

Depending on the severity of hearing loss and age of onset, a hearing-impaired person may not be able to communicate verbally. Few congenitally profoundly deaf individuals have fully intelligible speech. These individuals may read lips. When talking, you should always face the patient directly and remove any clothing covering your mouth. When in doubt, it is perfectly acceptable to write notes, passing a paper and pencil back and forth. This is a very good way to obtain SAMPLE information, especially medications. Another method is to text back and forth on smartphones. If a companion is present who knows sign language, have the person be a translator.

You may need to talk to a deaf *relative* of a patient on the phone. To do this, call 7-1-1 for the Relay System. Using any phone, you can access this service anytime. You will talk to an operator, who will type your words for display to the deaf person's visual receiver on the other end of the call. The deaf person will type back to the operator, who will give you a voice response. Relay services also may be available communicating with American Sign Language by Internet video conference software.

PATIENT ASSESSMENT OF ADAPTIVE ATHLETES

The evaluation of trauma or illness in adaptive athletes will present OEC technicians with unique challenges (**Figure 32-25**). Respect for the patient, patience, and common sense are an OEC technician's best tools for performing a useful and accurate evaluation. The physical exam might require

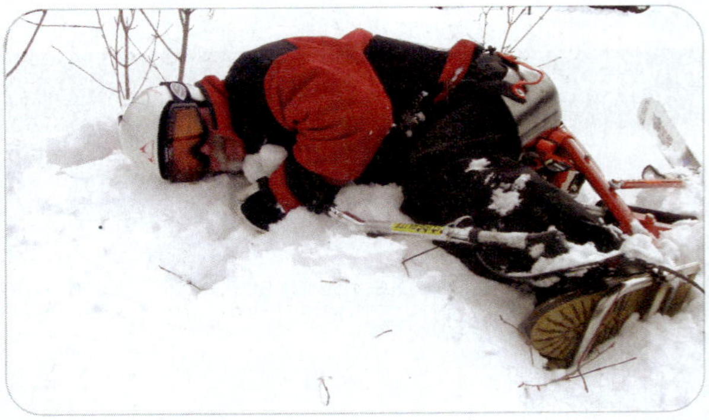

Figure 32-25 OEC technicians can be presented with unique first-aid and transportation challenges when assessing injured adaptive athletes.

© Greg Bala.

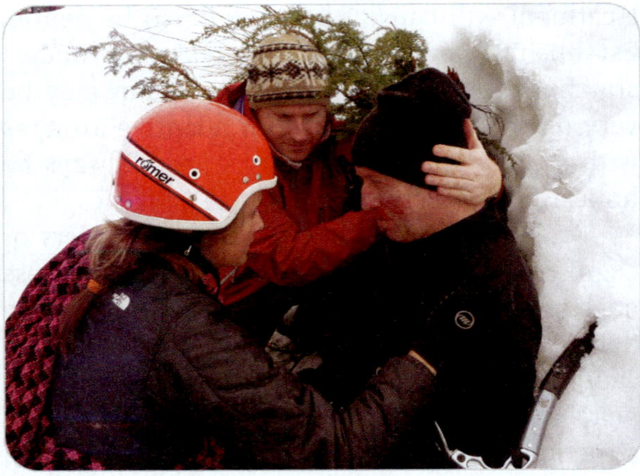

Figure 32-26 Good communication skills when assessing adaptive patients include making appropriate eye contact and using good listening skills.

© Brigitte Schran Brown.

modification or special considerations for unique injuries. The principles of a good assessment, however, apply to all adaptive athletes, whether their disability is physical, intellectual, or sensory. Always use body substance isolation (BSI), as many adaptive athletes have body fluids in bags attached to their bodies.

After the scene is safe, begin with a scene size-up, followed by a primary assessment, and the correction of significant bleeding and ABCD-related problems. Here *D* represents *new* disability problems. OEC technicians should take particular care to check for medic alert tags. Because adaptive patients with spina bifida and others with latex allergies can go into anaphylactic shock if exposed to natural latex rubber, OEC technicians should always use latex-free disposable gloves and equipment.

Start by introducing yourself as a patroller or OEC technician using your first name. Speak directly to adaptive athletes, not through their guides or companions, using a clear voice and calm demeanor. Do not assume that the patient knows your role or can read your name badge. Ask if you can help. OEC technicians should quickly reassure patients that the scene is safe and they are there to help them. Remaining calm is essential in helping an adaptive athlete with an intellectual disability. If the adaptive athlete is unable to provide this information, ask the athlete's guide or companion how you can help. Consider the level of stress that injured or ill adaptive athletes are experiencing. Pain from an injury or anxiety caused by being separated from a companion or guide may reduce their ability to communicate with you.

Be an especially good listener and use the responses of the adaptive athlete and the companion to guide your assessment and management (**Figure 32-26**). Refer to the person by name, not by condition. Do not say, "Please take vitals on the paralyzed man." Appreciate that you may not be familiar with the impairments or the equipment of an adaptive athlete and that the encounter may be stressful for you as well. Be willing to ask the patient and companions about their condition and equipment. Usually they will be happy to help you.

Calling for additional assistance when starting an encounter with an adaptive athlete is often indicated. A rescuer may need additional help with crowd or traffic control, a patient's equipment, of lifting in preparation for transport. Calling ahead alerts the aid room staff that a patient with special needs is en route and may allow time for notification of chaperones, staff interpreters, or family members who can assist in caring for the adaptive athlete.

Begin the secondary assessment by obtaining a medical history using SAMPLE and OPQRST (onset, provocation, quality, radiation, severity, and time), if available. When necessary, ask the patient's guide or companion for information such as the individual's "baseline" mental status and ability to communicate. A new headache or a change in responsiveness should alert a rescuer to the possibilities of a closed head injury or the development of autonomic dysreflexia. Some adaptive athletes take multiple medications, and medical conditions such as seizure disorders are associated with certain physical disabilities.

Perform a complete physical exam using DCAP-BTLS (deformity, contusions, abrasions/avulsions, punctures/penetrations, burns/bleeding/bruises, tenderness, lacerations, swelling). To help reduce the patient's anxieties, as you perform the physical exam, be sure to explain in detail what you are doing. Abnormal blood pressure, muscle wasting, spasticity, loose joints, and skeletal deformities may be preexisting. Patients who lack sensation and normal muscle movement due to central or peripheral nerve damage may have decreased sensitivity or no pain at injury sight. Patients with sensory deficits may not realize they have a broken bone. Thermoregulation problems may be present in many adaptive athletes. Watch for hypothermia, frostbite, and poor circulation in limbs.

Neuromuscular irregularities such as hypertonia (an abnormally high level of muscle tone), hypotonia, and rigidity can facilitate injury. Sit-skiers' legs may be partially protected within the ski frame in a fall or collision, but lower extremity injuries can happen due to the osteoporotic nature of their leg bones. Osteoporosis is a condition where bones can weaken, in this case by lack of exercise. A thorough physical exam is a crucial part of the assessment, but it should not outweigh the risks of prolonging the patient's exposure to cold or hot temperatures when outside. Obtain a complete set of vital signs, repeating at regular intervals as needed.

Occasionally, the mechanism of injury involves the patient's adaptive equipment (**Figure 32-27**). Three-track skiing puts all the force and weight on the skier's one leg, so be sure to check for knee injuries. Falls while using tall outriggers or sit-skis and short outriggers tend to cause more injuries to the upper extremities of sit-skiers. Extremities can also be injured at the site of amputation by the pressure and twisting of a prosthetic limb. If there is pain or swelling at the site where the prosthesis attaches, check for trauma. In most cases unless there is bleeding, remove prostheses only in the aid room, and never without asking permission. Treat these carefully as they are custom made and

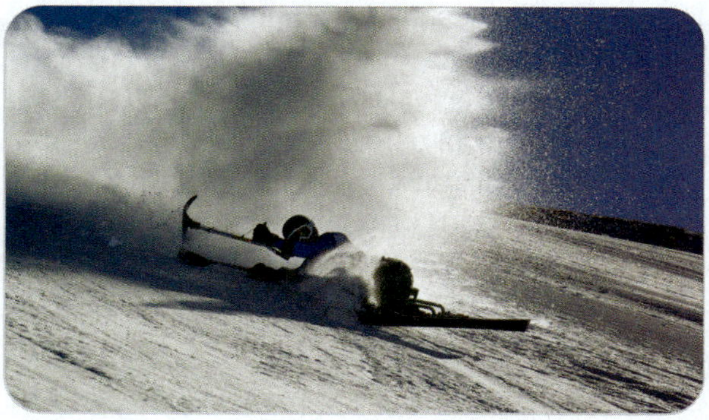

Figure 32-27 The adaptive equipment that an athlete uses can contribute to the mechanism of injury.

very expensive. If they become removed by a fall, they should be transported (usually in the toboggan) with the patient.

Ostomy bags and tubing should be examined for damage or associated bleeding from the stoma site. The adhesive tape securing the bag to the stoma site can be pulled loose. Tubing can become blocked during extrication or when packaging the patient for transport. Do not put pressure on an ostomy or bladder bag while securing the patient on a litter or in the toboggan. Always observe standard precautions when inspecting or handling a collection bag or inspecting an ostomy site.

Lack of responsiveness when communicating, inability to follow commands, inappropriate emotional responses, and abnormal physical movements may be part of the patient's preexisting condition. To determine if the behavior is emergent from the accident or is preexisting, it is important to ask the patient's caregivers or companions what is considered "normal" functioning for the athlete. *When treating cognitively impaired athletes, the OEC technician should assume that any deficit in mental status could be the result of a new injury or illness, or that an established intellectual disability may mask an emergent condition.*

The calm, easy-going manner of adaptive athletes with Down syndrome can be deceiving because they tend to minimize pain or complaints, or they may have a serious injury that could be overlooked without a careful exam. Additionally, loose ligaments in the upper cervical spine or apparent joint instability should prompt rescuers to carefully evaluate the mechanism of injury and related physical findings.

Adaptive athletes with ASD also tend to minimize complaints of pain. Because ASD is a disability of communication, these patients may appear to ignore questions or repeat what you have said. They may avoid eye contact or attempt to move away from you. Using simple, concrete phrases can help direct the assessment.

MANAGEMENT AND TRANSPORT OF ADAPTIVE ATHLETES

Most medical or trauma problems that adaptive athletes have are treated the same as other patients. However, some of these injuries are cared for differently based on the impairment. Splinting may require adaptation, and certain preexisting problems may need to be addressed.

If time permits, it may be necessary to demonstrate how to put a splint on another patroller before putting it on the patient. When managing adaptive athletes' injuries, how you communicate with the patient is key.

Stabilization of injuries in amputees often means splinting in a position of comfort. Using traction for a midshaft femur fracture in a below-the-knee amputee is not practical in outdoor environments. In general, immobilize this fracture above and below the fracture, using a quick splint. Use extra padding to avoid pressure on areas without sensation, whether those areas are close to the injury or not. Modify splints and strapping if needed, but never force an injured extremity into a rigid splint. For patients with muscle spasticity as in CP, traction splints used for a femur fracture may aggravate muscle spasticity, so use a quick splint or other immobilization technique if necessary.

In patients with preexisting spinal cord problems, OEC technicians should be alert for potential causes of autonomic dysreflexia, a true medical emergency, during both assessment and management. Simply unblocking an obstructed catheter or loosening restrictive clothing may prevent or relieve autonomic dysreflexia. An injury below the level of the previous spinal cord problem may cause autonomic dysreflexia. Often, SCI patients can assist you in determining the cause. In many cases, these patients can tell you their normal blood pressure and pulse rate. Normal systolic blood pressure levels in SCI patients typically range from 90 to 110 mm Hg at rest.

Many syndromes or traumas causing cognitive impairment may also include other neurologic conditions, so be prepared to treat for seizures if necessary. Disabilities from stroke or traumatic brain injury often cause specific motor and/or sensory deficits. Signs such as muscle wasting (the weakening, shrinking, or loss of muscle mass) or flexor tendon contractures (which can cause permanent contortion of a joint or limb) may be evident in patients with preexisting brain injuries. These conditions can make assessment and immobilization more difficult.

Getting a physically disabled athlete out of their specialized equipment and caring for the injury requires gentle care, planning, coordination, common sense, a lot of help, and ingenuity. For example, if someone in a "bucket seat" with the legs attached to a frame has injured a lower leg, it will be necessary to leave the patient in the device (which immobilizes the leg) until more help arrives on scene. Evaluate the situation and do what is easiest and safest for the patient. OEC technicians should never attempt to assist an injured patient down the hill in the patient's sit-ski or ski stander. Nor should they keep injured adaptive athletes in their sit-ski when placing them into a toboggan or on a litter. To perform a thorough patient assessment and adequately splint and bandage any injuries, adaptive skiers need to have their adaptive equipment removed.

Be sure to ask the adaptive athlete and/or their guide how the various buckles and straps on their equipment operate. It will take several patrollers to extricate a skier from a sit-ski for loading into a toboggan or litter, so the OEC technician should plan accordingly. When removing a sit-skier from their sit-ski, it is best to do a limited "test" pull before fully removing the patient from their bucket, to make sure that all straps have been loosened. The same principles apply to other to other adaptive equipment such as a bucket seat tricycle.

Remember, sit-skiers with an SCI, spina bifida, or other neurologic disorders may have a high pain tolerance and/or serious injuries that they cannot feel below the level of the spinal cord problem. A thorough patient assessment is mandatory before moving these patients. Based on the mechanism of injury, be sure to check for deformities, swelling, or bleeding before moving. Osteoporosis in these patients can sometimes lead to fractures and dislocations from relatively minor falls or collisions. Be sure to fully support these patients when transferring. Patients with muscular dystrophy or CP may not be able to assist with their transfer, and the OEC technician will need extra patrollers to help move them since they may be stiff, floppy, and/or "dead weight."

Adaptive equipment and prosthetic limbs often cost thousands of dollars. Adaptive equipment needs to be transported along with the patient to the aid room during "clean-up," and at the end of a rescue, make sure all items are accounted for. Reassure adaptive athletes that their equipment will be cared for appropriately and waiting for them in the first-aid room. For injured adaptive athletes who depend on a wheelchair, inquire how to secure their equipment so that you can make it available to them when they are ready to leave an aid station or clinic. Be aware that wheelchairs are typically very expensive. Motorized chairs can be extremely heavy and awkward to transport.

Adaptive athletes may be accompanied by service animals, especially at base areas. Make every effort to maintain the normal relationship between injured adaptive athletes and their service animals, including proximity. Doing so will comfort both the patients and their service animals during an obviously stressful situation. A service dog is not a pet. The OEC technician should make sure the animals are not petted or distracted by bystanders in the aid room.

When lifting, transferring, or transporting a cognitively impaired adaptive athlete, be sure to show them in advance the steps that will be taken and the equipment that will be used. Explain to them the role of all the persons who are there at the scene assisting and the procedure to be followed to move them. Explain the need for the restraints to safely secure them in the toboggan for transport, and demonstrate how they will work in advance.

Be sure to explain *in advance* what you are doing when loading and transporting visually impaired individuals in the toboggan. Be sure to communicate clearly the action to be taken. Explain to them the scene, the persons who are there assisting, and the procedure to be followed. Speak directly to them and not through their guide. If

KEY POINT

Service Animals

Under the ADA, service animals are dogs (and in some rare cases miniature horses) that have been trained to help their owner overcome a disability (**Figure 32-28**). Common examples are seeing eye dogs or dogs trained to detect seizures. Emotional support dogs or other animals that provide comfort just by being with a person are *not* considered service dogs under the ADA because they have not been trained to perform a specific job or task. However, some state or local governments have laws that allow people to take emotional support animals into public places. You may check with your state and local government agencies to find out about these laws.

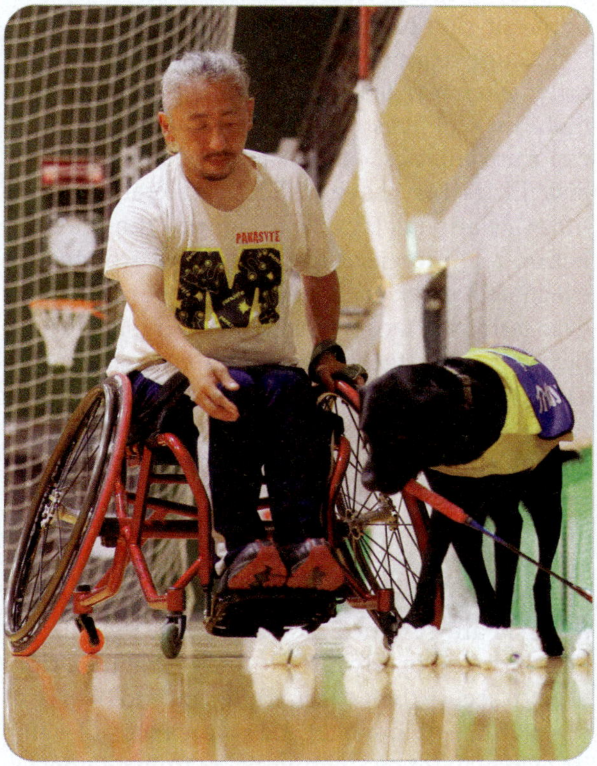

Figure 32-28 Service animals help their owners overcome disabilities.

a blind person is mobile and needs to be guided while walking, offer your upper arm to hold onto and walk to the side. Come to a complete stop before steps, curbs, and other such objects. When lifting, transferring, or transporting a deaf adaptive athlete, be sure to show them in advance what you are going to do and the equipment that will be used.

Lift Evacuation

Patrollers in North America are trained to evacuate adaptive athletes from ski lifts. Gondolas, trams, and chair lifts are designed for this purpose. Gondolas and trams must have doors wide enough to accommodate disabled athletes. Chair lifts may be accompanied by a sign that indicates how high the lift's seat is, so adaptive sitting athletes can adjust the heights of their buckets to get on the lift. Every time an adaptive athlete in a sit-ski gets onto a chairlift, a safety strap should be attached to the back of the chair (**Figure 32-29**). The strap, which prevents the adaptive athlete from falling out of the chairlift, is necessary because the safety bar may not fully close due to the size of the seat or the sit-ski's bucket.

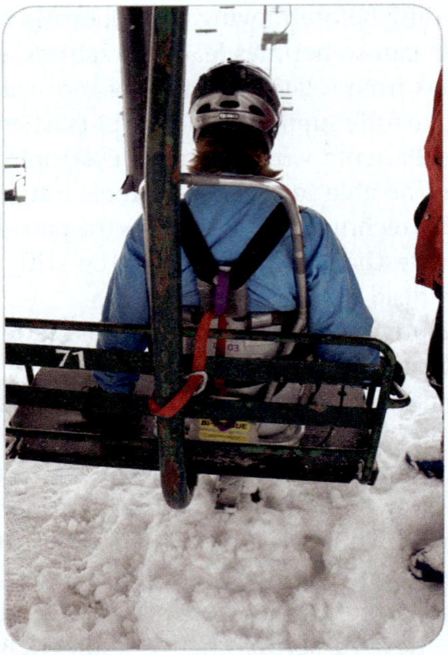

Figure 32-29 A safety strap should be secured to the back of the chairlift seat after loading the sit-ski.

© Craig Brown.

Adaptive athletes should always be given priority when evacuating chairlifts. Athletes with mobility problems have an increased risk of cold exposure injuries, and athletes with intellectual disabilities may have difficulty tolerating chairlift evacuation delays. Working with the lift evacuation team to ensure that adaptive athletes are evacuated early is standard practice during lift evacuations in most resorts. Sit-skis typically have factory-built attachments to an evacuation line. These evacuation straps are generally placed between the person's legs and on either side of the bucket. However, every style of sit-ski can be different. Adaptive athletes should inspect all webbing on their bi-ski or mono-ski to be sure it is in operating condition (and accessible) before riding the lift. They should know how the straps on their ski are designed to operate, and they should also carry a properly rated locking carabiner, to be used to secure their evacuation straps to the area's evacuation equipment. Each ski area must develop its own plan for evacuating skiers from all nonsurface ski lifts.

Skiers or snowboarders who are blind or have cognitive impairments will need additional oral coaching and reassurance during an evacuation, even if they have a guide with them in the same chair. During chair evacuation, OEC technicians must communicate clearly with cognitively impaired skiers and riders, because the evacuation process may be difficult to understand and could cause anxiety. It will be very important to clearly demonstrate all the steps to be taken and to speak in a clear but reassuring tone. If three or more individuals are on the lift, it may be helpful to evacuate one of them first, so that the cognitively impaired athlete can witness the procedure. *Always evacuate a cognitively impaired skier or rider before the person's companion.* In this way, the companion can assist with the process, and it ensures that the adaptive athlete is not left alone on the lift. Because cognitively impaired skiers may be anxious until their companion can join them on the ground, have someone remain with and talk to them so that they can feel safe.

Deaf or hard-of-hearing skiers and snowboarders will present challenges for the OEC technician who is assisting with a chairlift evacuation, as they may not be able to hear verbal directions. They may be skiing or riding with a hearing friend, who can act as a translator. Also, you could communicate with the adaptive athlete with a cell phone using text on your phone. Regardless, be sure to clearly visually demonstrate how the evacuation will work. If three or more people are on the lift, it may be best to take another person off the lift first if they are available, so that the hearing-impaired person can see the procedure.

CASE Outcome

Because the patient has remained confused and unresponsive to questioning, you are not sure of her mental status. You explain in detail to her and the coach that you are going to apply a cervical collar while the patient is still on the ski slope. You transport her using spinal motion restriction with the cervical collar in place. During transport in the toboggan down the slope, one patroller skis beside the toboggan, reassuring the patient and watching to make sure she does not vomit. You've radioed ahead to the patrol room, and EMS will be waiting for your arrival to transport the patient to further medical care. A family member and the coach meet the patient in the patrol room. The ambulance takes her away. X-ray imaging at the hospital of the patient's cervical spine shows no evidence of injury, but a computed tomography scan of her brain shows a new small subdural hematoma. Even though the patient had a history of seizures, you made the correct decision to have her evaluated for a new condition, which probably saved her life.

CHAPTER REVIEW

In Summary

- All adaptive athletes with disabilities are people and are not solely defined by their impairment.
- Altered mental status is the result of a new injury or illness until proven otherwise.
- Do not speak to mentally disabled adults as if they are children, but do use simple words. Be calm and reassuring, and explain actions in advance.
- Ask adaptive athletes how you can assist them. Also ask the athlete's skiing guide, chaperone, or caregiver for information and assistance.
- Describe and demonstrate how you will help or move an adaptive athlete before doing a procedure.
- Ask about medications and medical history. Look for medical alert jewelry or other alerts to help identify preexisting medical conditions. Ask the athlete's skiing guide, chaperone, or caregiver for information.
- Request additional rescuers when caring for athletes with disabilities.
- Collect an adaptive athlete's equipment and transport it with the athlete. Treat the items with care, as most of this equipment is expensive, is very personal, and will take a long time to replace if lost or damaged.
- Paraplegics and athletes with neuromuscular disorders are at an increased risk for hypothermia and frostbite.
- Patients with spina bifida are commonly allergic to latex. Always use latex-free gloves when treating these patients to avoid an anaphylactic reaction.
- Adaptive athletes with neurologic disorders may have serious injuries without self-awareness of pain, deformity, or bleeding.
- Special consideration will need to be made when extricating, transporting, or evacuating adaptive athletes.
- Some adaptive athletes have syndromes that include multiple physical and cognitive impairments. They may also be susceptible to seizures.
- Many "legally blind" persons have some residual vision of limited acuity and/or field of view, or at least perception of motion or light/dark.
- OEC technicians should convey respect for adaptive athletes and for their disability by using the basics of good communication.
- Adaptive athletes appreciate that you're trying to help, so enjoy the challenge and give them the best care possible.

Key Terms

Adaptive athlete A person with disabilities participating in competitive or recreational sports.

Attention-deficit/hyperactivity disorder (ADHD) A behavioral syndrome that causes short attention span, impulsive behavior, and restlessness.

Autonomic dysreflexia Abnormal function of the nervous system associated with spinal cord injuries; can lead to dangerously high blood pressure.

Bi-ski A molded bucket seat mounted on two skis (with or without a suspension system).

Bucket The seat of a sit-ski, handcycle, or hockey sled in which the adaptive athlete is secured.

Cochlear implant A small, surgically implanted electronic device for deaf persons that works like an artificial human cochlea in the inner ear, helping to send sound from the ear to the brain.

Cognitive disability Impairment of brain function that limits the ability to process information and reach reasoned conclusions.

Dyslexia Impairment of information processing that makes learning new information difficult.
Expressive aphasia Inability to express speech normally.
Four-track adaptive skier An adaptive skier with two legs who also uses two outriggers.
Guide A trained person who assists an adaptive athlete (such as a blind skier or a bi-skier) in the field.
Mono-ski A molded bucket seat mounted on suspension bindings to a single ski.
Ostomy bag A pouch worn over the stoma created by an ostomy to collect stool or urine.
Outrigger Adaptive ski poles with short ski tips attached to crutch-like handles that are used by three-track and four-track adaptive skiers to assist with balance and agility.
Paraplegics People who do not have use of the legs from paralysis caused by illness or injury; the loss is usually sensory and motor.
Prosthetic An artificial device designed to replace a missing or impaired part of the body; also called an artificial limb.
Quadriplegics People who do not have use of the legs and arms from paralysis caused by illness or injury.
Sit-ski A device consisting of a "bucket" or seat in which the adaptive skier sits. It has one or two skis attached to the bucket.
Ski bra A device that attaches to the front of each ski and holds the skis a fixed distance apart, so that the tips do not cross or spread apart.
Ski spreader A bar placed under the heels of adaptive skiers to keep the rear of the skis separated and fixed. Often used in conjunction with ski tip tethers to facilitate a stable wedge ski position.
Ski stander A device that attaches to skis and utilizes a waist harness and arm rests to help support an adaptive skier in a standing position.
Sliding board A flat board that is used to help an adaptive athlete transfer to or from a wheelchair.
Snow slider A device like a walker with small ski tips attached that allows a standing adaptive skier to shuffle on the snow.
Stoma A surgical port created in the body by surgery to allow the elimination of stool or urine. For ostomies, it is located on the abdomen and is dark pink in color. A pouch (ostomy bag) is worn over the stoma to collect stool or urine.
Tether A strap used by adaptive ski guides to help control the speed and direction of adaptive skiers.
Three-track adaptive skier An adaptive skier using one ski with two outriggers.
Two-track adaptive skier A skier who uses two skis without outriggers.

Chapter Questions

1. Handicap is defined as:
   a. a condition that markedly restricts a person's ability to function physically, mentally, or socially.
   b. a loss of a specific physical, physiological, or psychological ability.
   c. any physical or mental condition that allows normal function or daily activity.
   d. All of the above
2. Impairment is best defined as:
   a. a condition that markedly restricts a person's ability to function physically, mentally, and socially.
   b. a loss of physiological or psychological ability.
   c. any physical or mental condition that prevents normal daily activity.
   d. a disorder characterized by hyperactivity, impulsive behavior, and restlessness.
3. Disability is best defined as:
   a. a condition that markedly restricts a person's ability to function physically, mentally, or socially.
   b. a loss of a specific physical, physiological, or psychological ability.
   c. any physical or mental condition that prevents a normal function or daily activity.
   d. a disorder characterized by hyperactivity, impulsive behavior, and restlessness.

4. When performing an assessment of an adaptive athlete, it is helpful to:
   a. refer to the patient in terms of his or her condition rather than by name.
   b. speak directly to the guide or companion rather than the adaptive athlete.
   c. use respect, patience, and common sense as your best tools.
   d. assume that deficits in mental status are the result of a previous condition.
5. When caring for an adaptive athlete who is injured or ill, it is important to keep in mind that:
   a. patients with neurologic disorders may have a high tolerance for pain.
   b. patients with preexisting spinal cord problems my develop autonomic dysreflexia.
   c. communication is key.
   d. All of the above
6. An adaptive ski pole with a short ski tip that assists the adaptive athlete with balance is called a(n):
   a. outrigger.
   b. ski bra.
   c. tether.
   d. sit-ski.
7. How should you communicate with a person who has an intellectual disability?
   a. Remain calm and be patient.
   b. Present one question or statement at a time.
   c. Use simple, polite, and direct sentences.
   d. All of the above
8. What is the phone number to dial to allow you to talk to a deaf person?
   a. 9-1-1
   b. 8-1-1
   c. 7-1-1
   d. 4-1-1

Answers: 1. a, Objective 32-1, p. 739; 2. b, Objective 32-1, p. 739; 3. c, Objective 32-1, p. 739; 4. c, Objective 32-5, p. 757; 5. d, Objective 32-6, p. 760; 6. a, Objective 32-8, p. 740; 7. d, Objective 32-9, p. 756; 8. c, Objective 32-13, p. 757

CHAPTER 33

BEHAVIORAL EMERGENCIES AND CRISIS RESPONSE

OBJECTIVES

Upon completion of this chapter, the OEC technician will be able to:

33-1 Define the following terms:
- Behavior
- Behavioral emergency

33-2 Describe the main difference between a mood, adjustment, or affective disorder and a psychotic disorder.

33-3 List the signs and symptoms of the common behavioral emergencies.

33-4 Identify ways to maintain rescuer safety when responding to a behavioral emergency.

33-5 Describe and demonstrate how to assess a patient with a behavioral emergency.

33-6 Describe and demonstrate the treatment of a patient with a behavioral emergency.

33-7 Define when to restrain a patient.

33-8 Describe and demonstrate how to properly restrain a patient.

33-9 Describe critical incident stress debriefing.

KEY TERMS

Agitation, p. 771
Anxiety, p. 770
Bipolar disorder, p. 771
Crisis, p. 768
Depression, p. 771
Mood, adjustment, or affective disorder, p. 770
Paranoia, p. 771
Psychosis, p. 770
Reasonable force, p. 780
Schizophrenia, p. 772
Stress, p. 769
Suicidal gesture, p. 772
Suicide, p. 772

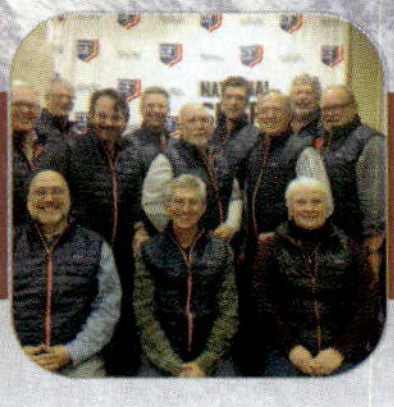

HISTORICAL TIMELINE

2018. The National Board approves a proposal to allow EMTs and paramedics to become OEC technicians by passing the OEC Modified Challenge course.

CHAPTER OVERVIEW

As an OEC technician, you will encounter emergencies with difficult interpersonal relationships. You may encounter people who are in **crisis**, behaving in an unexpected, unusual, or possibly dangerous manner. This behavior may be caused by a variety of conditions ranging from relatively minor to immediately life threatening. Regardless of the cause, scene safety remains your first concern (**Figure 33-1**). Failure to recognize abnormal behavior or an unsafe situation could result in serious injury to you, the patient, or others.

Behavior is the way one acts or conducts oneself, especially toward others. The environment, other relationships, and internal feelings contribute to behavior. Some behaviors come from underlying emotions, such as laughing, crying, or yelling. Whether one's behavior is considered normal or abnormal is subjective and largely depends on social norms, which vary from region to region and from culture to culture. Therefore, what is acceptable behavior in one community may not be acceptable in another. When a person's behavior differs from accepted norms, the person's actions are considered abnormal. If the shift in behavior is severe enough, the person is experiencing a behavioral emergency.

A behavioral emergency is a situation in which a person acts in a way that is unacceptable or intolerable to others and may pose a danger to self or others. Others see the behavioral emergency, but the person does not realize there is problem, with the noted exception of suicidal patients who may call for help for themselves. A key concept in this definition is that the behavior must be taken into *context within the situation*. For example, the mother of a missing child might yell, scream, cry, or display other emotional outbursts. In the context of this situation, this behavior might not be considered unusual. However, if she were to become uncontrollable or she appeared to have no reaction at all, her behavior might be considered abnormal. Likewise, if she behaved in the same way without any apparent cause, the situation might be considered a behavioral emergency.

As an OEC technician, you must carefully approach patients who exhibit abnormal behavior to evaluate them in the circumstances presented.

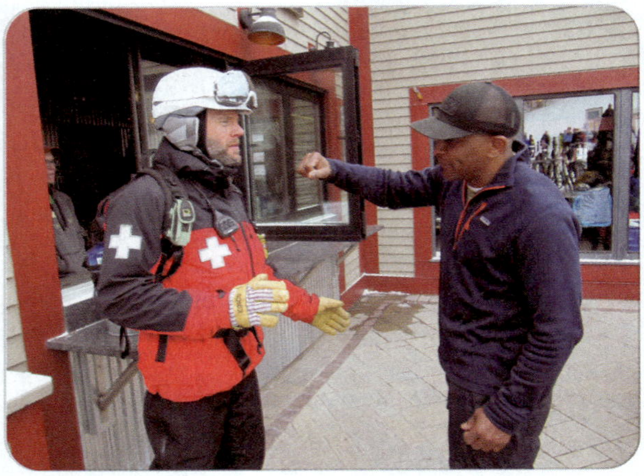

Figure 33-1 Safety is the primary concern for an OEC technician who is interacting with an individual showing atypical behavior.

CASE Presentation

You receive a call to respond to a person "having an anxiety attack." Upon your arrival, you find a visibly upset male who appears to be in his 40s sitting on a bench along one of the area's popular trails. The man, who is wild-eyed and appears to be anxious, is yelling at a nearby female, who identifies herself as the man's wife. Upon identifying yourself, the man yells angrily at you to "Get away or I'm going to punch you!" while repeatedly clenching and unclenching his fists.

What should you do?

The underlying cause may be a medical, chemical, traumatic, or psychiatric disorder. It is important that you quickly recognize the existence of a behavioral emergency and implement effective strategies for safeguarding the patient and others while addressing any threats to life.

This chapter presents a basic introduction to behavioral emergencies, their causes, and general management principles. In addition, this chapter describes the death and the grieving process, as well as the potential effects and available care for acute or cumulative stress on OEC technicians.

ANATOMY AND PHYSIOLOGY

The human body can adapt to various internal and external stimuli. This ability is controlled by the brain and nervous system. In response to various situations, whether social or physical, the brain initiates a variety of corrective actions to return the body to homeostasis (a state of stability) as quickly as possible.

Stress is defined as a person's response to strain, environmental demands, or pressures. When exposed to stress, the body responds by making a physical, mental, or emotional adjustment (**Table 33-1**). Stress is caused by a stimulus, a perceived threat or a stress-inducing factor known as a stressor.

In humans, stress results from interactions between individuals and/or their environment that are perceived as straining or exceeding their adaptive capacities and threatening their well-being. Stress is a normal part of life and may be caused by internal or external factors.

When the body is stressed, its "fight, flight, or stand" system (or simply "fight-or-flight system") automatically triggers a series of responses throughout the body, including the release of the neurologic chemicals (neurotransmitters: epinephrine, norepinephrine, and dopamine). In addition to preparing the body for stress, these chemicals activate a part of the brain known as the amygdala, which triggers an emotional response to the stressor.

The fight-or-flight system is highly effective for short periods of time. However, when the body receives too much stress at one time or suffers prolonged stress, serious imbalances alter mental processes, causing abnormal behavior. How a person responds to stress depends on a variety of factors, including age, overall health, genetics, individual physiology, personality, attitude, and self-image (**Figure 33-2**).

A small amount of stress may be desirable, beneficial, and even healthy. An example of this is when an OEC student is preparing for an evaluation, and stress encourages the person to study. Too much stress, in this example, could impair the student while taking the evaluation.

Table 33-1 Warning Signs of Stress

- Irritability toward coworkers, patients, family, and friends
- Inability to concentrate
- Difficulty sleeping, nightmares
- Aggressive behavior
- Inability to make decisions
- Feeling of helplessness
- Difficulty adjusting

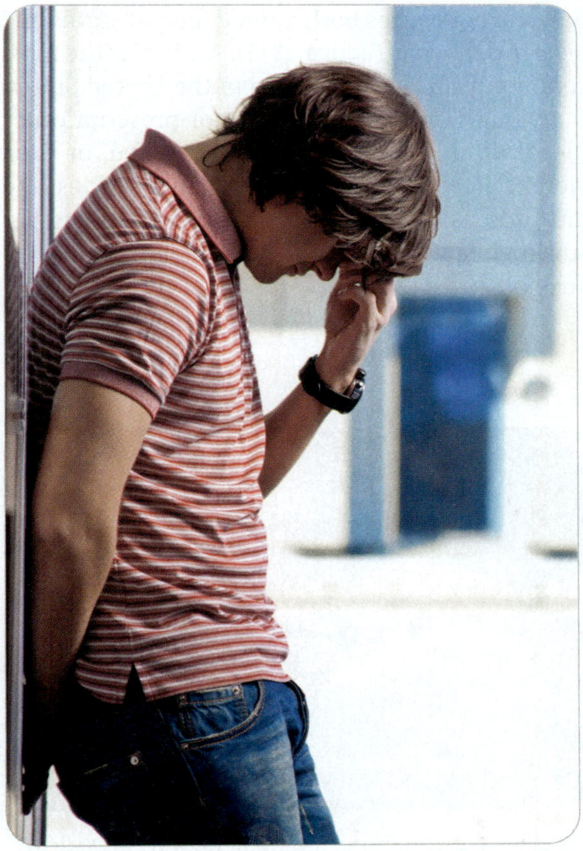

Figure 33-2 How each individual reacts to stress depends on a variety of factors.

CAUSES OF BEHAVIORAL EMERGENCIES

Medical Disorders

In some instances, the source of a person's apparent behavioral emergency can be traced to an underlying medical condition. Whenever you detect an alteration in mental status, *always* consider potential medical conditions first. The brain requires a steady supply of oxygen and glucose and quickly malfunctions when levels of either of these crucial nutrients become too low causing hypoxia or hypoglycemia. Other possible medical causes of abnormal behavior include, but are not limited to, epilepsy, seizures, cardiopulmonary disorders, hypotension, dehydration, electrolyte imbalance, medication overdose, illegal drug overdose, head trauma, and carbon monoxide poisoning.

Chemical Exposures

The use of mind-altering substances such as alcohol or drugs causes both altered mental status and bizarre behavior (**Figure 33-3**). Alcohol is the most commonly abused substance in the United States. Individuals who abuse alcohol or prescription or illegal drugs can be depressed, agitated, or even violent. In addition, many wild plants, berries, and mushrooms can also produce adverse effects, resulting in a wide range of symptoms that may invoke bizarre behavior.

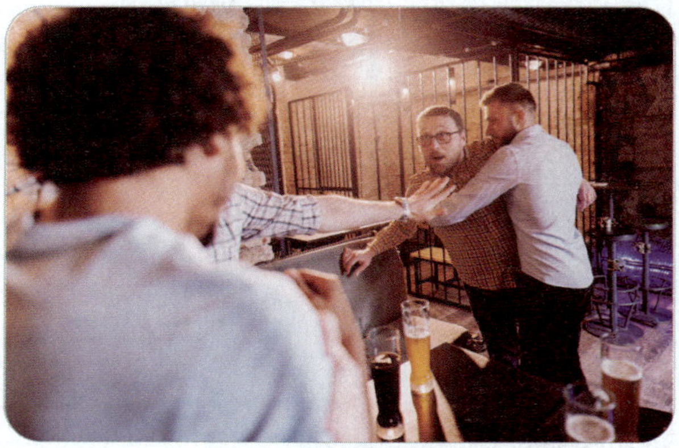

Figure 33-3 The ingestion of alcohol or drugs can alter mental status, at times mimicking the signs and symptoms of a behavioral emergency.

Trauma

Traumatic brain injuries can cause altered responsiveness and behavioral disorders. These may initially appear to be an underlying psychiatric disorder. Patients with a head injury can present with confusion, irritability, agitation, verbal outbursts, irrational behavior, and personality changes. Some can be violent. Brain hypoxia from acute blood loss causing hypovolemic shock may cause abnormal behavior, producing many of these same signs and symptoms. Environmental conditions, including hypothermia and hyperthermia, are also associated with bizarre behavioral changes.

Behavioral Conditions

The human psyche is highly complex, and a full discussion of specific psychiatric disorders goes well beyond the scope of this text. Many different psychological conditions can cause abnormal behavior. However, it is important for the OEC technician to recognize if a person understands reality (the way things really are).

A **mood, adjustment, or affective disorder** (previously known as neurosis) is characterized by abnormal behavior in a person who remains firmly in touch with reality. Anxiety, depression, paranoia, agitation, and bipolar disorder are considered mood, adjustment, and affective disorders. This sharply contrasts with **psychosis**, or a psychotic disorder, which is characterized by abnormal behavior and altered perceptions of reality. Psychotic individuals often have visual or auditory hallucinations, which can lead the person to engage in dangerous, suicidal, or homicidal behaviors. Many patients with a psychosis-based emergency are generally considered more dangerous than those with a mood, adjustment, or affective disorder–based emergency due to their increased tendency to exhibit violent behavior.

Mood, Adjustment, or Affective Disorders

Previously called neuroses, mood, adjustment, and affective disorders are now defined separately. People with these commonly seen conditions understand what is real and not real.

Anxiety is a feeling of worry, nervousness, or unease, typically about an imminent event or something with an uncertain outcome. It is a common emotional disorder in the United States,

KEY POINT

Causes of Behavioral Alterations

- Reduced oxygen to the brain (hypoxia)
- Very low blood pressure
- Low blood sugar (hypoglycemia)
- Illnesses such as a seizure disorder, Alzheimer disease, or infections
- Dehydration
- Abnormal electrolyte levels
- Situational stress (e.g., witnessing the death of a loved one)
- Head injuries
- Environmental exposures (hypothermia or hyperthermia)
- Accidental ingestion of mind-altering substances such as wild herbs, berries, or mushrooms
- Ingestion of drugs or alcohol
- Psychiatric disorders

affecting more than 40 million people over age 18. Anxiety is a normal reaction that occurs when one is faced with a stressful situation. Not all anxiety is harmful. In fact, certain amounts of anxiety can make a person more alert or careful or prompt a person to take purposeful action. Excessive anxiety, however, can result in feelings of impending doom and an inability to function. Over time, anxiety can lead to clinical depression and other health problems. Acute episodes may cause panic attacks that often look like heart attacks. In such cases, a person experiences acute anxiety, palpitations, shortness of breath, chest pain, and a sense of impending doom.

Depression is defined as having feelings of sadness, worthlessness, hopelessness, or despair, and can become so severe that it interferes with normal living. The National Institute of Mental Health states that over 16 million US adults had at least one major depressive episode in 2016. It is estimated one in six adults in the United States will have a major depressive episode in their life. Depression is most common in ages 18 to 25 years and it is characterized by low self-worth, guilt, loss of interest in once-pleasurable things, sleep or appetite disturbances, and poor concentration. Most episodes of depression are brief, lasting only a few days. Severe depression, however, can last for months or even years and can lead to self-destructive behaviors or suicide attempts.

Paranoia is a condition in which individuals believe that they are in imminent danger of being harmed (e.g., physically, emotionally, financially) by others who are plotting against them. The condition is characterized by feelings of deep suspicion, irrational fear, severe distrust of others, delusions, and eccentric behavior. Paranoid individuals often believe that they are being unfairly persecuted. Paranoia is often associated with other behavioral conditions and can present by itself as a symptom of a deep-rooted psychosis such as schizophrenia.

Agitation is defined as excessive restlessness and increased mental or physical activity. It can occur suddenly or develop gradually over time and is characterized by irritability, tension, heightened sensitivity, and excessive motion. The causes of agitation are numerous. Sudden development of agitation can be seen in a traumatic brain injury, hypoglycemia, and shock. When associated with a mental disorder, agitation often precedes more aggressive behavior and is considered a warning sign for impending violence.

Bipolar disorder formerly known as manic-depressive illness, is a psychiatric disease that has been likened to an emotional rollercoaster of highs and lows. It is characterized by alternating intermittent periods of euphoria, known as mania, and periods of depression. During the manic phase, a person experiences an emotional high that may be exhibited as increased excitability, increased energy levels or activity, elevated mood, restlessness, or impulsive behavior (such as hypersexuality or compulsive spending). During this phase, the person can become physically violent or dangerous. The depression phase is characterized by increased irritability, frustration, feelings of worthlessness, and thoughts of suicide. People with bipolar disorder can become psychotic if symptoms become extreme.

Psychotic Disorders

Psychotic individuals can experience anxiety, depression, paranoia, or agitation. However, psychotic people do not understand the difference between what is real and not real.

Schizophrenia is a complex mental disorder in which a person cannot differentiate between what is real and what is not real. It is characterized by impaired reasoning, emotional instability, paranoia, auditory or visual hallucinations, delusions, and (in many cases) violent behavior. Schizophrenia is a serious, lifelong mental disorder that in many cases can be effectively managed with medication, provided the person continues to take it. People who have schizophrenia and discontinue their medications can pose a danger to themselves and others. Other causes of relapse include use of alcohol, marijuana, and other drugs and exposure to emotional trauma and loss.

Suicide

Suicide, the intentional taking of one's life, is a problem that affects thousands of individuals each year. In 2017, it was the tenth leading cause of death in the United States and was the second leading cause of death among people ages 10 to 34 years. Anyone, regardless of race, sex, or socioeconomic background, can become suicidal if the level of emotional distress is severe enough. Among the many reasons a person might attempt suicide are depression, a high-stress lifestyle, mental or physical pain, family trauma or abuse, legal problems, and social, economic, or psychiatric problems. People who have tried suicide before, have a family history of suicide, are depressed, or take illegal drugs, especially opioids, are at greater risk for suicide.

Individuals who have made a very superficial wound on the body or have taken pills and then immediately tell someone they did so have committed a **suicidal gesture**. Such gestures indicate a serious situation, and even if the results of the suicidal act are not life threatening, psychiatric care is urgently needed. A patient who has made a suicidal gesture *cannot be left alone or allowed to refuse medical care*. These individuals are indirectly asking for help.

KEY POINT

Hallucinations and Delusions

Hallucinations are perceptions of things that are not present in the real world by a person who is awake and responsive. Hallucinations may involve any of the five senses (hearing, sight, smell, touch, or taste) and may be caused by any number of medical, chemical, traumatic, and psychotic conditions (especially schizophrenia). Auditory (hearing) hallucinations are more common than visual hallucinations with psychiatric disorders, whereas visual hallucinations are more commonly associated with an underlying medical or traumatic condition.

Delusions are abnormal thoughts not based in reality. Most commonly, these individuals experience paranoid delusions, feeling people are plotting against them, conducting mind control, or wanting to hurt them. This can result in violent behavior as they try to protect themselves.

Violence

Violence, the use of force to abuse, damage, or injure, is an unfortunate by-product of numerous disorders, including mental illness. Violence may be directed inward (a suicidal individual), or it may be directed outward, toward others. It may be intentional, or it may be unintentional, as occurs in patients who are severely hypoxic or have suffered a traumatic injury. Violence is also associated with several forms of mental illnesses. It may also occur independent of a mental illness, most often in the form of physical assault. Patients who exhibit violent behavior may be sociopathic (anxious or depressed and fully aware of their surroundings) or psychotic (psychopathic) and completely out of touch with reality. Not all violent patients are sociopathic or psychopathic.

Abusive Behavior

Abuse is a complex legal, social and psychological act, affecting millions of people around the world. Often the bully/bullied and victim/abuser have underlying emotional and abuse problems. Abuse can take several forms. Verbal abuse, the most common form, involves the use of hurtful words and may include sarcasm, verbal humiliation, name calling, and personal attacks on a person's character or abilities. Verbal abuse may lead to physical abuse, which involves force or violence that results in pain, physical humiliation, or bodily injury. Sexual abuse involves forcing a sex act on another person against their will. Rape is a particularly heinous form of sexual abuse that involves unlawful sexual intercourse or sexual penetration carried out against a person without the person's consent.

Grief

Following a loss, it is common for people to experience a period of grief—an emotional, often painful, reaction. Grief is especially likely when individuals lose a loved one or someone they have known. Yet people can experience grief after other losses; for example, going through a romantic breakup, losing a job or a home, having a body part, such as an arm or leg, removed, being diagnosed with a terminal illness, or having to drop out of college could cause grief.

Grief is a normal response to loss, and can result in a wide range of reactions that were documented and categorized by Dr. Elisabeth Kübler-Ross. She refined her model to include seven stages of loss. This model is a more in-depth analysis of the components of the grief process. According to Kübler-Ross, a person who has experienced a loss may go through the following seven stages of grief:

1. Shock
2. Denial
3. Anger
4. Bargaining
5. Depression
6. Testing
7. Acceptance

At first there is shock; this could not have happened. The person experiencing the loss feels paralyzed and emotionless. During the denial phase, a person refuses to believe that a loss has occurred or will occur, or to acknowledge the events leading up to the loss. This phase is followed by the anger phase, in which the person becomes enraged by the circumstances. Next, the person enters the bargaining phase, which involves attempts to negotiate with oneself or one's higher power to postpone or undo the loss. The fourth phase, depression,

CASE Update

Your immediate concern is for your own safety and for that of others near the irate man. As other OEC technicians clear bystanders from the scene, you attempt to defuse the situation using a calm and caring tone. You assure the man that you are there to help him. Within a few minutes, he begins to settle down, and then he starts to cry.

After obtaining his permission, you carefully approach the man in a nonthreatening manner. As you begin to build trust, you learn that the patient's brother died 1 year ago today. The man and his wife were hiking up to the top of their brother's favorite ridge, where they planned to release his ashes into the wind. Today is the patient's first time hiking in over 5 years. He is still upset and repeatedly says, "I can't believe that he's gone."

The patient is now breathing deep and hard and continues to cry intermittently, but he is alert and oriented to place, date, and time. During your assessment, you learn that the patient has not eaten since last night, and that he never eats breakfast. The patient is not diabetic. It is now midday. With prompting, you get the patient to agree to eat an energy bar while you continue your assessment. He denies chest pain. He complains that his lips and hands are tingling and that he feels like he may "pass out." The physical assessment is unremarkable for obvious trauma, although the patient's fingers are now tightly contorted. He begins to become agitated because he cannot open his hands. He denies that this has ever happened before or having used any mind-altering substances. He agrees to let you take his vital signs. His heart rate is 108 beats per minute, his blood pressure is 126/72 mm Hg, and his respiratory rate is 26 breaths per minute. His skin is somewhat sweaty and warm to the touch.

What should you do now?

occurs when the person realizes that nothing can change the situation. In the testing stage, the person tries to find realistic solutions for coping with the loss and rebuilding his or her life. This phase is followed by the acceptance phase, during which the person comes to terms with the loss and becomes ready to move forward.

The phases of loss occur in no specific time frame, and not every grieving person goes through every stage or experiences the stages in the order listed. In fact, people may remain stuck in one phase for months or even years. In addition, a person may revert to a previous phase during the healing process, as often occurs during evocative times such as holidays, birthdays, or anniversaries.

Post-traumatic Stress Disorder

Post-traumatic stress disorder, or PTSD, is an anxiety-related condition that may occur following exposure to a traumatic incident such as a critical injury, an extremely emotional event, a violent event, or an unexpected death. In 2019, according to the US National Center for PTSD, about 7% to 8% of the US population will have PTSD at some point in their lives. After returning from war, many US military personnel suffer from this condition. The condition can affect the patient, family members, and rescuers.

Symptoms are highly individualized and may either occur immediately following the incident or not become apparent for weeks, months, or even years afterward. The condition is characterized by feelings of helplessness, difficulty adjusting, sleep or eating disturbances, heightened awareness, aggressive behavior, interpersonal relationship challenges, and an inability to cope with normal, everyday situations. Untreated, the condition can cause long-term health problems, including depression and suicidal thoughts.

PATIENT ASSESSMENT OF BEHAVIORAL EMERGENCIES AND CRISIS RESPONSE

Maintaining the safety of rescuers and others is of paramount importance. This is *especially* true in any situation involving people exhibiting abnormal behavior. It is therefore essential that OEC technicians rapidly identify potentially dangerous situations and remember that individuals experiencing a behavioral emergency can become violent. If there is a violent person, even though medical personnel should not initiate patient care until law enforcement personnel have secured the scene, it is not always possible to wait until someone arrives on scene. In these instances, always follow your "gut" instinct. If something doesn't feel right, it probably isn't right. If a weapon is present, *do not* put yourself in danger by going near the patient. Talking to the person at a distance may defuse the situation.

> **KEY POINT**
>
> **Weapons**
>
> Never approach a patient who has a weapon.

When approaching a patient who may be having a behavioral emergency, make mental notes about the scene and look for at least two escape routes. Whenever possible, remain near an escape route, and never let the patient get between you and it. Approach patients from a direction that enables them to see you so that you do not surprise them. Announce that you are a patroller or an OEC technician and are there to help. Always attempt to speak to the patient at eye level. Speak in a normal but firm voice. Avoid yelling or raising your voice even if the patient does not reciprocate. Maintain a comfortable distance from patients until they have given you permission to approach them. Avoid sudden movements, which may startle patients and invoke an aggressive or violent response. Assume that patients could be dangerous, and act accordingly. If at any time the scene becomes unsafe, evacuate to a safer location and await additional assistance (**Figure 33-4**).

If you have a portable communications device, use it to quickly summon any needed help, especially the police if needed. Some two-way radios are equipped with a distress button that, when activated, alerts others on the same frequency that you are in trouble. Be aware that radio static and loud radio traffic can agitate an emotionally unstable individual. A high-powered flashlight not only can illuminate the scene but also can temporarily blind a person who is acting aggressively or

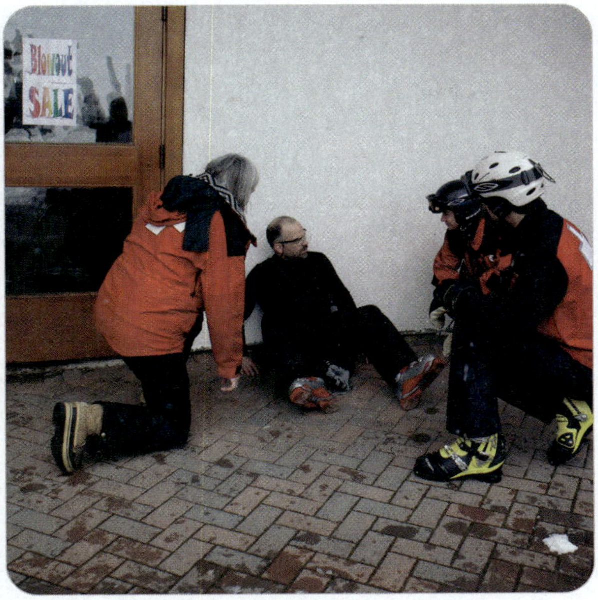

Figure 33-4 Scene safety is especially important when someone exhibiting abnormal behavior is involved.

charging toward you. Be prepared to quickly drop your equipment or pack and evacuate the scene if it suddenly becomes unsafe.

Situational stressors, such as witnessing the death or injury of a loved one, can cause a person to respond with fear, anger, or grief. Remember that these responses are typical under the circumstances. Often, as you take control of the situation, the patient will begin to calm down. It is important to keep your emotions under control while you give patients time to gain control of their emotions. Be honest with patients, explaining what you are going to do before you do it, and continue to observe them for any changes in their behavior.

The primary patient assessment begins with a rapid evaluation of the patient's ABCDs and checking for severe bleeding. If the patient has been speaking to you, the person's airway, breathing, and heartbeat (circulation) are not compromised. If there is an ABCD problem and the scene is safe, correct the problem. Realize that the patient's condition can change physically. For example, the respirations of a patient who overdosed in a suicide attempt or is high on opioids may be normal at first but may then become compromised later. For this reason, regularly monitor the ABCDs (airway, breathing, circulation, disability) of any patient with documented altered mental status.

Table 33-2 Signs and Symptoms of a Behavioral Emergency

- Agitation
- Paranoia
- Speech that appears stressful
- Bizarre thinking or actions
- Self-destructive behavior or attempted suicide
- Mental confusion
- Hostility, anger, or uncontrolled rage
- Uncontrolled crying

Patients with a behavior-related problem can range from withdrawn and quiet, to agitated and overly talkative, to hostile and threatening (**Table 33-2**). In some cases, the patient is simply "not acting right." A patient's behavior may change quickly or slowly, and some changes may not be immediately obvious. For this reason, patients with any behavior considered abnormal, bizarre, or unacceptable must be evaluated by a physician. Although this chapter teaches the basics of mental disease, OEC technicians are discouraged from attempting to diagnose the underlying cause of a patient's behavior and instead should protect the patient from harm. OEC technicians should be able to determine whether patients are in touch with reality, are suicidal, or are anxious, depressed, or dangerous.

Once the scene is secured, approach the patient carefully, identifying yourself and then stating why you are there (**Table 33-3**). When evaluating a patient who appears to be having a behavioral emergency, it is important to determine if the patient is in touch with the real world. Observe the patient's appearance and overall demeanor. Does the person exhibit poor judgment? Is the person wearing clothing that is appropriate for the prevailing conditions? Does the person appear calm, or does the person instead exhibit signs of aggression such as tensing muscles (especially the jaw muscles), clenching the fists, pacing back and forth, or punching the air or inanimate objects? Does the person appear happy, sad, angry, or emotionless? Is the patient alert and oriented?

Individuals who have certain chronic mental diseases, such as schizophrenia, do not function within the normal boundaries of reality. When in crisis, these individuals are often not oriented to the situation, place, or time and appear confused

Table 33-3 Approaching and Caring for the Behavioral Emergency Patient

- Always maintain your safety; always have an escape route.
- Approach patients in a way that they can see you.
- Avoid unnecessary physical contact with patients.
- Try to calm patients.
- Take time to talk to patients and to listen to their responses.
- Never lie to patients.
- Never play along with any auditory or visual hallucinations.
- Consider the medical conditions that might resemble a behavioral emergency.
- Treat any life-threatening problems you encounter.
- Monitor patients for signs of agitation or worsening of their condition.

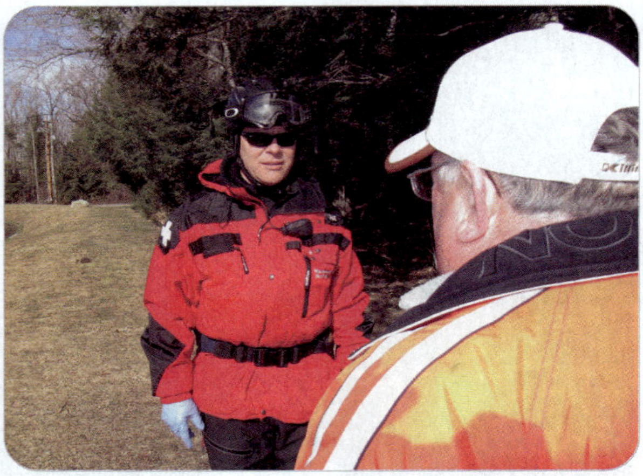

Figure 33-5 Approach a person who may be having a behavioral emergency carefully; identify yourself and explain your purpose.

and disorganized. They may not even know who they are. People who have underlying mood or behavioral disorders can also exhibit bizarre behavior, but they generally function within reality and know who they are, what date it is, where they are, and what has happened, unless other factors such as alcohol or drug use are involved.

As the patient speaks, listen to both the words and the tone of voice. Is the patient yelling and using obscenities? Does the person express homicidal or suicidal thoughts? Is the patient's speech fast or slow? Are the words slurred, pressured (i.e., the speaker can't get them out fast enough), or threatening? Does the person raise or lower his or her voice by an octave? Does the person make sense? Is the patient oriented to time, situation, people, and place? Does the person appear to be functioning within the realm of reality?

Maintain a safe distance until the patient calms and encourage the patient to talk. Calming a patient having a behavioral emergency is essential before performing a secondary assessment. Explain to the patient, in simple terms, what you are doing before assessing them or rendering treatment. Do not make physical contact at this point because doing so could invoke an aggressive or violent response. Unless the patient requires emergent treatment, proceed without hurrying to avoid upsetting the patient (**Figure 33-5**).

If the patient is yelling, it is imperative that you do not yell, argue, or raise your voice in return because doing so will only increase the patient's level of agitation. Instead, ask questions in a calm, reassuring voice. Acknowledge and validate that the patient seems upset and repeat that you are there to help. Continue to encourage patients to discuss what is troubling them. Listen carefully to what they say, because verbal clues may be subtle. From time to time, demonstrate active listening skills by acknowledging what the patient has said by using words such as "If I understand you correctly . . ." or "So what you're saying is . . ." Be honest with the patient, but avoid being judgmental, accusatory, or confrontational. If the patient is hallucinating, do not play along. Instead, redirect the patient's focus to you and to what you are asking.

Begin the secondary assessment by obtaining a complete SAMPLE history (signs and symptoms, allergies, medications, past medical history, last oral intake, events leading up to the problem), including a history of prior treatment for any medical, traumatic, or mental health disorders that might cause the patient's altered mental status, such as diabetes, epilepsy, or head injury. Look for a medical alert tag. If the patient has a history of mental illness, ask whether the patient has been prescribed any medications for that illness, and whether the

KEY POINT

Patient Assessment of Behavioral Emergencies

As you assess the patient, note the presence of any signs or symptoms that might suggest a behavioral emergency, including the following:

- Agitation: repetitive motions, threatening actions
- Paranoia: thoughts that someone or something is going to harm them; often accompanied by anxiety and fear
- Pressured speech: a very rapid, difficult-to-understand speech pattern; can be also seen in patients on stimulants such as cocaine or methamphetamine
- Bizarre thinking or actions: a frequent reason why someone calls for help or is concerned about a behavioral emergency
- Self-destructive behavior or attempted suicide: physical actions or verbal statements indicating that the patient is trying or did try to hurt himself or herself
- Mental confusion: disorganized words or thoughts that are difficult to follow during a conversation
- Hostility/anger/uncontrolled rage: can pose a danger to the patient, the rescuers, and those around them
- Uncontrolled crying: inconsolable despite the rescuer's attempts at calming
- Unusual appearance: withdrawn stance, clothing in disorder, poor personal hygiene, too many or not enough clothes for the ambient temperature

patient is taking those medications as directed. If the patient may have overdosed on a medication or some other substance, gather as much information as possible about the ingested product, including the name of the substance, the quantity ingested, and when the ingestion occurred.

Patients with anxiety exhibit a wide range of signs and symptoms that may include fear, apprehension, agitation, crying, and hyperventilation.

Patients who are depressed are often withdrawn and relatively quiet. They exhibit apathy toward their appearance, health, or general well-being. Patients who are willing to talk may express feelings of worthlessness, despair, or profound sadness. They may reveal that they have experienced one or more life changes such as the loss of a loved one, the loss of a job, or some other personal tragedy. Such patients may describe a host of symptoms, such as a loss of appetite, problems sleeping, or frequent somatic complaints such as headaches or stomachaches.

Patients who are chronically depressed frequently take medication to control their depression. Patients who stop taking their medications or experience more severe depression may begin thinking about suicide. Even though the role of OEC technicians does not include diagnosing suicidal intent, briefly assess the patient's suicide risk by noting whether the patient exhibits or articulates indications that they could harm themselves. This is especially important in interacting with individuals who are refusing medical care. As part of the exam process, note the presence of current wounds or old scars, especially over arterial sites such as the wrist, inside the elbow, and neck. Do not be afraid to ask the patient directly, "Are you trying to hurt yourself?" because many patients are relieved that someone has heard their cry for help.

Patients with paranoid tendencies can be difficult to assess because they are typically suspicious of anyone who attempts to help them. Some patients may accuse you of attempting to harm them; others may openly seek your protection. The irrational fears of paranoid patients often lead these patients to refuse a physical examination or the use of medical equipment such as a blood pressure cuff on them. Paranoid patients who are psychotic may complain of hearing voices that feed their anxieties.

Patients who have a psychotic disorder such as schizophrenia are among the most difficult behavioral emergency patients to assess, especially if they are concurrently paranoid. These patients often have auditory hallucinations of voices that instruct them to harm themselves or others or to engage in bizarre or dangerous activities. It is

> **KEY POINT**
>
> **Frequently Used Medications for Mental Illness**
>
> Anti-anxiety (can cause addiction, sedation, decreased level of consciousness and death)
> - Xanax (alprazolam)
> - Ativan (lorazepam)
>
> Antidepressants (can cause headaches, gastrointestinal upset, sedation, suicidal thoughts)
> - Zoloft (sertraline)
> - Lexapro (escitalopram)
> - Wellbutrin (bupropion)
> - Prozac (fluoxetine)
> - Cymbalta (duloxetine)
>
> Antipsychotics (can cause sedation, muscle spasm, weight gain, hypertension, diabetes)
> - Seroquel (quetiapine)
> - Risperdal (risperidone)
> - Abilify (aripiprazole)
> - Zyprexa (olanzapine)
>
> Mood stabilizers (can cause sedation, lack of coordination, severe skin rash, tremor)
> - Depakote (valproic acid)
> - Lamictal (lamotrigine)
> - Lithium (lithium carbonate)
>
> Attention deficit hyperactivity disorder (ADHD) (can cause hypertension or hypotension, tachycardia, weight loss, insomnia)
> - Concerta (methylphenidate)
> - Adderall (amphetamine)
> - Tenex (guanfacine)

important to ask schizophrenic patients if they have taken their medications as prescribed, because schizophrenic attacks are often precipitated by the patient's noncompliance with their medications. Patients who appear to be psychotic do not think or act rationally, so reasoning with them can be extremely difficult, if not impossible. Besides being paranoid, psychotic patients can also be depressed or anxious, or have mania (periods of great excitement and overactivity).

Table 33-4 Signs of Physical Abuse

- Bruises or injuries of various ages, especially in young children
- Injuries that are not age appropriate (e.g., a long-bone fracture in a child)
- Fear of physical contact
- Exaggerated startle reflex
- Obvious fear of a spouse, significant other, parent, guardian, or sibling
- Suspicious injuries that are "explained away" by the patient or a significant other

Table 33-5 Signs and Symptoms of Sexual Abuse

- Frequent, unexplained somatic complaints (e.g., headaches, stomachaches)
- Description of inappropriate touching or physical contact of a sexual nature
- Self-mutilation
- Poor personal hygiene

Any patient who has been abused, whether only recently or over a long period of time, may exhibit numerous behavior-related signs and symptoms (**Tables 33-4** and **Table 33-5**). Abuse is a crime that, if suspected, must usually be reported to those who will be caring for the patient and to law enforcement officials. Abuse should be suspected whenever any tell-tale signs or symptoms are present.

Complete the secondary patient assessment as you would for any patient, using the OPQRST (onset, provocation, quality, radiation, severity, and time) and DCAP-BTLS (deformity, contusions, abrasions/avulsions, punctures/penetrations, burns/bleeding/bruises, tenderness, lacerations, swelling) mnemonics, noting all pertinent signs or symptoms and documenting them on the patient care report. Obtain a complete set of vital signs and monitor them frequently, especially if the patient has ingested any drugs or alcohol. Continue to treat patients in

KEY POINT

OPQRST for Behavioral Emergency Patients

O: Is this a new mental illness or worsening of a preexisting one?

P: What brought it on? Is substance abuse involved? Is there a medical illness or injury causing this?

Q: What is the quality of the patient's thinking? Is it reality based or is the patient responding to hallucinations, delusions, or other abnormal thinking?

R: Is this mental illness causing other problems? For example, is anxiety causing hyperventilation with shortness of breath or chest pain?

S: We can rate anxiety, depression, worry, and suicidal or homicidal thoughts on a severity scale of 0 to 10, like we rate pain. The severity of these emotions may determine the urgency of patient care.

T: Are the symptoms getting better or worse?

a dignified, caring manner, regardless of their appearance, attitude, or behavior, and document all assessment findings on the patient care report. Be ready to protect yourself if you detect even the possibility of aggressive or violent behavior.

MANAGEMENT OF BEHAVIORAL EMERGENCIES

First, make sure the scene is safe. As with any patient, treatment begins by correcting any potential threats to life, including any external hemorrhage resulting from self-inflicted wounds. Until proven otherwise, assume that the patient's abnormal behavior results from an underlying medical condition. The treatment of patients having a behavioral emergency is both preventive and supportive. Prevention efforts center on keeping patients safe and away from hazards or potential weapons and on preventing them from harming themselves or others.

Continue to calm and reassure the patient as you provide treatment. Be empathetic to the patient's feelings and redirect the patient's attention as needed to reduce anxiety, paranoia, or suicidal thoughts. Remember that special patient situations warrant additional help in the form of additional patrollers, area management, and (if appropriate) security or police. Call EMS early, and if needed, ALS for drug intervention to assist patients with severe symptoms.

Consider restraining patients who exhibit violent behavior or present a danger to themselves or others, following all local protocols and procedures. This is especially important for any patient who presents with psychosis. Continue to provide supportive care as needed and transport the patient to the nearest definitive-care facility for further evaluation and ongoing treatment. Be sure to carefully document the patient encounter on the patient care report, including the patient's behavior and response to treatment. Use direct quotes as appropriate to convey the patient's feelings.

Restraints

When a patient's behavioral emergency escalates to the point at which words are no longer calming and the patient poses an imminent threat of violence, physical restraint is needed. Restraint is a process that restricts a patient's normal movement; its goal is to prevent the patient from harming self or others. OEC technicians should be familiar with two forms of restraint: physical restraint, which involves directly holding onto a patient, and mechanical restraint, which involves the use of equipment such as a flexible band, strap, or cuff. Only patients who are clearly demonstrating an imminent danger to themselves or others should be restrained. It is best to seek the patient's cooperation to avoid the need for restraint. Unfortunately, this may not always be possible.

Under these circumstances, there is no alternative but to protect the safety of the patient, the rescuers, and bystanders. The most common indication for the use of restraints is a violent psychotic patient. It is always best to ask for the assistance of area security or law enforcement personnel and have them restrain or isolate the individual, both for your safety and for the safety of others. When a patient is violent, it is best not to enter the scene and to wait for police.

Restraining a patient, if necessary, is *always* best done by law enforcement officials. Law enforcement personnel can restrain anyone if they have probable cause; this is not true for medical personnel. Most states and provinces have specific laws governing the use of restraints by those outside of law enforcement. In many states, EMS personnel have protocols to physically and chemically restrain patients. When permitted, the prevailing tenet is to use only **reasonable force**, the minimum amount of force required to keep the patient from hurting self or others. Many factors contribute to determining this level of force, including the patient's size, strength, mental attitude, and degree of agitation; the type of abnormal behavior; and the availability of restraint equipment and personnel. OEC technicians must be familiar with their local protocols regarding the use of restraints and the procedures for restraining a combative patient. They should also be aware that use of excessive force can have both civil and criminal legal consequences.

If it becomes necessary to restrain a patient, all on-scene personnel must work together. Ideally, a minimum of five people is required to safely restrain a patient: one person to hold each extremity and one person to hold the patient's head in neutral alignment. If the patient must be mechanically restrained, a sixth person is needed to apply the mechanical restraints. The patient and/or the rescuers are more likely to be injured when too few personnel are available to properly restrain a patient. A team leader should be designated, and that leader should brief all personnel involved on their respective roles.

Once a plan is established, the team should move into position upon receiving a preestablished signal. A simple show of force will often prompt a patient to submit peacefully. The team leader should always attempt to seek the patient's cooperation and consent to treatment. If the patient remains noncompliant, then it becomes necessary to restrain the patient. Throughout the restraining process, continue to talk to the patient, providing instructions in a firm voice. Be polite always. Use statements such as, "Sir, please stop fighting us," "We are here to help you," and "Please lie down." Once the patient is physically restrained, use only enough force to keep the patient submissive; any additional force may be considered excessive.

Patients should be placed supine on a backboard to facilitate safe transport and the monitoring of vital signs. The exact method by which you mechanically restrain a patient should be consistent with local protocol as approved by your medical director. In one widely accepted technique, one of the patient's arms is secured to the board above the patient's head to prevent the patient from sitting up. The patient's other arm should be extended alongside the torso and tied to the board. The legs, too, should be securely tied to the lower end of the board while remaining a neutral alignment. Additional straps may be secured across the patient's hips and chest to further increase restraint. Be ready to tip the board on its side should the patient vomit. Never stick your finger in a restrained patient's mouth. Additionally, *never restrain a patient in a prone position because death can result due to asphyxia*. To physically or mechanically restrain a patient, follow the steps in **OEC Skill 33-1**.

Under most circumstances, any patient who required physical restraint to be brought under control should be mechanically restrained until examined by a physician (**Figure 33-6**). Handcuffs may be used *only* by law enforcement personnel, who should physically accompany the patient to the hospital. Restrained patients often try to persuade medical personnel to remove the restraints.

Be sure to provide thorough documentation of both the patient's behavior before, during, and after the application of restraints and your reasons for using restraints. Documentation should also include what efforts were taken to avoid restraining the patient, the restraint method(s) used, the total time the patient was restrained, and all ongoing CMS (circulation, movement, sensation) exams.

Mandatory Reporting

You may be required to report abuse of a child, elder, or any person who is in immediate danger of being further harmed. Check with your management and go by what your state or provincial laws mandate.

Critical Incident Stress

As an OEC technician, you are not immune to the emotional and psychological consequences of managing ill or injured patients and witnessing

OEC SKILL 33-1 Physical/Mechanical Restraint of a Patient

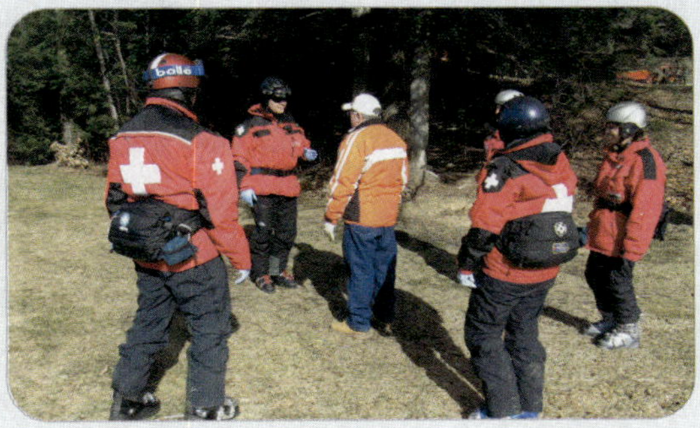

1 Make a plan involving all the rescuers and then have one person speak calmly with the patient.

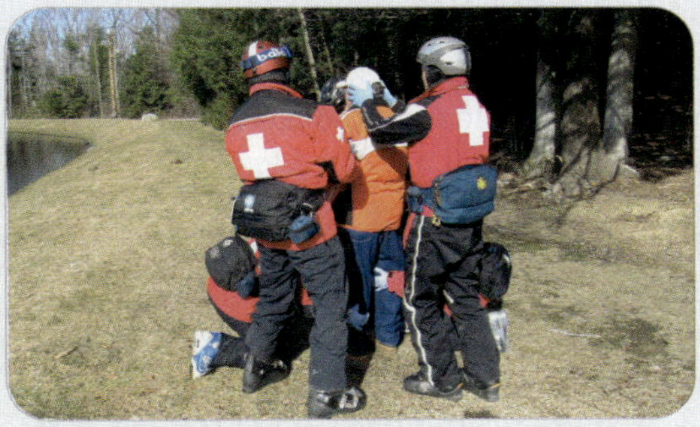

2 The team moves into position upon receiving a preestablished signal. Each member of the team should restrain either a single limb or the head.

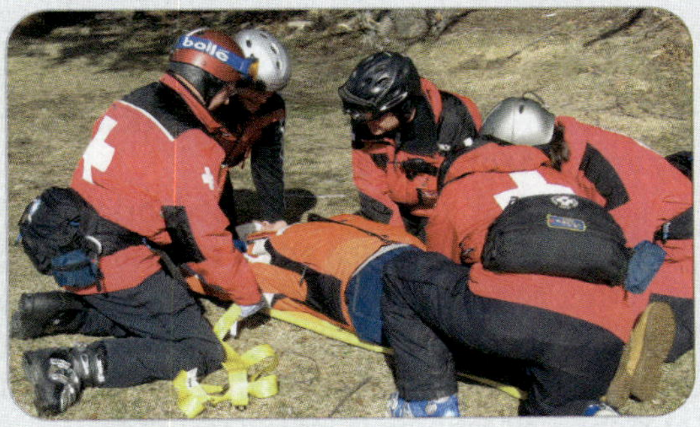

3 Firmly support the patient as you lower the person to the ground or onto a backboard.

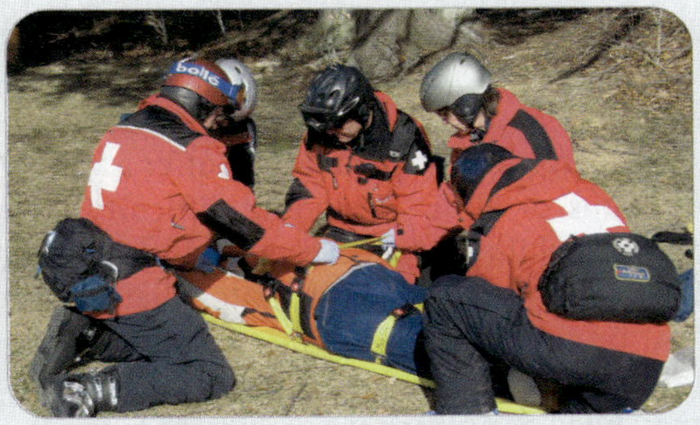

4 Secure the patient with the right arm over the head and the left arm along the torso.

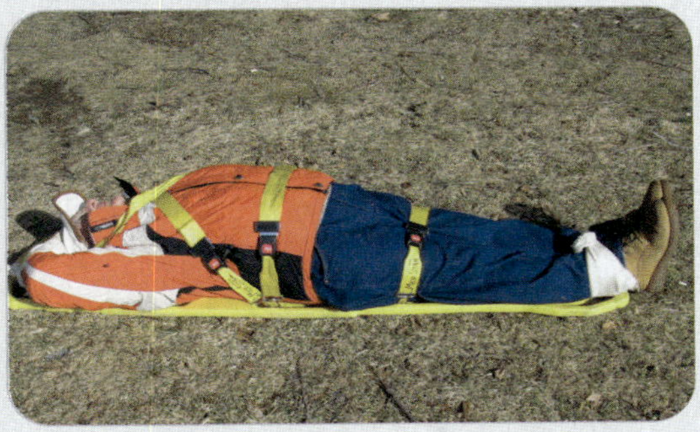

5 Tie the patient down completely, using as many straps as needed; be prepared to tilt the board if the patient should vomit.

KEY POINT

Behavior and Injury

One of the most difficult situations is handling the head-injured patient who is aggressive, will not listen to reason, and yet needs spinal immobilization due a traumatic injury. You will need help from trained rescuers to provide careful handling for this person who is exhibiting behavioral issues. Aggressive restraint in order to immobilize this patient to a spine board may be necessary; however, it is important to exercise care and not cause more harm to the patient.

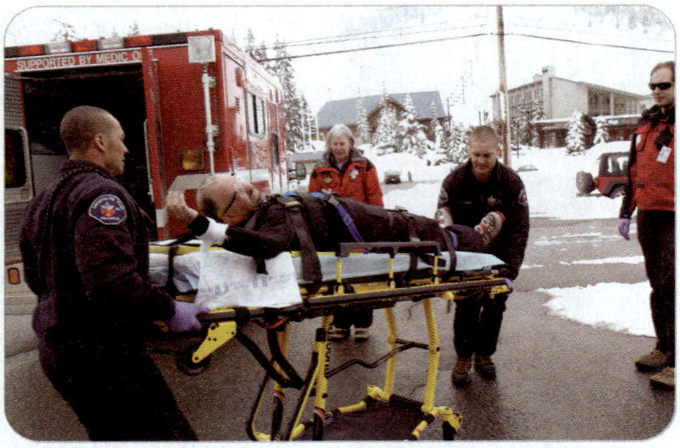

Figure 33-6 Individuals who exhibit abnormal behavior should be considered to have a medical illness and transported to a medical facility for further evaluation.

death. The consequences may be either short lived or long term. Rescuers and others involved in extraordinary circumstances can be adversely affected by such encounters and can suffer a variety of symptoms of PTSD, including difficulty concentrating, inability to sleep, repeatedly replaying the incident, headache, gastrointestinal abnormalities, profound sadness, and depression. Fortunately, professional help is available to rescuers who may need assistance in working through the aftermath of a traumatic incident, and many agencies have formal agreements with a local critical incident stress management (CISM) team created for this very purpose. If you find yourself disturbed by an incident, seek assistance.

A critical incident stress debriefing (CISD) brings OEC technicians and a trained professional together to talk about the rescuers' feelings. CISD may help OEC technicians understand the signs and symptoms of stress and receive reassurance and coping techniques from a trained professional.

CASE Outcome

You try to calm the patient by having him breathe in a slow, controlled fashion. After several minutes, he calms down and stops crying. Shortly thereafter, the tingling subsides, so he now has full use of his hands and no longer feels faint. He drinks a bottled sports drink from his backpack. Embarrassed, he tells you that he has been very stressed since his older brother died, and he thanks you for your kindness. You and another OEC technician accompany the patient and his sister to the top of the ridge, which is only a quarter mile away. From a respectful distance, you watch as the pair open an urn and throw ashes off the ridge. As the two hug each other, you smile, knowing that the healing process has begun.

This behavioral emergency was likely brought on by the combination of anxiety and grief. The techniques used to manage the patient and his behavior enabled the OEC technician to determine it was not a medical emergency and deescalate what could have been a potentially difficult situation.

CHAPTER REVIEW

In Summary

- Scene safety is the top priority when managing a behavioral emergency.
- A behavioral emergency exists when a person exhibits abnormal thoughts or actions.
- The cause of a behavioral emergency may be medical, chemical, traumatic, or behavioral.
- Signs and symptoms of a behavioral emergency include panic, agitation, violence, and self-destructive behavior.
- Anxiety, depression, paranoia, agitation, and bipolar disorder are considered mood, adjustment, and affective disorders.
- The seven stages of grief are shock, denial, anger, bargaining, depression, testing, and acceptance.
- As you approach a patient experiencing a behavioral emergency, if appropriate, call for help, including area security personnel and police authorities.
- The treatment of patients having a behavioral emergency is both preventive and supportive. Prevention efforts center on keeping patients safe and away from hazards or potential weapons, and on preventing them from harming themselves or others.
- Contact critical incident stress debriefing professionals to help OEC technicians who have stress following a difficult rescue.

Key Terms

Agitation Excessive restlessness and increased mental or physical activity.

Anxiety A feeling of worry, nervousness, or unease, typically about an imminent event or something with an uncertain outcome.

Bipolar disorder A serious mental illness characterized by extreme mood swings, which range from depression to mania. If severe, psychosis can result.

Crisis A state of emotional turmoil within an individual in which the balance between thoughts and emotions is lost.

Depression A clinical state marked by feelings of sadness and self-loathing.

Mood, adjustment, or affective disorder Abnormal behavior in a person who remains firmly in touch with reality; specific disorders of this type include anxiety, depression, paranoia, agitation, and bipolar.

Paranoia A condition in which individuals believe they are in imminent danger of being harmed (e.g., physically, emotionally, financially) by others who are plotting against them.

Psychosis A condition in which a person exhibits abnormal behavior and has altered perceptions of reality.

Reasonable force The minimum force needed to keep a patient from hurting himself or others.

Schizophrenia A psychiatric disorder in which a person cannot distinguish what is real from what is not real.

Stress A person's response to environmental demands or pressures. When exposed to stress, the body responds by making a physical, mental, or emotional adjustment.

Suicidal gesture An action taken by someone that leads others to believe it was a suicide attempt to communicate that the person is in distress or to influence the behavior of others in some way.

Suicide The intentional taking of one's own life.

Chapter Questions

1. Behavior is the way a person acts, especially in relation to others. A behavioral emergency occurs when a person's behavior:
   a. is intolerable to others.
   b. puts themselves or others in danger.
   c. is considered out of context within the situation.
   d. All of the above

2. Which of the following is always associated with a psychotic disorder?
   a. Anxiety
   b. Paranoia
   c. Inability to differentiate between what is real and what is not real
   d. Depression

3. You are responding to a call for a person "out of control" in the lift line. What are some of the behaviors you might expect to find upon your arrival?
   a. Someone moving around with jerky movements, appearing agitated
   b. A guest calmly talking to a lift attendant
   c. Loud, angry shouting
   d. Both a and c

4. Scene safety for the rescuer and others in the vicinity can be challenging when responding to a behavioral emergency. What are some best practices that OEC technicians should follow?
   a. Never approach a patient who has a weapon.
   b. Ensure you always have two escape routes.
   c. Avoid sudden movements or raising your voice.
   d. All of the above

5. Restraining a patient by physical or mechanical means is needed:
   a. when a patient's behavioral emergency deescalates.
   b. when a patient poses an imminent threat of violence.
   c. to protect the safety of the patient, the rescuers, or bystanders.
   d. Both b and c

6. To properly restrain a patient *physically*, a minimum of how many people is recommended?
   a. Four
   b. Five
   c. Six
   d. Seven

7. Last weekend, your team responded to a scene that involved a collision between an adult and a small child. The child was unresponsive at the scene and despite the efforts of the OEC technicians, EMS providers, and hospital personnel, the child did not survive his injuries. Your patrol leader sets up a critical incident stress debriefing for all the OEC technicians involved and includes your local EMS team. What is the purpose of this meeting?
   a. For trained professionals to guide the rescuers in how to deal with their post-incident feelings
   b. To identify potential reactions that are normal after a stressful incident
   c. To understand the signs and symptoms of stress and how to cope with them
   d. All of the above

8. Which of the following statements about stress is *true*?
   a. The fight-or-flight response is highly effective for long periods of time.
   b. A small amount of stress may be desirable, beneficial, or even healthy.
   c. Everyone responds to stressors in the same way.
   d. Stress is *not* a part of normal life and is caused by external factors only.

Answers: 1. d, Objective 33-1, p. 768; 2. c, Objective 33-2, p. 771; 3. d, Objective 33-3, p. 775; 4. d, Objective 33-4, p. 774; 5. d, Objective 33-7, p. 779; 6. b, Objective 33-8, p. 780; 7. d, Objective 33-9, p. 782; 8. b, Objective 33-9, p. 769

Design Credits: Mountain: © thianchai sitthikongsak/Getty Images; Honeycomb Texture: © Erlon Silva - TRI Digital/Getty Images.

CHAPTER 34

SPECIAL OPERATIONS AND AMBULANCE OPERATIONS

OBJECTIVES

Upon completion of this chapter, the OEC technician will be able to:

34-1 Define special operations.
34-2 List several activities that are classified as special operations.
34-3 Describe one disaster response agency that OEC technicians are encouraged to join.
34-4 Explain the meaning of "try before you pry."
34-5 List the words that make up the term HAZWOPER.
34-6 Identify the purpose of the NFPA hazard identification system.
34-7 List and describe the three hazard control zones.
34-8 Describe the purpose of and the mechanism of action for the contents of a nerve agent antidote kit.
34-9 Describe and demonstrate how to properly self-administer the contents of a nerve agent antidote kit.
34-10 Describe the actions you should take in the event of an active shooter.
34-11 Describe what a Recco system is.
34-12 Name three of the four functions of avalanche rescue.
34-13 Describe what the term "silence is golden" refers to in SAR response.
34-14 Describe crew resource management.

KEY TERMS

CBRNE, p. 791
Cold zone, p. 795
Crew resource management (CRM), p. 806
Extrication, p. 789
HAZWOPER, p. 793
High-angle rescue (HAR), p. 802
Hot zone, p. 794
Low-angle rescue (LAR), p. 802
Rescue, p. 799
Search, p. 799
Special operations, p. 786
Terrorism, p. 791
Warm zone, p. 795

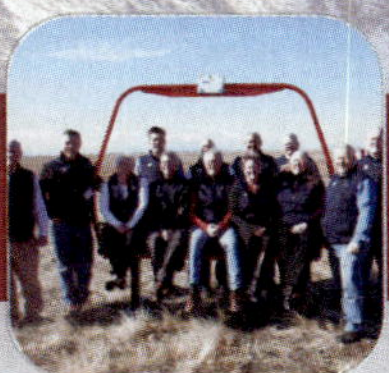

HISTORICAL TIMELINE **2020.** *Outdoor Emergency Care, Sixth Edition,* is published.

CHAPTER OVERVIEW

OEC technicians are educated and prepared to manage medical and trauma emergencies. They can identify and mitigate hazards, direct the actions of other rescuers at an emergency scene, and triage patients. Despite their rigorous training, OEC technicians occasionally encounter incidents that exceed the scope of their education and expertise. In these rare situations, OEC technicians may need to summon rescuers with specialized skills and equipment to assist in managing the situation.

This chapter provides an overview of the **special operations** situations (infrequently performed activities requiring specialized education and equipment in remote and/or difficult settings) in which OEC technicians are most likely to become involved: natural and human-caused disasters, hazardous materials (hazmat) incidents, and searches. This chapter also includes a basic overview of ambulance operations. Although most OEC technicians do not operate with an ambulance, many of the principles presented apply to other equipment that OEC technicians operate and maintain. Other topics covered in this chapter are community-based emergency response groups, rope rescues, terrorism, and basic fire ground operations. Additionally, the chapter covers indications for and the self-administration of nerve agent auto-injectors.

The material in this chapter is intended to keep OEC technicians safe when working on an incident involving specialized response personnel; it is not intended to either be all-encompassing or to replace specialized training. Additionally, the material presented is intended to encourage OEC technicians to obtain additional training to meet the needs of their respective resort areas and communities, and it is included so that patrollers can meet the requirements for achieving emergency first-responder status. Some ski patrollers may find the information on avalanche rescue particularly valuable.

AMBULANCE OPERATIONS

OEC technicians frequently interact with EMS personnel and other health care practioners. Depending on the design of the emergency care system, OEC technicians may even be asked to assist in a patient's care during transport to the hospital. It is important that OEC technicians have a basic understanding of ambulance operations and a familiarity with some of the nuances of working within such a confined environment.

OEC technicians may encounter three basic ambulance designs:

- A type I ambulance has a truck-style chassis with a separate driver's compartment and a modular, box-style patient's compartment (**Figure 34-1**).
- A type II ambulance has a van-style design that has a long wheelbase and direct access between the patient's compartment and the driver's compartment.
- A type III ambulance has a van-style driver's compartment with direct access to an integral, modular patient's compartment.

CASE Presentation

A call comes in to respond to a four-wheeler accident just off a mountain bike racecourse. One of the racers was injured. Upon your arrival, you find a four-wheeler in a ditch, with a teenage girl strapped to a stretcher on the back of the vehicle. The driver had hit a large rock and was thrown clear and is complaining of shoulder pain. Quite angry and yelling, the 16-year-old racer who has a splint on her lower leg is bleeding from a small cut on the top of her head caused by a branch of a tree near the trail. A small crowd has assembled.

What should you do?

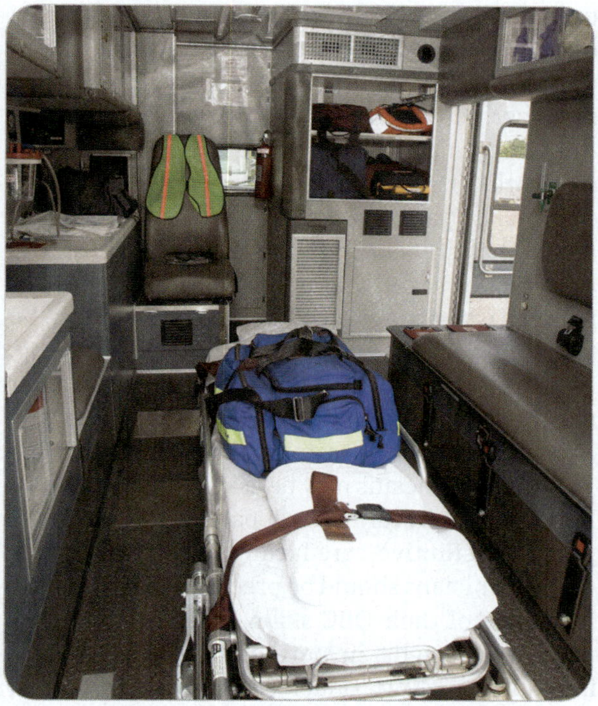

Figure 34-1 Equipment and supplies are stored in accordance to how urgently they might be needed and/or how often they are used.

Individual states, counties, and cities impose rules and regulations regarding ambulance operations, including essential equipment requirements, minimum crew configurations and certification requirements, and who may operate an ambulance. The next sections describe basic operational tasks and objectives for ambulance operations.

Preparing for a Call

An ambulance must always be maintained in a state of readiness and be fully stocked. Such readiness is made possible by regular maintenance, equipment checks, and routine cleaning. Quality EMS systems perform equipment inspections daily or at the beginning of each work period. Additionally, durable equipment (e.g., a stretcher, long spine boards) is cleaned after each use, and disposable equipment is replaced as needed to maintain minimum supply levels.

Ambulances generally should be strategically positioned within their geographic response area to reduce the response time to a request for assistance.

Responding to a Call

When an OEC technician requests an ambulance to transport a patient, many events must occur if the ambulance is to arrive in a timely manner. For instance, the ambulance crew must receive accurate information regarding the location and nature of the emergency, and the crew must safely navigate to the scene despite possible dense traffic, hazardous road conditions, and/or inclement weather.

As a rule, ambulance operators must obey all traffic laws, regardless of whether or not lights and siren are in use, although some exceptions may exist. The driver of an emergency vehicle must always observe "due regard for the safety of others," including that of the ambulance crew, the patient, passengers, other motorists, and the public at large. The following standard driving rules apply:

- Observe all traffic laws, except as allowed by law.
- Use the most appropriate route to and from the scene of the emergency.
- Maintain a safe distance from other vehicles.
- Use warning devices (e.g., lights and siren) only as authorized by law or policy.

Intersections are the location of most ambulance accidents; most collisions occur during daylight hours and in dry conditions. When approaching an intersection, the ambulance crew must visually "clear" the intersection by ensuring that all other vehicles have come to a complete stop before the ambulance enters the intersection (**Figure 34-2**). Ideally, the ambulance operator should make eye contact with other drivers before proceeding through the intersection.

Arriving at the Scene

The location in which an ambulance is parked depends on the circumstances. Whenever possible, the ambulance should be parked in a designated parking space, away from traffic. If law enforcement personnel or fire equipment are at the scene, the ambulance should be parked approximately 100 feet *beyond* the scene; if the scene has not yet been secured, the ambulance should be parked approximately 50 to 100 feet *before* the scene, using the ambulance to protect the scene, the rescuers, and bystanders. The parking brake should be set after the vehicle is

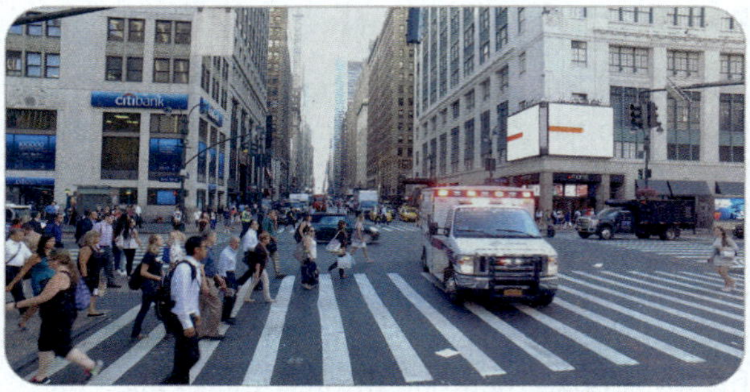

Figure 34-2 Intersections are the most dangerous to ambulance crews, especially during daylight hours.

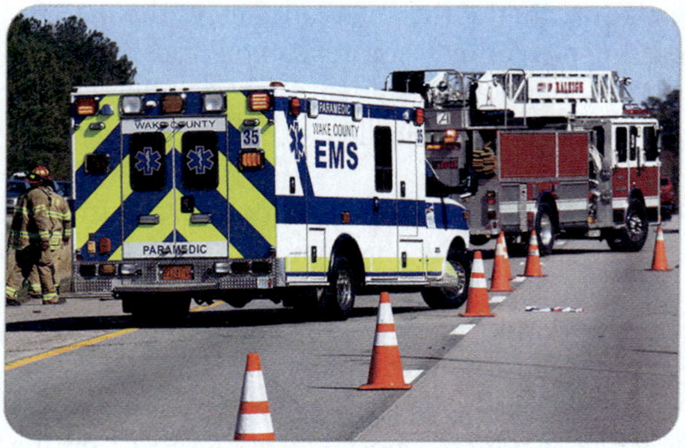

Figure 34-3 Proper placement of the ambulance at an accident scene will greatly reduce the risk of the crew being injured by traffic going by the scene.

placed in "Park," and warning lights should be left on to visually alert drivers to the presence of an accident scene.

The area around the ambulance and accident scene is known as the "ambulance operation zone" and is designed to provide a safety barrier. When moving back and forth between the ambulance and the scene, walk along the side of the ambulance that is *farthest* from traffic (**Figure 34-3**).

Loading and Assisting with Patients

Patients are generally moved to and from an ambulance on a wheeled ambulance stretcher, which typically can be raised and lowered by as few as two people. Newer types of electric stretchers may often be seen on ambulances and can be raised and lowered by one person. Specific ambulance stretcher operations vary, so check the manufacturer's instructions or contact the EMS agencies you work with to obtain training on the use of this device. The patient is secured to the stretcher by straps that are usually placed over the chest, the abdomen or upper thighs, and the lower legs. For patients who are agitated, the strap buckles can be turned toward the patient to prevent unbuckling. Loading and unloading an ambulance stretcher may be performed by one or two people, typically by the ambulance operator and an assistant.

OEC technicians may be asked to assist an ambulance crew in caring for a patient during transport to a definitive-care facility. When this occurs, OEC technicians should be prepared to provide the full range of their OEC skills, including CPR, airway management, hemorrhage control, bandaging, and splinting. Under certain circumstances, they also may be asked to *assist* an advanced life support (ALS) provider, such as an advanced EMT or a paramedic.

The patient's compartment of ambulances is organized so that essential equipment is close at hand. For instance, airway equipment and oxygen are typically stored near the head of the stretcher, whereas bandaging supplies and splints are usually placed in cabinets near the middle of the stretcher.

Working in the back of a moving ambulance is extremely dangerous and is much different than providing care on a stable, stationary surface. Accordingly, OEC technicians asked to assist in the back of a moving ambulance must be very careful when standing or moving around because of the risk of losing their balance and becoming seriously injured. Unless absolutely necessary, remain seated at all times, either at the patient's head or side, or as instructed by the ambulance crew. While seated, use restraining devices. Stand only long enough to perform the required task and then sit down and put on your seat belt. In some locales, ambulances are equipped with track-mounted harnesses that facilitate standing while the vehicle is in motion. These devices do not seem to be gaining popularity.

Be aware of any sharp objects (e.g., needles, edges) that may be present. Secure or stow loose objects and equipment to prevent them from becoming projectiles in the event of a sharp turn or sudden braking. Always keep your center of gravity low. If you have any questions regarding how to operate safely in the back of a moving ambulance, consult a member of the ambulance crew.

KEY POINT

Anatomy of a Vehicle

- Front
- Driver's side of vehicle
- Passenger's side of vehicle
- Rear of vehicle
- Working area (inner circle; 10 feet around outside of vehicle)

Extricating a Patient from a Vehicle

Extrication is the process of removing a trapped person (as from a vehicle that has been involved in a collision) when the removal of the person via a conventional exit (e.g., a door, a window) is impossible or inadvisable. Examples in which OEC technicians may become involved in extrication from a vehicle include an automobile crash, an overturned snowcat or groomer, or an airplane or helicopter crash.

Vehicle extrication is a time-consuming process involving several basic operational tasks and objectives, including assessment, stabilization, gaining access to the patient, and the initial care and removal of the patient.

Scene Size-up

Conduct a scene size-up to identify potential hazards and to form a general impression of the situation. During this step, assess the vehicle's position (e.g., upright, on its side, upside down), stability (e.g., what is needed to keep the vehicle from inadvertently moving), and overall condition (e.g., leaking fuel, smoking, fire possible or already present). Mitigate all hazards (e.g., sharp edges, fuel or chemical leaks, undeployed airbags, high-voltage batteries) before beginning extrication efforts. Gather basic patient information during this step (e.g., the total number of patients, priority of extrication, triage status).

To prevent injuries during extrication efforts, all rescuers must use proper personal protective equipment (PPE). Ski patrollers should keep their helmets, goggles, and gloves on at all times. Other OEC technicians should wear, at a minimum, an approved safety helmet, impact-resistant glasses, and heavy leather work gloves.

Vehicle Stabilization

A vehicle that has been involved in a crash must be properly stabilized. Stabilization is especially important if the vehicle is found on its side or, worse, upside down. Even a vehicle that is upright must be stabilized to prevent accidental movement during rescue operations.

Standard vehicle stabilization-related tasks include shutting down the vehicle's engine, de-energizing the electrical system by disconnecting the battery cables, engaging the parking brake, and cribbing the vehicle (i.e., placing 4-inch by 4-inch or 6-inch by 6-inch wood blocks at strategic points to stabilize the vehicle and keep it from moving). If needed, a vehicle may be further stabilized using chains or come-alongs attached to nearby trees, rocks, or rescue vehicles.

Gaining Access to the Patient

Whenever a patient must be extricated from a vehicle, rescuers create an imaginary 10-foot radius around the vehicle known as the "working area" or "inner circle." Access into this area is generally restricted to personnel who are directly involved in the extrication process or who are providing lifesaving interventions to the patient.

As a rule, experts recommend that rescuers "try before you pry"—that is, check all the vehicle's doors before attempting a forcible entry to reach a patient. A door on the opposite side of the vehicle is often undamaged and fully functional. Using this door may save precious minutes or even hours of unnecessary extrication efforts.

Gaining access to a patient can involve moving or cutting away parts of the vehicle so that rescue personnel can make physical contact with the patient. This action also provides an exit through which the patient may be removed from the vehicle. A variety of tools may be used, ranging from simple hand tools such as a spring-loaded punch, a screwdriver, or a crowbar to complex hydraulic tools such as cutters, spreaders, or saws. Additionally, chains, ratchet straps, come-alongs, airbags, and winches may be used, especially if large parts of the vehicle must be moved, lifted, or pulled away. OEC technicians should be familiar with and be able to appropriately use a variety of simple hand tools (**Table 34-1**).

If extrication is required, all windshield, rear window, and side window glass in the immediate area should be carefully removed. In addition, any vehicle restraint devices such as seat belts or harnesses should be cut away. If necessary, the vehicle's door(s) or top may be removed, a third "door" may be cut, or the dashboard may be moved.

Initial Care and Removal of the Patient

The care of a patient follows the general principles described in other chapters and centers on correcting threats to life and protecting the patient's spine. Care may need to be initiated while the patient is still inside the vehicle. Long backboards are commonly used to remove a patient from a vehicle if spinal motion restriction is indicated (**Figure 34-4**).

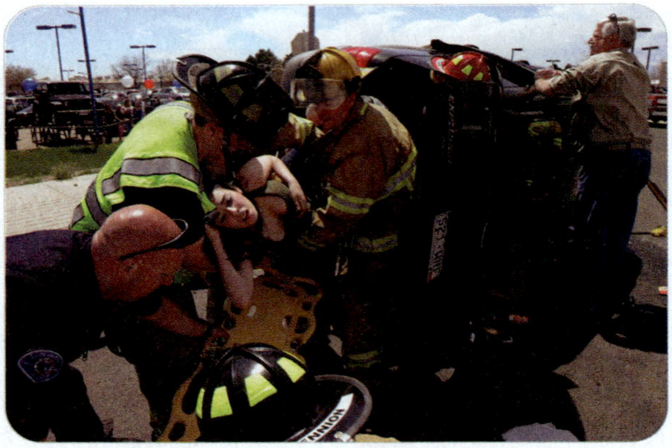

Figure 34-4 A backboard can be used to transfer a patient from a vehicle to an ambulance.

Table 34-1 Simple Hand Tools

Tool	Use(s)
Belt cutter	To cut seat belts, restraining straps, or other cloth materials
Bolt cutter	For cutting thick metal objects such as locks, Nader pins, hinges, or thick wires
Center punch	To break safety glass to gain access through a window
Chock/step chock	To stabilize the wheels of a vehicle; may incorporate multiple "steps" for wheels of different heights
Come-along	To provide a mechanical advantage in pulling apart metal and gaining access to the patient compartment
Cribbing (a set of wood blocks)	To stabilize a vehicle or provide support to an unsteady object
Hacksaw	To cut metal, typically small metal objects or sheet metal
Hammer/sledge hammer	To make sharp edges blunt; to pound parts of the vehicle to gain access to the inside
High-lift jack	To provide a mechanical advantage for lifting heavy or unstable objects
Pry bar/crowbar	To serve as a fulcrum to open doors or to move twisted metal aside
Screwdriver	To remove screws or to pry open narrow spaces
Wedge	To mechanically hold a door open
Wire cutters	For cutting thin metal objects such as retaining clips or wires

CASE Update

You immediately assess the situation and make sure the scene is safe by instructing bystanders to continue to have the race stopped 100 feet up the trail. You make sure the four-wheeler is turned off. There is no gasoline leaking from the vehicle. The injured teen is still yelling, so you calm her down. You control the bleeding on her head. Following your initial assessment, you call on the radio for help, management, and additional EMS transport, and ask a responsible bystander to keep the crowd back. The driver of the vehicle is up walking and comes over apologizing, still holding his shoulder. Another OEC technician arrives, and you instruct him to take care of the driver. The other OEC technician sits the driver down, assesses him, and applies a sling and swathe. Other race officials arrive to help.

What should you do now?

DISASTER RESPONSE

Chapter 4, *Incident Command and Triage*, discussed the management of multiple-casualty incidents (MCIs), including the structure of the National Incident Management System (NIMS), the process of utilizing the Incident Command System (ICS), and methods for triaging patients into treatment priorities. Most MCIs can be managed using local resources or by enlisting the assistance of resources from the surrounding areas. However, when an incident becomes so large that outside resources are needed, the situation is considered a disaster. Although rare, disasters often have serious consequences. The key to effective disaster management is preparedness.

Disasters are typically grouped into two broad categories: natural disasters and human-caused disasters. Examples of natural disasters include floods, tornados, hurricanes wildland fires, and earthquakes. Human-caused disasters can be subdivided into unintentional or intentional disasters. Examples of unintentional disasters include failure of an electrical power grid, an explosion at a power plant requiring mass evacuation of the local population, or a fire in a warehouse. Intentional disasters often are due to an act of **terrorism** and are typically classified by the substance involved using the mnemonic **CBRNE** (pronounced "SEE-burn"), which represents chemical, biological, radiological, nuclear, and explosive.

Whether natural or human-made, a disaster often brings temporary chaos to a local or regional community. Fortunately, an organized system is in place in the United States to respond to disasters, whether local or national in scale. Trained individuals who are not part of this organized system often want to volunteer to help in the response to disasters, but because organized disaster teams have specific tasks and procedures that typically require specialized training, the presence of unofficial disaster responders can impede the overall mission. Therefore, if you wish to participate in disaster response, consider becoming a member of an established disaster response team, such as a local Community Emergency Response Team, a local Disaster Medical Assistance Team, a regional Medical Resource Corps, or the national Urban Search and Rescue (US&R or USAR) group. These groups are part of the country's National Response Framework (NRF).

Developed by the Department of Homeland Security, the NRF provides guidelines for the all-hazards response to any incident within the United States, identifies the key principles to the response, and delineates the responsibilities of all entities that may participate in the response. The NRF is supported by five principles: engaged partnerships, a tiered response, scalable operational capabilities, a unified command, and readiness to act.

The backbone of the NRF consists of the following 15 specialized groups, called Emergency Support Function (ESF) annexes:

ESF #1: Transportation
ESF #2: Communications
ESF #3: Public works and engineering

ESF #4: Firefighting
ESF #5: Information and planning
ESF #6: Mass care, emergency assistance, housing, and human services
ESF #7: Logistics management and resource support
ESF #8: Public health and medical services
ESF #9: Search and rescue
ESF #10: Oil and hazardous materials response
ESF #11: Agriculture and natural resources
ESF #12: Energy
ESF #13: Public safety and security
ESF #14: Long-term community recovery
ESF #15: Cross-sector business and infrastructure

National Disaster Medical System

The Office of the Assistant Secretary for Preparedness and Response (ASPR) within the US Department of Health and Human Services (DHHS) oversees the administration of ESF #8, public health and medical services. The mobilization and operation of ESF #8 is largely carried out by the National Disaster Medical System (NDMS). The primary purpose of NDMS is to supplement local and regional public health and medical resources in dealing with the medical effects of major disasters. NDMS has three primary components:

1. Medical response to a disaster
2. Movement of patients from a disaster site to an unaffected area
3. Definitive medical care at participating hospitals in unaffected areas

Disaster response within NDMS is carried out through the following five types of specialized response teams:

1. Disaster Medical Assistance Teams
2. Disaster Mortuary Operational Response Teams
3. National Veterinary Response Teams
4. National Nurse Response Teams
5. National Pharmacy Response Teams

Of the five response teams within NDMS, Disaster Medical Assistance Teams (DMATs) are responsible for the medical aspects of disaster response. DMATs are trained to deploy to disaster sites and are equipped with supplies to be self-sustainable for 72 hours. Each team consists of physicians, nurses, paramedics, pharmacists, mental health professionals, communication specialists, logistics specialists, and administrative support personnel. To ensure continuous availability for disaster medical response, DMAT members are employed part-time by DHHS and dedicate a portion of their professional time to disaster response.

Although a fully deployed team typically consists of 35 members, the team may also deploy in five-member strike teams. DMATs can set up and run a self-supporting field hospital. They may also supplement local health care resources by providing staff at first-aid stations and/or within hospitals.

Given their expertise in providing emergency care in outdoor settings, OEC technicians are encouraged to join a DMAT. For more information about DMATs, visit the DHHS Public Health Emergency website.

Medical Reserve Corps

In addition to the formalized structure of the NDMS, another asset available for the local, regional, and national disaster response is the volunteer Medical Reserve Corps (MRC). On a national level, MRCs are organized through the Readiness Division, Office of Emergency Management and Medical Operations, of the DHHS.

At the unit level, MRCs are community based and composed of volunteer medical professionals who have agreed to help in the event of a disaster. Although the training and time commitment are not as intense as that for a DMAT, MRC team members are required to complete basic disaster training and maintain a minimum set of credentials. Many MRCs are given specific goals for strengthening the national public-health infrastructure. Because the OEC curriculum is accepted by MRCs, OEC technicians are encouraged to join their local or regional MRC. For more information about MRC or to find a local unit, visit the Medical Reserve Corps webpage.

Community Emergency Response Team

Each local community needs citizens trained in basic disaster response, and these needs extend well beyond medical care. Communities affected by disasters need assistance with evacuation, search and rescue, fire suppression, communications, and other forms of basic assistance (**Figure 34-5**). A Community Emergency Response Team (CERT)

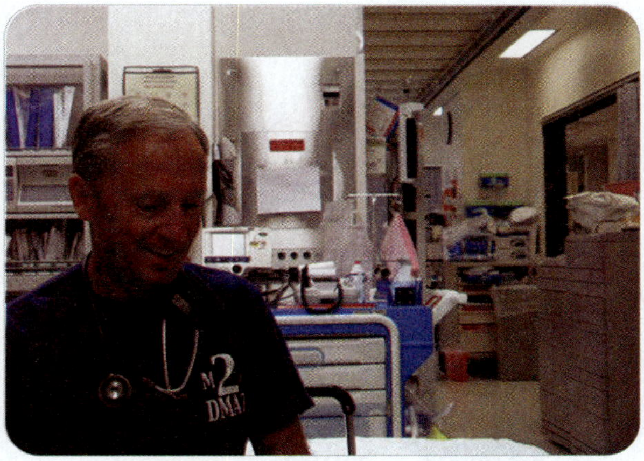

Figure 34-5 OEC technicians can be a valuable resource for your local Community Emergency Response Team, Medical Reserve Corps, and DMAT organizations.

is designed specifically for this purpose. Although organized through the Federal Emergency Management Agency (FEMA), CERTs are composed of local volunteers that support local public-safety officials and provide immediate assistance to victims during a disaster. Members receive basic training in emergency response, search and rescue, and other topics specifically related to disaster management. The federal CERT program and the NSP have been working together for several years to encourage patrollers to join their local CERT teams. For more information about CERT or to find a local unit, visit Ready.gov.

The NSP encourages ski patrollers and OEC technicians to serve on their local MRC or CERT so they can be mobilized to aid in the event of a national, regional, or local disaster. In serving in this capacity, OEC technicians continue the legacy of volunteerism established by NSP founder Charles "Minnie" Dole.

HAZARDOUS MATERIALS RESPONSE

A hazardous material is any substance that, because of its quantity, concentration, or physical or chemical characteristics, is capable of harming people, property, or the environment. Hazardous materials can be solids, gas, or liquids. Control of hazardous materials in the United States is under the authority of the US Department of Transportation (DOT), which uses an international hazard classification system to distinguish the following nine classes of hazardous materials:

- Class 1: Explosives
- Class 2: Gases
- Class 3: Flammable liquids (and combustible liquids in the United States)
- Class 4: Flammable solids, spontaneously combustible materials, and dangerous-when-wet materials/water-reactive substances
- Class 5: Oxidizers and organic peroxides
- Class 6: Toxic substances and infectious substances
- Class 7: Radioactive substances
- Class 8: Corrosive substances
- Class 9: Miscellaneous hazardous materials/products, substances, or organisms

As required by the DOT and the National Fire Protection Association (NFPA), each hazardous material that is in transit must be identified by a specific placard, known as the NFPA safety diamond (**Figure 34-6**). This diamond-shaped placard contains four smaller, color-coded diamond-shaped fields, each of which identifies the known hazards for a given material—flammability (red), health hazard (blue), chemical reactivity (yellow), and special precautions (white).

Hazmat incidents are managed using the ICS. Within the ICS structure, a hazmat safety officer reports directly to an incident commander and ensures the safety of personnel responding to the incident. The hazmat ICS operations branch includes a hazmat entry team, with backup decontamination personnel, and medical sector personnel (**Figure 34-7**). Fortunately, most hazmat incidents in the United States are unintentional. However, there is always the potential for an intentional hazmat incident, which is considered an act of terrorism. Management of a hazmat terrorist event also utilizes the ICS structure, with the addition that all terrorist events are considered criminal acts and fall under the jurisdiction of the federal government.

The response to and decontamination of a hazmat site are conducted in accordance with Occupational Safety and Health Administration standards. These standards are referred to as **HAZWOPER**, which stands for **HAZ**ardous **W**aste **OP**erations and **E**mergency **R**esponse.

The federal government mandates HAZWOPER training for any worker (paid or volunteer)

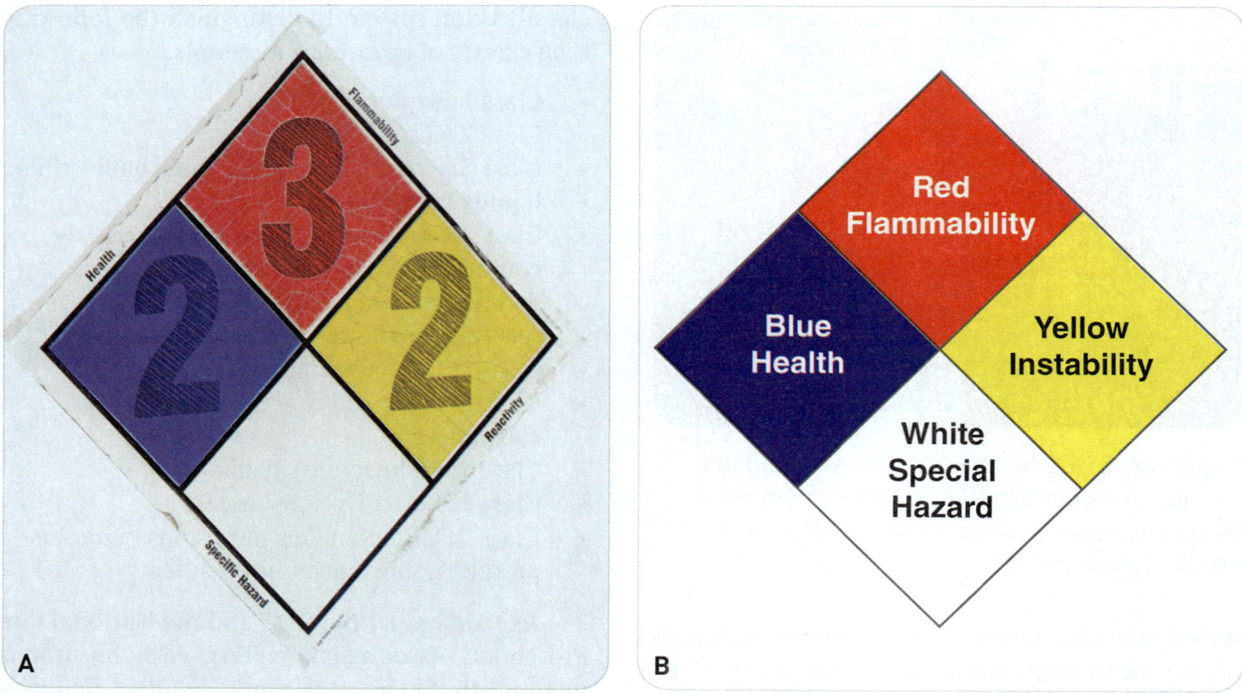

Figure 34-6 **A.** A diamond-shaped NFPA hazard identification system placard. **B.** Each color used in the diamond represents a particular property or characteristic.

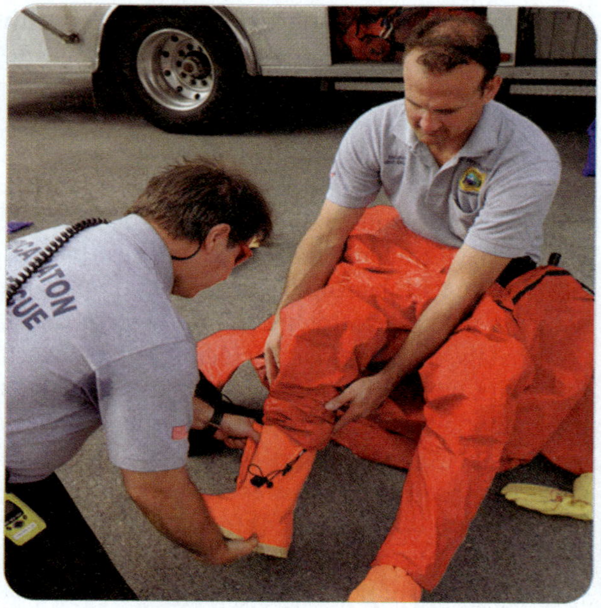

Figure 34-7 Placing hazmat protective equipment on a member of a response entry team.

who works in an environment in which uncontrolled hazardous materials may be encountered. Training and certification needs depend on the type(s) of substances to which an employee may be exposed and the worker's expected duties when responding to a hazmat-related incident. Typical training covers the types of hazardous materials present and their associated risks, recognition of hazardous materials, and procedures relating to hazmat response, PPE, and containment and decontamination. Training requirements generally include classroom and practical training, formal certification, and annual refresher training.

The most important step in the initial management of a hazmat incident is to prevent members of the public from contacting the hazardous material by establishing an isolation perimeter to prevent their entry. The boundary may be established by placing traffic cones at street intersections or by stringing barrier tape around buildings. Emergency responders may need to enforce the boundary with their physical presence.

Once the isolation perimeter is set, the next step is to establish three hazard-control zones, which establish the working areas of the incident. The zone surrounding the incident, which is the most dangerous and the most contaminated, is known as the **hot zone** (**Figure 34-8**). As for the hot zone, only personnel with training in decontamination techniques are permitted to enter

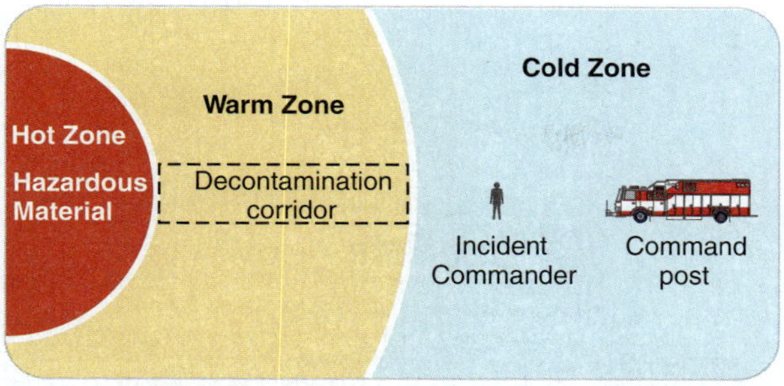

Figure 34-8 The safety control zones at the site of a hazmat emergency.

this zone. It is designated for personnel with specialized training and equipment. The **warm zone** surrounds the hot zone and is a transition zone in which decontamination occurs. The outer **cold zone** is that part of the incident area that contains support personnel and equipment; it is considered safe to operate in this zone without specialized protective equipment. Located within the cold zone are the command post and the triage, treatment, and transport areas to which OEC technicians are typically assigned to assist in the medical care of ill or injured patients. Once a patient has been removed from the hot zone and has been decontaminated in the warm zone, medical treatment can begin in the cold zone.

KEY POINT

HAZWOPER

Several levels of HAZWOPER training and certification are available, and they include the Awareness, Operations, Technician, and Commander levels. Awareness-level personnel receive an overview of hazmat response and typically perform tasks in the outer "safe" zone. Operations-level personnel receive more specialized training and typically operate within the warm zone. Technician-level personnel are trained to function in any of the hazard zones, whereas Commander-level personnel supervise the overall management of response and cleanup efforts.

At times, a member of the incident response team will require treatment due to exposure to a hazardous material. One potential hazard is organophosphate poisoning. As discussed in Chapter 12, *Substance Abuse and Poisoning*, organophosphates cause excessive pulmonary secretions that can lead to respiratory failure. Signs and symptoms of organophosphate poisoning can be remembered using the acronym DUMBELS or SLUDGEM. These mnemonics are covered in more detail in Chapter 12, *Substance Abuse and Poisoning*. The treatment for organophosphate poisoning is the administration of IV atropine, often in large doses, and pralidoxime and diazepam by ALS providers. The treatment for organophosphate exposure in mass-casualty settings, in which IV access is often impractical, is self-administration of a nerve agent antidote kit. Two common kits are the Mark I kit and the DuoDote kit.

If you have been exposed to an organophosphate or a chemical nerve agent, OEC technicians may need to self-administer a nerve agent antidote. Administration of the antidote kit can be lifesaving. Each kit contains two medications: atropine and pralidoxime chloride (2-PAM Cl). The Mark I kit administers the medications in two auto-injectors, whereas the DuoDote kit administers the medications in a single auto-injector. The kits also include step-by-step directions (**Figure 34-9**).

Mechanism of Action of Nerve Agents

The nervous system controls bodily functions by secreting various chemical transmitters, which act as "instructions" to nerves, muscles, and glands. These neurologic instructions are of two types: those that stimulate activity by muscles and glands and those that signal inactivity in those structures. The presence of a nerve agent interferes with the normal instructions of chemical transmitters in a way that overstimulates the nerve endings, so muscles and certain glands overreact. The results are excessive salivation, tearing, airway secretions, respiratory distress, and depressed mental status. The initial treatment for a nerve agent exposure consists of a two-part antidote: atropine (to dry up secretions) and 2-PAM Cl (to reverse the action of the nerve agent).

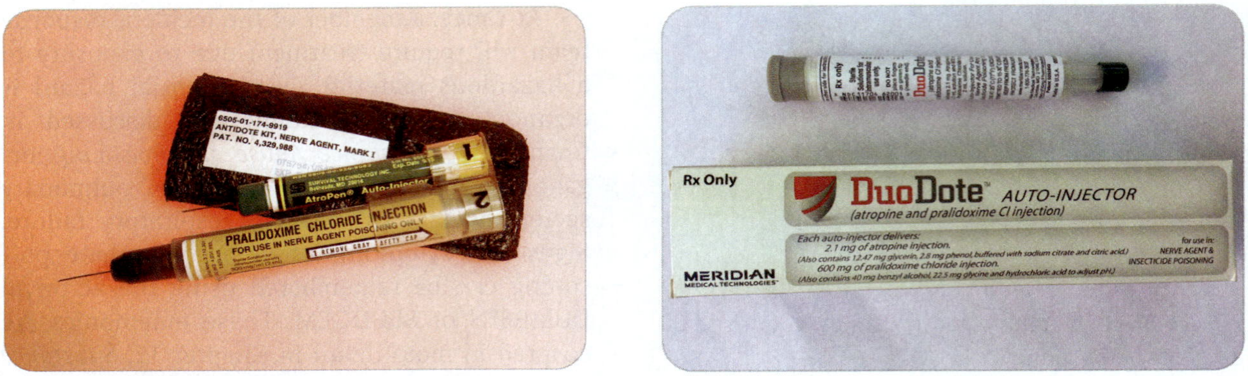

A B

Figure 34-9 The Mark I kit administers the medications in two auto-injectors (**A**), whereas the DuoDote kit administers the medications in a single auto-injector (**B**).

Recommended Dosing Schedules for Exposure to a Nerve Agent

If you have been exposed to a nerve agent and have mild symptoms, self-administer one kit containing both drugs. If excessive salivation and mental status changes become present, self-administer two atropine auto-injectors and one 2-PAM Cl injector. In assisting with a patient who has been exposed, start by ensuring that you have on the correct PPE, then remove secretions (using suction if necessary) and maintain the patient's airway. The need for PPE is necessary even if the patient has been removed to a safe zone to protect you from off-gassing (release of airborne particulates or chemicals) from the nerve agent. If severe signs and symptoms are present, the EMS providers will administer three atropine auto-injectors and three 2-PAM Cl injectors in rapid succession. Note the following information concerning the administration of nerve agent antidote medications:

1. The medications are administered in a similar manner as used for an EpiPen. Follow the directions on the nerve agent antidote kit.
2. When assisting with another patient support ventilations with a bag-valve mask, if needed.
3. Repeat dosages will be administered by EMS as needed.
4. If signs and symptoms resolve, then only continued monitoring is necessary.
5. Premeasured doses of auto-injectors should be safe in most adults. Note, however, that auto-injectors were designed for a "standard military profile"—that is, for an individual who is healthy, is approximately 18 to 35 years old, weighs about 70 kg (154 pounds), and has no preexisting medical conditions.
6. Pralidoxime chloride (2-PAM Cl) is most effective, especially for severe exposures, if administered immediately after poisoning and *following* (not before) the administration of atropine.
7. When the nerve agent has been ingested, exposure may continue for some time due to slow absorption from the lower bowel, and fatal relapses have been reported after initial improvement. In such cases, continued medical monitoring and transport are mandatory.
8. If dermal exposure has occurred, decontamination is critical and should be done using standard decontamination procedures. Monitoring should be directed to the observation of the same signs and symptoms seen with all exposures to nerve agents.

TERRORISM

Individuals today with extreme religious beliefs, severe mental illness, a grudge, or other antisocial behavior can inflict tragedy in public locations. "Lone wolf" terrorists with weapons or bombs can make a concert, church, shopping center, or school a place of mass destruction, with multiple casualties. Our society today facilitates many of these beliefs in people who may or may not have preexisting mental illness with television shows and video games that promote violence and websites promoting antisocial behavior. Most of these individuals are not associated with terrorist groups directly, but have antisocial personalities and decide to "become infamous" by killing people. Following their act, the media make them well known in their own mind.

If you are responding to a terrorist attack involving an act of violence, first make the scene safe for as many people as possible and yourself. Notifying law enforcement is an early necessity. Your first inclination is to rush in and help the injured. However, do not approach an active violence scene until law enforcement says it is safe. Becoming a victim yourself is never good. As of 2019, the Federal Bureau of Investigation and US Department of Homeland Security advocate the Run, Hide, Fight program during active shooter situations (**Figure 34-10**). The following description of this program is modified from the Ready.gov website:

1. *Run.* Evacuate if possible.
   - If there is considerable distance between you and the gunfire/armed person, quickly move away from the sound of the gunfire/armed person. If the gunfire/armed person is in your building and it is safe to do so, run out of the building and move far away until you are in a secure place to hide.
   - Leave your belongings behind.
   - Keep your hands visible to law enforcement.
   - Take others with you, and do not stay behind, if others will not go.
   - Call 9-1-1 when it is safe to do so. Do not assume that someone else has reported the incident. The information that you can provide law enforcement may be critical (e.g., number of shooters, physical description and identification, number and type of weapons, location of the shooter).
2. *Hide.* Hide silently in the safest place possible.
   - If the shooter is close and you cannot evacuate safely, hide in an area out of the armed person's view.
   - Choose a hiding place with thicker walls and fewer windows, if possible.
   - Lock doors and barricade with furniture, if possible.
   - Turn off lights.
   - Silence phones and turn off other electronics.
   - Close windows, shades, and blinds, and avoid being seen from outside the room, if possible.
   - If you are outdoors and cannot *run* safely, find a place to hide that will provide protection from gunfire, such as a brick wall, large trees, or buildings.
   - Remain in place until you receive an "all clear" signal from the police.
3. *Fight.* Take action to disrupt or incapacitate the shooter.
   - As a last resort, fight. If you cannot evacuate or hide safely and only when your life is in imminent danger, take action.
   - Attempt to incapacitate or disrupt the actions of the shooter.
   - Act with physical aggression toward the shooter.
   - Use items in your area such as fire extinguishers or chairs.
   - Throw items at the shooter if possible.
   - Call 9-1-1 when it is safe to do so.
4. Immediately after an incident:
   - Wait for local law enforcement officers to assist you out of the building, if inside.
   - When law enforcement arrives, you must display empty hands with open palms.
5. Additional information:
   - Understand that gunfire may sound artificial. Assume that any popping sound is gunfire.
   - If there are two or more persons in the same place when a violent incident begins, you should spread out in the room to avoid offering the aggressor an easy target.
   - Be mindful that violent attacks can involve any type of weapon, not just a

HOW TO RESPOND
WHEN AN ACTIVE SHOOTER IS IN YOUR VICINITY

Quickly determine the most reasonable way to protect your own life. Customers and clients are likely to follow the lead of employees and managers during an active shooter situation.

1.Run
- Have an escape route and plan in mind
- Leave your belongings behind
- Keep your hands visible

2. Hide
- Hide in an area out of the active shooter's view.
- Block entry to your hiding place and lock the doors

3.Fight
- As a last resort and only when your life is in imminent danger.
- Attempt to incapacitate the active shooter
- Act with physical aggression andthrow items at the active shooter

CALL 911 WHEN IT IS SAFE TO DO SO

HOW TO RESPOND WHEN LAW ENFORCEMENT ARRIVES ON THE SCENE

1. How you should react when law enforcement arrives:
   - Remain calm, and follow officers' instructions
   - Immediately raise hands and spread fingers
   - Keep hands visible at all times
   - Avoid making quick movements toward officers such as attempting to hold on to them for safety
   - Avoid pointing, screaming and/or yelling
   - Do not stop to ask officers for help or direction when evacuating, just proceed in the direction from which officers are entering the premises
2. Information you should provide to law enforcement or 911 operator:
   - Location of the victims and the active shooter
   - Number of shooters, if more than one
   - Physical description of shooter/s
   - Number and type of weapons held by the shooter/s
   - Number of potential victims at the location

RECOGNIZING SIGNS OF POTENTIAL WORKPLACE VIOLENCE

An active shooter may be a current or former employee. Alert your Human Resources Department if you believe an employee exhibits potentially violent behavior. Indicators of potentially violent behavior may include one or more of the following:
- Increased use of alcohol and/or illegal drugs
- Unexplained increase in absenteeism, and/or vague physical complaints
- Depression/Withdrawal
- Increased severe mood swings, and noticeably unstable or emotional responses
- Increasingly talks of problems at home
- Increase in unsolicited comments about violence, firearms, and other dangerous weapons and violent crimes

U.S. Department of Homeland Security · National Tactical Officers Association · Police Fairfax County Virginia · National Retail Federation® The Voice of Retail Worldwide · RILA Retail Industry Leaders Association Retail's Future...Educate, Innovate, Advocate

Contact your building management or human resources department for more information and training on active shooter response in your workplace.

Figure 34-10 Run from shooter if possible; hide in a secure location, locking doors, pulling shades down and turning off lights; and block doors with furniture or files if possible. Fight as a last resort; look around for items you could use as a weapon such as a letter opener, scissors, or spray items like keyboard cleaner and hair spray.

Reproduced from How to Respond When an Active Shooter Is in Your Vicinity. Department of Homeland Security. Retrieved from https://www.cisa.gov/sites/default/files/publications/active-shooter-poster-2017-508.pdf.

> **KEY POINT**
>
> **Active Shooter**
>
> Stay out of an area with an active terrorist until law enforcement says the scene is safe.

gun. Knives, blunt objects, physical force, or explosives can be just as deadly as a gun. The suggested actions provided here are applicable in any violent encounter.
- Plan ahead: Visualize possible escape routes, including physically accessible routes for staff with disabilities and others with limited mobility.

Once the scene is safe, and the perpetrator(s) are in custody, treat the scene as a triage exercise.

There has not been a terrorist attack at a ski area as of 2020. However, management, security, the medical advisor, and the patrol may want to consider putting a plan of action in place in case one does occur, much like many school systems have done.

SEARCH AND RESCUE

A search-and-rescue (SAR) operation has two interrelated components: a **search**, the methodical process of actively gathering information about and then physically looking for one or more individuals in distress or imminent danger, and a **rescue**, the process of extracting such individuals from distress or danger. Efforts can quickly shift from one component to the other. For instance, upon locating a missing individual, the search portion of the mission is terminated, but if the individual is trapped and/or injured, the focus of the mission shifts to rescue operations.

Among the many SAR disciplines are combat, mountain, urban, ground, air, and sea operations. Even though the term *search and rescue* is used generically, each SAR discipline has distinctly different missions, roles, training and staffing requirements, equipment needs, and operational procedures.

SAR work is dangerous. Among the countless challenges a SAR team faces are difficult terrain, inclement weather, extremes of temperature, time of day, size of the area to be searched, and the total number of people missing. Additionally, natural or human-caused hazards can further complicate a SAR team's mission. These variables, and others, must be considered whenever a SAR team organizes its plan of action because they can turn a relatively simple search into a technical evacuation that requires additional personnel, advanced training, and specialized equipment.

Ski patrollers and other OEC technicians at many ski resorts routinely engage in the most basic type of search—that is, looking for a person who has become separated from family or friends. Many ski areas have developed a protocol manual that specifically identifies the steps to be taken when searching for a lost person. Because of their backcountry expertise, OEC technicians are often asked to join a SAR team or to assist a team during a mission.

Because many ski and recreational areas around the country are typically close to or adjacent to state or federal lands, SAR efforts often require assistance from multiple local emergency management and response agencies. Under these circumstances, the need for cross-jurisdictional coordination and common procedures and systems becomes critical. Accordingly, SAR teams within the United States operate under the federal NIMS structure and use the ICS to manage SAR-related incidents.

Although complex, SAR operations can be broken down to five basic tasks:

1. *Mobilization.* Once the team is informed of a mission, it assembles and responds to the site of the incident. Each team member has a specific role; team leaders are typically cross-trained in multiple roles.
2. *Intelligence gathering.* Team members gather information about the lost person(s), typically by asking the following questions:
    - Where was the person last seen? (This helps to narrow the search area.)
    - What was the person's intended destination? (This helps to establish a search grid and identify possible travel routes the person may use.)

- How physically fit is the person? (A person who is fit can travel farther and faster than one who is not.)
- What is the person's mental status? (Does the person have a known mental illness? Is the person in a rational state of mind? Is the person depressed or suicidal?)
- What equipment does the person have? (A person who is well equipped can survive longer than one who has minimal supplies.)
- What type of terrain exists within the search area? (A person can travel faster and farther on flat ground than in mountainous terrain.)

3. *Containment.* Using the information gathered, the team establishes a containment area, an area with defined boundaries within which the party was last seen and might still be located. For ski patrollers, containment may include patrolling the boundaries of the ski area to look for tracks or signs that the missing person left the containment area.
4. *Search.* Once the search area has been defined, it is divided into a search grid consisting of smaller areas. Based on available information, search teams are deployed to search the grid(s) in which the person is most likely located.
5. *Rescue.* A person who has been found may require medical care, evacuation, or other assistance. In the event of a fatal outcome, the body must be recovered and removed.

SAR skills are something that every patroller and OEC technician should acquire through additional training. It is not a matter of *if* patrollers or OEC technicians will be asked to participate in an SAR operation, but *when* they will be asked to participate (**Figure 34-11**). SAR training can be acquired through NSP Mountain Travel and Rescue and Avalanche courses or through local SAR teams, which are usually operated by a local law enforcement agency.

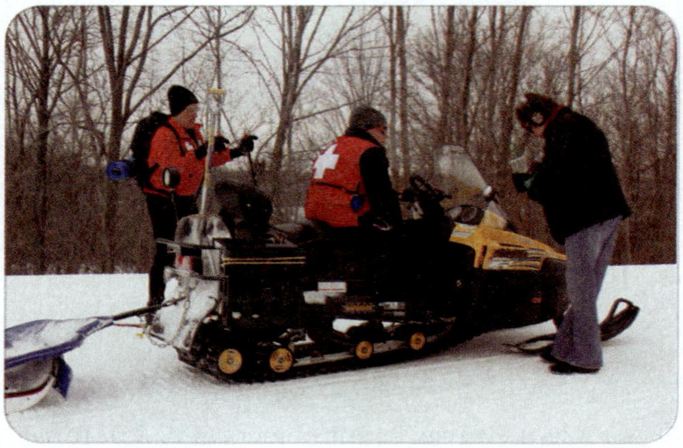

Figure 34-11 Patrollers working together on a search-and-rescue operation.

Avalanche Rescue

Burial in an avalanche is a true medical emergency, and small avalanches can be just as deadly as large ones. Although most avalanches occur primarily during winter, they have claimed lives during every month of the year and in every kind of weather. What's more, they are not confined to remote, high alpine terrain and can occur on any steep, snow-covered slope, even rooftops. Because the chances of surviving complete burial decrease rapidly with time, dropping to 50% within the first 30 minutes, rescue operations must be initiated as soon as possible, preferably by a companion who was not caught in the avalanche. However, companion rescue efforts alone are not often successful without the additional resources provided by organized rescue operations. There is minimal likelihood of survival when avalanche victims are buried for more than 35 minutes with an obstructed airway and in cardiac arrest upon extrication.

Avalanche rescue operations within the United States are conducted using the ICS. Operational effectiveness is greatly enhanced by using technology, including wireless communications, which enable rescuers to quickly learn of incidents, and helicopters, which enable rescuers to reach the scene within minutes. Avalanche transceivers and the Recco system (a highly effective avalanche rescue system) have also improved rescue efforts by dramatically reducing search time. The use of rescue dog teams has also shortened search times. Specially trained and equipped rescuers, including OEC technicians, can provide lifesaving emergency medical care in the field.

> **KEY POINT**
>
> **Recco**
>
> Recco is a highly effective avalanche rescue system that enables rescuers to quickly locate an avalanche victim using harmonic radar. The system consists of two parts: a small reflector that is usually sewn into a person's clothing, and a handheld detector that enables rescuers to locate a buried avalanche victim.

An organized avalanche rescue consists of four basic functions:

- *The immediate search.* Get rescuers to the site as quickly as possible to find and uncover the victim(s).
- *Medical care.* Provide emergency care for the victims.
- *Transport/evacuation.* Get the victims out of the field and to advanced medical care, if needed.
- *Support (logistics).* Care for the rescuers in the field (provide food, shelter, rest, and replacements).

These functions are not sequential and may be performed simultaneously, depending on need and the availability of resources.

Although many variables affect avalanche incidents and the resulting response, most rescue operations follow a similar sequence of events.

1. *The incident is reported.*
   - If physically present, a team member interviews the reporting party and, if the reporting person is a witness, arranges for transport back to the site.
   - If the report was patched through from a 9-1-1 call, a team member gets as much detail as possible on the location and number of buried victims as well as a callback number.
2. *The team is alerted and responds.*
   - Rescue headquarters is notified.
   - A predesignated incident commander takes charge and initiates the rescue operation according to preestablished plans.
   - The immediate search team is assembled (including witnesses), equipped (including a dog team, avalanche receivers, and a Recco detector, if available), and dispatched.
   - A permanent site leader is appointed and dispatched.
   - A medical team is assembled, equipped, and dispatched.
   - Logistics support for dispatched teams and incoming resources is organized.
   - Additional teams are assembled and dispatched to perform a variety of functions as needed.
3. *The victim(s) are located/extricated.*
   - The immediate search team leader determines and marks a safe route to the incident site, assesses scene safety, initiates the search, and incorporates resources (personnel and equipment) into the search effort as they arrive. As the operation grows, this team member may be replaced by a permanent site leader.
   - When located, the victim is dug out as quickly and safely as possible. (Spine injuries are presumed until proven otherwise.) Snow is quickly removed from around the victim's face and an airway is established, followed by excavating around the chest to enable chest wall expansion. The rest of the victim's body is then dug completely free to allow extrication and other emergency care.
4. *Medical care is provided.*
   - Basic life support (and ALS if needed and available) is provided.
   - The patient is moved to a safer location, if necessary.
   - The patient's other injuries are treated.
   - The patient is assessed and treated for hypothermia.
   - The patient is protected from further injury or cooling.
   - The patient's condition is continually monitored.

5. *The victim(s) is/are evacuated.*
   - The patient is prepared for transport (in a litter or sled).
   - The patient is transported to an appropriate medical facility for more definitive care.
6. *The operation is given logistical support.*
   - Additional searchers are made available.
   - Additional equipment is made available.
   - Care for rescuers (e.g., food, water, shelter, sanitation) is arranged.
   - Transport of rescuers and equipment back to base is arranged.

As with any incident, rescuer safety is the top priority. The fact that an avalanche has occurred should strongly suggest a high probability for similar conditions along the route and on the slopes adjacent to the incident site. Upon arrival, the immediate search team leader, who is highly educated and experienced in managing avalanche-related incidents, assesses overall site safety. If there is a significant residual avalanche hazard at the site, the hazard must be mitigated before the team proceeds.

During prolonged operations, team leaders must ensure that rescuers are properly cared for and supported. Because rescuers who are dehydrated, cold, or exhausted could divert precious resources from the rescue effort by becoming additional casualties, all members of the avalanche rescue team must be physically fit, thoroughly educated and trained, and properly equipped for the operation

Buried avalanche victims often have life-threatening conditions associated with asphyxia, trauma, and hypothermia. Cardiac problems can occur also, either immediately or subsequently because of asphyxia, shock, or hypothermia. OEC technicians should assess and manage these injuries in the usual fashion, as described in previous chapters.

Whenever possible, a helicopter equipped with ALS providers and equipment should be dispatched and landed close to the incident site. If multiple patients are buried or injured, standard triage methods are employed in which patients with vital signs take priority over those without vital signs.

Rope Rescue

A rope rescue is any technical rescue operation involving static ropes, anchors, belaying devices, and other equipment that provides a mechanical advantage. The ski patrol recognizes two types of rope rescue: high-angle rescue and low-angle rescue. A **high-angle rescue (HAR)** is any rescue work performed by ascending or descending a slope of approximately 45 degrees or steeper. A **low-angle rescue (LAR)** is any rescue work performed by ascending or descending a slope that is less than approximately 45 degrees.

Given that patrollers and rescuers often find themselves in terrain that is not conducive to an easy rescue or evacuation, knowing how to safely remove a patient from sloped terrain is a skill that all OEC technicians should possess.

Of the many sources of information regarding LAR, some are geared toward crevasse rescue for mountaineering and climbing, whereas others focus on emergency rescue for SAR teams or fire departments. The information in these LAR guidelines covers the basics: raising and lowering systems; setting up anchors, pulleys, and Prusiks; and safety concerns.

One of the first decisions that rescuers must make in a LAR is whether to lower or raise the patient out of the incident zone, the area in which the patient is located. As with all rescue operations, the safety of the rescuers and the patient is the primary concern in LAR operations, but the simplicity of the rescue system should also be considered. Generally, if it is a viable option, it is easier to lower a patient to a safe zone while letting gravity do some of the work. If the incident zone does not allow for the patient to be easily lowered to a safe zone, additional rescuers and equipment may be required to pull the patient up to a safe zone. For more information about LAR, contact the National Ski Patrol or your local SAR team.

Rope rescues, which fall under the Operations section, should be performed using the ICS. Ideally, you should have two teams: a technical rope team that is responsible for providing safe access to the patient and for extricating the patient and rescuers, and a second team that is responsible for providing medical care to the patient. The technical rope team and the medical team should each have a team commander.

Depending on the situation, it may be necessary to initiate medical treatment for a patient before a completed rope system is in place. Providing rapid medical treatment requires that members of the medical team can safely access the patient.

Safe access may be accomplished by rappelling down to the patient using a separate rope, and then tying off to a tree or some other natural anchor near the patient.

Confined Space and SAR Rescue Dogs

A confined space rescue is a type of rescue involving an enclosed area that has limited or restricted means of entry or exit. The confined space may be natural or human-made. Rock caves, ice caverns, and fissures, for instance, are natural confined spaces, whereas underground pipes, tunnels, mine shafts, wells, storage tanks, and trenches are human-made confined spaces. A confined space may also be created in the rubble following a building collapse.

Many confined space rescues may be facilitated not only by equipment, but also by a specially trained search dog. The exceptional sense of smell and trainability of dogs makes them ideally suited for finding objects or people. Search dogs can be trained to "alert" when they detect the odor of almost anything, including humans, even when that odor is part of a complex mixture of odors. Avalanche dogs are probably the most common search dogs that ski patrollers may encounter.

A well-trained avalanche dog can be a great asset in a search operation, especially if buried victims lack avalanche transceivers (**Figure 34-12**). Under favorable conditions, dogs can easily search an area much faster than is possible using a probe line, and in cases involving large search areas, dogs work faster than transceiver searches. Many patrols at ski resorts in avalanche country have dogs on duty so that they can respond quickly to incidents within and near the resort's boundaries. Many alpine SAR groups also have dog teams with handlers on call so that they can be deployed into the field quickly. If an area or a rescue agency does not have a dog team on staff, its alerting and rescue plan should identify available local dog resources and the procedures for mobilizing them.

Several avalanche dog training organizations and certification standards are in place within the United States. Because these organizations have slightly different training methods, the ways search dogs behave in the field can vary. An initiative to establish international standards for the training and certification of avalanche rescue dogs is currently underway.

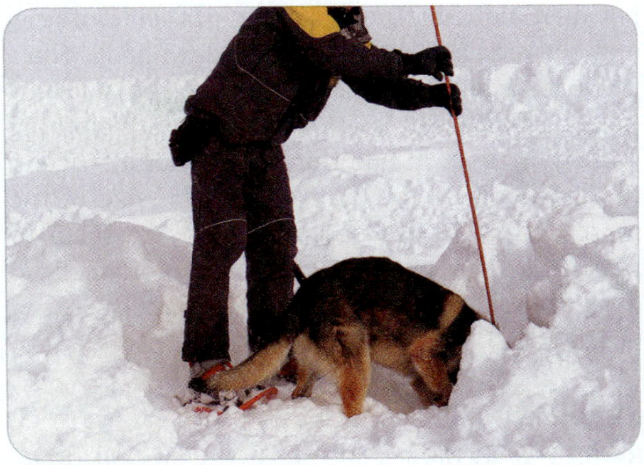

Figure 34-12 Avalance dogs are invaluable members of the search-and-rescue team at ski areas.

Scent Factors

Dogs follow a cone-shaped scent trail in the air to the victim or to some other source of the scent. To be detected, the scent of a person buried in an avalanche must first reach the surface of the snow. The time it takes for a scent to reach the surface depends on both the depth of burial and the scent's rate of diffusion through the snow, which in turn depends on the temperature and density of the snow. In general, colder snow temperatures speed the diffusion rate, whereas greater snow density slows the diffusion rate. These rates can vary from less than 1 min/meter in dry powder snow to 15 min/meter in wet packed snow.

A scent does not always travel in a straight line up through the snow—it follows the path of least resistance. Scent may move horizontally between blocks of snow or rocks or be channeled by running water or trees to emerge a significant distance from the actual burial location. A dog will "alert" wherever this scent emerges from the snow, which is not necessarily directly over the victim. Steady winds of low to moderate velocity provide ideal conditions for dogs; strong, gusty winds make searching more difficult. Dogs are best positioned downwind of the search area before the search begins.

Dog Capabilities

A dog's sense of smell is so sensitive it can not only discriminate among individuals, but also between individuals and articles of their clothing, and between a live victim and a dead body. Thus, in alpine avalanche rescue situations, it is advantageous for dogs to "alert" on the victim's clothing and equipment, in addition to the victim's scent, to provide clues that can reduce the size of the search area. Air temperature does not seem to affect the sensitivity of a dog's sense of smell, so dogs are a huge asset in alpine avalanche rescue operations.

Simplifying the Search

Because dogs detect all the scents around them, they must in effect ignore every scent but that of the buried victim to earn a reward for their search. Their task can be made easier by reducing as many competing scents as possible, and thus rescuers should keep bystanders and nonessential personnel out of the search zone. It is more difficult for a rescue dog to detect the scent of a buried victim in an avalanche runout zone if the area contains distracting scents. For this reason, rescuers should stage equipment and food away from the area (preferably downwind), should avoid leaving any kind of litter or body wastes (including saliva or urine) in the search area, and should even avoid sitting on the snow.

Search Dog Etiquette

Even though dog teams are trained to work around other rescuers and equipment, the only person giving commands to a dog should be the dog's handler, who often uses hand signals to communicate with the dog. During an avalanche rescue, obey the rule "silence is golden" to avoid distracting the dog. If the dog comes over to investigate you, it is only doing so to rule out your scent; ignore it and stay focused on your job. Never approach, touch, or feed a rescue dog without its handler's permission.

Dog Alerts

A dog "alerts" when it locates the source of a human scent coming off the surface of the snow. It communicates this alert to the handler in different ways—sometimes by barking, sometimes by digging, sometimes by both. It is up to the handler to decide whether the dog's behavior constitutes an alert. When a dog alerts, immediately spot probe the area. Because the scent may leave the surface some distance from the actual burial site, shoveling before attaining a probe strike may waste precious time and should be avoided unless the probe pole is shorter than the depth of the debris.

It usually does not hurt for a dog to dig aggressively where it alerts, but the dog's handler should call the dog off as soon as a probe strike is made so that rescuers can dig out the victim using appropriate shoveling techniques. This course of action protects the dog and allows rescuers to safely excavate, extricate the patient, and provide emergency medical care.

Incidents Involving Structures

In situations involving multiple casualties of people trapped in buildings such as resort structures, urban search dogs certified by FEMA may be superior to dogs trained specifically for alpine avalanche SAR. FEMA-trained dogs are familiarized with scents found in buildings and are trained to alert to live humans only, rather than to dead bodies, clothing, or other items. These dogs are trained to explore cavities, and they work without wearing harnesses, which makes them less likely to be caught on wreckage debris in tight spaces.

Water Rescue

Water rescue is another type of specialized rescue operation and includes swift-water rescue, flood rescue, ice rescue, and dive rescue. The basic principles of water rescue are covered in Chapter 29, *Water-Related Emergencies*.

FIRE GROUND OPERATIONS

Fire ground operations (e.g., fire operations at a structure fire, brush fire, or hazmat incident) are usually conducted in accordance with NFPA standards because most fire departments adopt NFPA standards as part of their standard operating procedures. On occasion, OEC technicians may be requested to provide medical support at the scene of a fire, most often to triage, treat, and transport patients, including injured firefighters. OEC technicians also may be asked to assist with firefighter rehabilitation, a process that involves monitoring the medical condition of firefighters following a work period and identifying those who are medically fit to return to duty. According to NFPA standards, firefighter rehabilitation should occur at any fire or prolonged rescue scene in which on-scene activities potentially exceed a safe level of physical or mental endurance.

Fire ground operations focus on the following key tasks, which are listed from highest priority to lowest priority:

1. *Size-up.* Identifying building size and type of construction and whether flames are visible
2. *Accountability.* Identifying the locations of people within the scene
3. *Rescue/life safety.* Helping people
4. *Confinement.* Keeping the fire contained and from damaging other structures
5. *Control.* Extinguishing the fire
6. *Ventilation.* Making an opening in the structure to allow flames, smoke, and toxic vapors to exhaust
7. *Property conservation.*

If called to a fire scene, you will likely be requested to report to one of possibly several staging areas until needed. The staging area may be located near the incident or several miles away. In the United States, fire ground operations are managed using the NIMS, which is described in Chapter 4, *Incident Command and Triage*.

You can do several things to assist fire personnel if you arrive at the scene of a fire before they do. First, report the fire, including its exact location and the type of structure involved, using the following standard terminology:

- Residence (including general size, such as large or small)
- Apartments (includes multi-unit dwellings)
- Commercial (such as warehouses, stores, or office building)
- High rise (four floors or taller)

In addition, provide basic information about the current fire conditions using the following common terms:

- Fire showing (flames are visible)
- Smoke showing (smoke is visible)
- Nothing showing (neither flames nor smoke is visible)

While you await the arrival of firefighters, attempt to gather information from witnesses or people evacuating the building. Among the questions to ask are the following:

KEY POINT

Fire Ground Anatomy

As you stand directly in front of a building, each of its sides is given a designation:

- Side A is the front of the building.
- Side B is the left side of the building.
- Side C is the back of the building
- Side D is the right side of the building.

- Is everyone out of the building? How do you know?
- How many people are still inside the building? How do you know?
- Where in the building are the people located? How do you know?
- Exactly where in the building is the fire located? How do you know?

Provide this information to the first fire officer to arrive on scene because it can save precious time and might save lives.

Firefighting is strenuous, even life-threatening work. According to the NFPA, tens of thousands of firefighters are injured each year, and approximately 100 firefighters are killed in the line of duty. From 2010 through 2014, an average of 30,290 injuries occurred each year. In 2018, a reported 60 firefighters were killed in the line of duty.

When firefighters are injured, they will be evacuated as quickly as possible, and as an OEC technician, you may be asked to help care for them. Firefighters wear PPE, including a self-contained breathing apparatus (SCBA). To effectively treat an injured firefighter, you will likely need to remove this equipment. To remove the PPE and SCBA of a firefighter who has suspected spinal injuries, perform the following procedure:

1. Rescuer 1: Manually stabilize the patient's head and neck in neutral anatomic alignment.
2. Rescuers 2 and 3: Logroll the patient onto his or her side.
3. Rescuer 4:
   a. Remove the regulator mounted on the face piece.
   b. Unstrap and remove the patient's helmet.

c. Slide the flame-resistant hood back.
d. Loosen the straps on the face shield.
e. Remove the firefighter's face shield.
f. Open the throat strap of the patient's turn-out coat.
g. Loosen the shoulder and waist straps on the SCBA, and remove the SCBA.
h. Remove the patient's uppermost arm from the sleeve of the turn-out coat.
i. Roll the remaining portion of the jacket toward the ground.

4. Rescuers 1, 2, and 3: Logroll the patient into a supine position on a long backboard.
5. Rescuer 4:
   a. Gently remove the patient's other arm from the turn-out coat.
   b. Remove or cut the patient's suspenders.
6. Rescuers 2 and 3:
   a. Remove the patient's boots.
   b. Unfasten and remove the patient's pants.

Crew Resource Management

Crew resource management (CRM) is a program that began in the early 1970s to attempt to decrease the number of airline crashes. There are many components to the program, but most can be applied to all emergency scenes. CRM looks at four human factors referred to as the SHEL model. The SHEL model examines software, hardware, environment, and liveware:

- *Software* refers to the basics of standard operating guidelines that are followed during emergency response.
- *Hardware* is the equipment used during emergency response.
- *Environment* includes weather, noise, terrain, and temperature.
- *Liveware* refers to the people involved in the emergency response at all levels.

CRM utilizes the principles of open communication and the ability of anyone at any skill level to communicate a concern to the incident commander. The idea of everyone taking an active role in situational awareness to prevent the occurence of one small error may make a huge difference in the outcome of the emergency. Often catastrophic errors result from the culmination of many small errors, whereas the prevention of one single error may prevent the domino effect and resulting disaster.

In order for CRM to work, everyone must be diligent in their awareness and be open with communications of any deviations from safe practice. Remember that weather conditions, including high winds, bitter cold, and heavy precipitation, can all be a distraction during a rescue. Having equipment that everyone on the team is not familiar with can also negatively affect the outcome of an emergency event. Practicing with new equipment and being familiar with its use during both fair-weather and poor-weather scenarios will allow the rescuer to develop a comfort level to operate equipment during the worst conditions. Practicing as a team and using good teamwork will also help to prevent issues that can arise from rescuers working with individuals they are either not familiar with, or don't know well. CRM needs to become a culture within the organization to maximize situational awareness, enhance communications, improve teamwork, strengthen decision making, and minimize errors.

KEY POINT

Everyone Has a Voice

Three patrollers/OEC technicians are operating at a serious accident at a ski area. One of the individuals is a new patroller and just completed the OEC class. The lead patroller has 20 years experience and is directing the rescue. At some point, the new patroller notices a serious safety concern relative to the use of the LAR equipment. According to the principles of CRM, it is incumbant on the new patroller to point out the issue immediately to the senior patroller, who should consider the comments and make adjustments as necessary to ensure the safety of the rescuers and the patient. While a new patroller may find it uncomfortable to voice a concern that is seemingly critical of a more experienced provider, doing so is important for the safety of all personnel.

CASE Outcome

With the help of the race officials, you carefully unstrap the stretcher from the vehicle, leaving the teenage girl in the stretcher with the splint on her lower leg and moving her away from the vehicle. You conduct a full patient assessment of the girl and fortunately find she has only sustained a small laceration of the scalp, in addition to the lower leg injury. A third OEC technician arrives, and you instruct him to find the girl's parents. Management arrives. The girl's parents are found in the stands and come to the scene. You explain to them what happened. While the mother accompanies her daughter to the hospital via ambulance, you return to the aid room and complete your paperwork. The next day, the mother calls the patrol room to tell you her daughter broke her leg, is in a cast, and is now home. She received four stitches in her head. The driver fractured his clavicle but is otherwise okay. Management thanks you for your quick action in managing a difficult situation.

CHAPTER REVIEW

In Summary

- Special operations require specialized training, skills, and equipment. Special operations situations include infrequently performed activities requiring specialized education and equipment in remote and/or difficult settings.
- OEC technicians need a basic understanding of basic special operations-related tasks and objectives so that they can safely assist EMS crews.
- When encountering a victim trapped in a vehicle, always "try before you pry."
- OEC technicians are encouraged to join a CERT, MRC, DMAT, or USAR team.
- The care for organophosphate exposure is self-administration of nerve agent antidote medications available in a kit (Mark I or DuoDote).
- The National Response Framework (NRF) is the organized system for disaster response in the United States.
- Remember to "run, hide, fight" during a terrorist incident.

Key Terms

CBRNE A mnemonic for the common types of human-caused disasters; represents chemical, biological, radiological, nuclear, and explosive.

Cold zone The area outside the warm zone, in which it is safe to operate without specialized equipment.

Crew resource management (CRM) A program that uses the principles of open communication and the ability of anyone at any skill level to communicate a concern to the incident commander.

Extrication The process of removing a trapped person (as from a vehicle that has been involved in a collision) when conventional means of exit are impossible or inadvisable.

HAZWOPER A abbreviation for **HAZ**ardous **W**aste **OP**erations and **E**mergency **R**esponse; refers to federally mandated training for anyone who may encounter uncontrolled hazardous materials.

High-angle rescue (HAR) Any rescue work done by ascending or descending a slope steeper than approximately 45 degrees.

Hot zone The area closest to the center of a CBRNE incident; the most dangerous and most contaminated area.

Low-angle rescue (LAR) Any rescue work done by ascending or descending a slope that is less than approximately 45 degrees.

Rescue The process of extracting a person or group from distress or danger.

Search A methodical process of actively gathering information about a person or group in distress or danger and then physically looking for them.

Special operations Infrequently performed activities requiring specialized education and equipment in remote and/or difficult settings.

Terrorism A human-caused event that is intended to inflict fear and can involve hazardous materials.

Warm zone A transition area surrounding the hot zone; the zone in which decontamination occurs.

Chapter Questions

1. Which of the following best describes special operations?
   a. A system to maximize situational awareness, enhance communications, improve teamwork, strengthen decision making, and minimize errors
   b. A methodical process of actively gathering information about and then physically looking for one or more individuals in distress or imminent danger
   c. Infrequently performed activities requiring specialized education and equipment in remote and/or difficult settings
   d. The response to and decontamination of a hazmat site
2. The NSP encourages OEC technicians to join which of the following local groups of volunteers that support local public-safety officials and provide immediate assistance to victims during a disaster?
   a. Urban Search and Rescue
   b. Community Emergency Response Team
   c. Disaster Medical Assistance Team
   d. All of the above
3. The response to and decontamination of a hazmat site are referred to as HAZWOPER, which is an abbreviation for:
   a. HAZardous Waste OPerations and Emergency Response.
   b. HAZardous Waste OPportunities and Emergency Rescue.
   c. HAZardous Waste OPERations.
   d. None of the above
4. The purpose of the NFPA safety diamond placard system is to:
   a. establish hazardous control zones.
   b. identify which ICS officer the hazmat safety officer reports to.
   c. identify from which community a chemical originated.
   d. identify hazardous materials that are in transit.
5. At a hazmat-related incident, only personnel with specialized training and equipment are permitted to enter the most dangerous and most contaminated zone, referred to as the:
   a. cold zone.
   b. warm zone.
   c. hot zone.
   d. dry zone.
6. You are assisting with the extrication of a patient from an automobile that has been involved in a crash. You know that the term "try before you pry" refers to:
   a. attempting entry with a simple hand tool prior to using a complex hydraulic tool.
   b. placing 4-inch by 4-inch or 6-inch by 6-inch wood blocks at strategic points to stabilize the vehicle.
   c. checking all the vehicle's doors before attempting a forcible entry to reach a patient.
   d. removing the vehicle's windows prior to the doors or top.

7. Exposure to a nerve agent causes overstimulation to the nerve endings, so muscles and certain glands overreact. A nerve agent antidote kit will:
   a. dry up secretions and reverse the action of the nerve agent.
   b. dilate the bronchi and reduce secretions.
   c. stop the patient from bleeding.
   d. stimulate the patient's heart.

8. During a search-and-rescue effort, "silence is golden" refers to:
   a. limiting your speech to avoiding distracting a search dog.
   b. limiting sounds that may disturb an unstable structure.
   c. the communication method that search dogs use to alert their handler to a scent.
   d. the communication method that handlers use to reward dogs.

Answers: 1. c, Objective 34-1, p. 786; 2. d, Objective 34-3, p. 791; 3. a, Objective 34-5, p. 793; 4. d, Objective 34-6, p. 793; 5. c, Objective 34-7, p. 794; 6. c, Objective 34-4, p. 789; 7. a, Objective 34-8, p. 796; 8. a, Objective 34-13, p. 804

APPENDIX A

EMERGENCY CARE EQUIPMENT

The equipment needs of an OEC technician vary widely according to the activity being supported, the environment in which that activity takes place, and the unique skills required when participating with special teams. One of the main limitations in providing prehospital care in outdoor settings is that a rescuer cannot have access to unlimited supplies or personnel. When deciding what will be included in a rescue pack, each OEC technician must decide what must be carried and what is too much to carry. The basic question that should guide the selection and preparation of the gear you take is "What injuries or illnesses do I expect to treat?" Another consideration is proximity to a higher level of care, which may be as nearby as a patrol room, or may be much farther away. Decreasing proximity (longer transport time) almost always requires an increase in a patroller's load.

The equipment specified in each of the following lists represents the minimum that OEC technicians need to treat the majority of injuries or illnesses they are likely to encounter in the most common outdoor activities: thus lists are provided for an alpine pack, a universal survival kit, a bike kit, a white water kit, and a Nordic kit. Working in some environments and terrains requires specialized gear; accordingly, equipment needed in areas with high avalanche risk is listed in a separate list.

ALPINE PACK

Suggested Items (**Figure A-1**)

- Two to four (2-4) pairs disposable non-latex medical gloves
- SAM™ splint
- Four (4) cravats
- Six (6) or more 4-inch by 4-inch gauze pads
- Two (2) 2-inch gauze wraps (or Kling)
- Hard candy (for diabetic emergencies)
- 3-inch roller bandage
- Two (2) abdominal pads
- Two (2) large trash bags (for use as a full body covering to prevent hypothermia)
- Pocket mask
- Roll of 1-inch adhesive tape
- Various sizes of adhesive bandages (e.g., Band-Aids™)
- Trauma shears (small enough to fit in the pack but strong enough to cut what you need to cut)
- A fine-tipped permanent marker (to write patient information on tape; is freeze- and smear-resistant)
- Multi-tool (Leatherman™ style, including pliers, knife, screwdriver (both flat and Phillips head) for binding anchors
- Sandwich bags (used for occlusive bandage, as a cooling pack when filled with snow or cool water, or to transport small, amputated body parts)
- Four (4) sizes of airways
- Small flashlight (with extra batteries)
- Space blanket
- Aspirin/Tylenol (for personal use)

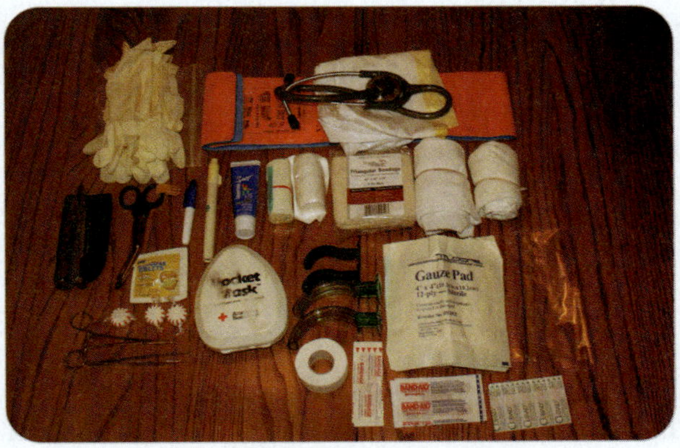

Figure A-1 An alpine pack.

Optional Items

- Stethoscope
- Forceps
- Hemostats
- Small pipe cutter
- Topical antibiotic packet
- Small tube of sun block

UNIVERSAL SURVIVAL KIT

A survival kit should be lightweight, small enough to throw in a bag or a car or to hook to a belt, and useful in any outdoor environment.

Suggested Items

- One (1) 1-liter water bottle
- Multi-tool (with knife blade)
- Waterproof matches or butane lighter
- Poncho (small pouch)
- Small flashlight or head lamp (with extra batteries)
- Space blanket (keep in original package)
- 50 feet of parachute (#550) cord
- Hard candy
- Aspirin/Tylenol (for personal use)
- Whistle
- Candle (survival-specific type)
- Signal mirror
- Small compass
- Water purification tablets
- Wire saw
- Commercial tourniquet

(Depending on the size of items, the items listed above can be stored in a 1-liter Nalgene™ bottle.)

Optional Items

- Water filter
- Plastic table cloth (may be used as a tarp or a shelter)
- Power bars
- Cell phone and/or GPS
- Commercial fire starter
- 50 feet of #20 fishing line

BIKE KIT

Because a bike rider will likely not want to carry much weight, this list is shorter than that for an Alpine pack. Still, these items will cover most injuries (Figure A-2).

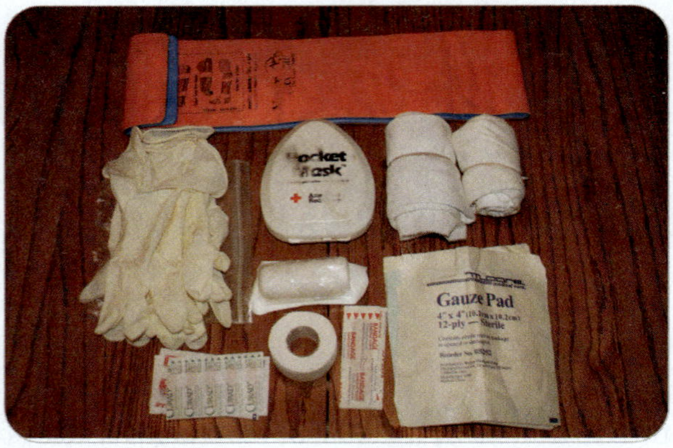

Figure A-2 A bike kit.

Suggested Items

- Two to four (2-4) pairs of disposable non-latex medical gloves
- SAM™ Splint
- Two (2) cravats
- Six (6) 4-inch by 4-inch gauze pads
- Kerlix wrap (or Kling)
- Roll of 1-inch adhesive tape
- Various sizes of Band-Aids™
- Pocket mask
- Commercial tourniquet

Optional Items

- Cell phone and/or GPS
- Sun block

WHITE WATER KIT

Items for a white water kit should be kept in a waterproof container that floats (Figure A-3).

Suggested Items

- Two to four (2-4) disposable non-latex medical gloves
- SAM™ Splint
- Four (4) cravats
- Three (3) 2-inch gauze wraps (or Kling)
- Pocket mask
- Roll of 1-inch adhesive tape
- Various sizes of adhesive bandages (Band-Aids™)
- Trauma shears
- Penlight
- Permanent marker
- Multi-tool, with knife blade
- Ziplock™ plastic bags

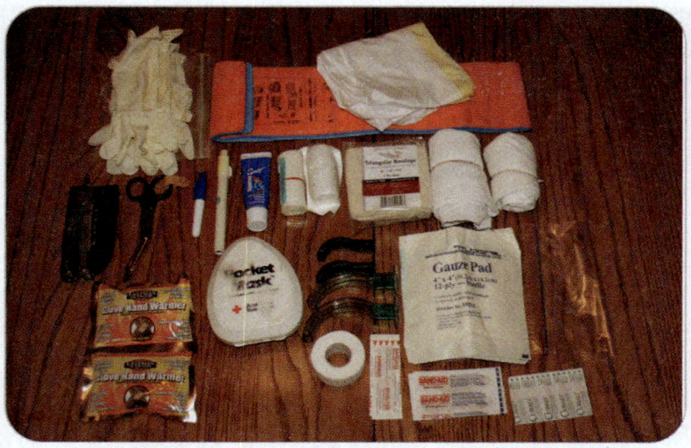

Figure A-3 A white water kit.

- Two (2) heat packs
- Sun block (with SPF of 30 or higher)
- Three or four sizes of airways
- Commercial tourniquet

NORDIC KIT

Suggested Items (**Figure A-4**)

- Two to four (2-4) disposable non-latex medical gloves
- SAM™ Splint
- Four (4) 4-inch by 4-inch gauze pads
- Four (4) cravats
- Two (2) 2-inch gauze wraps (or Kling)
- Pocket mask
- Roll of 1-inch adhesive tape
- Various sizes of adhesive bandages (Band-Aids™)
- Trauma shears
- Penlight/headlamp
- Permanent marker
- Thermometer
- Multi-tool, with knife blade
- Plastic bag
- Kendrick traction device (KTD) or adapter for ski poles
- Commercial tourniquet

Optional Items

- One (1) 1-liter water bottle
- Tube tent
- Waterproof matches or butane lighter
- Small compass
- Small poncho
- Wire saw

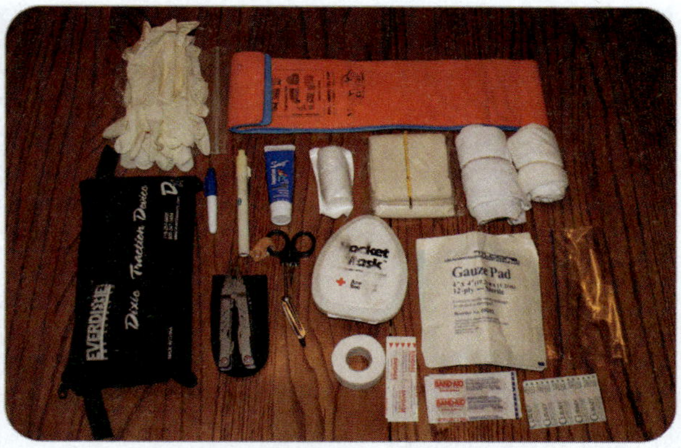

Figure A-4 A Nordic kit.

- Small flashlight (with extra batteries)
- Space blanket (keep in original package)
- 50 feet of parachute (#550) cord
- Whistle
- Candle (survival-specific type)

Additional Equipment to Consider in an Avalanche Risk Area (Alpine or Nordic)

- Snow shovel
- Transceiver
- Snow probe
- Radio or cell phone

MEDICATIONS

The medications to consider for inclusion in your personal wilderness kit are listed in **Table A-1**. The National Ski Patrol does not recommend dispensing or administering any medication to an injured patient.

Before you take any medicines, seek the advice of a licensed provider. Your medical advisor can provide information regarding limitations on the use of medications. Although many of these medications are available by prescription only, they can be obtained for self-use through your personal physician. Other medications are controlled medicines and can only be obtained from a licensed provider registered with the Drug Enforcement Agency.

As a rule, all medications should be kept in their original containers to avoid errors in dispensing. For many prescribed medications, it is a legal requirement that the medication remain in the original container so that the prescriber's information can be read on the container's label.

Table A-1

High Altitude			
Medication	**Dose**	**When Taken**	**Indication**
Acetazolamide*	250 mg	Twice a day	Mountain sickness
Albuterol inhaler*	As needed		Respiratory distress
Ciprofloxacin*	500 mg	Twice a day	Diarrhea/urinary infection
Ondansetron*	4 to 8 mg	Every 6 hours	Nausea
Cyclopentolate opth*	1%	1-2 drops	Snow blindness
Dexamethasone*	4 mg	Every 6 hours	Mountain sickness
EpiPen*	0.3 mg	As needed	Severe allergic reaction
Nifedipine*	30 mg	Twice a day	Pulmonary edema
Tylenol	500 mg	Every 4 hours	Pain
White Water			
Medication	**Dose**	**When Taken**	**Indication**
Augmentin*	875 mg	Twice a day	Skin/respiratory infection
Ciprofloxacin*	500 mg	Twice a day	Diarrhea/urinary infection
Diphenhydramine	50 mg	Every 6 hours	Allergies/itch
EpiPen*	0.3 mg	As needed	Severe allergic reaction
Hydrocodone**	5 mg	Every 6 hours	Severe pain
Nordic			
Medication	**Dose**	**When Taken**	**Indication**
Albuterol inhaler*	As needed		Respiratory distress
Ciprofloxacin*	500 mg	Twice a day	Diarrhea/urinary infection
Cyclopentolate opth*	1%	1-2 drops	Snow blindness
EpiPen*	0.3 mg	As needed	Severe allergic reaction
Tylenol No. 3**	30 mg	Every 4 hours	Pain
Bike			
Medication	**Dose**	**When Taken**	**Indication**
Albuterol inhaler*	As needed		Respiratory distress
EpiPen*	0.3 mg	As needed	Severe allergic reaction
Hydrocodone**	5 mg	Every 6 hours	Severe pain
Tylenol No. 3**	30 mg	Every 4 hours	Pain

* Medication available only by prescription.
**Controlled medication that can be obtained only from a licensed provider registered with the Drug Enforcement Agency.

GLOSSARY

30–2-Can Do A mnemonic for remembering the assessment findings of the START triage system: *30* respirations per minute, capillary refill of *2* seconds, and ability to follow simple commands (*can do*).

A

Abandonment The act of withdrawing one's support or help from, especially in spite of duty, allegiance, or responsibility.

Abdominal evisceration A tear in the abdominal wall exposing the intestines and/or other organs to the external environment.

Abduction Motion of a limb away from the midline.

Abruptio placentae The premature separation of a normally situated but improperly implanted placenta; usually occurs late in pregnancy but may occur during labor.

Absence seizure A sudden, temporary loss of mental awareness and physical activity lasting a few seconds to several minutes; also known as a petit mal seizure.

Absorption The way in which a substance or poison enters the body. The four routes of absorption are ingestion, inhalation, transdermal absorption, and injection.

Acclimatization The body's physiological process of *gradual* adjustment to changes in altitude. (Term also can be used for adjustment to light or temperature.)

Acromioclavicular (A/C) joint A joint of the shoulder in which the acromion (top of the scapula) and the clavicle articulate.

Acute abdomen A condition of sudden onset of pain within the abdomen, usually indicating peritonitis; immediate medical or surgical treatment is necessary.

Acute mountain sickness (AMS) A medical condition that is caused by exposure to high altitude.

Acute myocardial infarction (AMI) The interruption of blood supply to part of the heart from a blocked artery, causing death of heart muscle. Also known as a heart attack.

Adaptive athlete A person with disabilities participating in competitive or recreational sports.

Adduction Motion of a limb toward the midline.

Advanced emergency medical technician (AEMT) An intermediate-level technician who has successfully completed an NHTSA-approved Advanced EMT course or its equivalent and is authorized to provide both basic and intermediate life support.

Advanced life support (ALS) A level of EMS care for which providers are trained and authorized to insert advanced airway devices, initiate intravenous lines, and give medications.

Afterdrop A continued drop in core body temperature after removal from exposure to the cold.

Agitation Excessive restlessness and increased mental or physical activity.

Airway The natural passageway that allows air to enter and exit the lungs.

Allergen A foreign substance (antigen) whose presence in the body stimulates an allergic reaction.

Allergic reaction A series of signs and symptoms that occur in response to exposure to an allergen.

Allergy An exaggerated immune response to a substance that does not normally cause a reaction.

Altered mental status A condition in which a person's level of awareness or responsiveness has changed.

Altitude illness Any type of illness caused by exposure to high altitude.

Ambient temperature The temperature in the immediate environment.

Amputation The complete or nearly complete separation of a body part or limb.

Anaphylactic shock A type of distributive shock that occurs when a person reacts violently to a substance to which he or she has become sensitized.

Anaphylaxis A severe allergic reaction that can result in serious cardiac or respiratory compromise.

Aneurysm Ballooning of an artery that weakens it and predisposes it to rupture.

Angina pectoris Sudden chest pain due to an inadequate supply of oxygen to the heart muscle; also called angina.

Angioedema Swelling that occurs beneath the skin or mucosa because of an allergic reaction.

Angulation A sharp bend in a broken bone; a broken bone that is visibly crooked.

Anisocoria Unequal size of the pupils.

Anoxia A condition characterized by the lack of an oxygen supply.

Antegrade amnesia Loss of memory of events that occurred *after* a traumatic event to the brain; an inability to recall new information.

Antibody A protein that is produced by the body to neutralize or destroy specific antigens.

Anticoagulants Medications that prevent blood from clotting; "blood thinners."

Antivenom A biological material (antibodies) administered to a patient to counteract exposure to a specific kind of venom; produced by injecting the venom into an animal and then harvesting the antibodies that the animal makes against the venom.

Anxiety A feeling of worry, nervousness, or unease, typically about an imminent event or something with an uncertain outcome.

Aorta The largest artery in the body, carries blood out of the left side of the heart to smaller arteries that travel through the entire body.

Aortic aneurysm An aneurysm that occurs anywhere along the length of the aorta.

Aortic rupture Development of a leak in the largest blood vessel in the body; results in massive bleeding that is usually fatal.

Arrhythmia Abnormal heart rhythm.

Arterial gas embolism (AGE) A condition that occurs immediately after rapid ascent in which air bubbles enter the bloodstream from a ruptured alveolus and lodge in an artery.

Artery A tubular vessel that carries blood from the heart to the lungs and body.

Articular cartilage The cartilage that is affixed to the end of a bone within a joint.

Articulation The site at which the ends of two or more bones come together to form a joint.

Assault The act of making a person reasonably fear that battery will occur.

Asystole A complete absence of a heartbeat due to a lack of electrical activity within the heart.

Ataxia Uncoordinated muscle movements; at high altitudes, it is associated with high-altitude cerebral edema.

Atherosclerosis A form of arteriosclerosis in which cholesterol and lipid plaques form within the walls of arteries.

Attention-deficit/hyperactivity disorder (ADHD) A behavioral syndrome that causes short attention span, impulsive behavior, and restlessness.

Aura A subjective sensation that precedes a seizure.

Automated external defibrillator (AED) A medical device used to deliver an electrical shock to a patient to restore an effective heart rhythm.

Automatic implantable cardioverter defibrillator (AICD) A defibrillator that recognizes common lethal heart rhythms and then delivers an electrical shock to the heart to restore an effective heart rhythm.

Autonomic dysreflexia Abnormal function of the nervous system associated with spinal cord injuries; can lead to dangerously high blood pressure.

AVPU scale A mnemonic for assessing neurologic function; represents awake and alert, responds to verbal stimuli or pain, or unresponsive.

Avulsion The incomplete separation of the soft-tissue layers where the injured tissue is left dangling as a flap.

Axon Long, slender projection of a nerve cell (neuron) that conducts electrical impulses away from the neuron's cell body.

B

Bag-valve mask (BVM) A manually operated resuscitator consisting of an oxygen reservoir, a self-expanding squeezable bag, a one-way valve, a universal adaptor, and a face mask; used to assist patient ventilations.

Bandage A strip or roll of gauze or other material used for wrapping or binding a body part.

Barotrauma Trauma that is caused by differences in pressure between the body and the environment.

Barrier device A personal protective device that provides a nonporous layer between the provider and the patient to prevent the transmission of communicable diseases.

Basic life support (BLS) A basic level of EMS care for which providers are trained and authorized to provide basic interventions, including noninvasive airway devices, application of oxygen, CPR, and basic first aid.

Battery The act of touching someone without his or her consent.

Bipolar disorder A serious mental illness characterized by extreme mood swings, which range from depression to mania. If severe, psychosis can result.

Bi-ski A molded bucket seat mounted on two skis (with or without a suspension system).

Bladder infection A condition in which bacteria enter the bladder, potentially causing a serious infection with fever and chills.

Blood pressure The pressure of the blood on the interior walls of the arteries.

Blowout fracture An injury caused by direct trauma to the eye or face that fractures the bony eye socket; can entrap the muscles that enable normal eye movement.

Body mechanics The relationship between the body's anatomic structures and the physical forces associated with lifting, moving, and carrying; the ways the body moves to achieve an action.

Body substance isolation (BSI) The practice of isolating all bodily substances (blood, urine, tears, feces, and so on) of patients from rescuers in order to decrease disease transmission.

Body system A group of organs and other structures that work together to perform specific functions.

Bone crepitus A noise or palpable feeling of crackling when fractured bone ends rub together.

Bradypnea A decreased respiratory rate; in adults, less than 10 breaths per minute.

Brain The organ in the nervous system responsible for the control of all the body systems. The brain coordinates the function of sensation; controls muscles; keeps body organs functioning automatically; and integrates consciousness, memory, emotions, and the use of language.

Breach of duty The failure to perform a promised act or obligation of due care.

Breath sounds An indication of air movement in the lungs, usually assessed with a stethoscope.

Bronchospasm The involuntary contraction of the bronchioles.

Bucket The seat of a sit-ski, handcycle, or hockey sled in which the adaptive athlete is secured.

Burn A lesion of the skin caused by thermal or frictional heat, chemicals, electricity, or nuclear radiation.

C

Capillaries Tiny blood vessels that connect arteries to veins. They provide nutrients and oxygen to and remove waste from cells.

Cardiogenic shock A type of shock caused by inadequate function of the heart, or pump failure, resulting in poor cardiac output.

Cardiopulmonary resuscitation (CPR) A procedure to revive a patient who is pulseless and not breathing.

Cardiovascular system Organs and structures that circulate blood around the body using the heart, arteries, and veins, delivering oxygen and nutrients to organs and cells. This system carries chemical waste products away from the cells and helps equalize body temperature. May also be referred to as the circulatory system.

Carry The act of lifting and moving the patient, usually a short distance.

Cartilage A tough, elastic, fibrous connective tissue found in various parts of the body, including the joints, outer ear, and end of the nose.

CBRNE A mnemonic for the common types of human-caused disasters; represents chemical, biological, radiological, nuclear, and explosive.

Cells The basic units of all living tissue.

Central nervous system The part of the nervous system that includes the brain and spinal cord.

Cerebral contusion A bruise involving the brain.

Chain of command A rank structure for management.

Charles Minot "Minnie" Dole The founder and creator of the National Ski Patrol.

Chief complaint The symptom or group of symptoms about which the patient is concerned.

Child abuse Any act or failure to act on the part of a parent, a caregiver, or any adult that results in serious physical or emotional harm or imminent risk of harm to a child.

Child neglect A failure to act on the part of a parent, a caregiver, or other responsible adult to provide for the physical, emotional, educational, safety, or social needs of a child to the extent that emotional, developmental, or physical harm may occur.

Chronic obstructive pulmonary disease (COPD) A chronic inflammatory lung disease that causes obstructed airflow by causing constriction of bronchi that carry air into and out of the lungs.

Clonic activity The spasmodic jerking of muscles during a seizure.

Closed chest injury A chest injury without penetration of the chest cavity.

Cochlear implant A small, surgically implanted electronic device for deaf persons that works like an artificial human cochlea in the inner ear, helping to send sound from the ear to the brain.

Cognitive disability Impairment of brain function that limits the ability to process information and reach reasoned conclusions.

Cold zone The area outside the warm zone, in which it is safe to operate without specialized equipment.

Coma An abnormal loss of responsiveness during which the patient cannot be aroused by external stimuli.

Commotio cordis Sudden cardiac death due to blunt chest trauma without any observable chest or cardiac damage.

Communication A process whereby information is transmitted from one person to another.

Compartment syndrome A condition in which the swelling of injured muscles within their connective tissue coverings causes pressure that can damage tissue and cut off blood flow.

Compression (pressure) dressing A dressing that closes bleeding blood vessels by compressing the wound.

Concussion Temporary unconsciousness (unresponsiveness) or confusion caused by a blow to the head.

Congestive heart failure (CHF) Failure of the heart to efficiently pump blood to body tissues.

Consent Permission or approval to perform a proposed or requested action.

Contamination Soiling of an object, water, or air by foreign material such as dirt, debris, bodily fluids, or radiation.

Core body temperature The temperature in the part of the body that contains the vital organs.

Cornea The clear but highly sensitive surface of the eye that refracts light entering into the visual system.

Coronary arteries Two arteries that come off the first part of the aorta, that provide oxygenated, nutrient rich blood to the heart muscle.

Coronary artery disease Narrowing of the coronary arteries, which supply blood and oxygen to the heart muscle.

Cortex The hard, outer layer of a bone.

Coup-contrecoup brain injury Dual-impacting of the brain into the skull; coup injury occurs at the point of impact; contrecoup occurs at the opposite side of impact, as the brain rebounds.

Cranium The skull.

Crepitus A "crackling" feel of the skin of the chest that is detected by palpation; is caused by the presence of air trapped beneath the skin.

Crew resource management (CRM) A program that uses the principles of open communication and the ability of anyone at any skill level to communicate a concern to the incident commander.

Crisis A state of emotional turmoil within an individual in which the balance between thoughts and emotions is lost.

Crush injury A compression injury in which a great amount of force is applied to the body.

D

DCAP-BTLS A mnemonic for assessing trauma-related injuries; represents deformity; contusions; abrasions and avulsions; punctures and penetrations; burns, bleeding, and bruises; tenderness; lacerations; and swelling.

Decerebrate posturing Abnormal extension of the arms and legs, downward pointing of the toes, and arching of the head due to an injury to the brain at the level of the brainstem.

Decompression sickness (DCS) Formation of nitrogen bubbles in tissues from being underwater too long or ascending too rapidly.

Decontamination The process of rendering an object, person, or area free of harmful substances such as bacteria, poison, gas, and radiation.

Decorticate posturing Abnormal flexing of the arms, clenching of the fists, and extending of the legs; due to an injury along the nerve pathway between the brain and spinal cord.

Defibrillation The restoration of a normal rhythm of the heart by electrical shock.

Delirium A state of mental confusion and/or excitement characterized by disorientation with respect to time and place; may be associated with delusions and hallucinations.

Dementia A broad impairment of intellectual function (cognition) that usually is progressive and that interferes with normal social and occupational activities.

Depression A clinical state marked by feelings of sadness and self-loathing.

Dermal poisons Harmful substances that are absorbed through the skin.

Designer drugs Drugs that are constructed by a chemist to produce unique and specific effects.

Diabetes mellitus A disease in which the body's ability to produce or respond to the hormone insulin is impaired, resulting in abnormal metabolism of carbohydrates (sugars) causing elevated levels of glucose in the blood and urine.

Diaphragm The large, thick, flat muscle between the chest and abdomen that is used for breathing.

Digestive system Also known as the gastrointestinal system, a group of organs and other structures that use mechanical and chemical processes to break down food and absorb nutrients into the body. This system also eliminates waste or unused material that is eaten.

Disease transmission The transfer of illness from an infected individual to a healthy individual.

Dislocation A separation or displacement of the bones of a joint.

Distributive shock A type of shock resulting from widespread dilation of the small arterioles, venules, or both.

Doctrine of public reliance A reasonable expectation held by the general public that an OEC technician can and will provide first-aid services.

Dorsal Toward the back of the body or of a body part.

Dorsiflex To move a part of the body dorsally (toward the back).

Drag A method of pulling a patient on the ground to another location.

Dressing Any material (preferably sterile) used for covering and protecting a wound.

Drowning The process of respiratory impairment caused by submersion or immersion in a liquid.

Duty to act A person's legal obligation to perform an action.

Dyslexia Impairment of information processing that makes learning new information difficult.

Dyspnea Difficult or labored breathing accompanied by feeling short of breath.

E

Ecchymosis A bruise; discoloration of the skin associated with a closed wound; signifies bleeding within the skin.

Eclampsia A potentially life-threatening disorder in pregnant women characterized by hypertension, generalized edema, and proteinuria (protein in the urine); involves the seizures of the convulsive stage of preeclampsia-eclampsia syndrome, which are not attributable to another cerebral condition such as epilepsy.

Ectopic pregnancy A condition in which the fertilized egg attaches outside of the uterus.

Emergency medical care system A network of specially trained personnel, equipment, facilities, and other resources that respond to medical emergencies. See EMS.

Emergency medical dispatcher (EMD) A person who has been trained to provide emergency medical advice and instructions over the telephone.

Emergency medical responder (EMR) A prehospital provider who is specially trained to provide medical care to patients in prehospital settings. There are many types of EMRs, each with various training requirements and scopes of practice. OEC technicians are trained at EMR level.

Emergency medical services (EMS) A network of services, including rescue operations, prehospital emergency care, ambulance transportation, emergency department services, and public education, for treating victims of illness or injury.

Emergency medical technician (EMT) A basic-level technician who has successfully completed an NHTSA-approved EMT course or its equivalent and is authorized to provide basic life support.

Endocrine system A collection of glands that produce chemical substances, called hormones, that travel through the bloodstream influencing target organs.

Envenomation Poisonous effects caused by bites or stings.

Epidural hematoma a traumatic brain injury in which a buildup of blood occurs between the dura mater and the skull.

Epiglottis A thin, leaf-shaped structure posterior to the tongue; covers the larynx when swallowing, preventing food or liquid from entering the airway.

Epilepsy A disorder in which abnormal electrical discharges occur in the brain, causing seizure and possible loss of responsiveness.

Epistaxis Nosebleed.

Ethics The science (study) of morality or behavior that defines what is "good" or "right."

Exhalation The act of expelling breath or air out of the lungs.

Expressed consent Consent given when a competent injured person gives permission to provide first-aid treatment and transport.

Expressive aphasia Inability to express speech normally.

Exsanguination Massive blood loss resulting in death; the process of bleeding to death.

Extension The straightening of a joint.

External auditory canal The passageway through the outer ear that ends at the tympanic membrane (eardrum).

Extrication The process of removing a trapped person (as from a vehicle that has been involved in a collision) when conventional means of exit are impossible or inadvisable.

F

Face shield A clear, usually rectangular, plastic sheet that includes a mouthpiece through which rescue breaths are administered.

Facility Any primary work area in or around an incident in which incident-related activities are planned, organized, directed, or conducted.

Fainting A loss of consciousness that results from a lack of blood flow to the brain. This condition may occur suddenly, resulting from the temporary dilation of the body's veins and pooling of blood in those vessels. May also be referred to as syncope.

False movement Motion that occurs at the site of a fracture of a long bone that is not present when the bone is intact.

Field care notes Notes written by OEC technicians at the scene of a patient rescue; may include a timeline, vital signs, witnesses' names, and other pertinent information.

Finger sweep A method of clearing the airway when a foreign body is seen in the mouth of an unresponsive patient.

Flail chest A condition in which two or more adjacent ribs are fractured in two or more places, causing a free-floating segment (paradoxical movement) of the chest wall.

Flexion The bending of a joint.

Flowmeter A device on oxygen cylinders used to control and measure the flow of oxygen.

Fontanels The unfused sutures between the bones of the skull of a newborn that allow expansion of the growing brain; the fontanels have closed by approximately 18 months of age.

Four-track adaptive skier An adaptive skier with two legs who also uses two outriggers.

Fracture A break in a bone's cortex.

Frostbite Damage to tissues from freezing due to the formation of ice crystals between and within cells, rupturing the cells and leading to cell death.

Frostnip (chilblains) A relatively minor, local cold injury that results from local vasoconstriction of blood vessels in response to cold.

G

Gamow bag A portable hyperbaric chamber that is used to treat altitude illness.

Gastric distention Inflation of the stomach with air; can lead to vomiting.

General impression Initial findings based on the patient's chief complaint, the scene size-up, the mechanism of injury or nature of illness, and the patient's initial appearance.

Generalized seizure A seizure consisting of the sudden onset of unresponsiveness, tonic contraction of muscles, loss of postural control, and a cry caused by contraction of respiratory muscles that forces an exhalation; clonic contractions of muscles occur, followed by a period of somnolence.

Geriatric Pertaining to elderly persons or to the aging process.

Gestational period The time from the first day of a woman's last normal menstrual period before fertilization, which is about 2 weeks before fertilization, until birth.

Glucose A simple sugar that is the product of carbohydrate digestion in the body and the chief source of energy for most cells, especially neurons.

Golden hour The first 60 minutes following a serious traumatic event, during which prompt medical treatment may prevent death.

Good Samaritan laws Laws that protect a person from legal liability when the person volunteers to perform an act to help someone else.

Gross negligence An intentional failure to perform a manifest duty in reckless disregard of the consequences as affecting the life or property of another. It also implies a thoughtless disregard of the consequences without the exertion of any effort to avoid them.

Guarding An involuntary action in which the abdomen becomes rigid upon examination. Guarding may also occur in the form of holding an injured arm or leg in a protective position to prevent further injury.

Guide A trained person who assists an adaptive athlete (such as a blind skier or a bi-skier) in the field.

H

Handoff report An oral or written report given at the transfer of a patient from one provider to another.

Hazardous materials Substances that have the potential to harm people, animals, or the environment. The term hazmat is often used adjectively (e.g., "hazmat incident").

HAZWOPER A abbreviation for **HAZ**ardous **W**aste **OP**erations and **E**mergency **R**esponse; refers to federally mandated training for anyone who may encounter uncontrolled hazardous materials.

Head tilt–chin lift maneuver A method used to open the airway when there is a possible cervical spine injury. The head is tilted as the chin is lifted.

Health Insurance Portability and Accountability Act (HIPAA) A law requiring that medical personnel who are compensated for the services they provide maintain patient confidentiality during the electronic transmission of medical records, among other requirements.

Heat acclimatization Adaptation of the body over time to a hot environment.

Heat index A measure of the risk for heat illness; combines the effects of increasing ambient temperature and increasing humidity.

Hematemesis Vomit that contains blood in it.

Hematoma A localized collection of blood inside the body that has leaked from a blood vessel.

Hemoptysis Coughing up blood.

Hemorrhage The escape of blood from the vessels; bleeding.

Hemostatic dressing A surgical gauze/mesh impregnated with a material that stops arterial and venous bleeding in seconds.

Hemothorax An accumulation of blood in the pleural space.

High-altitude cerebral edema (HACE) A potentially deadly condition in which the brain swells in individuals at high altitude.

High-altitude pulmonary edema (HAPE) A condition in which fluid accumulates in the lungs of individuals at high altitude.

High-angle rescue (HAR) Any rescue work done by ascending or descending a slope steeper than approximately 45 degrees.

Histamine A chemical that is released in the body because of an allergic reaction.

Hot zone The area closest to the center of a CBRNE incident; the most dangerous and most contaminated area.

Human anatomy The study of structures that can be seen with the unaided eye and structures visible only through a microscope in humans.

Human physiology The study of the mechanical, physical, bioelectric, and biochemical functions of humans.

Humidity The amount of water vapor in the air.

Hyperglycemia An excess of glucose in the blood; when severe, may be associated with confusion or changes in mental status.

Hypersensitivity An exaggerated immune response to an allergen, drug, or other foreign substance.

Hypertension Abnormally high blood pressure.

Hyperthermia Elevated core body temperature.

Hyperventilation syndrome (HVS) Abnormally low levels of carbon dioxide in the blood.

Hyphema Blood in the anterior chamber of the eye.

Hypoglycemia An insufficient amount of glucose in the blood; may be associated with a myriad of signs and symptoms such as tremor, diaphoresis, drowsiness, headache, confusion, and lack of responsiveness.

Hypotension Abnormally low blood pressure.

Hypothermia An abnormally low body temperature; below 35°C (95°F).

Hypovolemic shock A type of shock caused by an inadequate amount of fluid or volume in the circulatory system.

Hypoxemia Insufficient oxygenation of the blood.

Hypoxia A decreased amount of oxygen reaching the tissues.

I

Immobilization The process of holding an object in place, as for a fracture by a cast or internal orthopedic hardware.

Immune response The body's response to a substance foreign to the body, such as bacteria.

Immunity The state of being protected from a disease, especially an infectious disease.

Impaled object A foreign object that remains in the body in a puncture wound.

Implied consent A form of consent that is not expressly granted by a person, but instead is inferred from a person's actions and the facts and circumstances of a particular situation.

Incident Anything out of ordinary day-to-day activities that necessitates a response (e.g., emergencies, disasters, outbreaks, vaccination programs, important meetings, conferences).

Incident commander (IC) The person who provides overall leadership at an incident.

Incident command system (ICS) A formal, organized method for managing an incident, regardless of its cause, size, scope, or complexity.

Incident investigation (II) team A group of personnel, usually including representation of management at a resort, who evaluate and document any accident that needs further legal documentation.

Incident report form A form provided by the National Ski Areas Association, a ski resort, or an insurance carrier, used by OEC technicians to document an incident; the forms include patient information and the circumstances leading to injury.

Incision A cut caused by a sharp object; has clean, smooth edges.

Informed consent Consent a person gives based on an appreciation and understanding of the facts, implications, and possible future consequences of an action.

Ingested poisons Harmful substances that enter the body through the mouth.

Inhalation The act of drawing breath or air into the lungs.

Inhaled poisons Harmful substances that are absorbed through the lungs.

Inhaler A device that contains respiratory medicine and is used to improve breathing.

Injected poisons Harmful substances that are injected into a vein or another tissue.

Injury pattern A combination of injuries commonly seen in a patient based on the mechanism of injury.

Insulin A hormone produced in the pancreas that regulates blood sugar levels.

Integumentary (skin) system Specialized tissues covering and protecting the body. The skin helps retain fluids, regulates temperature, transmits information from the environment to the brain, and protects the body from the outside environment.

Intracerebral hematoma A hematoma inside the brain from bleeding inside the brain's tissue.

Intracranial pressure The pressure within the skull; can also be exerted on the brain tissue and cerebrospinal fluid.

Ischemia A deficiency in blood supply (and thus a deficiency of oxygen and nutrients) to a tissue; if prolonged, may result in death of tissue.

J

Jams and pretzels A phrase that refers to the process by which someone who is injured and an awkward position is returned to normal supine anatomic position while maintaining spinal motion restriction.

Jaundice A dull, yellow color of the skin, whites of the eyes, and mucous membranes caused by an excess of bilirubin; usually indicates liver disease.

Jaw-thrust maneuver The primary technique used to open a patient's airway, where the jaw is thrust forward.

Joint A site at which two or more bones meet.

Joint capsule A sheet of fibrous connective tissue enclosing a synovial joint.

K

Khumbu cough A dry, persistent cough caused by inhaling excessively cold, dry air that is typical at high altitude; also known as high-altitude bronchitis and "dry hack cough."

Kinetic energy The energy generated by a body in motion.

Kyphosis Abnormally increased dorsal curvature of the thoracic spine.

L

Laceration A cut caused by forces that tear or crush the skin; tends to have *jagged* edges.

Lacrimal glands The glands that produce tears, which irrigate the surface of the eye.

Landing zone (LZ) An area picked for the landing of aircraft that meets specific size and safety requirements.

Laryngospasm Spasm of the vocal cords that prevents air movement through the respiratory tract.

Level of responsiveness The degree of cognitive function and arousal of the brain; ranges from fully alert to unresponsive.

Lift A way of moving the patient by raising the person from a lower position to a higher one.

Ligament Tissue that connects a bone to another bone; connective tissue that provides structure for a joint.

Lordosis Abnormally increased anterior curvature of the spine (usually the lumbar spine).

Low-angle rescue (LAR) Any rescue work done by ascending or descending a slope that is less than approximately 45 degrees.

Lucid interval A state in which the patient is relatively alert and then becomes increasingly less responsive and eventually unresponsive.

Lymphatic system Organs and other structures that remove extra fluid from tissues, absorb and transport fats from the cardiovascular system, and make white blood cells and transport them from the lymph nodes.

M

Mammalian diving reflex A protective response when the body is immersed or submerged in extremely cold water whereby the metabolic and heart rates slow significantly, reducing oxygen demand and conserving oxygen.

Mandible The jawbone.

Maxillae The bones of the midface that form the upper jaw.

Mechanism of injury The type of force that acts on the body to cause injury; the method of trauma causing an injury.

Meconium Fecal stool found in amniotic fluid.

Medical director A physician who is responsible for ensuring and evaluating the appropriate level and quality of care throughout an emergency care system. Also referred to as a medical advisor or physician supervisor.

Medical oversight The process by which a physician monitors the quality of medical care rendered to patients and provides assistance and guidance to prehospital providers and emergency care systems.

Melana Stools that appear black and tarry due to digested blood in the bowel.

Meningitis Inflammation of the membranes covering the spinal cord and brain; may be caused by viruses or bacteria.

Meniscus A specialized cartilage found in some joints, such as the knee and the acromioclavicular joint.

Menstruation The process in a woman of discharging blood and other materials from the lining of the uterus at intervals of about 1 month; occurs from puberty until menopause.

Metabolism The chemical processes occurring within a living cell or organism that are necessary for the maintenance of life.

Minor consent Consent a parent or legal guardian gives for the treatment of a minor, because legally the minor is not competent to give consent to medical treatment. The ability to provide such consent varies among states.

Miscarriage A common term for a spontaneous abortion; the spontaneous termination of a pregnancy before about 20 weeks of gestation, at which time the fetus is not yet sufficiently developed to survive.

Mono-ski A molded bucket seat mounted on suspension bindings to a single ski.

Mood, adjustment, or affective disorder Abnormal behavior in a person who remains firmly in touch with reality; specific disorders of this type include anxiety, depression, paranoia, agitation, and bipolar.

Move The transport of a patient from one location to another.

Mucous membranes The linings of body cavities and passages that are in direct or indirect contact with the outside environment.

Multiagency coordination system (MACS) A process for managing an incident in which multiple agencies that have different command structures and communication capabilities are participating.

Multiple-casualty incident (MCI) An incident involving two or more patients and in which the number of patients exceeds the capability of local resources.

Muscular system Tissues that allow movement of the body, beating of the heart, and movement within the organs of the digestive system and other tubular structures (e.g., helping move food through the intestines, allowing blood vessels to contract to raise blood pressure).

Musculoskeletal system The combination of the bony skeleton, the voluntary muscles, and other supporting structures that gives the body form and enables movement.

Myocardial contusion A bruise of the heart muscle.

Myocardium Heart muscle tissue.

N

Nasal cannula An oxygen delivery device consisting of plastic tubing with two open prongs that are inserted into the patient's nostrils; provides low-flow oxygen when connected to an oxygen source.

Nasopharyngeal airway (NPA) A trumpet-shaped airway adjunct made from soft rubber or silicone inserted into the nostril to maintain a patent airway.

National Highway Traffic Safety Administration (NHTSA) The federal agency tasked with overseeing the development of emergency care systems in the United States. It is an agency of the executive branch of the US government and is part of the Department of Transportation. Its mission is "Save lives, prevent injuries, reduce vehicle-related crashes."

National Incident Management System (NIMS) A federally mandated "all-hazards" approach for responding to and managing an incident. It was created as a result of Homeland Security Presidential Directive 5.

National Medical Advisor A licensed physician with an interest in outdoor/wilderness medicine and ski patrolling who is appointed by the National Ski Patrol's chairman and approved by the National Ski Patrols board of directors to advise the NSP in all matters of medical concern; chairs the National Medical Committee.

National Medical Committee A group of physicians that includes the Division Medical Advisor from each division of the National Ski Patrol, the National OEC Program Director, and other physicians selected at large as approved by the National Board and the National Medical Advisor.

National OEC Program Committee A committee composed of all Division OEC Supervisors and the National Medical Advisor, and chaired by the National OEC Program Director; provides insight and guidance to the board of directors annually on matters related to the functioning of the OEC program.

National OEC Program Director A National Ski Patrol (NSP) member who is responsible to the board for the effective management and operation of the national OEC program. This individual is an active specialist in the field of outdoor medicine and is appointed by the NSP chairman and confirmed by the NSP board of directors. The National OEC Program Director also chairs the national OEC Program Committee and serves as a member of the National Education Committee and the National Medical Committee.

National OEC Refresher Committee A committee responsible for developing the annual OEC Refresher program. It is appointed and supervised by the National OEC Program Director.

National Ski Patrol System, Inc. (NSP) The largest winter rescue group in the world, as recognized by the US Congress under Title 36 of the US Code; the premier snow sports rescue organization in the United States.

Nature of illness The type of medical illness present.

Necrosis Death of most or all the cells in an organ or tissue due to disease, injury, or failure of the blood supply.

Negligence The failure to exercise the care that a reasonably prudent person with similar training would exercise in a similar circumstance.

Nervous system A group of organs and other structures that regulate all body functions by collecting and processing information, using the brain and a complicated wiring system to all organs.

Neurogenic shock A type of distributive shock that is caused by disruptions of the central nervous system, most often from a spinal cord injury.

Neuron A specialized cell that conducts electrical impulses; a nerve cell.

Nonrebreather mask An oxygen delivery device that has a mask, a one-way flow valve, and a reservoir bag; when connected to an oxygen source, provides a high concentration of supplemental oxygen.

Nutrition The body's process of utilizing food substances needed for growth and the maintenance of life.

O

Obstructive shock A type of shock caused by a blockage that prevents oxygenated blood from reaching vital organs.

Occlusive dressing A dressing made of Vaseline gauze, aluminum foil, or plastic wrap that prevents air and liquids from entering or exiting a wound.

Occupational exposure An event in which a worker comes into contact with a bodily fluid or hazardous material while on the job.

Open chest injury (sucking chest wound) A chest injury that involves penetration of the chest wall.

Opioids Drugs that are derived from opium or opium-like compounds; sometimes referred to as narcotics.

OPQRST A mnemonic that is used in the assessment of a patient's chief complaint; represents onset, provocation and palliation, quality, radiation, severity, and time.

Orbit The bony socket of the eyeball.

Organs Structures containing similar tissues that act together to perform specific body functions.

Oropharyngeal airway (OPA) A rigid plastic airway adjunct inserted into the oropharynx to maintain a patent airway.

Osteoporosis A disease process that leads to a reduction in bone mass, allowing fracture to occur more easily.

Ostomy bag A pouch worn over the stoma created by an ostomy to collect stool or urine.

Outdoor Emergency Care (OEC) A course of medical instruction developed and taught by the National Ski Patrol.

Outdoor Emergency Care (OEC) technician A provider who has successfully completed the NSP's OEC course and met the annual refresher requirement. This person must complete CPR training, including AED training.

Outdoor First Care (OFC) provider A person who has completed the NSP's Outdoor First Care course and is trained to render basic first aid in outdoor, nonurban environments.

Outrigger Adaptive ski poles with short ski tips attached to crutch-like handles that are used by three-track and four-track adaptive skiers to assist with balance and agility.

Ovarian cyst A fluid-filled sac or pocket in an ovary or on its surface.

P

Palpation The act of touching a patient during an examination to feel for any abnormality.

Pancreatitis A painful condition in which the pancreas becomes inflamed.

Paradoxical motion Inward movement of a flail chest segment upon inhalation.

Paraesthesia A sensation of tingling, pricking, or numbness of the skin, or the feeling of "pins and needles" or a limb being "asleep."

Paramedic An allied health care professional who has successfully completed an NHTSA-approved paramedic course or its equivalent and is trained to deliver both basic and advanced life support.

Paranoia A condition in which individuals believe they are in imminent danger of being harmed (e.g., physically, emotionally, financially) by others who are plotting against them.

Paraplegic A person who does not have use of the legs from paralysis caused by illness or injury; the loss is usually sensory and motor.

Patent A descriptive term for an airway that is open and clear.

Pathogen An infectious agent that can cause disease or illness.

Patient assessment The procedure performed to determine a patient's condition, especially any immediate life-threatening injuries or conditions; forms the basis for decision about emergency medical care and transport.

Patient care report (PCR) A report documenting a patient's complaints and past medical history, plus a chronological (timeline) account of the examination and treatment of the patient, including vital signs. The PCR is a legal document.

Patient privacy The practice of maintaining the security and confidentiality of patient records. It includes the conversational discretion of health care providers and the security of all medical records.

Pediatric assessment triangle An assessment tool that utilizes a pediatric patient's appearance (mental status, body position, and muscle tone), work of breathing (visible movement, effort, and audible sounds), and circulation (skin color) to assess the patient's well-being.

Pelvic inflammatory disease An infection of the organs of a women's reproductive system.

Perfusion The circulation of blood within an organ or tissue in adequate amounts to meet the cells' current needs for oxygen, nutrients, and waste removal.

Pericardial tamponade The accumulation of blood or other fluid within the pericardial sac.

Pericarditis Inflammation of the pericardium or sac surrounding the heart, causing chest pain.

Periosteum The thin vascular outer covering of the cortex of a bone.

Peripheral nervous system The part of the nervous system outside the central nervous system.

Peripheral vascular resistance The tightening of the smaller-diameter blood vessels in the extremities, enabling increased blood flow to the vital organs.

Peritoneum A membrane that covers the organs of the abdomen and also lines the inner wall of the abdominal cavity.

Peritonitis Inflammation of the peritoneum of the abdominal cavity, typically caused by leakage of hollow organ contents; it is usually worse if caused by bacteria from inside the intestines.

PERRL A mnemonic for assessing the eyes; represents pupils equal, round, reactive to light.

Personal protective equipment (PPE) Items worn by medical providers, including gloves, mask, safety eyeglasses (or mask with shield), and gown, to protect them from bodily fluids.

Personnel accountability system A system that readily identifies both the locations and the functions of all members operating at an incident scene.

Placenta previa Low implantation of the placenta where it partially or completely covers the internal opening of the uterus. Upon the onset of any contractions and cervical dilation, or when the cervix begins to dilate at the onset of labor, the placenta is stretched and pulled from the uterine wall, producing painless bleeding that may be life threatening to both mother and fetus.

Plantarflex Movement of the foot or toes downward, toward the sole of the foot.

Pleural space The potential space that lies within the pleura covering the outside of the lungs and the inside of the chest wall.

Pleura The thin transparent membrane covering the outside of the lungs and the inside of the chest wall.

Pneumothorax An abnormal collection of air within the pleural space.

Pocket mask A triangular or pear-shaped barrier device made from clear, soft plastic or silicone.

Poison Any substance that can cause severe organ damage or death if ingested, inhaled, injected into the body, or absorbed through the skin.

Polydipsia Excessive thirst and fluid intake.

Polypharmacy The simultaneous use of several medications in combination.

Polyuria Frequent urination.

Popliteal fossa The posterior part of the knee.

Preeclampsia A toxemia during pregnancy characterized by high blood pressure and edema of the hands or face; also called pregnancy-induced hypertension.

Prehospital care Any medical care rendered by trained personnel prior to arrival at a hospital.

Prehospital providers People who are specifically trained to render medical care to patients outside of a hospital or medical care facility.

Primary patient assessment A step within the patient assessment process that identifies and initiates treatment of immediate and potential life threats.

Prosthetic An artificial device designed to replace a missing or impaired part of the body; also called an artificial limb.

Protocols Written procedures for assessing, treating, and transporting a patient. Protocols are generally written by a team of emergency care professionals and managed by a medical director.

Pruritus Severe itching; frequently occurs in the skin during mild and moderate allergic reactions.

Psychosis A condition in which a person exhibits abnormal behavior and has altered perceptions of reality.

Pulmonary contusion A bruise of the lung tissue.

Pulmonary edema An accumulation of fluid in the lungs.

Pulmonary embolism A condition where a blood clot becomes stuck in and blocks a pulmonary artery. May also be referred to as thromboembolism.

Pulse A rhythmic throbbing of the artery caused by the movement of blood.

Pulse oximeter A device that attaches to a patient's finger, toe, or earlobe and photoelectrically measures blood oxygen content as a percentage of oxygen saturation.

Puncture An injury that is caused by a pointed object that penetrates the skin.

Q

Quadriplegic A person who does not have use of the legs and arms from paralysis caused by illness or injury.

R

Reasonable force The minimum force needed to keep a patient from hurting himself or others.

Referred pain Pain that originates in one part of the body but is felt in another part of the body.

Refresher Annual required continuing education training, usually given each year in the fall, that covers one-third of topics taught in the OEC curriculum.

Reproductive age The years when a woman can become pregnant, approximately age 12 to 49 years.

Reproductive system Organs and other structures responsible for human reproduction.

Rescue The process of extracting a person or group from distress or danger.

Resource management Under NIMS, a response component that includes mutual-aid agreements; the use of special federal, state, local, and tribal teams; and resource mobilization protocols.

Respiratory system Organs and structures that bring air containing oxygen into the body and eliminate carbon dioxide to the environment through the process of breathing, or ventilation.

Retinal detachment Separation of the retina from the posterior wall of the inside of the eyeball.

Retrograde amnesia Loss of memory of events that occurred before a traumatic event to the brain; an inability to recall old information.

RISE Rest, ice, splint, elevate, the sequence of actions that providers should take when caring for contusions.

S

Safety data sheet (SDS) A form that contains relevant information pertaining to a specific substance, with a focus on the hazards it poses to workers.

SALT triage system A triage system developed as an all-hazards method of triaging all patients regardless of age or special need. The acronym SALT stands for *s*ort, *a*ssess, *l*ifesaving interventions, and *t*reatment and/or *t*ransport.

SAMPLE A mnemonic used to obtain medical history information during the patient assessment process; represents signs/symptoms, allergies, medications, past medical history, last oral intake, and events leading up to the present incident.

Scald An injury caused by a hot liquid or a hot, moist vapor.

Scene safety The process of identifying any hazards or possible hazards that could harm you or others and mitigating them prior to attending to the patient.

Scene size-up A general overview of the incident and its surroundings.

Schizophrenia A psychiatric disorder in which a person cannot distinguish what is real from what is not real.

Scoliosis Abnormal lateral curvature of the spine.

Scope of practice A set of rules, regulations, and ethical considerations that define the extent, boundaries, and limitations of a prehospital provider's duties.

Search A methodical process of actively gathering information about a person or group in distress or danger and then physically looking for them.

Secondary patient assessment The thorough, systematic physical examination that follows primary patient assessment, any immediate resuscitation, and history taking; includes taking the patient's vital signs.

Section chiefs The heads of the functional areas within the incident command system.

Span of control The total number of individuals or resources supervised by a single person; usually three to seven individuals or resources. The optimal number is considered to be five.

Seizure A neurologic episode caused by a surge of electrical activity in the brain; can be a convulsion characterized by generalized, uncoordinated muscular activity, and can be associated with loss of responsiveness.

Sepsis A serious medical condition caused by the presence of pathogenic organisms or their toxins in the blood, leading to a systemic inflammatory response.

Septic shock A type of distributive shock that is caused by severe systemic infection.

Shaken baby syndrome A condition in which an infant or toddler is picked up and violently shaken, causing a traumatic brain injury.

Shock Inadequate perfusion, or flow of blood to the cells, causing cellular and tissue hypoxia due to reduced oxygen delivery.

Sign Any objective finding that can be seen, heard, smelled, or measured (e.g., a bruise, the patient's blood pressure); typically discovered during a physical exam.

Sit-ski A device consisting of a "bucket" or seat in which the adaptive skier sits. It has one or two skis attached to the bucket.

Skeletal muscle The type of muscle that attaches to the bony skeleton and is controlled voluntarily by the nervous system; functions to move joints to perform physical activities.

Skeletal system The bones and other supporting tissues that provide structure to the body, provide attachment points for muscles, protect internal organs, allow movement, store minerals, and constitute the major site where blood cells are made.

Ski bra A device that attaches to the front of each ski and holds the skis a fixed distance apart, so that the tips do not cross or spread apart.

Ski spreader A bar placed under the heels of adaptive skiers to keep the rear of the skis separated and fixed. Often used in conjunction with ski tip tethers to facilitate a stable wedge ski position.

Ski stander A device that attaches to skis and utilizes a waist harness and arm rests to help support an adaptive skier in a standing position.

Sleeping altitude The altitude to which a climber *descends* to sleep when climbing at high altitude; typically 500 to 1,000 feet below the highest elevation of that day's ascent.

Sliding board A flat board that is used to help an adaptive athlete transfer to or from a wheelchair.

Sling and swathe A soft splint used to immobilize many upper extremity injuries.

Snow slider A device like a walker with small ski tips attached that allows a standing adaptive skier to shuffle on the snow.

Special operations Infrequently performed activities requiring specialized education and equipment in remote and/or difficult settings.

Spinal motion restriction Restricting the entire spine to limit spinal motion, protecting the spinal cord from injury.

Splint A mechanical device used to prevent a part of the body from moving, protecting it from further injury.

Sprain A stretched or torn ligament.

Squeeze Severe pain when the pressure inside an organ or body cavity cannot adjust to increased external pressure.

Stabilized extrication Keeping a patient's spine anatomically aligned during removal from an accident, therefore preventing any neurologic damage.

Standard of care A level of care an OEC technician must render based on OEC training, local medical protocols, and the requirements of a state's EMS system.

Standard of training The training of National Ski Patrol OEC technicians as set forth in the OEC course, using this text as a reference.

Standard precautions Practices used by health care workers to protect themselves from exposure to bodily fluids based on the assumption that all patients are potentially infectious.

START triage system A triage system commonly used by public safety personnel. The acronym START stands for *s*imple *t*riage *a*nd *r*apid *t*reatment.

Sternocleidomastoid muscles Powerful muscles at the sides of the neck that facilitate turning of the head.

Stoma A surgical port created in the body by surgery to allow the elimination of stool or urine. For ostomies, it is located on the abdomen and is dark pink in color. A pouch (ostomy bag) is worn over the stoma to collect stool or urine.

Straddle injury An injury to the pelvis and the internal organs between the genitals and anus that results when a patient forcefully straddles a fixed object.

Strain A stretched or torn muscle or tendon.

Stress A person's response to environmental demands or pressures. When exposed to stress, the body responds by making a physical, mental, or emotional adjustment.

Strike team A group of resources of the same size or type that is managed by a strike team leader (e.g., a group of Nordic patrollers).

Stroke An interruption of blood flow to the brain that results in the loss of brain function; also called a cerebrovascular accident (CVA).

Stroke volume The amount of blood pumped out of the left ventricle into the aorta during one heartbeat.

Subcutaneous emphysema Air-filled bubbles that are palpable underneath the skin, indicating an injury to an airway structure.

Subdural hematoma An accumulation of venous blood between the outer covering of the brain (dura mater) and the surface of the brain.

Subluxation An event in which a joint partially dislocates and returns to its normal anatomic position.

Substance abuse The intentional misuse of a substance that results in impairment or physical harm.

Subungual hematoma A painful collection of blood under a nail.

Suctioning The process of creating a vacuum to clear foreign material that is obstructing the airway.

Sudden cardiac arrest (SCA) The abrupt cessation of an effective heartbeat.

Sudden infant death syndrome (SIDS) The sudden, unexplained death of an infant in which a postmortem examination fails to determine the cause of death.

Suicidal gesture An action taken by someone that leads others to believe it was a suicide attempt to communicate that the person is in distress or to influence the behavior of others in some way.

Suicide The intentional taking of one's own life.

Symphysis pubis The site on the anterior pelvis at which the two pubic bones are joined together.

Symptom A subjective finding or a departure from normal function or feeling that is noticed by a patient (e.g., pain, blurred vision), reflecting the presence of a medical problem.

Synovium The inner layer of the joint capsule whose cells make a viscous fluid that lubricates joints.

T

Tachycardia A heart rate greater than 100 beats per minute in adults.

Tachypnea A respiratory rate greater than 20 breaths per minute in adults.

Task force A combination of different resources with common communications that is managed by a task force leader (e.g., a sheriff's deputy, an NSP Alpine patrol, a search-and-rescue team).

Tendon The dense tissue that connects a muscle to a bone.

Tension pneumothorax The accumulation of pressurized air within the pleural space; causes the displacement of the great vessels, tracheal deviation, distention of the jugular veins, and compression of the other lung.

Terrorism A human-caused event that is intended to inflict fear and can involve hazardous materials.

Tether A strap used by adaptive ski guides to help control the speed and direction of adaptive skiers.

Thermoregulation The process of maintaining normal body temperature.

Three-track adaptive skier An adaptive skier using one ski with two outriggers.

Tissue A collection of cells acting together to perform a specific body function.

Tonic activity A general stiffening of the muscles.

Tourniquet An instrument that when tightened around an arm or leg temporarily arrests the flow of blood through a large artery.

Toxicological event An event in which a patient has been exposed to a harmful substance *or* an incident in which the intentional or unintentional use of a substance or poison endangers public safety and/or results in a medical emergency.

Toxin A noxious or poisonous substance that is produced by an organism.

Traction The amount of force required to straighten a limb and keep it in alignment; for a fractured femur, typically 10% of the patient's body weight, or approximately 15 pounds.

Traction splint A splint used on a lower extremity to align a fracture, such as a midshaft fracture of the femur.

Trauma Physical injury caused by an external force.

Trauma center A specialized hospital providing 24-hour trauma care, including stabilization, critical care, subspecialty care, and nursing care.

Traumatic asphyxia The inability to breathe and hypoxia that results from the inability of the chest wall to expand due to external pressure or massive crushing trauma.

Traumatic brain injury Physical trauma to the brain.

Triage A process of prioritizing patients for treatment and transportation based on their clinical signs and symptoms. It operates under the philosophy of "Do the most good for the most people."

Two-track adaptive skier A skier who uses two skis without outriggers.

U

Ultraviolet radiation (UVR) Waves of solar energy that are beneficial in small amounts but harmful to the skin and eyes upon overexposure.

Universal dressing A sterile, soft, highly absorbent, individually wrapped dressing that provides superior padding and protection for major wounds; usually measures 9 inches by 36 inches; also called *trauma dressing*.

Urinary system Organs and structures that remove wastes and toxins from the blood and excretes them as urine. This system maintains the body's water and electrolyte balance.

Urticaria Hives or rashes that accompany an allergic reaction.

V

Vein A tubular vessel that carries blood to the heart.

Venom A specific toxin or poisonous secretion of an animal, most commonly from a snake, spider, or scorpion, usually transmitted by a bite or sting.

Ventilation The process by which air moves into and out of the lungs, so that oxygen can be exchanged for carbon dioxide in the alveoli.

Ventricular assist device (VAD) A device implanted into the chest that assists the heart's ventricle circulate blood to the body.

Ventricular fibrillation (VF) Chaotic and ineffective contraction of the ventricles that leads to cardiac arrest.

Ventricular tachycardia (VT) Rapid regular contraction of the ventricles that can lead to ineffective blood flow to body tissues and eventually cardiac arrest.

Vital capacity The maximum amount of air that can be expired following a maximum inhalation.

Vital signs The key objective findings used to evaluate a patient's overall condition; includes pulse rate, respiratory rate, blood pressure, temperature, and level of responsiveness.

W

Warm zone A transition area surrounding the hot zone; the zone in which decontamination occurs.

Wheezing A high-pitched respiratory sound caused by a narrowing of the tubular airways.

Wind chill The apparent temperature felt on exposed skin; is a function of the air temperature and wind speed.

Winter Emergency Care A textbook, developed by Dr. Warren Bowman, that was the precursor to the *Outdoor Emergency Care* text.

Withdrawal The physical and mental readjustment that accompanies the discontinued use of an addictive substance.

Z

Zone of injury The area that is close to or surrounding an injury of an extremity, such as a sprain or fracture.

INDEX

Note: *Page numbers followed by "f" and "t" indicate figures and tables respectively.*

B

C

E

F

G

H

I

J

K

L

M

N

P